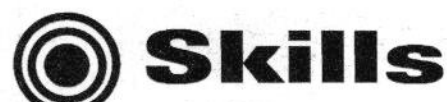

Skills

FUNDAMENTAL NURSING

Concepts and Skills

SECOND EDITION

Grace Cole, RN
Coordinator/Instructor
Department of Vocational Nursing
Grayson County College
Denison, Texas

with 383 illustrations, with 204 in color

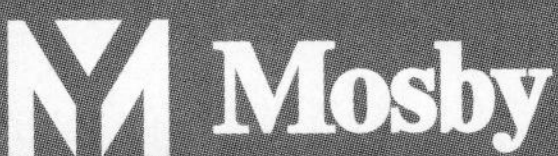

St. Louis Baltimore Boston Carlsbad Chicago Naples New York Philadelphia Portland
London Madrid Mexico City Singapore Sydney Tokyo Toronto Wiesbaden

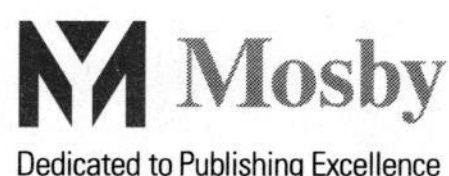

Dedicated to Publishing Excellence

A Times Mirror Company

Publisher: Nancy L. Coon
Senior Editor: Susan R. Epstein
Associate Developmental Editor: Laurie K. Muench
Project Manager: Carol Sullivan Weis
Senior Production Editor: Pat Joiner
Designer: Sheilah Barrett
Manufacturing Supervisor: Karen Lewis

SECOND EDITION

Printed in the United States of America
Composition by The Clarinda Company
Printing/binding by Von Hoffmann Press, Inc.

Mosby–Year Book, Inc.
11830 Westline Industrial Drive
St. Louis, Missouri 63146

Library of Congress Cataloging in Publication Data

Fundamental nursing concepts and skills / [edited by] Grace Cole.—
2nd ed.
p. cm.
Rev. ed. of: Basic nursing skills and concepts. c1991.
Includes bibliographical references and index.
ISBN 0-8016-7884-6
1. Practical nursing. I. Cole, Grace. II. Basic nursing skills and concepts.
[DNLM: 1. Nursing Process. 2. Nursing Care. WY 100 F977 1996]
RT62.F86 1996
610.73—dc20
DNLM/DLC
for Library of Congress 95-44621
CIP

95 96 97 98 99 / 9 8 7 6 5 4 3 2 1

CONTRIBUTORS

Eileen Colon, RN, BSN
Nurse Specialist I
Guilford County Public Health
Greensboro/High Point, NC

Faith Darilek, RN, BSN
Director/Instructor
The Victoria College School of Vocational Nursing
Gonzales, Texas

Sharon Duncan, RN, BSN, MSAC, MSN
Nursing Instructor
Ivy Tech State College
Evansville, Indiana

Jody Lambright Eckler, RN, BSN
Public Health Nurse
Huron County Health Department
Castalia, Ohio

Larita Kaspar, RN, MSN
Associate Professor of Nursing
Lorain County Community College
Elyria, Ohio

Sandra Kirkland, RN, MSN, CETN
Manager, Orthopaedic Services
Mobile Infirmary Medical Center
Mobile, Alabama

Patricia A. Knecht, RN, BSN
Practical Nursing Instructor
Center for Arts and Technology
Coatesville, Pennsylvania

Elizabeth Mahoney, RN, MS, EdD
Professor of Nursing
The Sage Colleges
Troy, New York

Sandra McKelvie, RN
Director, Practical Nursing Program
John Wood Community College
Quincy, Illinois

Michelle Morrison, RN, BSN, MHS, FNP
Nurse Educator/Consultant
Health and Educational Consultants
Williams, Oregon

Carol Ormond, RN, MSN, CNAA, CS, FNP
Assistant Professor
Georgia College School of Nursing
Milledgeville, Georgia

Judith Pulito, RN, MSN
Instructor of Nursing
Lorain County Community College
Elyria, Ohio

Lois White, RN, BSN, MS, PhD
formerly Chairperson, Department of Vocational Nurse Education
Del Mar College
Corpus Christi, Texas

REVIEWERS

Mary Arnold, RN, BSN, MA
VOCN Program Director
Blinn College
Bryan, Texas

Wendy Wilson Bauer, RN, BSN, MSN, LNHA
Nursing Home Administrator
St. Luke Hospital
Ft. Thomas, Kentucky

Sharon Beasley, RN, BSN, MSN
Nursing Instructor
Rend Lake College
Ina, Illinois

Marti Burton, RN, BS
Nursing Instructor
Metrotech Vocational-Technical Center
Oklahoma City, Oklahoma

Jan Camargo, RN, CRRN
Nursing Instructor
South Plains College
Lubbock, Texas

Betty R. Coffman, RN, BS, MEd
Practical Nursing Instructor
Coosa Valley Technical Institute
Rome, Georgia

Cynthia M. Davis, RN, BA, BSN, MEd
Associate Professor of Nursing
Bainbridge College
Bainbridge, Georgia

Kathleen Reilly Dolin, RN, BSN
Nursing Instructor
Monroe County Area Vocational-Technical School
Bartonsville, Pennsylvania

Judy A. Donaldson, RN
Nursing Instructor/Coordinator
North Seattle Community College
Seattle, Washington

Dot Eastin, RN, BSN, MS
Nursing Instructor
Panola College–Marshall Center
Marshall, Texas

Ruth Ann Eckenstein, RN, BS, MEd
Nurse Educator
Francis Tuttle Vocational-Technical School
Oklahoma City, Oklahoma

Kathleen Fraker, RN, BSN, MA
Associate Professor of Nursing
Berkshire Community College
Pittsfield, Massachusetts

Cheryl Fries, RN, BSN, MSEd
Associate in Occupational School Supervision
New York State Education Department
Albany, New York

Helene R. Frigen, RN, BS, MS
Coordinator, Allied Health
S.W. BOCES
Valhalla, New York

Hayward S. Gill, Jr, RN, BS, MS, AAS
Nursing/Community Health Education Faculty and Consultant
NYC BOE Adult and Continuing Education
Brooklyn, New York

Barbara M. Jorenby, RN, BSN, MA
Nursing Instructor
Dakota County Technical College
Rosemount, Minnesota

Karen D. Meyer, RN, BSN
Assistant Professor, Practical Nursing Program
North Central Technical College
Mansfield, Ohio

Elizabeth K. Michel, RNC, BSN, MSN
Assistant Dean, Health Occupations
Galveston College
Galveston, Texas

Candace Moore, RN, BSN, CNOR
Nursing Instructor
Pinellas Technical Education Center
Clearwater, Florida

Linda North, RN, BSN, MSN, EdS
ADN Faculty
Athens Area Technical Institute
Athens, Georgia

Anita Norton, RN, BSN, MSN
Instructor and Chairperson
Department of Nursing
Jefferson State Community College
Birmingham, Alabama

Joann Elaine Potts Peuterbaugh, RN, BSN, MSN
LPN Coordinator
F.W. Olin Vocational School of Practical Nursing
Alton, Illinois

Joyce Robertson, RNC, BSN
Nursing Instructor
Asheville-Buncombe Technical Community College
Asheville, North Carolina

Judith D. Sawyer, RN, BSN, MS
Director, Isabella Graham Hart School of Practical Nursing
Rochester General Hospital
Rochester, New York

Susan R. Seager, RN, MSN, EdD
Director, School of Practical Nursing
Baptist Hospital
Nashville, Tennessee

Shirley Stamford, RNC, BSN
Nursing Faculty
Erwin Technical Center
Tampa, Florida

Cynthia A. Steury-Lattz, RN, BSN, MSN
Nursing Instructor
Kankakee Community College
Kankakee, Illinois

Janice A. Traylor, RN, BSN, MEd, MSN
Nurse Educator
Casper College
Casper, Wyoming

Lori Walton, RN, BSN
Nurse Instructor
Glasgow School for Health Occupations
Glasgow, Kentucky

Barbara Washington, RN, BSN, MSN
Training Specialist/LPN Instructor
Kennedy-King College/Dawson Technical Institute
Chicago, Illinois

Teresa E. Wilkins, RN, BSN
Head, Department of Practical Nursing
Macon Technical Institute
Macon, Georgia

This edition is lovingly dedicated to my beautiful daughters, **Karen and Sharon,** *who have so enriched my life.*

PREFACE

Fundamental Nursing Concepts and Skills has been refocused, revised, and expanded to provide comprehensive coverage of the basic concepts and skills that practical and vocational nursing students must master. Two goals remained foremost in the minds of all who participated in this revision: (1) address the realities of current practice, including patient needs, changes in the delivery of health care, and the expanding roles of practical and vocational nurses; and (2) present this information in a clear, consistent format that engages students and promotes learning and understanding.

ORGANIZATION

The text is logically organized in four units that cover foundations of nursing practice, factors that influence health and illness, basic nursing skills, and basic patient needs. Chapters also follow a logical format, beginning with Learning Objectives, Key Terms, and a list of Skills to help students focus on the material to be covered. Clinical chapters are designed to help students learn to use the nursing process. Each chapter includes an overview of the application of the nursing process to the specific chapter content. Nursing care plans demonstrate how to select and customize interventions to address specific patient problems. All the skills for each chapter follow discussions of principles and interventions. This approach enables students to read through the narrative of the chapter without interruption, and then turn their attention to the performance of specific skills.

FEATURES

- Clear, concise writing style is easy to read and comprehend.
- Hundreds of large, clear illustrations clarify important concepts and demonstrate essential techniques.
- Numerous skills are presented in a logical, consistent, two-column format that features rationales for each step.
- Chapters begin with Learning Objectives, Key Terms and a list of Skills to help students identify and focus on essential content.
- Chapters conclude with a Summary, Key Concepts, and Critical Thinking Questions to help students reinforce and apply learning.
- Numerous boxes and tables present material in an easy-to-digest format.
- A glossary at the end of the book allows quick access to important nursing and medical terminology.
- References and Suggested Readings for each chapter highlight up-to-date research and point students to further areas of study.

NEW FEATURES

- Expanded coverage throughout of basic concepts, principles, and nursing interventions makes this revision a comprehensive fundamentals text.
- Discussions of home care and care in community settings address the growing trend of providing health care outside the hospital.
- A new chapter on skin integrity provides current guidelines on the care and treatment of pressure ulcers.
- The nursing process focus helps students learn to apply knowledge to patient care:
  - Each clinical chapter includes an overview of the application of the nursing process to provide a consistent context for the information that follows.
  - Nursing process overviews and care plans focus on expected outcomes and evaluative measures related to NANDA diagnoses to reflect current practice.
- Patient Teaching boxes highlight knowledge and skills that patients and family members need to master.
- Gerontologic Considerations boxes summarize the special considerations and needs of this important patient population.
- A new streamlined skills format clearly presents step-by-step instructions with rationales to guide students through each action and explain why every step is performed.
- All the skills for each chapter are presented *after* the discussions of principles and interventions to eliminate disruption of the narrative and facilitate access to the skills.
- New two-color design and large, clear type make the text easy to read and follow.

- Many new illustrations and the addition of a contrast color to virtually all drawings add both instructional value and visual appeal.

TEACHING-LEARNING PACKAGE

An unsurpassed array of material has been developed to enhance teaching and learning and to provide support for busy educators:

- Instructor's Manual with skills checklists and test bank
- NEW two-color Transparency Acetate package (48 total) to enhance lectures
- NEW Skills Performance Checklist booklet available for student purchase either separately or packaged with the text
- Mosby's Instructor's Resource Kit for Practical/Vocational Nurse Educators, a tabbed binder that provides handy storage for all teaching materials
- Mosby's Nursing Skills Video Series

Grace Cole

ACKNOWLEDGMENTS

I could not realize as we began work on the second edition that it would be as exciting as the first. Perhaps it is meant to be. If it occurs because of the people with whom I have had the pleasure of working, I look forward with anticipation to the next project.

Suzi Epstein, Senior Editor, and Laurie Muench, Developmental Editor, understand my gratitude for having been there when I needed them. Without them, I would not have been able to create the type of text I wished for my students. Suzi's wonderful humor tempered with enough reality to help keep us on track was so calming. Thanks, Suzi. Laurie is so capable and positive, always helping me look forward to the next part of the project. No one could ask for a better person with whom to work so closely. Thanks, Laurie. Pat Joiner, Senior Production Editor, made my work easy to accomplish because of the organized schedule planned for us. Thanks, Pat. Sheilah Barrett, Designer, brought our words to life, combining function and style. Thanks, Sheilah.

I would like to acknowledge Wilson N. Jones Memorial Hospital for allowing the use of important hospital forms to provide students with illustrations necessary for their learning.

My thanks to the contributors who added so much to the second edition and for the timely submission of chapters. I would also like to thank the reviewers who made me aware of helpful suggestions for needed improvement.

Most important, thank you to my students who are drawn to our nursing program, for being so caring and dedicated to the nursing care of their patients. I continue to learn from all of you.

A very special thanks to Wayne.

Grace Cole

CONTENTS

FUNDAMENTAL NURSING

Concepts and Skills

CHAPTER 1

The Profession of Nursing

Learning Objectives

After studying this chapter, the student should be able to . . .

- Define the key terms.
- Describe at least one major contribution of the following nursing pioneers: Florence Nightingale, Dorothea Dix, Linda Richards, Mary E.P. Mahoney, Lillian Wald, and Mary Adelaide Nutting.
- State the modern definition of *nursing.*
- Describe the purpose of nursing theories.
- Define four theories of nursing.
- Explain the purpose of nurse practice acts.
- Identify four members of the health care team.
- Discuss the role of the practical/vocational nurse.
- Describe five roles of a nurse.
- Explain holistic nursing.
- Describe the educational program for practical/vocational nursing.
- Describe the different types of educational preparation for professional nurses, including the associate degree, diploma, and baccalaureate degree programs.
- List three types of nursing actions.
- Identify three kinds of preventive nursing actions to promote wellness.
- Explain at least two methods available to the licensed nurse for continuing nursing education.
- List six major employment opportunities available for a licensed practical/vocational nurse.
- Discuss three styles of leadership that may be used by nurses.
- Describe the four phases of the therapeutic helping relationship.

Key Terms

Autocratic leadership
Clinical nurse specialist
Continuing education
Democratic leadership
Dependent nursing action
Endorsement
Health care team
Holistic care
Independent nursing action
In-service education
Interdependent nursing action
Laissez-faire leadership
Licensure
Nurse administrator
Nurse anesthetist
Nurse educator
Nurse midwife
Nurse practice act
Nurse practitioner
Nurse researcher
Nursing
Practical/vocational nursing
Registered nursing
Standards of practice
Theory
Therapeutic nurse-patient relationship

Welcome to nursing—a challenging, exciting, and evolving profession. The nurse of today does more than merely care for the sick and injured. The nurse serves as a nurse educator, researcher, advocate, role model, and activist. The nurse is also instrumental in shaping health care and social policy.

HISTORY OF NURSING

Although an exact description of the origin of nursing has not survived from early civilization, much evidence supports "the premise that *nurturing* has been essential to the preservation of life. Survival of the human race, therefore, is inextricably intertwined with the development of nursing" (Donahue, 1985). The word *nursing* itself evolved from the Latin word *nutrire,* which means "to nourish."

Primitive Health Care

From the earliest days, social, economic, and political forces helped to shape the history of the nursing profession. Mystical and occult beliefs led primitive people to believe that illness and accidents were caused by evil spirits. Later, explanations of life and death evolved into religious concepts. Medicine men, priests, and shamans developed complex herbal and ritualistic treatments that would drive the evil spirits out of the body and thus restore health. "Wise women" assisted medicine men with treatments, dressed wounds, and gathered herbs for medicines. Although the care of the sick varied with tribal customs, "primitive societies sowed the seeds of hygiene, sanitation, and public health as well as medicine, psychiatry, midwifery, and nursing" (Donahue, 1985). As man domesticated plants and animals, nomadic lifestyles ceased, and civilizations emerged in China, India, Babylonia, Persia (Iran), Egypt, and the Mediterranean. Egypt and the eastern Mediterranean civilizations had the greatest influence on the modern Western world.

Egypt

Written records in Egypt date back to 3000 BC. As the Egyptian civilization evolved, care of the sick consisted of folk practice and magic, which later included ideas about anatomy, the cause of disease, and preventive health measures. "Living in a tropical region, the Egyptians developed strict rules about such matters as cleanliness, exercise, food, drink, and sexual relations" (Shryock, 1959). Doctors and priests treated the sick, whereas nursing care was left to female family members or slaves. Ritual and religious beliefs played an important role in health care, but many ideas were based on scientific observation.

Ancient Civilizations

The Greeks were keen observers and philosophers with a love for beauty. They erected temples to their gods near springs. These places later became religious baths and lodgings. The sick were also cared for at these health resorts, although no maternity or terminally ill patients were admitted. Nursing care was not provided in early Greece.

During the golden age of Greece (600 to 400 BC), the school of "natural philosophy" was born. Philosophers such as Socrates, Plato, and Aristotle used close observation and clear thinking to identify the fundamental principles of good living.

The ancient civilizations of Greece, Rome, and India all recognized the need for trained nurses. Standards and qualifications for nurses may be traced to Indian writings dating back to 800 BC.

Early Christian Era

As Greece and Rome declined (AD 50 to 476), Christianity grew. Care of the sick was considered an expression of charity, and wealthy women such as Phoebe of Cenchreae, Fabiola, Marcella, and Paula devoted their lives to forming religious orders dedicated to caring for the sick and poor. The first organized nursing began with the crude education programs and hospitals established during this era.

Middle (Dark) Ages

Although little is known about nursing during the Dark Ages (AD 477 to 1450), it is clear that nursing was strongly influenced by religion and the military. Religious orders that trained monks to fight and care for the sick were established. The Knights Hospitalers, Knights Templars, and Teutonic Knights are examples of nursing and fighting orders.

The political system known as *feudalism,* along with primitive living conditions, contributed to high death rates during the Dark Ages. Nursing duties were usually the responsibility of the head mistress and servants of the manor. Physicians were rare because the Church did not emphasize medicine as much as nursing.

Monasteries, however, established hospitals outside their walls. The Hotel Dieu in Paris was founded in 650 and offered shelter for the poor, orphans, and pilgrims and nursing care for the sick or infirm. Nurses were recruited from penitents (fallen women) and widows. Men also assisted with nursing care. Eventually the staff was organized into a religious order called the *Augustinian Sisters and Brothers,* which is thought to be the oldest order of nurses in existence. They are still practicing today.

During the Middle Ages, concepts such as sanitation, cleanliness, ventilation, and disease transmission were not practiced. People lived with their animals, dumped sewage in the street, and obtained water from contaminated sources. Hospitals took care of people who were ill because of these factors. Plagues, such as the black death of the fourteenth century, and epidemics swept throughout Europe.

Toward the end of the Middle Ages, feudalism began to deteriorate. As the Church lost much of its power, it no longer attracted people to care for the sick.

Renaissance to Nineteenth Century

In 1517 a faction known as Protestantism split from the Catholic Church, thus ending religious domination and opening the way for many new ideas. These changes affected nursing profoundly. Monasteries were closed and religious orders disbanded, so there were few trained nurses. As a result, there was little care for women, the sick, and the poor, even though epidemics continued to periodically ravage Europe and plague and famine brought these people to the cities. Pitiful sanitary conditions prevailed in hospitals. Nurses were "usually the *dregs* of society, those individuals who were immoral, drunken, and illiterate" (Donahue, 1985). For example, a bad image was created in 1843 by the character of Sairey Gamp in Charles Dickens' *Martin Chuzzlewit.* Mrs. Gamp was depicted as a drunken, uncaring, and slovenly nurse (Fig. 1-1). Needless to say, characters such as Mrs. Gamp created a bad image of nurses that was difficult, almost impossible, to overcome.

During this time, however, one notable priest, St. Vincent de Paul, established the Sisters of Charity, an order whose members care for the poor and ill even today.

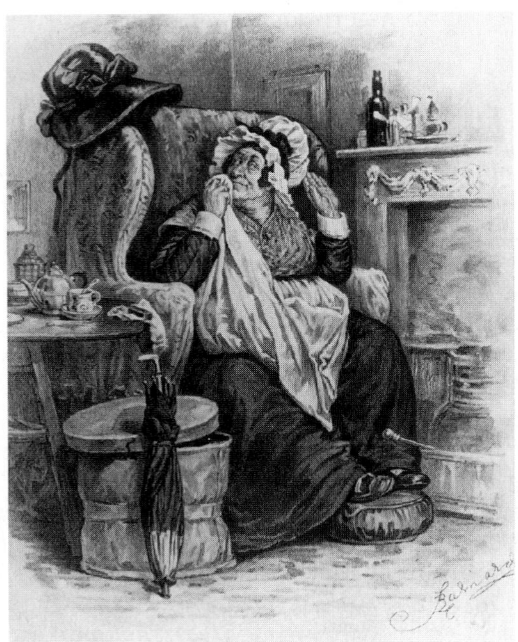

Fig. 1-1 Mrs. Gamp.

Nineteenth Century

Nursing had reached a low point by the end of the eighteenth century, but the need for nurses was growing. In 1836, Europe's first nursing school, Kaiserwerth Deaconess Institution, offered a 3-year training course for nurses, with topics such as pharmacology, theoretic and bedside nursing, visiting nursing, religious doctrine, and ethics. Graduates of the institution established similar programs throughout the world and set the stage for the emergence of modern nursing.

Florence Nightingale

One of the most significant figures in nursing history is Florence Nightingale: reformer of hospitals, pioneer of public health care, and founder of modern nursing.

Florence Nightingale was born to wealthy, upper-class English parents on May 12, 1820, in Florence, Italy. She was educated in England and had mastered higher mathematics, literature, philosophy, religion, history, science, economics, and several languages by the age of 17. During her travels to Rome, Egypt, Greece, and Germany, she studied hospitals and the training of nurses. Nightingale was the first to believe that nursing should include classroom theory as well as experience in nursing the patient at the bedside. These beliefs are still evident in nursing programs today. Finally, in 1852 at 31 years of age and much against the wishes of her family, Nightingale enrolled for a 3-month course of study at Kaiserwerth, Germany.

During her first position as superintendent of a London women's hospital, her exceptional administrative abilities were revealed. When the Crimean War began (1854 to 1856), England had no nurses for its wounded. On invitation from the Secretary of War, Nightingale led a group of 38 women to care for the wounded in Scutari, Turkey. Conditions were deplorable—filth, poor diet, little nursing care, and drunkenness were common, and administrators were appalled by the idea of women in war zones.

Through sheer determination and hard work, Nightingale transformed the hospitals in the Crimean from filthy pesthouses into havens for the sick and injured. She is credited with putting into effect many of the first public health measures. Improvements in housing, sanitation, nutrition, and nursing care were immediately successful. "Deaths dropped dramatically from 420 per 1000 to 22 per 1000" (Kurzen, 1993).

Nightingale had begun to break down age-old prejudices and change the face of nursing. In Longfellow's poem *Santa Filomena,* she became known as the "Lady with a Lamp" because she would walk among the injured soldiers in the camp hospital and say a word or two of comfort and encouragement, giving hope to the men.

While working in hospitals along the Black Sea, Nightingale contracted "Crimean fever" and nearly died. In July 1856, after she returned to England as a semiinvalid, Nightingale began her fight to improve military health care. By 1857 her first book about hospital administration, complete with statistical records, was published. Five years later the Army recognized its health care delivery system, developed a sanitary code, and established a military medical college. Nightingale soon became recognized as an authority on hospital administration and statistical record keeping. She was frequently consulted about plans for hospitals throughout the world.

By 1860 the first nursing school in England admitted its first 15 students. Financing through the Nightingale Fund allowed nurses to be formally trained for 3 full years. Graduates of this first school at St. Thomas' Hospital in London would establish new nursing schools wherever they were needed, but all were based on "the Nightingale system," which was adapted from Nightingale's book, *Notes on Nursing* (1859).

In 1862, Nightingale established the Training School and Home for Nurses of the Royal Infirmary, a program dedicated to providing private duty, hospital, and district nurses. This project was the beginning of today's public health (and home health) nursing.

Nightingale died in 1910 at the age of 90 years. During her lifetime she had a profound impact on the health of people. She was a scholar, nurse, hospital administrator, researcher, author, teacher, founder of nursing schools and public health nursing, sanitation expert, social reformer, and women's rights advocate.

Nursing in America

Florence Nightingale's influence would have brought many rapid changes to nursing in the United States if the Civil War had not begun. Few nursing schools were available at this time, making for few trained nurses to help in the war. However, many untrained women volunteered to serve as nurses. Dorothea Dix (1802 to 1887) was appointed by the Union government to supervise all women nurses in the Union forces. Although she encountered strong opposition and incompetence, Dix set the standards for recruitment, volunteer selection, and training for thousands of women. Outstanding nurses of the Civil War included Clara Barton (1821 to 1912), founder of the American Red Cross; Ella King Newsom, Confederate Army nurse and hospital organizer; Mary Ann Bickerdyke (1817 to 1901), who fought for the comfort of the common soldier; Louisa May Alcott (1832 to 1888), who published *Hospital Sketches,* a book based on her experiences as a volunteer nurse; Walt Whitman (1819 to 1892), a poet who described his nursing work in Washington, DC; and Harriet Tubman (1820 to 1913), who after leading more than 300 slaves to freedom, served as superintendent of a Virginia hospital.

Still, nursing schools did not appear until the 1870s. Linda Richards (1841 to 1930), who was America's first trained nurse, graduated from Boston's Womens' and Childrens' Hospital in 1873. Other women who had an influence on nursing include Isabell Hampton Robb (1860 to 1910), who advocated licensure, 3-year training programs, and an 8-hour work day for nurses and founded the *American Journal of Nursing;* Mary E.P. Mahoney (1845 to 1926), America's first black graduate nurse, who devoted her life to improving working and health care conditions; Lillian Wald (1867 to 1940), who established the first public health nursing service with the Henry Street Settlement for New York City's poor in 1893; Lavinia Dock (1858 to 1956), author of the classic text *History of Nursing,* who became superintendent of Johns Hopkins Nursing School and was a nursing reformer; and Mary Adelaide Nutting (1858 to 1947), graduate of the first class of Johns Hopkins School of Nursing, who raised the standards for nursing education and founded the first college-level nursing program at Columbia Teachers College.

Anne Goodrich (1876 to 1955) planned the Army School of Nursing for World War I in 1918 and advocated raising nursing to professional status. Mildred Montag researched, developed, and implemented a new educational model for nurse technicians that later evolved into associate degree nursing programs at community colleges. Montag continues to contribute to the associate degree nursing program.

Practical/Vocational Nursing

Before 1892, women who were not formally trained but experienced in caring for the sick were referred to as *practical nurses.* As society shifted toward urban living, the need for capable bedside nurses grew. By 1892 the Ballard School opened a formal 3-month training program at the Young Women's Christian Association in Brooklyn, New York. Because few controls existed, early practical nursing schools varied widely in education, supervision, and practice. "It was not until 1941 that a national association for practical nursing was formed" (Kurzen, 1989). The National Association of Practical Nursing Education was opened for membership in 1942. By 1945 a program for accreditation of practical/vocational nursing schools was begun. In 1951 the *Journal of Practical Nursing* was published. Today the organization is known as the National Association for Practical Nurse Education and Services, Inc. (NAPNES). Membership is open to anyone interested in furthering practical/vocational nursing, and the organization is considered a leading voice in practical/vocational nursing education. Today, the official organization for the licensed practical/vocational nurse (LPN/LVN) is the National Federation of Licensed Practical Nurses (NFLPN), which was founded in 1949 by Lillian Kuster. Only LPNs/LVNs are allowed to join NFLPN. Both organizations educate the public about the importance of practical/vocational nursing. Texas and California are the only two states that call their programs and licensed graduates *vocational nursing* and *licensed vocational nurses.*

Nursing today, more than ever before, faces many challenges. Knowing and appreciating the rich and varied history of the profession encourages nurses to continue to strive for excellence and for autonomy for the four levels of licensed nursing, which are practical/vocational nursing, associate degree nursing, diploma nursing, and baccalaureate degree nursing. The nurse may also choose to receive a master's degree in nursing (MSN) and a doctorate in nursing or another area (PhD).

NURSING TODAY

Nurses of today strive to meet the needs of patients ***holistically,*** which means caring for the total human being. Nurses work with patients to meet physiologic, psychologic, psychosocial, emotional, and spiritual needs. Nurses are sensitive to the patient's family, significant others, and cultural and social background. In short, nurses treat the "whole" patient—a unique individual of great worth and dignity functioning within a dynamic environment.

Definition of Nursing

The definition of ***nursing*** from the American Nurses Association, which is the national association for registered nurses (RNs), or professional nurses, is the diagnosis and care of human responses to actual or high-risk health problems.

Nurse Practice Acts

Nurse practice acts regulate the licensure and practice of nursing in all states of the United States and all provinces of Canada. The scope of nursing practice is defined by each state or province; similarities exist in all respective practice acts. The scope of practice for the LPN/LVN and RN is defined in these acts. The nurse practice act of each state also includes designated sections of the law that covers professional and practical/vocational definitions, educational qualifications, requirements, licensure, fees, appropriate use of RN or LPN/LVN titles, examinations, renewal of license, grounds for denial or revocation of a license, and other important areas governing the practice of nursing.

It is important to become familiar with the local nurse practice act. The act provides the legal definition for nursing in each state. Texas is the only state using a Title Act instead of a practice act.

Standards of Nursing

Standards of practice are statements that define the qualifications, functions, and principles of practice. These definitions provide criteria for evaluating the effectiveness of nursing care. Standards for LPNs/LVNs have been developed by the NFLPN and NAPNES. Legal definitions of *nursing* usually include standards of practice.

It is the responsibility of each nurse to work within the state practice or title act and function at levels defined by standards of nursing care.

Nursing Education

To be called a *nurse,* one must have graduated from an education program approved (accredited) by the state board of nursing. All programs for RNs and LPNs/LVNs must be accredited by state boards of nursing. Programs are analyzed for theory, practice, and instructor qualifications. Once a nursing program meets all criteria established by the board, it is allowed to educate nurses, who on completion of the program, are eligible to apply to take the licensure examination.

The time that a student spends in a basic nursing program ranges from 1 to 4 years. All nursing graduates must pass a national examination to receive licensure. This test is now being administered on computers. The LPN/LVN takes the National Council Licensure Examination for Licensed Practical/Vocational Nurses (NCLEX-PN). The RN takes the National Council Licensure Examinations for the RN (NCLEX-RN).

Practical/Vocational Nursing Programs

The goal of **practical/vocational nursing** is to provide a state-board–approved (accredited) program that provides the theoretic knowledge and physical skills needed to safely perform entry-level nursing care directed by the RN or physician, to meet patient needs, and to practice health maintenance and disease prevention. The program of study includes theory and clinical practice supervised by program faculty. Courses include practical/vocational nursing adjustments (fundamentals), anatomy, nursing skills, mental illness, nutrition, pharmacology, microbiology, maternal-child nursing, medical-surgical nursing, and clinical laboratories. Programs range from 6 to 18 months in length, and more nursing courses are taught in some states than in others. Practical/vocational nursing graduates may be allowed to enter an RN program and receive varying amounts of credit from the previous program toward registered nursing licensure. These programs are called *transitional entry* and *career-ladder* or *career-mobility programs.*

Registered Nursing Programs

The **registered nursing** program includes an associate degree, diploma, or bachelor degree.

The associate degree program is a 2-year academic program in which the graduate receives an associate degree in applied science. The program is usually found in technical schools and community and junior colleges. The student receives a knowledge of nursing theory as well as clinical practice. In some programs, the student is eligible for LPN/LVN licensure on completion of the first year.

The graduate with a nursing diploma comes from a 3-year program often affiliated with a college to allow credit for academic courses. Private institutions and hospitals also sponsor this program.

The baccalaureate degree nursing program, referred to as a bachelor's of science in nursing (BSN), lasts four years and is associated with 4-year colleges or universities. The curriculum emphasizes the physical and social sciences. Managerial theories and leadership skills are studied in relation to nursing.

Each type of program prepares the nurse for the licensing examination and licensure as an RN. Today, advanced degrees such as master's degrees and doctorates are available for nurses who choose to continue their studies beyond the baccalaureate level. Nurses may also choose to go into research.

Nursing Theories

A **theory** is a set of ideas based on observable behaviors and facts. The theory is developed to explain the nature or behavior of something. "Theories are ideas that help to explain reality, predict actions, and provide guidance for their users" (Morrison, 1993). Many theories have been developed to explain nursing. See Table 1-1 for a summary of nursing theories.

Today, nurses are men and women who are graduates of approved (accredited) programs. Too often, people hold a negative image of nurses as docile, dependent followers. Because of these incorrect images, it is important to educate the public about caring, competent professional nursing care.

NURSING ROLES

Because the nursing profession is affected by social and scientific forces, it is dynamic—changing, growing, and evolving. Consequently, the *role* of the nurse changes and evolves. The nursing specialties of today were almost unheard of 25 years ago. Nursing was once a passive, subservient occupation, but nursing is now a profession of competent, decisive professionals who participate as valued members of the health care team. As nursing continues to grow, new roles will be developed, and nurses will continue to contribute to the health care policies of the future. Health care needs will see the LPN/LVN performing more in a leadership role than in the past. Management techniques should be included in all nursing curricula.

Nursing service

The National League for Nursing, the highest accrediting body for nursing, is concerned with improving nursing education, nursing service, and health care delivery in the United States. The league has identified basic roles for the nurse. Situ-

Table 1-1 SUMMARY OF NURSING THEORIES

Theorist	Goal of Nursing	Framework for Practice
Nightingale (1860)	To facilitate "body's reparative processes" by manipulating patient's environment (Torres, 1986)	Patient's environment is manipulated to include appropriate noise, nutrition, hygiene, light, comfort, socialization, and hope.
Peplau (1952)	To develop interaction between nurse and patient (Peplau, 1952)	Nursing is significant, therapeutic, and interpersonal process (Peplau, 1952). Nurses participate in structuring health care systems to facilitate natural ongoing tendency of humans to develop interpersonal relationships (Marriner-Tomey, 1989).
Abdellah (1960)	To provide service to individuals, families, and society. To be kind and caring but also intelligent, competent, and technically well prepared to provide this service (Marriner-Tomey, 1989)	This theory involves Abdellah's 21 nursing problems (Abdellah et al, 1960).
Orlando (1961)	To respond to patient's behavior in terms of immediate needs. To interact with patient to meet immediate needs by identifying patient behavior, reaction of nurse, and nursing action to be taken (Torres, 1986; Chinn, Kramer, 1987)	Three elements, including patient behavior, nurse reaction, and nurse action, compose nursing situation (Orlando, 1961).
Levine (1966)	To use conservation activities aimed at optimal use of patient's resources	This adaptation model of human as integral whole is based on "four conservation principles of nursing" (Levine, 1973).
Rogers (1970)	To maintain and promote health, prevent illness, and care for and rehabilitate ill and disabled patient through "humanistic science of nursing" (Rogers, 1970)	"Unitary man" evolves along life process. Patient continuously changes and coexists with environment.
Orem (1971)	To care for and help patient attain total self-care	This is self-care deficit theory. Nursing care becomes necessary when patient is unable to fulfill biologic, psychologic, developmental, or social needs (Orem, 1985).
King (1971)	To use communication to help patient reestablish positive adaptation to environment	*Nursing process* is defined as dynamic interpersonal process between nurse, patient, and health care system.
Travelbee (1971)	To assist individual or family to prevent or cope with illness, regain health, find meaning in illness, or maintain maximal degree of health (Marriner-Tomey, 1989)	Interpersonal process is viewed as human-to-human relationship formed during illness and "experience of suffering."
Neuman (1972)	To assist individuals, families, and groups to attain and maintain maximal level of total wellness by purposeful interventions	Stress reduction is goal of systems model of nursing practice (Torres, 1986). Nursing actions are in primary, secondary, or tertiary level of prevention.
Leininger (1978)	To provide care consistent with nursing's emerging science and knowledge with caring as central focus (Chinn, Kramer, 1987)	With this transcultural care theory, caring is central and unifying domain for nursing knowledge and practice (Leininger, 1980).
Roy (1979)	To identify types of demands placed on patient, assess adaptation to demands, and help patient adapt	This adaptation model is based on physiologic, psychologic, sociologic, and dependence-independence adaptive modes (Roy, 1980).
Watson (1979)	To promote health, restore patient to health, and prevent illness (Marriner-Tomey, 1989)	This theory involves philosophy and science of caring. Caring is interpersonal process comprising interventions that result in meeting human needs (Torres, 1986).
Parse (1981)	To focus on man as living unity and man's qualitative participation with health experience (Parse, 1981) (Nursing as science and art [Marriner-Tomey, 1989])	Man continually interacts with environment and participates in maintenance of health (Marriner-Tomey, 1989). Health is continual, open process rather than state of well-being or absence of disease (Parse, 1981; Marriner-Tomey, 1989; Chinn, Kramer, 1987).

Adapted from Potter PA, Perry AG: *Fundamentals of nursing: concepts, process and practice,* ed 3, St Louis, 1993, Mosby.

ations may vary, but all nurses perform in these basic roles.

Provider of care

This role depicts the traditional nursing role. The nurse assesses and diagnoses patient health problems, plans (using expected outcomes) and implements solutions (nursing care or interventions), and last, evaluates the patient care administered to determine the effectiveness of the interventions and the patient's satisfaction of the care given. Although LPNs/LVNs do not usually assume final responsibility for patient care planning, they contribute significantly by assessing patient problems and administering much of the care to solve the problems. In some institutions the LPN/LVN may use the entire nursing process, including appropriate documentation.

Communicator

In the communicator role, the nurse assesses the communication patterns of patients and their families, plans effective communication strategies, and documents important information. The success of the therapeutic nurse-patient relationship depends on the quality of communication. The nurse must also communicate effectively with members of the health care team in other disciplines to provide overall effective care for the patient.

Teacher

Health care is a complex system that requires extensive knowledge. Patients undergoing diagnostic procedures or treatments need appropriate information to help them cope. The nurse defines the patient's learning needs and develops, implements, and evaluates teaching plans to assist the patient in coping successfully with problems. The LPN/LVN provides and reinforces patient teaching methods. In some institutions the LPN/LVN is allowed to perform patient teaching.

Manager

The RN usually assigns nursing personnel, sets priorities for care, and evaluates the effectiveness of the nursing care administered. The LPN/LVN assists in assigning and monitoring auxiliary workers under the direction of a registered nurse. In some institutions the LPN/LVN manages other workers and serves as a nursing team leader by assisting and supporting workers such as nursing assistants.

Member of the nursing profession

All levels of nurses are expected to recognize the limits of their own formal education, seek out professional growth, practice within the legal and ethical framework of nursing, and assume individual responsibility for self-development.

Nurses practice in a variety of settings, although hospital nursing still remains one of the favorite work settings. Many nurses are becoming clinical specialists and pursuing advanced education. However, all nurses function as caregivers, communicators, teachers, and managers within the framework of professional nursing.

NURSING SPECIALTIES

Because so much information exists today, many nurses choose to specialize—limit practice to a certain area of expertise in nursing. In this way the nurse has the opportunity to become extremely knowledgeable and competent within the specialty. The nurse may choose career roles such as clinical specialist, practitioner, midwife, anesthetist, educator, researcher, and administrator.

Clinical nurse specialist

The nurse with specialized education and expertise is called a ***clinical nurse specialist.*** Areas of practice include pediatrics, gerontology, psychiatric nursing, intensive or cardiac care, emergency care, and management of various disease processes. Although a master's degree is required, LPNs/LVNs may assist within defined areas of practice and become knowledgeable in this area.

Nurse practitioner

"A **nurse practitioner** has the knowledge and skills necessary to detect and manage limited acute and chronic stable conditions" (Potter, Perry, 1993). This professional must maintain special certification to continue to practice in this capacity. Practice areas include pediatrics, adult and family practice, obstetrics/gynecology, and gerontology.

Nurse midwife

Care of women during pregnancy, labor, delivery, and the postpartum period is the specialty of **nurse midwives.** Certified nurse midwives are usually associated with a group of physicians or a hospital or health care agency.

Nurse anesthetist

The nurse who receives special advanced training in administering anesthesia is a **nurse anesthetist.** This nurse provides general and local anesthesia with physician supervision. LPNs/LVNs also work as scrub nurses in the operating room of hospitals.

Nurse educator

The nurse with a background in clinical nursing and advanced education may work as a **nurse educator** in patient, staff, or nursing education. Patient educators develop plans to teach patients to cope with disability or illness. Staff development educators focus on improving the skill knowledge of agency nurses. Nursing program educators concentrate on providing information necessary to become a licensed nurse.

Nurse researcher

The nurse may also choose to go into research to help find ways to improve nursing care through problem solving and working with others. These professionals are **nurse researchers.**

Nurse administrator

Management of patient care and its delivery of nursing services is the responsibility of the **nurse administrator.** Special education in management, supervision, and leadership is necessary. In addition to nursing care delivery services, departments such as quality assurance, risk management, discharge planning, and infection control may be staffed with nurse administrators.

Health care team

Nurses are usually members of a **health care team**—a group of specially trained health care workers who meet the common goal of providing individualized quality care for patients. The team members and their functions are listed in Table 1-2.

Within the past decade the role of the nurse has greatly expanded, and the nurse's responsibility within medicine has thus increased. The future of today's nurse is based on self-motivation and knowledge of current nursing trends. Some points of interest follow:

1. The success of a licensed nurse is obtained through unity in the profession. There is a significant demand for nursing to meet the unlimited needs of society.
2. Various registered nursing programs are available to the LPN/LVN to allow advancement to a higher level of education in the nursing profession. Some of these programs offer competency entrance examinations to help the nurse enter at a level consistent with experience.
3. Employment opportunities available for the LPN/LVN are unlimited. The variety of specialty areas in medicine offers the nurse many choices.

Table 1-2 HEALTH CARE TEAM

Health Care Team Member	Function
Physician	Collaborates with other members, but retains final responsibility
RN	Implements and evaluates nursing care plan and coordinates all nursing activities
LPN/LVN	Provides nursing care and treatments, administers medications, and acts as team leader in some agencies
Dietician	Works with physician and nurses to provide optimal patient nutrition
Allied health specialist Respiratory therapist Occupational therapist Physical therapist Speech therapist Rehabilitation therapist Social worker Pharmacist Spiritual advisor	Collaborates with other members of team to improve patient's condition and coordinates specialized information for the nursing care plan

4. It is the nurse's responsibility to meet the expectations of the nursing profession. This includes not only abiding by the nursing code of ethics and standards, but also complying with the Patient's Bill of Rights (see Chapter 3) and knowing the legal aspects of nursing.

Continuing education

The nurse must remain current in knowledge and skills because new advancements are continually being made in medicine. This may be accomplished through **continuing education** by attending formal and informal educational programs, conferences, and workshops and by becoming a member of the nursing organization representative of the chosen level of nursing. The programs are organized and structured in short-term periods and are offered by specialized groups or health care institutions. Of particular interest to the LPN/LVN is the *Journal of Practical Nursing,* published quarterly by NAPNES. On completion of one of the studies from this journal the nurse earns a certificate and accumulates continuing education credit. Some states require a certain number of hours or credits for renewal of the license.

There are other ways to earn continuing education credit. **In-service education** programs are offered in hospitals and other places of employment. Each facility offering in-service programs usually does so to meet specific needs. Conventions and workshops for specific groups of nurses are offered by universities, community colleges, and private educational organizations. Most courses offer continuing education units for relicensure. The nurse should keep a record of all continuing education activities to show proof for relicensure.

NURSING ENVIRONMENT

Nursing care is focused on encouraging the highest level of patient functioning and providing the highest sense of well-being possible for the patient. Nursing activities must promote high-level wellness.

Types of Nursing Care

Primary prevention

A nursing intervention that applies to healthy patients and that is designed to decrease the probability of or actually prevent dysfunction is known as *primary prevention.* Examples are nursing education classes, immunizations, and nutritional assessment.

Secondary prevention

Secondary prevention focuses on early diagnosis and prompt treatment. It also focuses on preventing or limiting disabilities. The nurse who works in an acute care unit in a hospital practices secondary preventive care.

Tertiary prevention

Restoration and rehabilitation are the goals of tertiary prevention. Care is designed to minimize the effects of a permanent disability and prevent complications or further deterioration. Even though the disability is permanent, this type nursing care is also preventive, since its goal is to prevent further disability. Nurses who work in rehabilitation centers or help newly blind or diabetic patients adapt to their conditions are practicing tertiary nursing care.

Types of Nursing Intervention

As nursing responsibilities grow so do the strategies or actions used to implement nursing care. Nursing actions are classified as independent, dependent, and interdependent.

Independent nursing actions

Nursing interventions that require no direction or supervision from others are classed as **independent nursing actions.** These actions do not require a medical order, but the nurse is accountable to practice within the boundaries of formal education received and the legal limitations of the state. An example of independent interventions is patient teaching regarding appropriate personal hygiene and the importance of receiving immunizations.

Dependent nursing actions

"**Dependent nursing interventions** are based on the instructions or written orders of another professional" (Potter, Perry, 1993). For example, it is not within the legal parameters of the nurse to order medications, treatments, or diagnostic procedures. However, it is the responsibility of the nurse to know the procedure, the clinical skills needed, expected outcomes, and possible side effects. The nurse is also expected to prepare the patient for the procedure and to communicate information to those involved in the patient's care. Examples of dependent nursing actions include sterile dressing changes, preparation for diagnostic tests, and medication administration.

Interdependent nursing actions

Interdependent nursing actions are the result of collaboration with other professionals. Examples include nursing care plans developed by an interdisciplinary team, which includes professionals from the physical therapy and respiratory therapy departments.

NURSING PRACTICE

The practice of nursing is regulated by each state board of nursing. Members of the board are usually appointed by the governor of the state. Both nurses and members of the public are appointed to serve 2- to 4-year terms.

Licensure

The process of **licensure** serves three purposes. First, it defines the standards for entry into the profession. Second, it defines and limits the professional scope of practice. Third, it allows for some type of disciplinary action. Nurses are initially licensed by a national examination and thereafter by endorsement, or licensure, in another state.

A graduate of an accredited nursing program is eligible to apply to take the national NCLEX-PN or NCLEX-RN examination. After successfully completing the examination the nurse is granted a license to practice nursing in that state. Currently the graduate takes a Computerized Adaptive Testing (CAT) examination, and the state board notifies the nurse in 2 to 3 weeks regarding the results.

Once a nurse is actively licensed in one state, licensure in other states is available through the process of **endorsement.** Endorsement is a process by which it is verified that the nurse is a member of the profession, is currently licensed, and is in good standing in the state in which licensure is currently held. The nurse thus applies to the state board to which licensure is needed and completes the criteria for licensure in that state. This allows the nurse to receive licensure in that state without having to take the licensing examination again.

Employment Opportunities

The LPN/LVN has a variety of employment opportunities because of the expanding role and the increasing responsibility given to this nursing level. Nursing positions are usually available in all communities and areas of the country. Because skilled nursing care is transferrable to many different positions, employment is rarely unavailable to the nurse. Although there are many more options than those listed, one of the seven general categories is often chosen by the nurse.

Hospital nursing

The hospital still remains the most popular place in which to work. Within the hospital, specialized areas such as intensive care, obstetrics, pediatrics, medical-surgical nursing, and psychiatry are available. These areas may require additional preparation for many members of the health care team but many require only on-the-job training for the nurse.

Extended care facility

The extended care facility today differs from those of years past. Some examples are nursing homes, residential homes for the ambulatory, and skilled nursing homes. They admit patients who are not ill enough to stay in the hospital but need care that may not be provided at home. In this setting, the LPN/LVN has a leadership role and should acquire management along with nursing skills. Generally, the nurse supervises other health workers and uses decisions relating not only to the patient but also to those under supervision as well.

Private duty nursing

Private duty nursing may be performed in the home, hospital, or other facilities. The nurse is employed usually at the request of a family member or patient or perhaps with a medical order. The nurse is considered self-employed and must work within local policies governing nursing. Salary and schedule are decided between the nurse and family or patient.

Community health nursing

Community health nursing relates to any available health services within the community. Examples include public health nursing, home health services, school nursing, and other services that recognize and meet the needs of the community.

Occupational health nursing

The nurse employed by an occupational or industrial organization cares for employees who become ill at work, administers immunizations to employees, and provides first-aid treatment to injured employees. The nurse also has a large role in performing nursing physical examinations and providing educational programs regarding exercise, smoking cessation, and alcohol and drug addiction.

Physician's office and clinic

Many physicians employ the LPN/LVN to perform outpatient care. Some nurses may work in specialty areas with the physician. The physician or charge nurse may supervise the work of the nurse. The role of the nurse is to assist in examinations, treatments, patient teaching, and office management.

Rehabilitation center

For the patient who requires long-term rehabilitation, the rehabilitation center offers the chance to practice psychosocial and physical nursing care. The nurse is able to give special, individualized attention.

▪ ▪ ▪

The nurse of today must have appropriate personal skills as well as knowledge of theory to be successful. The nurse must be courteous, have a positive attitude, be cooperative, be a good listener, and and be assertive. Because nursing is a profession, the nurse must behave in a professional manner at all times.

LEADERSHIP AND MANAGEMENT

As the cost of health care continues to soar, the nurse must develop financial responsibility. Financial responsibility is practiced through the judicious use of materials and supplies for nursing care. This concept has been included in the curricula for nurses for many years. For example, becoming adept with sterile technique decreases opportunities for contamination, thus saving money for both the patient and the facility. Using the oldest dated, yet current sterile packages first saves the cost of resterilizing and restocking supplies. Taking care not to waste supplies that are disposable also reduces the cost of patient care. The nurse who is financially responsible in practice is aware of health care costs for all people.

The leadership role of the nurse requires special skills in management techniques. This is becoming more evident in the responsibility of the nurse. Management courses are offered in the workplace, and many educational institutions offer these courses. The nurse may be promoted to a leadership role. As leaders, nurses are responsible for ensuring the delivery of quality nursing care by all health care workers under their supervision. Leadership methods vary, and each individual is educated in a certain philosophy or uses a type of leadership comfortable for that person. Methods for leading people range from extreme control to total permissiveness. These approaches are known as *leadership styles.* The three most common leadership styles are autocratic, democratic, and laissez-faire. The nurse who develops an awareness of the best style for each situation becomes an effective leader.

No single leadership style is best for every situation. Assessing the environment, task, group, and the self as leader will help in choosing the most appropriate style of leadership in any situation.

Autocratic Leadership

A situation in which the leader controls all the information and makes all decisions is known as ***autocratic leadership.*** The leader decides what to do, how it is to be done, and who will do it. Staff members are expected to conform and follow directions. The autocratic leadership style is appropriate in situations in which a crisis or emergency exists or in which a quick decision must be made. Staff members with high security needs and limited knowledge or skills usually respond well to an autocratic leadership style.

Democratic Leadership

Democratic leadership is a people-oriented leadership style that builds an effective group by stressing the value of the worker. Leaders using this method encourage group members to participate in making decisions and voicing opinions. The democratic leadership style is more effective in situations in which staff members work well together and communicate effectively and in which no rapid critical decisions need to be made.

Laissez-Faire Leadership

The **laissez-faire leader** is passive, permissive, and nondirective. Decisions are made by the group, and the leader provides no suggestions or direction. This leadership style works well with mature, cooperative group members such as professional researchers, but for most situations this may not be an effective style.

Team Leadership

A student may be given the opportunity to be a student team leader. This role entails assisting and guiding the nursing team in providing care for a select group of patients. The team leader assigns patients to each team member and takes responsibility for the delivery of care to patients as well as for supervision of all members of the team, including nursing assistants. The licensed nurse follows this same plan. Duties of a team leader include the following:

1. Receiving reports on assigned patients
2. Making assignments for team members
3. Making rounds and assessing all assigned patients
4. Giving team members a report on assigned patients
5. Assisting in administering medications and treatments
6. Providing time in the early part of the shift to have a conference with team members on priority patients (those with the most urgent needs) to keep everyone informed of progress in patient care, provide continuity of care, and allow the team leader to answer questions and resolve problems

The nurse with leadership and management skills is better able to provide quality nursing care in an ever-changing profession.

THERAPEUTIC NURSE-PATIENT RELATIONSHIP

The **therapeutic nurse-patient relationship** establishes "rapport (harmony and unity in a relationship) that is the basis for an ongoing resolution of the patient's health problems" (Potter, Perry, 1993). This relationship is focused on the patient. It is a valuable tool for helping the nurse give the patient the best possible nursing care. The four phases of the helping relationship are preinteraction, orientation, working, and termination.

Preinteraction Phase

The purpose of the preinteraction phase is to prepare the nurse to meet the patient. All information relating to the patient is reviewed, and possible problems or concerns are identified. The nurse then plans an approach to the patient based on the data. This helps avoid stereotyping. Finally, the nurse determines the location and setting for meeting the patient.

Orientation Phase

The first meeting between the patient and the nurse sets the tone for the remainder of the relationship. This is the "getting to know you" time in which each person closely assesses the other. Conversation is casual and superficial at first. The patient may frequently test the nurse by questioning competency and reliability or by becoming silent. As the patient's concerns begin to be addressed, trust is built. Genuine caring and concern, as well as respect, help the nurse develop a trusting relationship with the patient and evolve to the point where identification of problems and goals may begin. Once the nurse and patient mutually agree on goals, they mutually decide who will do what. In this way both the patient and nurse are aware of the patient's needs, the necessary nursing care measures, and the patient's responsibilities. This clarification of roles sets the stage for establishing a contract with the patient. In this situation a contract is usually a brief verbal exchange of information that outlines the frequency, duration, and length of contacts with the patient. It is important for the patient to be informed of when the relationship will terminate or end.

Working Phase

During the working phase, the patient and nurse work to achieve the goals. Frequently the patient expresses emotions and begins to engage in self-exploration. Respect and understanding is communicated by the nurse's support and encouragement. If the working phase results in success, the patient will be able to act on the newly acquired knowledge and begin to change behaviors.

Termination Phase

The goal of the termination phase is to prepare the patient and nurse for the end of the relationship. This may cause the patient anxiety or feelings of being deserted, which must be openly discussed before the relationship may successfully conclude. Ideally, the patient and nurse enjoy a sense of accomplishment and fulfillment during this phase. The nurse assists the patient in becoming less dependent.

SUMMARY

Florence Nightingale paved the way for nursing by sacrificing her health, time, and money to further nursing. The nursing leaders of Nightingale's time and those who came later have all helped to make nursing a profession of which to be proud.

Practical/vocational nursing can be an entry level position into the profession of nursing. Graduates may further their education or remain at this level by choice.

Nurse practice acts regulate licensure and practice to protect the public. They also regulate fees, educational requirements, use of the titles *RN* or *LPN/LVN*, examination for licensure, licensure, renewal, and revocation of license.

Nursing theory is a set of ideas based on observable behaviors and facts. A summary of nursing theories is listed in Table 1-1.

Nursing roles are expanding, and each level of nursing is being used in areas once held only by physicians. As health care in the United States changes there will be an even larger expansion of nursing duties and more changes in the workplace of physicians.

Continuing education is an important aspect of quality care. Many states now mandate a certain number of continuing education hours to renew the nursing license.

The nursing environment focuses on the highest possible functioning level for the patient. Types of nursing care in this area include primary, secondary, and tertiary prevention. Types of nursing intervention include independent, dependent, and interdependent nursing actions.

Initial licensure is issued to a graduate of an accredited nursing program on successful completion of the licensing examination. Licensure by endorsement is the method by which a nurse becomes licensed in other states without having to retest.

Types of management and leadership styles include autocratic, democratic, and laissez-faire leadership. Team leadership is used in nursing to assist other workers in administering quality care to patients.

The therapeutic nurse-patient relationship is the basis for an ongoing resolution of the patient's health problems. The four phases of the relationship are the preinteraction, orientation, working, and termination phases.

Key Concepts

- Florence Nightingale was the founder of modern nursing.
- Nursing pioneers assisted in making nursing what it is today. These pioneers include Dorothea Dix, Clara Barton, Louisa May Alcott, Ella King Newsomn, Mary Ann Bickerdyke, Harriet Tubman, Mildred Montag, Linda Richards, Isabell Hampton Robb, Mary E.P. Mahoney, Lillian Wald, Lavinia Dock, and Mary Adelaide Nutting.
- Practical/vocational nursing began in 1887. The National Association Practical Nurse Education and Services, Inc., was formed in 1942. The first accredited practical/vocational nursing program was begun in 1945.
- A state nurse practice act regulates licensure and practice.
- Nursing standards are statements that define the qualifications, functions, and principles of practice. Legal definitions of nursing usually include standards of practice.
- Nursing roles are ever changing, and there are many nursing specialties today.
- The health care team works together for the good of the patient.
- Continuing education is the responsibility of each nurse.
- Nurse licensure defines the standards for entry into the profession, defines and limits the professional scope of practice, and allows for disciplinary action.
- Many employment opportunities are open to the nurse today.
- Hospital nursing remains a favorite for nurses.
- Leadership skills are more important today in nursing than ever before.
- The therapeutic nurse-patient relationship establishes rapport, harmony, and unity in a relationship.

Critical Thinking Questions

1. Why is it important for a profession such as nursing to be regulated? Discuss at least three methods of professional regulation that you understand from reading this chapter.
2. You are a new nurse working in an acute medical-surgical health care setting. Describe some of the health care colleagues that you would encounter in your daily care management for your patients. How critical is your role as "communicator" when working with so many health care colleagues?

REFERENCES AND SUGGESTED READINGS

Abdellah FG et al: *Patient-centered approaches to nursing,* New York, 1960, Macmillan.

Becker BG, Fendler DT: *Vocational and personal adjustments in practical nursing,* ed 7, St Louis, 1994, Mosby.

Burke MM, Walsh MB: New opportunities in gerontologic nursing, *Nursing 93* 23(12):40, 1993.

Chinn PL, Kramer MK: *Theory and nursing: a systematic approach,* ed 4, St Louis, 1994, Mosby.

Clinton HR: Nursing in the front lines, *Nursing and Health Care* 14(6):286, 1993.

Donahue MP: *Nursing: the finest art, an illustrated history,* ed 2, St Louis, 1995, Mosby.

Hull M: Your nursing image: tending the flame, *Nursing 93* 23(5):116, 1993.

Johnson JE: Health care reform and nursing, *Nursing and Health Care* 14(2):59, 1993.

Kurzen CR: *Contemporary practical-vocational nursing,* ed 2, Philadelphia, 1993, Lippincott.

Leininger MM: Caring: a central focus of nursing and health care services, *Nursing and Health Care* 1(3):135, 1980.

Levine MC: *An introduction to clinical nursing,* ed 2, Philadelphia, 1973, Davis.

Marriner-Tomey A: *Nursing theorists and their work,* ed 3, St Louis, 1994, Mosby.

Morrison M: *Professional skills for leadership: foundations of a successful career,* St Louis, 1993, Mosby.

Orem DE: *Nursing: concepts of practice,* ed 3, New York, 1985, McGraw-Hill.

Orlando IJ: *The dynamic nurse-patient relationship: function, process, and principles,* New York, 1961, Putnam.

Parse RR: *Man-living-health: theory of nursing,* New York, 1981, Wiley.

Peplau HE: *Interpersonal relations in nursing,* New York, 1952, Putnam.

Potter PA, Perry AG: *Fundamentals of nursing: concepts, process, and practice,* ed 3, St Louis, 1993, Mosby.

Rogers ME: *An introduction to the theoretical basis of nursing,* Philadelphia, 1970, Davis.

Roy C: The Roy adaptation model. In Riehl JP, Roy C, editors: *Conceptual models for nursing practice,* New York, 1980, Appleton-Century-Crofts.

Schull PD: Specialization: the choice is yours, *Nursing 94* 23(1):75, 1994.

Shryock RH: *The history of nursing: an interpretation of the social and medical factors involved,* Philadelphia, 1959, Saunders.

Torres G: *Theoretical foundations of nursing,* Norwalk, Conn, 1986, Appleton-Century-Crofts.

Zuker E: Five tips for managing a stressful job, *Nursing 93* 23(5):126, 1993.

CHAPTER 2

The Practice of Nursing

Learning Objectives

After studying this chapter, the student should be able to . . .

- Define the key terms.
- Discuss the importance of prevention, health promotion, and education in maintaining health.
- Define the role of culture in health maintenance.
- Participate in a health team approach to the delivery of health care in the community.
- Examine the various roles of the nurse in community health care.
- Discuss governmental influences on the practice of community health nursing.
- Define the role of primary care in health maintenance, health promotion, and improvement of access to health care.

Key Terms

Centers for Disease Control and Prevention (CDC)
Communicable disease
Community
Community health nursing
Culture
Enculturation
Primary care
Primary health care

The definition of nursing has remained in a state of change through the years because it is not easily defined. In 1965 the American Nurses Association (ANA) presented a broad definition of nursing that, unlike previous definitions, depicts nursing as an independent profession:

> Nursing is a helping profession and, as such, provides services which contribute to the health and well-being of people. Nursing is a vital consequence to the individual receiving services; it fills needs which cannot be met by the person, by the family, or by other persons in the community. The essential components of professional nursing are care, cure, and coordination. The care aspect is more than "to take care of," it is "caring for" and "caring about" as well. It is dealing with human beings under stress, frequently over long periods of time. It is providing comfort and support in times of anxiety, loneliness, and helplessness. It is listening, evaluating, and intervening appropriately. The promotion of health and healing is the cure aspect of professional nursing. It is assisting clients to understand their health problems and helping them to cope. It is the administration of treatments and the use of clinical nursing judgment in determining, on the basis of clients' reactions, whether the plan for care needs to be maintained or changed. It is knowing when and how to use existing and potential resources to help clients toward recovery and adjustment by mobilizing their own resources. Professional nursing practice is this and more. It is sharing responsibility for the health and welfare of all those in the community, and participating in programs designed to prevent illness and maintain health. It is coordinating and synchronizing medical and other professional and technical services since these affect patients. It is supervising, teaching, and directing all those who give nursing care.

PRACTICE SETTINGS

The role of the nurse has expanded in the health care system, causing an increase in practice settings. The different types of nursing care open to the nurse allows a choice in employment.

Hospital nursing remains the most popular place of employment for nurses. Within the hospital there are many areas from which to choose. For example, medical-surgical nursing units provide care for patients with medical or surgical diagnoses. The registered nurse and the practical/vocational nurse are employed in many of these areas.

Hospital nursing also allows the nurse to participate in different approaches to providing nursing care. These approaches include functional nursing, team nursing, specialty nursing, total patient care, primary nursing, and modified primary nursing.

The people of the United States face massive changes in health care. Because of increasing health care costs, many people have little or no health monitoring or health care. These problems make it difficult to imagine the future of health care. These changes in the health care system are causing a shift in nursing practice from the hospital to the community. Nurses from every level must be ready to accept this and other changes while providing quality care.

Historically, nursing care was provided by nurses in the homes of their patients. Many nurses (for example, Lillian Wald) lived and provided nursing care in the same community. Wald wrote a book, *The House on Henry Street,* in which she described problems with basic sanitation and illnesses caused by poverty and communicable diseases (Wald, 1915). Wald and nurses like her charged for their services based on their patients' ability to pay. Currently, health care is preparing to return to community-based care. ***Primary health care*** is a term used to describe essential health services that are universally accessible. This type of health care is community based and includes health promotion, illness prevention, monitoring of chronic diseases, and education of patients to help them live healthy, productive lives. **Primary care** is a strategy for providing primary care whereby medical care is provided to patients at the point of contact with the physician (McElmurry, 1992).

Community Health Concepts

According to the World Health Organization (WHO), a **community** is as a social entity that may be within a specific geographic boundary or is a social group sharing common interests and values. The ANA (1980) defines ***community health nursing*** as "a synthesis of nursing and public health practice applied to promoting and preserving the health of populations." The ANA further states that community health nursing is "directed to individuals, families, or groups" and that "the dominant responsibility is to the population as a whole." The responsibilities of the community health nurse are education, counseling, and collaboration with other members of the health care team as well as provision of nursing care to patients.

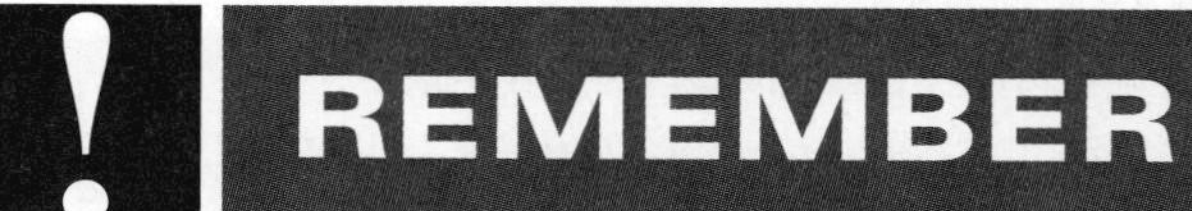

- The role of the community health nurse is education, counseling, and collaboration with other members of the health care team as well as administration of nursing care.
- The nurse must be culturally sensitive to work in the patient's home.
- The nurse must deal with frustrations such as reduced funding in areas in which patient need is the greatest.

Communities are composed of groups of people from different cultural backgrounds. A **culture** is the socially inherited characteristics of a human group that are transmitted from one generation to the next (Fejos, 1959). The nurse working in community nursing must be culturally sensitive and informed to provide relevant nursing care. (Chapter 8 discusses cultural influences on health care.) As discussed by Krebs (1994), nurses also come from a variety of cultural backgrounds, and they must be aware of their own biases before administering nursing care to a multicultural community. Through **enculturation** (the process of learning the concepts, values, and behavioral standards of a particular culture), individuals develop a world view. This world view permeates every aspect of life, including ways of thinking and behaving and the values that guide a person's life.

Nurses can become culturally sensitive by reading about other cultural beliefs, assessing individual biases, and listening and developing other communication techniques. By also knowing ethnic customs and beliefs, conducting assessments based on the needs of particular cultural groups, and planning population-based interventions, the nurse makes health care services more relevant and responsive to cultural groups and to the individuals in them.

Community nurses should also acknowledge traditional healing practices that do not injure the individual's health or interfere with treatments. This practice demonstrates respect for patients as well as their culture.

Infection-Control Practices

Historically, public health problems were related to poor sanitation and health practices. With the advent of antibiotics, immunizations, and improvements in sanitation, many infectious diseases were controlled. The greatest public health challenges today stem from unhealthy life styles that lead to the development of chronic diseases such as heart disease, lung disease, some cancers, and various genetic disorders. Public health efforts to control the development of chronic disease focuses on prevention. Preventive measures include education regarding the benefits of a healthy diet, smoking cessation, weight control, exercise, and early detection of health problems, including cancer.

The **Centers for Disease Control and Prevention (CDC)** in Atlanta, Georgia, distributes information about research findings to health care providers, both in the public health and private sectors. In addition, the CDC provides guidelines for the care, treatment, and prevention of disease to health care providers. The CDC also maintains a monitoring system to track outbreaks of **communicable disease,** or contagious disease.

Some infectious diseases must be reported to public health departments. Tuberculosis; meningitis; and syphilis, gonorrhea, and other sexually transmitted diseases (STDs) are a few examples of reportable diseases. Individual states may add to this list of reportable diseases depending on risk factors within a particular area of a state. These reports are the means by which communicable diseases are monitored.

Health care providers are facing new challenges regarding infectious and communicable diseases. Some infectious diseases have no cure and can only be controlled. Two examples are herpes genitalis caused by type 2 herpes simplex virus and acquired immunodeficiency syndrome caused by the human immunodeficiency virus. New communicable diseases continue to develop, and infectious diseases believed to be controlled are recurring because of breakdowns in sanitation, crowded living conditions, and poverty. Some microorganisms are also becoming resistant to antibiotics. Thus nurses working in community settings must teach sanitary practices and use disease-prevention strategies to control the occurrence of infectious disease.

Home Health Nursing

Community health nursing is a term encompassing many employment settings. The settings include public health, rural health, school health, occupational health, correctional, and home health nursing. Nurses practice in a community health role when the focus is on groups and populations. It is estimated that most employment opportunities will be in home health care. Many practical/vocational nurses are currently employed in this area.

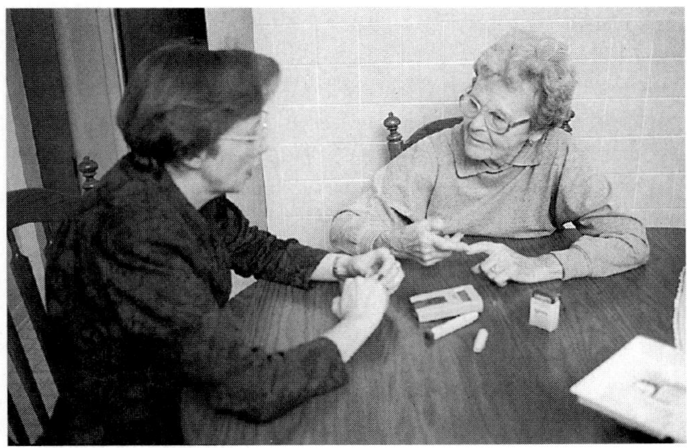

Fig. 2-1 Nurses teach skilled procedures in the home. (From Potter PA, Perry AG: *Basic nursing: theory and practice,* ed 3, St Louis, 1995, Mosby.)

Home health nurses must remember that they are guests in the patient's home. The therapeutic nurse-patient relationship is replaced by a partnership that develops as the nurse assumes a consultant role (Fig. 2-1). In addition, the opportunity to assess a patient in the family setting and to assess the support systems of the patient allows the nurse to identify the unmet needs of the patient and the family. For this reason the family is considered the focus of nursing care in the community.

A network of services is available in many communities to meet the needs of the family that is caring for the ill member. The home health nurse is often advises, educates, and cares for the family through the use of these services.

The family member directly responsible for care of the patient often needs time away from the stress of the full-time care. The home health nurse may fill this need and also identify unhealthy relationships, disease in other family members, and symptoms of family stress. The home health nurse should assess all of these factors and obtain care for any problems. Referrals should also be made to available services. A list of common services can be found in Appendix A. For example, the American Heart Association, American Lung Association, and National Arthritis Foundation offer educational materials and can direct patients to support services.

Future of Nursing

Community-based health care recognizes the effects of the environmental, occupational, societal, cultural, and biologic factors affecting health. With the trend toward this type of health care, the nurse and other health care professionals will need to develop a broader understanding of community health concepts to maximize the effectiveness of and to appropriately use available services. Educational institutions are already beginning to prepare graduates who have basic skills for effective practice in the community.

SUMMARY

Early nursing care was administered in the homes of patients, and now, nursing (health) care is beginning to return to community-based care. Primary health care is community based and includes health promotion, illness prevention, monitoring of chronic diseases, and education of patients to prepare them to live healthy, productive lives. Nurses today are being prepared to provide nursing care in community-based centers. Many practical/vocational nurses are now employed in community areas. This trend is expected to continue.

The community health nurse must become culturally sensitive and informed to provide relevant nursing care. The nurse must learn about other cultural beliefs and work within patients' value systems. The health care industry must also deal with new diseases, diseases resistant to antibiotics, and diseases for which there is no cure.

Key Concepts

- The American Nurses Association's definition of nursing has been broadened to encompass all aspects of nursing care and nursing roles.
- Nursing is returning to the community setting.
- Nurses are being educated to work in community health nursing.
- The responsibilities of the community health nurse include education, counseling, and collaboration as well as administration of nursing care.
- The nurse must become culturally sensitive when working in the patient's home.
- Health care providers will face new challenges in disease control and prevention.
- The Centers for Disease Control and Prevention distributes information about research findings to health care providers.
- Community health nursing includes public, rural, school, occupational, correctional, and home health nursing.

Critical Thinking Questions

1. With the decreasing length of hospital stays for people needing acute care, what are the kinds of things that you could do as a new nurse to keep up with these changes and maintain your quality of care but also stay sensitive to the needs of patients who come through your hospital so quickly?
2. Mrs. Phillips is a 55-year-old woman newly diagnosed with diabetes. You visit her twice a week to evaluate blood glucose measurement and insulin administration. Today, her blood glucose level is high, and she tells you she cannot afford her medicine. She has barely enough income to cover living expenses. Identify a diagnosis and one goal and describe interventions for Mrs. Phillips.
3. An 18-year-old healthy college student arrives at the clinic complaining of sunburn. He just returned from 12 hours on the beach playing volleyball. What alterations in vital signs would you expect? What nursing interventions are indicated?

REFERENCES AND SUGGESTED READINGS

American Nurses Association Committee on Education: *A position paper,* New York, 1965, The Association.

American Nurses Association: *ANA standards of community health nursing practice,* Kansas City, 1980, The Association.

Bernal H: A model for delivering culture-relevant care in the community, *Public Health Nursing* 10:4, 1993.

Crow K: Multiculturism & pluralistic thought, *Journal of Nursing Education* 32:5, 1993.

Fejos P: Man, magic, and medicine. In Goldstone I, editor: *Medicine and anthropology,* New York, 1959, International Universities Press.

Fry S: *Ethics in community health nursing practice.* In Stanhope M, Lancaster J, editors: *Community health nursing: promoting health of aggregates, families, and individuals,* ed 2, St Louis, 1995, Mosby.

Krebs G, Kunimoto E: *Effective communication in multicultural health care settings,* Thousand Oaks, Calif, 1994, Sage.

McElmurry BJ et al, eds: *Women's health and development: global perspective,* Boston, 1992, Jones & Bartlett.

Mitchell P, Grippando G: *Nursing perspectives and issues,* ed 5, Albany, NY, 1993, Delmar.

Potter PA, Perry AG, *Basic nursing: theory and practice,* ed 3, St Louis, 1995, Mosby.

Smith S, Duell D: *Clinical nursing skills,* ed 3, Norwalk, Conn, 1992, Appleton & Lange.

Stanhope M, Knollmueller RN: *Handbook of community and home health nursing: tools for assessment, intervention, and education,* ed 2, St Louis, 1995, Mosby.

Wald L: *The house on Henry Street,* New York, 1915, Holt.

CHAPTER 3

Legal and Ethical Considerations

Learning Objectives

After studying this chapter, the student should be able to. . . .

- Define the key terms.
- Describe four principles that provide the basis for ethical behavior.
- Discuss the role of ethics in nursing practice.
- List six points addressed in the Code of Ethics from the National Association for Practical Nurse Education and Services, Inc.
- Explain the purpose of the Patient's Bill of Rights.
- Describe three ethical dilemmas and give a solution for each.
- List the five steps of the ethical decision-making model.
- Explain how laws contribute to legal changes in nursing.
- State the difference among nursing licensure, suspension, and revocation.
- Explain the purpose of Good Samaritan laws.
- List four nursing responsibilities relating to the patient's medical record.
- Discuss the importance of obtaining an informed consent.
- Name two legal implications relating to the use of restraints.

Key Terms

Accountability
Assault
Autonomy
Battery
Bioethical committee
Code of ethics
Confidentiality
Crime
Defamation of character
"Do not resuscitate" (DNR)
Duty
Ethical dilemma
Ethics
False imprisonment
Felony
Fidelity
Fraud
Good Samaritan law
Incident report
Informed consent
Invasion of privacy
Justice
Libel
Living will
Maleficence
Malpractice
Misdemeanor
Moral
Negligence
Nurse practice act
"A Patient's Bill of Rights"
Principle
Responsibility
Slander
Standard
State board of nursing
Tort
Value
Veracity

ETHICAL CONSIDERATIONS

The word *ethics* comes from a Greek word that means "custom." Today, ***ethics*** is defined as "principles and standards that govern 'right' from 'wrong' behaviors" (Morrison, 1993). Ethics reflects what a society defines as good or worthy and bad or undesirable. Ethics may differ from individual to individual, and conflict may arise because the foundation for ethics is deeply rooted in values and morals.

Values

A **value** is "a personal belief about the worth of a given idea or behavior upon which a person acts" (Potter, Perry 1993). What people believe is important is what they value, and these important beliefs (values) develop into standards for action. For example, if people value honesty, they do not lie or cheat.

Strong personal beliefs about the absolute right or wrong of an issue are **morals.** Culture, religious beliefs, and traditions form the basis for morals. Usually, people are unwilling to change their viewpoints relating to moral issues. For example, abortion is a highly publicized issue today. A nurse must make decisions about personal views on this issue and decide whether these views would interfere if the nurse is requested to assist in the performance of an abortion procedure. This is referred to as an ***ethical dilemma,*** or a situation involving a choice between equally unsatisfactory alternatives.

Responsibility and Accountability

Doing what you say you will do simply defines **responsibility.** The nurse is responsible for safe nursing practice, obtaining knowledge about new procedures and theories, and performing within ethical guidelines and standards. One example of taking responsibility is to be dependable at work.

Ethics also includes **accountability,** which is defined as taking responsibility for one's actions. The nurse is answerable for personal actions and may demonstrate accountability by practicing within the professional code of ethics. Being accountable means that the nurse cannot wrongly abandon care of a patient. The nurse has a **duty** (responsibility) to make certain that the patient receives the best care available. For the student nurse, it is a duty to attend class and clinical laboratories on time.

PRINCIPLES OF ETHICAL BEHAVIOR

The Florence Nightingale pledge was created in 1893 for the registered nurse. Its purpose is to provide "a framework for clarifying moral and ethical values and principles needed for delivering health care and promoting the standards of nursing" (Calhoun, 1993). The Nightingale pledge, like many others, is based on ethical **principles,** or guidelines for the conduct of the nurse. The nurse who practices seven principles—autonomy, prevention of maleficence, beneficence, justice, confidentiality, fidelity, and veracity—is an ethically responsible professional.

The principles of **autonomy** (independence or self-government), prevention of **maleficence** (the act of committing harm or evil), beneficence (quality or state of being kind and charitable), and justice help define the foundation of nursing practice (Table 3-1). The nurse also follows the principles of confidentiality, fidelity, and veracity. **Confidentiality** deals with the ethical responsibility to protect the patient's privacy by respecting privileged, personal information. Sharing information about a patient with only those involved in that person's care

Table 3-1 ETHICAL PRINCIPLES

Definitions	Nursing Implications
Autonomy	
Personal liberty of action, self-determination	Promote patient decision-making. Support patient's right to informed consent. Make decisions when patient's choice poses harm. Exercise autonomy when members of health care team agree to importance of autonomy.
Prevention of maleficence	
Duty to do no harm	Avoid deliberate harm, risk of harm, and harm that occurs during performance of nursing actions. Consider degree of risk permissible. Determine whether use of technologic advances provides benefits that outweigh risks.
Beneficence	
Doing or active promotion of good	Provide health benefits to patients. Balance benefit and risks of harm. Consider how patient is best helped.
Justice	
Fairness or equity	Ensure fair allocation of resources, such as appropriate staffing or mix of staff to all patients. Determine order in which patients should be treated (for example, priority treatment for patients in pain).

From Potter PA, Perry AG: *Fundamentals of nursing: concepts, process, and practice,* ed 3, St Louis, 1993, Mosby.

helps ensure confidentiality. The nurse may be held liable for talking about the patient with anyone except those on the health care team. **Fidelity** is loyalty to something to which one is bound by a pledge or duty. **Veracity** means "truthfulness" or "honesty," and the nurse is obligated to tell the truth. Licensed practical/vocational nurses (LPNs/LVNs) may have several pledges based on these values and principles. Some nursing programs say a pledge at the capping or graduation ceremony.

ETHICS IN NURSING

Because the quality of life is highly valued, the nurse and other health care workers are committed to strong ethical principles. One of the most important commitments made by the student nurse involves the obligation to uphold the profession's ethical principles.

A **standard** is a measure or guide established by authority for measuring quality. Standards for nursing practice provide guidelines for ensuring quality patient care. The nurse is ethically obligated to practice according to standards.

A principle governing standards of conduct for a profession is frequently referred to as a code. A **code of ethics** involves statements that describe the values, goals, and standards of conduct to be maintained. The code acts as a guideline for nursing behavior and offers a framework for making ethically sound decisions. Codes of ethics for the nurse have been developed by the American Nurses Association (ANA); the Canadian Nurses Association (CNA); the International Council of Nurses (ICN); the National Association for Practical Nurse Education and Service, Inc. (NAPNES); and the National Federation of Licensed Practical Nurses (NFLPN). Although each code may vary in language and emphasis, they all share the same underlying principles of autonomy, prevention of maleficence, justice, confidentiality, fidelity, and veracity.

Ethical Codes for Licensed Practical/Vocational Nursing

Both national LPN/LVN organizations (NAPNES and NFLPN) have developed similar codes of ethics. For NAPNES' code of ethics, see the box.

NAPNES CODE OF ETHICS

The licensed practical nurse shall:

1. Consider as a basic obligation the conservation of life and the prevention of disease.
2. Promote and protect the physical, mental, emotional, and spiritual health of the patient and his family.
3. Fulfill all duties faithfully and efficiently.
4. Function within established legal guidelines.
5. Accept personal responsibility for his/her acts and seek to merit the respect and confidence of all members of the health team.
6. Hold in confidence all matters coming to his/her knowledge in the practice of his/her profession and in no way at any time violate this confidence.
7. Give conscientious service and charge just remuneration.
8. Learn and respect the religious and cultural beliefs of his/her patient and of all people.
9. Meet his/her obligation to the patient by keeping abreast of current trends in health care through reading and continuing education.
10. As a citizen of the United States of America, uphold the laws of the land and seek to promote legislation which shall meet the health needs of its people.

From National Association for Practical Nursing Education and Service, Inc: *NAPNES code of ethics,* New York, 1988, The Association.

Patient's Bill of Rights

The ethical practice of nursing involves a primary consideration of others. The ethical principle of autonomy requires the nurse to consider and support the rights of patients to freely make decisions based on accurate and current knowledge. Twelve of these principles relating to rights of patients were published in 1975 by the American Hospital Association. This document, entitled **"A Patient's Bill of Rights,"** recognized the existence of the rights of people to make informed, confidential decisions about their health care (see box). It is the ethical duty of the nurse to consider the rights of the patient when providing nursing care.

ETHICAL ISSUES

In today's complex health care delivery system, social and technologic changes have compelled the nurse and other caregivers to consider many ethical issues. Special groups of patients, such as children, older adults, the dying, and the mentally and physically challenged, bring with them ethical questions of many varieties. Other major ethical issues focus on informed consent, confidentiality, the behavior of health care professionals, and allocation of resources.

A PATIENT'S BILL OF RIGHTS

1. The patient has the right to considerate and respectful care.
2. The patient has the right to obtain from his physician complete current information concerning his diagnosis, treatment, and prognosis in terms the patient can be reasonably expected to understand. When it is not medically advisable to give such information to the patient, the information should be made available to an appropriate person in his behalf. He has the right to know by name the physician responsible for coordinating his care.
3. The patient has the right to receive from his physician information necessary to give informed consent prior to the start of any procedure and/or treatment. Except in emergencies, such information for informed consent should include but not necessarily be limited to the specific procedure and/or treatment, the medically significant risks involved, and the probable duration of incapacitation. Where medically significant alternatives for care or treatment exist or when the patient requests information concerning medical alternatives, the patient has the right to such information. The patient also has the right to know the name of the person responsible for the procedures and/or treatment.
4. The patient has the right to refuse treatment to the extent permitted by law and to be informed of the medical consequences of his action.
5. The patient has the right to every consideration of his privacy concerning his own medical care program. Case discussion, consultation, examination, and treatment are confidential and should be conducted discreetly. Those not directly involved in his care must have the permission of the patient to be present.
6. The patient has the right to expect that all communications and records pertaining to his care should be treated as confidential.
7. The patient has the right to expect that within its capacity a hospital must make reasonable response to the request of a patient for services. The hospital must provide evaluation, service, and/or referral as indicated by the urgency of the case. When medically permissible a patient may be transferred to another facility only after he has received complete information and explanation concerning the needs for and alternatives to such a transfer. The institution to which the patient is to be transferred must first have accepted the patient for transfer.
8. The patient has the right to obtain information as to any relationship of his hospital to other health care and educational institutions insofar as his care is concerned. The patient has the right to obtain information as to the existence of any professional relationships among individuals, by name, who are treating him.
9. The patient has the right to be advised if the hospital proposes to engage in or perform human experimentation affecting his care or treatment. The patient has the right to refuse to participate in such research projects.
10. The patient has the right to expect reasonable continuity of care. He has the right to know in advance what appointment times and physicians are available and where. The patient has the right to expect that the hospital will provide a mechanism whereby he is informed by his physician or a delegate of the physician of the patient's continuing health care requirements following discharge.
11. The patient has the right to examine and receive an explanation of his bill regardless of source of payment.
12. The patient has the right to know what hospital rules and regulations apply to his conduct as a patient.

From American Hospital Association: *A patient's bill of rights,* Chicago, 1992, The Association.

Ethical Dilemmas

Complicated questions frequently evolve into ethical dilemmas—conflict or uncertainty about the moral principles that support a course of action (behavior). Caring for patients with human immunodeficiency virus, for example, may conflict with the nurse's value system, resulting in a conflict between personal values and the ethical principles of beneficence and justice. In fact, so many ethical dilemmas exist that groups of health care providers have been formed specifically to study the complex ethical issues relating to patients and their care. An example of an ethical dilemma is when Nurse A drops a medication tablet on the floor, picks it up, and administers it to the patient. Nurse B witnesses this behavior and knows that it is against policy but the nurse is a friend of Nurse A. The ethical dilemma lies in what Nurse B should do about this situation.

Bioethics Committee

As ethical issues become more complicated, hospitals and other health care institutions have developed committees to clarify and assist with ethical problems. **Bioethics committees** are groups of health care workers who routinely meet to address ethical issues. These specialized committees have four basic functions (Potter, Perry, 1993) (see box).

FUNCTIONS OF A BIOETHICS COMMITTEE

- *To educate:* to provide knowledge about ethical issues and principles for health care workers
- *To develop policies:* to construct, review, and evaluate ethical responsibilities (for example, policies regarding abortions or resuscitation)
- *To advise:* to serve as a resource for specific patient care situations or decisions
- *To evaluate:* to review the outcomes of the ethical decisions made

Ethics in Nursing Practice

The nurse practices ethical behavior in two basic manners: the incorporation of ethical principles into daily behavior and the use of the ethical decision-making process when faced with a dilemma. The ethical decision-making process is a systematic arrangement of principles used to motivate and guide ethical actions (Husted, Husted, 1994).

Nursing Conduct

The first concern of the nurse on duty is the patient. Consideration for the patient includes working quietly and efficiently, not talking or laughing loudly in the immediate patient care area, and protecting the privacy of the patient.

Truthfulness, honesty, and loyalty are important qualities of a nurse. Nurses are responsible for human lives because other human beings depend on them to provide physical, emotional, and spiritual care. The nurse is obligated to report a mistake immediately to the supervisor and describe in detail what happened to cause the error. The temptation to cover up a mistake or take an error lightly is never justified in nursing because it involves the life of another human being. The nurse is also responsible for reporting the unprofessional care of others, an action that must be performed with discretion.

Loyalty to the nursing profession and the institution is one of the most essential values of ethical conduct. One who is loyal exemplifies dedication and commitment to the profession, its ethics and standards, and the employing institution. Loyalty to the welfare of the patient is exemplified by complying with the Patient's Bill of Rights. Loyalty to oneself is demonstrated by using ethical principles in daily nursing practice.

Ethical Decision Making

Although each ethical issue is unique, the nurse may consider several guidelines for making ethical decisions or coping with ethical dilemmas (Potter, Perry, 1993) (see box). Making ethical decisions in an orderly, systematic manner increases the ability to deal with the dynamic and sometimes complex issues relating to ethics. The quality of nursing care depends on the skills and ethical integrity of the practitioner.

GUIDELINES FOR MAKING ETHICAL DECISIONS

- *Identify important factors:* The nurse gathers as many facts, opinions, and viewpoints as possible. Every person involved in the process (physician, nurse, family, and spiritual advisor) is identified.
- *Presume good will:* Usually all people involved wants what they feel is "best" for the patient, provider, and agency.
- *Gather relevant information:* The nurse assesses patient's and family's preferences, support systems, wishes, and daily lifestyle. Factors such as medical treatments, expenses, resources, and the staff's opinions also affect the decision. The nurse should try to form an "ideal picture" as a resolution for the dilemma.
- *State and rank values:* Using the seven ethical principles (autonomy, prevention of maleficence, beneficence, justice, confidentiality, fidelity, and veracity), the nurse decides which principles are the most important and places them in order, with the highest priority first. The nurse then determines a plan of action.
- *Take action:* The plan of action should be followed. The nurse should monitor changes and evaluate the effectiveness of the plan.

LEGAL CONSIDERATIONS

Each nurse is expected to use reasonable care in the practice of nursing. *Reasonable care* means providing the same level of care as would another nurse who has a similar education and experience. Therefore laws apply to the student nurse, the LPN/LVN, and the registered nurse. A nurse's background and experience are considered when reasonable care is determined. For example, an LPN/LVN would not be expected to perform to the standards of a registered nurse.

As a health care provider, the nurse must be aware of the problems that may arise when administering care to the patient. The patient places great trust in the nurse, and any violations of this confidence may be considered an illegal or unethical act. Because the nurse is a professional, some behaviors and actions (for example, gossiping about a patient) are unacceptable. A nurse has a moral and legal obligation to perform as expected. The patient has the right to expect reasonable care. This is referred to as a *duty of care.*

The concept of basic human rights is widely accepted among health care providers. The Patient's Bill of Rights serves as a guideline for reasonable care and is supported by hospitals and other health care agencies. For example, the Patient's Bill of Rights provides, in writing, the moral and legal obligations for nursing care and defines the responsibility of the agency or institution providing nursing service. It also outlines the type of relationship that a patient may expect with the physician. These legal considerations must be used in the practice of nursing.

Principles of the Role of Law

Some general principles govern the role of law and its contribution to the practice of nursing. These principles help the student gain an understanding of the differences in law that occur from state to state. These general points follow:

1. The definitions in this chapter are general. Each state has variations explaining how these definitions are interpreted and applied.
2. These terms should give the nurse a general understanding of legal terms and are not intended to be a complete study of the law.
3. The law constantly changes, and what is true today may not necessarily be true tomorrow. It should not be assumed that the laws are understood because the nurse attends a workshop. The nurse should attend workshops as often as possible to keep abreast of the many changes.
4. Any questions regarding the law should be answered by a person competent in law. Misinterpretation or ignorance of the law is not usually a defense.

LEGAL PRINCIPLES

A *law* is "the controls that a society imposes upon itself to maintain order" (Morrison, 1993). Western society established its system of laws on four basic principles: justice, change (process of making different), standards, and individual rights and responsibilities. **Justice** is concerned with fairness. Laws will change as society changes. An individual's actions are compared to the standard of what a similarly educated, reasonable, and prudent person would do in a similar situation. Last, each person is entitled to the rights and privileges of living in a society, but this person also has responsibilities as a citizen of that society. For example, after graduating, the nurse will be a professional but will still be a citizen in the community and will be expected to perform obligations within that group.

Types of Laws

The law assists in governing relationships. Changes within the relationship between society and its health care system will contribute to legal changes that automatically affect nursing. The nurse is responsible for learning about these legal changes and applying them to practice. Basically, two types of law deal with relationships: public and private law.

Public law

The relationship between the government and its citizens is the focus of public law. The division of public law that concerns nursing is called *criminal law.*

Criminal law The purpose of criminal law is to protect the public. A **crime** is a violation of the laws of society, and a person who commits a crime is punishable by law. There are two types of crime: felony and misdemeanor.

Serious crimes against society, such as arson, armed robbery, and homicide, are known as **felonies.** Penalties for felonies usually include lengthy imprisonment or death. **Misdemeanors** are less serious crimes. Fines and prison terms of less than a year are the usual penalties for these crimes.

Private law

Often referred to as *civil law,* private law deals with relationships among individuals within a society. Two important types of civil (private) law for the nurse are contract and tort law.

Contract law Agreements between an individual or institution defines contract law. Agreements (contracts) may be written or implied. The nurse who begins work for an agency enters into implied (unspoken) or written contracts.

Tort law A **tort** is a legal wrong that is committed against the person or the property of another individual (Morrison, 1993). Tort law relates to the rights of the individual. Several types of torts are of special importance for the nurse and are discussed later in this chapter.

LEGAL PRINCIPLES FOR THE NURSE

The profession of nursing is regulated by several legal mechanisms. Criminal and civil laws as well as mandatory licensure procedures help define and govern the practice of nursing.

State Board of Nursing

Every state in the United States and province of Canada has a **state board of nursing.** The size of the group may vary, but each board consists of registered nurses, LPNs/LVNs, lay members of the community, and other members such as a physician and nursing home administration. All board members are appointed by the state governor.

Functions of the state board

Primary functions The primary functions of state and provincial boards are to define and regulate the practice of nursing through the use of administrative and licensing procedures.

Administrative functions The board of nursing enacts rules that define the minimal standards and curricula for all nursing programs. Once accredited by the board, each program is then periodically surveyed to ensure that the standards are being met.

The board of nursing also writes rules and regulations that further define nursing. This document is referred to as the state ***nurse practice act.*** It is important for the nurse to become familiar with the local nurse practice act. The board also regulates nursing practice by denying or closing nursing programs or suspending individuals who do not meet the defined standards. Texas has a nursing title act instead of a nurse practice act and is the only state in which the name differs.

Licensing functions To practice nursing the nurse must be granted a legal license. Licensure is mandatory in all states. To become licensed, an individual must graduate from an accredited school of nursing and must successfully pass a standardized national examination, the National Council Licensure Examination for Licensed Practical/Vocational Nurses (NCLEX-PN). In 1994, the licensing examination was changed to Computerized Adaptive Testing (CAT). The results of the computerized test are returned much sooner than the former pencil-and-paper test. This process allows the individual to be employed as a licensed nurse soon after graduation from the nursing program. Once the nurse is licensed in one state, licensure may be received in another state by endorsement (see Chapter 1).

Other functions The board of nursing also has the power to deny, suspend, or revoke a license or accreditation of a program. A license may be denied because of unsuccessful completion of the licensing examination, a conviction for a felony, or documented inability to perform the duties of a nurse.

Suspension and revocation of an active nursing license is another method that the board of nursing uses to protect the public. Suspension of licensure involves the loss of a nursing license for a specified time or until the nurse can prove that the deficiencies are corrected. Once the license is reinstated, the nurse can return to work. Revocation is the permanent loss of licensure because of serious unethical or illegal behavior. Each state or provincial board defines the requirements for nursing licensure. Failure to meet these requirements may lead to the suspension or revocation of the license. Some of the more common reasons for losing a license include failure to pursue continuing education requirements (maintain or develop current knowledge), drug abuse (including alcohol), and patient abuse. State and provincial boards of nursing play an important role in protecting the public and the nursing profession from unscrupulous or unsafe practice.

Guidelines for Practice

The nurse is ethically and legally accountable for individual actions. Following sound principles helps ensure quality nursing care.

Standards of Practice

A standard is a model or example by which to compare and measure something. Standards of nursing practice provide exact criteria against which patients, nurses, and employers may evaluate nursing care for effectiveness and excellence (Kozier, 1993). Medical-surgical nursing standards were first developed by the American Nurses Association in 1974. Since then most specialties have established specific standards for nursing practice.

Agency Practices

The policies, procedures, job descriptions, and contracts of an employing agency influence nursing practice. Policies define a course of action. For example, the policy of one hospital may be to perform a physical assessment on all patients at least every 8 hours. The way that a task of skill is to be performed is found in the agency's procedure manual. Job descriptions define the job, its functions, its qualifications, and the person to whom the nurse reports. The nurse has a right to learn and carry out written agency policies. Written policies and procedures protect the nurse in the employing agency. For this reason, it may be unsafe for the nurse to work in an agency that has no written policies.

The nurse enters into a contract with the employer. A contract may be written, verbal, or implied. An agency's application for employment may include a contractual agreement. The nurse should make certain that the contractual obligations are understood before signing because a contract is legally binding once it is signed. The nurse should also ask pertinent questions about legal and ethical implications of any policies. It is not a good practice to sign the contract, thinking that the situation will work out once employment has begun.

Reasonable Nurse Principle

The law judges a nurse by asking the question, "What would a reasonable and prudent nurse do under similar circumstances?" and then making a comparison between the behaviors. The nurse who consults with others and seeks new information before acting follows the principle of the reasonable and prudent nurse. Another application of this principle is seen in the Good Samaritan laws.

Good Samaritan Laws

The **Good Samaritan law,** enacted in most states, protects persons who perform emergency care in a reasonable and prudent manner without appropriate equipment and supplies. Some states do not have these laws to protect nurses. Therefore familiarity with state laws is a necessity. The reasonableness of the actions of the nurse is related to the circumstances of the event. A higher standard of medical care is expected of an individual with special training, such as a physician, a professional nurse, an LPN/LVN, an emergency medical technician, paramedics, or any person trained in basic first aid. The person performing immediate assistance is expected to release responsibility of care to a person with more training if one becomes available.

The nurse may practice "reasonably and prudently" by following the state nurse practice act, professional standards of practice, the policies of the agency, and contracts. Safe nursing practice is based on knowledge of theory and the application of accurate theory and skills to nursing care.

HEALTH CARE RECORD

In addition to the duty of nursing care the nurse has several other legal responsibilities. The medical record, commonly called a *patient chart, chart,* or *client care record,* is just one of these. The medical record is used for the legal documentation of a patient's level of care in a health care agency. *Chart* is the informal term for the patient's medical record and the process of entering data into a patient's record. The nurse is responsible for accurately describing the patient's condition and response to treatment. In a court of law the medical record is sometimes the determining factor of the quality of a patient's care. The patient has a right to view the medical record. Each agency usually has a policy for carrying out this request.

Documentation (Charting) Guidelines

The nurse may be protected legally by making certain that every patient's chart is accurate by signing all entries immediately, leaving no blank spaces or lines, not signing another nurse's entries, not entering false information, and not attempting to cover up an incident. Doing any of these may be grounds for fraud. Fraud is the act of intentionally misleading or deceiving another person by any means so as to cause legal injury, usually the loss of something valuable or the surrender of a legal right.

The use of the nursing process should result in completeness in documentation. The nurse should document identified patient problems, nursing actions taken to solve the problems, and the patient's response to nursing care. Documentation should provide evidence that standards of care were met and actions were taken to prevent complications.

Correctness may deal with actions such as correcting a documentation error: crossing out the entry with a single line, writing "error in charting" above the incorrect section, and signing the nurse's initials. The nurse should never erase an entry, use correction fluid, or obliterate any entry. In court it would be difficult or perhaps even impossible for the nurse to prove what information was written in an obliterated entry.

The nurse should write the date and time on every entry. This is especially important in an emergency situation.

Follow-through deals with documenting communication with a physician, treatments, and the patient's response to them. Any change in the patient's condition is reported to the charge nurse, supervisor, or physician and documented.

Documentation must be legible (readable) and permanent. Entries must be written only in black ink. Black ink is usually used because it appears clearly when the record is placed on microfilm. Entries must include the correct spelling and correct grammar. You may need to carry a small dictionary while learning the process of documentation.

The nurse should document objectively, using facts, not judgments, which are subjective. The nurse should use objective data to support nursing actions. The nurse should also document as soon as possible after nursing care administered. A rule to follow is, "if it was not charted, it was not done." In court, a nurse must prove that care was administered, and documentation helps prove this.

Special Considerations

To prevent the possibility of legal problems, it is important to examine areas of potential liability. These include abuse, confidentiality, and gerontologic and home health nursing.

Abuse affects people of all ages and social classes. It is a legal responsibility for health care providers to report suspected cases of physical abuse. Children and older adults are the most common victims of abuse. Signs indicating abuse include long bone fractures in various stages of healing, burns, bruises, numerous scars, welts, head injuries, starvation, or a history of fractures. The LPN/LVN should immediately report any signs or symptoms of suspected abuse to the charge personnel. Any member of the health care team may report suspected abuse. However, some agencies have policies regarding the reporting of abuse, and a person is designated to handle such cases. Usually the cases are reported to the appropriate law enforcement agency or the health care welfare agency of the area. If a nurse is suspected as the abuser, the board of nursing should be notified. The nurse should be familiar with the procedure for reporting abuse, since it varies from state to state. The person who reports the abuse is given legal protection or immunity from the parties involved. If the suspected abuse is not reported, the health care worker may be held liable.

Confidentiality is the patient's right to privacy and is a legal and an ethical responsibility. The nurse must practice confidentiality by discussing patients with only the health care workers directly involved in their care. The nurse must not reveal information about a patient to friends or family. If any questions arise regarding confidentiality, the charge nurse should be contacted.

Gerontologic nursing relates to people over 65 years of age, an ever-increasing segment of our population. The most important legal question for older adults is that of competency. Unless legally judged otherwise by a court, older adults are considered competent and able to make decisions regarding their health care.

Home health nursing is becoming more important because of changes in the health care system. Most home health and hospice programs are regulated by states, but federal laws define the standards of care that must be met. The nurse who works in home health or hospice settings may avoid legal problems by following the policies and procedures of the agency, providing quality nursing care, and documenting thoroughly.

Incident Report

Descriptions of unusual occurrences such as patient falls, a medication administration error, an accidental needlestick, or an illness of a visitor are recorded on an **incident report** form. Accidents, especially those that result in injury, must be reported. Incident reports are data-gathering tools that help prevent future occurrences. They are internal (kept within the agency) documents that should be filled out accurately, objectively, and completely. This form is used only within the agency to help prevent similar problems. Subjective judgments (for example, "He looked confused") should be avoided. The nurse should document objective facts such as the following: "Patient said, 'Where am I?' and then fell on left side." The nurse should not document in the medical record that an incident report was completed.

Informed Consent

When special invasive procedures, such as surgery, chemotherapy, or certain diagnostic procedures, are required, a consent form must be signed by the patient or legal guardian giving permission to perform the procedure. This is referred to an **informed consent** and gives proof that the patient consents to having the procedure. Informed consent helps prevent misunderstandings and thus protects the patient and health worker performing the procedure. Four factors make the consent valid (see box). The physician who orders the procedure is responsible for obtaining informed consent. The nurse is responsible only for being a witness to the patient's signature and not for providing the information needed by the patient. If the patient does not understand and asks questions, the nurse must contact the physician to talk to the patient again before witnessing the signature.

Living Will

"The **living will** is a directive from competent, seriously ill persons to medical personnel and family or those responsible for their care regarding the treatment they wish to receive when they become in-

ENSURING THE VALIDITY OF INFORMED CONSENT

For the informed consent form to be valid, four factors are necessary:

- The patient must be mentally and physically *competent* and of legal age.
- The patient must freely *volunteer* the consent without coercion.
- The patient must be informed and *understand* the procedure and benefit from the procedure, potential complications associated with the procedure, and possible alternative procedures.
- The patient has a right to have all *questions* answered satisfactorily and in understandable terminology.

competent to make decisions for themselves" (Creighton, 1986). The nurse who is presented with a living will should place the document in the patient's medical record (chart) and then notify the attending physician and nursing supervisor. State laws vary considerably regarding the living will. Consulting the supervisor helps protect both the patient and nurse.

Pediatrics

The specialty of medicine and nursing that focuses on children is pediatrics and has much potential for legal problems. The most common causes for liability are medication errors, burns, accidents, abandonment, inappropriate use of restraints, failure to detect life-threatening signs and symptoms, and failure to report child abuse. Nurses who specialize in pediatric nursing protect themselves by practicing with the specialty's standards of care, by keeping skills and knowledge current, and by not caring for patients who require procedures and subsequent care for which the nurse has not had formal education.

Resuscitation Orders

The purpose of cardiopulmonary resuscitation and other resuscitation efforts is to establish effective circulation and ventilation to prevent irreversible cerebral damage resulting from anoxia. **"Do not resuscitate" (DNR)** or "no code" orders allow the patient to die without receiving life-prolonging measures. Many agencies define levels of life support. One example is the "chemical code" (medications only). With a "slow code" the health care team takes longer to initiate life-support measures or do not arrive in time to carry out such measures. A slow code is illegal and could be punishable by law.

Unless it is otherwise written as a medical order in the patient's medical record, full resuscitation measures must be carried out to protect everyone involved. The decision to be resuscitated lies, first and foremost, with the patient. Agency policies governing DNR orders have been adopted by most hospitals, long-term facilities, and hospices. The nurse, especially one caring for critically ill patients, must be familiar with the agency's DNR or code policy.

Patient Teaching

One role of the nurse is that of teacher. Two basic legal responsibilities relate to the this role: the duty to know and the duty to instruct (teach). The duty to know includes the duty of the nurse to maintain current knowledge and skills as well as the duty to know the learning abilities of the patient. Teaching is most effective when the patient is ready and willing to learn as well as capable of learning.

The duty to teach patients relates to maintaining current teaching materials, references, learning objectives, time tables for teaching, and evaluation tools. Orally giving the patient directions and medication instructions may be legally hazardous. Instead, the nurse provides written instructions. All teaching activities as well as the patient's response should be documented because appropriate documentation provides legal protection. Many agencies have formal materials for patient teaching such as those for the patient with newly diagnosed diabetes mellitus. However, the nurse must still accurately present the materials to the patient.

Crimes Relating to Nursing

The most common criminal acts seen in the health care setting involve homicide and assisted suicide, controlled substance violation, and theft. The difference between homicide and murder is the intent of the person committing the crime. Legally, homicide is the killing of a human being, whereas murder is killing with forethought. For example, unknowingly giving a patient a wrong drug that causes death may be homicide, but knowingly administering a lethal drug may be murder.

Suicide is the killing of oneself. Mercy killing, euthanasia, and assisted suicide are active or passive acts that assist a person in committing suicide. Many legal and ethical questions regarding a person's right to die are now being considered in U.S. courts. The nurse still has a duty to protect the patient from harm. The nurse is legally and ethically obligated to exercise care to prevent suicide by the patient. When suicidal thoughts are expressed, the nurse must take action to prevent the act and then carefully document patient behavior and nursing actions. A nurse who knowingly participates in an assisted suicide may be tried for a crime.

In 1970 congress instituted the Controlled Substance Act, which regulates the supply and distribution of certain types of potent drugs. Controlled drugs are narcotics, stimulants, depressants, hallucinogens, and some tranquilizers. The nurse administers controlled drugs. See Chapter 15 for rules about ordering, administering, documenting, and disposing of controlled substances.

Robbery, theft, and larceny all describe the taking of another person's personal property. Patients who lose valuable items may hold the agency liable for theft. Making certain that a disposition list for valuables is completed for every patient is an important protection against theft and the involvement of hospital staff.

Torts Relating to Nursing

A violation against an individual is called a *tort.* The nurse works with people and must know about several types of torts such as assault and battery; false imprisonment; fraud; invasion of privacy; libel, slander, and defamation of character; and negligence and malpractice.

Assault and battery

Assault is an act that intentionally provokes fear in a victim. An example of assault is demonstrated by the following comment, which was made to a patient by a health care worker: "If you don't eat your food, we will have to put a tube in your stomach to feed you."

Battery is an act of forcing people to do something against their will. This charge may also include touching someone without consent. For example, if a health care worker tries to force a patient to do something, such as sitting in a chair or walking, it is an act of battery.

False imprisonment

Detaining a competent patient against personal will constitutes **false imprisonment.** For example, locking a patient in a room or detaining a patient for nonpayment is considered false imprisonment. Health care workers may confine a mentally ill patient to ensure safety and prevent injury, but authority for confinement must be obtained as soon as possible.

The application of protective devices and restraints may also constitute false imprisonment. The nurse must be very careful to know when and how to correctly use restraints. A restraint may be applied in some agencies for protection, but the physician and family must be notified immediately. Restraints should be used only for the protection of the patient and not for the convenience of the staff. The least restrictive measure should be tried first and documented. Once a restraint is applied, the nurse is required to assess and monitor the site restrained every 15 minutes and to perform range-of-motion exercises every 2 hours. The nurse must also document assessments and nursing actions. The nurse must make certain that a current written order is on file in the patient's medical record.

Fraud

Fraud is giving false information, knowing that it will be acted on. For example, a nurse documents a medication that was not administered, so the physician bases a decision on the patient's lack of response. The nurse would be guilty of fraud. Practicing nursing with honesty is the best protection against being charged with fraud.

Invasion of privacy

People in society have the right to protect themselves from public scrutiny. "The right to privacy includes privacy related to the body, confidential information, and the right to be left alone" (Morrison, 1993). The nurse must be continually vigilant to protect the patient's privacy and to protect against **invasion of privacy.**

Libel, slander, and defamation of character

Libel is a written statement that may injure a person's reputation. A false statement documented on a patient's medical record that raises questions about the reputation of the person is an example of libel.

Slander is an oral statement that may injure a person's reputation. A nurse who gossips is at risk of being sued for slander.

Defamation of character is any form of communication that may injure a person's reputation. Whether harm is done to one's reputation is the factor that must be proved in court. A nurse accusing another nurse of misconduct while on duty is an example of defamation because doubt of one's professional conduct could harm the person's reputation. It should be noted that this situation is different from a situation in which incompetent nursing care is reported. Incompetence should always be legally reported.

Negligence and malpractice

The concepts of negligence and malpractice are rooted in the "reasonable and prudent person"

REQUIREMENTS FOR MALPRACTICE

- The nurse owed a *duty* to the patient.
- The nurse did not carry out the duty *(breach)*.
- The patient was injured as a result of the action or inaction of the nurse *(proximate cause)*.
- Loss or *damage* resulted from the action of the nurse.

For example, the medical order states to administer a hot pack for 15-minute applications three times a day. The nurse prepares the hot pack (duty to perform the treatment according to safe and accepted standards). The hot pack was applied, and the patient received burns and blisters. In this case the nurse failed to assess the temperature of the soak before applying it to the patient (breach of duty) who was burned (damage) as a direct result of the inaction of the nurse (proximate cause).

theory. **Negligence** applies to the public and is defined as the omission (or commission) of an act that a reasonable and prudent person would (or would not) do. For example, a child care worker who did not prevent a serious injury to a child could be guilty of negligence.

The concept of **malpractice** applies to professionals. Malpractice is the failure to exercise an accepted degree of professional skill or education by one rendering professional services, such as medicine or nursing, that results in injury, loss, or damage. The nurse is commonly involved with negligent acts that relate to medication administration, patient injuries such as falls and burns, perioperative care, equipment problems such as those involving intravenous feedings and catheters, record keeping, and abandonment.

Malpractice criteria are the four requirements that must be met before an incident can be designated as one involving professional misconduct (see box).

Avoiding Liability

To avoid malpractice and other legal wrongdoings, the nurse should keep several guidelines in mind when caring for patients (see box). The best way to avoid the danger of malpractice is to follow standards, administer competent nursing care, and develop an empathetic rapport with the patient. If a nurse expresses genuine concern and provides appropriate nursing care, it is less likely that a patient will file a lawsuit.

AVOIDING LIABILITY

- Remember the principle of the reasonable and prudent nurse: What would a reasonable and prudent nurse do, given the same situation?
- Know and follow the local state nurse practice act.
- Use professional standards of nursing practice.
- Follow agency policies, procedures, and job descriptions.

A nurse should also have malpractice or liability insurance. Most health care institutions carry malpractice insurance that covers employees, but there may be some limitations on protection of the nurse. Therefore it is wise for each nurse to carry personal insurance.

Labor Laws

The Labor Management Relations Act was amended by Congress in 1974. The act stipulates that an employer cannot interfere with or discriminate against any employee who is instrumental in organizing or one who joins a union or similar association. This amendment also includes collective bargaining, which covers areas such as staffing, equipment, wages, fringe benefits, staff-development programs, grievance procedures, the ability to voice views about health care without fear of retribution, and provision of support personnel to free the nurse from nonnursing functions. If this law is violated by either the employer or employee, the violation may be brought before the National Labor Relations Board.

Civil Rights

The Civil Rights Act, amended in 1964, provides for equal job opportunities. Discrimination on the basis of color, religion, gender, pregnancy, or national origin is prohibited by the act. Any complaints in regard to possible discrimination of an employer may be filed with the Equal Employment Opportunity Commission. This agency has the authority to investigate and file a lawsuit. Retaliation of an employer against an employee who files a complaint of discrimination is prohibited by state and federal law.

SUMMARY

Ethics helps the nurse use values that develop into appropriate standards for actions. Morals deal with the absolute right or wrong of an issue. The nurse must strive for these qualities in nursing care and other dealings with people.

Responsibility is doing what one says will be done. The nurse must be accountable for personal actions. The nurse also has a duty or responsibility to the patient in delivering quality patient care.

Using confidentiality, the nurse protects the privacy of the patient in all areas and prevents others from invading that privacy.

Ethical standards must be upheld by the nurse in daily activities. Codes of ethics are available for each level of nursing and describe standards of conduct to be maintained. The National Association for Practical Nurse Education and Services, Inc., has a code of ethics and supports licensed practical/vocational nurses in their right to provide quality care to patients.

The Patient's Bill of Rights dictates that the nurse consider the rights of the patient when administering nursing care.

Ethical dilemmas cause conflict in nursing today. The nurse must be aware that patients may have different values, morals, and codes of ethics than the nurse. The nurse must deal with these differences when caring for these patients.

Legally, the nurse must use reasonable care in the practice of nursing. The nurse must know the principles of law and use them in providing nursing care. Types of law are public (criminal) and private (contract and tort).

The state board of nursing defines and regulates the practice of nursing through the use of administrative and licensing procedures. The nurse's employing agency influences the practice of nursing by drafting policies and procedures for nursing care.

The reasonable-nurse principle expects the nurse to consult with others and seek new information before acting.

Nurses should know whether the Good Samaritan law is active in the state in which they are employed.

The medical record is used for legal documentation of the level of care that a patient received in a health care agency. The nurse must follow documentation guidelines to ensure accuracy.

The nurse must also ensure informed consent. The nurse only witnesses the signature for informed consent.

Patients have living wills when they do not prefer to undergo specific treatments when they become incompetent or physically unable to make choices about care.

Patient teaching is a role of the nurse. Teaching must be competent and thorough. The nurse must ensure that the patient learned the information taught.

Crimes relating to nursing include homicide and assisted suicide, controlled substance violation, and theft. Torts relating to nursing are assault and battery; false imprisonment; fraud; invasion of privacy; libel, slander, and defamation of character; and negligence and malpractice. The nurse must become aware of labor laws and civil rights in regard to possible discrimination toward others.

Key Concepts

- To be known as a professional the nurse must honor the ethics of nursing by living by these standards of right and wrong.
- Doing what one says will be done defines responsibility.
- Accountability is taking legal responsibility for one's own actions.
- The nurse has a duty (responsibility) to make certain the patient receives quality care.
- The Florence Nightingale pledge was created for the registered nurse. It provides a framework for clarifying the moral and ethical values and principles needed for delivering health care and promoting the standards of nursing. Pledges for the licensed practical/vocational nurse also provide the same concepts.
- Ethical standards for nursing practice ensure quality nursing care.
- A code of ethics depicts the values, goals, and standards of conduct for nursing.
- The Patient's Bill of Rights must be considered when providing nursing care.
- Ethical issues are more complex now than ever before. The nurse must make decisions today that raise questions for which there are no clear-cut answers.
- Complicated questions frequently evolve into ethical dilemmas—conflict or uncertainty about moral principles that support a behavior. In some agencies, a bioethics committee has been established to help deal with these problems.
- Nursing conduct must include duty to the patient, consideration by working quietly and efficiently, truthfulness, honesty, loyalty, and caring for the physical, emotional, and spiritual aspects of the patient.

- The nurse must know and use the guidelines for making ethical decisions.
- The nurse must follow the legal aspects of nursing by providing reasonable care.
- The nurse must become aware of the types of laws such as public and private law.
- The state board of nursing performs functions that assist the nurse and protect the public (patient).
- Nursing care must include standards of practice.
- The nurse must abide by the reasonable-nurse principle.
- Nurses must know the Good Samaritan laws of the state in which they are employed.
- The medical record is a legal document, so the nurse must document patient care and teaching legally and accurately.
- The nurse must legally report suspected patient abuse.
- Informed consent is obtained by the physician. The nurse only witnesses the patient's signature.
- Patient teaching is a role of the nurse.
- The nurse must be aware of the requirements for malpractice.
- The nurse must know the guidelines for avoiding liability.
- The nurse must be aware of labor laws and civil rights.

Critical Thinking Questions

1. Determine your position on a common ethical issue (for example, abortion, assisted suicide, euthanasia). Then pose as many arguments as you can against your own position.
2. You are arriving at work and are in a crowded elevator. The conversation in the elevator revolves around a college student who was admitted during the night with a drug overdose. You realize that you know the patient. How has the patient's right to confidentiality been breached? What are your actions?
3. Mr. James is admitted to your division after surgery for an abdominal injury. He received a narcotic analgesic 45 minutes ago. The physician has decided that a computed tomographic scan with contrast is needed, and you need to obtain the patient's consent to the procedure. What factors must be considered before obtaining consent?

REFERENCES AND SUGGESTED READINGS

Calhoun J: The Nightingale pledge: a commitment that survives the passage of time, *Nursing and Health Care* 3(14):130, 1993.

Creighton H: *Law every nurse should know,* ed 5, Philadelphia, 1986, Saunders.

Haddad A: Ethics in action: What would you do? *RN* 56(11):23, 1993.

Husted GL, Husted JH: *Ethical decision making in nursing,* ed 2, St Louis, 1994, Mosby.

Kowalski S: Assisted suicide: where do nurses draw the line? *Nursing and Health Care* 2(14):70, 1993.

Kozier B: Concepts and issues in nursing practice, Redwood City, Calif, 1993, Benjamin-Cummings.

Meyer J: "End of life" care: patients' choices, nurses' challenges, *American Journal of Nursing* 93(2):40, 1993.

Moore GM: Surviving a malpractice lawsuit: one nurse's story, *Nursing 93* 23(10):55, 1993.

Morrison M: *Professional skills for leadership: foundations of a successful career,* St Louis, 1993, Mosby.

Potter PA, Perry AG: *Fundamentals of nursing: concepts, process, and practice,* ed 3, St Louis, 1993, Mosby.

Schmidt J: John had A.I.D.S.—and one romantic wish, *Nursing 93* 23(1):54, 1993.

Toevs A: Creating an environment of ethics, *American Journal of Nursing* 11:60, 1993.

CHAPTER 4

Nursing Process

Learning Objectives

After studying this chapter the student should be able to . . .

- Define the key terms.
- Identify the five steps of the nursing process.
- Describe all of the actions to be used in each step of the nursing process.
- Describe the responsibility of the nurse in writing a plan of nursing care.
- Identify the purpose of the nursing care plan.
- Explain three methods of collecting data.
- Differentiate between objective and subjective data.
- Describe the three parts of a nursing diagnosis statement.
- Give examples of independent, dependent, and interdependent nursing interventions.
- Explain the interaction among the steps of the nursing process.
- Write an appropriate nursing order, including all details necessary for effective intervention.
- List the benefits of evaluation in nursing care.

Key Terms

Assessment
Data clustering
Etiology
Evaluation
Goal
High-risk problem
Implementation
Medical diagnosis
Nursing diagnosis
Nursing intervention
Nursing process
Objective data
Planning
Problem
Subjective data
Validation

The **nursing process** serves as the organizational framework for the practice of nursing. It is a problem-solving plan that assists nurses in providing effective, systematic, and scientifically based nursing care. The process consists of five steps: assessment, diagnosis, planning, implementation, and evaluation (Fig. 4-1). The nursing process steps provide the framework for collecting and analyzing data, making a nursing diagnosis, setting outcome goals with the patient, planning nursing care, implementing care, and evaluating the results of nursing care. All five steps should be performed by the nurse when providing patient care.

The nursing process is accepted as the standard for providing competent nursing care. Although the registered nurse is often responsible for ensuring its use in written patient care plans, the licensed practical/vocational nurse is taught to use the process. In some institutions, the practical/vocational nurse implements the entire process in developing a care plan, whereas in other facilities the practical/vocational nurse may develop only certain parts of the care plan. The five steps of the nursing process are discussed separately (see box).

NURSING ASSESSMENT

Assessment is the first step of the nursing process. During this step, the nurse gathers data to make nursing judgments about the patient's health status and to identify patient needs, preferences, and abilities. Assessment is the most important step of the nursing process because the information gathered allows the nurse to provide appropriate and individualized nursing care. The other steps of the nursing process depend on the accuracy and completeness of assessment data.

There are three areas of concern in assessment: collecting data, validating data for correctness and

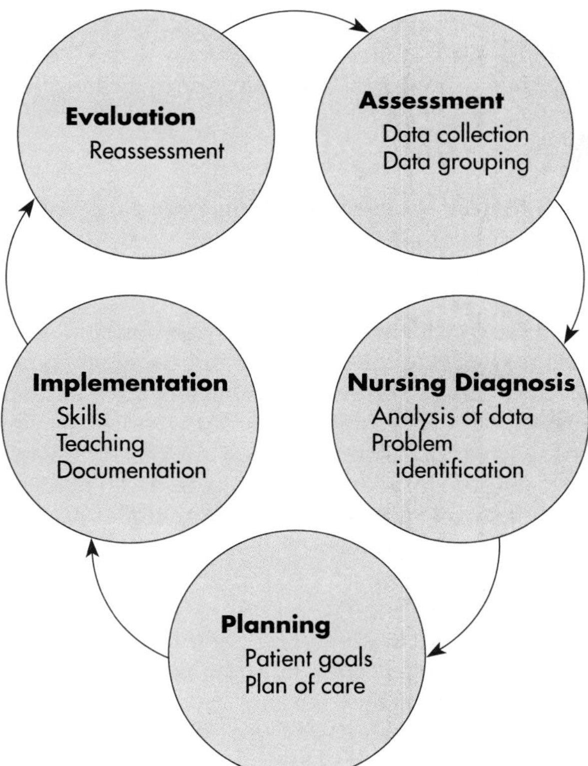

Fig. 4-1 The nursing process.

detail, and organizing data. Collecting data is the main focus.

Data Gathering

Assessment begins when the patient enters the health care facility and continues until the need for health care is no longer necessary. Data should be gathered in a planned, organized, and comprehensive pattern. Data gathering should focus on the patient's physical and mental health as well as social interaction, social circumstances (resources and living conditions), and community life.

Types of data

The nurse collects objective and subjective data. **Objective data** are data that are collected through the senses and that can be perceived by others. In other words, objective data are signs that the nurse can hear, see, feel, touch, and smell. Examples of objective data are an elevated temperature and the observation that the patient did not eat all the food on the tray. **Subjective data** are symptoms that the patient relates to the nurse and that can be perceived and validated only by the patient. Examples of subjective data include information such as headache, itching, and pain. These data pertain to the patient's perceived feelings, fears, and reactions to the internal and external environment.

FIVE STEPS OF THE NURSING PROCESS

- *Assessment:* Assessment is the collection of patient information, such as age, weight, medical diagnosis, health history, family history, social history, and past illnesses, which is used in the formulation of a nursing diagnosis.
- *Nursing diagnosis:* The nursing diagnosis is a statement of a health problem or a high-risk health problem that a nurse is licensed to treat. Four steps are required in the formulation of a nursing diagnosis: (1) analyzing and clustering data to determine problems and their defining characteristics, (2) comparing findings to normal function or standards, (3) determining the problem or unmet need and formulating a tentative nursing diagnosis, and (4) prioritizing the problem after validation of data indicates the priority of need. Each diagnostic statement has three parts: the problem, the etiology (cause), and the defining characteristics (signs and symptoms) of the problem.
- *Planning:* Planning is the setting of goals and selection of appropriate nursing interventions to meet the patient's needs. This includes input from the patient and significant others.
- *Implementation:* Implementation is putting the plan of interventions into action by giving nursing care to the patient as designed for goal attainment.
- *Evaluation:* Evaluation is the determination and recording of the results of nursing actions (that is, the extent to which the established goals of care have been met). To make this judgment, the nurse estimates the degree of success in meeting the goals, evaluates the effectiveness of each nursing intervention, investigates the patient's compliance with the plan and therapy, and records the patient's responses to therapy. If the goals were not met, the plan is modified and continued. If goals are met and new assessment data confirms the resolution of the problem, the plan is discontinued.

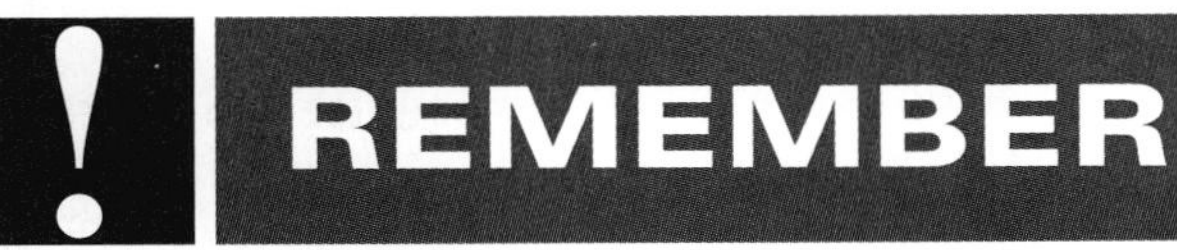

- Data should be collected every time that contact is made with the patient or significant others.

Methods of data gathering

The nurse collects data using three methods: interview, observation, and physical assessment.

Interview An interview is an information-gathering conversation in which the nurse is seeking specific information from the patient and significant others. It should be held in a comfortable environment, and nurses should introduce themselves to the patient and explain the purpose of the interview. If the nurse explains how the information is to be used to identify the patient's needs and to provide nursing care, most individuals cooperate readily. To perform an effective interview the nurse should use the principles of communication discussed in Chapter 5.

Observation Observation is gathering data through the five senses (vision, hearing, smell, touch, and taste). Examples of inspection include using the sense of hearing for listening to a cough, voice control, and breath sounds and using the sense of touch to reveal the temperature and roughness of the skin. Observation is a continual process that takes place every time that contact is made with the patient. Further observations are conducted when treatments are administered, other methods of assessment are performed, and the patient is interacting with others.

Physical assessment Many nurses use the head-to-toe method for physical assessment, whereas others use a body systems approach. Nurses should master the following skills to perform an accurate physical assessment (see Chapter 12):

1. Inspection is a systematic, intensified observation to note any abnormal areas of function.
2. During auscultation, a stethoscope or other monitoring devices are used to systematically listen to sounds within the patient's body. Using auscultation, the nurse listens to an apical pulse, bowel sounds, or respiratory action.
3. Palpation is a systematic examination in which the nurse uses the hands and fingers to press on or feel body parts. One method of palpation is a light touch, which is used to examine for tenderness, peripheral pulses, and skin changes. Deep palpation is to check the abdomen for masses or organs.
4. Percussion is a method of examining the density of a part by tapping the body's surface with an instrument (a percussion hammer) or the fingertips. For example, the nurse taps on the abdomen to determine the sound created: If fluid or a solid mass is present, the sound is dull, but if the sound is hollow, it usually indicates that air is present.

Sources of data

The nurse obtains information from primary and secondary sources. The primary source of information is the patient. Secondary data are obtained from sources other than the patient, including the medical record, Kardex, health team members, and family or significant others. The medical record provides information from diagnostic studies, including clinical laboratory findings; other therapy areas; reports from other disciplines; and community resources.

Data Validation

Validation is the verification that data are free from misinterpretation, error, and bias. As assessment data are gathered, the nurse may suspect that a problem exists. However, the nurse must seek more data in this area to verify whether this suspicion is correct. Validation is also indicated when only subjective data are present and no objective data are found. In this case, data from one source are compared with those from another source. The nurse may validate data during the gathering phase or may do so after assessment is completed.

Data Organization

Assessment data should be organized into groups or categories. This is commonly called ***data clustering.*** Clustering of data assists the nurse in identifying a specific problem and the strengths of the patient. Clustering of data may be developed according to Maslow's hierarchy of needs or according to body systems. Maslow believed that as humans we strive to be everything we can become. He developed an order of needs (Fig. 4-2).

The base of Maslow's hierarchy of needs consists of physiologic or basic needs such as oxygen, food, water, elimination, sleep, and sex. These basic needs are necessary to survive. Each step, including safety, love and belonging, self-esteem, and eventually self-actualization (the fulfillment of one's human potential), moves upward in rank. According to Maslow's theory, the highest step cannot be achieved unless the lower needs are met.

A need is something necessary, practical, or yearned for in order to have a good life and a feeling of well-being. Humans strive to use their greatest potential (strengths) to meet their needs in both wellness and illness.

NURSING DIAGNOSIS

Establishing a nursing diagnosis is the second step in the nursing process. The nurse carefully analyzes the data gathered during assessment and compares it to normal function and standards. As data are compared and evaluated with normal function, patterns that indicate a problem or an unmet need begin to form. Strengths and abilities also present

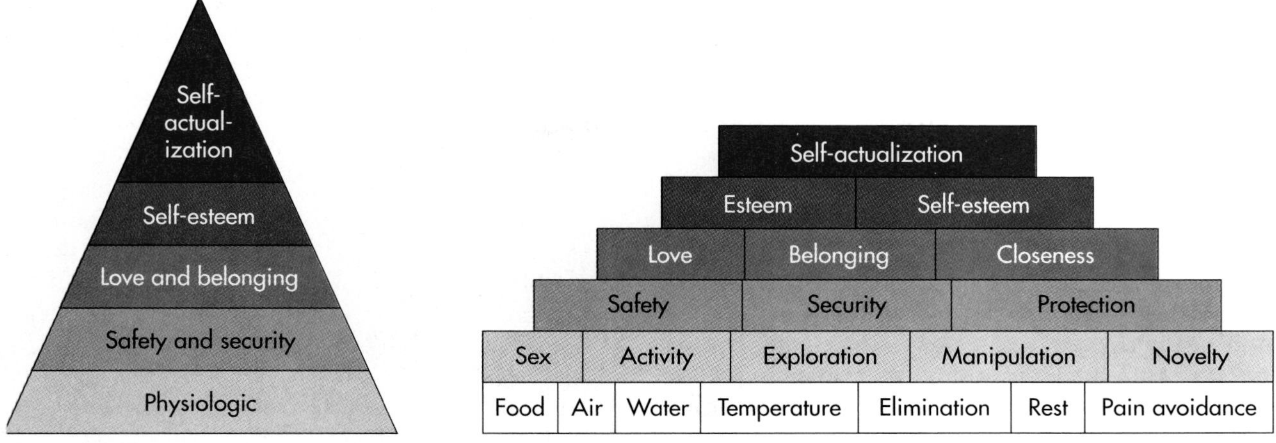

Fig. 4-2 Maslow's hierarchy of needs and Maslow's needs as adapted by Kalish. (From Kalish RA: *The psychology of human behavior,* ed 5, Pacific Grove, Calif, 1983, Brooks/Cole.)

themselves. Thus analysis of data enables the nurse to draw conclusions about the patient's needs, problems, or concerns and about strengths that the patient can use to resolve the problems. These conclusions are nursing diagnoses.

A **nursing diagnosis** is a statement about a health problem that the nurse is qualified and licensed to treat. The nursing diagnosis deals with the patient's response to illness or an unmet need that may respond to nursing interventions. It is not the same as a medical diagnosis. A **medical diagnosis** is a physiologic impairment, disease, or pathologic condition. Patients with the same medical diagnosis may have different nursing diagnoses. The purpose of a nursing diagnosis is to identify a patient problem so that specific nursing interventions may be planned to solve the problem or meet the patient's needs.

After analyzing the assessment data carefully, the nurse may conclude that the patient may be at risk for developing a problem. This **high-risk problem** may be prevented by a plan of care initiated to support the patient's health. Interventions may include a healing diet, fluids, and activity.

Parts of the Nursing Diagnosis

The nursing diagnosis statement has three parts. The first part of the statement specifies the **problem** (for example, *altered nutrition: less than body requirements*). The appropriate terminology for this part of the nursing diagnosis is found in the list of accepted nursing diagnoses established by the North American Nursing Diagnosis Association (NANDA). NANDA is responsible for the developing and updating a classification system for nursing diagnoses.

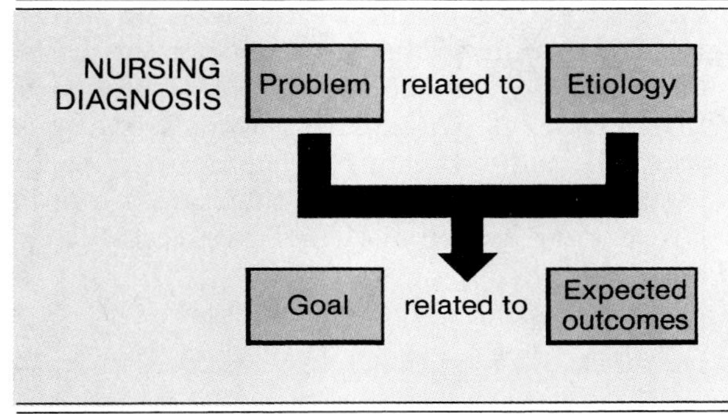

Fig. 4-3 Relationships of parts of the nursing diagnosis to the goals and expected outcomes. (Redrawn from Hickey P: *Nursing process handbook,* St Louis, 1990, Mosby.)

Each NANDA nursing diagnosis has (1) a definition of the problem, (2) a list of defining characteristics (symptoms) and clustered data associated with the nursing diagnosis, and (3) related or risk factors that may cause or relate to the problem. To determine a nursing diagnosis, the nurse compares acquired patient data to the defining characteristics. If they correspond, a nursing diagnosis is made. A list of NANDA-approved nursing diagnoses may be found on the inside cover of the text. The list is revised approximately every 2 years.

The second part of the nursing diagnosis statement is the **etiology** (the cause of the problem). The etiology should not be a medical diagnosis but should reflect the *cause* of the problem or *pathologic* condition that a nurse is qualified to treat (for example *R/T nausea, weakness, and inability to feed self*). The first two parts are connected by the words *related to* or the abbreviation *R/T* (Fig. 4-3).

The third part of the statement is *as evidenced by (AEB)*. It is a list of signs and symptoms from the assessment data (defining characteristics) that support the diagnosis (for example, *AEB weight loss of 5 pounds since admission (1 week), inability to reach mouth (casts on both arms), nausea, and fatigue when up*).

PLANNING

Once data are collected and analyzed, problems are identified, and a nursing diagnosis is made, the nurse is ready to plan nursing care. **Planning** is the selection of appropriate nursing interventions to be taken to meet the patient's needs or to resolve the problem. Planning involves prioritizing the problems, setting goals, selecting appropriate interventions, and recording the plan of care.

Planning for nursing care is based on the nursing diagnosis statement and prioritization of each diagnosis according to its importance or the critical need for intervention. According to Maslow's hierarchy, physiologic (life-threatening) needs are the most important. If patients can participate in the planning step, it is vital to include their ideas and desires to ensure cooperation and a successful outcome.

Prioritizing the Problem

Patients usually have more than one nursing diagnosis (problem). Therefore the nurse must determine which diagnosis requires *immediate* attention and list all diagnoses in order of priority for patient safety. Health problems that endanger life or that cause pain take top priority (Table 4-1). Problems of lesser priority are ranked lower and are treated immediately after the prioritized problems.

Table 4-1 PRIORITY SETTING

Nursing Diagnoses	Rationale
High priority	
Diarrhea related to unknown cause	Prompt resolution of diarrhea and its cause prevents further decline in physiologic and emotional status.
Risk for ineffective individual coping related to unknown medical diagnosis	Prompt intervention for ineffective coping will help client prepare for diagnostic test, treatment, or diagnosis.
Risk for ineffective airway clearance after surgery related to abdominal incisional pain	Because of risk of postoperative pulmonary complications, nurse will institute preventive client education early in nursing care.
Intermediate priority	
Risk for altered nutrition: less than body requirements related to chronic diarrhea for 3 weeks	This nursing diagnosis does not affect client's immediate physiologic or emotional status. Possible surgery will also assist nurse in resolving diagnosis.
Low priority	
Risk for chronic infections related to history of smoking for 20 years	This nursing diagnosis reflects client's long-term needs.

From Potter PA, Perry AG: *Fundamentals of nursing: concepts, process, and practice,* ed 3, St Louis, 1993, Mosby.

The reasons for developing a plan of care for each patient follow:

1. Individualization of care: The nurse meets individual needs and uses the patient's strengths.
2. Prioritization: The nurse gives attention to the most immediate need.
3. Facilitation of communication with all team members: The nurse ensures continuity of patient care.
4. Coordination of care: The nurse prevents interruption of therapeutic interventions.
5. Evaluation of nursing care: The nurse evaluates the positive and negative responses to interventions.

Setting Goals

A **goal** is the result or expected outcome of nursing care and teaching (see Fig. 4-3). The terms *goal, objective,* and *expected outcome* are used interchangeably. The goal statement acts as a guide for the selection of appropriate interventions and the evaluation of the patient's response to nursing interventions. The goal statement should describe the change in patient's behavior or condition that is expected after nursing intervention. Goals should be patient oriented, realistic for the patient, and mutually set with the patient. They should also have a time frame (time and date for goal to be reached).

Characteristics of a Goal

Goals assist the nurse in determining appropriate nursing interventions, give direction to interventions, and provide a means for measuring the outcome of a specific diagnosis. A well-written

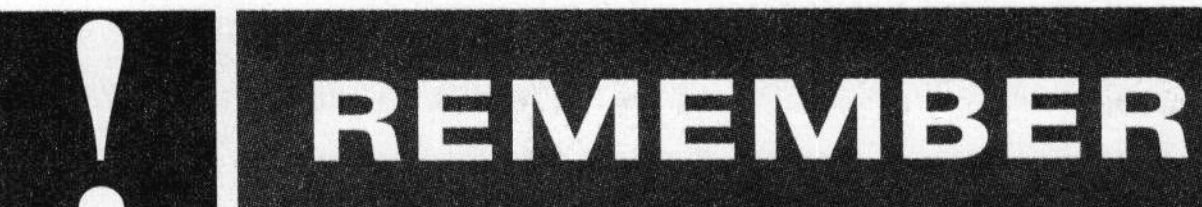

- Assess each goal to ensure that it is realistic for the patient. Use a measurable verb when writing a goal statement.
- The patient helps to set the goals to be accomplished.
- Patient involvement helps ensure the patient's participation in attainment of the goals.

goal should describe a change in the patient's behavior or in the patient's condition. Thus the goal is patient centered (individualized) and realistic.

For completeness, the goal statement should reflect three areas of evaluation. The goal should be observable (that is, have an expected behavior), should be measurable (that is, include factors such as distance and time), and should have conditions (that is, special circumstances, restrictions, or requirements under which the behavior should be accomplished). An example of a well-written goal follows: "The patient will be able to walk to the foot of the bed with the assistance of one nursing assistant and a walker by 4/5 at 0800."

Each goal should have only one behavior and have a time and date for measurement and evaluation. The behavior desired should be very specific so that the goal can be easily evaluated. The verb indicating the behavior should be clear so that the behavior can be easily measured. Terms such as *will understand* refer to behavior that is difficult to measure, but specific verb phrases such as *will state the basic reasons for* are clear and concise and reflect understanding.

Types of Goals

Two types of goals are set. Short-term goals are to be met in 24 to 48 hours. Long term goals are to be met 48 to 72 hours or by discharge. Time commitments for goals may be extended, depending on the situation. A short-term goal may be as long as a week, and a long-term goal may be set for a month after discharge or may be ongoing (for example, "patient *will maintain weight*").

Selecting Interventions

Nursing interventions are actions taken by the nurse to solve problems. These interventions are communicated to other nursing team members in the form of nursing interventions on the written patient care plan. The written intervention is designed to resolve the parts (problem, etiology, and signs and symptoms) of the nursing diagnosis statement and to meet the set goals. Each intervention should be clear and concise (for example, "Encourage patient to rest 15 to 30 minutes before meals"). It should include timing (for example, "before meals") and conditions *("rest 15 to 30 minutes")*. It should answer the following questions: what, when, where, how much, how long, and how often? A well-selected and planned intervention is effective only if nurses understand exactly what is expected of them.

IMPLEMENTATION

Implementation is putting the plan of care into action to achieve goal attainment. This is the action phase of the nursing process and includes hands-on nursing care. The purpose of this fourth step is to assist the patient in achieving the goals written in the plan of care and in resolving the problem. To do this, the nurse uses independent, dependent, and interdependent nursing interventions.

Independent nursing interventions are actions that are completely within the responsibility of nursing practice and that require no directions from other members of the health care team. Examples of independent nursing actions include assisting the patient with activities of daily living, teaching health care, and supervising the nursing care given by others.

Dependent nursing interventions are actions taken by the nurse that are based on the written instructions of a physician who is licensed to practice medicine. Examples of dependent nursing interventions include administering prescribed medications, inserting urinary catheters, and scheduling diagnostic studies.

Interdependent nursing interventions are actions that the nurse performs with other members of the health care team. For example, a patient goes to physical therapy every other day to learn to use a leg prosthesis. On alternate days the nurse applies the prosthesis and assists the patient with ambulation while reinforcing the teaching of the physical therapist.

Documentation of nursing care is a major responsibility of the nurse, who records the patient's responses to the plan of nursing care and documents goal attainment. Procedures for the accurate documentation of care (charting) are discussed in Chapter 5. The patient's record not only is an important tool for communication among members of the health care team, but is also a legal document.

NURSING CARE PLAN GUIDELINES

Nursing Diagnosis/Problem (Prioritize)

Do's

1. The nursing diagnosis or problem is an actual or high-risk problem statement.
2. The statement has three parts: Problem/need related to (R/T): cause/etiology as evidence by (AEB): signs and symptoms from assessment cluster.
3. The nursing diagnosis statement should be used from NANDA.
4. Only one patient problem should be stated in each nursing diagnosis statement.
5. The problem should be a patient's response to the illness.
6. The nurse should not use a medical diagnosis as an etiology but should use the actual cause.

Examples

- Altered nutrition (less than body requirements)
- R/T nausea, weakness, and inability to feed self
- AEB weight loss of 5 pounds since admission (1 wk), inability to reach mouth (cast on both arms) complains of (c/o) nausea, and fatigue.

Goals/Expected Outcomes

The goal/expected outcome is the new behavior or change the nurse and patient want as a result of planned nursing interventions. A *short-term goal* should be accomplished in 24-48 hr. A *long-term goal* should be accomplished in 72 hr, or on discharge, or after a longer time.

Do's

1. The goals should be realistic to the patient's ability to achieve.
2. The patient should be involved in setting goals.
3. Each goal should have only one behavior.
4. Each time frame should have a date and time for the nurse to measure the outcome.
5. Goals may be stated with the expected outcomes.

Examples

- *STG:* Patient will eat 50% of food with no nausea by 11/24.
- *STG:* Patient will eat all snacks and retain by 11/24.
- *LTG:* Patient has 5-pound weight gain by 11-30 (0600).

Nursing Interventions (Prioritize)

Do's

1. An intervention is a statement of the nursing interventions to be performed to solve the problem and meet expected outcomes.
2. Each intervention should be specific and individualized to the patient's capabilities. It should be realistic for the patient.
3. Each statement should answer the questions what, how often, how long, how much, when, and where.
4. Each statement should be written for the three parts of the nursing diagnosis and checked against expected outcomes.

Examples

- Encourage patient to rest 15-30 minutes before meals.
- Give ginger ale (4 oz) 20 minutes before meals.
- Encourage patient to eat small amounts during meals with rest periods between.
  - Encourage 2-3 bites and then a rest.
  - Encourage fluids with each bite.

Evaluation of Goals/Expected Outcomes

Do's

1. Evaluation is an assessment of how the patient is or is not meeting the goals/expected outcomes.
2. All goals and expected outcomes should be evaluated for changes or a continuation of the plan.
3. The nurse evaluates goals and expected outcomes for whether they can be attained and whether they address the etiology and signs and symptoms of the problem.
4. The nurse evaluates the interventions according to whether it offers the appropriate approach and whether the patient and health care team are following through with interventions.

Examples

- The goal and expected outcome were met as evidenced by patient meeting all criteria of goal statement.
- The goal and expected outcome was partially met as evidenced by patient progressing slower than timeframe. Goal time will be advanced to 72 hr.

STG, Short-term goal; *LTG,* long-term goal.

EVALUATION

Evaluation is the fifth step of the nursing process. Its focus is to assess the patient's responses to nursing care and the extent to which the established goals have been met. The nurse evaluates the effectiveness of the interventions used, the need for changing the goals of care, the skill with which the nursing interventions were implemented, and the need for change in the patient's environment or the equipment or procedures used.

During the evaluation phase of the nursing process, the nurse first measures how well the patient's goals were met. To do this, the nurse reassesses the present status of the patient and compares the new data to those indicated by the nursing diagnostic statement and goals to be met. If the patient's goals were not met or only partially met, the care plan must be revised, or time frames may need to be extended. The plan is continued. If all goals of the nursing care plan are met, the problem is considered resolved, and the plan for that specific nursing diagnosis is discontinued.

APPLYING THE NURSING PROCESS

The nursing process is dynamic and continuous. The nurse uses the steps of the nursing process in every interaction with the patient. After assessing the patient's status and making a diagnosis, the nurse determines outcomes and nursing interventions to correct the problem. The situation is then evaluated for resolution. The following example indicates the way in which the nursing process works:

> If the nurse finds *(assessment)* the patient trying to get up while on bedrest restrictions *(goal),* the nurse immediately intervenes *(intervention)* to assist the patient back to bed and pull up all siderails. The nurse then asks the patient to explain what is needed *(assessment),* and meets the need *(intervention).* Together the nurse and patient determine how the patient will get help next time something is needed *(planning).* The patient is then given an explanation as to how to call the nurse for help and the importance of bedrest *(intervention).* Later the patient rings for help and greets the nurse with "See, I remembered not to exert myself" *(evaluation).*

Assessment and evaluation are integral parts of the nursing process. Accurate data are necessary for identifying problems and making correct nursing diagnoses. A valid nursing diagnosis is vital for establishing realistic and measurable goals. Ongoing collection of data and evaluation of nursing care are necessary to determine the effectiveness of the nursing care plan. The nursing process is a continuous, flexible model for providing the best possible nursing care for the patient (see box).

SUMMARY

The nursing process enables the nurse to provide individualized nursing care to resolve an unmet need. During the assessment phase, the nurse gathers data about the patient's condition. A nursing diagnosis describes an unmet need that a nurse may treat independently. Each diagnosis is prioritized according to Maslow. When planning, the nurse selects goals with the patient's input and assesses motivation toward goal attainment. Short- and long-term goals are realistically written, and a time frame is determined for each. Each intervention communicates the care given and facilitates continuity of nursing care. Interventions must be compatible with the medical plan and realistic for the patient's condition. Evaluation measures determine whether the goals are met. If goals are met, the problem is considered resolved, and the plan is terminated.

Key Concepts

- The nursing process is a problem-solving approach and aids the nurse in providing effective, systematic, and scientifically based nursing care.
- The steps in the nursing process provide a framework for collecting and analyzing data, formulating a nursing diagnosis, setting outcome goals and planning nursing care, implementing nursing care, and evaluating the results of nursing care.
- Involving the patient with planning encourages compliance.
- Data are gathered in an orderly, organized, and comprehensive manner.
- Objective and subjective data are collected during assessment.
- A nursing care plan serves as a communication tool for providing continuity of care and consistent nursing care.

Critical Thinking Questions

1. Take the following narrative and identify subjective and objective data: Mr. Kantor is lying on his side, grimacing and rubbing his abdomen, and complaining of pain. His vital signs are as follows: BP, 140/100; P, 120, and R, 22. He is pale and diaphoretic, and his skin is warm to touch. Oral temperature is 102° F.
2. List the components of the planning phase of the nursing process.
3. Discuss the relationship of the planning phase to the other steps of the nursing process.
4. Correctly write the following incorrect nursing interventions:
   a. Irrigate nasogastric tube with normal saline.
   b. Suction client every 2 hours.
   c. Change client's dressing at 0600, 1400, and 2200 hours.

REFERENCES AND SUGGESTED READINGS

Alfaro-LeFevre R: *Applying nursing process: a step by step guide,* ed, 3, Philadelphia, 1994, Lippincott.

Carpenito IJ: *Nursing care plans and documentation: nursing diagnosis and collaborative problems,* Philadelphia, 1991, Lippincott.

Carpenito IJ: *Nursing diagnosis: application to clinical practice,* ed 5, Philadelphia, 1993, Lippincott.

Gordon M: *Manual of nursing diagnosis: 1995-1996,* St Louis, 1995, Mosby.

Potter PA, Perry AG: *Basic nursing: theory and practice,* ed 3, St Louis, 1995, Mosby.

Zerwekh J, Claborn J: *Nursing today: transition and trends,* Philadelphia, 1994, Saunders.

CHAPTER 5

Communication, Documentation, and Reporting

Learning Objectives

After studying this chapter, the student should be able to . . .

- Define the key terms.
- Explain the importance of communication to the nurse-patient relationship.
- Differentiate between verbal and nonverbal communication.
- Give examples of therapeutic techniques of communication.
- Describe blocks to communication.
- Describe ways to communicate effectively with children.
- List considerations the nurse should use in communication with older adults.
- Discuss the three primary purposes of the medical record.
- Explain how the patient's medical record is used as a legal document.
- State the general rules for documentation and give an example of each.
- Demonstrate use of common nursing forms by correctly completing forms such as the Kardex, a nursing data sheet, a flow sheet, and a graphic.
- Identify appropriate abbreviations and symbols used in documentation and give the meaning for each.
- Indicate common ways in which nurses exchange information regarding nursing care.
- Explain the acronyms SOAPIE, PIE, and DARE.
- Indicate specific types of patient information to be documented and give an example of each.
- Illustrate appropriate documenting of at least five specific types of information by documenting the patient's mental status and clinical appearance, changes in behavior, symptoms, procedures and nursing measures for patients.

Key Terms

Charting by exception
Communication
DARE
Documentation
Focus charting
Incident report
Kardex
Kinesics
Medical record
Nonverbal communication
PIE
Problem-oriented medical record (POMR)
Process recording
Reporting
SOAPIE
Verbal communication

COMMUNICATION

Communication is any process in which a message is transferred, especially from one person to another. This interchanging of ideas, information, attitudes, and emotions is a nearly constant human activity, since everything one does, thinks, and feels has communicative value. Communication is the most vital skill the nurse needs to function as a nurse. Effective communication is the basis of all nursing situations and is necessary in the development of all therapeutic relationships.

Communication occurs in many forms, such as writing, speech, signals, sign language, gestures, music, pictorial art, theater, and dance. It includes anything perceived by our senses: the ring of a telephone, the aroma of a Christmas tree, the touch of a puppy's tongue, the taste of a favorite food, and the nod of a teacher's head. We refer to communication skills as *interpersonal relations* skills. There are two kinds of communication: verbal, which is spoken, written, or recorded, and nonverbal, which is transmitted by gestures, facial expression, eye contacts, or body actions or positions.

Components of the Communication Process

All communication consists of six basic aspects (Fig. 5-1):

1. The sender is the initiator, the individual who has something to share with others.
2. The message includes information (ideas, attitudes, emotions) perceived by one individual and passed to another, verbally or nonverbally. The person's vocabulary, tone of voice, volume, and body language are all a part of the message.
3. The receiver is the intended target (person) for the information.
4. The environment is the physical, cultural, social, and personal (life experiences) context in which the transmission occurs.
5. Feedback is the process that denotes a response to a transmission and the initiation of a new message.
6. Context is the setting, meaning, and language of a message. If a message is interpreted without strict regard for these limits, it will be taken out of context.

To communicate effectively, the sender and receiver must be able to perceive, interpret, and transmit information. The message must be phrased in terms understandable to the receiver. The receiver must be ready and willing to receive the message, or the receiver may be in denial and not wish to hear the message. Errors in communication may result from a problem with any one of these five basic aspects.

Perception requires correct sensory response to the environment and the capacity for comprehension. This includes the senses of hearing and sight, sensory stimulation, and language skills. An individual may perceive a brown, warm mass, but it is only through past experience that this mass is perceived as a lovable puppy.

Interpretation involves understanding, linking sensory perceptions to recognizable messages. If the sender erroneously interprets a perception, the message is not comprehended as it was intended. The transmission, as well as the perception, of the message is influenced by the environment, cultural or ethnic background, and social and personal experiences.

Communication is the nurse's link with the patient, the health team, and people in general. It is a basic skill in all human activities. Effective communication requires practice, but the rewards for improved communication are numerous.

Dimensions of Communication

Knowing oneself For communication between the nurse and patient to be therapeutic, the nurse must first have insight into personal feelings. Knowing oneself is not an easy task. It is a lifelong process. Nevertheless, self-knowledge is the first step of effective communication and human relations. To increase effective communication, the

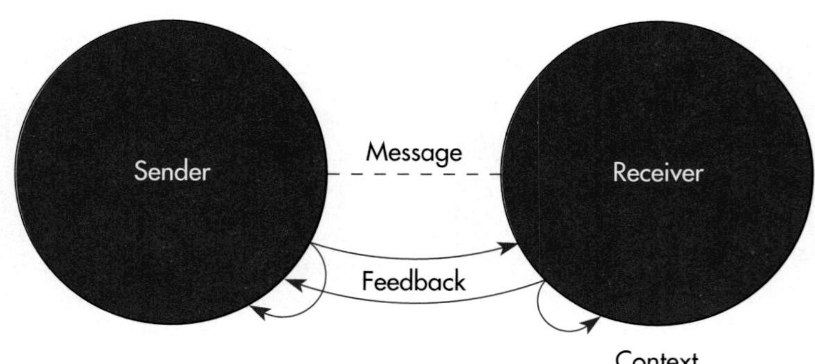

Fig. 5-1 Components of the communication process. (Redrawn from Sundeen SJ et al: *Nurse-client interaction: implementing the nursing process,* ed 5, St Louis, 1994, Mosby.)

nurse should request feedback from others to determine whether messages are being received and comprehended.

Empathy Empathy is the act of putting oneself in another situation and perceiving that person's feelings. Empathy is the key to expressing concern and understanding to the patient. Empathy is easier when the sender and receiver share similarities in life experiences. If the nurse has experienced surgery, it is more likely that understanding of the patient's fear, pain, or nausea will be reflected in the nurse's caring and sensitivity.

Although the nurse may not share the patient's perception, the situation still must be viewed from the patient's perspective, and the nurse must show that an attempt is being made to perceive the patient's view. Empathy assists the nurse in making positive judgments by using restating and reflection to verify the patient's perception of the situation.

Observation Observation is one of the most important skills that a nurse can develop. Active observation should be used every moment that the nurse is in contact with the patient. The process uses not only sight but also all of the senses to perceive the patient's changing condition. For example, the nurse may sense the odor of infection during a dressing change. An increase in body temperature may be perceived through touch. The tone of voice that an angry patient uses may reveal the real meaning behind the statement "Sure, I love cold eggs." Observation is a skill that must be sharpened daily. It is the nurse's guide to the patient's needs, changes in condition, and effective communication.

Verbal Communication

Verbal communication is the interchange of information using spoken or written words. Since verbal communication is a voluntary activity, the sender chooses the written or spoken message. The choice of words should be based on the receiver's sociologic background and psychologic state. Characteristics of the receiver that the sender should consider include educational level, language skills, knowledge of technical terms, and attentiveness. The message will not be understood if the sender uses terms or language with which the receiver is unfamiliar or if the sender transmits a message that the receiver is not ready to hear. The nurse should avoid using medical terminology when talking with patients. The timing of the interaction must be right to facilitate perception and internalization of new information. If the patient is anxious and preoccupied, the nurse should recognize and minimize these problems before trying to convey the intended message.

The message should be clear, brief, and simple and, for the nurse, should be presented in a way that keeps personal opinions and values in perspective. The nurse should also address the patient with respect and use formal names unless asked by the patient to do otherwise. The nurse should avoid using terms of endearment (for example, honey, sweetheart) when talking with patients and families. The nurse should talk with people face to face, maintain eye contact, and use an appropriate tone of voice, rhythm, volume, and inflection (Fig. 5-2).

Talking is the most common form of verbal communication. Some factors to consider when speaking include the sound of the voice, volume, kinesics, inflection, speech habits, and tone. These factors may alter the meaning of the message and even discourage the receiver from listening. For example, saying "Tell me how you feel Mrs. Travis," may communicate interest. However, the nurse's monotonal voice and simultaneous assessment of the intravenous line may contradict the verbal statement. The nurse's tone and actions may be interpreted as lack of interest or lack of time to listen.

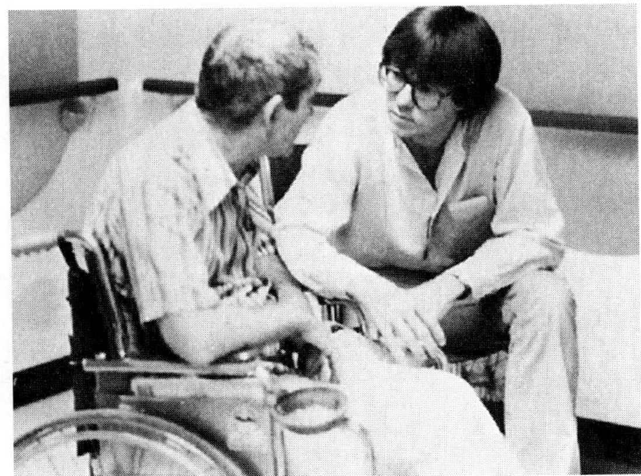

Fig. 5-2 Effective communication and listening skills enhance the nurse-patient relationship. (From Burnside I: *Nursing and the aged: a self-care approach,* ed 3, St Louis, 1988, Mosby.)

! REMEMBER

- If the message intended is not understood by the receiver, communication does not take place.
- Not all that is said is what is heard. Patients may say one thing and mean another.

Nonverbal Communication

How the message is conveyed is just as important as what is said. **Nonverbal communication** is the interchange of information without the use of words and encompasses observation, gestures, body language, touch, physical appearance, territory and personal space, and intrapersonal and environmental factors. Nonverbal communication confirms, strengthens, adds emotion to, or contradicts verbal messages.

Since nonverbal communication tends to be unconscious, it represents the true feelings of the sender, perhaps more honestly than verbal communication. For example, if the sender grimaces while complimenting a person's new hairstyle, the sender probably thinks that the hairstyle is not attractive. The study of the way that such expressions and other nonverbal communication relates to verbal communication is **kinesics.**

Nonverbal communication is affected by the sender's and receiver's culture, geographic region, socioeconomic status, and education level. Understanding this aspect of communication may help the receiver interpret messages and may help the sender convey messages more accurately. For example, the receiver is more likely to understand when the sender's nonverbal and verbal messages match. It is important for the nurse to be able to communicate both verbally and nonverbally and thus make communication more effective (Table 5-1).

Gestures Gestures are nonverbal signals, such as movement of the hands, head, or other body parts, used to communicate information. Gestures may be effectively used in communication and are especially useful when the patient is unable to speak. If the patient uses sign language or another type of nonverbal communication, the nurse should confirm the meaning with verbal questioning. The nurse may instruct patients who are unable to speak to use one finger or one blink to indicate *yes* and two fingers or two blinks to indicate *no.* Then questions should then be designed for *yes*-or-*no* answers.

Body language Body language, another form of nonverbal communication, may add to the conversation or completely change the meaning of the message. Body language assists communication only when it is observed and interpreted correctly. Position, posture, and distance between individuals all communicate more than words alone. A patient who faces away from the door may desire privacy or comfort. A stooped posture may indicate depression or orthopedic problems. The patient who moves away when touched may not desire physical contact or fears that body odors may be detected. The nurse should ask for feedback from the patient to ensure correct interpretation.

Touch Touch is an important aspect of nonverbal communication, especially for the nurse. Touch has different meanings for different people. The nurse should be aware of the patient's personal feelings about touch. Some people are not comfortable being touched or when touching others. Other people may need touch. Sometimes, it will be requested verbally ("Please hold my hand.") or nonverbally (reaching out). The nurse must let the patient's reaction be a guide in the use of touch. Tactile contact may help some patients feel the nurse's sincerity or honesty.

Physical appearance Physical appearance and dress are nonverbal statements about self-

Table 5-1 FUNCTIONS OF NONVERBAL COMMUNICATION

Function of Nonverbal Communication	Verbal Behavior	Nonverbal Behavior
Confirms verbal message	"I'm upset about telling my parents that I want to move out."	Voice shaky, words haltingly stated, hands wrung, no eye contact established
Strengthens or emphasizes verbal message	"I don't like to be treated that way."	Loud voice, harsh tone, emphatic statement of words, forward leaning, direct eye contact, hands on hips
Adds emotional color to verbal message	"I like you so much."	Words sing, tone is modulated, smiles, direct eye contact is established, arm of other person is touched
Contradicts or confuses verbal message	"Well . . . sure . . . I think I'm free."	Affirming words, low tone of voice, loss of eye contact, slumped posture, forehead rubbed

From Haber J et al: *Comprehensive psychiatric nursing,* ed 4, St Louis, 1992, Mosby.

concept, health, socioeconomic status, and culture. Clean, worn-looking clothes may communicate positive self-image, comfort, and economic status. Grooming and accessories may call attention to oneself, indicate concern about detail, or cause one to blend into the surroundings. Ethnic attire may communicate cultural pride and the need for the nurse to validate the influence of cultural beliefs in patient interactions and treatments.

Territory and personal space Territory and personal space provide information about power and the personal characteristics of the participants. In meetings the seating may be arranged to reflect control such as the boss or teacher sitting at the head of the table or behind a desk. Allegiance or support is indicated when those with similar ideas or feelings sit together, whereas equality may be reflected by sitting in a circle or at the same level.

Personal size can reflect dominance or weakness. If the nurse is large and dominant in gesture, the patient may be overwhelmed and resist all communication. The nurse should consider the patient's physical position and sit before communicating. In a group, sitting in a circle reduces dominance, promotes equality among the members, and encourages group participation.

Intrapersonal and environmental factors Intrapersonal factors relate to individual development, skill mastery such as language and decision making, differences in perception, self-concept, and values. Any of these areas may affect interpretation of the communicated message. A patient with limited finances may not hear the reasons for a treatment after the cost is mentioned. If a relative is causing trouble in the family a patient may be unable to follow the therapeutic regimen because of the distraction.

Environmental factors include temperature, ventilation, lighting, furniture type and arrangement, formality, isolation, and mood. A warm room may cause physical discomfort—perspiration and feelings of faintness—and may thus interfere with communication. A positive tone for effective communication may be facilitated with a well-lighted, well-ventilated room with no clutter. Avoiding distractions in the environment fosters sound understanding and acceptance.

Effective and Therapeutic Techniques

Effective communication is necessary for the development of a therapeutic nurse-patient relationship. To be an effective communicator, the nurse must consider the patient's mental and physical capabilities, culture, socioeconomic background, interests, educational level, language skills, and knowledge of technical and medical terms because these factors influence nurse-patient communication. The nurse must use such information to individualize communication.

Therapeutic communication is goal oriented: It meets the patient's needs and helps the nurse provide optimal care. Therapeutic communication promotes sharing between the nurse and patient and allows the nurse to effectively gather data from the patient and develop the plan of care *with* the patient. Nontherapeutic communication interferes with nurse-patient interaction. Communication remains on a social level, preventing the gathering of pertinent assessment data and patient participation in planning nursing care.

Three ways of developing effective communication tools are to speak in front of a mirror, record the voice, and write nurse-patient dialogue for analysis. These techniques may help the student identify positive and negative aspects of speech and interactions. The last technique, a **process recording,** is a 5-minute nurse-patient conversation that is written down and analyzed for the patient's response, technique of communication, analysis of therapeutic technique, and changes in technique that would facilitate the communication (Table 5-2).

Therapeutic techniques

Several communication techniques are described in Table 5-3. A few are highlighted in the text that follows.

Listening and hearing are different aspects of communication. Hearing is the reception of sound, whereas with listening, the receiver actively thinks about and gives meaning to any sound that is heard. The receiver must be a good listener to effectively interpret the message. Listening is a skill that can be learned. The process involves two steps: One must pay attention to receive the sound and then interpret what is heard and in some cases what was omitted from the statement. When listening to a patient's complaint, the nurse should focus on the patient and assess the patient's facial expressions. The heart of the matter may not be the complaint but underlying feelings of fear, insecurity, and other unconscious motivators. Awareness of the ever-changing needs of the patient is the nurse's goal and responsibility. The nurse must give complete attention as the patient communicates personal needs or feelings. Eye contact and gestures of understanding are vital to therapeutic communication.

Silence, another nonverbal communication skill, is very useful because it gives both the nurse and patient time to think about what is happening and

Table 5-2 SAMPLE PROCESS RECORDING

Student Statement	Patient Response	Techniques Used (Name)	Analysis of Techniques	Recommended Change of Techniques
Is something wrong?	"No" (eyes fill with tears).	Closed question	Nontherapeutic	Omit. Use next statement.
You look sad, as if you're about to cry.	(Cries)	Reflecting and supporting	Therapeutic	Use technique.
I'll sit here a while with you (sits down). (After 30-second pause) Sometimes its hard to share the things you're concerned about with someone you don't know well. I'd like to be able to help you.	(Angrily) "You can help me by telling me the truth."	Supporting	Therapeutic	Use technique.
Leaning forward and maintaining eye contact.	"Everyone beats around the bush when I ask them what's wrong. The head nurse said, 'What do *you* think is wrong?' That kind of put-off drives me up the wall!"	Attending	Therapeutic	Use technique.

Courtesy Ivy Tech State College, Evansville, Indiana.

Table 5-3 **SUMMARY OF THERAPEUTIC COMMUNICATION TECHNIQUES**

Technique	Definition	Therapeutic Value
Listening	Active process of receiving information and examining one's reaction to messages received	Nonverbally communicates to patient nurse's interest in patient
Silence	Periods of no verbal communication among participants	Nonverbally communicates nurse's acceptance of patient
Establishing guidelines	Statements regarding roles, purpose, and limitations for particular interaction	Helps patient to know what is expected
Open-ended comments	General comments asking patient to determine direction interaction should take	Allows patient to decide what material is most relevant and encourages patient to continue
Reducing distance	Diminishing physical space between nurse and patient	Nonverbally communicates that nurse wants to be involved with patient
Acknowledgment	Recognition given to patient for contribution to interaction	Demonstrates importance of patient's role within relationship
Restating	Repeating to patient what nurse believes is main thought or idea expressed	Asks for validation of nurse's interpretation of message
Reflecting	Directing back to the patient own ideas, feelings, questions, or content	Attempts to show patient importance of own ideas, feelings, and interpretations
Seeking clarification	Asking for additional input to understand message received	Demonstrates nurse's desire to understand patient's communication
Seeking consensual validation	Attempts to reach mutual denotative and connotative meaning of specific words	Demonstrates nurse's desire to understand patient's communication
Focusing	Questions or statements to help patient develop or expand idea	Directs conversation toward topics of importance
Summarizing	Statement of main areas discussed during interaction	Helps patient to separate relevant from irrelevant material and serves as review and closing for interaction
Planning	Mutual decision-making regarding goals and direction of future interactions	Reiterates patient's role within relationship

From Sundeen SJ et al: *Nurse-client interaction: implementing the nursing process,* ed 5, St Louis, 1994, Mosby.

what is being said. Although silence is a helpful therapeutic technique, the patient needs nonverbal cues that the nurse is focused on the message and considers it important. The nurse's facial expressions should be calm and friendly during times of silence so that the patient feels at ease. The nurse must be able to use silence without becoming anxious. The patient should also be allowed to remain silent without feeling the need to socially entertain the nurse.

The nurse should begin all communication interactions by establishing a purpose for the conversation. In this way the nurse sets guidelines for the conversation. Setting the guidelines permits the patient to understand the outcome of the interaction and the nurse's expectations for it. The interaction helps the nurse to establish rapport with the patient and set the stage for data gathering or teaching.

Open-ended questions are used to gather data while allowing the patient to decide what is important to reveal. This type of questioning uses a statement or question that cannot be answered with one word or a short sentence. Using words like *tell me about, describe,* and *explain* indicate to the receiver that a broader explanation is expected. Another example of an open-ended question is for the nurse to state, in the form of a question, the last word of a patient's comment such as "Worried?," or "You say you are worried?"

Direct questions require for short, specific answers and are used to gain specific data. This type of question is usually answered with one word or a short sentence. The nurse must use caution in using closed questions, since patients may feel as if they are being grilled. Direct questions may be very appropriate if the nurse needs specific information.

Closure, or bringing the conversation to a close, is very important to facilitate understanding and validate the conclusions reached. The nurse should summarize the highlights of the conversation and cover the planning decisions made from the interaction.

Blocks to communication

Blocks to communication include any activity that interferes with the reception of an intended message.

One block alone should not destroy effective communication, but all blocks should be recognized and avoided to keep the lines of communication open. The nurse should recognize blocks in communication to improve communication skills when working with the patient. Some common blocks include the following:

1. Using cliches. Cliches are overused phrases that have lost their meaning and instead indicate lack of interest, minimize the problem, or offer false hope (for example, "Everything will be OK" or "everyone feels that way").
2. Changing the subject. The presentation of a new topic blocks communication by telling the patient not to continue talking about the previous topic. Changing the subject usually indicates that the topic makes the person uncomfortable. For example, when the patient asks, "Am I going to die?" the nurse says, "Are you ready for breakfast?"
3. Challenging responses. Rejecting the patient's view blocks communication. Rejection occurs when the receiver is defensive or denies statements made by the patient. For example, the patient states, "Dr. Jones must not be a very good doctor. He hasn't been to see me today." The nurse replies "Dr. Jones is an excellent doctor. All of his patients like him."
4. Giving opinions. Opinions expressed by the receiver block communication because they may indicate a mind closed to new ideas. The nurse should convey a neutral attitude when hearing opinions to avoid discouraging the speaker (patient).
5. Giving advice or directions. Giving advice or directions interferes with the patient's identification of options to solve problems. The nurse should ask for the patient's suggestions and allow involvement in problem solving.
6. Failing to listen. Not attending (listening) to what the patient is saying. Giving nonverbal indications of listening but thinking of other things will block communication and the progress in meeting the needs of the patient.
7. Using closed-ended statements or questions. Comments or questions that ask for one- or two-word responses limit the patient's ability to express concerns, understanding, and needs and conversely restrict the nurse's opportunity to know more about the patient. For example, the nurse might ask "How did you sleep last night?" instead of "Describe how you slept last night." The answer to the latter question provides more information about the patient's sleep pattern.

Communication with children

Children have special needs in communication because of their age, limited life experiences, and limited language ability. The nurse should try to communicate with children on their intellectual and physical level. The nurse should sit or kneel so as not to tower over the child and use language at the child's level of understanding. Children often have names for bodily functions or parts. Parents and children should be asked to identify these names during the admission interview. Dolls can be used to show a child the steps of procedures to be performed. Since children are just as afraid of the unknown as adults and do not always possess the necessary verbal skills to express their fear and understand explanations, they require extra help from the nurse. The nurse must always be honest with the child. Telling a child, "you will feel a little sting with the needle" helps build a trusting relationship more than saying, "This won't hurt." Such honesty may increase cooperation from the child and decrease the child's stress.

Communication with the older adult

Communication with the older adult may be challenging. The older adult may have vision and hearing losses, slower thought processes, and different interests. Sometimes, lifestyles limit opportunities for the older adult to communicate, but the need for communication is very real. When communicating with the older adult, the nurse should remember that older adulthood is not synonymous with impaired thought processes. Each person must be assessed and treated individually and with respect (see gerontologic box).

A loud voice should never be used, even for the hearing impaired. The nurse should get closer to the patient and speak slowly and distinctly. The nurse should use the patient's formal name unless instructed to do otherwise. Terms of endearment should not be used because they do not show respect. Trust and confidence should be inspired by the nurse's calm attitude in both verbal and nonverbal communication. The nurse should be especially patient in requesting information because the response time of the older adult may be longer than

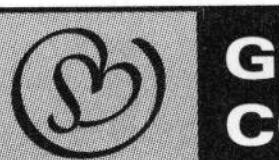

GERONTOLOGIC CONSIDERATIONS

- The nurse should use short, simple sentences.
- Moving quickly from one subject to another should be avoided.
- The environment needs to be quiet. Background noise should be eliminated.
- It is important to include the patient's family and friends in conversations.
- The nurse should never use a loud voice, even for the hearing impaired. Instead, the nurse should speak slowly and distinctly.

that of a younger person. Patronizing or condescending approaches should be avoided.

Written communication

Written communication is a form of verbal communication because words are used for the exchange of information. Thus writing requires all considerations as speaking but with some additions. Written communication should be clear, easy to read, spelled correctly, precise, and complete. Written communication should stand alone without the benefit of nonverbal signals, and therefore it often must be longer so that it is as complete as verbal communication. If abbreviations are used, they must be familiar to the recipient. Words with unclear meanings should be avoided. Even with these precautions, written communication may be misunderstood, and some written or verbal follow-up of the receiver's responses should be available.

NURSING PROCESS IN COMMUNICATION

Assessment

Before planning ways to promote communication, the nurse must assess the patient's developmental level, perceptions, emotions, cultural orientation, and knowledge. This may be difficult if a patient has physical impairments that affect communication such as shortness of breath or speech problems resulting from a stroke or brain tumor. In this instance, the nurse should consult the patient's family, friends, or significant others. The nurse should also consider whether the patient is taking any medications that could impair speech or communication abilities.

Nursing Diagnosis

The nursing diagnosis should focus on the cause of the patient's inability to communicate. This will provide the basis for selecting the appropriate interventions. Possible nursing diagnoses for impaired communication include the following:

Impaired social interaction
Impaired verbal communication
Ineffective family coping: disabled or compromised
Ineffective individual coping
Powerlessness

Planning

Goals of care are mutually set by the patient and nurse. When possible, the nurse collaborates with the patient, family, friends, and health care team members (see care plan on p. 54). The nurse's communication style and ability to establish a therapeutic relationship with the patient are important factors in achieving established goals. Those goals could include the following:

Goal #1: Patient appropriately responds to stimuli.

Outcome

Patient is oriented to time, person, and place within 24 hours of admission.

Goal #2: Patient establishes effective communication with family and health care team members by day 4 of hospitalization.

Outcome

Patient participates in problem solving by day 4 of hospitalization.

Implementation

It is important for the nurse to facilitate activities that provide the patient with health promotion, maintenance, and restoration. These activities, such as health screenings or auditory testing, should be designed to maximize the patient's ability to communicate. The nurse may need to use special techniques when communicating with patients with special needs such as children and older adults. It is important for the nurse to identify barriers that may restrict effective communication with these patients.

Evaluation

The nurse should continuously evaluate the success of interventions. Systematic evaluation requires the nurse to determine whether expected outcomes have been met. Examples of goals, outcomes,

■ NURSING CARE PLAN ■

NONCOMPLIANCE

Mrs. J, age 67, refuses to practice prescribed health-related behaviors. The nurse has discovered that the medical orders interfere with the patient's personal beliefs.

NURSING DIAGNOSIS

Noncompliance related to patient's value system as evidenced by patient's refusal of treatment, failure to adhere to treatment regimen, and refusal to set personal goals regarding treatment

GOAL

- Patient will follow treatment regimen by day 3 of hospitalization.

EXPECTED OUTCOMES

- Patient will keep appointments with nursing staff.
- Patient will practice teaching measures to perform daily personal care and activities within the limits of strength.

NURSING INTERVENTIONS

- Listen and support patient's fears and anxieties to help patient vent and begin to trust.
- Emphasize positive factors to help patient focus on problem instead of herself.
- Assist patient to understand teaching regarding treatment measures.

EVALUATION

- Patient describes factors that influence compliance with treatment.
- Patient performs personal care with minimum assistance.

and corresponding evaluative measures include the following:

Goal #1: Patient appropriately responds to stimuli.

Evaluative measure

Ask patient to identify time of day, name, and location.

Goal #2: Patient establishes effective communication with family and health care team members by day 4 of hospitalization.

Evaluative measure

Conduct a discussion with the patient and family regarding discharge plans.

DOCUMENTATION

The **medical record** provides an accurate description of a patient's nursing and medical care from the time of admission to the time of discharge. The informal term commonly used to refer to the medical record is the *chart,* and making an entry in the chart is referred to as *charting* or ***documentation.***

Purposes of the Medical Record

Legal documentation The chart contains written legal documentation of the patient's health status and the approach for meeting the patient's health care needs. The medical record provides a "total picture" of the patient's nursing care.

Communication The medical record is a means of communication among nursing personnel on different shifts, as well as among other members of the health care team. Notations on the chart are made by all members of the team. Some agencies designate specific sections for each discipline, or all may document on the same progress notes.

Protection The patient's record provides protection for the institution and the employees responsible for recording. For example, in the event that a patient accuses an individual of malpractice or negligence, the patient's record should prove or disprove the accusation. It is imperative to remember that, in essence, if it was not documented, it was not done.

Education Documenting may also be used for educational purposes, such as statistical data for research. Findings may indicate a need for continuing education for the nursing staff or other members of

> **! REMEMBER**
>
> - All information in the medical record is confidential. No information may be revealed without the consent of the patient.

the health care team. Educators in the health field use the patient's record as a source of teaching (for example, as a case study). Students use the medical record to compare textbook cases, including symptoms, to actual patient situations or diagnoses.

Statistical and research data The patient's medical record may provide vital statistics and data for certain research projects. This information includes the frequency of certain diseases, causes of death, longevity, carcinogenic factors relating to lifestyle, births, and other statistics. These projects may provide useful information both locally and nationally.

Continuity of standards Periodic auditing of patient medical records is performed by the Joint Commission on the Accreditation of Healthcare Organizations to maintain standards of information to be included in documentation. To comply with these standards, many agencies have a designated person or committee that regularly performs internal audits throughout the year.

Legal Aspects of Documentation

The law requires that a medical record of each patient's nursing and medical care be maintained. Therefore the medical record is a legal document providing proof of quality care because all entries refer to events relating to a particular patient. Medical records are often used in hearings for malpractice, mental status of the patient, personal injury, and disability. What is documented or not documented may mean the outcome of winning or losing a court case for the nurse or employer.

Legal guidelines for documentation

1. All the information in the chart refers to the patient, and therefore it should be unnecessary to use the identifier *patient*. The word *patient* may be used for correct sentence structure or clarity of description.
2. Only the correct color of ink should be used.
3. The nurse should never erase a word or statement entered into the medical record. This may provide an opportunity for a lawyer to question the competency of the documenter or may be construed as deliberate concealment of facts by the documenter.
4. When an error is made, one line should be drawn through the incorrect word or statement, and *error in charting* is written above the erroneous word or sentence. Then, the correct word or sentence is printed next to the error. An example follows:

   error in charting
   Voided ~~2000~~ 200 ml dark amber urine.

5. Legal action may be taken against a person who falsifies or helps to falsify information in a patient's medical record.
6. The nurse should never leave a blank space or skip lines when documenting. This will prevent the possibility of someone adding information that is incorrect or inconsistent with other remarks.
7. If a statement must be finished in the middle of a line, a line should be drawn through to the end of the line, leaving enough room for the signature. Next, the nurse signs the name and title at the end of the line.
8. If it is necessary to recopy a whole page of the nursing progress record or nurse's notes draw an X through the entire page from corner to corner. The nurse must not obscure the original documentation and must keep the original sheet in the medical record because it is a part of the medical record. Otherwise, agency policy should be followed. The person recopying the page must sign the name and title and write *recopied* and record the date of the copy at the top of the page.
9. Headings that identify the patient should be complete and placed on each medical record page. Most agencies use address-o-graph machines that hold a premade plastic card with vital information of the patient such as name, age, physician's name, and other information according to the agency policy. The nurse would not know where to place a lost page if it did not contain a completed heading.
10. All special forms requiring a patient's signature and witnesses are part of the legal document.
11. The nurse should be specific about the time that changes or specific events occurred or procedures were performed.
12. Entries should be documented only by the nurse who performed the nursing care. The person who documents is accountable for the information written in the medical record.
13. Treatments, medications, observations, and as-

Table 5-4 DO'S AND DON'TS FOR FILING AN INCIDENT REPORT

Do's	Don'ts
Accurately record time, date of incident, patient's name, name of family member notified, time and manner of notification (that is, in person, by phone).	—
Record name of physician who was notified and time report was made.	—
Include names of witnesses.	Do not list addresses or phone numbers of witnesses.
Give objective description of incident. For example, if medication error occurred, note only dose, medication given, and route.	Do not give reason, such as in hurry or short staffed.
Use quotation marks with *direct* quotes to convey information from another source (for example, description of incident by patient or aide's comments). Record name and title, if appropriate, of person being quoted.	—
Include patient assessment in clinical terms of what is seen and heard and what patient says. Record symptoms appropriately, and if form includes diagram, mark this.	Do not surmise or speculate about what injuries may have been sustained. Do not write about follow-up care because that information belongs in medical record.
Document immediate action, such as putting patient back to bed, assessing injuries, and getting orders.	Do not mention actions taken to prevent recurrence of incident. Omit references to investigation or report to insurance carrier. These could be misconstrued in court case.
Write signature and title legibly when completing incident report.	—

sessments are never documented before the nursing care is administered. Something, such as patient refusal of an intervention, may prevent the care from being administered.

14. Agency policy and procedure regarding documentation should be followed.

Incident report

An **incident report** is a confidential document that describes any patient accident or incident, such as a fall, injury, medication error, or omission of prescribed therapies, that occur while a nurse or other health care personnel are providing care. An incident report is also completed when an employee or visitor is injured or falls. Any statements that may infer blame or express opinions or conclusions could have impact on a court case. It is imperative that an incident report explain exactly what occurred, avoiding the use of conclusions, assumptions, opinions, judgments, or blame. Incident reports are not stored in the medical record. Some "do's and don'ts" are found in Table 5-4.

Patient access to the medical record

A patient may be allowed access to the personal medical record under certain conditions. It may be the responsibility of the nurse to inform the appropriate authority of the request. The medical record remains stored in the agency after dismissal of the patient from the agency.

Suggested Rules of Documentation

The methods and forms used for documenting may vary from one health care institution to another, but the principles of documentation remain the same wherever a medical record is required. Therefore it is important for the nurse to remember the following general rules of documentation:

1. Make statements legible and grammatically appropriate:
   a. Make each entry neat and print or write legibly.
   b. Use appropriate spelling and punctuation and only accepted abbreviations and symbols. If necessary, refer to a dictionary for the correct spelling. Know that misspelled words can cause confusion and promote lack of professionalism.
   c. Sign the name and title after each entry. Use the first initial, last name, and title (for example, G. Nurse, RN, LPN, or LVN).

MILITARY TIME

0700 = 7:00*	1900 = 7:00 PM
0800 = 8:00 AM	2000 = 8:00 PM
0900 = 9:00 AM	2100 = 9:00 PM
1000 = 10:00 AM	2200 = 10:00 PM
1100 = 11:00 AM	2300 = 11:00 PM
1200 = 12:00 noon	2400 = 12:00 midnight
1300 = 1:00 PM	0100 = 1:00 AM
1400 = 2:00 PM	0200 = 2:00 AM
1500 = 3:00 PM	0300 = 3:00 AM
1600 = 4:00 PM	0400 = 4:00 AM
1700 = 5:00 PM	0500 = 5:00 AM
1800 = 6:00 PM	0600 = 6:00 AM

*0701 = 7:01 AM, 0702 = 7:02 AM, and so on.

2. Make statements following an appropriate time sequence and using military time (see box):
   a. Record events in a logical time sequence.
   b. If information was unintentionally omitted make a late entry by stating "late entry" and noting the specific time the treatment was performed or follow guidelines of agency policy and procedure.
   c. Document after the fact, using the past tense after completing a treatment or nursing measure or administering medication:
      (1) Use the verb that designates past tense.
      (2) Do not use future tense because this is a legal issue and all documentation must be in past tense. (The nurse could not prove whether the nursing care was administered if documented in the future tense.)
3. Use clear, concise, accurate, and factual statements. Describe the problem, nursing actions performed, and the patient's response:
   a. Choose words carefully and record them in an organized manner (follow the steps of the nursing process).
   b. Condense information briefly yet completely. Remember that a lengthy report with unnecessary wording tends to obscure pertinent information. For common abbreviations of terms, see Table 5-5.
   c. Be *exact* about time, actions, observations, assessments, effects and the results of nursing interventions.
   d. Ensure that the page reflects the current date and time as well as the patient's name and vital information. Record the date once at the top of the page.
4. Follow agency policy for documentation:
   a. Document with an appropriate colored ink. (Some agencies require black ink so that all information can be microfilmed.)
5. Place appropriate forms in the designated sections of the chart (for example, a section on physician's orders or nurse's notes would be found in separate sections of the chart). When reading each section of the medical record, place the most current information first in each section.

Since documentation represents a written picture of events and situations pertaining to the nursing care of a patient, clear recording is important. Documentation leaves no doubt in the reader's mind about what is being expressed. Students might ask themselves the following questions:

1. Is the information understandable?
2. Is the information clear and concise?
3. Can you picture the patient and the response to a certain activity or intervention?

The information necessary to record includes the patient's problems and needs, reactions and responses (both positive and negative) to treatments, nursing interventions, medications, and changes in condition. The agency's policies and procedures dictate the format, style, and order of documentation.

Documentation Formats

Problem-oriented medical record A **problem-oriented medical record (POMR)** was introduced in the 1960s to facilitate documentation of pertinent information in an organized fashion. Each person of the health care team contributes to a given list of patient problems. The team may consist of a physician, nurse, dietitian, and other health professionals. The format used was called *SOAP* and later ***SOAPIE.*** Each letter represents a step in the approach (Table 5-6).

Another part of the POMR is a flow sheet used to record simple data and recurring activities in treatment or responses such as vital signs, neurologic assessments, diabetic treatments, and intravenous assessments and piggyback.

Charting by exception Charting by exception is performed for exceptions to the norm. The information may be narrative, but several standardized flow sheets may be used to simplify documentation of the patient's health status and nursing interventions. A standardized care plan serves as a baseline (a known value or quantity with which an unknown is compared) for assessment, intervention, and documentation. In this way, standards of practice are established, and the standardized form indicates the nursing assessments and interventions that are routinely performed. When a standardized statement is not met, the nurse writes a description of it in the patient's progress notes.

If the same data are to be used, they are not rewritten, but they are indicated, using * or *ck* on the

Table 5-5 ACCEPTED ABBREVIATIONS AND SYMBOLS

Abbreviations and Symbols	Meanings	Abbreviations and Symbols	Meanings
$\overline{aa}$	Of each or in each	OU	Both eyes
a.c.	Before meals; ante cebum	P	Pulse
		$\overline{p}$	After
ad lib	As desired	p.c.	After meals; post cebum
ADL	Activities of daily living	P.I.	Present illness
AM	Morning	po	By mouth; per os
amb.	Ambulatory; walking	PM	Afternoon
@	At	p.r.n.	When necessary; as desired
b.i.d.	Twice a day	$\overline{q}$	Every
BM	Bowel movement	qd	Every day
BP	Blood pressure	qh	Every hour
BRP	Bathroom privileges	q.i.d.	Four times a day
$\overline{c}$	With	q.o.d.	Every other day
cc	Cubic centimeters	q.s.	Quantity sufficient
gtt	Drop	q2h	Every 2 hours
h.	Hour	q3h	Every 3 hours
H_2O	Water	q4h	Every 4 hours
hs (h.s.)	Hour of sleep	q6h	Every 6 hours
I & O	Intake and output	q8h	Every 8 hours
IM	Intramuscular	R (resp)	Respirations
IV	Intravenous	RR	Recovery room
kg	Kilogram	$\overline{s}$	Without
l	Liter	S.S.E.	Soap suds enema
lb	Pound	stat	Immediately
m	Minim	t.i.d.	Three times a day
ml	Milliliter	TL	Team leader
NPO	Nothing by mouth	TLC	Tender loving care
O_2	Oxygen	TPR	Temperature, pulse, and respiration
OD	Right eye	TWE	Tap water enema
OOB	Out of bed	UA	Urinalysis
OR	Operating room	wt	Weight
OS	Left eye		

flow sheet, that they are unresolved or will be carried in the nursing care plan as nursing diagnoses with follow-up documentation.

A **PIE** format is used for charting by exception. This format is similar to the SOAPIE format because it is a problem-solving approach. It was designed to provide an ongoing plan of nursing care with daily documentation. The care and assessment flow sheet consists of standardized assessment criteria (human needs categories) and interventions. The nurse assesses all areas within normal standards. There are several ways that APIE format may be written (see Fig. 5-6). The nurse should use the format according to agency policy or according to the area assigned. Each shift evaluates each patient problem at least once, and if the problem remains unresolved, it is carried until resolution is reached. After the patient problem is resolved it is no longer covered by the daily documentation.

A variation of the PIE format is sometimes used to include assessment data by placing an *A* (assessment data) before the *PIE* (APIE). This helps the nurse follow the steps of the nursing process.

Focus charting **Focus charting** is a format that focuses on patient needs that deviate from the norm. A flow sheet of standardized human needs and interventions is used with multiple flow sheets to facilitate assessment and intervention documentation. After a complete assessment at the beginning of the shift the nurse assesses all normal areas and separately handles any deviations from the norm. The nurse further describes any deviation in the flow sheet. This form consists of three columns: date/time, focus, and narration (progress notes). The problem is written in the focus column using the NANDA statement list for nursing diagnoses. Documentation is written using the data, action, response, education or evaluation **(DARE)** format:

Table 5-6 SOAPIE DOCUMENTATION

Letter	Description	Example
S—Subjective symptom	This is symptom patient expresses to nurse: pain, needs, headache, likes, or dislikes.	Patient reports headache and feeling warm.
O—Objective information	This is observation by nurse: anything nurse sees, hears, feels, smells, or touches. Items must be measurable: laboratory results, vital signs, or information from x-ray examinations.	Nurse observes that patient's face is flushed and skin is warm. Oral temperature 102° F.
A—Assessment	This is evaluation of subjective and objective symptoms obtained. Nursing diagnosis comes from this data. Example of such data is patient problem.	Nurse assesses and recognizes that patient needs medication to reduce temperature.
P—Planning	This is plan of care necessary to meet patient needs. Planning includes goals for patient care.	Nurse reads medical orders and prepares medication if it is ordered or notifies physician.
I—Implementation	This is statement of how plan of care was implemented. Plan is implemented by putting into action necessary steps to resolve or meet patient's needs.	Nurse implements plan and administers medication. Nurse notifies team leader or charge nurse and charts implementation (administration of medication).
E—Evaluation	This is record of plan's results. Evaluation measures how well goals of plan were reached. If plan does not work, nurse must replan.	Nurse evaluates action taken, such as reassessing patient's temperature 30 min after medication was administered, and documents evaluation (that is, effectiveness of medication).

D Objective and subjective assessment data that support the focus or nursing diagnosis
A Nursing intervention provided
R Patient's responses
E Patient teaching, evaluation, or both

Once documentation indicates that the problem is resolved, it no longer appears in documentation.

Narrative notes Narrative documentation is an established format used to tell the story of the health status of the patient, interventions and treatments performed for the patient, and reactions to overall care. Flow sheets have been adopted to use with this format to simplify and decrease the amount of time the nurse spends performing documentation. The narrative format usually involves the documenting of a complete head-to-toe assessment when the patient is admitted to the health care facility, at the beginning of each shift, and after any incident or change of the patient's health status occurring during the shift (Fig. 5-3).

Documentation Forms

Several methods of documentation are being used to describe a patient's concerns or problems. The format used is determined by procedure and policy and may be altered to fit the needs of the agency. Descriptions of the following forms are provided to assist the student to become familiar with commonly used forms.

An admission form, commonly called *admission data base,* provides general information about the newly admitted patient. The information includes the patient's name, address, telephone number, age, gender, social security number, marital status, religious preference if desired, name and phone number of the nearest relative, insurance number, medical record number, and name of the attending physician. This form is usually completed by admitting personnel.

An *initial nursing assessment* contains a head-to-toe assessment (nursing physical examination) and is performed by the nurse. The assessment form provides information about the patient at the time of admission to the nursing unit, at the beginning of each shift, and after any incident or change in the patient's health status. It usually includes additional information such as allergies, weight, height, presenting symptoms or chief complaint, prosthesis, prominent marks or deformities, food preferences, pressure sores, and a nursing physical and mental

NARRATIVE DOCUMENTATION (DARE)		
Date	Time	Progress Notes
Current	1000	F- Pain related to surgical intervention
		D- States has moderate pain in RUQ,
		guarding abd. incision c̄ depicting
		facial grimace.
	1010	A- Demerol 75mg. c̄ Vistaril 50mg given
		IM Z-tract in (L) ventrogluteal region.
	1050	R- States has pain relief.
		E- Explained importance of ambulation
		to prevent complications. Verbalizes
		understanding. — M. White, LVN

Fig. 5-3 Narrative documentation (DARE).

assessment. The date and time (military) are recorded at the beginning of each assessment. Many agencies now photograph pressure ulcers for legal purposes. This form is usually completed by a nurse (Fig. 5-4). Specific information to document in a head-to-toe assessment include the following:

1. *Mental status:* Level of consciousness, such as orientation to person, place, and time; disorientation, confusion, or memory loss
2. *Head and face:* Hair, skin color, eyes, nose, mouth, dental status, ears, and swallowing
3. *Neck and trunk:* Assessment of the neck, condition of breasts, lung sounds, chest shape, rib cage, skin color, and back and spinal column
4. *Abdomen:* Distention, shape (flat, hard, rigid, boardlike), palpation (firm, soft), bowel sounds
5. *Extremities:* Symmetry, edema, joint pain, weakness, tremors, and range of joint motion
6. *Motor ability:* Ataxia, muscle strength, and muscle tone
7. *Character of respirations:* Regular, irregular, deep, shallow, labored, use of accessory muscles
8. *Vital signs:* Temperature, pulse, respirations, and blood pressure
9. *Elimination:*
   a. *Urine:* Amount, color, consistency, odor, bladder distention, frequency, pain
   b. *Bowel:* Amount, color, consistency, odor, constipation, impaction, last bowel movement (date), abdominal distention, bowel sounds, flatus, pain
10. *Skin:* Turgor, condition, color, temperature, edema, lesions
11. *Sensory:* Hearing, seeing, smelling, tasting, touching, and emotions
12. *Position and comfort:* Pain, position assumed, position placed in, and supports used to position
13. *Environment:* Room temperature, safety, signal bell within reach
14. *Pain:* Onset, location, duration, intensity (mild, moderate, severe), level (1 to 5, 1 to 10, ratio with one being the least), description (sharp, dull, knifelike, stabbing, aching)
15. *Symptoms:* Time of onset, location, duration, intensity, and other body parts or areas involved

1020 States having a stabbing pain in center of anterior chest lasting 5 minutes and becoming worse on movement. "My shoulder hurts and it goes down my left arm to my elbow." Pointed to inner aspect of left arm. ________________ Nurse's Signature, LPN.

16. *Procedures and nursing measures:* Time the nursing intervention was implemented and what action was taken

1105 Warm sterile water compresses applied to right dorsal foot; specimens collected, labeled, and sent (or taken) to lab. ____________ Nurse's Signature, LPN

17. *Medications:* Date; time; and name, dose, and route of administration of drug; also, location of administration

1330 Demerol 75 mg. given IM Z-tract in left ventrogluteal region for severe pain in abd. surgical incision. ________________ Nurse's Signature, LPN.

Text continued on p. 65.

WILSON N. JONES MEMORIAL HOSPITAL • SHERMAN, TEXAS

ADMISSION NURSING DATA BASE

1 ADMISSION INFORMATION

DATE OF ADMISSION 1-2-95	TIME 0948	AMBULATING ✓	IN WHEELCHAIR	ON STRETCHER

HT.	WT.	RACE	SEX	TEMP	PULSE	RESP.	BLOOD PRESSURE LEFT ARM	RIGHT ARM
5'6"	141	C	F	98² (ORAL) RECTAL TYMP	94 APICAL (RADIAL) IRREG.	22	REG. ✓	

2 ALLERGIES TO FOOD/DRUGS/OTHER

NKDA

3 PERSONAL HISTORY

PRE-HOSPITAL STATE

ADMITTED FROM: HOME ☒ NURSING HOME ☐ HOSPITAL ☐ NAME OF FACILITY: ____ LIVES: ALONE ☐ WITH SPOUSE ☒ OTHER ☐ ____ ☐ SUPERVISED LIVING

PERSON TO BE NOTIFIED RE: DISCHARGE PLANS ▶ NAME: John G. Smith HOME PHONE 892-6094 WORK PHONE 893-2314

WAS PATIENT RECEIVING HELP AT HOME? ☐ YES ☐ NO ☒ UNDETERMINED | IF YES, SPECIFY ACTIVITIES REQUIRING HELP: ☐ SHOPPING ☐ MEALS ☐ HOUSEKEEPING ☐ LAUNDRY OTHER:

SPECIFY PROVIDER OF SERVICE: NAME: TELEPHONE: | IS PROVIDER WILLING AND ABLE TO HELP AFTER HOSPITALIZATION? ☐ YES ☐ NO

HEALTH RISKS

CIGARETTE SMOKING: ☐ NEVER ☒ EX-SMOKER DATE STOPPED: 10 yrs. | ☐ SMOKES: | SMOKING HISTORY #/DAY - #/YEARS - | ALCOHOL INTAKE: ☐ NONE ☒ OCCASIONAL ☐ FREQUENT USUAL AMT. 1 | DATE/TIME OF LAST INTAKE:

SLEEP PATTERN: ▶ DESCRIBE USUAL PATTERN: Some insomnia | ROUTINE EXERCISE ☒ YES ☐ NO DESCRIBE: walk daily

SPIRITUAL NEEDS EXPRESSED ☒ YES ☐ NO | CONTACT CLERGYMAN: ☐ YES – NAME ☒ NO

COMMUNICATION

MAKES NEEDS KNOWN: ☒ VERBALLY ● ENGLISH ○ OTHER LANGUAGE ☐ NON-VERBALLY – METHOD: | ☐ DOES NOT COMMUNICATE

SPEECH ☒ NO IMPAIRMENT ☐ IMPAIRMENT (DESCRIBE): | ☐ DOES NOT SPEAK

AWARE OF SURROUNDINGS AND REACTS TO ENVIRONMENTAL STIMULI: ☒ YES ☐ NO – IF NO, CHECK IF RESPONSIVE TO: STIMULUS: ☐ VISUAL ☐ AUDITORY ☐ TACTILE ☐ PAINFUL ☐ NO RESPONSE

MENTAL STATUS ☒ ORIENTED: ☒ YES ☐ NO – IF NO, DISORIENTED TO: ☐ TIME ☐ PLACE ☐ PERSON ☐ EVENT DATE OF ONSET:

VISION ☐ WITHOUT GLASSES/LENSES ☐ SEES NEWSPRINT ☐ SEES OBSTACLES ☐ CAN TELL LIGHT FROM DARK ☐ DOES NOT SEE

☒ WITH GLASSES/LENSES ☒ SEES NEWSPRINT ☒ SEES OBSTACLES ☒ CAN TELL LIGHT FROM DARK ☐ DOES NOT SEE

HEARING ☐ WITHOUT HEARING AID ☒ HEARS NORMAL VOICE ☐ HEARS LOUD VOICE ☐ HEARS ONLY LOUD NOISES ☐ DOES NOT HEAR

☐ WITH HEARING AID ☐ HEARS NORMAL VOICE ☐ HEARS LOUD VOICE ☐ HEARS ONLY LOUD NOICES ☐ DOES NOT HEAR

NUTRITION

LAST FOOD INTAKE: ▶ DATE Previous day TIME 6:30 p.m. | LAST FLUID INTAKE ▶ DATE Current TIME a.m. | RECENT CHANGE IN: ☐ WEIGHT +/– LBS. | APPETITE ☒ YES ☐ NO

DIET HABITS DESCRIBED BY PATIENT: 3 meals/day

DENTITION: ☒ ALL/MOST TEETH | DIFFICULTY CHEWING ☐ YES ☒ NO | DENTURES: ☐ UPPER ☐ LOWER ☐ OTHER:

ELIMINATION

BOWEL FUNCTION ☒ CONTINENT ☐ INCONTINENT ONSET: | ☐ OSTOMY – SELF-CARE: ☐ YES – EXPLAIN: ☐ NO

LAST B.M.: previous date / / / / USUAL PATTERN: Daily

BLADDER FUNCTION ☒ CONTINENT | GET UP AT NIGHT TO URINATE? ☒ YES - HOW OFTEN? once ☐ NO

☐ INCONTINENT ONSET: | ☐ DIALYSIS ☐ CATHETER | ☐ EXTERNAL DEVICES | ☐ OSTOMY – | SELF-CARE: ☐ YES ☐ NO

4 CHECK PROSTHETIC DEVICES BROUGHT TO HOSPITAL

☐ HEARING AID ☒ GLASSES ☐ CONTACT LENSES ☐ GLASS EYE ☐ PROSTHETIC LIMBS ☐ DENTURES OTHER:

5 ADMISSION CHECK

I.D. BAND ON: ☒ YES | ORIENT TO HOSPITAL ENVIRONMENT: ☒ YES ☐ NO | PRE-ADM ORDERS WRITTEN? ☒ YES ☐ NO | PHYSICIAN NOTIFIED? ☐ YES ☐ NO | NAME OF M.D. Miller

6 VALUABLES LIST

Wristwatch, eyeglasses, purse

DISPOSITION OF ☐ SENT HOME ☐ HOSPITAL SAFE ☒ PATIENT RETAINED AT REQUEST ☐ SECURITY

DO YOU HAVE ANY ADVANCE DIRECTIVES? ☐ YES ☒ NO DO YOU PLAN TO BE AN ORGAN DONOR? ☐ YES ☐ NO

Fig. 5-4 Initial nursing assessment. (Courtesy Wilson N. Jones Memorial Hospital, Sherman, Texas.)

Continued.

7 FUNCTIONAL STATUS

BATHING	PRE ADM	AT ADM	TOILETING	PRE ADM	AT ADM	WALKING	PRE ADM	AT ADM
WITHOUT HELP OF ANY KIND	✓	✓	WITHOUT HELP OF ANY KIND	✓	✓	WITHOUT HELP OF ANY KIND	✓	✓
USING ASSISTIVE DEVICE(S)			USING ASSISTIVE DEVICE(S)			USING ASSISTIVE DEVICE(S)		
WITH HELP OF ANOTHER PERSON			WITH HELP OF ANOTHER PERSON			WITH HELP OF ANOTHER PERSON		
DEVICE AND HELP OF ANOTHER			DEVICE AND HELP OF ANOTHER			DEVICE AND HELP OF ANOTHER		
IS BATHED BY OTHERS			DOES NOT USE TOILET ROOM			CONFINED TO BED/CHAIR		
DRESSING/UNDRESSING	**PRE ADM**	**AT ADM**	**TRANSFERRING**	**PRE ADM**	**AT ADM**	**EATING**	**PRE ADM**	**AT ADM**
WITHOUT HELP OF ANY KIND	✓	✓	WITHOUT HELP OF ANY KIND	✓	✓	WITHOUT HELP OF ANY KIND	✓	✓
USING ASSISTIVE DEVICE(S)			USING ASSISTIVE DEVICE(S)			USING ASSISTIVE DEVICE(S)		
WITH HELP OF ANOTHER PERSON			WITH HELP OF ANOTHER PERSON			WITH HELP OF ANOTHER PERSON		
DEVICE AND HELP OF ANOTHER			DEVICE AND HELP OF ANOTHER			DEVICE AND HELP OF ANOTHER		
IS DRESSED BY OTHERS			IS TRANSFERRED BY OTHERS			TUBE FED		
IS NOT DRESSED			IS NOT TRANSFERRED			FED INTRAVENOUSLY		

DESCRIBE DEVICES AND ASSISTANCE NEEDED:

SIGNATURE OF INDIVIDUAL COMPLETING SECTIONS 1-7: G. Grasslow, RN DATE: 1-2-95 TIME: 10:15

INFORMANT: Patient DATE: 1-2 RELATIONSHIP TO PATIENT:

RN MUST COMPLETE SECTIONS 8-19.

8 HEALTH HISTORY

ADMITTING DIAGNOSIS: DJD, CHF DRG: ______ LOS: ______ REASON FOR ADMISSION: heart DESCRIBED BY: ☒ PATIENT ☐ FAMILY

PAST MEDICAL HISTORY:
A. SURGERIES vag. hyst. – BTL – D+C
B. MEDICAL PROBLEMS
C. FRACTURES Ⓡ foot 1962

9 MEDICATIONS

☒ PRESCRIBED ☐ OTHER
☒ OVER-THE-COUNTER ☐ NONE
☐ ADMINISTERED BY: ☐ SELF ☐ OTHER
BROUGHT TO HOSPITAL: ☐ YES - IF YES, ☐ NO ☐ SENT HOME ☐ TO PHARMACY ☐ RETAINED BY PT

LIST MEDICATIONS, DOSE, FREQUENCY AND OF THOSE TAKEN TODAY, THE TIME:

Clinoril 200 mg. bid
Inderal 20 mg. bid
Tylenol Sinus prn

10 BIOPHYSICAL: COMPLETE ASSESSMENT FLOW SHEET

11 DISCHARGE PLANNING NEEDS

A. WILL YOU RETURN HOME AFTER DISCHARGE? ☒ YES ☐ NO COMMENTS:

B. FAMILY/SO SUPPORT PRESENT FOR POST DISCHARGE ASSISTANCE: ☒ YES ☐ NO
WHO: Husband

C. AT HOME CARE: SELF/SO (LIVE-IN: ☒ YES ☐ NO) ☐ OTHER: ______

D. ANTICIPATED DISCHARGE NEEDS: ☒ NONE ☐ EQUIPMENT/SUPPLIES: ______

E. ANTICIPATED AGENCIES FOR FOLLOW-UP: ☒ NONE ☐ HOME HEALTH ☐ MEALS ON WHEELS ☐ HOME HOSPICE ☐ TRANSPORTATION ☐ OTHER:

12 EDUCATION NEEDS

A. ANTICIPATED PT/SO LEARNING NEEDS: ☐ DIET ☐ MEDICATION ☐ ILLNESS ☐ HEALTH MAINTENANCE RISK FACTORS
COMMENTS: ______

B. THE PATIENT REQUIRES OR MAY REQUIRE THE FOLLOWING SUPPORT SERVICES:
☐ DIETARY ☐ CLERGY ☐ PT ☐ OT ☐ RT ☐ ET ☐ OTHER: ______
REFERRAL MADE: ☐ YES ☐ IF NOT, WHY ______

DSU Staff Signature ______

Fig. 5-4, cont'd Initial nursing assessment. (Courtesy Wilson N. Jones Memorial Hospital, Sherman, Texas.)

13 SKIN RISK ASSESSMENT

IF >10 IMPLEMENT "ALTERATION I SKIN/TISSUE INTEGRITY PROTOCOL" (POTENTIAL)

PARAMETERS	0	1	2	3
Physical Condition	Good ✓	Fair	Poor	Seriously Deteriorated
Mental Status	Alert ✓	Lethargic	Semiconsc.	Unconscious
Nutrition Status	Good ✓	Fair	Poor	Serious problem
Activity*	Self ✓	With Assistance	Chair Only	Bedrest
Mobility*	Full	Slightly Limited ✓	Vert Limited	Immobile
Incontinence*	Never ✓	Occasional	Frequent	Always

*Double Source

Total Score

14 FALL RISK ASSESSMENT SCALE

IF >15 IMPLEMENT "FALLS RISK MGT. PROTOCOL"

PARAMETERS	RISK POINTS	SCORE
Confused, disoriented, hallucinating	15	0
Recent hx of syncope/seizure disorder	15	0
Recent hx of falls	15	0
Unstable gait/balance	15	4
Use of orthopedic devices (walker, cane, crutches)	10	0
Post-op condition or sedated	10	0
Drug or alcohol withdrawal	10	0
Postural hypotension	10	0
Poor eyesight - hearing	5	4
Mental/Physical changes due to medications: cardiac, antihypertensives	5	0
Age 70 or older	5	0
Uncooperative attitude (resistant, belligerent, conbative)	5	0
Urinary – bowel frequency or incontinence	5	0

Total Score 8

15 R.N. VALIDATION

The RN assigned to the patient has determined that based on this admitting information, the following Standards are appropriate for this Pt. at this time:

A. Standard of Care: ______

B. Associated protocols: Pain

C. Additional protocols: ______

The Standards chosen for this patient's care have been briefly reviewed with the patient/SO for understanding/participation.

The RN assigned to the patient has seen the patient and reviewed the completed NDB to validate that the information is accurate and complete.

Tisha Fleming RN 1-2-95 1000

Signature Date Time

Fig. 5-4, cont'd Initial nursing assessment. (Courtesy Wilson N. Jones Memorial Hospital, Sherman, Texas.)

Continued.

NURSING DISCHARGE SUMMARY

16 SOCIAL SERVICES

☐ REFERRED TO SOCIAL SERVICES ☒ NO ONGOING NEEDS; NO NEED FOR REFERRAL ☐ OTHER ______

17 DISCHARGE STATUS

VITAL SIGNS	TEMP	PULSE	RESP	BLOOD PRESS.	TRANSPORTATION
	98²	76	16	128/78	☐ OTHER ☒ CAR ☐ AMBULANCE

MOBILITY & FUNCTIONING

MOBILITY	WITHOUT HELP	USES A DEVICE	HELP OF ANOTHER	DEVICE & HELP	DONE BY OTHERS	IS NOT DONE
WALKING	✓					
WHEELING						✓
STAIR CLIMBING	✓					
GOES OUTSIDE	✓					CONFINED TO: BD/CHR BED

XINCLUDES DRESSINGS, APPLIANCES, CRUTCHES, PACEMAKER, ETC.

ADL	WITHOUT HELP	USES A DEVICE	HELP OF ANOTHER	DEVICE & HELP	DONE BY OTHERS	IS NOT DONE
BATHING	✓					
DRESSING	✓					
TOILETING	✓					
TRANSFERRING	✓					
EATING/FEEDING	✓					

PLEASE MARK AREA OF INTEREST

R L   L R

SKIN CONDITION: ☐ REDDENED ☐ INTACT ☐ OPERATIVE SITE ☐ DECUBITUS

DESCRIBE: warm ē dry ē smooth skin. No pressure sores.

ELIMINATION

BOWEL FUNCTION	☒ CONTINENT ☐ OSTOMY	☐ INCONTINENT FREQ.: SELF-CARE: Y N
BLADDER FUNCTION	☒ CONTINENT ☐ CATHETER	☐ INCONTINENT FREQ.: ☐ EXTERNAL DEVICE ☐ OSTOMY SELF-CARE: (Y)/ N

MENTAL

ORIENTED: (Y)/ N — IF NO, DISORIENTED TO: ☐ TIME ☐ PLACE ☐ PERSON — AWARE OF SURROUNDINGS AND REACTS TO ENVIRONMENTAL STIMULI? (Y)/ N — IF NO, CHECK IF RESPONSIVE TO: STIMULUS – ☒ VISUAL ☒ AUDITORY ☒ TACTILE ☒ PAINFUL ☐ TOTALLY UNRESPONSIVE

BEHAVIOR APPROPRIATE (Y)/ N — IF NO, DESCRIBE BEHAVIOR EXHIBITED:

18 DISPOSITION

DISCHARGE DATE: 1-2-95 TIME: 1040 ☒ HOME ☐ SUPERVISED LIVING

☐ CONVALESCENT/NURSING HOME ☐ HOSPITAL ☐ AMA

PHYSICIAN NAME: TO FOLLOW Pierce M.D. — BODY TO FUNERAL HOME TIME

☐ EXPIRED TIME: A.M. P.M. PRONOUNCED BY: M.D. AT: — NAME OF FUNERAL HOME

19 DISCHARGE STATUS

1015 3 medication prescriptions given. No restrictions on diet. No activity restrictions. Given written appt. for follow up visit ē Dr. Pierce. Color pink. Ambulatory. Denies chest pain. Alert. Vital Signs stable.

SIGNATURE – NURSE: M. White, LVN DATE: current

Fig. 5-4, cont'd Initial nursing assessment. (Courtesy Wilson N. Jones Memorial Hospital, Sherman, Texas.)

18. *Patient responses:* Response to treatments, medications, pain relief, nursing interventions, and patient's refusal to take medication or to allow procedure to be performed

The medical history contains the health history and initial physical and mental assessment of the patient. It also includes the diagnosis and plan of action for the illness or disorder. This form is usually dictated by the physician admitting the patient.

The medical order form contains all medical orders written by the physician. Any physician participating in the care of a patient may write medical orders on this form.

Progress notes are usually written by the physician to record observations, plans for continuation or change of therapy approach, and the patient's condition and progress during hospitalization. Other health team members may also record their progress notes on the same form according to agency policy and procedure. The nursing staff may use their own progress notes.

The graphic form (or just "graphic") is used to record vital signs, weight, bowel movements, voidings, and other pertinent information from repeated assessments or measurements. The form is a type of flow sheet. Many hospitals use this form as a checklist for all types of care administered to the patient. Some facilities use only the graphic sheet for both nurses' notes and statistical data, whereas others use it with the narrative nurses' notes.

A flow sheet is used for routine assessments, observations, medications, treatments, and specific measurements of nursing activities. These forms may include a diabetic form, intake and output form, preoperative and postoperative records, tube feedings form, and intravenous fluid form. Some facilities may include this form as a separate sheet or as part of the graphic form (Fig. 5-5).

Nurses' progress notes are the nursing documentation of assessments, observations, interventions, and the patient's responses. The notes are recorded as the agency policy indicates.

A medication profile is used to document all medications administered to the patient. It includes the name of the medication, dose, time, date, and signature of the nurse administering the medication. Some facilities use this type of form for routine medications, one-time orders, and medications ordered as needed. As-needed medications may also be recorded in the nurses' progress notes according to agency policy and procedure.

The health-related discipline records include entries from consulting health team members about their contributions to the patient's nursing care. Some of the disciplines using a special form are respiratory therapy, physical therapy, nutrition or dietary specialties, radiology, social services, and clinical laboratories. In some agencies, these records may appear in separate sections of the medical record.

A discharge summary and planning form includes information about the patient's health status, prognosis, follow-up care, and rehabilitative measures and instructions, as well as the patient's understanding of instructions at the time of discharge.

Special forms may include informed consent forms and living wills. The nurse should be familiar with all special forms that may be used for patients.

The **Kardex** is a card filing system that is usually kept in a portable index file holder, in a notebook at the nurse's station, or on a computer. The system provides for quick reference of information about a patient without having to spend time searching through the medical record. The Kardex is used by the nurse as a means of communicating the current daily activities ordered for the patient. It also serves as a source of patient information for the nurse when giving the patient report at the change of shift.

In most facilities, the Kardex is usually not part of the patient's medical record and is not a legal document. Therefore entries are made in pencil. If the policy of an agency requires the Kardex to be kept, it may be placed in the patient's record or stored.

Organization of the medical record

The order in which forms are placed in a medical record varies in each agency. The traditional order of placement is found in the box.

REPORTING

Reporting is the transfer of information from the nurses on one shift to the nurses on the following

ORDER OF FORMS IN PATIENT'S MEDICAL RECORD

- Admission form
- Medical order form
- Progress notes
- History and physical examination forms
- Graphic
- Flow sheet
- Nurses' notes
- Medication profile
- Health-related disciplinary forms
- Discharge summary

ASSESSMENT FLOW SHEET

DATE: 1-2 SHIFT: 7-3

ASSESSMENT COMPLETED — TIME	7	8	9	10	11	12	13	14	15	16	17	18	19	20	21	22	23	24	1	2	3	4	5	6
INITIALS		GK																						
NEUROLOGICAL	7	8	9	10	11	12	13	14	15	16	17	18	19	20	21	22	23	24	1	2	3	4	5	6
A. Gen LOC	Alert, Drowsy, Stupor, Coma, Oriented, Disoriented, PEARL, Lethargic																							
	Confused, Answers: appropriate, inappropriate																							
B. Speech	Normal, Slurred																							
CARDIOVASCULAR	7	8	9	10	11	12	13	14	15	16	17	18	19	20	21	22	23	24	1	2	3	4	5	6
A. Pulses	Present, Absent (describe), Regular, Irregular																							
B. Extremities	Warm, Cool, Edematous, Cyanosis, Clubbing																							
C. Pacemaker/Tele	None, Monitor showing:																							
RESPIRATORY	7	8	9	10	11	12	13	14	15	16	17	18	19	20	21	22	23	24	1	2	3	4	5	6
A. Breath pattern	Regular, Nonlabored, Labored, Tachypnea, Cheyne-Stokes, Kussmall																							
B. Lung sounds	Clear, Crackles, Rhonchi, Wheezing, Location: ______																							
C. Chest Contour	Normal, Barrel																							
D. Cough	No, Productive, Nonproductive																							
E. Sputum	Clear, Yellow, Green, Frothy, Bloody, Amt: ______																							
GASTROINTESTINAL	7	8	9	10	11	12	13	14	15	16	17	18	19	20	21	22	23	24	1	2	3	4	5	6
A. Abdomen	Soft, Firm, Nontender, Tender, Distended																							
B. Stool	Last BM: (date) current, Brown, Black, Green, Yellow, Mucus																							
	Consistency: Soft formed, Frequency: daily																							
C. Bowel Sounds	Active, Hypoactive, Hyperactive, Absent, Quadrant: URQ, ULQ, LLQ, RLQ, ALL																							
D. Diet	Breakfast 90 % Lunch % Dinner % HS SNACK %																							
GENITOURINARY	7	8	9	10	11	12	13	14	15	16	17	18	19	20	21	22	23	24	1	2	3	4	5	6
A. Urine Char.	Continent, Incontinent, Clear, Yellow, Amber, Bloody, Voiding adequately																							
B. Catheter	Foley, Suprapubic, Urostomy, Other: (list)																							
INTEGUMENTARY	7	8	9	10	11	12	13	14	15	16	17	18	19	20	21	22	23	24	1	2	3	4	5	6
A. Skin	Jaundice, Dry, Diaphoretic, Turgor: elastic																							
B. Decubitus	NONE, Stage I, II, III, IV Location: ______																							
C. Description	Width: ______ cm., Length: ______ cm., Depth: ______ cm.																							
D. Special bed/pads	Eggcrate, Kinair bed, Fluid-air bed, Maxifloat mattress, Resque bed																							
E. Preventive Care	Heel/elbow protectors, Massage to pressure points, Pillows to position																							
F. ET consulting	Yes No Date: ______ Time: ______																							
G. IV	Infusing via Pump: YES NO																							
	Site: top (R) hand, Red, Hard, Sore, Swollen, Patent, Saline lock																							
H. Wound/Dressings	NONE, Site: ______, Drainage: NO, YES (describe); Appearance: (describe)																							
I. Drains	NONE, JP, Hemovac, Penrose, T-tube, Drainage: NO, YES (describe) ______ CC																							
PSYCHOLOGIC	7	8	9	10	11	12	13	14	15	16	17	18	19	20	21	22	23	24	1	2	3	4	5	6
A. Behavior	Relaxed, Restless, Angry, Elated, Depressed, Indifferent																							
B. Pain	Denies pain, c/o pain, Location: ______, Scale: 1, 2, 3, 4, 5, 6, 7, 8, 9, 10																							
MUSCULOSKELETAL	7	8	9	10	11	12	13	14	15	16	17	18	19	20	21	22	23	24	1	2	3	4	5	6
A. ROM	Paralysis: NO YES (describe) Partial Paralysis: NO YES (describe)																							
B. Gait	Steady, Unsteady, Requires assistance with ambulation/transfers																							
ADLs	7	8	9	10	11	12	13	14	15	16	17	18	19	20	21	22	23	24	1	2	3	4	5	6
A. Self-care	Baths self: NO, YES, WITH ASSIST; Feeds self: NO, YES, WITH ASSIST																							

Fig. 5-5 Assessment flow sheet. (Courtesy Wilson N. Jones Memorial Hospital, Sherman, Texas.)

NURSING PROGRESS RECORD		
Date	Time	
1-2	1120	3+ dependent edema both lower legs. Dyspnea ē
		fearful. Dr. Grant notified. — J. Gross, LVN

ADDRESSOGRAPH	NURSE'S INITIALS/SIGNATURE AND TITLE	
	M. White	LVN
	J. Gross	LVN
	SNF • MED/SURG • TELEMETRY • ONCOLOGY	

Fig. 5-5, cont'd Assessment flow sheet. (Courtesy Wilson N. Jones Memorial Hospital, Sherman, Texas.)

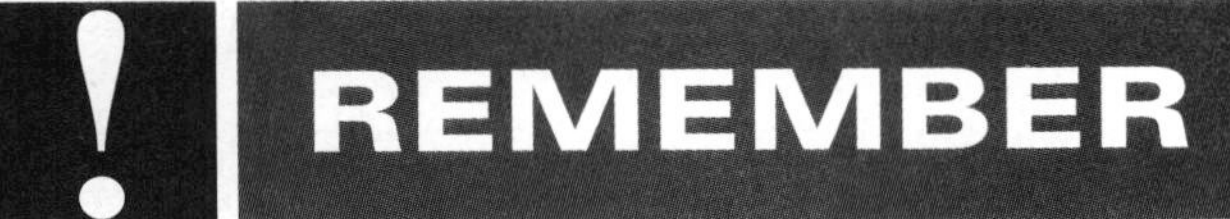

- Before reporting, nurses should make certain that they have all information that will be needed to give a complete description of the patient's condition or problem.

shift or from nurses to other members of the health care team. Reporting provides continuity of nursing care. The report occurs usually at 0700, 1500, and 2300. There are four occasions when reporting is necessary. These are:

1. Shift change
2. Telephoning a report regarding the patient's condition
3. Any sudden change or emergency situations needing immediate reporting
4. Nurse or students leaving the assigned area at different times

The nurse reporting for duty receives a report from the nurse going off duty. This type of report is usually given orally or by audiotape. Information about patient's status is given to the oncoming nurse before the shift is begun. The oral means of reporting seems to be preferred by many nurses because this permits immediate questions or verification. The audiotape saves time and may be heard repeatedly if verification or clarification is necessary. This method of reporting provides only one-way communication and no opportunity for feedback unless the nurse who made the recording is notified. An agency using this method may require the nurse going off duty to remain for questions about the audiotape report or be available for a certain period of time after leaving the agency.

Reports may be given in a designated area such as a conference room or the nurses' station. Some agencies use the "walking rounds" report. This type report is carried out as nurses from both shifts make rounds together, visiting each patient and discussing the patient's condition. This allows the patient to be involved and to meet the nurse coming on duty. A disadvantage of this type of report is that it may be time consuming.

Information to report

For a report to be successful it should be organized, concise, and efficient. The usual sequence of reporting is by order of room numbers or areas of

APIE DOCUMENTATION (SOAPIE)		
Date	Time	Progress Notes
Current	1000	S- States has moderate pain in RUQ.
		O- Guarding abd. incision RUQ ē depicting
		facial grimace.
		A- Pain related to surgical intervention.
	1010	P- Pain medication.
		I- Demerol 75 mg. c̄ Vistaril 50 mg.
		given IM Z-tract in Ⓛ ventrogluteal
		region.
	1050	E- States has pain relief. M. White, LVN

Fig. 5-6 APIE documentation.

patient care. The order may vary, but the following basic information is typical for an oral report:

1. Room number, patient's name, age, gender, and hospital day and postoperative day
2. Attending physician's name
3. Medical diagnosis
4. General physiologic and psychologic description
5. New orders concerning therapies or medications
6. Scheduled diagnostics procedures or special therapies (for example, surgery, chemotherapy)
7. Dietary modifications and fluid orders
8. Activities allowed
9. Patient's responses to therapies, nursing actions, or special medications or intravenous treatments
10. Instructions given to the patient or family regarding any procedures or treatments for home care.
11. Pertinent information regarding family members
12. Nursing diagnosis problems or recent changes in the patient's health status

Other information to document includes the following:

1. Safety restraints, dressings, or tubings inserted
2. Instructions to the patient and family
3. Visits made by the attending physician, consultant, or other health care personnel in relation to the special needs of the patient
4. Times when a patient must be absent from the room to go to other departments for special treatments or diagnostic studies
5. Patient transfer to another room or facility or patient discharged
6. Description of impending death and emergency measures taken, including significant others present or notified, any visits by a minister or chaplain, and the time the physician pronounced death

Telephone Reporting

A report given using the telephone is usually brief and concise. This report usually refers to only one patient. The nurse identifies the self by name and position and states the reason for calling:

> "This is Ms. Good Nurse, nurse on unit 3 West. I would like to report to Dr. Right about his patient, Mr. Dire, in room 3601."

When the physician responds to the call, the nurse should be prepared with all necessary information. When the nurse has related the information, the physician may give medical orders to the nurse. When orders must be taken over the telephone, the nurse repeats and verifies the orders.

Student Reporting

When a student is in the clinical setting, the assigned patient is the student's responsibility according to the accepted "mastery of clinical objectives." The staff nurse and clinical instructor also have a responsibility to the patient. Whatever the circumstances, the student nurse should always report to a designated nurse when going onto or leaving the unit. When the student leaves before a shift is finished, someone will need to know what has occurred while the student cared for the patient and what is still to be done for the rest of the shift. Giving a detailed but concise and pertinent report about nursing care and the responses of the patient is the responsibility of the student.

TECHNOLOGY AND DOCUMENTATION

The use of computers is increasing in health care facilities, and many institutions are encouraging the use of computers in nursing documentation. Formats vary and may be entered with manual keyboards, with electronic checklists with light pens, or using other equipment and programs. Terminals may be centrally located at the nurses' station or at the bedside. Small terminals may be hand carried or worn on the nurse's wrist. Computer technology helps reduce the time that the nurse must spend performing clerical duties.

Routine data and information are placed in the computer for quick reference. Some of the data that can be computerized are routine standing medical orders, flow sheets containing routine medications, nursing procedures or daily informational data, lists containing supplies and available equipment or equipment needing to be ordered, procedures for requisitioning supplies, orders for diagnostic tests, standard nursing forms such as care plans, policies and procedures, educational information, and hospital formulary and other pharmaceutical information helpful in maintaining a current knowledge of medications.

In the future, computer-generated data may help clarify the patient's nursing care and progress, improve reimbursement, and increase job satisfaction. Because of the wide use of computers, many schools of nursing are offering a computer-assisted instruction (CAI) program as part of the curriculum. The computer is also being used with the Board of Nursing licensing examination, and computers will undoubtedly be used in even more ways in the future.

Fax machines are becoming widely used in health care facilities. This technology allows the nurse to receive and send patient records, documentation forms, medication orders, and medical orders from their offices (eliminating need for telephone medical orders). Laboratory and test results may be faxed for immediate interpretation by the physician.

SUMMARY

Communication takes many forms. The nurse uses verbal communication to relay information to the patient, the family, and other members of the health care team. Verbal (written) communication includes documenting and reporting the changing circumstances of the patient. The use of nonverbal gestures assists the receiver and sender to interpret perceptions of, and responses to, the message. Communication is essential among nurses and members of the health care team for developing and improving professional standards and performance evaluations, coordinating patient care, and educating new professionals. Communication must be accurate, explicit, and supportive to improve nursing care.

Key Concepts

- Communication is any process in which a message is transferred from one person to another.
- Communication is anything perceived by our senses.
- Communication consists of five basic aspects: sender, message, receiver, environment, and feedback.
- People communicate one to one by verbal and nonverbal communication techniques.
- Verbal communication is the interchange of information using spoken or written words.
- Nonverbal communication is the interchange of information without the use of words.
- Communication is a vital skill that the nurse needs to function.
- Self-knowledge and understanding is the first step of effective communication and human relations.
- Therapeutic communication techniques assist the health care professional in acquiring detailed information from the patient and allows the patient to select data to be revealed.
- Written communication is a form of verbal communication because words are used to exchange information.
- It is the nurse's responsibility to document the

steps of the nursing process in the patient's medical record.

- Documentation is a means of accurately describing a patient's quality of nursing care.
- The medical record is a legal document.
- Various documentation formats may be used to communicate the same information.

Critical Thinking Questions

1. Develop examples of closed and open questions on a similar subject. Practice using them on a classmate and compare the information you gather.
2. Walter is a 34-year-old man brought to the emergency room with complaints of crushing chest pain, shortness of breath, and exercise intolerance. His wife is at his side, in tears, moaning that "He's dying." What elements of the communication process are needed to develop a helping relationship with Walter and his wife?
3. After administering all of a patient's medications you are informed by another nurse that they were already given 30 minutes before but not charted. What actions are indicated? What actions could prevent future occurrences?
4. Locate a chart on a nursing division and find six examples of nursing documentation that follow guidelines for accuracy and currentness.
5. Describe criteria to use in charting patient education, including subjective and objective data about a patient and evaluation of responses.

REFERENCES AND SUGGESTED READINGS

Arnold E, Boggs KU: *Interpersonal relationships: professional communication skills for nurses,* ed 2, Philadelphia, 1995, Saunders.

DeWit SC: *Rambo's nursing skills for clinical practice,* Philadelphia, 1994, Saunders.

Linton AD, Matteson MA, Maebius NK: *Introductory nursing care of adults,* Philadelphia, 1995, Saunders.

Potter PA, Perry AG: *Basic nursing: theory and practice,* ed 3, St Louis, 1995, Mosby.

Potter PA, Perry AG: *Fundamentals of nursing: concepts, process, and practice,* St Louis, 1993, Mosby.

Sundeen SJ et al: *Nurse-client interaction: implementing the nursing process,* ed 5, St Louis, 1995, Mosby.

CHAPTER 6

Patient Teaching

Learning Objectives

After studying this chapter, the student should be able to . . .

- Define the key terms.
- Describe formal and informal teaching.
- Identify three purposes for performing patient teaching.
- Practice the principles for effective teaching.
- Use the principles of effective teaching.
- Identify special considerations for teaching and learning based on developmental and physical capabilities.
- Describe the three types of learning: cognitive, affective, and psychomotor.
- Compare and describe the similarities of the teaching process and the nursing process.

Key Terms

Affective learning	Patient teaching
Cognitive learning	Psychomotor learning
Consumer	Teaching
Learning	

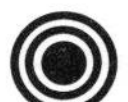 Skill

6-1 Patient Teaching

Patient teaching has always been a role of the nurse. However, teaching is emerging as one of the most vital responsibilities of the nurse. Shorter hospital stays require that the patient or family be able to continue prescribed care at home during convalescence. More people are living longer, and more people have a chance of acquiring a chronic disease. Chronic disease may require changes in lifestyle, especially diet and activity. Patient teaching is necessary to ensure continuity of care and to assist the patient in making lifestyle changes.

PATIENT

Society's view of the patient has changed. No longer is the patient a passive recipient of nursing care. The patient is now a **consumer** in the health care system. As a consumer the patient must make personal decisions based on accurate information and must accept some of the responsibility for personal and family health care. Considering these new views of the patient, the role of the nurse in patient teaching is more important related to legal issues now than ever before. Appropriate instruction on how to continue nursing care after hospital discharge allows the patient to continue therapy and to participate in the recovery process—perhaps preventing rehospitalization for the same condition. Also, patient and family teaching may reduce health care costs by providing information about how to remain healthy and how to recognize danger signs to report to the physician. The trend in health care is for the patient to take responsibility for staying healthy (wellness) instead of waiting until becoming ill and needing treatment. With teaching, people may be more independent and more in control of their lives.

GUIDELINES FOR PATIENT TEACHING

Some accrediting agencies have guidelines for health care facilities for providing patient teaching. These guidelines help ensure that patients and families have the necessary information to maintain the highest level of wellness. The Joint Commission on the Accreditation of Healthcare Organizations (JCAHO) has set two standards regarding patient teaching:

1. Education and knowledge of self-care are given special consideration for the patient and family in the nursing care plan.
2. As appropriate, patients who leave the hospital requiring more nursing care receive instructions and individual counseling before discharge. In fact, patient teaching should begin at admission and continue until discharge.

TEACHING AND LEARNING

Teaching and **learning** cannot be separated. While one person teaches, another learns. Teaching is effective when it meets the specific needs of the learner. The teacher facilitates learning by identifying those needs with the help of the learner. Communication of the information to meet those needs should change based on feedback from the learner. The learner has a responsibility to actively participate in the teaching-learning process.

Teaching may be formal or informal. A formal situation is planned and presented at a specific time and place. Many hospitals have formal classes for groups of patients with the same learning needs. For example, prospective parents need information about pregnancy, labor, delivery, and infant care. Cardiac (heart) patients need information about diet and exercise. A patient newly diagnosed with diabetes mellitus must learn to administer insulin, maintain the appropriate diet, and perform required exercise to follow the regimen ordered by the physician. Practical/vocational nurses may be responsible for teaching within their scope of knowledge or may reinforce information taught by the registered nurse. In many areas the registered nurse is responsible for the plan of teaching.

Informal teaching usually takes place spontaneously. Almost every nurse-patient interaction has the potential for informal teaching. The nurse should take advantage of every opportunity to help the patient learn. Most informal teaching occurs in response to questions asked by the patient or family and during nursing care as the nurse becomes aware of the need for teaching. Teaching often occurs from tactfully correcting inappropriate health habits.

The nurse must know the answer before responding to a question. The nurse must also know what the physician has told the patient. The nurse should not be fearful of saying, "I am not certain but I will try to find out for you" or "I will find someone who can answer your question." The patient will be grateful for this honesty. The nurse should also follow through by finding out the answer and appropriately communicating it to the patient or making certain the person who can help is obtained. If someone else is requested to respond, the nurse should follow up with the patient to ensure that the patient understands the information.

PURPOSES OF PATIENT TEACHING

Patient teaching is important for promoting health or preventing illness, restoring health, and helping the patient cope with impaired function or terminal illness. Society has become more health conscious as evidenced by the number of health or exercise clubs, nutrition centers, and health-screening programs sponsored by organizations. Employers often provide classes aimed at health promotion and illness prevention. Health care agencies offer classes on a variety of topics such as first aid, cardiopulmonary resuscitation, prenatal care, immunizations, nutrition, exercise, and parenting. These classes are generally open to the community. Some classes are free, whereas others require a nominal fee. The impact of these classes may be widespread because the information is often implemented by the participant's entire family and may be shared with others.

When the restoration of health is the purpose of patient teaching the topics generally include the cause of the disease or condition, the way that the body is affected, the prognosis, the reasons for the various treatments, the duration of care, patient participation in care, and the possible limitations to which the patient must adapt. Patients are not always interested in learning about their conditions and treatments. This may occur when the patient denies the reality of the diagnosed disease or condition. The nurse must be aware of the patient's and family's readiness for learning.

The nurse should include the family or significant others in the teaching plan so that everyone understands what is necessary for the patient to return to health. Conflicts between the patient and family may develop if both have not been taught what to expect or what to do for the patient. For example, it takes time for a patient who has a colostomy to be able to accept having a bowel movement through an opening outside the abdomen and learning care for the colostomy. A family member must be taught the care for a colostomy in case the patient cannot perform this routine.

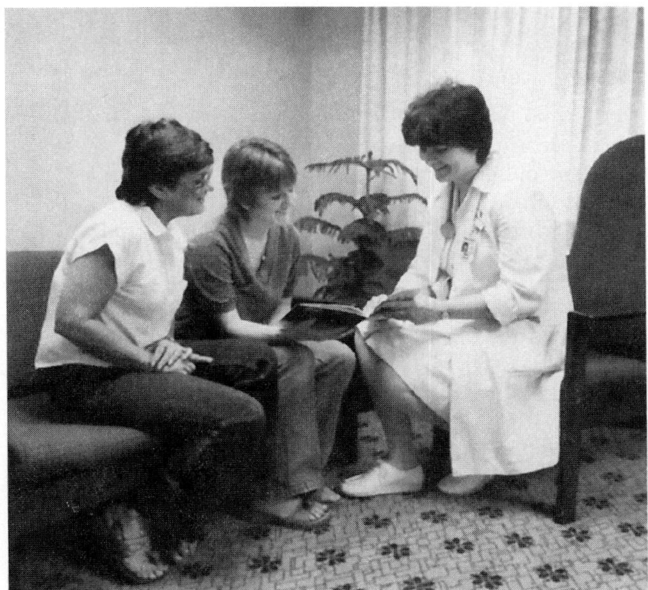

Fig. 6-1 Choosing a comfortable, pleasant environment enhances the learning experience. This nurse is using a teaching booklet to explain health care principles to the patient and a family member.

Teaching is also necessary to help patients cope with or adapt to permanent changes in health (Fig. 6-1). Everyone does not make a complete recovery from illness or injury. Some must be taught how to cope with a terminal illness. Patients often need to be taught to perform activities of daily living while dealing with the impaired functioning resulting from the injury or illness. Depending on the seriousness of the disability, the patient's role may change within the family unit. Teaching should begin as soon as the need is determined and the patient and family members are willing to learn. The nurse should be certain that the appropriate people are being taught.

NURSING PROCESS IN TEACHING

The teaching process and the nursing process are very similar. First, the assessment is made, goals (expected outcomes) are set, the plan is written, and an evaluation of the plan is performed (Table 6-1). Teaching is often part of the plan and interventions (implementation of the plan) in the nursing process.

The nurse begins the teaching process by assessing the patient's need for learning. Nursing diagnoses are identified based on the assessment. Specific nursing diagnoses help the nurse identify patient goals and the appropriate nursing interventions to assist the patient in attaining the goals.

Table 6-1 NURSING AND TEACHING PROCESSES

Nursing Process	Teaching Process
Assessment	
Determine care needs.	Determine teaching needs.
Goals	
Determine how patient's condition should change.	Determine what patient should learn.
Planning	
Decide what care is to be performed, when, and by whom.	Decide how teaching is to be accomplished.
Implementation	
Give care.	Perform teaching.
Evaluation	
Evaluate whether patient's condition has changed as planned.	Evaluate whether planned learning occurred.

Nursing interventions related to patient teaching include assessing the ability of the patient to learn and the ability of the nurse to teach. The effectiveness of teaching is evaluated after nursing interventions are completed. The sample nursing care plan on p. 77 shows how to plan, implement, and evaluate teaching for a specific patient.

Assessment

Several areas must be assessed for teaching to be the most effective.

Need for teaching

The patient must accept the reality of the disease or injury before learning can occur. Even if the nurse sees a need for patient teaching or the physician requests that teaching be performed, the patient may not be receptive to the new information. Assessment of this acceptance and the desire to learn are necessary before teaching is initiated. Teaching is begun when the patient or family asks a question or when the nurse identifies the need for learning. Sometimes the physician may write a medical order for specific teaching.

Disease process or injury

Consideration of the disease process or injury should guide the information taught. Teaching how the body works and how it has changed will aid the patient in understanding any needed lifestyle changes. Once patients understand what has changed about their bodies, they are generally more receptive to tests, treatments, medications, or the ways in which surgery will help.

Patient's ability to learn

For teaching to be successful, the learner's developmental ability to learn must be assessed. It would be inappropriate to give a 4-year-old child or an illiterate person a booklet to read. The nurse should assess the patient's base knowledge and build on it. Generally, age reflects the developmental capability for learning. Physical development and general physical health should also be considered.

Comfort for learning

The patient should be physically comfortable when teaching is performed. This allows the patient to focus on the teaching and not on physical discomfort. Any negative change in the patient's condition may be a reason to postpone teaching until the condition improves. The environment, such as room temperature, lighting, and noise level, should also be comfortable and not distracting.

Learning domains

Learning may take place in three different domains or areas: cognitive, affective, and psychomotor. **Cognitive learning** involves the acquisition and use of knowledge. Acquiring new or changing unhealthy attitudes, feelings, and values is **affective learning.** Learning to physically perform an act involves **psychomotor learning.** Teaching and learning may involve any one or all learning domains, depending on the topic. Many prenatal classes, for example, use all domains of learning. Information and facts are explained to the parents-to-be, leading to cognitive learning. Knowing the facts and information may change attitudes or feelings about the pregnancy and involves affective learning. Putting a diaper on a doll or holding a doll involves psychomotor learning. The patient's needs determine which learning domain is used.

Teacher's knowledge

The teacher should have a thorough knowledge and understanding of the material to be taught. Then the teacher may, with confidence, present the material in a logical sequence and readily answer questions. Knowledge of the learning process guides the teacher in planning a teaching session.

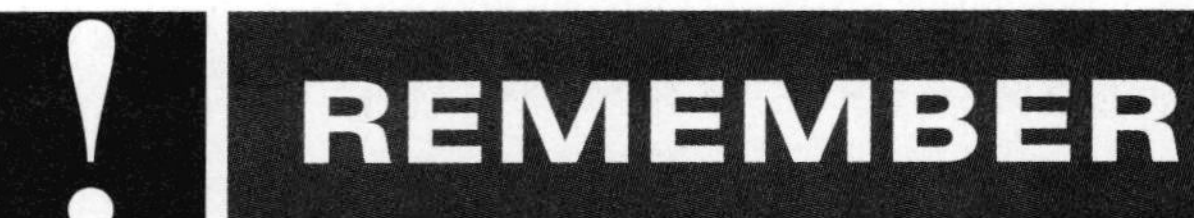

- Determine what the patient needs to know.
- Determine the best time and mood for patient learning.
- Assess the patient's self-confidence in regard to learning.

Nursing Diagnosis

The nurse interprets the information gathered during assessment to form diagnoses that reflect the patient's learning needs. This ensures that patient teaching is goal directed and individualized.

Some examples of nursing diagnoses related to learning needs include the following:

Knowledge deficit (affective) related to misunderstanding of prognosis

Knowledge deficit (psychomotor) related to inexperience with skill or lack of interest in learning

Impaired social interaction related to poor communication skills

Planning

When the patient's learning needs have been determined, the nurse and the patient work together in setting specific learning objectives. Each objective is a statement of a behavior that identifies the patient's ability to demonstrate learning. For instance, if a patient has a fractured leg, he or she will demonstrate the learned behavior by walking on crutches to the end of the hall.

The nurse must match teaching methods with the patient's learning needs and work with the patient to determine the most effective time to conduct a teaching session (see care plan on p. 77). For patients discharged early, home health nurses reinforce learning.

Implementation

Teaching techniques

Many teaching techniques may be used for patient teaching. For learning in the cognitive domain, pamphlets, videos, and discussions are useful. Placing the name of the patient on a pamphlet or underlining a phrase personalizes the information and enhances learning. Learning in the affective domain may be enhanced by using therapeutic communica-

TEACHING IN SPECIAL SITUATIONS

Blind
Identify self when approaching.
Use normal voice tone.
Make audiocassette of teaching session.
Guide patient's hand with nurse's.
Warn when touching patient.

Illiterate
Remember that these patients generally speak and understand very well.
Use discussion and visual methods.

Terminally Ill
Adapt teaching strategies to patient's abilities.
Focus on comfort, adapting, or coping.
Make sessions practical.

Hearing Impaired
Approach where patient can see nurse.
Use pamphlets, pictures, and videos.
Keep slate handy.
Face person when speaking.

Mute
Present information as best for topic.
Keep slate handy.
Watch nonverbal clues for frustration.

Another Culture and Language
Learn patient's values and beliefs.
Do not violate beliefs or values.
Use interpreter.

tion skills and role playing. Demonstration of a skill by the nurse and having the patient return the demonstration is one of the best ways to assist psychomotor learning.

The teacher should remember to praise the effort and success of the learner. The teacher's attitude affects all teaching techniques. Believing that patient education is an important part of nursing care is apparent in the the nurse's attitude. The nurse should show enthusiasm for teaching, be well prepared, and use appropriate techniques (Skill 6-1).

Teaching in special situations

Each teaching situation is unique. The teacher should competently prepare for each session. In some special situations, extra preparation or specific techniques should be used (for example, dealing with a blind patient, an illiterate patient, or a terminally ill patient) (see box). Any person involved in caring for the patient should also be involved in the teaching sessions. The teaching session should end with the learner giving a review of what was learned.

Teaching the patient who is blind

A person who is blind appreciates help from the nurse who is considerate in dealing with the problem and who treats the patient like everyone else except when help is necessary. When approaching a blind patient, nurses should identify themselves and explain what will be done for the patient. To prevent being startled, many blind people appreciate a touch on the hand or arm as the nurse begins to speak. The nurse should speak in a normal tone of voice, remembering that teaching will need to be performed verbally. The nurse may consider preparing a cassette tape of the session so it may be used later in patient teaching. The nurse should assist the patient in handling and exploring supplies or equipment. When teaching a skill, the nurse's hand should be placed over the patient's hand and the movements guided as necessary. It is important to explain that this will be done before touching the patient.

Teaching the patient who is hearing impaired

When speaking to the patient who is hearing impaired, the nurse must speak in a controlled, slightly slower, distinct tone of voice. A mistake often made with this patient is to speak in a high-pitched voice, almost shouting. This voice usually makes the patient nervous, and the patient usually cannot hear what is said. Printed materials, pictures, and videos are appropriate. A slate or paper and pencil should be kept on hand for suggestions and answers from the patient. If the person can read lips, the nurse should face the person and speak slowly and distinctly.

Teaching the patient who is illiterate

A person who cannot read is not necessarily below average in intelligence. The person may speak and understand very well. Discussion and visual methods of teaching may be used. The nurse may provide diagrams, pictures, videos, or cassette tapes for future review. The physician may be able to provide assistance in making arrangements to help the patient learn to read.

Teaching the patient who cannot speak

The teaching session should be presented in the manner best suited for the topic. A slate or paper and pencil should be made available for questions or comments. The paper should be placed on and the pencil affixed to a clipboard to prevent loss of an important means with which the patient can communicate. Nonverbal clues, especially facial expression, may indicate frustration or a lack of understanding or interest. Because this patient becomes frustrated at times, the nurse must be patient.

Teaching the patient with a terminal illness

Teaching strategies must be adapted to the abilities of the patient who is terminally ill. Strategy changes will be necessary as the condition of the patient changes. Most teaching focuses on comfort measures and ways of adapting to or coping with the increase in pain and the physical changes. The nurse should make certain that the patient is comfortable and as alert as possible before beginning a teaching session. All information should be practical and useful. The session should be stopped when the patient becomes tired.

Teaching the patient from another culture and who speaks another language

The nurse should learn as much as possible about different cultures, especially their values and beliefs (see Chapter 8). Teaching plans and strategies should be modified so that the patient's beliefs and cultural practices are not violated. If another language is involved, an interpreter may be used to make the patient less fearful and more cooperative regarding the nursing care administered. A two-language dictionary is very helpful, as are pictures, gestures, and other methods of nonverbal communication.

Teaching the child

Play may assist a child to learn about illness, procedures, and treatments. It may also help a child cope with the hospital experience, which often is one of the most frightening situations a child can encounter. The child may then be better able to communicate fears and concerns. After assessment of the child's developmental level and physical condition, appropriate play activities may be planned and implemented for use as teaching tools. Toys, games, and hospital equipment provide a nonthreatening way to introduce important information to the child. Opportunities may be provided to practice (role play) for future experiences. Word games or crossword puzzles may be created to assess the understanding of an older child.

Teaching the older adult

An older adult patient may be assisted by asking about concerns related to the illness and the nursing care required. The nurse may also learn about the lifestyle and usual activities of the patient. Many older adults accept and adapt to the gradual physical changes that occur with aging. Knowing how the patient has already adapted is important and may be used as a beginning point in teaching. Tips for teaching older adults are provided in the gerontologic box.

Hearing and eyesight tend to deteriorate with age but not in all aging patients. If the patient wears glasses, the nurse should make certain that they are on and are clean before beginning a teaching session. The nurse should ensure appropriate lighting and, if necessary, use large-print teaching aids. A cassette tape may be made of each session so that the patient can listen to the information several times for better understanding. Facing the patient helps the patient see the nurse's mouth. Many patients learn to lip read as hearing decreases. It is important for the nurse to speak slowly and clearly in a normal tone of voice.

Mental response time may slow in the older adult. The nurse needs to slow the pace of teaching and pause when necessary to assess patient comprehension. Sensitivity to the patient's feelings of frustration is important, especially if the nurse finds it necessary to repeat information several times. The nurse should present short teaching sessions and only one topic per session.

The nurse needs to assess the medications being administered to the patient. Some drugs may cause drowsiness. Teaching sessions should be scheduled when these medications are having the least effect. Other medications may cause visual disturbances. If these effects interfere with teaching, the problem should be reported to the physician. Patience is very important.

GERONTOLOGIC CONSIDERATIONS

- Information should be repeated frequently and should be based on the patient's previous level of learning.
- The nurse should allow more time for patients to express themselves, demonstrate learning, and ask questions.
- A slow presentation pace and the use of examples promote effective learning in the older adult.

The gradual loss of muscle strength and endurance and skeletal flexibility may cause difficulty in psychomotor learning. The problem is especially noticeable when tasks require fine motor skills. Sometimes patients have already adapted to these physical changes and may have suggestions on how the new skill may be performed. The nurse should listen to these suggestions.

Evaluation

The nurse evaluates success by observing the patient's performance of each expected behavior. Observation of patient behavior, role playing, use of questions, and discussions can be used to evaluate patients' knowledge. If a knowledge or skill deficit is indicated, the nurse may repeat or modify the teaching plan. Alternative teaching methods often help in clarifying information or strengthening skills the patient was originally unable to understand or perform.

■ NURSING CARE PLAN ■

KNOWLEDGE DEFICIT: SELF-INJECTION

Mrs. C, age 60, is to perform self-injection of insulin every morning after discharge from the hospital. She is anxious about performing the procedure.

NURSING DIAGNOSIS
Knowledge deficit related to self-injection as evidenced by her statement to the nurse.

GOAL
- Patient will self-administer insulin by 0830 today.

EXPECTED OUTCOME
- Patient will express confidence in self-administering insulin.

NURSING INTERVENTIONS
- Assess ability of patient to learn.
- Assess ability of nurse to teach.
- Determine the learning domains in which to teach required information.
- Teach self-injection of insulin.
- Supervise patient's self-administration of insulin.

EVALUATION
- Patient expresses confidence in self-administering insulin.

SKILL 6-1 PATIENT TEACHING

Steps	Rationale
1. Assess knowledge of material to be taught.	Identifies knowledge and ability of nurse to teach material.
2. Assess knowledge of patient regarding illness or condition, including health promotion and coping with impaired function.	Indicates what may or may not need to be taught.
3. Decide what information or skill needs to be taught.	Focuses on required information to be taught.
4. Assess patient readiness and ability to learn; acceptance of illness or condition; and language, visual and hearing acuity.	Allows for specific teaching plan to be developed.
5. Refer to medical record, care plan, or Kardex for special interventions.	Provides basis for teaching.
6. Obtain supplies and equipment: ▪ Materials related to teaching ▪ Clean gloves if needed ▪ Checklist for patient to review or for return demonstration	Organizes procedure.
7. Introduce self.	Decreases anxiety level.
8. Identify patient by identification band.	Identifies correct patient for procedure.
9. Explain procedure to be taught.	Seeks cooperation and decreases anxiety.
10. Wash hands and don clean gloves according to agency policy and guidelines from Centers for Disease Control and Prevention and Occupational Safety and Health Administration.	Helps prevent cross-contamination.
11. Prepare patient for intervention:	
a. Close door to room or pull curtain.	Provides privacy.
b. Drape patient for procedure if necessary.	Prevents exposure of patient.
12. Raise bed to comfortable working level.	Provides safety for nurse.
13. Arrange for patient privacy.	Shows respect for patient.
14. Implement teaching plan.	Helps patient begin learning process to meet need for learning.
15. Praise efforts and success of patient.	Increases patient's confidence and self-esteem.
16. End session with patient review of what was learned.	Increases retention of material learned.
17. Remove gloves and wash hands.	Helps prevent cross-contamination.
18. Document.	Documents procedure and patient's response.

SUMMARY

Patient teaching is necessary for continuity of hospital nursing care and for care after discharge. The patient's need for teaching and ability to learn should be assessed before teaching.

The nurse should also assess personal knowledge while preparing to teach.

Teaching children or older adults requires special techniques.

Key Concepts

- The teaching process is similar to the nursing process.
- Learning is effected by cognitive, affective, and psychomotor domains.
- Each session should end with the learner reviewing what was learned.
- The teacher should remember to praise the efforts and success of the learner.
- When the primary nursing caregiver is someone other than the patient, that person should be involved in the teaching sessions.
- Play is often used when teaching children.
- The nurse must listen to suggestions offered by the patient.

Critical Thinking Questions

1. Mr. Garcia is a 70-year-old man with a neurogenic bladder requiring self-catheterization. His vision is poor. He lives alone and is accustomed to being very independent. He has been shown the technique of self-catheterization. Identify a nursing diagnosis and one goal, and describe your approach to teaching this patient.
2. You are teaching a recently diagnosed 15-year-old diabetic about his diet when he says "I'm going to eat whatever I want. It doesn't matter anyway, since I have to take this insulin stuff." Regarding this situation, determine what value conflicts may be present, discuss this patient's moral/value developmental needs, and suggest how this nurse may demonstrate accountability and responsibility.
3. Joey Carter is a 6-year-old boy who was recently hospitalized for bronchial asthma. This was his first admission and initial diagnosis of asthma. He is being sent home, inhaled and nebulized bronchodilators have been prescribed, and he is to return to the clinic in 1 week. Design teaching plans for Joey and his parents.
4. Mrs. Jones, 38 years old, is scheduled for a breast biopsy. Her mother and sister have a history of breast cancer. They are both currently in remission and are in their sixth and seventh year after the initial diagnoses. Mrs. Jones has never had surgery. She is nervous and "scared of the diagnosis." List your teaching priorities for this patient.
5. Before your patient with a full-leg cast can go home, he or she must be taught to ambulate with crutches and a three-point gait. Develop a teaching plan for your patient.

REFERENCES AND SUGGESTED READINGS

Barnes L: Don't forget to play! *Maternal and Child Nursing* 17(4):183, 1992.

Barnes L: The illiterate client: strategies in patient teaching, *Maternal and Child Nursing* 17(3):127, 1992.

Cochrane K et al: Do they really understand us? *American Journal of Nursing* 92(7):19, 1992.

deWit S: *Rambo's nursing skills for clinical practice,* ed 4, Philadelphia, 1994, Saunders.

Earnest V: *Clinical skills in nursing practice,* ed 2, Philadelphia, 1993, Lippincott.

Joint Commission on the Accreditation of Healthcare Organizations: *Accreditation manual,* Chicago, 1994, The Commission.

Roe C: The muddy waters of clinical teaching, *American Journal of Nursing* 92(7):20, 1992.

Rousseau P: A painful lack of patient education, *Patient Care* 26:32, 1992.

Stewart K, Walton R: Teaching the elderly, *Nursing* 22(10):66, 1992.

Yawn B: Thinking patient education, *Patient Care* 26:37, 1992.

CHAPTER 7

Admission, Transfer, and Discharge

Learning Objectives

After studying this chapter, the student should be able to . . .

- Define the key terms.
- Identify principles for the admission, transfer, and discharge of a patient.
- Describe common patient reactions to hospitalization.
- Identify ways in which the nurse may respond to patient reactions to hospitalization.
- Identify the responsibilities of the nurse in admitting, transferring, and discharging a patient.
- Describe how to prepare a room for the admission of a patient to the hospital.
- Describe how the nurse prepares a patient for transfer to another unit or to another facility.
- Describe how the nurse prepares a patient for discharge, including teaching, from the hospital.
- Identify the role of the nurse when a patient chooses to leave the hospital against medical advice.

Key Terms

Admission
Against medical advice (AMA)
Consumer
Continuity of care
Discharge
Discharge planning
Empathy
Interagency transfer
Intraagency transfer
Orientation
Separation anxiety
Transfer

Skills

7-1 Admitting a Patient
7-2 Transferring a Patient
7-3 Discharging a Patient

Generally, accepted nursing interventions (procedures) are followed when a person enters or leaves a health care facility. These interventions are identified and explained in this chapter. The nurse should consider the following factors involving admission, transfer, and discharge:

1. The patient should be viewed as a **consumer** (user) in the health care system and as a human being who deserves to be treated with dignity, courtesy, and respect.
2. The patient's first impression after being admitted to the hospital usually persists for the entire hospitalization.
3. The attitude of the nurse may form the basis for the patient's feelings about nursing care received.
4. Coordination is the key to efficient and safe transfer.
5. Plans for discharge are started on the day of admission.

Admission to a hospital or another health care agency is an anxious time for most patients and families. The patient is usually very concerned about health problems or high-risk problems and the outcome of treatment. The patient often experiences pain or other discomfort. The patient's first contact with nurses and other health care workers is important. At this time, anxiety and fear may be lessened, and a positive attitude regarding nursing care is initiated.

A health care facility is very different from a patient's home. New sights, sounds (noises), and smells may interfere with patient comfort. The nurse assists the patient in maintaining dignity and a sense of control and in becoming comfortable in this new environment.

COMMON PATIENT REACTIONS TO HOSPITALIZATION

The reaction of each patient to hospitalization is unique. However, the nurse may anticipate some reactions such as fear of the unknown, loss of identity, separation anxiety, and loneliness. These reactions are related to some of the needs described by Maslow (1970).

The nurse helps reduce the severity of these reactions with a warm, caring attitude. Treating each patient with respect, helping the patient to maintain personal dignity, involving the patient in the plan of care, and adjusting hospital routine to meet the patient's desires when possible helps the patient adapt. Courtesy and empathy are also important. **Empathy** is the ability to recognize and to some extent share the emotions and states of mind of another.

Fear of the Unknown

Fear of the unknown may be the most common reaction to hospitalization. The patient feels insecure and may ask questions such as, "How do I call the nurse?" "How do I work the bed?" "How or when do I get some food?" "When can my family visit?" and "What are they going to do next?" These questions usually indicate anxiety and insecurity. A caring nurse may relieve anxiety by explaining the equipment and procedures, listing mealtimes, and orienting the patient to the unit. Explanations about hospital policies; information about medical orders and procedures; and simple, direct answers to questions help the patient feel more comfortable and more in control.

Loss of Identity

During admission to a health care facility, a patient may feel a loss of identity. This reflects the need for self-esteem and recognition described in Maslow's work. An identification (ID) band is placed around the patient's wrist, possibly causing the patient to feel recognized only as a number and name instead of a person. However, this is a necessary procedure for patient safety. Medications, anesthesia, pain, or emotional reactions may cause the patient to become confused or unresponsive, so the ID band may be the only means of positive identification. The nurse should explain the need for and importance of the band to the patient.

The nurse should learn the name of a new patient as soon as possible and call each patient by name. The nurse should use courtesy titles such as *Mr., Mrs., Ms.,* or *Miss* with the patient's last name, unless the patient requests otherwise. Calling a patient *honey, dear, gramps,* or *grandma* is not appropriate, and it does not show respect.

Separation Anxiety and Loneliness

Separation anxiety and loneliness reflect the patient's need to belong and to be loved, one of the "steps" in Maslow's hierarchy of needs. **Separation anxiety** is fear and apprehension caused by separation from familiar surroundings and significant persons. It is widely recognized in young children, but adults and older adults may also have this reaction. The problem is generally expressed in children by crying. Adults may be very quiet or very talkative. The older adult may exhibit disorientation, depression, or confusion.

Visiting hours in health care facilities are liberal, encouraging family and friends to visit. Many hospitals today allow even small children to visit relatives, especially their mother and a new sibling. Parents are encouraged to stay with their hospitalized children to prevent an emotional reaction to separation. This also helps the child feel secure. In some facilities, pets are allowed to visit. Pets even live in some nursing homes.

HEALTH CARE AGENCIES

Acute Care Facilities

Acute care facilities are also called *general hospitals.* They include many areas of service, such as the emergency, intensive care, coronary care, surgical and medical care, surgery, obstetrics, and pediatrics units. The skills in this chapter focus on this type of health care agency. Minor adaptations may be necessary for other types of health care agencies.

Outpatient Facilities

Outpatient services may be part of an acute care facility or may be a separate facility. In outpatient facilities, patients receive care for up to 23 hours. Services may include laboratory testing, respiratory therapy, physical therapy, and many types of surgery. In outpatient surgical settings the nurse admits, teaches, and prepares the patient for surgery. After surgery, the nurse monitors the patient for several hours until it is safe for discharge. The next day the nurse generally telephones the patient to ask how recovery is progressing.

Home Health Care Agencies

Home health care is one of the fastest growing health care agencies in the United States. Care provided by nurses in the patient's home may prevent a hospital or nursing home admission. Some patients need only temporary care or assistance with self-care. Home care helps control health care costs.

Extended Care Facilities

Extended care facilities are also called *nursing homes.* Extended care is often associated with older adults. Younger people who have chronic or rehabilitative health needs may also be residents of extended care facilities. Nursing homes are authorized by licensure to provide skilled, intermediate, and residential care. Skilled care requires 24-hour nursing services. Intermediate nursing care involves periodic assessment by a nurse but provision of care by a nursing assistant. Residential care provides only room and board. Social and recreational activities are often available.

Psychiatric Facilities

There are special types of admissions for patients who have mental illnesses: voluntary or involuntary. With a voluntary admission, a person realizes that there is a mental health problem and requests admission. That person retains the right to sign out of the institution at any time.

Involuntary admission occurs when one person legally requests that another person be admitted for psychiatric reasons. A judge must issue a court order for an involuntary admission. An emergency involuntary admission occurs when a person is dangerous to the self or to others. Generally, this admission expires after 48 or 72 hours. A temporary admission, lasting up to 60 days, follows a court hearing in which a psychiatrist proves a need for continued hospital treatment. An extended admission, lasting 60 to 180 days, follows another court hearing when the psychiatrist testifies about the need for longer treatment. The patient can testify about the situation, and generally, legal counsel is present.

ADMISSION OF A PATIENT TO A HOSPITAL

The **admission** procedure generally begins in the admitting department. There, the clerical staff gathers information to start the patient's record. This information usually includes the patient's name, address, telephone number, age, birth date, social security number, next of kin, insurance company and policy number, place of employment, and physician's name and the reason for admission. This information is primarily used in the business office for billing purposes. The ID band is prepared with the patient's name, age, ID number, physician's name, and room number. The admitting clerk usually places the band on the patient's wrist. The unit where the patient is assigned is notified, and the patient is escorted to the room.

Some hospitals have telephone admitting. The day before a planned admission, a clerk from the admitting office calls the patient at home and gathers all the information needed to begin the records. Instructions are given regarding a time for arrival at the hospital, items to bring to the hospital, and items that should not be brought to the hospital (for example, jewelry and large sums of money). When the patient arrives the following day, the records and identification band lack only the room number.

Persons brought to the emergency room may be admitted directly to a patient care room or a special care unit, such as the intensive care, coronary care, or burn unit. In these situations a family member provides the necessary information.

NURSING PROCESS FOR ADMISSION

Assessment

For the nurse, assessment of the patient begins at admission. Subjective and objective data about the patient's health history are collected. An initial health assessment is performed (see Chapter 12). Most patients are anxious about being admitted to a health care agency. The anxiety may be related more to family, work, or financial problems than to the actual health care problem or reason for the admission. Anxiety may cause the patient to be uncooperative.

Nursing Diagnosis

The nursing assessment identifies patient problems needing nursing care and discharge planning, since the latter begins at admission. Working with the patient during admission assists the nurse in planning care and later meeting patient needs. Some problems may need further attention after discharge. Nursing diagnoses for admission may include the following:

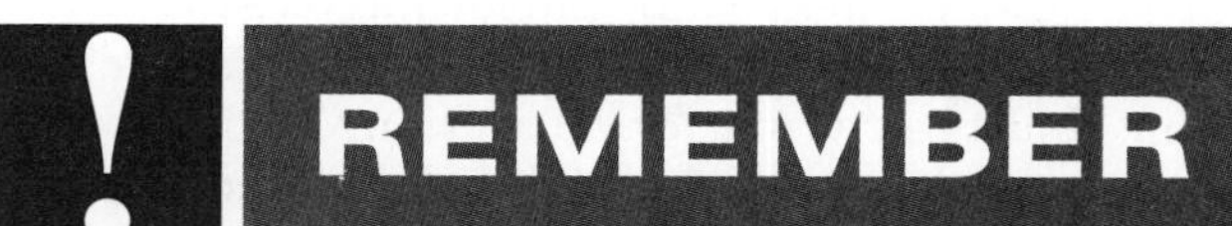

- Most patients are anxious about being admitted to a health care facility.
- Helping a patient to comfortably settle into the hospital and relieving fears usually make the patient more cooperative throughout hospitalization.

Altered health maintenance
Altered role performance
Fear
Ineffective family coping, compromised
Knowledge deficit (specify)
Noncompliance (specify)
Pain
Powerlessness
Risk for infection
Risk for injury
Self-care deficit (specify)

Planning

The plan of care for hospital admission of a patient should include nursing care measures for the patient's hospitalization and should lead toward resolution of the patient's problems (see care plan). To begin discharge planning, the nurse identifies problems that cannot be solved during the patient's hospitalization or that will need more time for resolution.

The admission plan should take into account the patient's personal preferences and may include the following:

Goal #1: Patient is more at ease after orientation to the hospital.

Outcome

Patient can relax and adjust to environment.

■ NURSING CARE PLAN ■

ANXIETY

Mr. T, age 23, is admitted for tests. He states that he has never been in a hospital and is nervous and concerned about what "goes on" in a hospital.

NURSING DIAGNOSIS

Anxiety related to first hospital admission as evidenced by verbalization of concern

GOAL

- Patient will be more at ease and will understand hospital routine by 1300 second day after admission.

EXPECTED OUTCOME

- Patient will express feeling more at ease and understand hospital routine by second day after admission.

NURSING INTERVENTIONS

- Orient patient to hospital policies and routine.
- Orient patient to room and equipment (bed, call light, television).
- Explain all procedures before performing them.
- Answer questions promptly.

EVALUATION

- Patient expresses feeling more at ease and understanding hospital routine.

Goal #2: Patient can operate equipment in the room such as the hospital bed, call light, and emergency button.
Outcome
Patient expresses confidence in using equipment.

Implementation

The nurse should **orient,** or acquaint, the patient to the hospital to put the patient at ease (Skill 7-1). Admission procedures include orientation to the hospital bed, call light system, and intercom; an explanation of how to obtain emergency assistance; information about mealtimes; and orientation to the patient unit. Other procedures include collection of patient information, specimens, and data about nutrition. The patient should be allowed to behave as independently as the condition warrants.

During the orientation, the nurse should also assess the patient's learning ability and readiness to learn. The nurse uses this information to plan teaching sessions.

Evaluation

On completion of patient orientation the nurse determines the effectiveness of the interventions by assessing whether the patient appears calm and verbalizes a relief of fear and anxiety. Examples of evaluative measures related to the goals established include the following:

Goal #1: Patient is more at ease after orientation to the hospital.
Evaluative measure
Ask about patient's comfort level regarding orientation to the hospital.

Goal #2: Patient can operate equipment in the room such as the hospital bed, call light, and emergency button.
Evaluative measure
Patient uses equipment and supplies with calmness and competency.

INTERVENTIONS

Preparation of a Patient Unit

When the unit is notified that a new patient is coming, a room will be made ready. A neat, clean room with appropriate lighting and temperature and with personal care items in place makes the patient feel expected and welcome. A room that is not prepared may make the patient feel that the arrival was unexpected or inconvenient. This makes a negative first impression—an impression on which the nurse-patient relationship is built.

If special equipment, such as that used to administer oxygen or provide traction, is required by the patient, it should be in place and ready for use when the patient arrives. A patient arriving on a stretcher needs the bed adjusted to the high position. The low position is best for a patient arriving by wheelchair or walking.

Patient Orientation

Greeting the patient by name and making the person feel welcome is one of the most important aspects of the admission procedure. The nurse should make an introduction by name and title (for example, Ms. Doe, student vocational nurse, or Mr. Doe, licensed vocational nurse). A person who is warmly welcomed will be more at ease in the new environment. An extra few minutes spent during admission may save time later during the hospital stay (Fig. 7-1).

The hospital routine should also be explained (see teaching box). Knowing when meals are served, when family and friends may visit, when laboratory tests or x-ray studies are scheduled, when the physician usually sees patients, and when side rails must be raised (usually at bedtime) will give the pa-

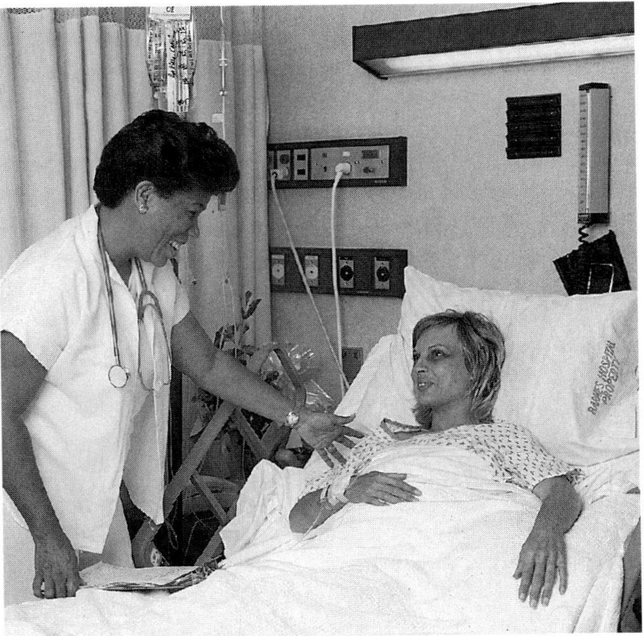

Fig. 7-1 Admitting a new patient. (From Potter PA, Perry AG: *Basic nursing: theory and practice,* ed 3, St Louis, 1995, Mosby.)

PATIENT TEACHING

- Describe the relationship of the patient's room to the nurse's station.
- Point out the location of the shower and bathroom.
- Demonstrate how to call the nurse when the patient is in bed or in the bathroom.
- Demonstrate how to use the intercom.
- Demonstrate how to adjust the bed and lights.
- Demonstrate how to operate the television.
- Demonstrate how to operate the telephone.
- Discuss policies related to the use of the telephone.

tient a sense of security and lessen anxiety. Many hospitals provide booklets explaining these routine activities to the patient. The patient can also refer to the booklets throughout hospitalization. Some of these booklets include information about various social, religious, and other services, such as the cafeteria, library, and gift shop.

The admitting procedure in the patient care unit is more extensive than that in the admitting department. The nurse should check the patient's ID band and verify the information with the patient. Other patients in the room should be introduced. Assessment of immediate conditions, such as pain, shortness of breath, or severe anxiety, should be made and documented.

NURSING CARE

The nurse begins the admission procedure with knowledge of common patient reactions to hospitalization. A nursing diagnosis affecting almost all patients being admitted is *anxiety.* Specific nursing diagnoses are formulated after data are gathered and the admission process is complete. The effectiveness of nursing care given during admission is evaluated after the interventions are completed. Examples of nursing diagnoses related to admission to a health care facility are listed on p. 84.

Valuables

Jewelry, money, and medications should be given to the family to take home. If no family member is present, the valuables may be put in the hospital safe or handled according to agency policy. Losing a patient's valuables may have serious legal implications for the hospital and nurse. Disposition of valuables must be documented on the medical record according to agency policy.

Assisting the Patient to Undress

The patient is usually asked to put on pajamas or a hospital gown. Sometimes the nurse must help the patient change clothes. If help is not needed, the patient should be given a few minutes of privacy to change. Clothing, as well as other personal items, such as glasses, contacts, dentures, prostheses, crutches, hearing aids, wigs, or Bibles, should be inventoried. Jewelry and money kept in the patient's room must also be recorded. A sample valuables form is shown in Fig. 7-2.

Initial Physical Assessment

Once the patient is settled the nurse should record the health history and perform an initial physical assessment (see Chapter 12). The health history generally includes the reason for admission, symptoms the patient is experiencing, past illnesses or hospitalizations, medications (prescription and nonprescription), allergies (food, medication, and other allergies), eating habits, elimination habits, sleep habits, and level and types of activity and exercise. The nurse ascertains the language that the patient speaks and understands as well as information about the patient's family members, home situation, and occupation.

The initial assessment should include the patient's level of consciousness, vital signs, height, weight, breath sounds, apical pulse, bowel sounds, range of motion, skin condition, vision, and hearing. Fig. 7-3 is an example of a record used to collect this information. The health history and initial physical assessment can be performed only by a registered nurse in some hospitals. In others, a registered nurse or a licensed practical/vocational nurse may collect this information.

The physician is generally notified when the patient has been admitted. If no orders have been received, the physician gives the nurse orders at this time.

When a patient is admitted while in critical condition, only the most pertinent information is collected immediately. The rest of the information may be obtained later.

Admission of Children

Admission of an infant or small child requires emotional support for the child and parents. Parents are generally encouraged to stay with the child. This prevents separation anxiety. The most reliable source of admission information is the parents.

Young children are very curious about what is

SPOHN HOSPITAL

VALUABLES FORM

VALUABLES BROUGHT WITH PATIENT TO HOSPITAL DATE ____________

Clocks ____________ Hearing Aids ____________

Dentures: no. of plates____________ Jewelry ____________

Bridgework: no. of pieces____________ Money (billfold) ____________

Eyeglasses ____________ Money (purse) ____________

Contact lens ____________ Radio ____________

Watches ____________ T.V. ____________

Electric toothbrush____________ Electric razor ____________

Prosthesis (any type)____________ Others ____________

I take entire responsibility for retaining in my possession the articles listed above. I am holding nothing in my possession which I have not declared here. I understand and agree that Spohn Hospital is not liable or responsible for any of the patient's property left in the care, custody and control of the Hospital at patient's or patient representative's request if items are not secured in the Valuables Storage Envelope or in the Hospital safe.

SIGNATURE OF PATIENT ____________

I have fully explained to this patient that Spohn Hospital takes no responsibility for articles retained by the patient.

SIGNATURE OF EMPLOYEE RECORDING ARTICLES ____________

VALUABLES STORAGE ENVELOPE

When Valuables Storage Envelope is used, record the following information:

Envelope Number ____________

Date property received ____________

Employee taking envelope to Cashier ____________

Fig. 7-2 Valuables form. (Courtesy Spohn Hospital, Corpus Christi, Texas.)

happening to and around them. Letting the child use equipment on dolls helps reduce anxiety. Children should be encouraged to tell how they feel. It is generally best to perform invasive procedures (that is, obtaining blood specimens or starting intravenous therapy) in a treatment room so that children associate their own rooms with safety.

Older children and adolescents are often self-conscious about the changes in their bodies. Nurses should be aware of their modesty and should provide privacy. Trust can be established by directing health-related questions to them instead of the parents.

Admission of the Older Adult

The nurse should speak slowly and clearly to older adults because their hearing may be less acute. The nurse should face the patient to enable the patient to read lips. Older adults should not be

SPOHN HOSPITAL
DEPARTMENT OF NURSING
PATIENT DATA BASE/ASSESSMENT

ARRIVED: DATE: 4/15/90 TIME 1445
BY: AMB ___ W/C X ARMS ___
STRETCHER ___
AMULANCE ___

HEIGHT: STATED ___ ACTUAL ___
WEIGHT: STATED ___ ACTUAL ___
TEMP 98⁶ PULSE 82 RESP 20 BP 118/76

LANGUAGE SPOKEN: ENG ___
SPANISH ___ OTHER ___

STATED ALLERGIES: NONE
DRUG: ___
FOOD: ___
OTHER: ___

REASON FOR HOSPITALIZATION AND DESCRIPTION OF SYMPTOMS:
(use Patient's or Significant Other's own words)
to have knee surgery in AM

ONSET OF SYMPTOMS: Twisted knee in basketball practice last week

HEALTH HISTORY: PAST SURGERIES/DATES: NONE

PREVIOUS DIET: Regular TUBE FEEDING YES ___ NO X COMMENTS

PREVIOUS ILLNESSES: COMMENTS

GLAUCOMA	YES ___ NO X	HYPERTENSION	YES ___ NO X
DIABETES	YES ___ NO X	PACEMAKER	YES ___ NO X
CANCER	YES ___ NO X	G.I. DISEASE	YES ___ NO X
LUNG DISEASE	YES ___ NO X	ARTHRITIS	YES ___ NO X
ASTHMA	YES ___ NO X	JAUNDICE	YES ___ NO X
HEART DISEASE	YES ___ NO X	NERVE DIS/PARALYSIS	YES ___ NO X
		OTHER	

MEDICATIONS NAME	DOSE	FREQ.	REASON FOR TAKING	LAST DOSE
NONE				

ASSISTANCE NEEDED WITH:
AMBULATION YES X NO ___
FEEDING YES ___ NO X
HYGIENE YES ___ NO X
ELIMINATION YES ___ NO X

EQUIPMENT BROUGHT:
EYEGLASSES YES X NO ___
CONTACTS YES ___ NO X
HEARING AID YES ___ NO X
CRUTCHES YES X NO ___
CANE YES ___ NO X
WALKER YES ___ NO X
DENTURES/UPPER ___ LOWER ___
BRIDGE
OTHER

PROSTHESIS:
EYE RT ___ LT ___
BREAST RT ___ LT ___
ARM/LEG RT ___ LT ___

PATIENT INSTRUCTIONS:
SIGNAL LIGHT ✓
BED CONTROLS ✓
LIGHT CONTROLS ✓
BATHROOM ✓
SHOWER ✓
T.V. ✓
TELEPHONE ✓
UNIT INTRODUCTORY/ WELCOME LETTER ✓
VISITING PRIVILEGES ✓
HIGH RISK PRECAUTIONS ___
I.D. BAND ON ✓
ALLERGY BAND ON ___
URINALYSIS:
OBTAINED ✓
INSTRUCTED ___

HIGH RISK FALL CHECKLIST

___ (2) AGE GREATER THAN 70
___ (5) HISTORY OF PREVIOUS FALLS
___ (3) FROM NURSING HOME
___ (3) HAS HAD SITTER/COMPANION AT HOME

STATUS: MENTAL/PHYSICAL
___ (5) CONFUSED/DISORIENTED
___ (5) SENSORY IMPAIRMENT
___ (5) SEDATED
___ (5) NONCOMPLIANCE/ UNCOOPERATIVENESS
___ (3) MOBILITY IMPAIRMENT/AMPUTEE
___ (3) WEAKNESS/DEBILITATION
___ (5) URGENT ELIMINATION NEEDS

MEDICATIONS
___ (3) DIURETICS
___ (3) LAXATIVES/G.I. PREPS
___ (3) ANTIHYPERTENSIVES
___ (3) ANTISEIZURES
___ (3) SEDATIVE/HYPNOTICS
___ (3) ANALGESICS
___ (3) CHEMOTHERAPY

___ TOTAL

IF SCORE IS 15 OR GREATER, INITIATE HIGH RISK MEASURES.

SKIN BREAKDOWN POTENTIAL CHECKLIST

GENERAL PHYSICAL CONDITION:
___ (1) FAIR (MAJOR BUT STABLE)
___ (2) POOR (CHRONIC/SERIOUS, NOT STABLE)

LEVEL OF CONSCIOUSNESS: (RESPONSE TO STIMULI)
___ (1) LETHARGIC (SLOW)
___ (2) SEMI-COMATOSE (VERBAL/PAINFUL STIMULI)
___ (3) COMATOSE (NO RESPONSE)

ACTIVITY:
___ (2) AMBULATORY WITH ASSISTANCE
___ (4) CHAIRFAST
___ (6) BEDFAST

MOBILITY:
___ (2) RESTRICTED MOVEMENT
___ (4) MOVES ONLY WITH ASSISTANCE
___ (6) IMMOBILE

INCONTINENCE:
___ (2) OCCASIONAL (<2 per 24 HRS.)
___ (4) USUALLY (>2 per 24 HRS.)
___ (6) TOTAL (NO CONTROL)

NUTRITION:
___ (1) FAIR (EATS/DRINKS 50% OR LESS)
___ (2) POOR (UNABLE/REFUSES DIET)
___ TOTAL

PTS. WITH A SCORE OF 8 OR ABOVE ARE HIGH RISK. INITIATE INTERVENTION PROTOCOL.

SIGNATURE & TITLE OF ADMITTING NURSE: J. Doe, LPN DATE: 4-15-90 TIME: 1500

PATIENT DATA BASE/ASSESSMENT

Fig. 7-3 Patient data base/assessment form.

SPOHN HOSPITAL
DEPARTMENT OF NURSING
PATIENT DATA BASE/ASSESSMENT

DISCHARGE PLANNING ADMISSION SCREEN

	YES	NO
Do you live in a nursing home?		X
Do you have a visiting nurse?		X
Do you have help at home with your daily care or needs?	X	
Do you have a dependent person at home with no one to care for him/her?		X

A yes answer to any of the above questions requires a referral to Social Services

ADDITIONAL COMMENTS: ____________________

SYSTEMS	YES	NO	COMMENTS
CNS			
L.O.C.			
- alert	✓		
- drowsy		✓	
- comatose		✓	
- disoriented		✓	
EYES			
- PEARL			
- vision normal	✓		
- prosthesis		✓	
EARS			
- responds to normal voice tone	✓		
- drainage		✓	
SPEECH			
- clear	✓		
- slurred			
- hoarse/raspy			
- aphasic			
INTEGUMENTARY			
SKIN - color normal	✓		
- warm, dry	✓		
- turgor good	✓		
- bruises, abrasions, lacerations		✓	
- rash, lesions		✓	
- scars		✓	
- decubitus		✓	
- dressing		✓	

SYSTEMS	YES	NO	COMMENTS
CARDIOVASCULAR			
PULSES			
- radial			82
- carotid		✓	
- pedal			80
APICAL RATE ____			
CHEST PAIN		✓	
RESPIRATORY			
RESPIRATIONS			
- rapid		✓	
- slow		✓	
- deep		✓	
- shallow		✓	
- labored		✓	
BREATH SOUNDS			
- clear	✓		
- wheezes		✓	
- rales		✓	
COUGH			
- present		✓	
- productive		✓	
GASTROINTESTINAL			
ABDOMEN			
- soft	✓		
- distended		✓	
- tenderness		✓	
ELIMINATION			
- bowel sounds	✓		
- diarrhea		✓	
- constipation		✓	
- incontinence		✓	
- ostomy		✓	
LAST B.M. this AM			

SYSTEMS	YES	NO	COMMENTS
MUSCLE/SKELETAL			
EXTREMITIES			
- moves all on command	✓		
- WEAKNESS (SPECIFY)			pain from injury
RA ____ LA ____			
RA ____ LA ____	✓		
- edema		✓	
- normal ambulation			c̄ crutches
- prosthesis (SPECIFY)			
GENITOURINARY			
VOIDING			
- normal	✓		
- frequency		✓	
- burning		✓	
- incontinence		✓	
- catheter		✓	
CATHETER INSERTION DATE ____			
DATE OF LAST MENSTRUAL PERIOD:			
PSYCHO-SOCIAL			
- cooperative	✓		
- agitated		✓	
- depressed		✓	
- frightened			anxious about surgery
- combative		✓	
HABITS			
- smoking		✓	
- alcohol		✓	
- drugs		✓	

After assessing this patient's physical condition, psycho-social needs, the Data Base and the Discharge Planning Admission screen, is Discharge Planning indicated at this time? ____YES ____NO

Referred to Social Services ____YES X NO

Reviewed for Discharge Planning: High Risk ____YES X NO

____________________ Signature of Registered Nurse ________ Date

____________________ Signature of Social Worker ________ Date

PATIENT DATA BASE/ASSESSMENT

Fig. 7-3, cont'd Patient data base/assessment form.

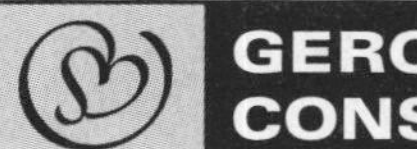

GERONTOLOGIC CONSIDERATIONS

- The older patient may have less acuity of senses, particularly sight and hearing. The nurse should assess for these problems.
- The older patient may become confused because of the change in environment and routine. The nurse should frequently orient this patient to time and place.

REMEMBER

- The nurse should assess the patient's reaction to being transferred to another unit. The transfer could signal progress in regaining wellness or regression of wellness.
- The patient's reaction could cause a change in physical or mental status.

rushed. The nurse should wait for them to answer rather than letting family members answer. The change in environment and daily routine may cause confusion, loss of appetite, or reversal of sleep patterns. Anxiety about hospitalization may also interfere with memory. Considerations for the admission of the older adult are listed in the gerontologic box.

TRANSFER OF A PATIENT

A patient may be transferred to another area for several reasons. The changing condition of a patient, whether for better or worse, may require **transfer** to another unit in the hospital or to another type of health care agency. For example, a patient may be transferred to a nursing home or a rehabilitation hospital. A patient whose condition becomes critical may be moved to special care areas such as an intensive care or a coronary care unit. A patient whose condition improves may be moved from a special care area to a general nursing care unit. A patient may be transferred to a nursing home for continued nursing care at a lower cost, since personal care needed does not require remaining in the hospital. A transfer may be performed at the patient's or physician's request. For example, the patient may prefer to move to a private from a double room.

Transfer combines admission and discharge. An **intraagency transfer** is a transfer within a health care facility. The patient is discharged from one unit and received on the new unit much like the initial admission.

An **interagency transfer** is a transfer to another health care facility. The family generally arranges transportation, either their car or an ambulance, to the new facility, or the physician orders the type of transportation according to the patient's condition. If appropriate, the patient dresses in street clothes. A nurse generally accompanies a critically ill patient when transferred. Financial arrangements with the new facility are made by the family.

A medical order is generally needed to begin the transfer process. The patient's family should be notified of the transfer.

NURSING PROCESS FOR TRANSFER

Assessment

The patient's condition is carefully assessed to ensure that is safe to move the patient to another area. The nurse takes vital signs and assesses the patient's physical condition.

Nursing Diagnosis

After the assessment is complete, the nursing diagnoses are identified and may include the following:

Altered health maintenance
Anxiety
Body-image disturbance
Pain
Powerlessness
Self-esteem disturbance

Planning

The plan for transferring a patient requires a decision about ways to transport the patient and ways to ensure that all personal belongings are taken with the patient. The nurse should also prepare the patient psychologically and emotionally for the transfer (see care plan). Goals and related outcomes follow:

Goal #1: Patient expresses comfort with the transfer.
Outcome
Patient can adapt to new environment.

Goal #2: Patient remains in stable condition after the transfer.
Outcome
Patient's condition does not worsen after transfer.

■ NURSING CARE PLAN ■

POWERLESSNESS

Mr. L, age 87, hospitalized with congestive heart failure, is ready for discharge to a nursing home. His wife died several years before, and his two sons work. The decision to put him in a nursing home was made by the sons. Mr. L will not eat or get out of bed and says, "Why should I? I'm no good for anything."

NURSING DIAGNOSIS

Powerlessness related to change of environment as evidenced by patient not eating or getting up and by verbal comments

GOAL

- Patient will feel in control of his life within 36 hours.

EXPECTED OUTCOME

- Patient will eat, get out of bed, and express control of daily activities within 36 hours.

NURSING INTERVENTIONS

- Assess reasons for lack of eating and mobility.
- Encourage patient to express feelings about going to a nursing home.
- Report changes in eating, mobility, and mental status to nurses at nursing home.
- Check with nursing home in 3 days about patient's status.

EVALUATION

- Patient is eating meals, getting out of bed, and expressing interest in and participating in nursing home activities.

Implementation

Patients are usually transferred by a stretcher but may be able to use a wheelchair for the short trip.

Evaluation

Before, during, and after patients are transferred to new areas and assisted into bed, the nurse should assess their physical condition. Evaluative measures follow for the established goals:

Goal #1: Patient expresses comfort with transfer.
Evaluative measure
Ask patient if he or she is experiencing discomfort or unease with new environment.

Goal #2: Patient remains in stable condition after transfer.
Evaluative measure
Monitor patient for any change in condition after transfer.

NURSING CARE

The nurse begins the transfer process by assessing the patient's reaction to the impending transfer. Patients often fear change, and adjusting to a new area of the hospital or a new facility may be difficult. Nursing diagnoses help the nurse identify specific patient goals and the appropriate nursing interventions to assist the patient in attaining those goals. The effectiveness of nursing care is evaluated after nursing interventions are completed. Examples of nursing diagnoses related to the transfer of a patient are listed on p. 90.

The nurse should assess the patient's current condition to verify that it has not changed since the medical order to transfer was written. The method of transportation is determined by the patient's condition. Assessing the patient's knowledge and feelings about the transfer identifies problems that may be encountered. The nurse determines whether the receiving unit or agency is ready for the patient. This ensures continuity of nursing care. **Continuity of care** means that care is planned and coordinated throughout hospitalization, during transfer to another unit or health care facility, and after discharge or referral to home health care.

Preparing for Patient Transfer

The nurse must ensure that the patient knows the reasons for the transfer. The family must be no-

PATIENT TEACHING

- Explain reasons for transfer.
- Discuss new unit and personnel.
- Assure patient that all personal belongings will also be transferred.
- Explain that nurse in new unit will orient patient and ensure comfort.

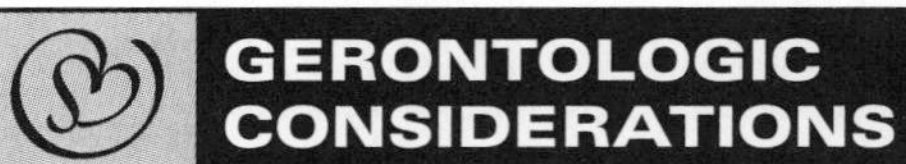

GERONTOLOGIC CONSIDERATIONS

- The nurse should explain the reasons for transfer.
- The nurse should also frequently discuss the anticipated transfer.
- The older adult's personal belongings are gathered so that the patient can see them.

tified. For an interagency transfer, the family needs some time to make transportation and financial arrangements. The nurse should describe the new unit to the patient. Positive statements should be made about the new environment and the personnel who will be there. The patient should be assured that all personal belongings will be moved as well. The teaching box highlights aspects of patient preparation.

Transfer

The nurse gathers all the patient's personal items, medications, and supplies and the Kardex and medical record (Skill 7-2). A means of transportation for the patient and a cart for flowers should also be procured. The nurse should accompany the patient on intraagency transfers. Introducing the patient to the nurses on the new unit begins a new nurse-patient relationship. Having to transfer to a new area may be difficult for the patient, so the nurse's presence and introduction prevents the patient from feeling abandoned.

Transfer of children

Infants are usually transported in a self-contained incubator bed that is returned to the health care agency. Parents usually accompany their child during transfer unless the move is by a care flight; parents then follow in family transportation. Older children may be transferred the same way as an adult.

Transfer of the older adult

Following agency policies and the requirements of third-party payors is important to prevent loss of benefits. Home care patients may be transferred for a few hours to a clinic or outpatient service unit for tests or treatments or transferred for admission to the hospital or nursing home. A nursing home patient may also be transferred to the hospital.

Another change in environment may cause increased confusion and anxiety. Often this interferes with the patient's memory. Tips to help the nurse prepare the older adult for transfer are listed in the gerontologic box.

DISCHARGE OF A PATIENT

When a patient is ready to be released from a health care agency the physician writes a **discharge** order. **Discharge planning** is a centralized, coordinated, multidisciplinary process that ensures that the patient has a plan for continuing care after leaving the hospital (AHA, 1983). It should begin at the time of admission so that all teaching is performed and referrals are made in time for the patient to feel confident to handle things at home. This also allows time for the family to make adjustments at home for the patient's return. Discharge planning thus ensures continuity of care. Planning for discharge must be individualized to the needs of the patient.

Throughout the hospital stay, patient teaching must be performed (see Chapter 6). Topics include medications, diet, activity, treatments, and any signs or symptoms that should be reported to the physician. General health teaching must also be performed.

Daily teaching allows the patient time to think about the information and to ask questions. It also gives the nurse a chance to verify the patient's understanding of the information. All teaching and the level of the patient's understanding must be recorded on the chart. Involving family members in this teaching ensures continuity of care at home.

At discharge, a review of the medications, diet, activities, and treatments to be continued at home should be conducted with the patient and family (Fig. 7-4). If the patient or family cannot manage this care, arrangements should be made for home health or nursing home care.

In many hospitals, the patient signs a form with written instructions and teaching documentation to acknowledge understanding of instructions (Fig. 7-5). The patient uses these instructions at home. The primary nurse may make a follow-up telephone call 1 or 2 days after discharge to discuss the patient's progress and any problems.

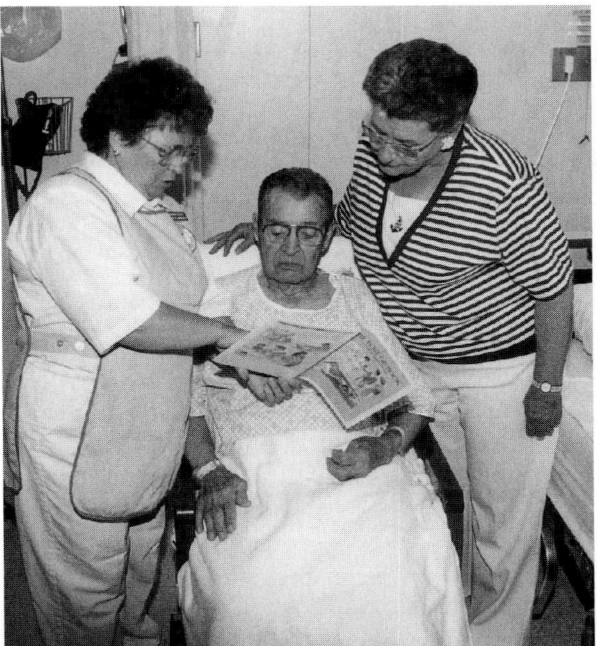

Fig. 7-4 Reviewing discharge planning instructions. (From Christensen BL, Kockrow EO: *Foundations of nursing,* ed 2, St Louis, 1995, Mosby.)

NURSING PROCESS FOR DISCHARGE

Assessment

After ensuring that there is a medical order for the discharge, the nurse should assess the patient's condition and feelings about being discharged to identify problems for which the patient is at high risk. The nurse also identifies medication administration and treatments that the patient can perform and diet and mobility restrictions that the patient must follow after discharge. Teaching goals are then specified. The nurse questions the patient and family to identify home environment problems that the patient may encounter so that the patient and family can make necessary plans or changes. The nurse also ascertains the identity of the patient's primary caregiver and includes that person in teaching sessions. The caregiver's feelings about the patient's discharge and the required care are assessed to help identify other high-risk problems and teaching goals.

Nursing Diagnosis

After the nursing assessment for discharge, the nurse ascertains whether additional nursing diagnoses are needed. These diagnoses indicate problems that may affect the patient at discharge. Even though teaching has been performed throughout hospitalization, the patient may still have some questions. The nursing diagnoses concerning discharge may include the following:

Altered family processes
Altered role performance
Anxiety
Impaired adjustment
Impaired physical mobility
Knowledge deficit (specify)
Powerlessness
Self-care deficit (specify)

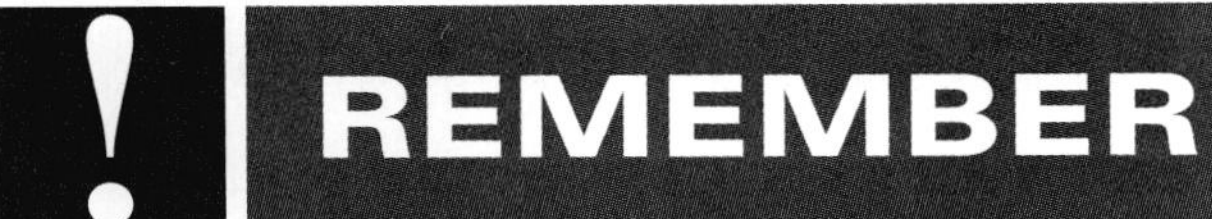

- The nurse should assess the patient's and caregiver's feelings about the discharge, since interventions depend on this information.
- The nurse should identify home environment problems that the patient may encounter
- Patients often have more than one physician. Each physician must discharge the patient.

Planning

The nurse begins planning for discharge by reassessing the patient's knowledge of the illness or disease, medications, diet, activity, and treatments to be continued at home. The nurse may need to review these items for the patient. Referrals for community services needed should be made, and family members who plan to assist the patient at home need to be taught any special care techniques (see care plan).

The plan of care focuses on achieving goals and outcomes that relate to the nursing diagnoses. An example of a goal and its outcomes follows:

Goal #1: Patient states or demonstrates understanding of information taught.

Outcomes

Patient demonstrates application of a dressing using sterile technique.

Husband demonstrates application of a dressing using sterile technique.

Implementation

On the day of discharge, all equipment, supplies, and prescriptions that the patient is to take home are gathered (Skill 7-3). The nurse verifies that the patient and caregiver understand the instructions for care (see teaching box). The nurse also determines whether the business office has given a release for discharge. The nurse reviews the list of clothing and valuables made on admission to ensure that the patient has all belongings when leaving. The nurse should assist the patient to dress and

SPOHN HOSPITAL
DEPARTMENT OF NURSING

DISCHARGE INFORMATION RECORD

PATIENT/FAMILY TEACHING AND INSTRUCTIONS

Diet: __X__ Regular ______ Bland

______ Diabetic ______________ (Specify)

______ Other ______________ (Specify)

______ Diet list given to patient

Comments: ______________

Activity: ____ Restricted __X__ Unrestricted

____ Ambulatory ____ With Assistance

Comments: ______________

Treatments/Self-Care: __X__ Not Applicable

Specify: ______________

MEDICATIONS	DOSAGE	FREQUENCY
Tylenol #3	1 tab	Every 4 hr. if needed for pain

OTHER: ______ ______ Not Applicable

Follow-up: To be seen in Dr Smith's (Dr. Name) office in 1 week 8-26-90 (Period of time/date).

______ Transferred to Nursing Home ______ (Specify).

______ Transferred to another hospital ______ (Specify).

______ Home Health/Hospice Services ______ (Specify)

______ Other ______ (Specify)

☒ Preprinted Instructions From Physician's Office Given to Patient/Family.

I understand the above information: ______________ (Patient/Family Signature)

Admission Date 4-15-90 Discharge Date 8-18-90 Via: Wheelchair Escorted by: J. Doe LPN

Time: 1 AM/PM Destination: Home

PATIENT DISCHARGE STATUS

Nursing Assessment of patient's condition at time of discharge: ______________

	Yes	No	N/A
Own meds from home returned to patient/family.	____ Yes	____ No	__X__ N/A
Prescription(s) given to patient/family.	__X__ Yes	____ No	____ N/A
Valuables returned to patient/family.	____ Yes	____ No	__X__ N/A

Signature/Title Discharge Nurse: J. Doe, LPN

Fig. 7-5 Patient discharge information record.

 **PATIENT TEACHING**

- Explain about medications, treatments, diet, and mobility restrictions.
- Instruct patient about when and how to call the physician if problems arise. Describe signs and symptoms of complications.
- Make sure teaching is understood. Have the patient and caregiver verbally verify understanding or give return demonstration of a skill.

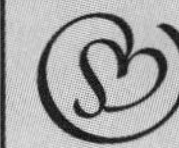 **GERONTOLOGIC CONSIDERATIONS**

- The older patient may not wish to be discharged from the health care agency. The nurse must be aware of and assess for this problem.
- The nurse should encourage the patient to be as self-sufficient as possible. Patient teaching should address this fact.

pack personal belongings. Most agencies require that patients be discharged by wheelchair even if they are able to walk. The patient should be escorted to the waiting vehicle and assisted into the vehicle.

Evaluation

During and after patient discharge, the nurse evaluates the effectiveness of teaching for the patient who must receive ongoing nursing care or follow-up at home. Examples of goals, outcomes, and evaluative measures include the following:

Goal #1: Patient states or demonstrates understanding of information taught.

Evaluative measure

Assess patient's ability to apply a sterile dressing.

NURSING CARE

The nurse begins the discharge procedure by knowing the patient's and family's reactions to the discharge and assessing the plan of care to identify additional high-risk problems or problems for which treatment must continue in the home. Possible nursing diagnoses related to discharge are listed on p. 93. The nurse confirms that the patient and family have all the information and equipment needed to continue care at home. If necessary, the nurse makes referrals to home health care or other agencies. At discharge, the nurse gathers the patient's belongings, helps the patient dress and pack, and escorts the patient to and assists the patient into the waiting vehicle. Throughout the discharge procedure, the nurse evaluates the measures taken to make sure that the patient is prepared to leave the hospital and that continuity of care is ensured.

Discharge Against Medical Advice

Sometimes a patient insists on leaving the hospital without the consent of the attending physician **(against medical advice [AMA])**. The patient's physician should be immediately notified about the patient's decision to leave. The physician should then inform the patient and family about the degree of risk in refusing treatment by leaving the health care agency. If the physician is unavailable, the head nurse or supervisor should explain the risks to the patient and family. If the patient still wishes to leave, a release form should be signed by the patient in which the person acknowledges leaving without the physician's consent (Fig. 7-6). This releases the physician, hospital, and hospital personnel from being held responsible for any problems or complications that might occur because of this action.

A rational adult patient who will not sign the form cannot be forcibly detained. Only if a court order was issued for the admission, as in some cases of mental illness, can a patient be detained forcibly. A lawsuit for false imprisonment could be filed against the physician, hospital, or hospital personnel for keeping patients in the facility against personal wishes. Documentation of the patient's refusal to sign the form and the information given by health care personnel about the risks of leaving should be made in the patient's medical record.

Discharge of Children

The parents should be included in all aspects of teaching and the entire discharge procedure. Some hospitals have a special form to be signed by the person legally responsible for taking the child away from the facility. The nurse should make certain, both for safety of the child and for legal implications involving the agency, that the person taking the child is entitled to do so.

Discharge of the Older Adult

Many older adults fear discharge. Often they are concerned about their care at home, especially if they live alone. Patient goals should focus on having the patient become as self-sufficient as possible before discharge (see gerontologic box). Necessary referrals should be made.

LEAVING HOSPITAL AGAINST MEDICAL ADVICE

Date____________________

This is to certify that____,
a patient in ________________________________, is leaving the hospital against the advice of the attending physician and the hospital administration. I acknowledge that I have been informed of the risk involved and hereby release the attending physician, and the hospital, from all responsibility and any ill effects which may result from this action.

____
Patient

____
Other Person Responsible

____
Relationship

Witness: ________________________

Witness: ________________________

Fig. 7-6 Form that patient must sign when leaving hospital AMA.

■ NURSING CARE PLAN ■

KNOWLEDGE DEFICIT: DRESSING CHANGE

Ms. K, age 32, has an open wound on the inside of the left lower leg. The dressing is to be removed and a sterile dressing applied each day. Ms. K is to continue this procedure at home. She states that she does not know how to do the dressing change the way the nurses do it.

NURSING DIAGNOSIS

Knowledge deficit related to sterile dressing application as evidenced by verbal comments

GOAL

- Patient will apply sterile dressing appropriately after return demonstration.

EXPECTED OUTCOME

- Patient will express confidence in applying sterile dressing.

NURSING INTERVENTIONS

- Gather needed supplies: sterile 4 × 4's, tape, and sterile gloves.
- Demonstrate removing old dressing.
- Demonstrate opening 4 × 4's to maintain sterility.
- Demonstrate donning sterile gloves.
- Demonstrate applying sterile 4 × 4's to wound and taping in place.

EVALUATION

- Patient correctly applies sterile dressing to wound and expresses confidence in doing so.

SKILL 7-1 ADMITTING A PATIENT

Steps	Rationale
1. Check assigned room. Open bed at appropriate height and turn light on.	Ensures that room is ready and makes patient feel expected and welcome.
2. Obtain equipment: ▪ Hospital gown ▪ Sphygmomanometer or Doppler ▪ Stethoscope ▪ Thermometer ▪ Scales ▪ Clean gloves ▪ Hospital admission form ▪ Note pad and pen ▪ Admission kit (if used) ▪ Written information regarding items in patient unit and basic agency policies	Helps organize procedure.
3. Introduce self.	Decreases anxiety.
4. Identify patient by ID band.	Identifies correct patient for procedure.
5. Wash hands and apply clean gloves according to agency policy and guidelines from Centers for Disease Control and Prevention and Occupational Safety and Health Administration.	Helps prevent cross-contamination.
6. Orient patient to unit, lounge, and nurses' station if condition warrants.	Provides sense of security.

Continued.

SKILL 7-1 ADMITTING A PATIENT—cont'd

Steps	Rationale
7. Orient patient to room and bathroom. Teach use of equipment such as call system, bed, telephone, and television.	Prevents accidents and allows some control over environment.
8. Explain hospital routines such as visiting hours, mealtimes, and wake-up time.	Decreases patient's fear of unknown and gives feeling of security.
9. Arrange patient privacy.	Shows respect for patient.
10. Assist patient to undress if needed.	Prevents fatigue and falling and allows for range-of-motion and skin assessment.
11. Follow agency policy for care of valuables, clothing, and medications.	Loss of valuables, clothing, or medications is upsetting to patient and family and could result in legal problems.
12. Obtain patient's health history and perform initial physical assessment following agency policy.	Provides information necessary for safe, effective, individualized management of health problems.
13. Provide for safety with bed in low position and side rails up.	Helps prevent accidents.
14. Review preadmission test results.	Acquaints nurse with patient's results to assist in data gathering.
15. Begin care as ordered by physician.	Gives positive impression of agency when care is begun immediately.
16. Invite family back into room if they left earlier.	Relieves family's anxiety to see patient settled.
17. Explain diagnostic studies and care that have been ordered.	Reduces fear of unknown.
18. Remove gloves and wash hands.	Helps prevent cross-contamination.
19. Document.	Documents procedure and patient's response.

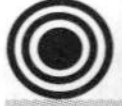

SKILL 7-2 TRANSFERRING A PATIENT

Steps	Rationale
INTRAAGENCY TRANSFER	
1. Obtain equipment: ▪ Patient's clothing ▪ Stretcher or wheelchair ▪ Utility cart ▪ Medications ▪ Kardex ▪ Medical record	Organizes procedure.
2. Refer to medical record, care plan, or Kardex for special interventions.	Provides basis for care.
3. Introduce self.	Decreases anxiety level.
4. Identify patient by ID band.	Identifies correct patient for procedure.
5. Explain procedure to patient.	Seeks cooperation and decreases anxiety.
6. Wash hands and don clean gloves according to agency policy and guidelines of Centers for Disease Control and Prevention and Occupational Safety and Health Administration.	Helps prevent cross-contamination.
7. Gather *all* patient's belongings and necessary care items, health records, Kardex, and medications.	Prevents loss of personal items.
8. Prepare patient for intervention:	
a. Close door to room or pull curtain.	Provides privacy.
b. Drape for procedure if necessary.	Prevents exposure of patient.

SKILL 7-2 TRANSFERRING A PATIENT—cont'd

Steps	Rationale
9. Raise bed to comfortable working level.	Provides safety for nurse.
10. Arrange for patient privacy.	Shows respect for patient.
11. Assist in transferring patient, usually by stretcher or wheelchair, and monitor condition.	Maintains patient safety.
12. Give personal belongings to nurse on receiving unit.	Prevents loss of patient's belongings.
13. Deposit medical record and medications at receiving nurses' station.	Prevents loss.
14. Introduce patient and family to nurses on new unit and to roommates and assist to bed.	Establishes beginning of new nurse-patient relationship and gives patient sense of belonging.
15. Explain equipment, policies, and procedures that are different in new unit.	Gives patient some control and reduces anxiety.
16. Record condition of patient and means of transfer. Ensure that new nurse records assessment of patient's condition on arrival.	Documents transfer and condition of patient.
17. Notify other departments such as radiology, laboratory, switchboard, dietary department, and business office of transfer and new room number.	Will allow patient's records to be kept straight, meals and medications to be brought to correct room, and errors to be avoided.
INTERAGENCY TRANSFER	
18. Complete interagency referral form. Telephone receiving agency to answer questions.	Ensures continuity of care.
19. Perform discharge procedure (see Skill 7-3).	Completes record with that agency.
20. Notify receiving agency that patient is being transported. Give nurse report on patient.	Prepares staff for arrival of patient and ensures continuity of care.
21. Send copy of medical record.	Ensures continuity of care.
22. Assist patient to transporting vehicle by wheelchair or stretcher and assess condition.	Maintains patient safety and ensures attention if condition changes.
23. Remove gloves and wash hands.	Helps prevent cross-contamination.
24. Document.	Documents procedure and patient's response.

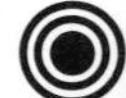

SKILL 7-3 DISCHARGING A PATIENT

Steps	Rationale
1. Obtain equipment: ▪ Discharge planning record ▪ Valuables form ▪ Written instructions for home care, if applicable ▪ Wheelchair or stretcher ▪ Utility cart ▪ Prescriptions, supplies, and equipment that patient is to take home	Helps organize procedure.
2. Refer to medical record, care plan, or Kardex for special interventions.	Provides basis for care and fact that patient can leave agency legally.
a. If there is no discharge order and patient insists on leaving, notify physician and have patient sign AMA form.	Patient's signature acknowledges full responsibility for what happens after patient leaves and releases hospital and physician from responsibility of patient's safety and welfare.
3. Introduce self.	Decreases anxiety level.
4. Identify patient by ID band.	Identifies correct patient for procedure.

Continued.

SKILL 7-3 DISCHARGING A PATIENT—cont'd

Steps	Rationale
5. Explain procedure to patient.	Seeks cooperation and decreases anxiety.
6. Wash hands and don clean gloves according to agency policy guidelines from Centers for Disease Control and Prevention and Occupational Safety and Health Administration.	Helps prevent cross-contamination.
7. Prepare patient for intervention:	
a. Close door to room or pull curtain.	Provides privacy.
b. Drape for procedure if necessary.	Prevents exposure of patient.
8. Raise bed to comfortable working level.	Provides safety for nurse.
9. Arrange for patient privacy.	Shows respect for patient.
10. Verify verbally that patient and caregiver understand instructions for care.	Ensures correct care of patient at home, since instructions are understood.
11. Determine whether business office has given release for discharge.	Prevents patient from undue waiting when ready to leave.
12. Check list of clothing and valuables made on admission according to agency policy.	Helps ensure that patient has all belongings when leaving facility.
13. Assist patient to dress and pack personal belongings.	Conserves patient's strength.
14. Transfer patient to wheelchair and escort patient and belongings to waiting vehicle. Assist patient into vehicle.	Ensures patient safety, which is responsibility of hospital personnel until patient has left the premises.
15. Remove gloves and wash hands.	Helps prevent cross-contamination.
16. Document.	Documents procedure and patient's response.

SUMMARY

Admission to a hospital or another health care agency is an anxious time for most patients and families. Measures should be taken to ensure a patient's comfort and to reduce anxiety. The nurse should orient the patient to hospital policies and routines.

It is important to ensure continuity of nursing care throughout the transfer and discharge processes. Daily teaching assists the patient and family in planning care at home after discharge.

Key Concepts

- Admission to a health care facility is usually an anxious time for patients and families.
- The nurse must refrain from calling a patient *honey, dear, gramps,* or *grandma.*
- A patient may not be kept in a health care facility against personal will unless the admission was ordered by the court.
- An introduction of personnel and orientation to the health care facility help establish a comfortable and trusting nurse-patient relationship.
- The transfer of a patient combines discharge and admission.
- Planning for discharge begins at admission.
- Each attending physician must write an order for a patient's discharge.

Critical Thinking Questions

1. Mr. Douglas is 66 years old, recovering from a stroke that has left his right side partially paralyzed. His physician has prescribed four medications to be taken after discharge from the hospital. As the nurse, what would you want to know about Mr. Douglas to plan his discharge from the hospital?
2. Mr. Stamm is an 86-year-old patient whose diagnosis includes vomiting and diarrhea presumed secondary to *Staphylococcus aureus*. Develop a discharge teaching plan.
3. You are conducting a health history on a 77-year-old man who tells you he is having an increasingly more difficult time with constipation. What normal, age-related physical changes are likely to be contributing to his constipation?

REFERENCES AND SUGGESTED READINGS

American Hospital Association: *Introduction to discharge planning for hospitals,* Chicago, 1983, American Hospital Publishing.

deWit S: *Rambo's nursing skills for clinical practice,* ed 4, Philadelphia, 1994, Saunders.

Earnest V: *Clinical skills in nursing practice,* ed 2, Philadelphia, 1993, Lippincott.

Iyer P: Documenting discharge AMA, *Nursing* 22(9):30, 1992.

Maslow AH: *Motivation and personality,* ed 2, New York, 1970, Harper & Row.

Meyer C: Discharged patients left with questions, *American Journal of Nursing* 92(10):16, 1992.

Tirk J: Determining discharge priorities, *Nursing* 22(7):55, 1992.

Tuazon N: Discharge teaching: use this MODEL, *RN* 55(7):19, 1992.

Tuazon N: Teaching patients about meds pays off (Clinical news: discharge planning), *American Journal of Nursing* 93(7):12, 1993.

UNIT II

FACTORS INFLUENCING HEALTH AND ILLNESS

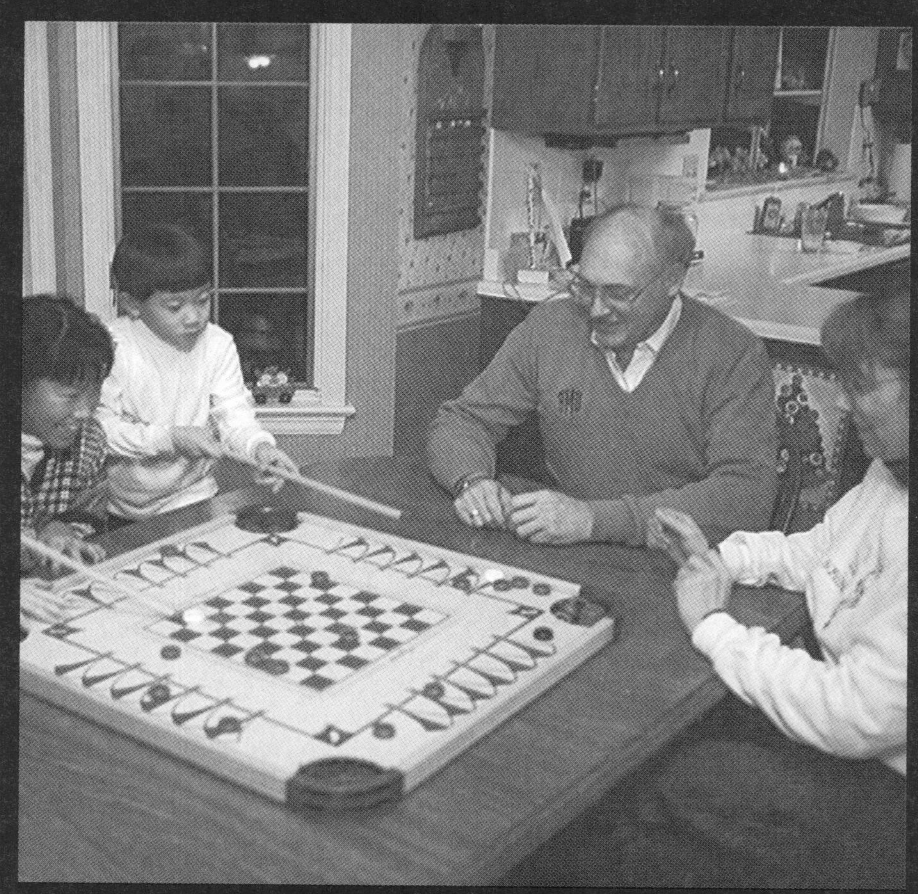

■ CHAPTER 8 ■

Family and Cultural Influences

Learning Objectives

After studying this chapter, the student should be able to . . .

- Define the key terms.
- Define and discuss family forms related to current family structures.
- Describe the characteristics and stages of family life.
- Describe and relate the impact of feelings about the self and childhood experiences on later adult family interaction patterns, including codependency aspects.
- List and describe factors that affect the relationship between parent and child as well as general family interactions, including step-parent, single-parent, and other families.
- Identify guidelines used for assessing the cultural background of a patient.
- Assess and evaluate effects of nursing interventions related to the ethnicity of the patient.

Key Terms

Codependency
Culture
Cultural assessment
Disengagement stage
Engagement stage
Establishment stage
Expectant stage
Extended family
Family
Family interaction
Matrifocal/martiarchal family
Multicultural nursing
Nuclear family
Parenthood stage
Patrifocal/patriarchal family
Single-parent family
Step-parent family

Family and cultural influences significantly influence people. Thus they can affect the ways in which patients approach health care and the ways in which the health care team provides nursing care.

The influence of the family is always with the patient. The nurse may not agree with all that occurs within the family unit, but despite all of its problems, the family remains the strongest force in the lives of its members.

FAMILY INFLUENCES

The **family** is a primary force in the lives of its members. The family unit is characterized by day-to-day contact; bonds of affection; a sense of loyalty and concern; a continuity of the past, present, and future; and shared goals, identity, values, and behaviors common only to the specific unit. The family is responsible for various roles, communication patterns, socialization, and physical and emotional care of the members in each developmental stage.

Healthy families are characterized by the following:

1. A sense of togetherness that promotes the capacity for change
2. A balance between mutual and independent action on the part of family members
3. Nurturing and use of resources for growth and sustenance
4. Stability and integrity of structure
5. Mastery of the developmental tasks leading to independence and the ability to meet the demands for survival and further development

The family in crisis may have some difficulty maintaining these characteristics. Assisting the family during illness helps them maintain togetherness.

FAMILY FORMS

Nuclear Family

Family consists of husband and wife and perhaps one or more children.

Presence of children affects family's time and economic resources.

Absence of children may lead husband and wife to seek counseling and health care.

Extended Family

Family includes relatives (aunts, uncles, grandparents, and cousins) in addition to nuclear family.

Closer the extended family, more influence it has on health care.

Family can provide diverse support base for members needing health care.

Single-Parent Family

Family is formed when one parent leaves nuclear family because of death, divorce, or desertion or when single person decides to have or adopt child.

Circumstances of separation influence its impact on family. It most commonly results from divorce today.

Reduced financial and emotional resources affect health of single-parent families.

Step-Parent (Blended) Family

Family is formed when parents bring unrelated children from prior relationships into new joint living situation.

Nature of prior living situations and rate of adapting to change affect health.

Stress of newly formed family patterns can affect mental health of family members.

Alternate Patterns of Relationships

These relationships may include multiadult households, "skip-generation" families (grandparents caring for grandchildren), communal groups with children, "nonfamilies" (adults living alone), cohabitating partners, and homosexual couples.

Health concerns focus on specific needs integral to each form but may include stability of relationships, child-rearing practices, and availability of community resources.

From Potter PA, Perry AG: *Basic nursing: theory and practice,* ed 3, St Louis, 1995, Mosby.

Forms

The family may take one of several forms (see box). One form is the **nuclear family** including the mother, father, and children of this couple. Another form is the **extended family,** which includes the nuclear family plus other relatives. Third and fourth forms are the **patrifocal/patriarchal family,** in which the father is the authority, and the **matrifocal/matriarchal family,** in which the mother is the authority. A fifth form is the **step-parent family** or blended family form whereby the family must try to adjust to having a different mother or father figure in the household. In the **single-parent family,** a parent is single, divorced, or widowed. Some different family forms have developed (for example, a man and woman living together without being legally married or a homosexual couple desiring to have a family and choosing to live together).

The nurse should be aware of the different family forms and consider the complexity of family relationships while performing nursing care and patient teaching. A deceased or missing family member may be remembered by other family members, which may affect the behavior of the family.

Today's family

The family of today differs in several aspects. First, today's family is decreasing in size. There used to be large families, but now families have fewer children. People are also marrying later in life, so some women have children after 35 years of age. Couples usually already have careers and homes and can often provide more for their families earlier than in the past. The divorce rate is higher, and a large percentage of people marry more than once. The wife and mother works outside the home, either in a chosen career or to help the family income because of economics. Despite these factors, marriage and family are still important.

People may not chose the traditional family form. Homosexuals are establishing homes and demanding the right to raise children through adoption. Grandparents may raise their grandchildren. Children may even be raised in a communal atmosphere.

People are also living longer. Many older adults are in the household, and many are in nursing homes. The children of these older adults must find ways to balance caring for their parents and caring for their children while caring for their own needs.

Stages of Development

Each family has a series of developmental stages that it must complete before moving successfully to

Table 8-1 STAGES OF THE FAMILY LIFE CYCLE

Family Life Cycle Stage	Emotional Process of Transition: Key Principles	Changes in Family Status Required to Proceed Developmentally
Between families: unattached young adult	Accepting parent-offspring separation	Differentiation of self in relation to family of origin Development of intimate peer relationships Establishment of self in work
Joining of families through marriage: newly married couple	Commitment to new system	Formation of marital system Realignment of relationships with extended families and friends to include spouse
Family with young children	Accepting new generation of members into system	Adjusting marital system to make space for children Taking on parenting roles Realignment of relationships with extended family to include parenting and grandparenting roles
Family with adolescents	Increasing flexibility of family boundaries to include children's independence	Shifting of parent-child relationships to permit adolescents to move in and out of system Refocus on midlife marital and career issues Beginning shift toward concerns for older generation
Launching children and moving on	Accepting multitude of exits from and entries into family system	Renegotiation of marital system as dyad Development of adult-to-adult relationships between grown children and their parents Realignment of relationships to include in-laws and grandchildren Dealing with disabilities and death of parents (grandparents)
Family in later life	Accepting shifting of generational roles	Maintaining own or couple functioning and interests in face of physiologic decline, exploration of new familial and social role options Support for more central role for middle generation Making room in system for wisdom and experience of older adults, supporting older generation without overfunctioning for them Dealing with loss of spouse, siblings, and other peers, and preparation for own death; life review and integration

From McGoldrick M, Carter E: *The stages of the family life cycle.* In Henslin J, editor: *Marriage and family in a changing society,* New York, 1985, Free Press; in Walsh F: *Normal family processes,* New York, 1982, Guilford Press.

the next stage (Table 8-1). Nurturing of the family goes on as does many other activities: employment, management of a household, participation in community groups, pursuit of leisure activities, and maintenance of friendships and family ties.

The **engagement stage** of family development usually precedes establishment of the family unit. During this time, the couple prepares for marriage and becomes free of parental domination. The main emotional tie is now with each other but the couple wants closeness with the parents. The couple commits to living together and working out developmental tasks.

The **establishment stage** begins when the couple lives together and works on deepening the relationship. They adjust to each other's needs and habits. The stage ends when the woman becomes pregnant or when the couple work out their living pattern and philosophy of life.

During the **expectant stage** (pregnancy), many domestic and social adjustments must be made. The couple learns new roles and gains new status in the community. Attitudes toward pregnancy and the physical and emotional status of the mother and father, as well as of significant others, affect future parenting abilities. Now the couple thinks in terms of "family" instead of "couple." They plan for the new member in terms of space, budget, and supplies.

The couple often has mixed feelings about the pregnancy. Both may experience similar physical and emotional symptoms such as nausea, indigestion, backache, distention, and depression. As time goes on the excitement of the new arrival takes over, and fears and concerns usually subside. In the man the symptoms are part of the couvade syndrome, or a man's physical and emotional reaction to his partner's pregnancy.

The woman needs encouragement from the partner and others during pregnancy. The man also needs extra attention and nurturing. The nurse should listen to couples' individual concerns and help them understand that what they are feeling is normal. Various teaching aids that explain what to expect are useful. Nursing care should be family centered and directed toward both parents-to-be.

In the **parenthood stage** the couple assumes a status that will never be lost as long as each has memory—that of parent. During the time after birth, parents are excited about the baby but also uncertain about parenting skills. A parent-child attachment is being formed for life. However, difficult adjustments must be made, and new roles and behaviors are learned by the parents. This will occur through each stage of the child's development. The parents are concerned about carrying out the tasks of the family and about the welfare of the child and family, and they must usually suppress their own desires for a while.

Sometimes the final or **disengagement stage** does not last too long. The stage occurs when the children become independent and move out to establish their own home and career. The young adult who is unemployed, a college dropout, or divorced may return home to live. If the young adult also brings one or more children, with or without a spouse, there is extra stress for the entire family unit: There are three generations living in the same household with desires of how they each want things done or with how they prefer doing them. This may cause serious problems unless the group can come to an agreement and understanding.

The aged parents may be unable to continue to live independently and then are included in the household of middle-aged offspring. Also, one of the spouses may die. With either of these situations, the tasks and relationships of the family must be reworked. Space and other resources must be redivided. Time schedules for daily activities may be reworked. Privacy, communication, and respectful use of possessions should be ensured.

Size

An only child may feel lonely but usually develops more rapidly and may seem older and more serious then peers who have siblings. The child may not share feelings with a peer unless very close to the person. The child is often brought into the conflicts of the parents and is likely the one to maintain harmony and preserve equilibrium in the household. This child often is forced to assume adult roles too soon. The child usually has a high need to achieve and prefers the novel or complex.

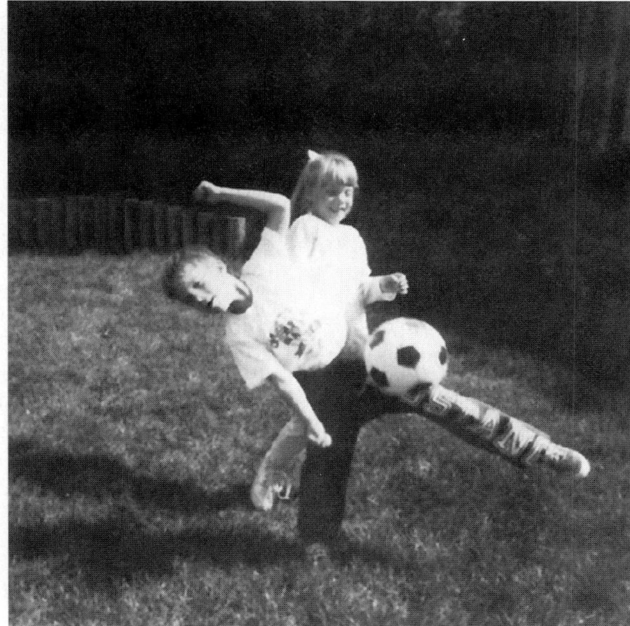

Fig. 8-1 Twins at play.

Fewer families have more than two children today. Each child has a place in the family unit. In a loving home, they have not only their parents, but also siblings, love, a listening ear, and help. They learn give and take, cooperation, and tolerance of and pull for one another.

Twins usually work and play with one another, since the mother has less time to deal individually with each child. Therefore twins tend to be slower to talk, and many have a slower intellectual growth unless parents work to prevent it. Multiple-birth children are likely to be closer to one another than other siblings (Fig. 8-1). Because of lower birth weight, twins must "catch up" in growth and some skills, usually by the end of the first year.

Developmental Tasks

The family is considered responsible for the child's growth and development as well as behavioral outcomes and for the welfare of its members. The family is expected to complete certain tasks (see

FAMILY DEVELOPMENTAL TASKS

- Provide for physical safety, daily routines, and economic needs of family members and obtain enough resources to survive.
- Create sense of family loyalty and security and mentally healthy environment for family's well-being.
- Reproduce and socialize children, teaching values and appropriate behavior.
- Teach members to effectively communicate their needs, ideas, feelings, and respect to each other.
- Provide social togetherness with division of labor, patterning of gender roles, and performance of family roles with flexibility and cooperation.
- Help members develop physically, emotionally, intellectually, and spiritually and develop personal and family identity while adjusting to demands of family life.
- Release family members into the larger society—school, church, organizations, employment, and eventually another family unit.
- Rework relationships, values, and philosophy of life throughout life span.

box). These tasks may be met in various ways, but the ability to complete them depends on the maturity of the adult members and the support given to them.

Interaction

Long before the child learns to speak, sensory, emotional, and intellectual exchanges are made between the child and other family members. Through such exchanges and later with words, the child learns how to live. The games and toys purchased for the child, the books selected and read, and the television programs allowed may provide key learning experiences. This **family interaction** is affected by the stage of family development and gender of the child (Fig. 8-2). The presence of an only child, of multiple births (such as twins), or of an adoptive child or step-child also influence interaction.

Parents tend to identify with their children and to treat them according to how they were treated as children. This does not mean that the parents do not love their children but that it is the only way that they know how to parent. In this case the parents can learn better methods through formal or informal education. A parent may identify best with the child who matches the same gender and sibling position. A man from a family of boys may not know how to interact with a daughter. The child also adopts many

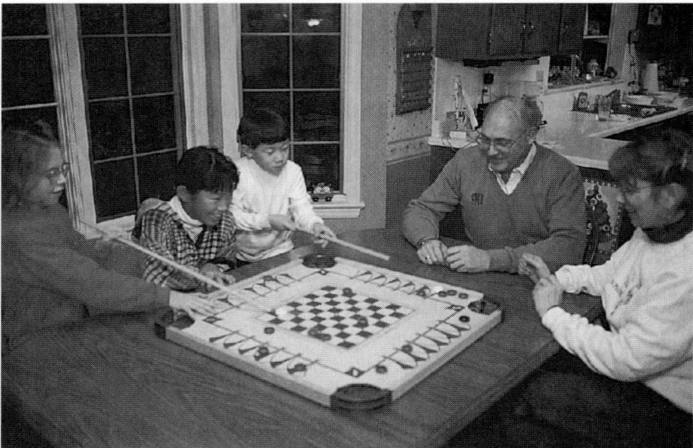

Fig. 8-2 Observing family interactions assists in understanding family functioning. (From Potter PA, Perry AG: *Basic nursing: theory and practice,* ed 3, St Louis, 1995, Mosby.)

of the parent's characteristics, especially if the child is the oldest or only child.

Relationships

Interaction between the husband and wife and other family members living in the same household is basic to the emotional, social, spiritual, and sometimes physical health of the adults and children. Children may be easily overlooked during times of problems and stress. The family may not think that the children are affected by the turmoil, but nothing could be farther from the truth. Children are often the most traumatized but go unnoticed and unaided in learning how to handle stress. Children should always understand that they did not cause the problems and that they continue to be loved by the parents.

Importance of self-esteem

A sense of self-esteem and love and a positive self-image evolve through interaction with parents from birth and in turn affects how the person interacts with others, including the spouse and children. The adult in the family who lacks self-acceptance and self-respect is not likely to be a loving spouse or parent, no matter how much the person desires it. The person may react in ways designed to defend the *self* from rejection. The person may criticize, become angry, brag, demand perfection from others, or withdraw. In turn, others are not likely to respond to the person's basic needs for love, acceptance, and respect. Remaining open and giving in such situations may be difficult for the nurse, but it may be the only way to elevate the person's self-esteem.

SIGNS OF STRAINED OR UNHEALTHY FAMILY RELATIONSHIPS

- Lack of communication between spouses or other family members
- Disregard shown by family members to each other, alternating with harassment through arguments or harshness with each other
- Lack of decision making or inability to cooperate with caregivers
- Overpossessiveness of children, mate, or other family members; extreme behavior or incest
- Derogatory remarks by children to parents or vice versa
- Blame placed among family members for difficulties
- High level of anxiety, tension, or insecurity present in interactions between family members
- Pattern of immature, regressive, or aggressive behavior in family members

Signs of strained or unhealthy relationships

During assessment, various behaviors indicate that the family is not relating in a constructive or harmonious manner. The behaviors listed in the box should be reported to a nurse manager. Family violence has reached an all time high, but few are seeking help and education on how to prevent it or about how to solve this problem.

Codependency

Codependency is a term applied to the individual in a family whose spouse is addicted to alcohol or other drugs. The family member enables the addicted spouse to continue the addictive behavior through caretaking activities instead of allowing the spouse to take responsibility. The addicted spouse thereby also becomes codependent. Family members may spend years "rescuing" the addict, waiting and hoping that the loved one will change. After a time the family members unconsciously encourage and even support the addiction. If and when the addicted family member seeks and receives help, the codependent family members cannot accept the change in behavior. Therefore the entire family should be treated along with the alcoholic to make the family well, and the term *codependency* is used to describe the personality characteristics of people involved in any unhealthy relationship from which they do not leave. Causes of codependency are listed in the box.

Family members who come from a dysfunctional family do not have stability because of the control, so the oldest child usually becomes the one who assumes responsibility to maintain order and care for the addicted and codependent parents. This causes the child to feel good about having control. However, the young person develops feelings that get in the way of forming relationships. Ways of helping families overcome codependency are listed in the box.

CAUSES OF CODEPENDENCY

- Traumatic event
- Abuse by a caregiver or spouse
- Involvement with or marriage to addicted person
- Personal involvement with addictive process
- Involvement in dysfunctional family or relationship

OVERCOMING CODEPENDENCY

- Evaluate personal behavior and lifestyle as honestly as possible. Listen to comments of person who is close that indicate codependency.
- Seek counseling from professional therapist who will be accepting and will look at all aspects of the self—physical, emotional, mental, social, and spiritual health.
- Admit that people or events outside the self cannot be controlled.
- Let go of defensive behavior.
- Write about feelings and behavior to help reshape thinking and behavior.
- Learn to recognize situations that trigger codependent reactions.
- Design ways to carefully assess situations. If necessary, say "no" to avoid becoming involved in situations that appear to call for someone to take control.
- Design ways to help others to help themselves.
- Identify and develop relationships in which esteem and happiness are felt and nurturing is given and received.
- Develop leisure activities that help release feelings of anger and that give feelings of control and security.

NURSING PROCESS FOR THE FAMILY

Assessment

The nurse begins assessment by considering family members and the patient's attitude toward family. Functions of the family should also be assessed. These include the ability to provide emotional support for family members, the ability to cope with the current health problem or situation, ways that goals are set, and progress made toward the achievement

GERONTOLOGIC CONSIDERATIONS

- Changes in roles and relationships present major developmental challenges to older adults.
- The older adult may need to seek social support within the community if a spouse or friends have died or are ill.
- The nurse should remember that the spouse of the older adult may suffer caregiver strain because of declining physical strength. The older adult's children may also be affected because they are trying to balance caring of their parent, children, and self.

of goals. The nurse attempts to work within the structure of the family when providing care.

Nursing Diagnosis

The nursing diagnosis often focuses on the family's ability to cope with the illness of the family member (see care plan at the top of p. 113). During times of acute illness, the family can become extremely distressed and may focus solely on the patient, neglecting the needs of other family members. While caring for a patient, the nurse may learn of such difficulties and may help the patient or refer the family to other resources. It is important for the nurse to maintain a family nursing perspective. Possible nursing diagnoses related to the family include the following:

Altered family processes
Altered growth and development
Altered parenting
Caregiver role strain
Ineffective family coping: compromised
Ineffective family coping: disabled
Ineffective individual coping
Risk for altered parenting
Risk for caregiver role strain

Planning

When planning nursing care of the patient, the nurse should work with the family in setting goals. It is important for the family to understand and agree on the goals being set. Ways that the older adult affects family structure should also be considered (see gerontologic box). The following is an example of a family-oriented goal and outcome:

Goal: The family understands and copes with the health problems of its members.

Outcome

The family is able to meet the needs of all members.

 PATIENT TEACHING

- Teach patient and family members about medications and treatments, especially those to be used after discharge.
- Provide information about community programs designed to aid families in problem solving and strengthening the family unit.

Implementation

After goals have been set, the nurse assists the family in learning health-promotion practices (see teaching box). Providing accurate health information about the patient's diagnosis and prognosis helps the family members understand the patient's experience and the best ways to be effective caregivers.

Evaluation

The nurse must be prepared to revise a plan of care depending on the findings of evaluation. The nurse determines whether expected outcomes have been met. An example of a goal and evaluative measure related to the family follows:

Goal: The family understands and copes with the health problems of its members.

Evaluative measure

Observe the abilities of family members to perform care measures correctly.

CULTURAL INFLUENCES

Health care in the United States is changing so rapidly that nursing will need to stay one step ahead in the delivery of nursing care into the new areas. Traditional nursing care is moving into the community as well as into other new areas. Many patients once brought to the hospital will be treated in the community, so hospital nursing will also change. Thus the practice of **multicultural nursing** (caring for people from all ethnic and cultural backgrounds) will be broadened. According to the U.S. Bureau of Census, one third of the U.S. population consists of individuals from ethnic and cultural subgroups. If current demographic trends continue into the twenty-first century, the cultural diversity will be 23% Hispanic American, 14% African American, and 12% Asian American. These groups will represent over 50% of the U.S. population. These statistics dramatize the need for health care professionals to understand and recognize cultural differences.

The health care team must develop culturally sensitive plans of care for these individuals, making certain that their needs are met.

Culture is a set of learned values, beliefs, customs, and behavior that is shared by a group of interacting individuals. Also included are their communication systems and norms that also guide and sanction the behavior of the group. An awareness of cultural backgrounds can allow the nurse to accurately assess patients. The nurse recognizes and treats patients according to their values, beliefs, and practices concerning health and illness. Culture encompasses areas such as diet, language and communication processes, religion, art, history, family, interactive patterns of social groups, value orientations, and healing beliefs and practices.

Trends or similarities among persons of a distinct cultural or ethnic group may be seen in their behavior in the clinical or community setting. Being unaware of a patient's cultural background may cause the health care team to misjudge the cultural effect on health care; make incorrect and inappropriate nursing care judgements; and provide inappropriate interventions.

When administering nursing care to patients from various cultural backgrounds, the nurse uses the same nursing process approach as with all other patients. **Cultural assessment** begins with awareness of the patient's culture and data that direct identification of nursing diagnoses and thus nursing intervention. The assessment promotes a better understanding of the patient as an individual and thus assists with administering appropriate nursing care to all patients. The nurse should know whether the patient prefers the traditional or modern approach to nursing care. Therefore effective intercultural communication must occur.

Specific Cultural Groups

The following sections highlight some general characteristics of specific cultural groups that may influence health-seeking behaviors. This information does not replace the necessity for the nurse to perform a personal cultural assessment. Communities with a similar ethnic background may vary, depending on geographic location and other influences. It is essential to remember that cultural variations may exist among the same cultural group.

Amish

There is a traditional old and new order of the Amish. The new-order Amish may live in larger communities and work in nearby towns while observing Amish customs. The Amish forbid ownership of autos, electricity, or telephones. They live in small congregations and usually are related by marriage or blood line. Monogamy is valued, and birth control is prohibited. They strive for self-sufficiency and oppose government aid. The Amish revere the elderly, and children are valued. Overall authority belongs to the man—woman is the helper to the man. They believe that God heals but are not forbidden to use medical services, including blood transfusions and immunizations. Healers exist in the community.

Asian American

Traditional home remedies and chants are used by healers. Politeness and formality are essential. Eye-to-eye contact and touching of strangers is considered inappropriate. Women do not shake hands with others. Silence is valued, and disagreements frequently are not verbalized. Many languages and dialects exist in this population, and translators are used when needed. Health depends on achieving a balance between the yin and yang. This is frequently referred to as the hot-and-cold theory. Medications and foods administered must achieve a balance or will be refused. They believe in good and evil spirits and in reincarnation.

African American

African Americans are close to family members. Family is extremely important to the group. Family roles are flexible. For example, the mother may be the decision maker. Religion is an integral part of their lives. Some illnesses are viewed as punishment from God or possession of evil spirits. The minister is important for supportive care. Modern health care is not forbidden, however. Folk medicine is practiced.

Hispanic American

Hispanic Americans touch frequently when speaking and require a small personal space. Modesty is valued, and open conversations about sex are not permitted. They have a strong sense of extended family values. The male is seen as dominant, elders are respected, and children are a priority. Illness is a result of physical imbalance resulting from God's will or evil spirits.

Native American

Early native American Indians lived in all the states. Many tribes now live on reservations or in towns and cities. They believe they must live in harmony and respect the surrounding environment and the earth. Many Native Americans are reserved and believe that it is disrespectful to make direct contact. An important belief is that the body, mind, and spirit must live in harmony to avoid illness. Other Native Americans include the Alaskans and Eskimos, who settled here thousands of years ago before immigrants from many other countries.

Gypsies

Gypsies have large extended families. Lighted candles around the bed of a dying family member is customary. Safety precautions must be followed.

NURSING PROCESS AND CULTURE

Assessment

The nurse must be aware of and sensitive to the health beliefs and practices of a patient's heritage. This awareness can be developed by carefully assessing the patient's beliefs and heritage. Cultural information includes ethnic origin, race, place of birth, customs, values, language, healing practices, and food and nutrition practices.

The nurse should also note educational status, family and community support systems, economic status, and religious influences. Assessment should also include growth and development patterns, body systems variations, and any diseases that may be prevalent in the patient's ethnic group.

Nursing Diagnosis

It is important for the nurse to be as specific as possible in identifying cultural variables when determining nursing diagnoses for a patient. This enables the nurse to individualize the plan of care for the patient. Examples of nursing diagnoses related to culture include the following:

Anxiety
Altered health maintenance
Impaired social interaction
Impaired verbal communication
Spiritual distress (distress of the human spirit)

Planning

Cultural beliefs and practices can be incorporated into the plan of care. The patient's cultural needs must be included when the nurse sets goals and expected outcomes. The patient and family members should actively work with the nurse and members of the health care team in establishing and carrying out a plan of care (see care plan, bottom right).

The health practices of the older adult may have a strong cultural basis and should be carefully examined by the nurse (see gerontologic box). The plan of care with cultural variables may include the following goal and outcome:

Goal: Patient and family understand the implications that health care beliefs have on health status.

GERONTOLOGIC CONSIDERATIONS

- Many older adults value home remedies and cultural practices in regards to health care. They may resist attempts by caregivers to change their practices even when they are harmful.
- Some older adults may persist in the religious practices of their youth. The older person's wishes should be respected if these practices are not harmful to their health.

Outcome

Patient and family are able to modify cultural and health practices to achieve an optimal level of health.

Implementation

Explaining all aspects of care is important if the patient is to understand and participate in the plan of care. The patient and family should be involved in all aspects of care. Any cultural questions related to care should be discussed so that the patient will understand how cultural variables relate to health beliefs and practices. The nurse must respect the patient's individuality and ethnic culture to avoid cultural conflicts and provide effective nursing care.

Evaluation

The nurse evaluates the success of interventions and determines the extent to which established goals have been met. This evaluation is made from feedback from the patient and family members. Nurses should evaluate their own attitudes toward multicultural nursing care. Self-evaluation can help the nurse be more at ease when giving care to patients.

The nurse uses specific evaluative measures when determining whether goals have been met. An example of a goal and evaluative measures related to cultural nursing care follows:

Goal: Patient and family understand the implications that health care beliefs have on health status.

Evaluative measure

Ask the patient how health care beliefs will affect self-care at home.

Role of the Nurse

The nurse should be aware of different cultures. Health care professionals may apply the concepts discussed in this chapter to help provide culturally

■ NURSING CARE PLAN ■

ALTERED PARENTING

Mrs. J, the mother of 4-year-old Jeremy, has had difficulty responding to the child's hospitalization and understanding explanations from the physician and the nurse regarding the child's condition.

NURSING DIAGNOSIS

Altered parenting related to lack of knowledge as evidenced by delay in growth and development of the child, inappropriate caretaking behaviors, inattention to child's needs, and lack of parental attachment behaviors

GOAL

- Parent establishes a beginning relationship with the child.

EXPECTED OUTCOMES

- Parent establishes eye, physical, and verbal contact with the child.
- Parent voices a willingness to have and work at a relationship with the child.

NURSING INTERVENTIONS

- Allow parent to take part in care of child.
- Act as role model when caring for child in front of parent.
- Praise parent when appropriate parenting skills are demonstrated to reinforce teaching and learning.

EVALUATION

- Parent makes appropriate physical, verbal, and visual contact with child.
- Parent demonstrates appropriate techniques for bathing, feeding, and other care.
- Parent uses community resources for help with parenting.

■ NURSING CARE PLAN ■

IMPAIRED SOCIAL INTERACTION

Mr. S, age 82, is admitted for hematuria (blood in the urine). He is having difficulty being understood by caregivers. A nurse who speaks Spanish has been notified to assist with communicating with Mr. S.

NURSING DIAGNOSIS

Impaired social interaction related to sociocultural dissonance as evidenced by patient's inability to communicate needs to make himself understood by health caregivers

GOAL

- Patient will express understanding of instructions.

EXPECTED OUTCOMES

- Patient explains needs to nursing staff.
- Family assists in planning care.

NURSING INTERVENTIONS

- Assign the same nurse for nursing care interventions to provide consistency of nursing care and relieve anxiety.
- Provide time to talk to patient when not performing nursing care to instill trust and show caring.
- Provide an interpreter as needed.

EVALUATION

- Patient expresses cultural and personal care needs.
- Patients copes with cultural differences.

sensitive health care. The following are ideas that the nurse may wish to use:

1. Conduct a cultural self-assessment.
2. Be aware of personal ethnocentric biases.
3. Conduct a cultural assessment.
4. Avoid idioms.
5. Be alert to changing trends in language.
6. Listen carefully.
7. Be aware of body language.
8. Ask patients how they would like to be addressed.
9. Identify the significant other and anyone else whom the patient wishes to participate in health care.
10. Examine the patient's health beliefs.
11. Integrate the patient's health beliefs as long as there are no negative consequences regarding the patient's health.

The nurse should respect and listen to all patients. Patients are the experts regarding their own bodies and health. However, their health beliefs are shaped by the cultures in which they were raised or are currently living.

SUMMARY

Family and culture influence people more than any other factor. Each family has its own characteristics that differ from those of other families. Today's family differs from that the past in makeup, authority figure, and size. Couples are marrying later in life, and women are bearing children at an older age. Cultural influences are becoming more diverse as people of different countries come to America. Because of these factors, the health care team must work out methods for communicating, treating, and supporting the family unit. Regardless of the changes, family and culture remain the strongest forces in the lives of patients.

Key Concepts

- Family affects its individual members and determines how its members approach life.
- Healthy families characteristically have positive attitudes.
- The family may take on many forms.
- The family goes through developmental stages of growth and maturity.
- Codependency occurs in many families, and the members need help in moving toward wellness.
- Nurses provide care to patients of diverse cultures.
- Specific cultural groups need understanding while obtaining medical assistance.

Critical Thinking Questions

1. Discuss the problems that ethnic stereotyping and ethnocentrism may cause for the nurse. Suggest some ways nurses can learn to recognize such tendencies in themselves.
2. Discuss different illnesses and their likelihood in different ethnic and cultural groups.
3. Describe societal factors that influence a family's health status.

REFERENCES AND SUGGESTED READINGS

Cassetta R: Emphasizing cultural diversity to improve nursing education, *American Nurse* 25(8):16, 1993.

Diaz-Gilbert M: Caring for culturally diverse patients, *Nursing* 23(10):44, 1993.

Eliason M: Ethics and transcultural nursing care, *Nursing Outlook* 41(5):225, 1993.

Fagan-Pryor E, Haber L: Codependency; another name for Bowen's undifferentiated self, *Perspectives in Psychiatric Care* 28(4):24, 1992.

Potter P, Perry A: *Basic nursing: theory and practice,* ed 3, St Louis, 1995, Mosby.

Roberson M: Defining cultural and ethnic differences to adapt to a changing patient population, *American Nurse* 25(8):6, 1993.

West E: The cultural bridge model, *Nursing Outlook* 41(5):229, 1993.

CHAPTER 9

Growth and Development

Learning Objectives

After studying this chapter, the student should be able to . . .

- Define the key terms.
- Describe Maslow's hierarchy of needs.
- Identify how Maslow's hierarchy of needs influences growth and development.
- Describe Freud's psychosexual theory of development.
- Describe Erikson's psychosocial theory of development.
- Describe Havinghurst's theory of developmental tasks.
- Compare and contrast Freud's, Erikson's, and Havinghurst's theories of growth and development.
- Assess patients and plan nursing care using appropriate stages of growth and development.
- Describe normal growth and development for age-groups throughout the life cycle.

Key Terms

Cephalocaudal	Libido
Cognitive	Menopause
Development	Menses
Developmental tasks	Osteoporosis
Ego	Proximodistal
Fixation	Psychosexual theory
Growth	Psychosocial theory
Heredity	Self-actualization
Hierarchy of needs	Superego
Id	

Growth and development are processes that span a person's lifetime, from conception to death. **Growth** is change in body size and structure. **Development** is a change in body function, including motor function, attitudes, beliefs, understanding, reasoning, values, emotions, and personal interactions. Although growth and development are separate processes, they occur simultaneously and are interdependent. For example, the legs must change in size and structure before a child can walk (change in function).

INFLUENCES

Growth and development are influenced by heredity and the physical and psychosocial environments (Table 9-1). The family plays the strongest influence and role on the child.

Heredity

Heredity is the genetic "plan" each person receives from both parents at conception. This predetermined plan guides the person's physical growth, function, organization, and integration. Ill health or inadequate nutrition may delay individuals from reaching their full potential. However, normal health and appropriate nutrition do little to increase the rate at which people reach their full potential.

Environment

Physical and psychosocial environments also influence growth and development. The physical environment includes water, food, air, noise, housing, home conditions, and community conditions and resources. These influences are positive when the individual has adequate food, clean air, low noise level, adequate housing with electricity, safe water, and

Table 9-1 MAJOR FACTORS INFLUENCING GROWTH AND DEVELOPMENT

Factors	Relevant Influences
Forces of nature	
Heredity	Genetic endowment includes gender, race, hair and eye color, physical growth, and stature.
Temperament	Temperament is characteristic psychologic mood with which child is born and includes behavioral styles of easy, slow-to-warm, and difficult.
External forces	
Family	Family purpose is to protect its members. Family functions include means for survival, security, assistance with emotional and social development, assistance with maintenance of relationships, instruction about society and world, and assistance in learning roles and behaviors. Family influences through its values, beliefs, customs, and specific patterns of interaction and communication. Ordinal position and gender influence individual's interaction and communication in family.
Peer group	Peer group provides new and different learning environment. Peer group provides different patterns and structures of interaction and communication, necessitating different style of behavior. Functions of peer group include allowing individual to learn about success and failure; to validate and challenge thoughts, feelings, and concepts; to receive acceptance, support, and rejection as unique person apart from family; and to achieve group purposes by meeting demands, pressures, and expectations.
Life experiences	Life experiences and learning processes allow individual to develop by applying what has been learned to what needs to be learned. Learning process involves series of steps: recognition of need to know task; mastery of skills to perform task; mastery of task; expertise in performing task, which expands capabilities; integration into whole functioning; and use of accumulated skills and experiences to develop repertoire of effective behavior.
Health environment	Level of health affects individual's responsiveness to environment.
Prenatal health	Preconception (for example, genetic and chromosomal factors, maternal age, health) and postconception (for example, nutrition, weight gain, use of tobacco and alcohol, medical problems, use of prenatal services) factors affect fetal growth and development.
Nutrition	Growth is regulated by dietary factors. Adequacy of nutrients influences whether and how physiologic needs, as well as subsequent growth and development needs, are met.
Rest, sleep, and exercise	Balance between rest or sleep and exercise is essential to rejuvenating body. Imbalances diminish growth, whereas equilibrium reinforces physiologic and psychologic health.
State of health	Illness or injury potentially hampers growth and development. Nature and duration of health problem influence its impact. Prolonged injury or illness leaves individual less able to cope and respond to demands and tasks of developmental stage.
Living environment	Factors affecting growth and development include season, climate, housing, and socioeconomic status.

From Potter PA, Perry AG: *Fundamentals of nursing: concepts, process, and practice,* ed 3, St Louis, 1993, Mosby.

heat. When the community provides adequate sewage and garbage disposal, transportation, appropriate health care, and cultural resources (for example, library, museum, concerts), the child's development is influenced by these important factors. If any of these aspects are absent or unavailable to the individual, a negative effect on growth and development may occur.

The physical connection between the fetus and the mother during pregnancy creates the infant's first environment. Mothers who smoke, use drugs, or drink alcohol negatively influence the growth and

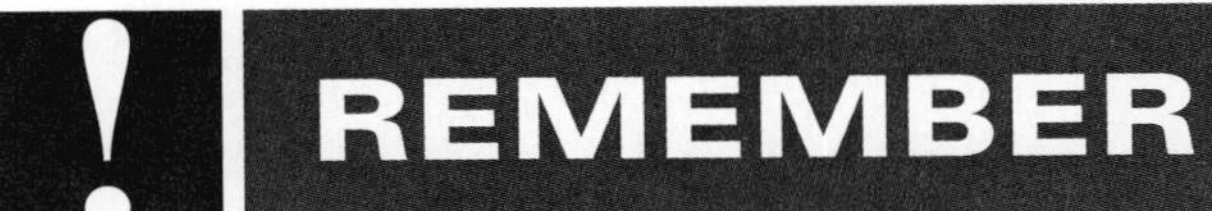

- Growth and development is relevant to persons of all ages, not only to children.

development of the fetus and the child's intellectual and emotional development after birth.

The psychologic experiences of the individual also influence development. Positive, open interpersonal relationships are advantageous to development. A person needs to have feelings of self-worth. The parent-child relationship is especially important in this area of development. Loving, caring parents meet the needs of their children and nurture them, providing a good foundation for meeting the world outside the home. Helping children meet the tasks of growing up gives them the security and confidence to handle situations that arise in life.

Social experiences within the family, peer group, and community greatly influence development. The child's gender and position in the family (oldest, middle, or youngest child) influence development. Parents generally treat boys and girls differently by providing gender-appropriate toys and having separate expectations of each gender. Generally, first-born children are greater achievers, and the rest of the children may be slower in motor and language development, usually because parents are more relaxed with each child's birth.

Family activities and outings and extended family get-togethers provide various social experiences. Peer groups such as Girl Scouts, Boy Scouts, school extracurricular activities, and church youth groups allow a child to experience different types of social situations. Community service and other volunteer service provide children and adults a chance to develop a much broader sense of their world. The use of the library or museum and attendance at theater productions and concerts develop another dimension of a person.

CONCEPTS

1. *Human beings are capable.* That is, human beings are born with the fundamental capabilities to survive and develop. A newborn is physiologically ready for breathing and taking nourishment. Crying brings assistance and care from parents through feeding, diaper changing, or cuddling. Responses between the infant and parent ensure the continuing parent-infant interaction needed for continued development.
2. *Human beings are similar.* Healthy children of the same age are generally at the same stage of growth and development. As age increases, the changes that occur in one child are very much the same as in other individuals of the same age-group. Fig. 9-1 depicts growth and development during the life-cycle.
3. *Human beings are individual.* Although persons of the same age are much the same in their growth and development, each person has an individual set of hereditary and environmental factors. A child may be ahead of the age-group because of heredity factors or parental interaction, interest, and stimulation. The child may also be behind the age-group because of heredity factors or lack of parental involvement. Older children have been influenced more by environmental factors than younger children.
4. *Growth and development are orderly and predictable.* Generally, growth and development are cephalocaudal, proximodistal (Fig. 9-2), and general to specific.

Cephalocaudal growth and development describes processes that begin at the head and move toward the feet. For instance, an infant controls the head before crawling and sits before walking.

Proximodistal growth and development describes the processes by which body parts near the midline develop before those distant from that point. For example, an infant learns to control arm movements before controlling finger movements.

General-to-specific growth and development is illustrated by infants who make sounds and noises before speaking. Another example is the fact that children walk before skipping or hopping.

Physical growth and development are easy to discern and gauge. Psychologic development occurs at the same time as physical growth and development, but it is much more difficult to see, measure, and nurture. Several theories are presented as a way to understand the influences on development.

Maslow

Abraham Maslow's theory of the **hierarchy of needs** is based on the premise that human beings have specific needs. If any of these needs remain unmet, they serve as a driving force or motivation for that individual. The individual then focuses energy and attention on attempting to meet the unmet need or needs. Meeting these needs help guide a person's behavior and thus development.

The needs identified by Maslow (1954) are physiologic, safety, belongingness and love, esteem, and self-actualization needs. Maslow organized these needs in a hierarchy of relative influence from the

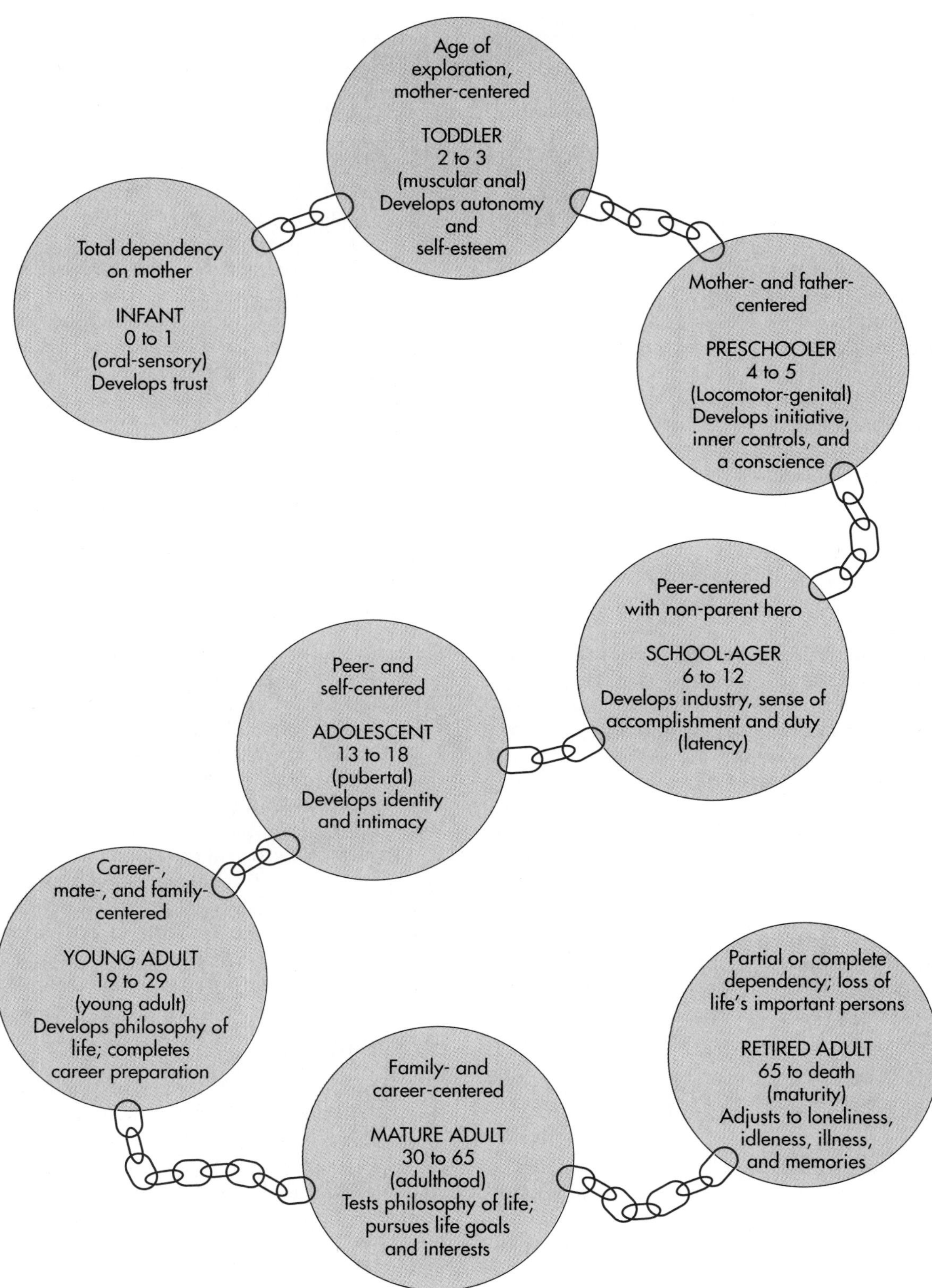

Fig. 9-1 The chain of life from infancy to old age. (Modified from the developmental theories of Freud and Erikson.)

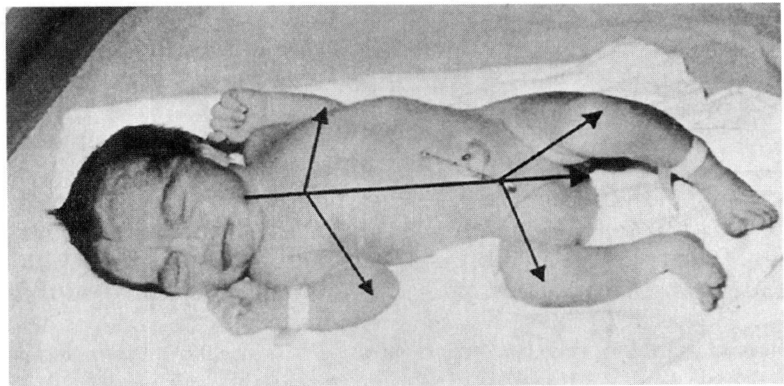

Fig. 9-2 Motor development is cephalocaudal and proximodistal.

most basic physiologic needs to the highest need for self-actualization. This highest need can be met only after the other needs have been satisfied.

Maslow did not identify the physiologic needs specifically. He felt that the list would be too long if every item was listed. However, in much of the literature, these needs are generally identified as oxygen, food, water, elimination, activity/rest/sleep, and sex. Sometimes these physiologic needs are called *survival needs.* Oxygen, food, water, elimination, and activity/rest/sleep must be met for the survival of the individual. The need for sex must be met for the survival of the human race. When the physiologic needs have been met, other, higher needs emerge and motivate the individual. A need that has been satisfied still exists as a potential need that may surface again if the person is deprived of that need. The individual is motivated only by unmet needs.

Maslow believes that most people have only partially satisfied their physiologic needs at any one time. Most individuals are less satisfied the higher one goes up the hierarchy of needs. The five needs are not met at a steadily progressive rate. Individuals may stay at one level for different lengths of time, depending on the situations in which they find themselves. In fact a person may go back to a lower level. An example of this would be a person who has reached self-actualization and who suddenly becomes ill and is having a great deal of difficulty breathing; meeting the physiologic need for oxygen becomes of prime importance to that individual. The need for safety is also partially unmet because of the disruption in the person's life.

When the physiologic needs have been relatively well met, a new need surfaces. That need is for safety. A person needs to feel secure in everyday life. To feel safe and secure, the individual must have structure, law and order, freedom from fear and anxiety, and stability in life. Illness is considered a threat to safety. It disrupts the order of a person's life and many times causes fear and anxiety.

If the physiologic and safety needs have been met fairly well, the need for belongingness and love emerges. Maslow stresses that love is not the same as sex. The individual wants affectionate relationships with other people. Participation in groups or organizations help meet these needs. The need for love requires both the giving and receiving of love to be met. Unmet love needs are often found in cases of mental illness.

The next need to emerge is the need for esteem. A person has a need for a stable and usually a high evaluation of the self—that is, for self-respect, self-esteem, and the esteem of others. Maslow divides these needs into two groups. One group includes the need for achievement, confidence, independence, and freedom. The second group includes the desire for reputation, status, recognition, attention, and appreciation. People need to feel good about themselves. They also need to know that others have good feelings about them. When esteem needs are met, the individual has feelings of self-confidence, worth, and capability and feels necessary in the world. Healthy self-esteem is based on deserved respect from others, competence, and adequacy for the task.

When all of these needs have been met, an individual may still feel discontented and restless. Maslow called this discontent the *need for self-actualization.* **Self-actualization** is self fulfillment, the need to become everything a person is capable of becoming. Self-actualized persons are content and satisfied with life. Their goals have been accomplished, and they are no longer motivated by their own personal needs but by the needs of society, by the good of the larger community. This need for self-actualization comes forth only after physiologic, safety, belongingness and love, and esteem needs have been satisfied.

Freud

The theory of development proposed by Sigmund Freud, who lived during the Victorian era, is called the ***psychosexual theory.*** Freud's work led him to believe that repressed sexual problems from childhood were the cause of problems later in life. According to Crain (1980), Freud's concept of sex was very broad. He included not only sexual intercourse but also anything that gives bodily pleasure. He called a person's general sexual energy ***libido.*** The libido begins developing at birth and goes through specific stages. Freud identified sexuality as the underlying motivation for behavior. Excessive gratification or excessive frustration at any stage may cause a **fixation** (a lasting preoccupation with the pleasures of that stage). Freud's theory includes psychosexual developmental stages. The stages identified by Freud follow:

1. *Oral stage (birth to 1 year of age):* All feelings are focused on and expressed by the mouth. Gratification and pleasure are gained through the mouth in the form of sucking, eating, and chewing. Sucking provides nourishment and so is necessary for life. Sucking needs vary in infants. Some are satisfied with sucking for nourishment; others suck fingers or pacifiers when they are not hungry. If a person's sucking needs are not met as an infant, the person may have habits centered on the mouth as an adult. Some of these habits are chewing gum, biting fingernails, and excessive eating or smoking.
2. *Anal stage (2 to 3 years of age):* When neuromuscular control over the anal sphincter begins to develop, the anal area is the focus of the child's sexual interests. The child becomes aware of the pleasurable sensations produced by a bowel movement. Children frequently take an interest in the products of their labors and enjoy smearing their feces. Toilet training is a crucial issue in this stage. A compromise between the pleasure of bowel function and the expectations of society must be reached. Crain believes that toilet training probably causes enough frustration to produce some measure of fixation in many children. For example, a child who fights toilet training and defecates when and where he pleases may become an impulsive, messy adult.
3. *Phallic stage (4 to 5 years of age):* A sexual identity begins to develop in this stage. The pleasure area changes from the anal sphincter to the genitals. Strong feelings develop toward the parent of the opposite gender, and a feeling of jealousy develops toward the parent of the same gender. This is called the *Oedipus complex* in males and the *Electra complex* in females. Children become aware of sexual differences in boys and girls during this stage. Freud believed that boys have a fear of castration and girls have "penis envy." Identifying with and imitating the parent of the same gender occurs at the end of this stage.
4. *Latency stage (6 to 12 years of age):* This is a quiet period for the libido. The child directs his energies toward socially acceptable activities such as school and sports. The refinement of roles and relationships is important in this stage.
5. *Genital stage (13 to 18 years of age):* Sexual interests are now renewed. Adolescence moves the child toward sexual maturity and toward adult sexual relationships. At this time, adolescents begin an emotional separation from parents and move toward independence.

Freud believed that the rest of a person's life was determined by the way that these early stages were handled as a child. Of course, parental care and influence during these stages is important.

Development of the mind was also important to Freud. He believed that the mind had three parts: the id, the ego, and the superego. The **id** controls the physical needs and instincts of the individual. The newborn is thought to have only id, wanting to have needs met immediately. The id has no sense of right or wrong. It is ruled by the pleasure principle and functions on the unconscious level.

The **ego** helps the individual deal with the world. It is the awareness of the conscious self that controls and guides the person's actions as it mediates between the physical needs and instincts of the id and the demands of society. Development of the ego begins in the first year of life through interactions with the environment. The ego continues to develop throughout childhood.

The **superego** begins to develop around 3 years of age and is fairly well developed by 10 years of age. It inhibits, regulates, and controls a person's impulses. The child gradually adopts behavioral, moral, and ethical standards learned from parents and society. The superego is often called the *conscience.* It helps the individual know right from wrong and functions on the conscious and unconscious levels.

Erikson

Erik Erikson (1963) sees human development as a continuous process taking place from birth to death and occurring in stages. His theory focuses on the psychosocial aspects of development and is known as the **psychosocial theory.** Each of Erikson's stages has a challenge or problem to be resolved. None of the problems is expected to be resolved in a totally favorable manner. Acceptable appropriate development is noted when the desirable alternative predominates over the undesirable alternative. Erikson's eight stages of development follow:

1. *Infancy—trust vs. mistrust:* During the first year, the challenge is to establish basic trust. Consis-

tent loving care by the parents or other caregivers is necessary for the development of trust. From trust in parents, the infant learns that the world is a safe and predictable place. Trust is necessary to develop the capacity to love others. When the infant's needs are not consistently met, mistrust is learned.

2. *Toddler—autonomy vs. shame and doubt:* Toddlers (2 to 3 years of age) who have learned to trust are ready to use their newly acquired motor skills to do things for themselves (for example, walking, climbing, feeding the self, and controlling bowel movements). Frequent use of the word *no* is the toddler's way of trying to control the environment. Family rules teach safety and acceptable behavior and thus increase independence. Constant disapproval of a toddler's efforts to be autonomous leads to feelings of shame and doubt.
3. *Preschool—initiative vs. guilt:* Having mastered trust and autonomy, preschool children (4 to 5 years old) are ready to explore the limits of their world. They are extremely curious and question everything. A vivid imagination is often evident. They begin to develop a conscience—the inner voice that warns and threatens. Guilt results when they are made to feel that their explorings, questions, or imaginings are bad.
4. *School-age—industry vs. inferiority:* School-age children (6 to 12 years of age) need and want achievement and are ready to develop social and scholastic skills. They learn to compete and cooperate with others when performing group assignments. Recognition for work well done is important to self-concept. Failure to achieve or to receive recognition for achievement results in feelings of inferiority.
5. *Adolescence—identity vs. role confusion:* During these years (13 to 18 years of age), rapid and marked physical changes occur. Adolescents become preoccupied with how they look. They struggle to find out "who they are," what they believe in, what their values are, and how they fit into society. They are influenced by their family and peers. Many times these influences are at odds with each other. Adolescents often feel that they must choose between their family and friends and are not comfortable choosing between these two important groups. Support from the family strengthens the adolescent's sense of identity and reinforces values. Selection of a career is also expected. Lack of support and difficulty in resolving conflicts may result in role confusion.
6. *Young adulthood—intimacy vs. isolation:* The development of an intimate love relationship and close relationships with friends, without fear of losing one's own identity, is the task of the young adult (19 to 29 years of age). Many times, the selection of a mate and marriage are the result of meeting the challenge of this stage. Establishing intimacy is affected by how the five earlier developmental tasks were accomplished. Without intimacy a person feels alone and isolated.
7. *Adulthood—generativity vs. stagnation:* Producing and nurturing the next generation is the primary way the challenge of this age group (30-65 years) is achieved. However, productivity at work, creative efforts, or caring for other groups are also ways of meeting this task. A lack of productivity, an uncharitable attitude, and self-absorption can result in stagnation.
8. *Old age—ego integrity vs. despair:* During this last stage (65 years of age and older) ego integrity is attained when a review of one's life brings feelings of satisfaction about and acceptance of one's past life. "Has my life been meaningful?" is the question to be answered at this stage. The question is not always answered positively. Disgust with oneself, bitterness about life, and fear of dying are characteristics of despair.

It would not be wise for a person to develop total trust with no mistrust. At times, mistrust is a healthy and safe response to a situation. In this way, a toddler learns autonomy. However, some doubt about individual abilities to handle certain situations may sometimes be a healthy and safe response. Indeed, learning to recognize such situations prevents accidents and injuries. Parental attitudes and the social environment affect the way an individual handles the challenges of each stage.

An individual's mastery of tasks can be altered at any time throughout life. For example, a child who is given little or no affection in infancy can grow up to be a normal adult if that child is given extra attention and affection at a later stage of development. This is important because the mastery of tasks is cumulative. That is, the way that a task is mastered in one stage affects the way that the person will be able to handle the task of the next stage.

Each of Erikson's eight stages has a specific challenge. Yet all the challenges are present throughout life. For example, trust is especially important to infants because they totally depend on others, but all through life a person must test the trustworthiness of others.

Every person must go through each stage, depending on the length of life. Usually, the forces of physical maturation and social expectations push an individual along whether success has been attained at earlier stages. Success at earlier stages increases the chance of success at later stages. That is why the first stage is so very important.

Havinghurst

Robert Havinghurst proposed that human individuals learn their way through life. At times the learning effort is strenuous. At other times, little effort is required. The tasks that an individual must learn are called ***developmental tasks*** (Havinghurst, 1953).

> They [developmental tasks] are the things a person must learn if he is to be judged and to judge himself to be a reasonably happy and successful person. A developmental task is a task which arises at or about a certain period in the life of an individual, successful achievement of which leads to his happiness and to success with later tasks, while failure leads to unhappiness in the individual, disapproval by society, and difficulty with later tasks.

Some of the developmental tasks arise mainly because of physical maturation. Examples include learning to walk, learning acceptable behavior toward the opposite gender, and (for women) adjusting to menopause.

Other developmental tasks arise primarily from the cultural pressure of society. Examples include learning to read and to be a socially responsible citizen.

A third source of developmental tasks are personal values and aspirations. As the self evolves, it becomes a force in the subsequent development of the individual. Examples include choosing and preparing for an occupation, achieving a scale of values, and developing a philosophy of life.

Thus developmental tasks may arise from physical maturation, cultural pressures, or the desires, aspirations, and values of the emerging personality. In most cases, the tasks arise from combinations of these factors acting together.

The developmental tasks that Havinghurst identified are listed. Most of the tasks still seem to apply. A few developmental tasks, especially those related to occupation and finances, would probably be listed under a different age group today.

Birth to 24 months
- Learning to walk
- Learning to take solid foods
- Learning to talk

18 months to 2 years
- Learning to control the elimination of body wastes
- Learning gender differences and sexual modesty
- Achieving physiologic stability
- Forming simple concepts of social and physical beauty
- Learning to relate oneself emotionally to others
- Learning to distinguish right and wrong and developing a conscience

6 to 12 years
- Learning physical skills needed for ordinary games
- Building wholesome attitudes toward oneself as a growing organism
- Learning to get along with age mates
- Learning an appropriate male or female role
- Developing skills to read, write, and calculate
- Developing concepts necessary for everyday living
- Developing conscience, morality, and values
- Achieving personal independence
- Developing attitudes toward social groups and institutions

12 to 18 years
- Achieving new and more mature relations with age mates of both genders
- Achieving a male or female social role
- Accepting the physical body and using it effectively
- Achieving emotional independence of parents and others
- Achieving ensurance of economic independence
- Selecting and preparing for an occupation
- Preparing for marriage and family life
- Developing the intellectual skills and concepts necessary for civic competence
- Desiring and achieving socially responsible behavior
- Acquiring values and ethics to guide behavior

18 to 40 years
- Selecting a mate
- Learning to live with a marriage partner
- Starting a family
- Rearing children
- Managing a home
- Getting started in an occupation
- Taking on civic responsibility
- Finding a congenial social group

40 to 65 years
- Achieving social and civic responsibility
- Establishing and maintaining an economic standard of living
- Assisting teenage children to become responsible and happy adults
- Developing adult leisure-time activities
- Relating oneself to one's spouse as a person
- Accepting and adjusting to physical changes
- Adjusting to aging parents

65 and older
- Adjusting to decreasing physical strength and health
- Adjusting to retirement and a reduced income
- Adjusting to the death of a spouse (or companion)
- Establishing explicit affiliation with one's age group
- Meeting social and civic obligations

Establishing a satisfactory physical living arrangement

Piaget

There are four major stages of human development according to Jean Piaget's theory of cognitive development. ***Cognitive*** refers to knowledge, perception or understanding. The spontaneous, automatic reflexes of the newborn begin this development. Habits formed by the young child continues the development. The older child uses knowledge and abstract thinking to solve complex problems. The four stages described by Piaget follow:

1. Sensorimotor (birth to 2 years old): A sense of cause and effect is developed. Learning evolves from tasting, touching, and feeling. The infant learns body movement control.
2. Preoperational (3 to 7 years old): Events and objects are interpreted in relation to the self.
3. Concrete operation (8 to 11 years old): Thinking becomes coherent and logical.
4. Formal operation (12 to 15 years old): Thinking is abstract, flexible, and adaptable. The child can solve complex problems.

STAGES

Newborn to 1 Year of Age

The first year of life is a time of rapid growth and development. Weight generally triples, and length increases approximately 9 inches by 1 year of age. The newborn (neonate) is unable to care for any needs and totally depends on parents or other caregivers. The reflex of sucking allows the neonate to receive nourishment. Other reflexes such as gagging, sneezing, and blinking are protective functions. Crying is the infant's means of communication.

All of the senses function at birth, with hearing and touch being the best developed. Infants have a great need to be touched. The neonate's response to the parents' voices and touch gives the parents confidence in their caregiving.

Controlling the head, rolling over, sitting, crawling, standing, and taking a few steps are all generally accomplished during this first year (Fig. 9-3). The diet changes from milk to solid foods, and communication changes from crying and noises to a few words.

This age closely parallels Freud's oral stage, as well as Erikson's infancy stage with the challenge of trust versus mistrust.

1 to 2 Years of Age

Growth slows considerably at this time. The appetite decreases in response to the slowing of growth. Parents sometimes worry about this change in appetite, but it is an expected change and should cause no problems. Walking alone with confidence is accomplished during this year. By the age of 2 years, a child can run and can climb stairs one at a time. The child begins self-feeding with a spoon and tries to help with dressing. The toddler is curious but has a short attention span. Safety in the environment should be foremost in the minds of those caring for children of this age-group.

Temper tantrums are common. This reaction to authority comes from the child's frustration at not being allowed to do what he wants to do. Tantrums may signal that the child is beginning to work on Erikson's challenge of autonomy versus shame and doubt. The vocabulary of a 2 year old is about 300 words, and the use of a pencil or crayon results in scribbles. Play is an individual activity at this age.

2 to 3 Years of Age

Weight increases about 5 lb, and height increases about 3 inches during this year. All 20 baby teeth have generally erupted by 3 years of age, and the child eats three meals a day with the family. Self-feeding is accomplished without too much mess.

Most authorities agree that toilet training should not be started until 2 years of age. Physical and psychologic readiness are not present until this time. By age 3, most children can take themselves to the toilet during the day, but they may need help at night. Freud's anal stage is usually associated with this age-group.

A vocabulary of about 900 words is established by 3 years of age. Several words may be joined together, but complete sentences are not yet used. The child can use scissors and can dress and undress without much help. Children of this age like to play near other children but not with them. This is called *parallel play.*

3 to 4 Years of Age

Growth in weight and height are about 5 lb and 3 inches during this year. Motor coordination greatly increases. The child buttons clothes, laces shoes, brushes teeth, and attempts to print letters (Fig. 9-4).

The 4 year old has a vocabulary of 1500 words. Mild profanities may be used, and name-calling often occurs. Children at this age ask questions almost constantly, many over and over.

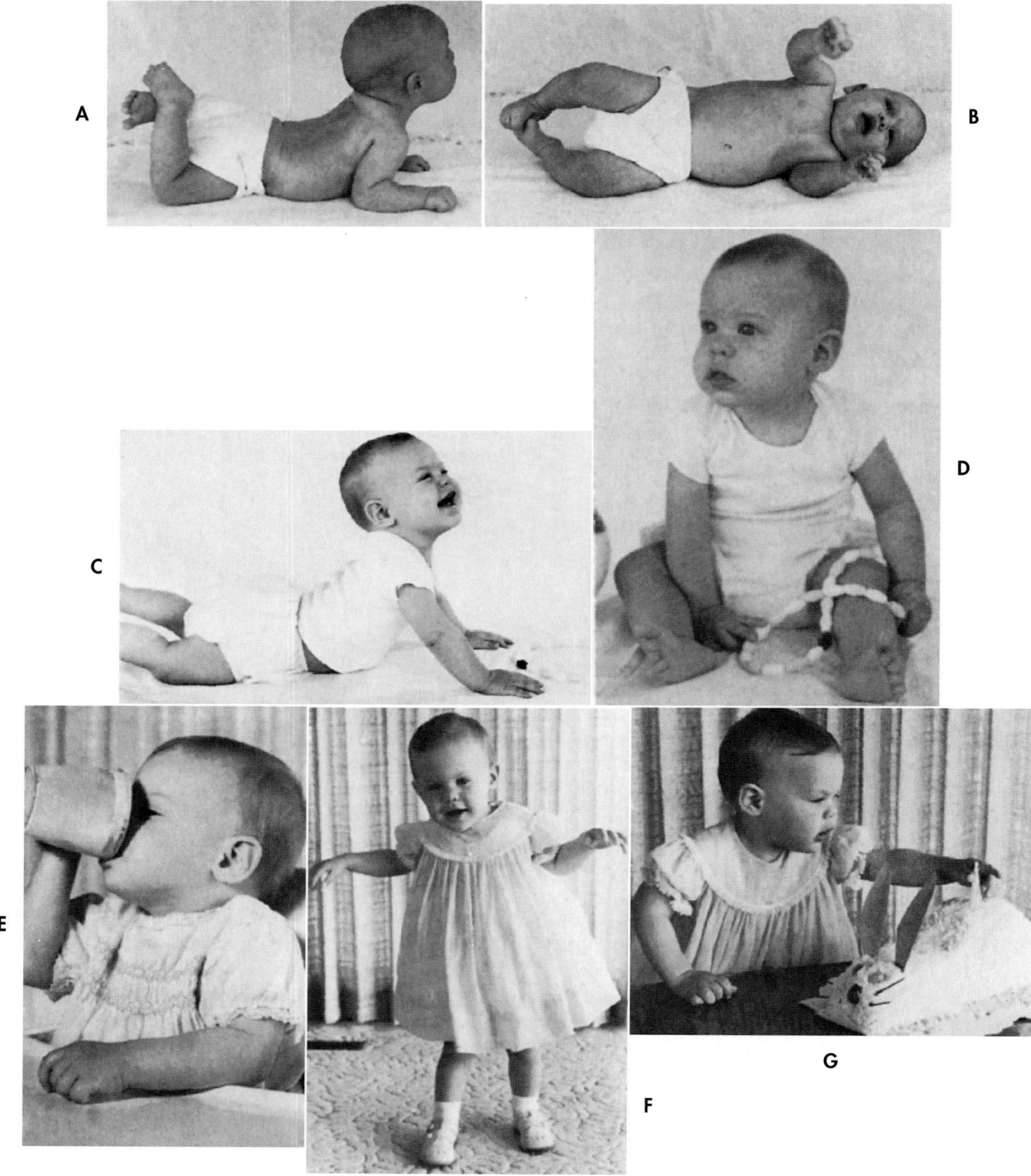

Fig. 9-3 Infant at 3 months: Raises head when prone, supports self on forearms **(A)** and turns from back to side **(B).** Infant at 7 months: Propels self forward on abdomen (crawling) **(C)** and sits alone without support **(D).** Infant at 12 months: Drinks from cup with ease **(E),** walks alone with wide stance and short steps **(F),** and has good finger-thumb opposition **(G).** (From Novak JC, Broom BL: *Ingalls and Salerno's maternal and child health nursing,* ed 8, St Louis, 1995, Mosby.)

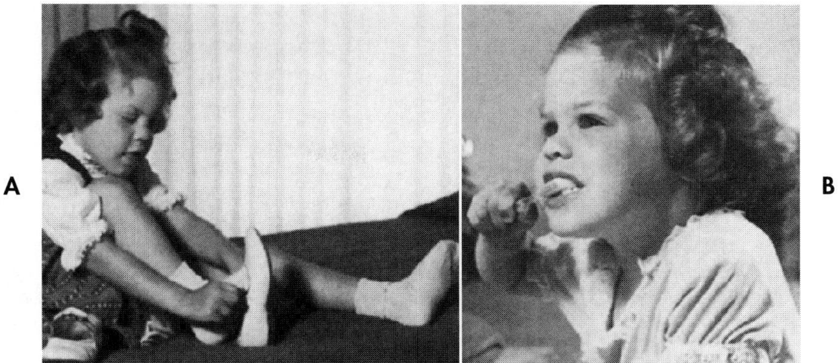

Fig. 9-4 Child 3 to 4 years of age. **A,** Can put shoes on. **B,** Can brush teeth. (From Novak JC, Broom BL: *Ingalls and Salerno's maternal and child health nursing,* ed 8, St Louis, 1995, Mosby.)

Number concepts develop, and the child can count to four. One or two colors can usually be named. Recognizable drawings are made but are without detail. Children of this age-group begin to imitate the activities of adults. They want to "help." Playing with other children and sharing toys begins. Imaginary playmates are common. Meeting Erikson's challenge of initiative versus guilt begins at this age and takes several years to be achieved. Freud's phallic stage is generally thought to also begin at this age.

4 to 5 Years of Age

Weight increases about 5 lb, and height increases 3 inches during this year. Fine motor coordination begins to develop, and children learn to print their own names and perhaps a few other words. They can tie shoelaces and wash their faces and hands without getting their clothing wet.

Vocabulary increases to 2100 words. The 5 year old talks constantly and in complete sentences. Fewer questions are asked, and they are more relevant.

Children can count to 10 and know four or more colors. They show interest in the relationship of relatives such as aunts, cousins, and grandparents. They enjoy having story books read to them.

The conscience begins to develop at this age. The child starts to accept values learned from parents. Right can be distinguished from wrong, and guilt is felt for actions that go against these values.

6 to 9 Years of Age

Weight increases 3 to 6 lb a year, and height increases 1 to 2 inches. Baby teeth are gradually lost and replaced by permanent teeth. The 6 year old is eager to try anything new but is easily distracted by things in the environment. The child of this age is clumsy and awkward at motor activities.

The 9 year old is independent, self-reliant, capable, and trustworthy. This child plays hard, works hard, and finishes jobs that are started. Eye-hand coordination is fully developed, as is good timing and control in motor activities.

Although unpredictable behavior is characteristic of the 6 year old, the 9 year old is sociable, understands empathy and sympathy, and has acceptable manners. School formally guides the increase in cognitive skills. The child's attention span increases with age, and work is evaluated in relationship to others.

All of the needs identified by Maslow are important to the child, with the exception of self-actualization. This period is the beginning of Freud's latency stage. Erikson's challenge of industry versus inferiority becomes important.

10 to 12 Years of Age

Boys usually grow at the same rate in weight and height as the previous age-group. Girls, however, may begin to develop sexually. This is characterized by a growth spurt, budding of the breasts, widening of the hips, growing of pubic hair, and sometimes the beginning of **menses** (menstruation).

Secret clubs and close friendships with others of the same gender are very important. Boys "hate" girls, and girls have no use for boys. Intense physical activity and competition are characteristic of this age-group. Generally, school is an enjoyable activity. Interests expand from family and community to nature, science, travel, and the world. The conscience is very well developed.

13 to 16 Years of Age

This is a period of transition characterized by the dramatic physical changes of puberty and the beginning of complex emotional and social development.

This transition takes time and is often a stormy period for the child and parent. Conflicting forces make it difficult for the child to work out a personal value system. Peer pressure is a great influence as independence from parental authority is attempted. Crushes on the opposite gender begin to occur.

Boys may begin to develop sexually at this age. This is characterized by an increase in genital size; beginning of rapid weight and height growth; broadening of the chest; swelling of the breasts; growing of chest, pubic and facial hair; production of spermatozoa; and nocturnal emissions (wet dreams). Voice changes also become noticeable. Full growth and maturity, however, have not been attained.

Growth for girls stops about 16 years of age, with a gain in weight during the past 4 years of 15 to 55 lb and an increase in height of 2 to 8 inches. Physical maturity is attained by most girls at this age.

Recreational activities, including competitive sports, are important in this age group. These activities provide a way to gain confidence and independence and to learn about team effort and cooperation.

This adolescent period is what Freud called the *genital stage.* Erikson described identity versus role confusion as the challenge to be accomplished.

17 to 20 Years of Age

Weight gain is about 15 to 65 lb during these years. Growth in height for boys generally stops about 20 years of age, after a growth spurt of 4 to 12 inches. Physical maturity is attained by most boys in this period. Becoming comfortable with physical growth is important.

Children usually attain emotional independence from their parents. More stable intimate relationships outside the family are established. A relationship with a specific person of the opposite gender often occurs. This is considerably different from the crushes of earlier ages.

Life goals and tasks are beginning to take shape. Young adults of this age begin to make decisions about careers, further education, and life styles. There is a definite move toward independence from the family.

21 to 25 Years of Age

Deciding on a career or vocation is the focus of much activity and time in this age group. Leaving the parents' home may also be a major decision. This decision is influenced by finances, education, and relationships. Some children leave home and do not move back. Other children leave and return once or twice. Sometimes the parents must force a child to leave their home. Occasionally, it may be acceptable or necessary for a child to live with the parents as an adult.

26 to 35 Years of Age

Being a productive member of society becomes important at this time. Activities in community functions increase. People with growing families spend a great deal of time involved in activities with their children. There is also pressure to advance in one's chosen career. Many people find it difficult to balance the time necessary to advance their career and the time and energy needed to meet family obligations. Stress on family relationships often results. The challenge of intimacy versus isolation, identified by Erikson, should be accomplished.

36 to 65 Years of Age

From the time a person reaches maturity, a gradual aging of all body tissues and organs occurs. The rate and extent of aging varies from person to person. Not much attention is paid to this stage until some tell-tale signs of aging appear. Things such as graying hair, a receding hairline, and glasses remind a person that he is growing older. Metabolism slows down, resulting in excess weight gain if one's diet is not changed (Table 9-2).

Menopause (the stopping of menses) is another change with which the older woman must cope. The change in hormone levels may result in hot flashes, mood swings, insomnia, or anxiety. **Osteoporosis,** the loss of calcium from the bone, may result in bones breaking easily.

Many people review their life's goals during this time. Some make deliberate, even drastic changes in their careers, lifestyles, and/or marriages. When children leave home, parents may find themselves alone and feeling useless. However, this can be a wonderful time for travel, creativity, and doing things the person wanted to do but never had time to do.

Planning for retirement should begin several years before the anticipated date. For instance, to prepare, a person should gradually give up some responsibilities in the workplace and begin interests in new activities or renew interests in cherished activities. The developmental challenge Erikson identified to be accomplished by this age group is generativity versus stagnation.

65 Years of Age and Older

People are living longer and have better health now than in the past. Without the pressures of a ca-

Table 9-2 NORMAL PHYSICAL CHANGES OF AGING

System	Normal Findings
Integument	
Skin color	Spotty pigmentation in areas exposed to sun; pallor even in absence of anemia
Moisture	Dry, scaly condition
Temperature	Cooler extremities; decreased perspiration
Texture	Decreased elasticity; wrinkles; folding, sagging condition
Fat distribution	Decreased amount on extremities; increased amount on abdomen
Hair	Thinning and graying on scalp; often, decreased amount of axillary and pubic hair and hair on extremities; decreased facial hair in men; possible chin and upper lip hair in women
Nails	Decreased growth rate
Head and neck	
Head	Sharp and angular nasal and facial bones; loss of eyebrow hair in women; bushier eyebrows in men
Eyes	Decreased visual acuity; decreased accommodation; reduced adaptation to darkness; diminished light reflex; sensitivity to glare
Ears	Decreased pitch discrimination; diminished hearing acuity
Nose and sinuses	Increased nasal hair; decreased sense of smell
Mouth and pharynx	Use of bridges or dentures; decreased sense of taste; atrophy of papillae of lateral edges of tongue
Neck	Nodular thyroid gland; slight tracheal deviation resulting from muscle atrophy
Thorax and lungs	Increased anteroposterior diameter; increased chest rigidity; increased respiratory rate with decreased lung expansion; increased airway resistance
Heart and vascular system	Significant increase in systolic pressure with slight increase in diastolic pressure; usually, insignificant changes in heart rate at rest; common diastolic murmurs; easily palpated peripheral pulses; weaker pedal pulses and colder lower extremities, especially at night
Breasts	Diminished breast tissue; pendulous, flabby condition
Gastrointestinal system	Decreased salivary secretions, which may make swallowing more difficult; decreased peristalsis; decreased production of digestive enzymes, including hydrochloric acid, pepsin, and pancreatic enzymes; constipation; reduced motility
Reproductive system	
Female	Decreased estrogen; decreased uterine size; decreased secretions; atrophy of epithelial lining of vagina
Male	Decreased levels of testosterone; decreased sperm count; decreased testicular size
Urinary system	Decreased renal filtration and renal efficiency; subsequent loss of protein from kidney; nocturia; decreased bladder capacity; increased incontinence
Female	Urgency and stress incontinence resulting from decrease in perineal muscle tone
Male	Urinary frequency and retention resulting from prostatic enlargement
Musculoskeletal system	Decreased muscle mass and strength; bone demineralization (more pronounced in women); shortening of trunk as result of intervertebral space narrowing; decreased joint mobility; decreased range of joint motion; enhanced bony prominences
Neurologic system	Decreased rate of voluntary or automatic reflexes; decreased ability to respond to multiple stimuli; insomnia; shorter sleeping periods

From Potter PA, Perry AG: *Fundamentals of nursing: concepts, process, and practice,* ed 3, St Louis, 1993, Mosby. Modified from Ebersole P, Hess P: *Toward healthy aging: human needs and nursing response,* ed 4, St Louis, 1994, Mosby.

reer, a person of this age-group has time for a productive life at a more leisurely pace. More physical changes take place as a person ages. Vision and hearing become less acute. There is some loss of muscle control. Often the chin and face sag, and the skin becomes wrinkled and dry.

Lifestyle may need to be altered as physical and income changes occur. It is important to be as active as possible. Development of interests or activities gives meaning to life and a feeling of self-worth (Fig. 9-5). Many older adults live on fixed incomes that may not meet their needs. Sometimes it is dif-

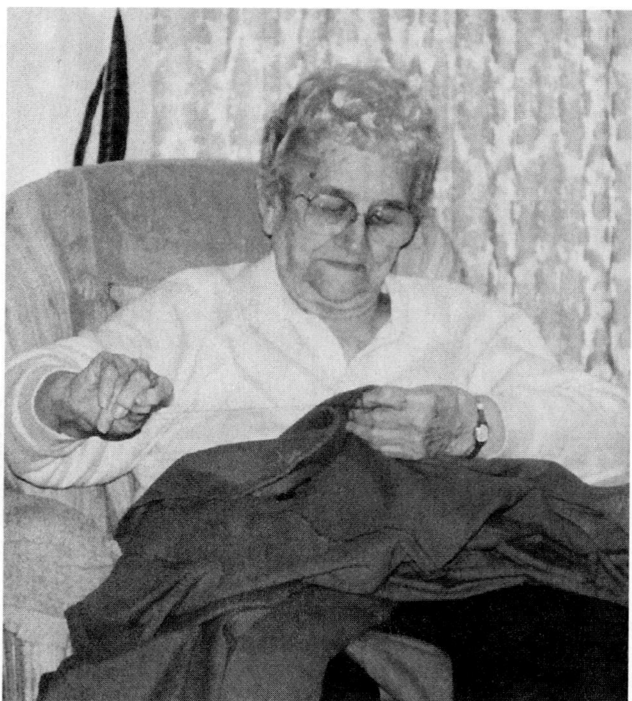

Fig. 9-5 Sewing is this older adult's favorite activity. (From Potter PA, Perry AG: *Fundamentals of nursing: concepts, process, and practice,* ed 3, St Louis, 1993, Mosby.)

ficult for an older person who has been independent to ask for or accept help from family or social service agencies.

As a person ages, interpersonal relationships change. Their children are adults and should be treated as such. The death of a spouse or peers brings the inevitability of death into focus. The older one becomes, the fewer peers are still alive. It is important to have friends of all ages.

Most communities have senior citizen centers with planned activities. Often a noon meal is served for a nominal fee. Many community colleges offer educational programs specifically for the older adult, often at no cost to the individual. Elderhostel programs offer travel and educational opportunities. Information about their programs can be requested from Elderhostel, 75 Federal Street, Boston, MA 02110. Staying active is a key to staying healthy.

Each person prepares for death in unique ways. Some are very open about plans for possessions and even plans for a funeral. It is important for family members to listen and not ignore the older person because of their own discomfort with the topic. Others prefer to give cherished items to family and friends while they are still alive.

NURSING PROCESS THROUGH THE LIFE SPAN

Assessment

Illness and hospitalization can be stressful experiences regardless of a patient's age. Assessment of the patient's developmental level enables the nurse to determine the patient's ability to understand, cooperate with, and if possible, assume responsibility for immediate and long-term care needs. A patient's previous experience with hospitalization and illness, coping skills, and the availability of support resources are also factors that should be considered during assessment.

Nursing Diagnosis

Nursing diagnoses are addressed in order of priority, with the most pressing problems being given attention first. Maslow's theory of human needs may be used to prioritize nursing diagnoses, which may include the following:

Altered family processes
Altered growth and development
Decisional conflict (specify)
Impaired social interaction
Ineffective family coping: compromised
Ineffective individual coping

Planning

The nursing care plan is based on the nurse's assessment of the patient's overall condition, as well as psychosocial factors and human growth and development. The degree to which a patient participates in planning care depends on developmental level and physiologic and psychologic status. Parents or caregivers of young patients must take part in planning care because young children may not be able to express their feelings and needs. The plan of care may include the following goal and expected outcome:

Goal: Patient progresses through normal growth and development levels.

Outcome

Patient accomplishes age-appropriate developmental tasks.

Implementation

When implementing the goals of care that have been established, the nurse should consider the patient's specific developmental status. A child's devel-

PATIENT TEACHING

- Encourage child to participate in bathing, dressing, and feeding.
- Promote social interaction with other children in the playroom.
- Provide play equipment and favorite toys from home to develop fine and gross motor skills.

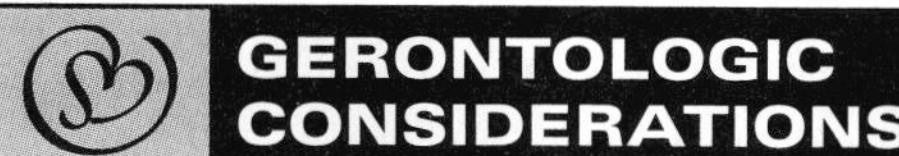

GERONTOLOGIC CONSIDERATIONS

- The steps of the nursing process should be implemented at a slower pace, depending on the older adult's functioning ability.
- When planning care, the older adult's own goals, desires, and coping skills should be considered.
- The nurse needs to have an awareness of how environmental factors affect the older person's function and health status.

■ NURSING CARE PLAN ■

ALTERED GROWTH AND DEVELOPMENT

Johnny, 4 years old, has ceased growing since having a debilitating disease and an extensive, long-term rehabilitation.

NURSING DIAGNOSIS

Altered growth and development related to physical disability as evidenced by altered physical growth, delay in developmental skills, lack of stimulation from parents, and inability to carry out self-care according to developmental level

GOAL

- Patient will assist in determining ability to participate in daily activities according to age and progress.

EXPECTED OUTCOMES

- Child performs skills appropriate to age.
- Patient participates in rehabilitative activities.

NURSING INTERVENTIONS

- Provide age-appropriate activities in which child may participate.
- Assess child by body systems to determine his ability to participate in activity.

EVALUATION

- Child performs skills appropriate to age.
- Child participates in play activities according to development.

opmental progress may be impeded by illness or hospitalization (see care plan). The nurse can implement interventions to promote growth and development (see teaching box). The needs of the older adult should also be considered during implementation, with special attention given to any limitations that a patient may have (see gerontologic box).

Evaluation

The nurse evaluates the patient's response to the interventions and thus determines the effectiveness of the plan of care. Since the patient's condition may change, the nurse must always be prepared to revise the care plan based on the evaluation. An example of a goal and evaluative measure follows:

Goal: Patient progresses through normal growth and development levels.

Evaluative measure

Conduct physical examination of select body systems.

SUMMARY

Knowledge of growth and development is especially important for the nurse in working with and providing nursing care for individuals in all age groups. In the same way that it is necessary to know the parts of the body and ways that they function, it is important to know the physical changes, thinking, and behavior appropriate for a patient's age.

This knowledge is used when assessing patients so that deviations from any norm can be identified. During an illness, a patient may regress to an earlier, more comfortable stage of development. The planning of appropriate nursing interventions is enhanced with this knowledge. Nursing care is then individualized to meet not only the physical needs, but also the developmental needs of the patient.

Key Concepts

- Growth and development are interdependent.
- Growth and development occur in an orderly and predictable manner throughout life.
- Maslow's theory of the hierarchy of needs states that unmet needs motivate behavior and that physiologic needs must be met first.
- Freud's psychosexual theory of development identifies sexuality as the motivation for behavior.
- Erikson's psychosocial theory of development has stages throughout life with a challenge to be met in each stage.
- Havinghurst's theory of developmental tasks is based on his belief that individuals learn their way through life.

Critical Thinking Questions

1. Discuss the concept of the family as patient. Suggest ways the nurse can focus on family development and assess family health.
2. Think of the family in which you grew up. Describe the values and attitudes you learned in this environment and the influence they may have on how you view your patient's family and health practices.
3. Sara is a 1-week-old newborn hospitalized for low birth weight. What measures can the nurse use to help develop attachment between Sara and her family (mother, father, and 4-year-old brother)?
4. Steven is a 4-year-old boy admitted for open heart surgery in 2 days. Describe the approach the nurse should use to prepare him for the procedures and care measures involved with surgery and to help him to cope with the required separation from his family and home.

REFERENCES AND SUGGESTED READINGS

Cole T: *The journey of life: a cultural history of aging in America,* Cambridge, 1992, Cambridge University Press.

Craig C: *Human development,* ed 6, Englewood Cliffs, NJ, 1992, Prentice-Hall.

Crain WC: *Theories of development,* Englewood Cliffs, NJ, 1980, Prentice-Hall.

Erikson EH: *Childhood and society,* ed 2, New York, 1963, Norton.

Havinghurst R: *Human development and education,* New York, 1953, Longmans, Green.

Kalman N, Waugfield CG: *Mental health concepts,* ed 3, Albany, 1993, Delmar.

Marks MG: *Broadribb's introductory pediatric nursing,* ed 4, Philadelphia, 1994, Lippincott.

Maslow A: *Motivation and personality,* New York, 1954, Harper & Row.

Novak JC, Broom BL: *Ingalls and Salerno's maternal and child health nursing,* ed 8, St Louis, 1995, Mosby.

Thompson E, Ashwill J: *Pediatric nursing: an introductory text,* ed 6, Philadelphia, 1992, Saunders.

Weiland S: Erik Erikson: ages, stages, and stories, *Generations,* 17:17, 1993.

CHAPTER 10

Loss and Grief

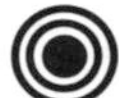

Learning Objectives

After studying this chapter, the student should be able to . . .

- Define the key terms.
- Discuss aspects of loss, grief, death, and dying.
- Describe the types and causes of loss.
- Discuss nurses' attitudes toward loss and caring for terminally ill patients.
- Explain the physical, psychosocial, and spiritual implications of loss.
- Discuss the physical, emotional, and spiritual needs of the terminally ill patient.
- Identify the signs and symptoms of impending death.
- Describe the measures used to provide emotional support to the grieving family.
- Discuss the nursing diagnoses related to patients and families experiencing loss.

Key Terms

Active euthanasia
Advance directive
Anticipatory grieving
Apnea
Autopsy
Cardiopulmonary resuscitation (CPR)
Coping
Death
Do not resuscitate (DNR)
Durable power of attorney for health care
Dying
Dysfunctional grieving
Euthanasia
Grief
Grieving process
Health care proxy
Hospice
Legal death
Living will
Loss
Passive euthanasia
Postmortem
Rigor mortis
Sudden death

Skills

10-1 Caring for the patient who is dying
10-2 Assessing the time of the patient's death
10-3 Caring for the body after death

CONCEPTS OF LOSS AND GRIEF

Loss and its major manifestations—grief, death, and dying—are encountered frequently, if not daily, in nursing practice. Therefore nurses must understand these concepts and their causes, ways that people experience them, and appropriate nursing interventions to help people deal with them.

Definitions

Loss is the lack or absence of something usually present (for example, a person, body part or function, role, emotion, or object). As with stress, loss may have a positive or a negative connotation. Parents are happy when a child graduates from high school, yet feel sad because the child has more outside interests and needs them less (maturational loss). Decreased mobility because of a fractured ankle limits freedom. Retirement from a job that was "one's life" can result in feelings of decreased self-esteem and aimlessness. Death can be the ultimate loss for the individual and a situational loss for persons who loved the deceased.

Grief

Grief is a set of physical and emotional responses to loss, separation, or bereavement. The physical symptoms of this nearly universal reaction are similar to those of stress because of sympathetic nervous system stimulation (increased heart rate, respiration, blood flow to muscles, and energy; dilated pupils; perspiration; and slowed digestion). Emotional responses range from alarm, denial, anger, and guilt to adjustment or acceptance.

Death

Death is the end of life and all vital processes. Advances in technology (for example, external stimulation to maintain heart and respiratory rates) have made the determination of death more complex and have raised many ethical and legal issues. **Legal death** is the total absence of brain activity as assessed and pronounced by a physician. **Sudden death** is the unexpected cessation of life.

Apnea, or absence of breathing, is a symptom of impending or actual death. An **autopsy** is a **postmortem** (after death) examination of the body and its organs to determine or confirm the cause of death. Autopsies are usually required in cases of unexpected death. ***Rigor mortis*** refers to the stiffening of muscles that results in fixed facial expressions and difficulty in moving joints after death.

Dying is the process of nearing death and the cessation of life. Frequently people are more afraid of dying, especially of being in pain, being dependent, or being alone, than of death itself.

Euthanasia, sometimes called "good death" or "mercy killing," is controversial. **Active euthanasia** is taking direct measures (such as an overdose of medication) to end life. **Passive euthanasia,** or letting one die, may involve withholding or withdrawing treatments that would prolong life unnecessarily. The intent is not to cause death but to allow the patient to be more comfortable and to die "naturally." Supportive interventions, such as comfort measures, should be given.

Nature of Loss

Loss may be described in many ways. One type includes the loss of external objects (books, jewelry, money), a familiar environment (school, neighborhood, place of work), a significant other (parent, sibling, spouse, friend, pet), a part of the self (limb, organ, sense, memory), or life itself. Losses may be physiologic (body structure, function), psychologic (identity, self-esteem, position), sociocultural (role, ethnic identity, divorce, death of significant other), or material (theft, misplacement of or damage to belongings). Losses may be natural or maturational (height, weight, graduation, teeth, hair color, death), accidental (natural disaster, automobile crash), or intentional (marriage, move to a new area, surgery, divorce, crime). Regardless of the cause, loss necessitates a change in a person's perception of and relationship with others and the environment. **Coping,** or how one deals with the loss, is influenced by many factors (see box), including previous coping behaviors.

FACTORS INFLUENCING LOSS EXPERIENCES

- Childhood experiences
- Significance assigned to the loss
- Physical and emotional state
- Accumulated loss experience
- View of loss as crisis
- Visibility
- Duration and timing
- Abruptness or suddenness
- Financial impact
- Availability of resources
- Cultural factors
- Personal attributes
- Relationship with the lost person

From Christensen BL, Kockrow EO: *Foundations of nursing*, ed 2, St Louis, 1995, Mosby.

Grieving Process

The **grieving process,** the physiologic and psychologic response to a loss, occurs over time. In chronic or terminal illnesses the process may begin before death and is called ***anticipatory grieving.*** This type of grief is not resolved until after life has ended. **Dysfunctional grieving** is an ineffective resolution of a loss.

Kübler-Ross' five stages of dying clearly illustrate the phases in dealing with loss: denial, anger, bargaining, depression, and acceptance. Behaviors indicating these stages are presented in Table 10-1. Many people do not progress in order from one stage to the next, some may return to a prior stage, and some may not resolve their grief. The nurse assesses the patient's and family's grieving response to best determine nursing interventions. For example, readiness to learn is a prerequisite for teaching. A person in denial is not ready to learn, so effective teaching cannot occur in this stage. In contrast, a person in the bargaining stage is a prime candidate for teaching.

Knowledge of these stages can help the nurse provide better emotional care for dying patients. After identifying the stage the patient is trying to work through, the nurse can understand and accept the patient's behavior and take appropriate nursing measures to help the patient cope. The patient works through these stages, ideally reaching acceptance of death.

Table 10-1 BEHAVIORS REPRESENTATIVE OF KÜBLER-ROSS' STAGES OF DYING

Stage	Behaviors
Denial	Avoids reality, cannot deal with decisions about treatment; may attempt activities for which one is no longer physically capable; isolates self from sources of accurate information; fails to comply with medical therapy; uses considerable emotional energy to deny truth; may appear artificially happy.
Anger	May retaliate against family members, nursing staff, or physicians; becomes demanding and accusing; anger may arouse guilt because patient is aware of dependence on caregivers; guilt may foster feelings of anxiety and low self-esteem.
Bargaining	Is fearful of losing body functions, experiencing uncontrollable pain, and losing control; is willing to do anything to change prognosis or fate; accepts new forms of therapies.
Depression	Recognizes potential loss of loved ones; may withdraw from important relationships to avoid painful feelings; may become quiet and noncommunicative when feeling loss of control; may express feelings of loneliness; does little to maintain appearance; may become suicidal when unrealistic hopes of a cure fade.
Acceptance	Accepts terms of death; begins to make plans for death (for example, writes a will, completes financial arrangements for the family, gives up personal possessions); is able to discuss feelings about death; reminisces about the past.

From Perry AG, Potter PA: *Clinical nursing skills and techniques,* ed 3, St Louis, 1994, Mosby.

NURSING PROCESS IN LOSS AND GRIEF

Assessment

The nurse begins providing care to the grieving patient by collecting subjective and objective data about the meaning of loss to the patient and family or significant others. The nurse interviews the patient and family, observing their responses and behaviors.

The nurse should recognize that each emotion helps the patient cope with loss. The patient's behaviors guide nursing interventions.

Nursing Diagnosis

The nurse gathers data to identify a pattern of characteristics that will lead to a diagnosis. Possible nursing diagnoses for loss and grief include the following:

Altered family processes
Anticipatory grieving
Hopelessness
Ineffective family coping: compromised
Sleep pattern disturbance
Social isolation
Spiritual distress (distress of the human spirit)

Planning

Nursing care is planned to meet the physiologic, emotional, developmental, and spiritual needs of the grieving patient. Whatever loss a patient has experienced or is facing, the nurse can use resources for the plan of care. Friends, family, clergy, support groups, and even legal consultants can assist (see care plan on p. 137).

The plan of care focuses on achieving specific goals and outcomes that relate to the identified nursing diagnoses. Examples of these include the following:

Goal #1: Patient resolves grief within 2 months.
Outcome
Patient participates in decision making and cooperates with recommended treatments within 1 month.

Goal #2: Patient maintains hope.
Outcome
Patient verbalizes finding meaning in life.

Implementation

Therapeutic communication is an important nursing intervention to assist the grieving and dying patient in coping with loss. The nurse's words and actions convey acceptance of the patient's and family's grief reactions. For example, if a patient begins to cry, the nurse quietly offers support and does

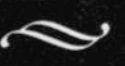 PATIENT TEACHING

- Describe ways the family can promote the patient's comfort, such as frequent rest periods and repositioning.
- Teach the family to recognize signs and symptoms to expect as the patient approaches death and information on whom to call in an emergency.
- Discuss ways to support the dying person and listen to needs and fears.
- Solicit questions from the family and provide information as needed.

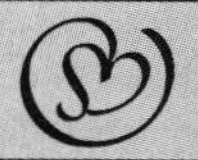

GERONTOLOGIC CONSIDERATIONS

- Many older adults have religious beliefs that may influence their responses to death and dying. Spiritual counselors should be available if one is desired.
- The older adult may experience many losses that result in a grief response. These include loss of job, possessions, home, friends, spouse, and autonomy. The older adult often needs emotional support to cope with grief.

not abandon the patient when comfort needs are the greatest.

Nursing care of the terminally ill patient can be demanding and stressful. It is important for the nurse to recognize the value of family members as resources and assist them in working with the dying person (see teaching box). The special needs of the older adult must also be considered (see gerontologic box).

Evaluation

Most patients are often under the care of a nurse for only a short time. It may help the nurse to remember that grieving is an individual process and that resolving loss does not proceed according to a set schedule.

The nurse refers to the goals and outcomes identified when planning care and performs measures designed to evaluate the achievement of those goals. Examples of goals, outcomes, and evaluative measures relating to the goals previously established include the following:

Goal #1: Patient resolves grief within 2 months.
Evaluative measures
Observe patient discussing loss with significant other.
Ask patient to talk about feelings of loss.

Goal #2: Patient maintains hope.
Evaluative measure
Ask patient to describe actions taken to achieve hope (for example, prayer).

DEATH AND DYING

The physician is usually responsible for informing the patient and family (at the patient's request) of the terminal nature of a condition and impending death. Ideally, the professional nurse is present when the patient and family are told. Thus the nurse can provide accurate clarification of the information, emotionally support the patient and family, and plan other appropriate nursing interventions (Skill 10-1).

Issues of Control and Power

Conflict arises about who should be told what information and when. The patient's right to know should be respected. If a patient asks, "Am I going to die?" the nurse should ask why the patient questions or thinks this. A "yes" or "no" answer should be avoided until more information is known about the reason for the question. Once the patient and family have been told the prognosis, the nurse works with them and other members of the health care team in planning for the death and in resolving grief.

People were once considered dead when their heartbeats and breathing stopped. The introduction of **cardiopulmonary resuscitation (CPR)** to restore circulation and respiration in a healthy individual who "suddenly died" created hope. However, the application of CPR and other advances in pharmacology, technology, and treatments have created ethical and legal issues related to control and power over death and dying and dying with dignity.

Advance directives are measures to enable persons to make decisions about their care when they may be incapacitated in the future. The Patient Self Determination Act, which became effective in December 1991, was created to provide for such decision making. This act mandates that health care agencies explain the individual's right to control decision making and offer the opportunity to make a written declaration on admission or to have a copy of an existing statement placed in the patient's chart. Several forms of written directives are available and, state laws vary regarding which are accepted as legal documents.

Do not resuscitate (DNR) means "do not restart a cardiac or respiratory function that has stopped." DNR orders usually do not address the withholding or stopping of nutrition, medications, fluids, comfort, or other measures.

The **living will** declares a person's wishes about withholding or withdrawing life-sustaining devices for a patient with a hopelessly terminal condition. A **health care proxy** assigns another person to act on behalf of a patient in making health care decisions. The patient can list restrictions that are desired. This latter directive also may be called a **durable power of attorney for health care.** It is important to remember that these directives apply only to health care decisions and only for times when the person is incapable of stating personal preferences. Ideally, people initiating these documents should review their wishes with family, significant others, and health care providers to avoid confusion and conflict in crises.

Nurses' Attitudes Toward Death

Attitudes toward death are influenced by age, family, religion, culture, and past experiences with illness and death. Nurses must explore their own feelings about death before they can more effectively assist patients and families in the grieving process.

Death is inevitable. However, a nurse's caring approach can affect how that person feels when he or she dies. Sensitive, quality care allows the patient to die with dignity. Nursing care must promote the patient's sense of identity and self-esteem. Appropriate communication skills are important in assisting the dying patient and the family during this time. The Dying Person's Bill of Rights ensures that the patient's right to die with dignity and to maintain and receive competent, compassionate care are respected (see box).

Caring for the dying patient is a critical part of nursing. Being with the patient at the time of death supports the patient and family during the last hours. However, many nurses find it overwhelming to care for the dying patient. If the nurse does not come to a personal understanding of death, a dying patient may benefit by having another nurse provide the necessary care. A wise nurse allows this exchange to occur.

THE DYING PERSON'S BILL OF RIGHTS

I have the right to be treated as a living human being until I die.
I have the right to maintain a sense of hopefulness, however changing its focus may be.
I have the right to be cared for by those who can maintain a sense of hopefulness, however changing this might be.
I have the right to express my feelings and emotions about my approaching death in my own way.
I have the right to participate in decisions concerning my care.
I have the right to expect continuing medical and nursing attention even though "cure" goals must be changed to "comfort" goals.
I have the right not to die alone.
I have the right to be free from pain.
I have the right to have my questions answered honestly.
I have the right not to be deceived.
I have the right to have help from and for my family in accepting my death.
I have the right to die in peace and dignity.
I have the right to retain my individuality and not be judged for my decisions which may be contrary to beliefs of others.
I have the right to discuss and enlarge my religious and/or spiritual experiences, whatever these may mean to others.
I have the right to expect that the sanctity of the human body will be respected after death.
I have the right to be cared for by caring, sensitive, knowledgeable people who will attempt to understand my needs and will be able to gain some satisfaction in helping me face my death.

From Barbus AJ: The dying person's bill of rights, *American Journal of Nursing* 75:99, 1975.

Physical Needs of the Terminally Ill

The dying patient has many physical needs that must be met by the nursing staff. Comfort is the major goal, so nursing care, not a cure, is the emphasis. The patient who is in pain requires pain medication and should be kept as comfortable as possible. The patient should be encouraged to remain active and maintain ambulation while avoiding fatigue. If the patient is on bedrest, skin care should be excellent to prevent skin breakdown (see Chapter 21). Adequate elimination must be maintained and incontinence managed appropriately, without causing embarrassment to the patient (see Chapters 30 and 31). Dieticians and nurses must effectively encourage the patient to eat.

Emotional Needs of the Terminally Ill

Patients differ in their emotional responses when recognizing that death is inevitable. Some quietly work through the process, whereas others are more vocal and involve others in the process. All patients should be encouraged to talk about their feelings. The terminally ill experience hope throughout the grieving process. The physician and nursing staff should be involved in giving hope while helping patients deal with reality. The dimensions of hope and implications for promoting hope are listed in the box. Nurses should accept patients' behavior, regardless of its manifestation, and view it as an expression of their needs during times of grief.

NURSING IMPLICATIONS FOR PROMOTING HOPE

Affective Dimension

- Convey an empathetic understanding of patient's worries, fears, and doubts. Reduce degree to which patient becomes immobilized by concerns. Build on patient and family strengths of patience and courage.

Cognitive Dimension

- Clarify or modify the hoping person's reality perceptions: Offer information about illness or treatment, correct misinformation, share experiences of others as a basis of comparison.

Behavioral Dimension

- Assist patient to use own resources and those of others in relation to hope. Balance levels of independence, interdependence, and dependence when planning care.
- Enhance person's self-esteem and capabilities. Give praise and encouragement appropriately.

Affiliative Dimension

- Strengthen or foster the relationships with others that are consistent with hope.
- Help patients know they are loved, cared for, and important to others.

Temporal Dimension

- Attend to a patient's experience of time. Apply patient's insights from past experiences to the present.

Contextual Dimension

- Provide opportunity to communicate about life situations that have an influence on hope.
- Encourage discussion of desired goals, reminiscing, reviewing values, and reflecting on the meaning of suffering, life, or death.

From Perry AG, Potter PA: *Clinical nursing skills and techniques,* ed 3, St Louis, 1994, Mosby.

Spiritual Needs of the Terminally Ill

Patients often deal with death in a spiritual nature. The nurse should follow the patient's cues and implement action according to those wishes and needs. Some terminally ill patients ask spiritual questions or talk to the nurse, and it is important

Table 10-2 RELIGIOUS PRACTICES RELATED TO DEATH

Religion	Death
Hinduism	Priest ties thread around neck or wrist and pours water into mouth. Only family touches and washes body before cremation.
Buddhism	Buddhist priest is present. Last rite is chanted.
Islam	Before death, patient confesses sins and asks forgiveness of family. Only family touches and washes body.
Judaism	Jews oppose autopsy and cremation. Fetus is buried. Ritual cleansing of body is done by members of ritual burial society.
Christianity	Last rites are optional for some Protestants and are mandatory for Eastern Orthodox Christians and Roman Catholics. Aborted fetus and stillborn infants are baptized by Roman Catholics.

Adapted from Potter PA, Perry AG: *Fundamentals of nursing: concepts, process, and practice,* ed 3, St Louis, 1993, Mosby.

that the nurse be willing to talk or just listen as needed.

In a multicultural society the nurse meets patients of various religious and ethnic backgrounds (see Chapter 8). The practices regarding death for five major religions are listed in Table 10-2. The nurse must remember that people vary in their adherence to religious rites and that not all patients actively practice their faith. The nurse should also be aware of and use the spiritual counseling services available in the agency and community.

Hospice Care

Many patients choose to die in a hospice instead of in a traditional hospital. A **hospice** is a caring environment where a person may die with dignity and the family may receive support for their grief. These facilities have homelike atmospheres and allow the family to stay with the loved one. Regardless of the setting, nursing care is provided around the clock so that all the patient's physical and emotional needs are met.

Care After Death

The nurse should treat with dignity the patient who has died. After assessing the patient's vital signs to determine that death has occurred (Skill 10-2), the nurse notifies the physician, who pronounces the time of death. The nurse offers the family the opportunity to view the body. After providing comfort measures for the family, the nurse then cares for the patient's body with respect (Skill 10-3).

■ NURSING CARE PLAN ■

DYSFUNCTIONAL GRIEVING

Mr. T, age 28, had an amputation below the knee after a crushing injury to his right lower leg 2 days before. He is employed on an oil rig and is angry that he may not be able to return to his job.

NURSING DIAGNOSIS

Dysfunctional grieving related to potential loss of work and altered lifestyle as evidenced by words, gestures, and facial expressions

GOAL

- Patient will reach acceptance of altered lifestyle in 1 month.

EXPECTED OUTCOME

- Patient will verbalize lifestyle options and hope and will participate in rehabilitation by discharge date.

NURSING INTERVENTIONS

- Ask patient about hopes and plans.
- Encourage patient to express anger and other feelings about situation.
- Look for signs of denial, bargaining, depression, or acceptance.
- Talk with patient, other health care providers, family, and employer about recovery potential and available options.

EVALUATION

- Patient verbalizes his concerns.
- Patient shows behaviors indicating progression from bargaining through depression to beginning acceptance by discharge.

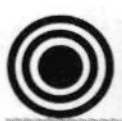

SKILL 10-1 CARING FOR THE PATIENT WHO IS DYING

Steps	Rationale
1. Obtain equipment for comfort measures: ▪ Pillows ▪ Pain medication	Helps organize procedure. Prepares for patient needs.
2. Refer to medical record, plan of care, or Kardex for special interventions.	Provides basis for care.
3. Introduce self.	Decreases anxiety level.
4. Identify patient by identification band.	Identifies correct patient for procedure.
5. Explain procedure to patient.	Seeks cooperation and decreases anxiety.
6. Wash hands and don clean gloves according to agency policy and guidelines from Centers for Disease Control and Prevention and Occupational Safety and Health Administration.	Helps prevent cross-contamination.
7. Prepare patient for intervention:	
a. Close door to room or pull curtain.	Provides privacy.
b. Drape for procedure if necessary.	Prevents exposure of patient.
8. Raise bed to comfortable working level.	Provides safety for nurse.
9. Arrange for patient privacy.	Shows respect for patient.
10. Assess patient needs.	Alerts nurse to patient's physical and emotional needs as they arise.
11. Provide comfort measures.	Helps patient cope.
12. Assess for signs and symptoms of approaching death (see box).	Provides a baseline for future assessment of patient needs.
13. Provide relief of pain.	Helps provide sense of well-being for patient.
14. Allow family members to assist in patient care when feasible (see box).	Helps prevent family from feeling helpless.
15. Assess spiritual needs. Initiate referral if requested.	Helps determine need for clergy. Provides support and helps patient communicate feelings.
16. Listen to patient and assess affect.	Communicates concern and interest. Provides information about patient's feelings.
17. Talk honestly to patient. Prevent telling patient anything physician has not shared.	Communicates caring and trust.
18. Explain to family about signs of death when applicable.	Provides family with information without revealing what physician has not told patient.
19. Remove gloves and wash hands.	Helps prevent cross-contamination.
20. Document.	Documents procedure and patient's response.

SIGNS OF APPROACHING DEATH

- Weak, thready pulse
- Falling blood pressure
- Labored respirations that may include Cheyne-Stokes respirations (period of apnea followed by period of overbreathing)
- Cyanosis of extremities, nail beds, and area around lips
- Diminished senses (Hearing is believed to be the last sense to fade. Therefore do not talk near patient about terminal condition.)
- "Death rattle" (rattling sound heard in throat caused by secretions that patient can no longer cough up)
- Coldness of extremities (caused from diminished peripheral vascular circulation)
- Possible coma
- Mottled extremities (discoloring from diminished circulation and purplish skin color)
- Possible drop in body temperature
- Eventual cessation of pulse, respiration, and blood pressure

INVOLVING THE FAMILY IN THE CARE OF A DYING PATIENT

- Assist in planning a visitation schedule for family members to prevent patient and family from becoming fatigued.
- Allow young children to visit a dying parent when the patient is able to communicate.
- Be willing to listen to family complaints about the patient's care, as well as positive or negative feelings about the patient.
- Help family members learn how to interact with the dying person (for example, using attentive listening, avoiding false reassurances, conducting conversations about normal family activities or problems).
- Allow family members to help with simple care measures such as feeding, bathing, and straightening bed linen. Family members are often more successful than nursing staff in persuading the patient to eat.
- When the family becomes fatigued with care activities, relieve them from their duties so that they can acquire needed rest and support. Refer them to resources for meals and lodging.
- Support the act of grieving between patient and family. Provide privacy when preferred. Do not discourage open expression of grief between family and patient.
- Provide information daily with regard to the patient's condition. Prepare the family for sudden changes in the patient's appearance and behavior.
- Communicate news of impending death when the family is together if possible. Members can provide support for one another. Convey the news in a private area and be willing to stay with the family.
- At the time of death, help the family stay in communication with the dying person through short visits, caring silence, touch, and telling the patient of their love.
- After death assist the family with decision making, such as selection of a mortician, transportation of family members, and collection of the patient's belongings.

From Potter PA, Perry AG: *Fundamentals of nursing: concepts, process, and practice,* ed 3, St Louis, 1993, Mosby.

SKILL 10-2 ASSESSING THE TIME OF THE PATIENT'S DEATH

Steps	Rationale
1. **Obtain equipment:** ▪ Stethoscope ▪ Sphygmomanometer ▪ Writing pad ▪ Pen ▪ Clean gloves	Helps organize procedure.
2. **Refer to medical record, plan of care, or Kardex for special interventions.**	Provides basis for care.
3. **Identify patient by identification band.**	Identifies correct patient for procedure.
4. **Wash hands and don clean gloves according to agency policy and guidelines from Centers for Disease Control and Prevention and Occupational Safety and Health Administration.**	Helps prevent cross-contamination.
5. **Close door to room or pull curtain.**	Prevents anxiety of other patients.
6. **Raise bed to comfortable working level.**	Provides safety for nurse.
7. **Assess cessation of pulse, respiration, and blood pressure, and report findings.**	Determines time to notify physician and report findings to appropriate personnel.
8. **Notify attending physician.**	Legally, the physician must pronounce death in most states.
9. **Remain in room until physician arrives and makes pronouncement of death.**	Shows courtesy and respect to deceased and to family.
10. **Allow family members to express feelings.**	Provides opportunity for family to verbalize grief. Communicates concern and interest.
11. **Remove gloves and wash hands.**	Helps prevent cross-contamination.
12. **Document.**	Documents procedure.

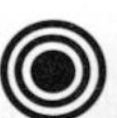

SKILL 10-3 CARING FOR THE BODY AFTER DEATH

Steps	Rationale
1. **Obtain equipment:** ▪ Clean gloves ▪ Bath towel ▪ Wash cloth ▪ Bath soap ▪ Bath basin ▪ Dressings ▪ Biohazard bag ▪ Plastic bag ▪ Clean hospital gown ▪ Valuables list ▪ Body bag (if body is to be transferred to morgue)	Helps organize procedure.
2. **Refer to medical record, plan of care, or Kardex for special interventions.**	Provides basis for care.
3. **Wash hands and don clean gloves according to agency policy and guidelines from Centers for Disease Control and Prevention and Occupational Safety and Health Administration.**	Helps prevent cross-contamination.
4. **Close door to room or pull curtain.**	Prevents anxiety of other patients.
5. **Raise bed to comfortable working level.**	Provides safety for nurse.
6. **Arrange for privacy and prevent other patients from seeing into room.**	Shows respect for patient and prevents anxiety of other patients.
7. **Explain to family regarding nursing activity and ask them to leave room unless religious beliefs determine their assistance with the body.**	Helps avoid further emotional stress or communicates respects for customs.
8. **Close patient's eyes and mouth if necessary.**	Provides a more normal appearance.
9. **Remove all tubes and other devices from patient's body.**	Makes patient look more peaceful.
10. **Place patient in supine position (Fig. 10-1).**	Provides easier access during procedures.

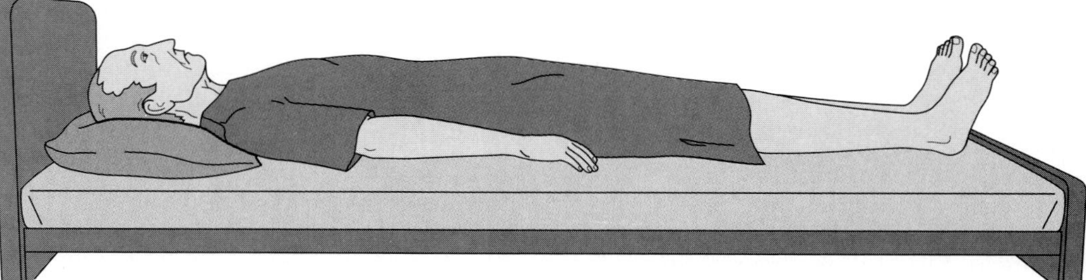

Fig. 10-1 Patient placed in the supine position.

Steps	Rationale
11. **Replace soiled dressings with clean ones.**	Avoids odor and provides neat appearance.
12. **Bathe patient as necessary.**	Reduces odor and removes secretions.
13. **Brush or comb hair.**	Provides more normal appearance.
14. **Apply clean gown.**	Provides better appearance.
15. **Care for valuables and personal belongings and document dispersement.**	Protects agency and staff legally.
16. **Allow family to view patient and remain in room.**	Provides emotional support.
17. **Attach special label if patient had contagious disease.**	Protects those who handle the body.
18. **Await arrival of ambulance or transfer to morgue (follow agency policy).**	Shows respect for body.
19. **Remove gloves and wash hands.**	Helps prevent cross-contamination.
20. **Document.**	Documents procedure.

SUMMARY

Knowledge of the concepts and theories concerning loss, death, and the grieving process provides a framework for the nursing process. The nurse's responses to and interactions with the grieving patient and family create a climate of openness in expressing grief. The nurse listens to the patient, offering support and showing respect for the patient's beliefs and values. This understanding promotes growth and paves the way for effective nursing care of grieving or dying patients and their families.

Key Concepts

- Loss, like stress, has positive and negative causes, and loss and stress have similar responses.
- Grief involves physical and emotional responses to a loss.
- Responses to death may vary with cultural and religious beliefs and prior coping behavior.
- The nurse must carefully collect data about the patient's and family's response to loss.
- Patient comfort (physical, emotional, and spiritual) is the major goal in caring for terminally ill patients.
- The family should be included in the care of the terminally patient when the patient and family desire.

Critical Thinking Questions

1. Mrs. James has been in the hospital for 4 months. You have taken care of her the last 4 weeks. You spend every free moment you have with her. When not at the hospital you worry about her and are concerned that no one else can give her as good care as you. Your supervisor has commented on your apparent overinvolvement with Mrs. James. What could some of the factors be that are influencing your reactions to Mrs. James?
2. Jim Jones, a 19-year-old victim of a traumatic injury, has become increasingly angry and noncooperative. He refuses all treatments. When approached he yells "Stay away from me. I just want to die." Describe how you would approach Mr. Jones and what you think you need to assess.
3. Jane is in the final phase of her terminal illness. It is clear she will die soon. Her family has asked you what they can do. Identify four needs of Jane and discuss what her family can do to help her.

REFERENCES AND SUGGESTED READINGS

Abner CS: Spousal death, a threat to women's health: paid work as a "resistance resource," *Image* 24(2):95, 1992.

Bolander VB: *Sorensen and Luckmann's basic nursing: a psychophysiologic approach,* ed 3, Philadelphia, 1994, Saunders.

Brown MA: Lifting the burden of silence, *American Journal of Nursing* 94(9):62, 1994.

Buehler JA, Lee HG: Exploration of home care resources for rural families with cancer, *Cancer Nursing* 15(4):299, 1992.

Christensen BL, Kockrow EO: *Foundations of nursing,* ed 2, St Louis, 1995, Mosby.

Craven RF, Hirnle CJ: *Fundamentals of nursing: human health and function,* Philadelphia, 1992, Lippincott.

Eakes GG: Grief resolution in hospice nurses, *Nursing and Health Care* 11(5):242, 1990.

Fina DK: A chance to say goodbye, *American Journal of Nursing* 94(5):42, 1994.

Harkness G, Dincher JR: *Medical-surgical nursing: total patient care,* ed 9, St Louis, 1996, Mosby.

Long BC, Phipps WJ, Cassmeyer VL: *Medical-surgical nursing:* ed 3, St Louis, 1993, Mosby.

McFarland GK, McFarlane EA: *Nursing diagnosis & intervention: planning for patient care,* ed 2, St Louis, 1993, Mosby.

Mosby's medical, nursing, and allied health dictionary, ed 4, St Louis, 1994, Mosby.

Potter PA, Perry AG: *Fundamentals of nursing: concepts, process, and practice,* ed 3, St Louis, 1993, Mosby.

UNIT III

BASIC NURSING SKILLS

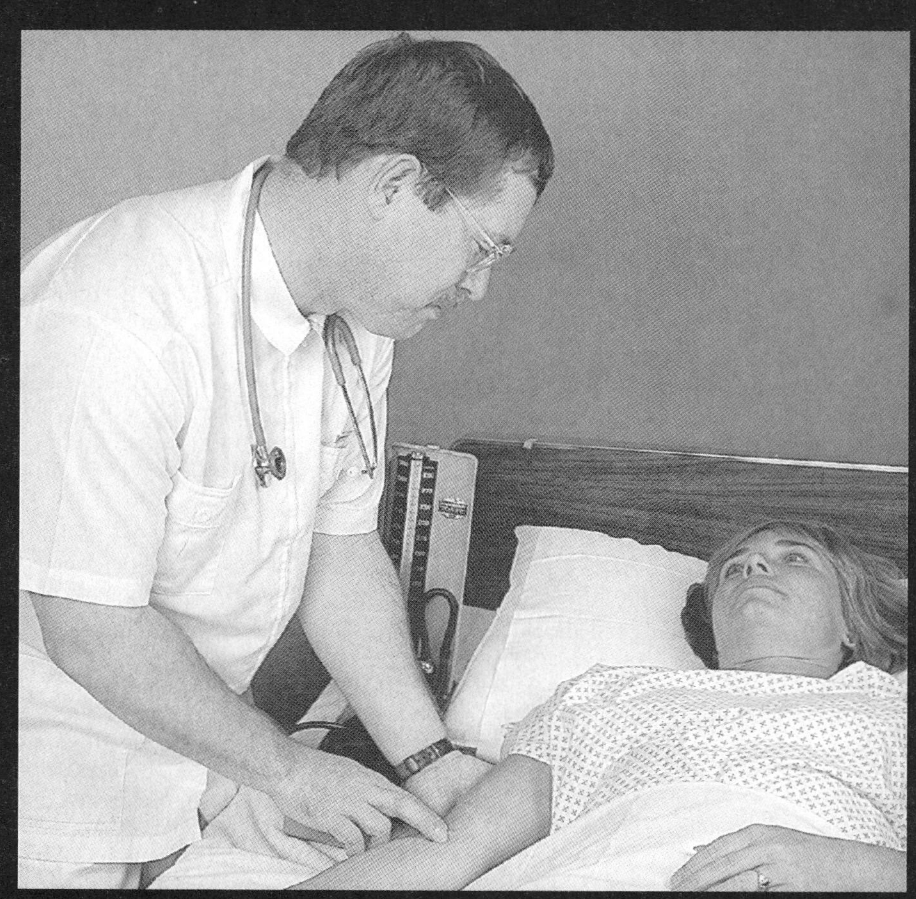

CHAPTER 11

Vital Signs

Learning Objectives

After studying this chapter, the student should be able to . . .

- Define the key terms.
- Explain the importance of accurately assessing temperature, pulse, and blood pressure.
- State the normal ranges for vital signs.
- Take an accurate oral, rectal, or axillary temperature.
- Take the following pulses accurately: radial, apical, carotid, pedal, and brachial.
- Take an accurate respiratory rate.
- Take an accurate blood pressure.
- Identify important guidelines for assessing vital signs.
- Discuss the rationale for each step of the vital sign procedure.
- Document vital signs.
- Communicate and document abnormal findings of vital signs to the appropriate team member.
- Discuss special considerations for assessing the vital signs of the pediatric patient and older adult.

Key Terms

Antipyretic
Apnea
Blood pressure
Body temperature
Bradycardia
Bradypnea
Celsius (C)
Cheyne-Stokes respirations
Core temperature
Diastolic pressure
Dyspnea
Dysrhythmia
Fahrenheit (F)
Febrile
Hyperpyrexia
Hypertension
Hypotension
Korotkoff sounds
Kussmaul's respirations
Obliteration
Orthostatic hypotension
Pulse
Pulse deficit
Pulse pressure
Respiration
Sphygmomanometer
Surface temperature
Systolic pressure
Tachycardia
Tachypnea
Vital signs

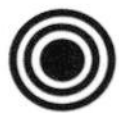 Skills

11-1 Measuring body temperature (oral, axillary, rectal)
11-2 Measuring pulse (radial, apical)
11-3 Measuring respirations
11-4 Measuring blood pressure

Vital signs are the measurements of pulse rate, respiration rate, and body temperature. Although not strictly a vital sign, blood pressure is also customarily included. The information obtained from vital signs provides important objective data used to assess a patient's condition and the need for intervention.

Vital signs are a part of the nursing data base collected when a patient is admitted to the hospital. Although the results of vital signs assessment at this time provide a baseline for future assessment, the nurse should remember that vital signs on admission are usually elevated because the patient is anxious about being admitted.

Vital signs normally vary during a 24-hour period. They are usually lowest during sleep and the early morning and gradually increase during the day and evening. The most accurate measurement of vital signs is made with the patient at rest or in bed and in a quiet environment.

Assessing vital signs is an important and frequently used skill. Accuracy is essential because subtle alterations may indicate a change in the pa-

GUIDELINES FOR ASSESSING VITAL SIGNS

- When patient is admitted to health care facility
- Before and after surgery
- Before and after invasive diagnostic procedures
- Before and after medications that could change patient's vital signs
- When patient's general condition changes
- When patient complains of specific symptom or comments on not feeling "right" or well

tient's condition. The nurse must never take vital signs assessment for granted or deviate from being accurate. For example, the pulse should be taken for a full minute. If the pulse skips a beat, the nurse should report the abnormality appropriately.

Changes in one vital sign often cause changes in another or in all of the vital signs. Thus in clinical practice all vital signs are monitored and documented together on the graphic sheet, on the nurse's flow sheet, or according to agency policy. Unexpected outcomes are documented in the nurses' notes or flow sheet and reported to the charge nurse or physician.

Health care institutions have policies that specify how often vital signs are to be taken. In addition, the physician may order vital signs to be assessed at certain times. The nurse also takes vital signs at other times (see box).

ASSESSMENT OF VITAL SIGNS

It is standard in nursing practice to group the assessment of body temperature, pulse, and respiration. There are three locations or routes for measuring body temperature (Table 11-1). When taking an oral temperature with a glass thermometer, the nurse assesses the patient's radial pulse and respirations while the thermometer is in the patient's mouth, keeping the fingers over the patient's radial artery while counting respirations. This practice focuses the patient's attention away from the respirations and allows the nurse to accurately assess respiratory patterns. When taking a rectal or axillary temperature, the nurse assesses the patient's pulse and respirations before or after taking the temperature to ensure that the necessary hold on the thermometer is maintained.

The following abbreviations are used for documentation of vital signs: oral temperature (T), radial pulse (P), respiration (R), and blood pressure (BP). The nurse should document that a temperature or pulse was taken in a location other than the normal site (orally and radially, respectively).

MEASURING BODY TEMPERATURE

Body temperature is the balance of heat produced by and heat lost from the body. Most body heat is a by-product of food metabolism. Heat production is influenced by the body's basal metabolic rate, hormone levels, nervous system control, and muscle activity and an increase in the temperature of body cells. Heat is lost from the body in many ways, some of which include sweating, breathing, and exposure of the skin to the environment.

Purposes

Body temperature provides a measurement of the current level of internal body heat. This assessment allows the nurse to determine whether nursing interventions are needed to reduce the patient's body temperature or conserve body heat. It also allows the nurse to monitor the patient's response to illness and treatments.

Types

There are two types of body temperature. The nurse measures the patient's **core temperature** (the temperature of the deep tissues of the body) when using a thermometer. This temperature remains relatively constant unless the patient is exposed to severe extremes in environmental temperature. The second type of temperature is **surface temperature** (the temperature of the skin), which may vary a great deal in response to the environment. The nurse may assess surface temperature by feeling the patient's skin for moisture and warmth.

The internal organs of the body function best within a relatively small temperature range. The standard normal temperature is 98.6° **Fahrenheit (F)** or 37° **Celsius (C),** which is considered the norm (normal). However, body temperature may differ according to age (Table 11-2).

The nurse may be asked to convert a Celsius reading into a Fahrenheit reading or vice versa. The following formulas are used:

1. Fahrenheit to Celsius: Subtract 32 from the Fahrenheit reading and multiply by $5/9$.

$$C = (\text{Fahrenheit temperature} - 32) \times 5/9$$

Table 11-1 LOCATIONS AND ROUTES FOR BODY TEMPERATURE MEASUREMENT

Common Uses	Advantages	Disadvantages and Contraindications
Oral		
Most adult	Is convenient Is easy to use Is not embarrassing to patient	Cannot be used in patient with confusion, chilling, shaking, combativeness, seizure disorders, mouth injury, or oral surgery Cannot be used in patient who is mouth breather Cannot be used in patient receiving oxygen via face mask Cannot be used in child under 5 years of age
Rectal		
Infants Small children	Can be used with crying infant	Cannot be used in patient with diarrhea, rectal surgery, or condition involving rectum or anus Is embarrassing or uncomfortable for patient May frighten children Provides inaccurate reading when stool is in rectum Can damage rectal mucosa Can slow heart rate (vagal stimulation)
Axillary		
Any patient	Is easily accessible Is most noninvasive method	Takes more time for accurate reading Cannot be used in patient in shock Cannot be used in patient with edema in axillary area

Table 11-2 NORMAL BODY TEMPERATURE BY AGE

Age	Temperature
Infant	35.5° to 37.5° C (96° to 99.6° F)
Adult	37° C (98.6° F)

For example, when the Fahrenheit reading is 100:

$$C = (100 - 32) \times 5/9$$
$$C = (68) \times 5/9$$
$$C = 37.7°$$

2. Celsius to Fahrenheit: Multiply the Celsius reading by 9/5 and add 32.

$$F = (\text{Celsius temperature} \times 9/5) + 32$$

For example, when the Celsius reading is 40:

$$F = (40 \times 9/5) + 32$$
$$F = 72 + 32$$
$$F = 104°$$

Types of Thermometers

Several types of thermometers may be used to take a patient's body temperature. The most common type is mercury in a glass thermometer that measures temperature on the Fahrenheit scale, Celsius scale, or both (Fig. 11-1). This is referred to as a *clinical thermometer.* This thermometer consists of a glass tube that is sealed at one end and that has a mercury-filled bulb at the other. Body heat causes the mercury to expand and rise into the tube. The mercury contracts and moves down the tube when cooled by a lower body temperature. A glass thermometer is inexpensive but breaks easily. It may be used to measure oral, rectal, or axillary temperatures. Standards for average adult temperature vary according to route and are as follows:

Oral	37° C (98.6° F)
Rectal	37.5° C (99.6° F)
Axillary	36.4° C (97.6° F)

There are three types of glass thermometers, and the bulb of each has a different shape (Fig. 11-2). Thermometers with long or slender tips are used to measure oral and axillary temperatures. Thermom-

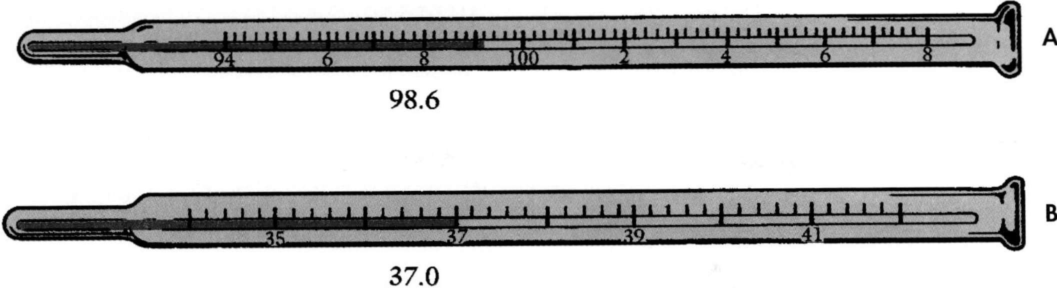

Fig. 11-1 **A,** Fahrenheit thermometer. The mercury level is at 99.2° F. **B,** Centigrade thermometer. The mercury level is at 37.0° C.

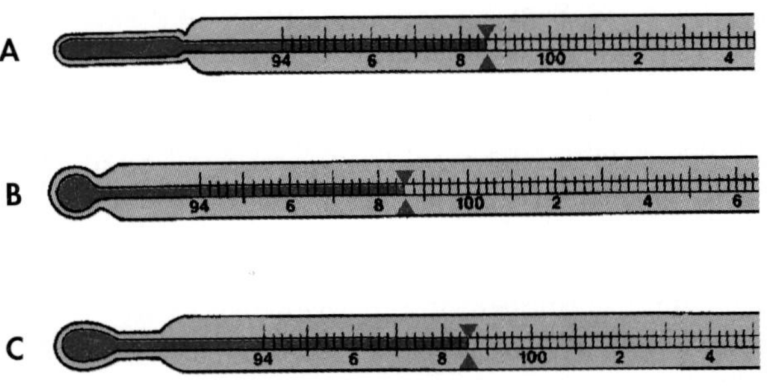

Fig. 11-2 Types of glass thermometers. **A,** Long or slender tip. **B,** Stubby-tip (rectal) thermometer. **C,** Pear-shaped tip.

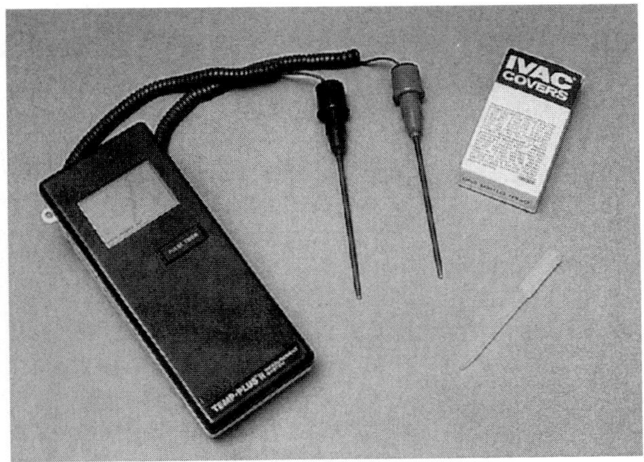

Fig. 11-3 Electronic thermometer with disposable plastic sheath. (From Perry AG, Potter PA: *Clinical nursing skills and techniques,* ed 3, St Louis, 1994, Mosby.)

eters with stubby and pear-shaped tips may also be used for oral and axillary temperatures. For the protection of the rectal mucosa, rectal temperatures must be taken with thermometers with stubby tips. The oral and rectal thermometers are usually color coded for use. For an accurate temperature reading the thermometer must be left in place according to procedure or agency guidelines: 3 minutes for oral, 5 minutes for rectal, and 10 minutes for axillary temperatures.

An electronic or digital thermometer consists of a battery-powered display unit connected to a temperature-sensitive probe with a thin wire cord (Fig. 11-3). An electrical charging unit recharges the thermometer when it is not in use. The nurse takes the digital unit to the patient's room, explains the procedure, and slips the probe into a disposable plastic sheath until it clicks, which indicates that the two are connected. The plastic sheath prevents transmission of organisms from patient to patient and prevents the nurse from having to touch a contaminated thermometer. Next, the covered probe is placed in the patient's mouth, under the tongue. The thermometer makes a sound and provides a digital readout of the body temperature.

The electronic thermometer registers body temperature in seconds to a minute and greatly reduces the amount of time the nurse must spend assessing vital signs. However, electronic thermometers are expensive and may give inaccurate readings if the unit has not been appropriately charged.

The tympanic membrane thermometer is yet another type of thermometer. It is inserted just inside the ear and takes only a few seconds to register body temperature (Fig. 11-4). There has been some concern regarding the accuracy with this type when it is not appropriately used.

A disposable, single-use thermometer has chemical dots that change color in response to body heat (Fig. 11-5). This thermometer measures body temperature in about 45 seconds. Some inaccuracy occurs when the thermometer is not appropriately used.

Another method of measuring body temperature is with temperature-sensitive tape. This tape, applied to the forehead or abdomen, changes color in response to increased body heat. It indicates whether the temperature is normal or above normal but does not measure exact body temperature. Neither this type nor the disposable, single-use oral

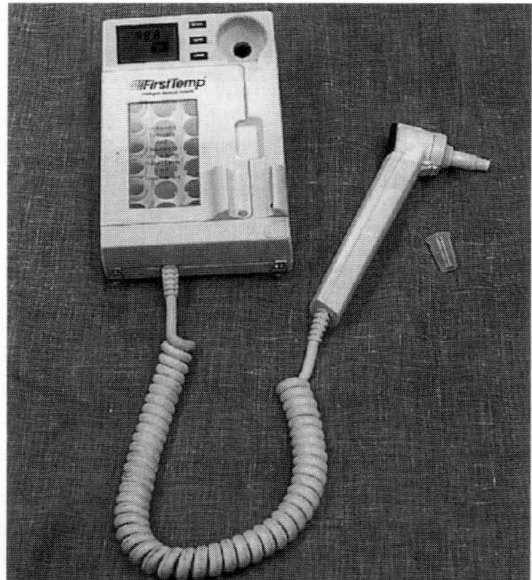

Fig. 11-4 Tympanic membrane thermometer. (From Perry AG, Potter PA: *Clinical nursing skills and techniques,* ed 3, St Louis, 1994, Mosby.)

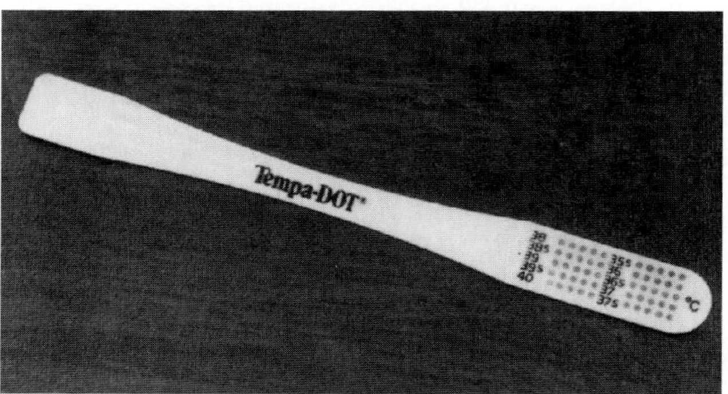

Fig. 11-5 Disposable, single-use thermometer. (From Perry AG, Potter PA: *Clinical nursing skills and techniques,* ed 3, St Louis, 1994, Mosby.)

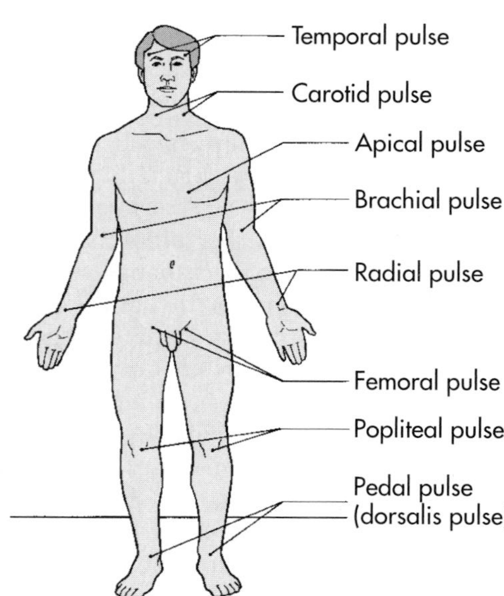

Fig. 11-6 Pulse sites.

FACTORS INFLUENCING PULSE RATES

- *Exercise.* Short-term exercise increases pulse rate. Long-term exercise strengthens heart muscle, resulting in lower-than-normal rate at rest and quicker return to the resting rate after exercise.
- *Fever and heat.* Fever and heat increase pulse rate because of increased metabolic rate.
- *Acute pain and anxiety.* Pain and anxiety increase pulse rate because of sympathetic stimulation.
- *Unrelieved severe and chronic pain.* Severe and chronic pain decrease pulse rate because of parasympathetic stimulation.
- *Medications.* Some medications alter pulse rate. For example, digitalis and beta blockers decrease pulse rate, whereas atropine increases it.
- *Age.* Pulse rate decreases as aging process progresses from infancy, through puberty, to adulthood. Newborn infant averages 100 to 180 beats/min, whereas adult averages 60 to 80 beats/min. Pulse rate in older adult may be greater than 80 beats/min to compensate for weakened heart muscle, and it can be higher because of medications.
- *Metabolism.* Certain diseases such as hyperthyroidism or cardiomyopathy can cause chronic elevated pulse rate. Hypothyroidism can cause slowing of pulse.
- *Hemorrhage.* Loss of blood increases pulse rate because of sympathetic stimulation.
- *Postural changes.* Lying down decreases pulse rate. Standing or sitting increases it.

From Potter PA, Perry AG: *Fundamentals of nursing: concepts, process, and practice,* ed 3, St Louis, 1993, Mosby.

thermometer is frequently used in health care settings. These thermometers are more commonly used in the home.

MEASURING PULSE (RADIAL AND APICAL)

The nurse obtains information about the circulatory status of the patient by assessing the pulse. The **pulse** occurs when the left ventricle of the heart contracts and sends blood into the arteries. This process creates a pulse wave that the nurse can palpate (feel). In a healthy person the pulse reflects the heartbeat or apical rate; that is, the pulse rate is the same as the ventricular contraction of the heart. However, in certain types of cardiovascular disease the heartbeat and pulse rate may differ. A person's

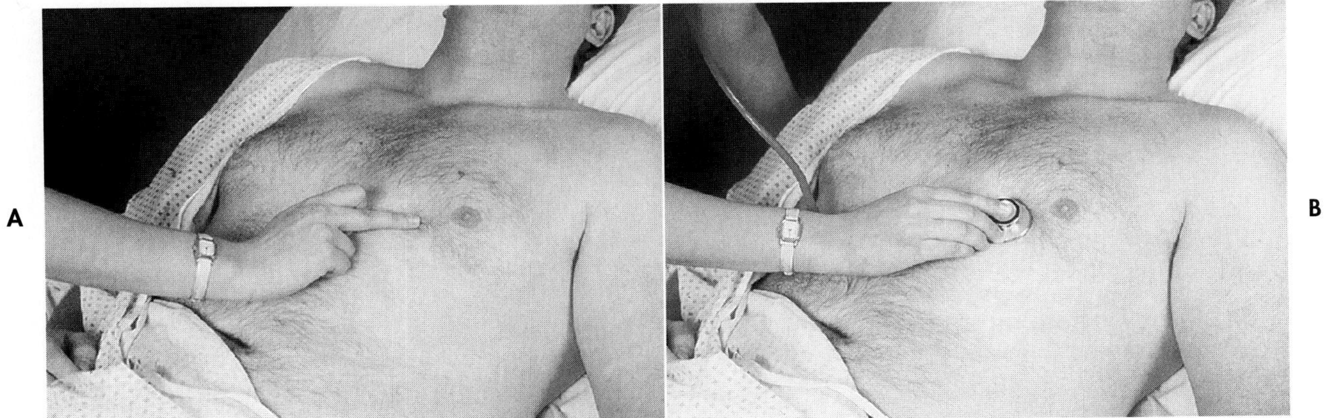

Fig. 11-7 **A,** Locating an apical pulse. **B,** Taking an apical pulse. (From Potter PA, Perry AG: *Fundamentals of nursing: concepts, process, and practice,* ed 3, St Louis, 1993, Mosby.)

heartbeat changes throughout the day to meet the circulatory needs of the body. Many factors change the pulse rate (see box).

Pulse rates also vary with age. The newborn has the fastest pulse rate, which may be as high as 180 beats per minute (beats/min). As a person ages the resting pulse gradually slows. The pulse range for adolescents and adults is 60 to 100 beats/min. The patient who has a pulse rate of below 60 beats/min is said to have **bradycardia.** The patient who is at rest and has a pulse rate above 100 beats/min has **tachycardia.**

Pulse Sites

The pulse may be assessed at a number of sites. Peripheral pulses are distant from the heart and are generally easy to palpate. The artery is near the surface of the skin and lies over a bone at these sites. Peripheral pulse sites are the temporal, carotid, brachial, radial, femoral, popliteal, and dorsalis pedis or pedal pulses. These pulse sites are found on both sides of the body.

The apical and radial sites are the most commonly used to measure pulse. Mastery of these sites is essential before attempting to use other sites (Fig. 11-6). The apical pulse is taken by auscultation (listening) with a stethoscope directly over the apex, or top or tip, of the heart (Fig. 11-7).

The radial site is the most often used peripheral pulse site because it is convenient and easily accessible. A radial pulse is measured on all patients except the following:

Newborns and children up to 2 or 3 years of age: Use apical site.

Patients whose radial pulse is difficult to palpate: Use apical site or use Doppler stethoscope to determine pulse rate.

Patients who need to have circulation to a specific body part assessed: Use the site near the body part (often the legs) and then assess the pedal pulse.

Patients with irregular radial pulses: Use the apical site.

Patients with known heart disease: Use the apical site.

Patients who are taking medications that may affect the pulse: Use apical site.

Patients whose radial pulses are not accessible because of a cast or dressing that prevents access to the site: Use apical site.

Assessment of the Pulse

When taking a pulse, the nurse should assess the pulse's rate, rhythm, and strength. The rate is the number of beats that occur in 1 minute. For peripheral pulses, this is the number of beats felt. For an apical pulse, it is the number of beats heard through the stethoscope. Each "lub-dup" sound is counted as one beat. The rhythm is the pattern of beats and the intervals between beats. Normally, successive beats occur at regular intervals. If the rhythm is not regular the patient is said to have a **dysrhythmia.** There are many kinds of dysrhythmias, some of which indicate serious cardiac (heart) problems. If a dysrhythmia is assessed when a peripheral pulse is palpated, it is important to take an apical pulse for 1 minute to gain more information about the dysrhythmia.

Table 11-3 PULSE STRENGTH

Scale	Description
0	Pulse is absent.
1+	Pulse is difficult to palpate, is weak, and is easily obliterated.
2+	Pulse is difficult to palpate, and light pressure will locate it.
3+	Pulse is considered normal, is easy to palpate, and is not easily obliterated.
4+	Strong pulse is easily palpated and is very difficult to obliterate.

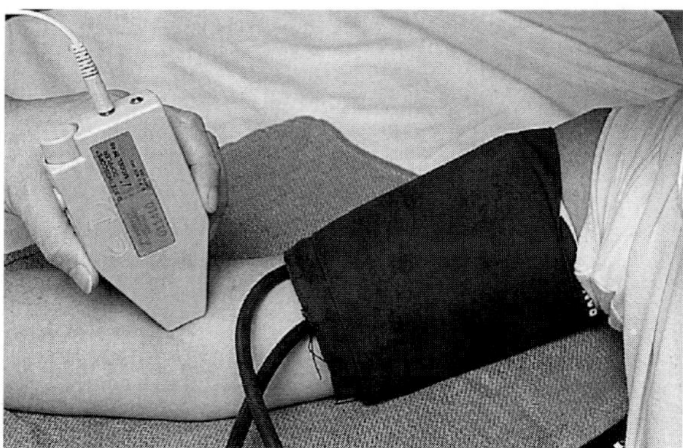

Fig. 11-8 Doppler stethoscope over brachial artery to measure the pulse. (From Perry AG, Potter PA: *Clinical nursing skills and techniques,* ed 3, St Louis, 1994, Mosby.)

In addition, the nurse may need to determine whether there is a **pulse deficit** (a condition that exists when the radial pulse rate is lower than the apical pulse rate). This is best performed simultaneously by two nurses. One nurse assesses the radial rate, and the other assesses the apical rate. Then the findings are compared. A pulse deficit may indicate inadequate blood circulation to the arms and legs with each contraction of the heart.

Assessing pulse strength is a skill that requires practice and experience. It is a subjective determination of the force of the blood being ejected against the arterial wall. The strength of a pulse is described as weak, normal (strong), or bounding. The concept of obliteration is central to these descriptions. **Obliteration** is the temporary disappearance of a palpable pulse when the examiner compresses the arterial pulse site. A normal pulse may be felt with moderate pressure over the arterial site, feels full, and is not easily obliterated. A weak pulse is more difficult to locate, is easily obliterated, and often feels "thready" (difficult to feel, like a piece of thread being softly pulled through material). A thready pulse may be found in a patient in shock. A bounding pulse is easy to find and almost "jumps through the skin" against the nurse's fingers. It is almost impossible to obliterate. Although there is no universally accepted standard, some agencies use a number system for measuring and describing pulse strength. According to Sunberg, this scale ranges from 0 to 4+ (Table 11-3).

The nurse may be unable to accurately palpate a peripheral pulse. At these times the nurse should first take the patient's apical pulse for 1 minute. If further assessment of a peripheral pulse is needed, the nurse may choose to use a Doppler ultrasonic stethoscope (DUS), which detects movement of red blood cells through a blood vessel (Fig. 11-8). In contrast, the conventional stethoscope amplifies only sound, not movement. The Doppler is particularly helpful in assessing blood flow to the arms and legs in situations in which decreased or inadequate blood flow exists.

MEASURING RESPIRATIONS

Respiration is the act of breathing air into the lungs (inhalation) and exhaling air out of the lungs (exhalation). This is a complex process that involves the intake of oxygen and the output of carbon dioxide. External respiration includes lung ventilation, absorption of oxygen, and elimination of carbon dioxide. Internal respiration, sometimes called *tissue respiration,* includes the use of oxygen by all of the body's cells for the production of heat through oxidation and the release of energy from food eaten. When measuring a patient's respirations, the nurse should assess their rate, rhythm, and depth (how deeply the patient breathes). A patient may have shallow breathing (a respiration pattern marked by slow, shallow, and generally ineffective inspirations and expirations). One inhalation and one exhalation equal one respiration.

Respiratory Rate

Respiratory rate refers to how fast a patient breathes, or the number of times that a patient breathes in 1 minute. Respiratory rates vary with age. Newborns breathe rapidly (35 breaths/min), even at rest. Throughout infancy and childhood, the resting respiratory rate declines. The normal rate for adults varies from 12 to 20 breaths/min while at rest. Respiratory rates below 12 breaths/min are called ***bradypnea,*** and those higher than 20 are referred to as ***tachypnea*** (abnormally rapid respiratory rate). ***Dyspnea*** is shortness of breath. Many factors alter the respiratory rate. The most common factor is activity, which increases the rate. Other factors include acute pain, fever, brainstem injury, smoking, anxiety, and certain medications.

Respiratory Rhythm

Respiratory rhythm refers to the regularity of inhalations and exhalations. Normal respirations are evenly spaced, but certain disease processes (for example, pneumonia) and other circumstances (for example, metabolic imbalances) may alter respiratory rhythm. **Apnea** is the absence of respirations. If the patient is not breathing, the nurse should begin resuscitation if appropriate. However, periods of apnea may occur as part of a respiratory pattern. An example of this is **Cheyne-Stokes respirations** (pattern characterized by alternating periods of apnea and deep, rapid breathing), which may indicate a life-threatening situation. Another serious respiratory pattern often seen in patients with diabetes mellitus is **Kussmaul's respirations** (abnormally deep, very rapid sighing type of respirations). Any periods of apnea, Cheyne-Stokes respirations, or Kussmaul's respirations need to be assessed, immediately reported, and accurately documented.

Respiratory Depth

Respiratory depth refers to the movement of the body during inhalation and exhalation. Respiratory depth is described in a range from shallow to deep. Shallow respirations are difficult to see, so the nurse should feel chest wall movement by placing the hand on the chest when counting the rate. Normal or moderate respirations involve some movement of the diaphragm but are easy and unlabored. Determining respiratory depth is subjective unless specialized respiratory equipment is used.

Breathing

The patient does not think about breathing, which is an automatic activity. It is important to count respirations for 1 minute and to determine rhythm and depth when the patient is not aware that the nurse is observing these processes. The patient who focuses on breathing may consciously or unconsciously alter the pattern, so the assessment does not reflect the patient's true respiratory status. Therefore respirations are usually counted immediately after the patient's pulse is taken. The patient is usually unaware of the procedure because many nurses leave their fingers in place after counting the pulse and then count respirations.

MEASURING BLOOD PRESSURE

Blood pressure is the force that the blood exerts on the walls of the arteries. The maximum amount of pressure on the arteries occurs when the left lower chamber of the heart—the left ventricle—contracts to eject blood. This is the **systolic pressure.** The **diastolic pressure** is the pressure exerted on the arterial walls when the heart muscle relaxes. Blood pressure is measured in millimeters of mercury (mm Hg) and is abbreviated *BP.* It is recorded using a fraction. The top number is the systolic pressure, and the bottom number is the diastolic pressure (that is $^{120}/_{80}$ millimeters of mercury [mm Hg]). The difference between the bottom and top numbers is the **pulse pressure.** For example, if a patient's blood pressure is $^{130}/_{70}$ mm Hg, the pulse pressure is $130 - 70 = 60$.

Factors Affecting Blood Pressure

Many factors alter blood pressure. As with other vital signs, age is a significant factor. Until a child reaches adolescence, blood pressure is assessed against standards of body size and age. An adolescent's blood pressure varies according to body size. An adult's blood pressure tends to increase with age. A healthy middle-aged adult has a normal blood pressure of $^{120}/_{80}$ mm Hg. However, a systolic pressure of below 140 mm Hg and a diastolic pressure below 90 mm Hg are also considered normal. The blood pressure must be taken over a period of time, even days, to learn a person's norm. A normal blood pressure range for an older adult is 140 to $^{160}/_{80}$ to 90 mm Hg. Blood pressure readings also vary according to gender. After puberty, male patients have higher readings than female patients, but the situation reverses in postmenopausal women. It is also significant to know that the black population has a higher rate of **hypertension** (elevated blood pressure) than the white population. Some other factors that may alter blood pressure are fever, stress, arteriosclerosis, obesity, hemorrhage, exposure to cold, eating, smoking, high blood cholesterol levels, heredity, and some medications.

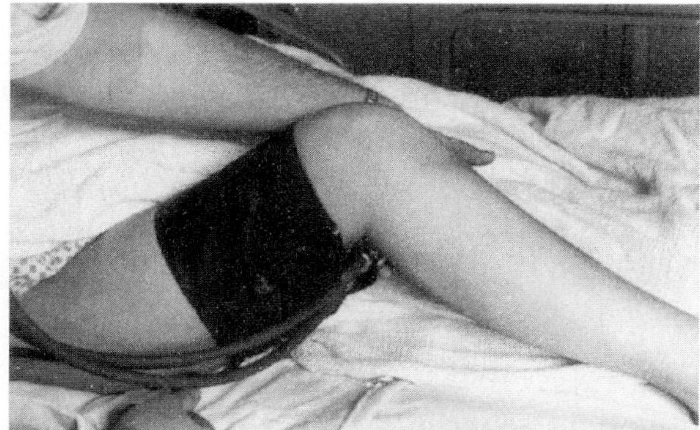

Fig. 11-9 Blood pressure cuff on thigh while nurse palpates patient's popliteal artery. (From Perry AG, Potter PA: *Clinical nursing skills and techniques,* ed 3, St Louis, 1994, Mosby.)

Hypotension

Hypotension is an abnormal condition in which the blood pressure is inadequate for the normal oxygenation of tissues. A change in body position may change blood pressure. The patient has **orthostatic hypotension** (postural hypotension) when the systolic pressure drops 15 mm Hg when moving from a lying to a sitting or standing position. People who are immobile or are on prolonged bedrest are at higher risk of having this condition. The drop in blood pressure may cause the patient to be dizzy or to faint. This may be prevented by slowly moving the patient from a lying to a sitting or standing position. For example, the nurse should assist a patient who has been on bedrest to a sitting or standing position using the following steps: elevating the head of the bed, allowing the patient to rest for a few minutes, assisting the patient to sit on the side of the bed (dangle), allowing the patient to sit for 1 to 2 minutes while the dizziness disappears, and then assisting the patient to a standing position.

The nurse frequently uses the upper arm and brachial artery for monitoring blood pressure. However, it may be necessary to use the thigh and popliteal artery when both arms have intravenous lines or saline locks, when the arms are edematous or injured, a severely burned patient, a patient who has a cast or bandage, or with a patient who has a shunt for dialysis (Fig. 11-9).

Equipment to Measure Blood Pressure

Special equipment is used to measure blood pressure. A **sphygmomanometer,** commonly called a *blood pressure machine,* consists of a cuff and a measuring gauge. There are two types of standard

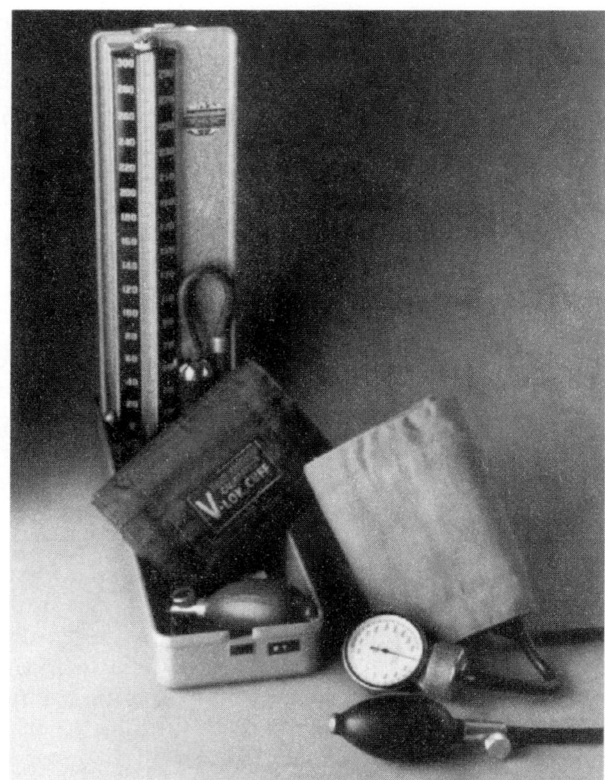

Fig. 11-10 Mercury *(left)* and aneroid sphygmomanometer. (From Potter PA, Perry AG: *Fundamentals of nursing: concepts, process, and practice,* ed 3, St Louis, 1993, Mosby.)

gauges. A mercury manometer consists of a calibrated vertical panel to which a glass tube containing the standardized column of mercury is attached (Fig. 11-10). An aneroid manometer is a calibrated, round dial unit with a needle pointer (Fig. 11-10).

The cuff is an airtight, flat, rubber bladder that is covered with an occlusive cloth. Cuffs come in many widths, from small sizes for infants to sizes large enough to fit large arms or thighs. For an accurate reading the width of the cuff should be 20% wider than the diameter of the upper arm or thigh at its midpoint. Two tubes are attached to the bladder within the cuff. One of the tubes is connected to the manometer, and the other is attached to a pressure bulb used to inflate the cuff. The bulb has an attached needle valve that, when closed, allows the bladder to be inflated as the bulb is being pumped. When the valve is turned in the opposite direction, the bladder is allowed to deflate. When learning to take blood pressure, the nurse should practice holding and manipulating the sphygmomanometer bulb and needle valve before concentrating on reading blood pressure on the manometer gauge.

When listening to blood pressure, the nurse hears a series of sounds through the stethoscope that are

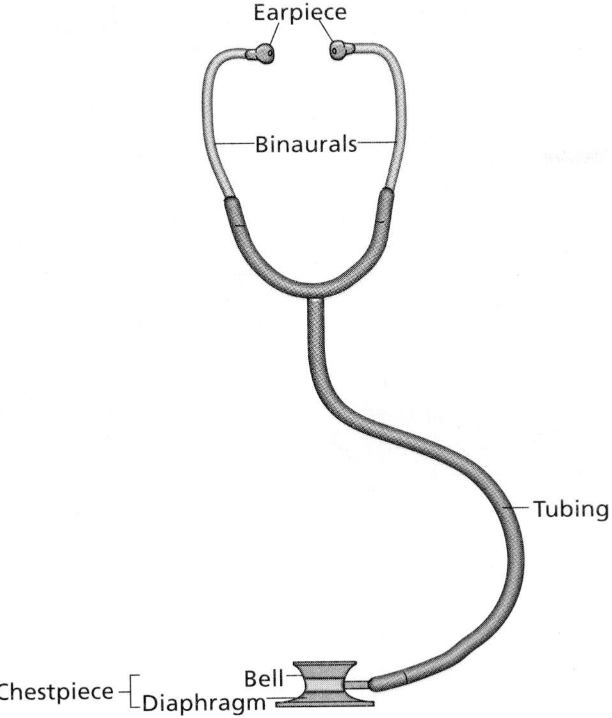

Fig. 11-11 Acoustical stethoscope. (From Potter PA, Perry AG: *Fundamentals of nursing: concepts, process, and practice,* ed 3, St Louis, 1993, Mosby.)

KOROTKOFF SOUNDS

- *First Korotkoff Sound:* This is the first in a series of clear rhythmical tapping sounds. This is the systolic pressure.
- *Second Korotkoff Sound:* As the cuff is further deflated, the sound changes to a murmur or swish. This is not recorded as part of a standard blood pressure reading.
- *Third Korotkoff Sound:* The sounds become crisper and more intense. This is not recorded as part of a standard blood pressure reading.
- *Fourth Korotkoff Sound:* The sounds become muffled and more low pitched as the cuff is deflated. This is recorded as the diastolic pressure only for infants and children and is not recorded as part of an adult blood pressure reading.
- *Fifth Korotkoff Sound:* This is the first time all sound disappears. This is recorded as the diastolic blood pressure for adolescents and adults.

created by the blood flowing through an artery (Fig. 11-11). These sounds are called **Korotkoff sounds.** These sounds and their significance to blood pressure readings are described the box.

In most clinical situations, the first and fifth Korotkoff sounds are recorded as a two-number blood pressure reading. However, if sounds are heard all the way to 0 during deflation of the cuff, the nurse records the reading with a three-number blood pressure reading (for example, 140/70/0 mm Hg). The first number is the first Korotkoff sound, the second number is the fourth Korotkoff sound (muffle point), and the last number is 0. Some agency policies or certain clinical situations dictate that the nurse record a three-number blood pressure reading. In this case, the three numbers are the first, fourth, and fifth Korotkoff sounds (that is, the first of the rhythmical sounds, the muffle point, and the point where all sound disappears).

When the nurse is unable to hear a blood pressure through a standard stethoscope because of a weak arterial pulse, a Doppler or ultrasonic stethoscope may be used to measure the systolic pressure (see Fig. 11-8). This allows the nurse to hear the fainter sounds.

NURSING CARE

Assessing vital signs is a routine part of nursing care. Vital signs provide important information about the health of the patient. Temperature, pulse, respirations, and blood pressure are measured as part of the initial patient assessment. These readings provide a baseline. Comparing subsequent measurements against these baseline data can reveal changes that may affect the health of the patient.

In addition, the nurse continuously assesses and observes the patient. These findings, along with any changes in vital signs, can help the health care team identify and correct the patient's medical problems.

The nurse ensures that the room environment is conducive for obtaining accurate vital signs. The nurse is also responsible for making certain that the equipment is in accurate working order. Inaccurate measurement of vital signs may occur from the use of faulty equipment, causing a change in the patient's condition to go unnoticed.

The nurse takes vital signs in a systematic order: for example, the temperature, pulse, respirations, and blood pressure. This routine is used unless there is an emergency. Significant changes in vital signs are reported and documented as appropriate according to agency policy.

In addition to measuring vital signs, the nurse is responsible the following aspects of nursing practice:

1. Palpating the patient's skin to determine its warmth or coolness. Looking for changes in the skin such as turgor to detect dehydration, flushed

skin, and moist skin. Variations may indicate an elevation in body temperature.
2. Determining the baseline temperature from the admission record.
3. Asking how the patient feels and describing any symptoms that could indicate fever.
4. Monitoring laboratory results especially for electrolyte imbalance.
5. Inspecting and palpating for dehydration.
6. Deciding whether vital signs need to be assessed.

NURSING PROCESS

Assessment

Vital signs indicate health status. Many factors can cause vital signs to change, sometimes outside normal range. A change in vital signs can indicate a change in physiologic functioning. After learning the physiologic variables that influence vital signs and recognizing the relationship of changes in vital signs and other physical assessment findings, the nurse can make an accurate determination of the patient's health problems.

Nursing Diagnosis

The nurse reviews all data gathered during assessment. Defining characteristics are clustered to reveal a diagnosis. Possible nursing diagnoses related to vital signs include the following:

Activity intolerance
Altered (specify) tissue perfusion (cerebral, cardiopulmonary, renal gastrointestinal, peripheral)
Decreased cardiac output
Fluid volume deficit
Hyperthermia
Hypothermia
Ineffective breathing pattern
Risk for altered body temperature
Risk for fluid volume deficit

Planning

The plan of care should focus on nursing care measures that the nurse can perform. For example, the care plan for patients with temperature alterations focuses on restoring normal body temperature, minimizing complications, and promoting comfort (see care plan on p. 156). The plan may include the following:

Goal: Complications of altered body temperature are minimized.

Outcome

Patient's blood pressure, pulse, and respirations are within normal limits.

PATIENT TEACHING 

- Give the patient information about normal or abnormal body temperature and rationales for corresponding nursing interventions.
- Children may be fearful of thermometers. Show them the thermometer and give age-appropriate calming explanations.
- Teach the patient to be his or her own advocate in having the correct size cuff used for monitoring blood pressure.

GERONTOLOGIC CONSIDERATIONS

- The basal metabolic rate decreases as a person ages.
- Because of normal age-related arterial changes, a pulse may be easily obliterated.
- As a person ages, it is normal for blood pressure to gradually increase.

Implementation

While implementing the plan of care, the nurse can also assess readiness to learn and teach health-promotion practices (see teaching box). Special considerations should be given to the older adult (see gerontologic box).

Evaluation

The nurse evaluates the success of interventions by comparing the patient's response to the outcomes of the plan of care. The evaluative process is ongoing because the patient's condition may change.

Goal: Complications of altered body temperature are minimized.

Evaluative measure

Assess vital signs after therapies for temperature alterations.

NURSING INTERVENTIONS

Preventing Body Temperature Elevation

The nurse should take measures to prevent **hyperpyrexia,** or fever (body temperature elevation above 98.6° F [37° C]) such as giving a tepid sponge and administering **antipyretics** (medications that

Table 11-4 COMMON FEVER PATTERNS

Type of Fever	Nature of Pattern	Possible Cause
Sustained	Little fluctuation	Scarlet fever Pneumococcal pneumonia Rickettsial fever Central nervous system problems
Intermittent	Wide temperature variations with return to normal at least once daily	Bacterial or viral infection Acute pyelonephritis Malaria
Remittent	Fluctuations less than intermittent; no return to normal	Endocarditis Pneumonia
Recurrent	Duration of few days; return to normal for 1 day or more and then return	Hodgkin's disease Rat-bite fever Yellow fever
Night	Occurrence late in evening or night	Tuberculosis

From Potter PA, Perry AG: *Fundamentals of nursing: concepts, process, and practice,* ed 3, St Louis, 1993, Mosby.

Table 11-5 SAMPLE EVALUATION OF INTERVENTIONS FOR HYPERTHERMIA

Goals	Evaluative Measures	Expected Outcomes
Patient will regain normal body temperature range by 3/21.	Monitor body temperature after intervention (for example, tepid sponge bath, antipyretic medications).	Body temperature will decline at least 1° C (18° F) after therapy
	Monitor body temperature every 4 hr.	Body temperature will remain in normal range for at least 24 hr by 3/20.
Fluid and electrolyte balance will be maintained by 3/21.	Assess skin turgor and texture. Monitor serum electrolyte values. Measure intake and output levels.	Skin will remain supple with normal texture. Electrolyte level will remain in normal range. Output will not exceed intake.
Patient will attain sense of comfort and rest by 3/21.	Question how patient feels. Observe for restlessness.	Patient will describe sense of relaxation with renewed energy. Patient will be able to rest or sleep quietly.

From Potter PA, Perry AG: *Fundamentals of nursing: concepts, process, and practice,* ed 3, St Louis, 1993, Mosby.

reduce fever). The physician indicates a temperature at which such medications are administered (for example, for fever above 102° F [39° C]).

Treatment for Fever

The nurse should always report fever to the physician. The physician may then request that specimens be obtained for diagnostic urine, blood, and sputum cultures. It is the nurse's responsibility to obtain the cultures and ensure that they are taken to the laboratory. The nurse also reports such test results to the physician.

Fever has common patterns that help the physician diagnose the patient's condition and thus direct treatment (Table 11-4). Some physicians say that a fever is not harmful if the patient's temperature is under 102° F (39° C). Thus the treatment of fever is still a topic of debate.

Independent nursing measures

The nurse may perform many independent nursing measures for patients who are **febrile** (have a fever) (Table 11-5). From these nursing measures the nurse may decide which, if any, symptoms need attention from the physician.

■ NURSING CARE PLAN ■

HYPOTHERMIA

Mrs. N, age 70, was found wandering in the snow and icy weather. When she was admitted to the emergency room, her body temperature was 92° F, her skin was cold, and she was shivering.

NURSING DIAGNOSIS

Hypothermia related to exposure to cold or cold environment as evidenced by cool skin, shivering, pallor, cyanotic nail beds, and tachycardia

GOALS

- Skin will be warm and dry to touch.
- Heart rate and blood pressure will be within normal limits.

EXPECTED OUTCOMES

- Body temperature is within normal limits.
- Patient is warm.

NURSING INTERVENTIONS

- Monitor vital signs at least every 2 to 4 hr.
- Provide supportive measures that provide body warmth and protect patient from heat loss.
- Follow prescribed treatment measures.

EVALUATION

- Patient's body temperature remains within normal limits.
- Patient voices feelings of comfort.
- Patient 's skin is warm and dry to touch.
- Patient describes measures to prevent episodes of hypothermia.

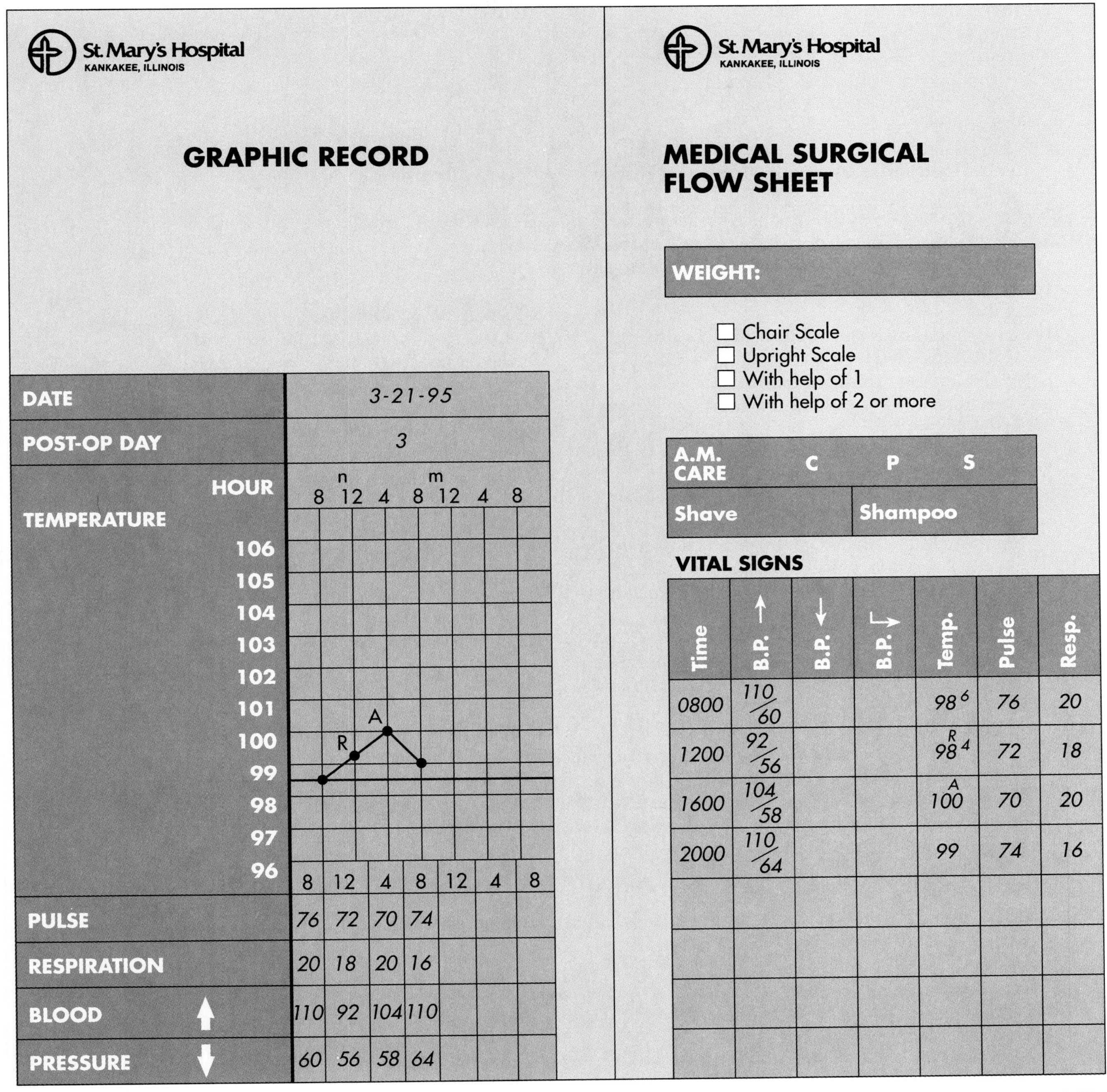

St. Mary's Hospital
KANKAKEE, ILLINOIS

GRAPHIC RECORD

DATE	3-21-95						
POST-OP DAY	3						
HOUR	8	n 12	4	8	m 12	4	8

	8	12	4	8	12	4	8
PULSE	76	72	70	74			
RESPIRATION	20	18	20	16			
BLOOD ↑	110	92	104	110			
PRESSURE ↓	60	56	58	64			

St. Mary's Hospital
KANKAKEE, ILLINOIS

MEDICAL SURGICAL FLOW SHEET

WEIGHT:

☐ Chair Scale
☐ Upright Scale
☐ With help of 1
☐ With help of 2 or more

A.M. CARE	C	P	S
Shave		Shampoo	

VITAL SIGNS

Time	B.P. ↑	B.P. ↓	B.P. ↳	Temp.	Pulse	Resp.
0800	110/60			98⁶	76	20
1200	92/56			R 98⁴	72	18
1600	104/58			A 100	70	20
2000	110/64			99	74	16

Fig. 11-12 Documentation of vital signs, temperature, pulse, respirations, and blood pressure. (Courtesy St. Mary's Hospital, Kankakee, Ill.)

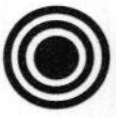

SKILL 11-1 MEASURING BODY TEMPERATURE (ORAL, AXILLARY, RECTAL)

Steps	Rationale
1. Obtain equipment: ▪ Appropriate thermometer ▪ Tissue or paper towel ▪ Clean gloves if necessary ▪ Water soluble lubricant for measurement of rectal temperature ▪ Pen and paper	Helps organize procedure.
2. Refer to medical record, care plan, or Kardex for special interventions.	Provides basis for care.
3. Wash hands and don clean gloves according to agency policy and guidelines from Centers for Disease Control and Prevention and Occupational Safety and Health Administration.	Helps prevent cross-contamination.
4. Introduce self.	Decreases anxiety level.
5. Identify patient by identification band.	Identifies correct patient for procedure.
6. Explain procedure to patient.	Seeks cooperation and decreases anxiety.
7. Prepare patient for intervention:	
a. Close door to room or pull curtain.	Provides privacy.
b. Drape if necessary.	Prevents exposure of patient.
8. Raise bed to comfortable working level.	Provides for patient's comfort and nurse's safety.
9. Arrange for patient privacy.	Shows respect for patient.
10. Measure oral temperature with glass thermometer:	
a. Remove clinical thermometer from container, being careful not to touch tip of thermometer.	Protects bulb end and keeps end clean for patient use.
b. Hold thermometer at eye level, rotate until mercury line is visible, and read.	Ensures reading accuracy.
c. Shake thermometer down to 96° F (35.5° C) using snapping motion of wrist while holding tip end of thermometer firmly between thumb and first two fingers.	Ensures accurate measurement.
d. Apply plastic sheath to thermometer.	Helps prevent cross-contamination.
e. Place thermometer tip gently under tongue in midline (right or left sublingual pocket) (Fig. 11-13).	Ensures that blood supply close to surface of mucous membrane will accurately record core body temperature.
f. Instruct patient to hold thermometer in mouth and to keep lips closed.	Helps ensure accurate reading.
g. Keep thermometer in place at least 2 to 3 minutes or according to agency policy.	Provides time needed to ensure accurate reading.
h. Remove thermometer carefully.	Prevents breakage of thermometer and patient injury.
i. Remove plastic sheath and discard.	Helps prevent cross-contamination.
11. Measure rectal temperature with glass thermometer:	
a. Place patient in left side-lying position.	Exposes anus for correct placement of thermometer.
b. Apply plastic sheath over thermometer with stubby or pear-shaped tip.	Prevents injury to rectal tissue.
c. Lubricate bulb of thermometer with water-soluble lubricant. For adult, lubricate 1 to 1½ inch, and for infant or young child, lubricate ½ to 1 inch.	Ensures safe and easy insertion of thermometer.
d. Uncover only rectal area and separate cheeks of buttocks, exposing anus.	Provides safe insertion of thermometer.
e. Ask patient to take deep breath.	Helps relax sphincter muscles for easier insertion.
f. Insert thermometer gently into anus (Fig. 11-14).	Minimizes risk of trauma to rectal area.

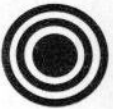

SKILL 11-1 MEASURING BODY TEMPERATURE (ORAL, AXILLARY, RECTAL)—cont'd

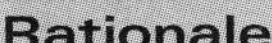

Steps	Rationale
g. Permit buttocks to fall in place and hold thermometer in place 3 to 5 minutes or according to agency policy.	Provides for patient safety.
h. Remove rectal thermometer gently, peel off plastic sheath, and discard.	Prevents patient injury.
i. Clean rectal area if necessary.	Ensures cleanliness and prevents skin breakdown.
12. Measure axillary temperature with glass thermometer:	
a. Place patient in prone position.	Provides easy access to axilla.
b. Apply plastic sheath over oral thermometer tip.	Prevents cross-contamination.
c. Place oral thermometer into center of axilla, lower patient's arm over thermometer, and place patient's arm across chest (Fig. 11-15).	Provides accurate measurement because central position of thermometer is against blood vessels in axilla.
d. Hold thermometer in place for 5 to 10 minutes or according to agency policy.	Provides time required to register temperature.
e. Remove thermometer carefully.	Prevents breakage of thermometer and patient injury.
13. Hold thermometer horizontally at eye level and read to 1/10° accuracy.	Ensures accurate reading.
14. Shake thermometer down.	Prepares thermometer for next use.
15. Return thermometer to container.	Avoids breakage.
16. Make patient comfortable.	Helps ensure patient's well-being.
17. Document (see Fig. 11-12).	Documents procedure and patient's response.

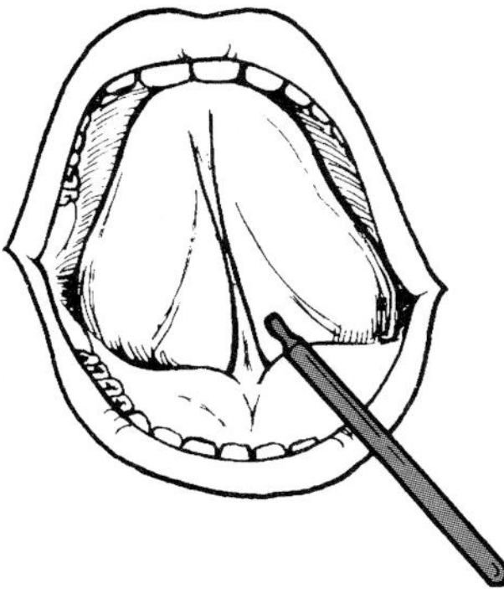

Fig. 11-13 Placement of oral clinical thermometer. (From Potter PA, Perry AG: *Fundamentals of nursing: concepts, process, and practice,* ed 3, St Louis, 1993, Mosby.)

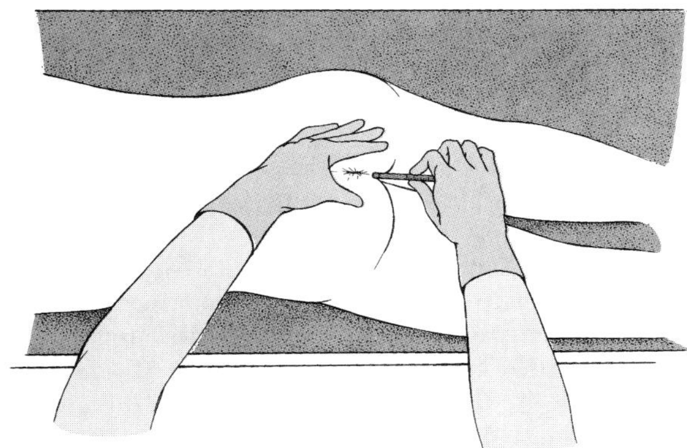

Fig. 11-14 Inserting a rectal thermometer. (From Potter PA, Perry AG: *Fundamentals of nursing: concepts, process, and practice,* ed 3, St Louis, 1993, Mosby.)

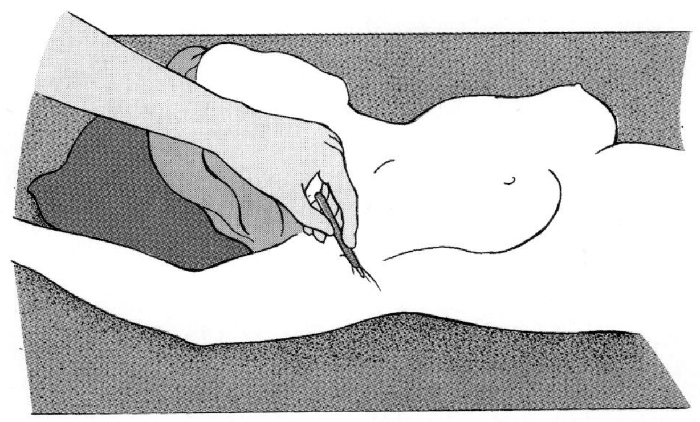

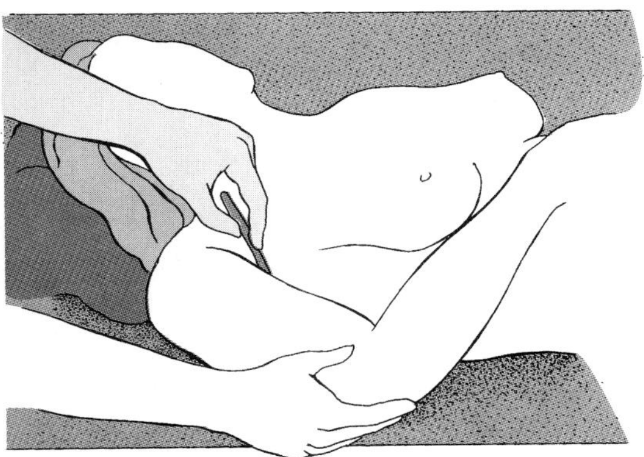

Fig. 11-15 Taking an axillary temperature. (From Potter PA, Perry AG: *Fundamentals of nursing: concepts, process, and practice,* ed 3, St Louis, 1993, Mosby.)

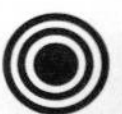

SKILL 11-2 MEASURING PULSE (RADIAL, APICAL)

Steps	Rationale
1. Obtain equipment: ▪ Pen and paper ▪ Wristwatch with second hand ▪ Clean gloves if necessary	Helps organize procedure.
2. Refer to medical record, care plan, or Kardex for special interventions.	Provides basis for care.
3. Wash hands and, if necessary, don clean gloves according to agency policy and guidelines from Centers for Disease Control and Prevention and Occupational Safety and Health Administration.	Helps prevent cross-contamination.
4. Introduce self.	Decreases anxiety level.
5. Identify patient by identification band.	Identifies correct patient for procedure.
6. Explain procedure to patient.	Seeks cooperation and decreases anxiety.
7. Prepare patient for intervention:	
a. Close door to room or pull curtain.	Provides privacy.
b. Drape if necessary.	Prevents exposure of patient.
8. Raise bed to comfortable working level.	Provides for patient's comfort and nurse's safety.
9. Arrange for patient privacy.	Shows respect for patient.
10. Measure radial pulse:	
a. Position patient's arm for comfort and for easy access.	Promotes patient's comfort and makes artery accessible to nurse.
b. Place first three fingers over and parallel to radial artery and lightly compress against radius (Fig. 11-16).	Helps ensure accuracy.
11. Measure apical pulse:	
a. Position patient on back.	Allows easy access to chest.
b. Move patient's gown to make upper chest visible without exposing patient.	Ensures access to apex of heart without exposing patient.
c. Palpate fifth intercostal space and move to left midclavicular line.	Locates where heartbeat is easiest to hear.
d. Place diaphragm of stethoscope in hand for 5 or 10 sec.	Promotes patient comfort.
e. Place diaphragm of stethoscope on apex of heart and listen for "lub dup" sounds (beats).	Allows identification of sounds that occur as blood flows through heart valves.
12. Count number of heartbeats for 1 min.	Helps ensure accuracy.
13. Note rate, rhythm, and strength of pulse.	Gives additional information about patient's cardiac status.
14. Make patient comfortable.	Helps ensure patient's well-being.
15. Remove gloves if necessary and wash hands.	Helps prevent cross-contamination.
16. Document (see Fig. 11-12).	Documents procedure and patient's response.

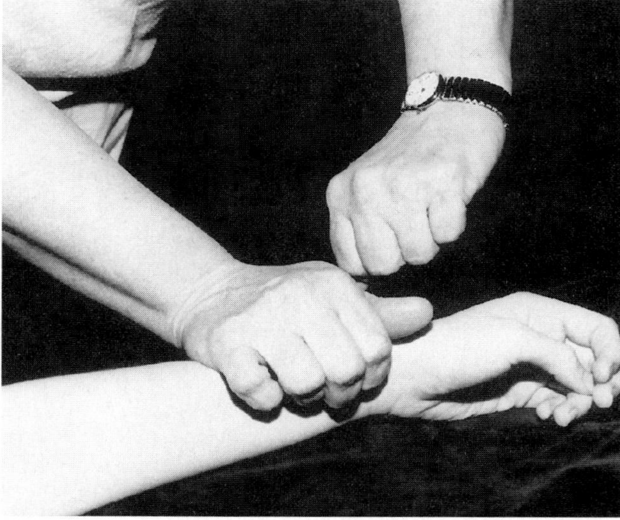

Fig. 11-16 Correct placement of fingers for taking a radial pulse.

SKILL 11-3 MEASURING RESPIRATIONS

Steps	Rationale
1. Refer to medical record, care plan, or Kardex for special interventions.	Provides basis for care.
2. Wash hands.	Helps prevent cross-contamination.
3. Introduce self.	Decreases anxiety level.
4. Identify patient by identification band.	Identifies correct patient for procedure.
5. Explain procedure to patient.	Seeks cooperation and decreases anxiety.
6. Prepare patient for intervention:	
a. Close door to room or pull curtain.	Provides privacy.
b. Drape if necessary.	Prevents exposure of patient.
7. Raise bed to comfortable working level.	Provides for patient's comfort and nurse's safety.
8. Arrange for patient privacy.	Shows respect for patient.
9. If assessing respirations immediately after assessing pulse rate, keep fingers in place after counting pulse.	Minimizes patient awareness of respiration assessment.
10. Count rise and fall of patient's chest for 1 min.	Ensures accuracy and allows assessment of abnormalities.
11. If unable to easily see breathing, move patient's arm across abdomen or lower chest or place own hand on patient's shoulder.	Enables nurse to count respirations by feeling respiratory movement.
12. While counting respirations, assess rate, depth, and rhythm.	Identifies abnormalities in respirations.
13. Make patient comfortable.	Helps ensure patient's well-being.
14. Document (see Fig. 11-12).	Documents procedure and patient's response.

SKILL 11-4 MEASURING BLOOD PRESSURE

Steps	Rationale
1. Obtain equipment: ▪ Sphygmomanometer ▪ Stethoscope ▪ Alcohol preps ▪ Pen and paper	Helps organize procedure.
2. Refer to medical record, care plan, or Kardex for special interventions.	Provides basis for care.
3. Wash hands and don clean gloves according to agency policy and guidelines from Centers for Disease Control and Prevention and Occupational Safety and Health Administration.	Helps prevent cross-contamination.
4. Introduce self.	Decreases anxiety.
5. Identify patient by identification band.	Identifies correct patient for procedure.
6. Explain procedure to patient.	Seeks cooperation and decreases anxiety.
7. Prepare patient for intervention.	
a. Close door to room or pull curtain.	Provides privacy.
b. Drape if necessary.	Prevents exposure of patient.
8. Raise bed to comfortable working level.	Provides for patient's comfort and nurse's safety.
9. Arrange for patient privacy.	Shows respect for patient.
10. Expose upper arm (Fig. 11-17).	Helps ensure accurate reading.
11. Palpate brachial artery in antecubital space (Fig. 11-18).	Locates appropriate area to position cuff.
12. Locate middle of inflatable bladder and position cuff 1 inch above brachial artery pulsation (Fig. 11-19).	Ensures that pressure applied during cuff inflation is centered over brachial artery.
13. Make certain cuff is fully deflated and wrap it evenly and snugly around arm (Fig. 11-20).	Prevents inaccurate reading caused by loose cuff.

Continued.

SKILL 11-4 MEASURING BLOOD PRESSURE—cont'd

Steps	Rationale
14. Position sphygmanometer at eye level.	Ensures accurate assessment.
15. Tighten screw valve but not too tight.	Closes system for inflation.
16. Place diaphragm of stethoscope over brachial artery (Fig. 11-21).	Denotes readiness to listen to sounds.
17. Place stethoscope ear pieces in ears.	Denotes readiness to listen to sounds.
18. Inflate cuff to 160 to 180 mm Hg.	Inflates cuff higher than blood pressure reading.
19. Release valve slowly, allowing mercury to fall two to three points per second (Fig. 11-22).	Allows time to correlate Korotkoff sounds with sphygmomanometer reading.
20. Note point on sphygmanometer at which first sound is heard and read pressure to nearest even number.	Identifies first Korotkoff sound or systolic reading when obliterated pulsation reappears.
21. Continue to deflate cuff gradually and note point at which muffled sound appears.	Identifies fourth Korotkoff sound and or diastolic reading for infants and children.
22. Continue to slowly deflate cuff and note point at which last sound is heard.	Identifies fifth Korotkoff sound and or diastolic reading for adults.
23. Complete deflation rapidly and remove cuff from arm.	Minimizes discomfort from cuff pressure.
24. If need to retake blood pressure, wait at least 30 sec before repeating procedure.	Permits blood trapped in veins to be released and prepares arm for measurement.
25. Fold cuff, store it, and clean earpieces of stethoscope with alcohol prep.	Prevents cross-contamination.
26. Make patient comfortable.	Helps ensure patient's well-being.
27. Document (see Fig. 11-12).	Documents procedure and patient's response.

Fig. 11-17 Exposing the upper arm fully. (From Potter PA, Perry AG: *Fundamentals of nursing: concepts, process, and practice,* ed 3, St Louis, 1993, Mosby.)

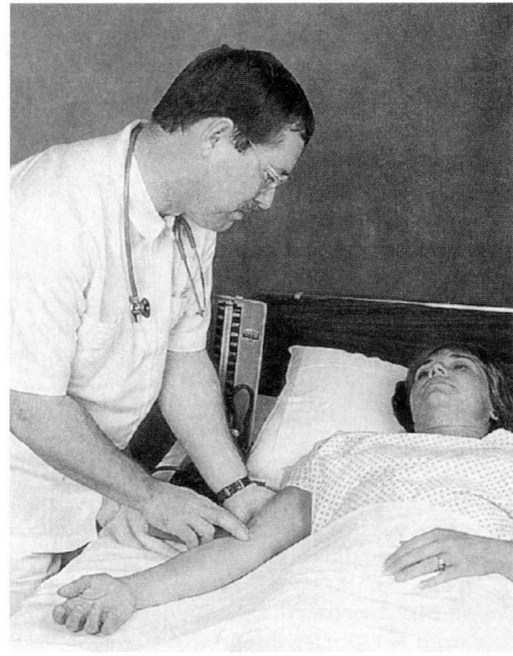

Fig. 11-18 Palpating the brachial artery in antecubital space. (From Potter PA, Perry AG: *Fundamentals of nursing: concepts, process, and practice,* ed 3, St Louis, 1993, Mosby.)

SKILL 11-4 MEASURING BLOOD PRESSURE—cont'd

Steps | Rationale

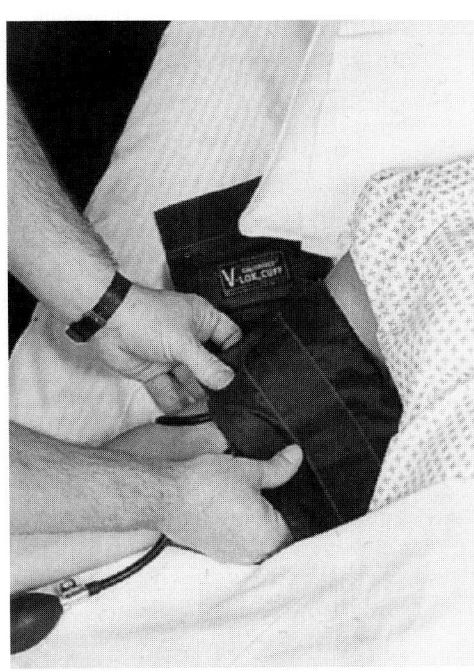

Fig. 11-19 Correct application of blood pressure cuff. (From Potter PA, Perry AG: *Fundamentals of nursing: concepts, process, and practice,* ed 3, St Louis, 1993, Mosby.)

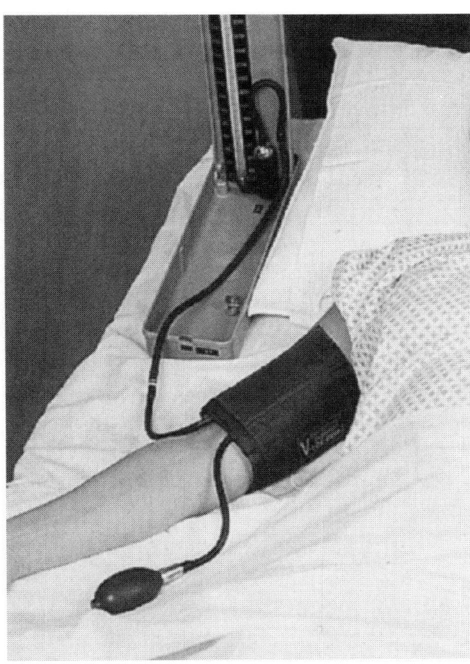

Fig. 11-20 Blood pressure cuff wrapped evenly and snugly around arm. (From Potter PA, Perry AG: *Fundamentals of nursing: concepts, process, and practice,* ed 3, St Louis, 1993, Mosby.)

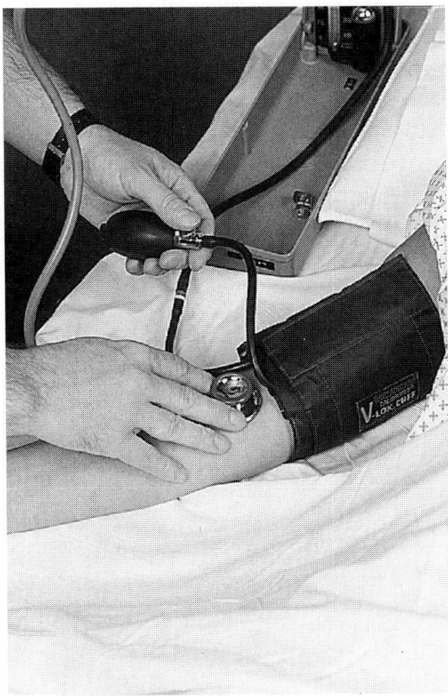

Fig. 11-21 Placement of diaphragm of stethoscope over brachial artery. (From Potter PA, Perry AG: *Fundamentals of nursing: concepts, process, and practice,* ed 3, St Louis, 1993, Mosby.)

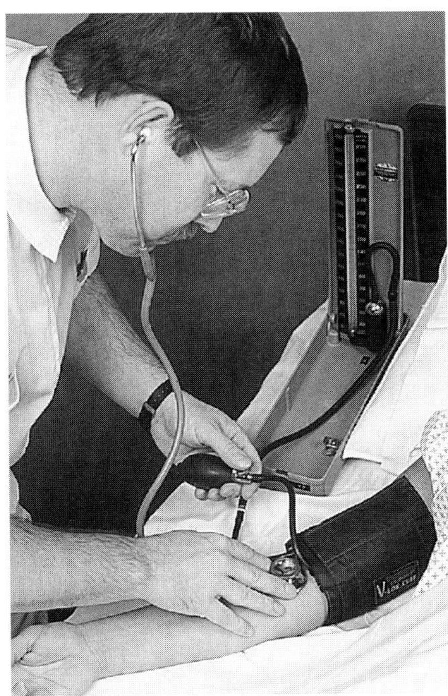

Fig. 11-22 Releasing valve slowly. (From Potter PA, Perry AG: *Fundamentals of nursing: concepts, process, and practice,* ed 3, St Louis, 1993, Mosby.)

SUMMARY

Vital signs provide important information about a patient's condition, so assessment of them is an important skill. Vital signs assessment should not be taken for granted, since the patient's life may depend on accurate assessment of body temperature, pulse, respiration, and blood pressure. Findings reported to the physician may mean early diagnosis and treatment of a patient's problem.

Key Concepts

- Vital signs must be assessed according to medical orders and agency policy but should also be assessed as soon as a change is manifested.
- Vital signs indicate the condition of the patient.
- Body heat must be kept within a certain range for organs to appropriately function.
- Core temperature remains relatively constant unless the patient is exposed to severe extremes in the environment.
- The axillary method is the least accurate measurement of body temperature.
- The nurse obtains information about the circulatory status of the patient by measuring the pulse rate.
- The pulse and respiratory rates vary with age.
- Assessment of the pulse includes rate, rhythm, and strength.
- Respiration involves the intake of oxygen and the output of carbon dioxide.
- One does not think about breathing, which is an automatic activity.
- The pulse pressure may be so low that it causes problems for the patient.

Critical Thinking Questions

1. A 69-year-old homeless person has been brought into the emergency department by police who report she was found wandering incoherently in the middle of the street. The temperature outside is −21.0° F, and it has been snowing for 2 hours. In what order should the nurse obtain vital signs? What method should be used to obtain each vital sign? What factors place this patient at risk for impaired temperature regulation?
2. A hospitalized patient, admitted for pneumonia, has a tympanic temperature of 100.2° F, pulse of 84 beats/min, blood pressure of 130/84 mm Hg, respirations of 22 breaths/min, and oxygen saturation of 98%. Explain the rationale for your anticipated interventions for this patient.
3. A 22-year-old patient sustained a fractured mandible, fractured right radius, and fractured left humerus during a motorcycle accident. He is admitted postoperatively with an intravenous line in an unaffectd extremity. What are the most effective methods for obtaining this patient's vital signs?

REFERENCES AND SUGGESTED READINGS

Beare PG, Myers JL: *Principles and practice of adult health nursing,* ed 2, St Louis, 1994, Mosby.

Carpenito JC: *Nursing diagnoses: application to clinical practice,* ed 4, Philadelphia, 1994, Lippincott.

Kozier B, Erb G, Buffalino PM: *Introduction to nursing,* Redwood City, Calif, 1993, Addison-Wesley.

Kozier B, Erb G: *Techniques in clinical nursing,* ed 4, Redwood City, Calif, 1993, Addison-Wesley.

Potter PA, Perry AG: *Fundamentals of nursing: concepts, process, and practice,* ed 3, St Louis, 1993, Mosby.

Sunberg MC: *Fundamentals of nursing with clinical procedures,* ed 3, Boston, 1993, Jones & Bartlett.

CHAPTER 12

Physical Assessment

Learning Objectives

After studying this chapter, the student should be able to . . .

- Define the key terms.
- Identify the purposes of physical assessment.
- Describe the techniques used in physical examination.
- Interview a patient.
- Identify equipment and supplies used during physical assessment.
- Identify various body positions used during physical assessment.
- Describe information obtained during a review of systems.
- Identify the steps needed in each of the skills described in physical assessment.
- Identify special concerns for special populations.
- Perform a physical assessment according to agency policy.

Key Terms

Auscultation
Breast self-examination
Bruit
Capillary refill
Cyanosis
Data base
Edema
Epistaxis
General survey
Health history
Inspection
Jaundice
Palpation
Percussion
Physical assessment
Testicular self-examination
Turgor

Skills

12-1 Performing a general survey
12-2 Assessing the skin
12-3 Assessing the hair and scalp
12-4 Assessing the nails
12-5 Assessing the eyes
12-6 Assessing the ears
12-7 Assessing the nose and sinuses
12-8 Assessing the mouth and pharynx
12-9 Assessing the structures of the neck
12-10 Assessing the thorax and lungs
12-11 Assessing the heart and vascular system
12-12 Assessing the abdomen
12-13 Assessing the breasts and axillae
12-14 Assessing the female genitalia and rectum
12-15 Assessing the male genitalia and rectum
12-16 Assessing the musculoskeletal system
12-17 Assessing the neurologic system

Physical assessment plays a major role in nursing care. Through physical assessment, information (data) about the patient's physical, emotional, and functional status is collected. Data collected during examination establishes a baseline and allows the nurse to identify patient problems and plan nursing care. Ongoing nursing assessment enables the nurse to evaluate the effectiveness of nursing care.

Physical assessment, which is a head-to-toe examination of each body system, along with the health history, provides a comprehensive picture of the patient's overall physical condition. Physical assessment is performed (1) on admission to a health care facility, (2) as a routine preventive measure, (3) to identify health problems or changes in health status, (4) to evaluate care, and (5) on a daily basis or during each shift.

TECHNIQUES

Techniques of physical assessment are skills every nurse should possess. Most physical examinations are conducted using a head-to-toe sequence. However, the patient's condition may require modifications in sequence or technique. For example, a patient admitted with severe gastrointestinal bleeding may be too ill to undergo a musculoskeletal system examination. Assessment of this system may be delayed until the patient's condition is stabilized.

Techniques used by nurses during physical assessment rely on the human senses of sight, touch, hearing, and smell. Skills necessary for physical assessment include inspection, palpation, auscultation, and sometimes percussion.

Inspection (looking or observing)

Inspection means "to look or observe." Inspection must be performed under good lighting conditions, with full exposure of the body part being assessed. Each body part is compared to its corresponding part. This comparison is extremely helpful in identifying abnormal changes. For example, when the nurse compares skin color of one hand to skin color of the opposite hand, an abnormality quickly becomes apparent.

Palpation (feeling or touch)

Using the hand and tips of the fingers because they are the most sensitive parts, the nurse gathers patient information through palpation. **Palpation** is using touch or feeling to determine temperature, moisture, movement, and shape.

During light palpation, the skin over the area to be examined is depressed about ½ inch. Light palpation is used primarily to determine areas of tenderness.

Deep palpation is used to examine organs, such as those in the abdomen. When deep palpation is used, the area being examined is depressed 1 inch. Deep palpation is sometimes applied using both hands (bimanually). An example of bimanual palpation is the palpation of a kidney.

The following guidelines and precautions that must be observed when using palpation:

1. The nurse should ensure that the patient is warm and relaxed.
2. The nurse should have very short fingernails and warm hands.
3. Palpation performed by one who is not appropriately trained can result in internal injuries.

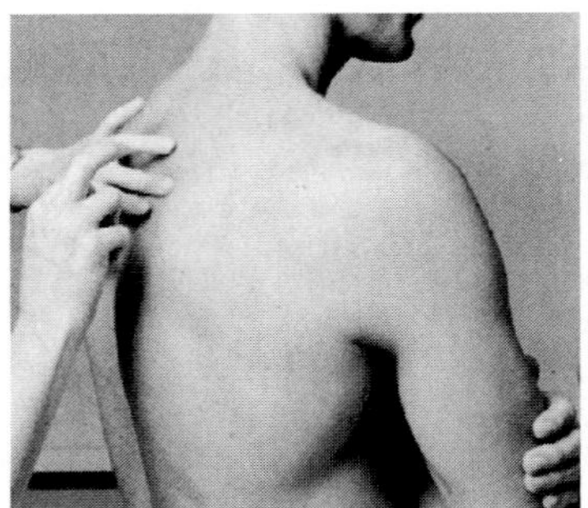

Fig. 12-1 Percussion of the intercostal spaces. (From Perry AG, Potter PA: *Clinical nursing skills and techniques,* ed 3, St Louis, 1994, Mosby.)

Percussion (tapping)

Percussion is used to assess the size of some internal organ or to determine the presence of air or fluid within body cavities. **Percussion** is performed by placing the nondominant hand over the area to be percussed, with the middle finger held firmly against the skin, and then striking that finger with the middle finger of the dominant hand (Fig. 12-1). This tapping action produces audible vibrations. With practice, several different tones may be identified. These tones follow:

1. Tympany. Sound heard when percussing an air-filled organ (for example, the stomach). It is a loud, drumlike sound similar to the sound heard when percussing a puffed cheek.
2. Resonance. A loud, low-pitched, hollow sound heard when the lungs are percussed.
3. Dullness. The high-pitched, thudlike sound heard percussing the liver is percussed. It is easily distinguished from the lungs.
4. Flatness. The soft, high-pitched sound that is heard when a muscle is percussed. This sound can be produced by percussing the thigh.
5. Hyperresonance. A very loud, booming, low-pitched sound. This sound can be heard when percussing the emphysematous lung.

Auscultation (listening)

Auscultation is listening to various sounds within the body, usually with a stethoscope. A stethoscope has two end pieces, a diaphragm, and a bell. To hear low-pitched sounds, such as those produced by the heart and vascular system, the nurse should use the bell. High-pitched sounds, such as those made by the lungs and intestines, are best heard with the diaphragm. The diaphragm should be pressed firmly against the skin, but the bell should be held lightly against the skin. Sounds heard during auscultation are assessed according to four characteristics: pitch, loudness, quality, and duration. Pitch is described from low to high. Loudness is described from soft to loud. Quality can be described in such terms as harsh, blowing, or swishing. Duration is described as short or long.

GATHERING A DATA BASE

The nurse uses the information from the health history, general history, and physical examination as part of the **data base** (a form that includes all the gathered information about a specific patient). This important information then is used to develop nursing diagnoses and a nursing care plan to help ensure quality nursing care.

Health History

The **health history** is data collected about a patient's level of wellness, changes in life patterns, sociocultural role, and mental and emotional reactions to illness. It is obtained by interviewing the patient. This is often the most important and most informative part of the examination. The nurse establishes a relationship with the patient during the interview. Only by establishing a relationship of trust and confidence will the nurse be able to obtain the information needed. Most agencies have their own form to use when obtaining a patient's health history. Often these forms are checklists or require only a word or two to complete each question.

A brief outline for obtaining a health history is shown (see box). This is intended to be a guide and should not limit the nurse. Suggestions for a more comprehensive history can be found in textbooks on physical examination.

If appropriate, information regarding the patient's religion, education, occupation, and lifestyle may also be obtained. The purpose of the history is to learn about the patient. Most of the information collected during the history is subjective data.

General Survey

The **general survey** begins with review of the patient's health problems (Skill 12-1). The nurse clinically observes or assesses the patient's general appearance. The nurse also determines whether the patient looks the stated age.

The nurse also includes a general information such as gender, ethnic origin, and age. After eliciting this information, the nurse begins the specific assessment, usually by asking the patient questions about the condition or functioning of each body system.

PERFORMING THE PHYSICAL EXAMINATION

The equipment and supplies used during the examination should be ready for use and conveniently arranged (see box). A stethoscope, sphygmomanometer, clinical or digital thermometer, scale, clean gloves, penlight, tongue depressor, and tape measure are commonly required.

Preparing for the Examination

The nurse should be prepared to perform the physical examination. Preparation includes the patient, environment, equipment, and supplies. Although examinations are sometimes performed in a patient's room instead of in a separate, specially equipped examination room, certain items are necessary. Privacy and organization are essential. Privacy curtains or dividers should be used to screen the patient. To prevent possible embarrassment and provide warmth, the patient should be covered with drapes and a gown. Drapes should be adjusted so that only the body part being examined is exposed. Adequate lighting is essential. The nurse should take steps to prevent interruptions during the examination. A *Do Not Disturb* sign on the door may be necessary.

Assessing the Skin

The skin is the first line of defense for the body. It protects, regulates temperature, and serves as a sensory organ for touch and pain. Skin can provide information about a patient's health status. The nurse assesses the skin's color and integrity (Skill 12-2). The color varies according to ethnic origin and exposure to the sun. Disease can also alter skin color. Flushing or redness is often associated with fever. **Cyanosis,** a bluish or dusky color, is associated with circulatory or respiratory problems. **Jaundice,** a yellowing of the skin, can indicate liver problems, whereas pallor or paleness can mean that the patient has a decrease in hemoglobin levels.

HEALTH HISTORY

Identifying data. Determine patient's name, age, gender, marital status, and identifying number if appropriate.

Source of information. Indicate whether information is provided by patient, relative, or friend. Indicate whether source is reliable.

Reason for seeking health care. Ask about patient's problem.

History of present illness. Ask when problem first appeared. Include date, specific symptoms, treatment, and results of treatment.

Past health status. Include past illnesses, surgeries, and injuries, as well as allergies and diagnostic tests. Also ask about and list prescription and over-the-counter medications patient is now or has recently taken.

Family health history. Ask whether anyone in patient's family suffers same or similar problems. Include immediate family (parents, grandparents, children, siblings, and spouse) and extended family (cousins, aunts, and uncles). Ask what other health problems have occurred in family.

Review of systems. Ask questions about patient's general health and about each body system.

General. Ask patient whether there have been any changes in weight or occurrences of weakness, fatigue, dizziness, or fever.

Level of consciousness. Assess orientation to time, place, person, and events.

Skin. Ask patient about rashes, lumps, itching, dryness, changes in color, bruising, changes in hair or nails, or changes in moles.

Head. Ask about headaches or injuries.

Eyes. Ask whether there been any vision changes or pain. Determine date of last eye examination and whether patient wears corrective lenses or contacts (and type).

Ears. Ask whether patient has problems with hearing. Determine whether patient has experienced ringing in ears, dizziness, signs of infection, earaches, or pain.

Nose and sinuses. Ascertain whether patient has had nosebleeds, stuffiness, frequent colds, drainage, or pain.

Mouth and throat. Determine whether patient has problems with teeth, gums, or throat.

Neck. Ascertain whether there has been pain, stiffness, swollen glands, or lumps.

Breasts. Determine whether there been pain, lumps, discharge from nipples, or changes in skin texture of breasts.

Respiratory system. Ascertain whether patient coughs or wheezes. Determine whether patient has any history of asthma, bronchitis, tuberculosis, or pneumonia; and history of coughing up blood or phlegm; shortness of breath, especially at night?

Cardiovascular system. Ascertain whether there is history of heart trouble, chest pains, or palpitations and history of rheumatic fever or heart murmurs. Determine whether patient has difficulty breathing at night? Edema?

Gastrointestinal system. Ascertain whether the patient has had problems with swallowing, heartburn, or vomiting. Are there problems with any foods? Any history of vomiting blood or of having bloody or black bowel movements? Any problems with constipation or diarrhea? Change in bowel habits? Indigestion?

Genitourinary system. How many times a day does the patient urinate? Determine the amount, frequency, and color of urine. Any problems with incontinence or blood in the urine? Any history of kidney stones? Any infections? Any burning or pain when urinating?

Female reproductive system. Ascertain date of last menses. Any pain or irregularities associated with periods? Any discharge or lesions? Number of pregnancies, living children, miscarriages.

Male. Ascertain whether there has been any scrotal pain, hernias, or unusual lumps? Any sores on or discharge from penis? Wake up at night to urinate?

Back and extremities. Does the patient have joint pain, swelling, or stiffness? Any limitation of movement? Any muscle pain or cramping? Any history of varicose veins?

Neurologic status. Has the patient experienced fainting or loss of consciousness? Any history of convulsions, tremors, or paralysis?

Normally the skin is smooth, without breaks, bruises, rashes, or lesions (areas of damaged skin) (Table 12-1). Rashes (eruptions on the skin) are assessed for type, color, size, location, and itching. The skin should be assessed continuously for pressure ulcers, especially over the bony prominences (see Chapter 21). These are assessed for size, color, location, type, and drainage, if any. If changes in the skin occur, the patient should see a physician (Table 12-2). Skin is assessed for **edema** (excess fluid in the tissue) and **turgor** (elasticity) (Fig. 12-2).

Assessing the Hair and Scalp

Hair is normally found on all parts of the body except for the palms of the hands and soles of the feet. Hair is inspected for color, texture, and distri-

Table 12-1 SKIN LESIONS

Type	Description	Example
Macule	Small, flat, nonpalpable skin discoloration, usually less than 1 cm	Freckle
Papule	Small, elevated, palpable mass, usually less than 0.5 cm	Nevus
Nodule	Larger, deeper, and firmer lesion than a papule	Wart
Tumor	Nodule larger than 1 to 2 cm and that may extend into subcutaneous tissue	
Wheal	Palpable, raised area of localized skin edema that is usually transient	Mosquito bite
Vesicle	Superficial elevation of skin, usually less than 0.5 cm and filled with serous fluid	Chicken pox
Bulla	Vesicle larger than 0.5 cm	Blister of second-degree burn
Pustule	Vesicle filled with pus	Acne
Erosion	Loss of skin surface in which area is moist but does not bleed	Broken blister
Ulcer	Deep erosion that may bleed	
Fissure	Crack in skin	Athlete's foot

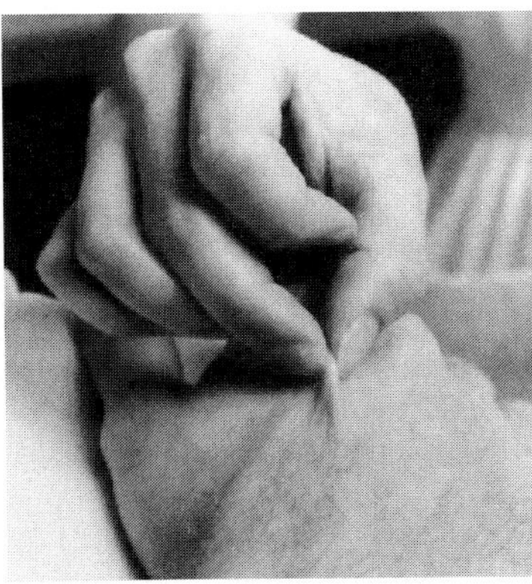

Fig. 12-2 Assessing skin turgor. (From Perry AG, Potter PA: *Clinical nursing skills and techniques,* ed 3, St Louis, 1994, Mosby.)

EQUIPMENT COMMONLY USED DURING PHYSICAL EXAMINATION

Ophthalmoscope. This instrument is used for examining interior of eye. It has two parts: handle or main body similar to flashlight, which contains light source, and detachable head, which contains adjustable magnifying lens.

Otoscope. This instrument is used for examining ear canal and ear drum (tympanic membrane). Otoscope head has speculum that directs light into ear canal. Otoscope head is used on same body as ophthalmoscope.

Percussion hammer. This instrument is used for testing reflexes. Also called *reflex hammer,* it consists of triangular rubber head attached to metal handle.

Snellen eye chart. This chart, used for testing vision, contains 11 lines of different-sized letters and numbers.

Nasal speculum. This instrument is used to inspect inside of nasal passages. Penlight or flashlight is needed as light source. Often, otoscope is used instead of speculum.

Vaginal speculum. This instrument is used to examine vagina and cervix. Physician usually examines vagina.

Tuning fork. This two-pronged instrument is used for testing hearing and vibration response.

Stethoscope. This instrument is used for assessing blood pressure and performing auscultation.

bution over the body (Skill 12-3). The nurse may examine the hair at once or at different points during examination of the body. For example, the hair and scalp may be examined when assessing all head and neck structures, whereas the pubic hair may be inspected during examination of the genitalia.

Assessing the Nails

Inspection of the nails provides clues to a patient's general state of health as well as the status of general circulation to the extremities (Skill 12-4). Normally, the nails are transparent and smooth, and the nail beds are pink (Table 12-3). **Capillary refill,** return of the nail bed's pink color after the application and release of pressure, is assessed. Cya-

Table 12-2 SKIN COLOR CHANGES

Condition	Related To	Location
Pallor (paleness)	Anemia, shock	Face, nailbeds, conjunctivae, palms of dark-skinned people
Jaundice	Liver disease, other conditions that cause destruction of red blood cells	Mucous membranes, sclerae of eyes, skin
Cyanosis	Decreased oxygen, heart or lung disease, cold environment	Nail beds, lips, face, hands, feet
Erythema (flushing)	Dilation of blood vessels or increased blood flow to skin, alcohol intake, fever, or infection	Face or any area of skin
Tan or browned color	Exposure to sun	Any area exposed to sun

Table 12-3 ABNORMALITIES OF THE NAIL BED

Type	Description	Associated Causes
Normal nail		
Clubbing (180 degrees; 180 degrees)	Change occurs in angle between nail and nail base; nail bed softens, with nail flattening. Eventually angle is greater than 180 degrees; fingertips often become enlarged.	Chronic lack of oxygen, heart disease, pulmonary disease
Beau's lines	Transverse depressions in the nails indicates that nail growth was temporarily disturbed; it grows out over several months.	Systemic illness such as severe infection, injury to nail
Koilonychia (spoon nail)	Concave curves occur.	Iron deficiency anemia, syphilis, use of strong detergents
Splinter hemorrhages	Red or brown linear streaks in nail bed occur.	Minor trauma, subacute bacterial endocarditis, trichinosis
Paronychia	Inflammation of skin occurs at base of nail.	Local infection, trauma

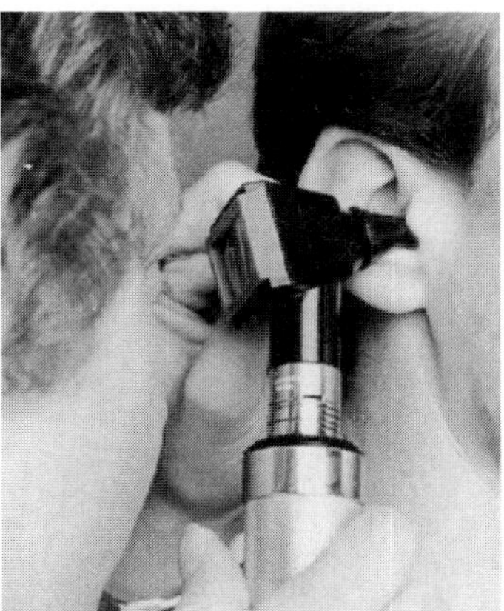

Fig. 12-3 Otoscope. (From Perry AG, Potter PA: *Clinical nursing skills and techniques,* ed 3, St Louis, 1994, Mosby.)

nosis of the nail beds should be reported immediately.

Assessing the Eyes

Examination of the eye includes assessing visual acuity, visual fields, eye movements, and structures (Skill 12-5). The nurse must be familiar with symptoms of eye disorders and be able to determine the extent to which visual impairment affects a patient's activities of daily living.

The internal structures of the eye—fundus, retina, optic nerve disc, macula, fovea centralis, and retinal vessels—are examined using the ophthalmoscope. The ophthalmoscopic examination is not usually part of the nursing examination.

Assessing the Ears

The nurse assesses the condition of ear structures and measures the patient's hearing acuity when performing an examination of the ear (Skill 12-6). The external ear, auditory canal, and tympanic membrane can be visualized using an otoscope (Fig. 12-3). Disorders of the middle ear may not be visualized but are sometimes reflected by the tympanic membrane.

Assessing the Nose and Sinuses

The nose and sinuses are examined to determine the presence of infection, allergies, or deformities (Skill 12-7). Inspection and palpation are the techniques of examination used. It is helpful to know whether the patient has a history of allergies, frequent colds, nosebleeds **(epistaxis),** or nose trauma.

Assessing the Mouth and Pharynx

Examination of the oral cavity may reveal information about the patient's oral hygiene and hydration. The best time to examine the patient's mouth is when giving oral care. The nurse uses a penlight and tongue depressor to perform a more detailed examination of the oral cavity (Skill 12-8). The lips are assessed for color and lesions. The oral mucosa is assessed for color, lesions, hydration, and texture. Other areas assessed are the gums, loose teeth, extraction sites, tongue, hard and soft palates, and pharynx. The nurse should also consider the patient's oral hygiene, the presence of tartar and dental caries, and the presence of dentures.

Assessing the Structures of the Neck

The structures of the neck are examined using the skills of inspection, auscultation, and palpation (Skill 12-9). The nurse assesses the neck for range of motion as well as size and position of the trachea, thyroid, and lymph nodes (Fig. 12-4). The carotid arteries, external jugular veins, and **bruits** (abnormal sounds or murmurs heard while auscultating a carotid artery, organ, or gland) may also be assessed at this time (Fig. 12-5).

Assessing the Thorax and Lungs

To adequately assess the chest and lungs, the nurse needs to understand the anatomy of the chest and underlying structures. Familiarity with the anatomic landmarks of the chest and the location of the lobes of the lungs enables the nurse to identify and document assessment findings. Techniques used for assessment include inspection, palpation, percussion, and auscultation (Skill 12-10). The nurse should be familiar with normal breath sounds (Table 12-4) and abnormal or adventitious breath sounds (Table 12-5).

Assessing the Heart and Vascular Systems

The nurse usually assesses the heart and vascular systems at the same time, since these two systems function together (Skill 12-11). Techniques used for assessment of the heart include inspection, palpation, and auscultation.

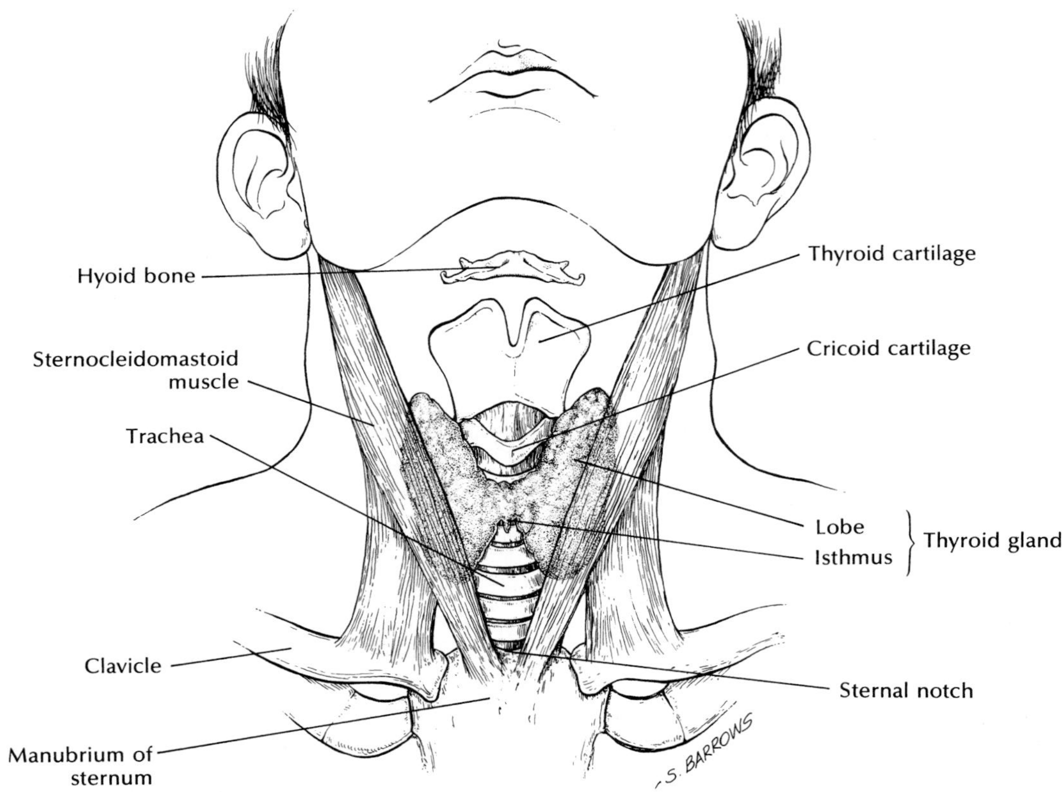

Fig. 12-4 Midline neck structures.

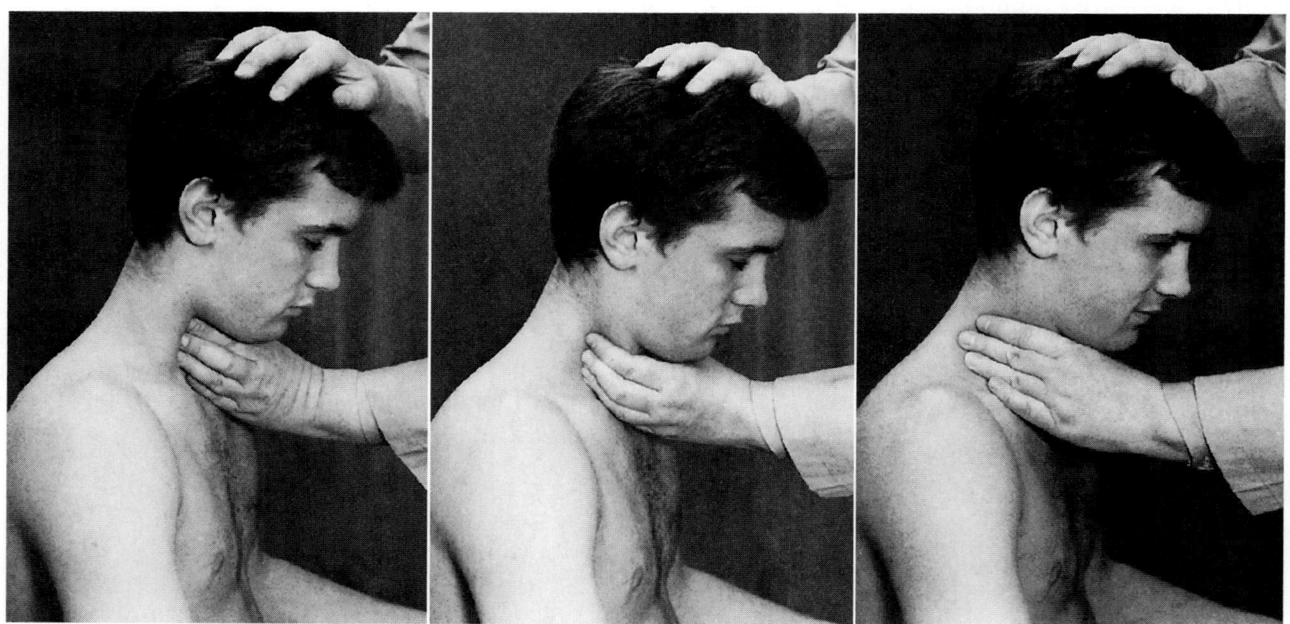

Fig. 12-5 Assessing the carotid artery by palpation.

Table 12-4 NORMAL BREATH SOUNDS

Sound	Where Heard	Characteristics
Bronchovesicular	Over large air passages, such as main bronchus (Stethoscope is placed over first and second intercostal spaces on anterior chest and between scapula on posterior chest.)	This sound represents movement of air through mainstem bronchus. Sounds are medium pitched and blowing, with inspiration equal to expiration.
Vesicular	Over normal lung tissue throughout lung fields	This sound represents movement of air through smaller air passages or bronchioles. Sounds are soft and low pitched, with inspiration longer than expiration.

Table 12-5 ADVENTITIOUS OR ABNORMAL BREATH SOUNDS

Sound	Characteristics
Crackles (also called *rales*)	Crackling sounds that vary in pitch, are best heard on inspiration, are caused by moisture in the small passageways and alveoli, may clear when patient coughs, and are similar to sounds heard when strands of hair are rolled between thumb and forefinger and held close to the ear
Wheezes	Squeaking, high-pitched sounds that are best heard on expiration, are caused by narrowed passage ways, and do not usually clear with coughing
Rhonchi	Course, gurgling, rattling, low-pitched sounds that are best heard on expiration, sound like air bubbling through water, and may clear with coughing
Pleural friction rub	Squeaking, grating sound that is heard along lower lateral lung fields, is heard best on inspiration, sounds like two pieces of leather rubbing together, and does not clear with coughing

As with assessment of the thorax, the nurse should be familiar with the anatomic landmarks used (Fig. 12-6). These landmarks include the following:

Aortic area. Second intercostal space on the right of the sternum

Pulmonic area. Second intercostal space on the left of the sternum

Tricuspid area. Fifth intercostal space on the left of the sternum

Apical area. Fifth intercostal space at the midclavicular line (halfway between the sternum and lateral edge of chest)

An understanding of these landmarks enables the nurse to accurately describe the location of findings.

Assessing the Abdomen

Several vital organs are contained within the abdominal cavity. To perform an accurate assessment, the nurse should know the location of each organ (Fig. 12-7).

To assist in identifying areas for examination, the abdomen is commonly divided into four quadrants or sections, with the umbilicus as the midpoint (Fig. 12-8). At times the abdomen is divided into nine regions (Fig. 12-9).

The order of the abdominal assessment differs slightly from the assessment of other systems in that the nurse begins with inspection, followed by auscultation, palpation, and percussion (if done) (Skill 12-12). Auscultation is performed before palpation because palpation may affect the frequency of bowel sounds.

Assessing the Breasts and Axillae

Examination of the breasts and axillae should be a routine part of any patient's health screening. Although examination of a woman's breasts is more detailed, the nurse should also examine a man's breasts and axillae to determine whether

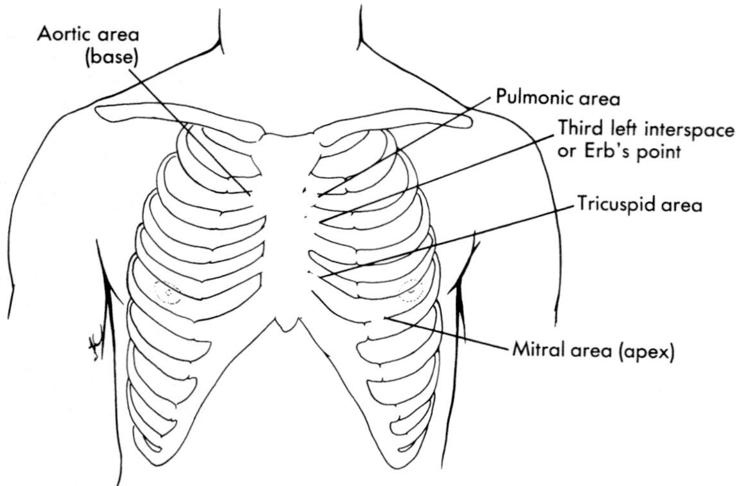

Fig. 12-6 Anatomic landmarks for cardiac auscultation.

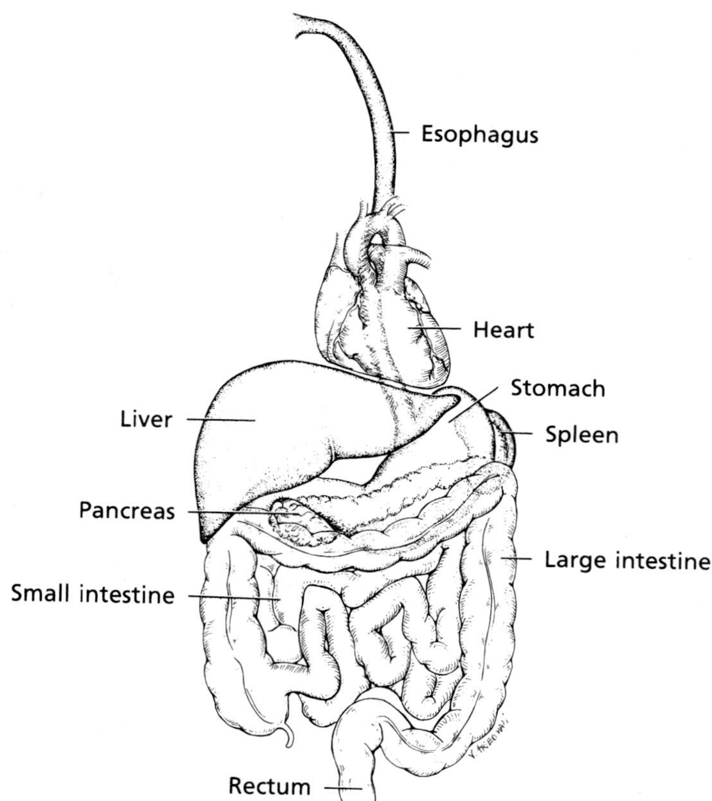

Fig. 12-7 Organs of the gastrointestinal system.

there are any tumors or other abnormalities (Skill 12-13).

The nurse should assess the breasts for position in relation to the chest wall and intercostal space. Breasts should be relatively symmetric, although slight variations may be normal (Fig. 12-10).

Since most breast masses are found by the patient, a woman should be familiar with the characteristics of her breasts (Fig. 12-11). One of the nurse's primary roles is to teach the female patient the technique of **breast self-examination,** in which a woman examines her breasts and their accessory structures for evidence of changes that could indicate a malignant process. Teaching should be performed during the examination.

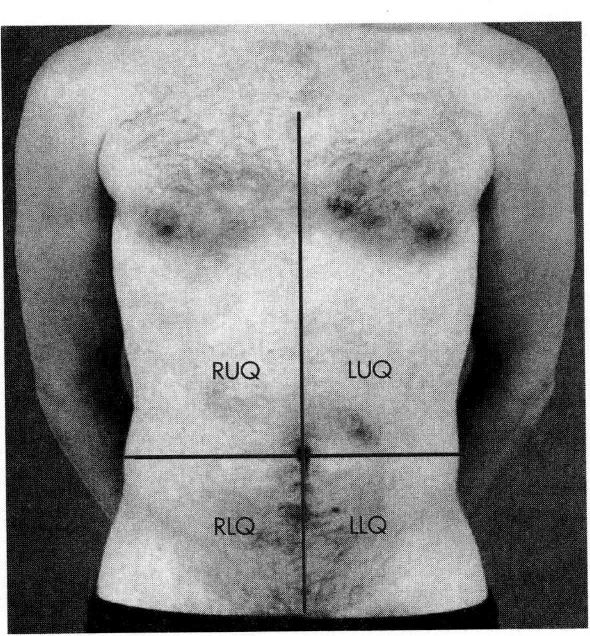

Fig. 12-8 Four quadrants of the abdomen. (From Christensen BL, Kockrow EO: *Foundations of nursing,* ed 2, St Louis, 1995, Mosby.)

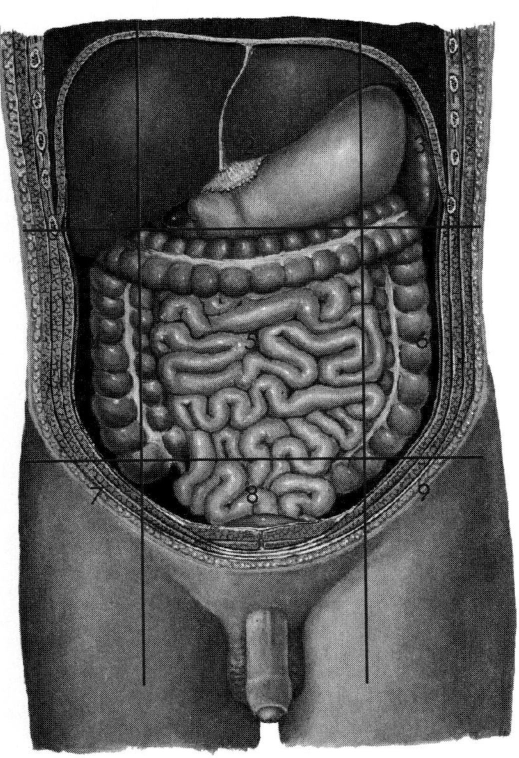

Fig. 12-9 Nine regions of the abdomen. *1,* Right hypochondriae. *2,* Epigastric. *3,* Left hypochondriae. *4,* Right lumbar. *5,* Umbilical. *6,* Left lumbar. *7,* Right inguinal. *8,* Hypogastric (pubic). *9,* Left inguinal. (From Christensen BL, Kockrow EO: *Foundations of nursing,* ed 2, St Louis, 1995, Mosby.)

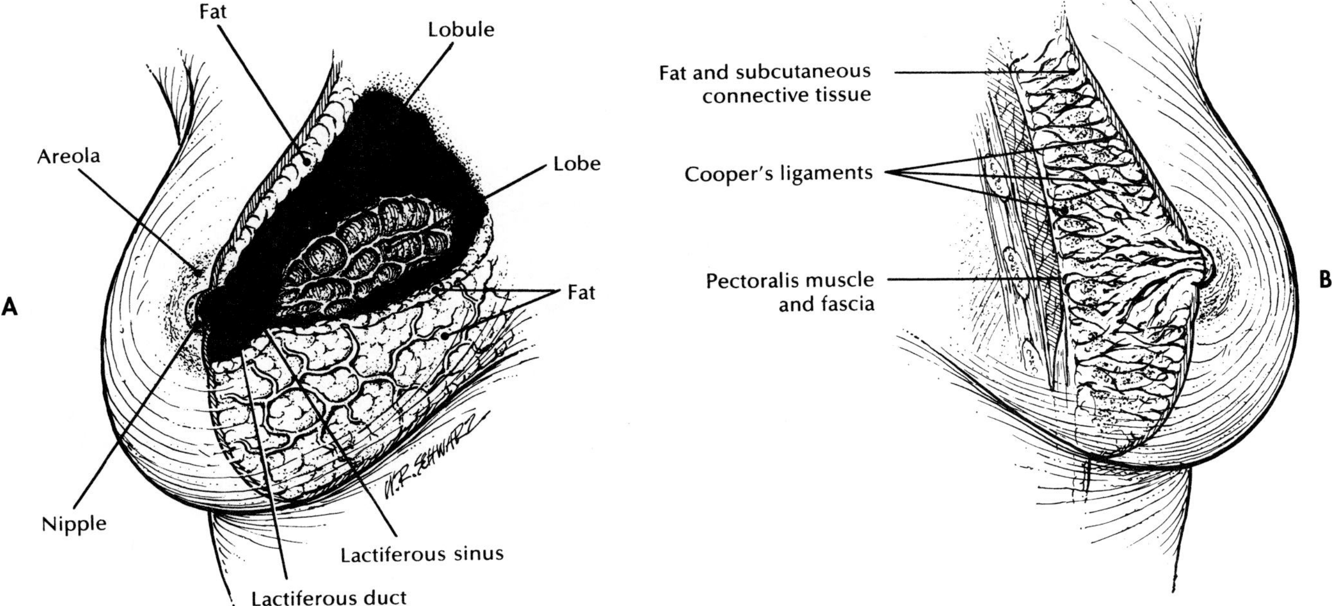

Fig. 12-10 Female breasts. **A,** Internal structures. **B,** Supportive tissue structures.

Assessing the Female Genitalia and Rectum

Examination of the external genitalia (Fig. 12-12) and rectum may be performed during hygenic care or during procedures such as insertion of a catheter (Skill 12-14).

Examination of genitalia may be very embarrassing to the patient. The nurse can do a great deal to promote relaxation and put the patient at ease.

Internal examination is performed only by those who have received special training in this technique and is not usually part of a nursing examination. Incorrect use of the speculum can cause trauma to vaginal walls. This technique is discussed briefly since nurses frequently assist with examination.

The patient should be given information about sexually transmitted diseases. The nurse should be available to answer questions.

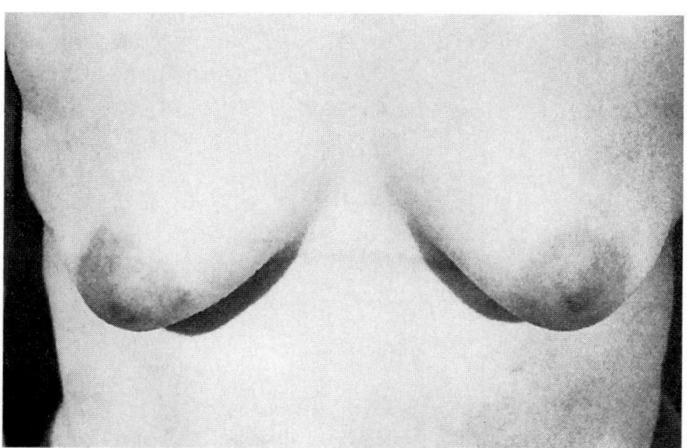

Fig. 12-11 Symmetric breasts.

Assessing the Male Genitalia and Rectum

Male patients are assessed to determine the condition of the external genitalia, which consists of the penis, scrotum, rectum, prostate, and inguinal ring and canal (Skill 12-15).

Assessment of the genitalia can be embarrassing for patients. Every effort should be made to preserve the patient's modesty. During examination, the patient's genitals should be handled gently to prevent discomfort or embarrassment.

At this time the patient may be instructed in techniques of **testicular self-examination,** in which a man examines his testicles and related structures for evidence of changes that could indicate a malignant process.

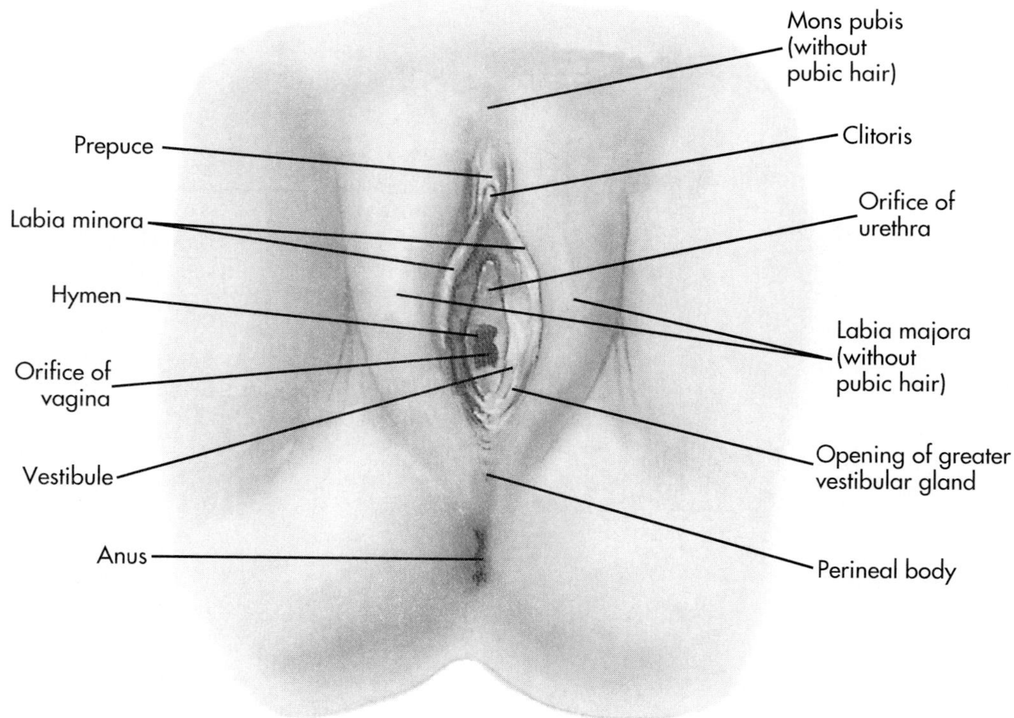

Fig. 12-12 External female genitalia (vulva). (From Christensen BL, Kockrow EO: *Foundations of nursing,* ed 2, St Louis, 1995, Mosby.)

The patient should also be given information on sexually transmitted diseases. The nurse should be available to answer questions.

Assessing the Musculoskeletal System

Musculoskeletal system assessment is often performed during examination of other body systems. For example, neck range of motion is assessed with other head and neck structures (Fig. 12-13).

Information obtained during musculoskeletal system assessment is used to determine a patient's ability to perform activities of daily living. Musculoskeletal disorders are frequently related to neurologic disorders. Therefore a neurologic assessment should be a part of the physical examination. This system is discussed later in the chapter.

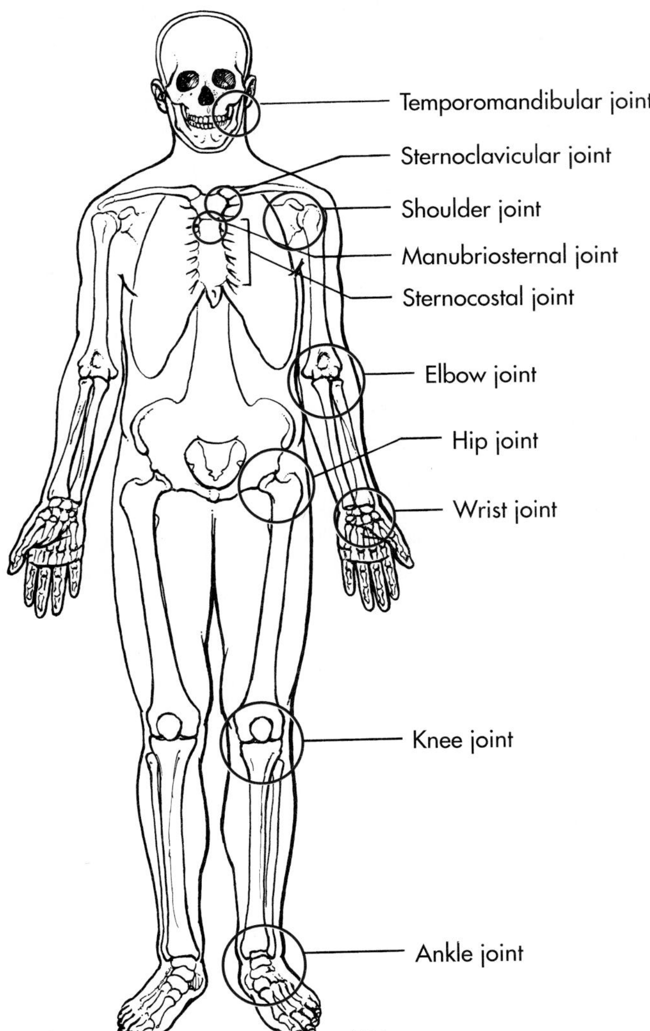

Fig. 12-13 Parts of the musculoskeletal system.

The techniques of inspection and palpation are used extensively throughout the musculoskeletal system assessment (Skill 12-16). A goniometer, an instrument used to measure angles, particularly the range-of-motion angles of a joint, may be used in the assessment of the musculoskeletal system (Fig. 12-14). A tape measure is used to determine muscle size.

Assessing the Neurologic System

The extent of the neurologic examination varies with the patient's condition or signs and symptoms. Patients who complain of frequent headaches or numbness require a more in-depth neurologic assessment than those with gastrointestinal problems.

Most nurses incorporate portions of neurologic assessment into assessment of other systems. For example, the function of many cranial nerves may be assessed during examination of the head and neck. Neurologic assessment of the extremities may be included in the assessment of the musculoskeletal system.

Examination of neurologic function is usually organized according to categories (Skill 12-17). These categories include mental and emotional status, cranial nerve function, motor function, reflexes.

Mental and emotional status Much can be learned about the patient's mental and emotional status when a health history is taken. Fully conscious patients respond to questions appropriately and quickly.

Cranial nerve function Cranial nerves are assessed in order of their number. To aid in remembering the order the nurse should remember this sentence: *O*n *o*ld *O*lympus *t*owering *t*ops *a* *F*inn *a*nd

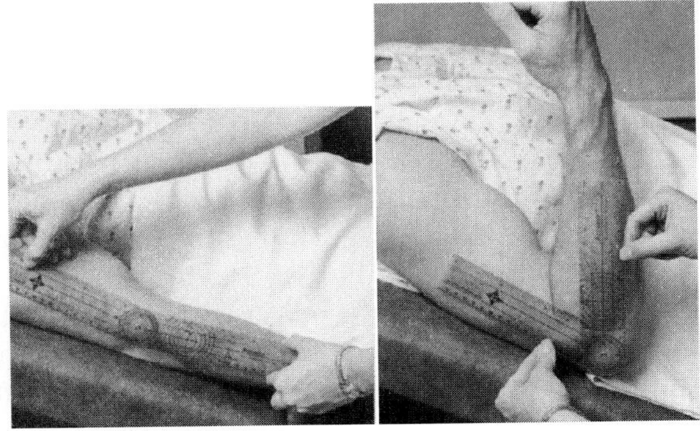

Fig. 12-14 Goniometer. (From Perry AG, Potter PA: *Clinical nursing skills and techniques,* ed 3, St Louis, 1994, Mosby.)

Table 12-6 METHODS OF CRANIAL NERVE ASSESSMENT

Nursing Action	Rationale	Nerve Assessed	
Ask patient to identify different smells, such as coffee or vanilla.	Assesses sense of smell	I	Olfactory
Use Snellen chart. Ask patient to read printed material.	Assesses vision	II	Optic
Assess patient's pupil response to light. Ask patient to follow movement of nurse's hand to test gaze.	Measures pupil response, evaluates parallel eye movements	III	Oculomotor
Evaluate directions of gaze.	Assesses upward and downward movement of eyeball	IV	Trochlear
Measure sense of pain and touch across face. Evaluate corneal reflex.	Evaluates sensation to skin of face	V	Trigeminal
Evaluate directions of gaze.	Assesses lateral movements of eyeball	VI	Abducens
Ask patient to smile, frown, puff cheeks, and raise eyebrows. Have patient identify salty or sweet tastes on front of tongue.	Evaluates facial expression, assesses sense of taste	VII	Facial
Whisper softly into patient's ear.	Assesses ability to hear whispered word	VIII	Auditory
Have patient stick out tongue. Evaluate ability to taste salty, sweet, and sour on back of tongue. Using tongue blade, stimulate gag reflex.	Evaluates sense of taste on back of tongue, evaluates ability to swallow and move tongue	IX	Glossopharyngeal
Ask patient to say "ah" and observe movement of pharynx. Use tongue blade to stimulate gag reflex. Assess hoarseness of voice.	Evaluates sensation of pharynx, ability to swallow, and voice	X	Vagus
Ask patient to shrug shoulders and turn head against nurse's hand.	Assesses movement of head and shoulders	XI	Spinal accessory
Ask patient to stick out tongue.	Assesses movement of tongue	XII	Hypoglossal

Table 12-7 TECHNIQUE FOR MOTOR FUNCTION ASSESSMENT

Nursing Action	Rationale
Nurse evaluates patient's posture, gait, and muscle strength as described in section on musculoskeletal assessment	Several neurologic disorders (for example, Parkinson's disease) are characterized by changes in gait, posture, or muscle strength.
Patient stands with feet together and eyes closed. Nurse notes swaying	This is known as the *Romberg test.* Slight swaying, especially among older adults, is normal. However, problems in keeping balance could indicate disease.

*G*erman *v*iewed some *h*ops. The first letter of each word corresponds with the first letter of the name of each cranial nerve (Table 12-6).

Motor function The nurse assesses motor function during the musculoskeletal examination. Coordination and balance are also assessed at this time (Table 12-7).

Reflexes Evaluation of reflexes requires skill and may not be a part of every nursing examination. Inappropriate technique may cause a great deal of discomfort. Reflexes should be symmetric and are reported using the following scale:

0	No response
1+	Low normal or hypoactive
2+	Normal
3+	Brisk
4+	Very brisk; hyperactive

Asymetry of reflexes indicates some defect of reflex pathway.

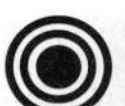

SKILL 12-1 PERFORMING A GENERAL SURVEY

Steps	Rationale
1. Refer to medical record, care plan, or Kardex for special interventions.	Provides basis for care.
2. Introduce self.	Decreases patient's anxiety level.
3. Identify patient by identification band.	Identifies correct patient for procedure.
4. Explain procedure to patient.	Seeks cooperation and decreases anxiety.
5. Wash hands according to agency policy and guidelines from Centers for Disease Control and Prevention and Occupational Safety and Health Administration.	Helps prevent cross-contamination.
6. Close door to room or pull curtain.	Provides privacy and shows respect for patient. Prevents exposure of patient.
7. Raise bed to comfortable working level.	Provides safety for nurse.
8. Review patient's health survey.	Helps determine priority problems for development of nursing diagnoses and care plan.
9. Assess patient's behavior, hair color and texture, emotional state, and general look of health.	Provides baseline for initial as well as daily nursing assessment and helps nurse make accurate decisions to meet patient's needs.
10. Note patient's gender, ethnic origin, and age. Assess for signs of distress or severe pain, posture, body type or build, gait, cleanliness, grooming, odor, speech, and possible patient abuse.	Helps nurse and other team members to get to know patient and personal needs.
11. Wash hands.	Helps prevent cross-contamination.
12. Ask patient questions about the condition and function of each body system (see box on p. 168).	Provides data about patient's health and present problem, as well as baseline data for future assessments.
13. Document.	Documents procedure and patient's response.

SKILL 12-2 ASSESSING THE SKIN

Steps	Rationale
1. Obtain equipment: ▪ Clean gloves	Helps organize procedure.
2. Refer to medical record, care plan, or Kardex for special interventions.	Provides basis for care.
3. Introduce self.	Decreases patient's anxiety level.
4. Identify patient by identification band.	Identifies correct patient for procedure.
5. Explain procedure to patient.	Seeks cooperation and decreases anxiety.
6. Wash hands and don clean gloves according to agency policy and guidelines from Centers for Disease Control and Prevention and Occupational Safety and Health Administration.	Helps prevent cross-contamination.
7. Prepare patient for intervention:	
a. Close door to room or pull curtain.	Provides privacy.
b. Drape for procedure if necessary.	Prevents exposure of patient.
8. Raise bed to comfortable working level.	Provides safety for nurse.
9. Arrange for patient privacy.	Shows respect for patient.
10. Inspect skin surfaces for color and lesions (see Table 12-2). Compare opposite body parts.	Identifies changes that may indicate disease.
11. Inspect color of lips, oral mucous membranes, nail beds, sclerae, conjunctivae, and palms.	Identifies changes, which may be observed in these areas more easily than in others.

Continued.

SKILL 12-2 ASSESSING THE SKIN—cont'd

Steps	Rationale
12. Palpate skin surfaces with fingers to determine moisture and texture of skin. Assess secretions.	Helps indicate changes in body temperature regulation and fluid imbalance.
13. Test for skin turgor: when skin is released, note how long it takes to return to normal position.	Determines elasticity of skin.
14. Assess temperature of skin by using back of hand. Compare opposite sides of body.	Detects subtle changes in temperature.
15. If lesions are detected, note size, location, and type. Palpate gently to determine shape, mobility, and character. Ask whether patient has pain or tenderness during palpation.	Describes characteristics of color and any abnormalities.
16. Assess for edema by inspecting feet, ankles, sacral area, and scapular areas. Assess degree of edema by pressing with thumb for 5 sec.	Determines degree of edema.
17. Remove gloves and wash hands.	Helps prevent cross-contamination.
18. Document.	Documents procedure and patient's response.

SKILL 12-3 ASSESSING THE HAIR AND SCALP

Steps	Rationale
1. Obtain equipment: ▪ Clean gloves	Helps organize procedure.
2. Refer to medical record, care plan, or Kardex for special interventions.	Provides basis for care.
3. Introduce self.	Decreases patient's anxiety level.
4. Identify patient by identification band.	Identifies correct patient for procedure.
5. Explain procedure to patient.	Seeks cooperation and decreases anxiety.
6. Wash hands and don clean gloves according to agency policy and guidelines from Centers for Disease Control and Prevention and Occupational Safety and Health Administration.	Helps prevent cross-contamination.
7. Prepare patient for intervention:	
a. Close door to room or pull curtain.	Provides privacy.
b. Drape for procedure if necessary.	Prevents exposure of patient.
8. Raise bed to comfortable working level.	Provides safety for nurse.
9. Arrange for patient privacy.	Shows respect for patient.
10. Inspect hair for color, thickness, distribution, and texture.	Determines condition of hair.
11. Inspect hair shaft and follicles to determine presence of lice.	Indicates need for treatment.
12. Inspect scalp for cleanliness and lesions by separating hair.	Determines whether patient has dandruff or other disorders.
13. Inspect hair distribution over lower extremities.	May indicate decreased arterial circulation.
14. Remove gloves and wash hands.	Helps prevent cross-contamination.
15. Document.	Documents procedure and patient's response.

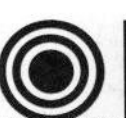

SKILL 12-4 ASSESSING THE NAILS

Steps	Rationale
1. Obtain equipment: ▪ Clean gloves	Helps organize procedure.
2. Refer to medical record, care plan, or Kardex for special interventions.	Provides basis for care.
3. Introduce self.	Decreases patient's anxiety level.
4. Identify patient by identification band.	Identifies correct patient for procedure.
5. Explain procedure to patient.	Seeks cooperation and decreases anxiety.
6. Wash hands and don clean gloves according to agency policy and guidelines from Centers for Disease Control and Prevention and Occupational Safety and Health Administration.	Helps prevent cross-contamination.
7. Prepare patient for intervention:	
a. Close door to room or pull curtain.	Provides privacy.
b. Drape for procedure if necessary.	Prevents exposure of patient.
8. Raise bed to comfortable working level.	Provides safety for nurse.
9. Arrange for patient privacy.	Shows respect for patient.
10. Inspect nails for color, thickness, shape, and curvature.	Indicates status of oxygenation of blood, nutritional status, disease, or trauma.
11. Assess capillary refill by applying pressure with thumb to nail beds.	Indicates normal status or impaired circulation.
12. Remove gloves and wash hands.	Helps prevent cross-contamination.
13. Document.	Documents procedure and patient's response.

SKILL 12-5 ASSESSING THE EYES

Steps	Rationale
1. Obtain equipment: ▪ Clean gloves ▪ Small ruler ▪ Cotton-tipped applicator ▪ Penlight ▪ Ophthalmoscope (not usually part of nurse's examination)	Helps organize procedure.
2. Refer to medical record, care plan, or Kardex for special interventions.	Provides basis for care.
3. Introduce self.	Decreases patient's anxiety level.
4. Identify patient by identification band.	Identifies correct patient for procedure.
5. Explain procedure to patient.	Seeks cooperation and decreases anxiety.
6. Wash hands and don clean gloves according to agency policy, and guidelines from Centers for Disease Control and Prevention and Occupational Safety and Health Administration.	Helps prevent cross-contamination.
7. Prepare patient for intervention:	
a. Close door to room or pull curtain.	Provides privacy.
b. Drape for procedure if necessary.	Prevents exposure of patient.
8. Raise bed to comfortable working level.	Provides safety for nurse.
9. Arrange for patient privacy.	Shows respect for patient.
10. Inspect external eye structures.	Allows detection of variations between eyes.
11. Examine eyes for position and alignment. Measure distance between pupils of eyes with small ruler.	May indicate neurologic or metabolic conditions.

Continued.

SKILL 12-5 ASSESSING THE EYES—cont'd

Steps	Rationale
12. Inspect eyebrows for position, hair growth, and movement.	Allows detection of hair loss or absence of hair, which may indicate metabolic disturbance, and loss of movement, which may indicate nerve damage.
13. Inspect eyelids for position by having patient open and close eyes.	Allows identification of abnormalities.
14. Inspect eyelids and sclerae for color, edema, inflammation, and lesions.	Allows detection of abnormalities.
15. Look for excess tears, signs of inflammation, infection, edema, or tumor. Use cotton-tipped applicator to invert upper eyelid to examine underside.	Allows identification of abscess, tumor, or infection.
16. Assess pupils for size and shape. Test pupillary response with ophthalmoscope or penlight.	Allows identification of neurologic injury.
17. Remove gloves and wash hands.	Helps prevent cross-contamination.
18. Document.	Documents procedure and patient's response.

SKILL 12-6 ASSESSING THE EARS

Steps	Rationale
1. Obtain equipment: ▪ Clean gloves ▪ Otoscope ▪ Penlight ▪ Tuning fork	Helps organize procedure.
2. Refer to medical record, care plan, or Kardex for special interventions.	Provides basis for care.
3. Introduce self.	Decreases patient's anxiety level.
4. Identify patient by identification band.	Identifies correct patient for procedure.
5. Explain procedure to patient.	Seeks cooperation and decreases anxiety.
6. Wash hands and don clean gloves according to agency policy and guidelines from Centers for Disease Control and Prevention and Occupational Safety and Health Administration.	Helps prevent cross-contamination.
7. Prepare patient for intervention:	
a. Close door to room or pull curtain.	Provides privacy.
b. Drape for procedure if necessary.	Prevents exposure of patient.
8. Raise bed to comfortable working level.	Provides safety for nurse.
9. Arrange for patient privacy.	Shows respect for patient.
10. Inspect opening of ear canal for edema, foreign body, or build up of cerumen (ear wax).	Identifies obstruction, which interferes with hearing acuity.
11. Assess patient's hearing acuity: Whisper in each ear or use a ticking watch from 1 to 2 feet while patient's eyes are closed.	Provides general screening of hearing.
12. Perform Weber's test if more precise assessment of hearing is needed:	
a. Holding tuning fork at base; strike it against hand so that it vibrates. b. Place base of fork on top of patient's head and ask patient to identify where sound is heard best.	Determines type of hearing loss. Assesses bone conduction of sound. (Patients with normal hearing hear sound equally in both ears.)

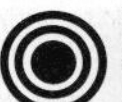

SKILL 12-6 ASSESSING THE EARS—cont'd

Steps	Rationale
13. Perform Rinne's test if more precise assessment of hearing is needed:	
a. Hold tuning fork at base and strike it against hand.	Determines type of hearing loss. Compares air conduction of sound to bone conduction. (Patient with normal hearing hear air-conduction sound better than bone-conduction sound.)
b. Place base of vibrating fork against mastoid process and ask patient to say when sound is no longer heard.	
c. Immediately move fork over ear canal and ask if sound can be heard.	
d. Ask patient which sound is heard best.	
14. Use otoscope to examine ear canals.	Allows detection of foreign body, drainage, and color.
15. Remove gloves and wash hands.	Helps prevent cross-contamination.
16. Document.	Documents procedure and patient's response.

SKILL 12-7 ASSESSING THE NOSE AND SINUSES

Steps	Rationale
1. Obtain equipment: ▪ Clean gloves ▪ Penlight	Helps organize procedure.
2. Refer to medical record, care plan, or Kardex for special interventions.	Provides basis for care.
3. Introduce self.	Decreases patient's anxiety level.
4. Identify patient by identification band.	Identifies correct patient for procedure.
5. Explain procedure to patient.	Seeks cooperation and decreases anxiety.
6. Wash hands and don clean gloves according to agency policy and guidelines from Centers for Disease Control and Prevention and Occupational Safety and Health Administration.	Helps prevent cross-contamination.
7. Prepare patient for intervention:	
a. Close door to room or pull curtain.	Provides privacy.
b. Drape for procedure if necessary.	Prevents exposure of patient.
8. Raise bed to comfortable working level.	Provides safety for nurse.
9. Arrange for patient privacy.	Shows respect for patient.
10. Inspect nose for placement, inflammation, and deformity.	Detects trauma.
11. Inspect mucosa for color, drainage, and edema using penlight.	Allows detection of abnormalities and need for intervention.
12. Using speculum, inspect inner nares for lesions, deviation of septum, and obstruction.	Reveals nasal obstruction that may interfere with breathing.
13. Examine frontal and maxillary sinuses by applying gentle pressure using thumbs.	Detects excessive pain, which indicates an abnormality.
14. Remove gloves and wash hands.	Helps prevent cross-contamination.
15. Document.	Documents procedure and patient's response.

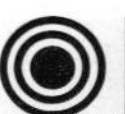

SKILL 12-8 ASSESSING THE MOUTH AND PHARYNX

Steps	Rationale
1. Obtain equipment: ▪ Clean gloves ▪ Penlight ▪ Tongue depressor	Helps organize procedure.
2. Refer to medical record, care plan, or Kardex for special interventions.	Provides basis for care.
3. Introduce self.	Decreases patient's anxiety level.
4. Identify patient by identification band.	Identifies correct patient for procedure.
5. Explain procedure to patient.	Seeks cooperation and decreases anxiety.
6. Wash hands and don clean gloves according to agency policy and guidelines from Centers for Disease Control and Prevention and Occupational Safety and Health Administration.	Helps prevent cross-contamination.
7. Prepare patient for intervention:	
a. Close door to room or pull curtain.	Provides privacy.
b. Drape for procedure if necessary.	Prevents exposure of patient.
8. Raise bed to comfortable working level.	Provides safety for nurse.
9. Arrange for patient privacy.	Shows respect for patient.
10. Inspect lips for color, contour, hydration, and lesions.	Allows detection of dehydration or dry mucosa.
11. Ask patient to open mouth slightly. Examine oral mucosa for color, moistness, and ulcers or lesions.	Allows detection of dehydration or ulcer.
12. Ask patient to open mouth wide. Using tongue depressor to retract cheek and penlight, inspect buccal mucosa: color, moisture, and lesions or patches.	Allows identification of white patches (leukoplakia).
13. Inspect patient's gums using tongue depressor to assess for color and edema.	Allows detection of lesions, masses, or bleeding tendencies.
14. Ask patient to open mouth wide and inspect all surfaces.	Determines need for intervention.
15. Remove gloves and wash hands.	Helps prevent cross-contamination.
16. Document.	Documents procedure and patient's response.

SKILL 12-9 ASSESSING THE STRUCTURES OF THE NECK

Steps	Rationale
1. Obtain equipment: ▪ Clean gloves ▪ Stethoscope	Helps organize procedure.
2. Refer to medical record, care plan, or Kardex for special interventions.	Provides basis for care.
3. Introduce self.	Decreases patient's anxiety level.
4. Identify patient by identification band.	Identifies correct patient for procedure.
5. Explain procedure to patient.	Seeks cooperation and decreases anxiety.
6. Wash hands and don clean gloves according to agency policy and guidelines from Centers for Disease Control and Prevention and Occupational Safety and Health Administration.	Helps prevent cross-contamination.
7. Prepare patient for intervention:	
a. Close door to room or pull curtain.	Provides privacy.
b. Drape for procedure if necessary.	Prevents exposure of patient.

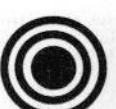

SKILL 12-9 ASSESSING THE STRUCTURES OF THE NECK—cont'd

Steps	Rationale
8. Raise bed to comfortable working level.	Provides safety for nurse.
9. Arrange for patient privacy.	Shows respect for patient.
10. Ask patient to move head and neck through full range of motion.	Identifies limited range of motion, which may indicate injury or disease. (This may also be assessed during assessment of musculoskeletal system.)
11. Inspect neck for scars or masses and ask patient to swallow, noting bulge.	Indicates enlarged thyroid gland).
12. Palpate for mass to determine size, shape, and mobility.	Aids in diagnosing mass.
13. Palpate each side of neck and under chin for lymph nodes.	Allows detection of tenderness or enlargement.
14. Palpate trachea at base of throat using first finger of one hand just above sternal notch.	Allows identification of edema or mass.
15. Palpate carotid pulse on each side of the neck (see Fig. 12-5).	Allows detection of unequal pulses.
16. Auscultate over carotid arteries for bruit.	Allows identification of a bruit resulting from narrowing or stenosis.
17. Remove gloves and wash hands.	Helps prevent cross-contamination.
18. Document.	Documents procedure and patient's response.

SKILL 12-10 ASSESSING THE THORAX AND LUNGS

Steps	Rationale
1. Obtain equipment: ▪ Clean gloves ▪ Stethoscope	Helps organize procedure.
2. Refer to medical record, care plan, or Kardex for special interventions.	Provides basis for care.
3. Introduce self.	Decreases patient's anxiety level.
4. Identify patient by identification band.	Identifies correct patient for procedure.
5. Explain procedure to patient.	Seeks cooperation and decreases anxiety.
6. Wash hands and don clean gloves according to agency policy and guidelines from Centers for Disease Control and Prevention and Occupational Safety and Health Administration.	Helps prevent cross-contamination.
7. Prepare patient for intervention:	
a. Close door to room or pull curtain.	Provides privacy.
b. Drape for procedure if necessary.	Prevents exposure of patient.
8. Raise bed to comfortable working level.	Provides safety for nurse.
9. Arrange for patient privacy.	Shows respect for patient.
10. Stand behind patient and inspect posterior thorax for shape; contour; and deformities of ribs, spine, or scapula.	Allows identification of abnormalities (Fig. 12-15).
11. Palpate posterior chest wall to determine masses, areas of tenderness, or deformities (Fig. 12-16).	Allows detection of abnormalities.
12. Assess for fremitus (vibrations) over intercostal spaces.	Allows identification of obstruction.
13. Percuss chest wall (may not be included in every assessment, depending on agency).	Allows detection of abnormalities.

Continued.

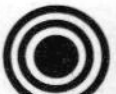

SKILL 12-10 ASSESSING THE THORAX AND LUNGS—cont'd

Steps	Rationale
14. Listen to lung sounds (Figs. 12-17 through 12-19).	Enables nurse to evaluate movement of air through lung fields.
15. Remove gloves and wash hands.	Helps prevent cross-contamination.
16. Document.	Documents procedure and patient's response.

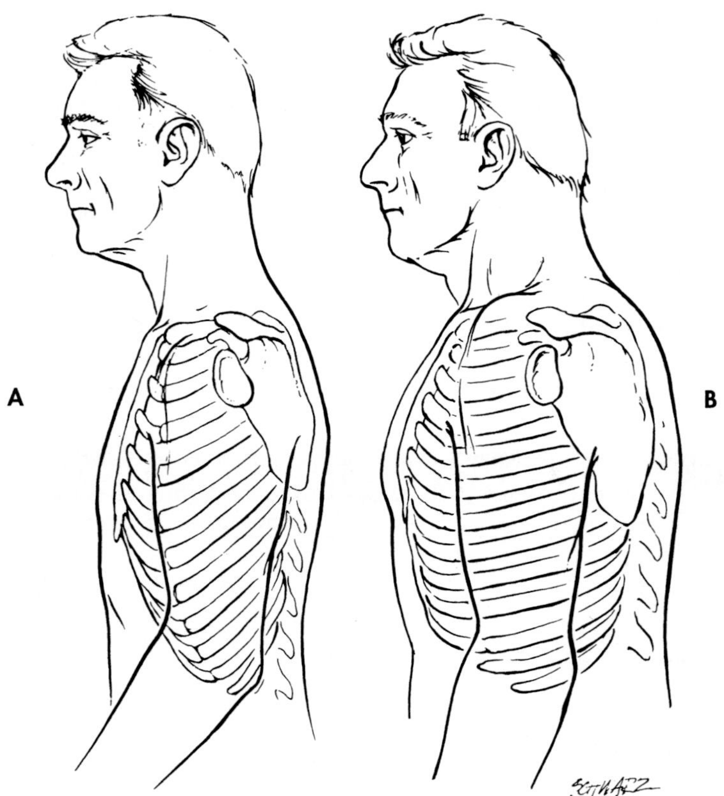

Fig. 12-15 **A,** Normal adult. **B,** Barrel chest.

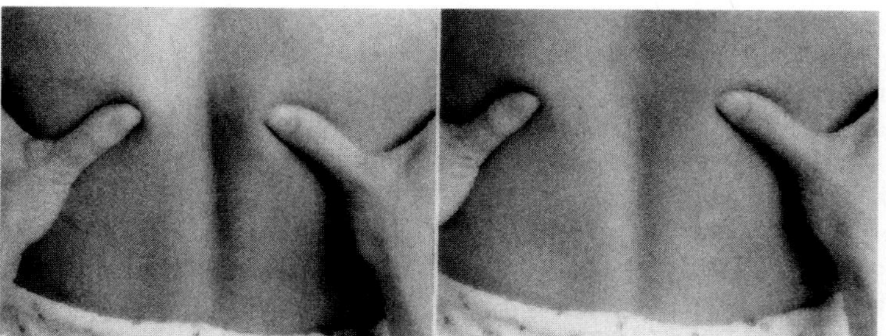

Fig. 12-16 Position of nurse's hands for palpation of posterior chest wall. (From Perry AG, Potter PA: *Clinical nursing skills and techniques,* ed 3, St Louis, 1994, Mosby.)

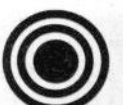

SKILL 12-10 ASSESSING THE THORAX AND LUNGS—cont'd

Steps	Rationale

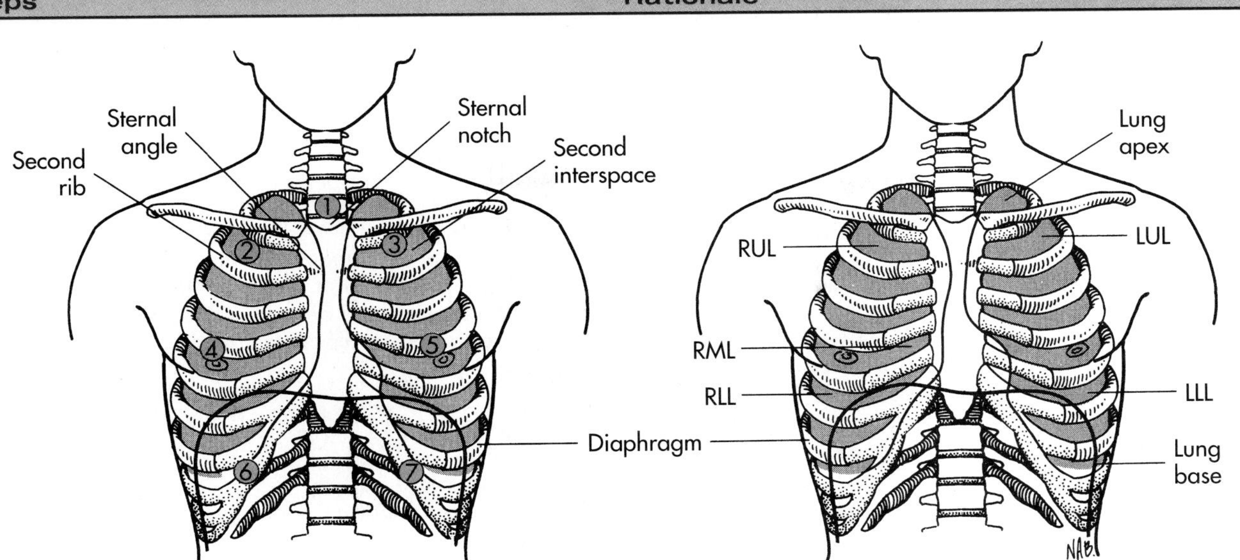

Fig. 12-17 Sites for anterior auscultation of intercostal spaces.

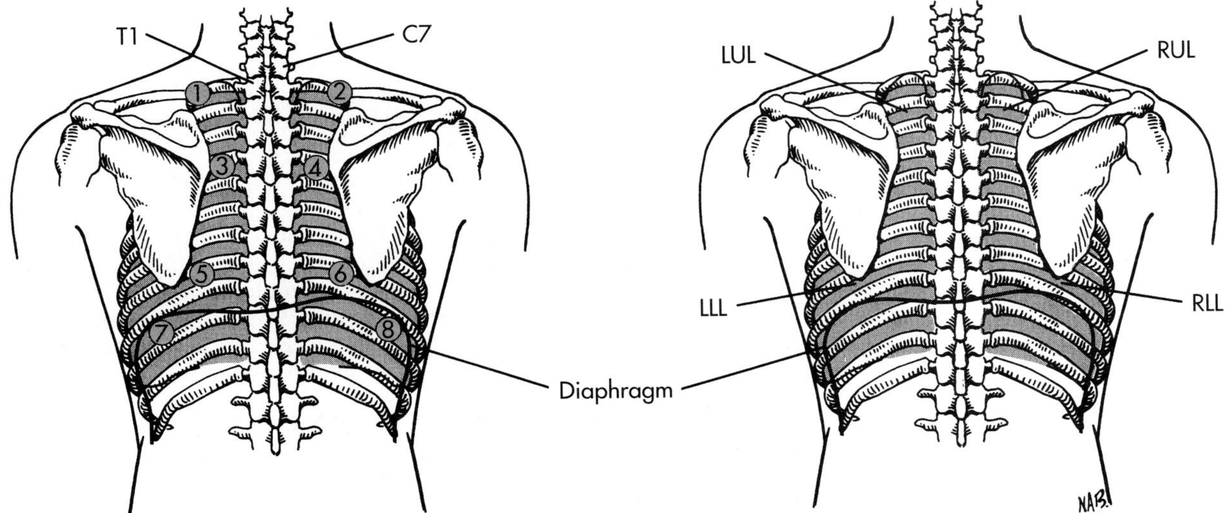

Fig. 12-18 Site for posterior auscultation of intercostal spaces.

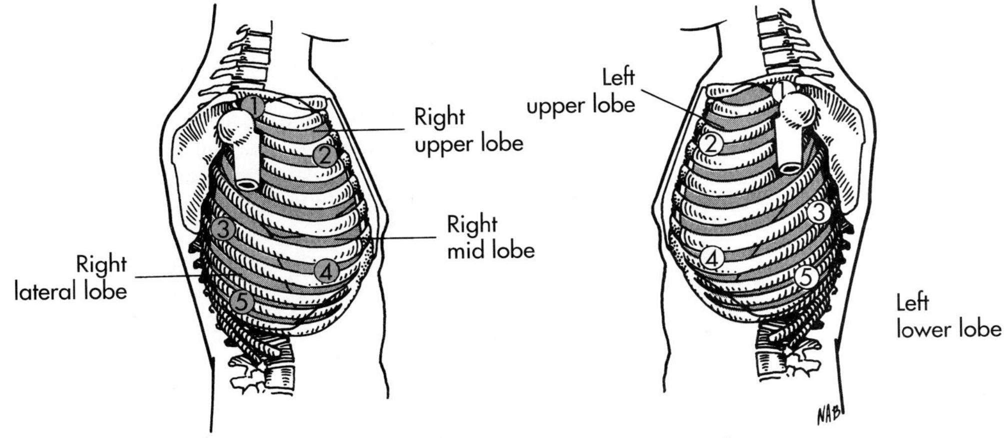

Fig. 12-19 Site for auscultation of intercostal spaces of the side.

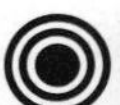

SKILL 12-11 ASSESSING THE HEART AND VASCULAR SYSTEM

Steps	Rationale
1. Obtain equipment: ▪ Clean gloves ▪ Doppler stethoscope ▪ Sphygmomanometer ▪ Stethoscope	Helps organize procedure.
2. Refer to medical record, care plan, or Kardex for special interventions.	Provides basis for care.
3. Introduce self.	Decreases patient's anxiety level.
4. Identify patient by identification band.	Identifies correct patient for procedure.
5. Explain procedure to patient.	Seeks cooperation and decreases anxiety.
6. Wash hands and don clean gloves according to agency policy and guidelines from Centers for Disease Control and Prevention and Occupational Safety and Health Administration.	Helps prevent cross-contamination.
7. Prepare patient for intervention:	
a. Close door to room or pull curtain.	Provides privacy.
b. Drape for procedure if necessary.	Prevents exposure of patient.
8. Raise bed to comfortable working level.	Provides safety for nurse.
9. Arrange for patient privacy.	Shows respect for patient.
10. Inspect neck and precordium for vein distention or pulsations.	Determines neck vein distention or noticeable pulsations and possible need for intervention.
11. Palpate chest over anatomic landmarks.	Determines normal closing of heart valves.
12. Auscultate heart sounds.	Allows nurse to recognize normal sounds.
13. Identify first (S_1) and second (S_2) heart sounds.	Allows identification of murmurs and bruits.
14. Auscultate for extra sounds.	Allows detection of murmurs and bruits.
15. Auscultate apical pulse and count beats for 1 min.	Allows identification of normal or irregular apical pulse.
16. Assess carotid, radial, brachial, femoral, popliteal, dorsalis, and posterior tibial pulses.	Allows detection of equal or unequal pulses.
17. Seek assistance if pulses are not present. Use Doppler stethoscope.	Helps determine need for medical intervention.
18. Remove gloves and wash hands.	Helps prevent cross-contamination.
19. Document.	Documents procedure and patient's response.

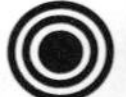

SKILL 12-12 ASSESSING THE ABDOMEN

Steps	Rationale
1. Obtain equipment: ▪ Clean gloves ▪ Measuring tape ▪ Stethoscope	Helps organize procedure.
2. Refer to medical record, care plan, or Kardex for special interventions.	Provides basis for care.
3. Introduce self.	Decreases patient's anxiety level.
4. Identify patient by identification band.	Identifies correct patient for procedure.
5. Explain procedure to patient.	Seeks cooperation and decreases anxiety.
6. Wash hands and don clean gloves according to agency policy and guidelines from Centers for Disease Control and Prevention and Occupational Safety and Health Administration.	Helps prevent cross-contamination.
7. Prepare patient for intervention:	
a. Close door to room or pull curtain.	Provides privacy.
b. Drape for procedure if necessary.	Prevents exposure of patient.

SKILL 12-12 ASSESSING THE ABDOMEN—cont'd

Steps	Rationale
8. Raise bed to comfortable working level.	Provides safety for nurse.
9. Arrange for patient privacy.	Shows respect for patient.
10. Inspect abdomen for venous patterns, white striae on skin, and artificial openings.	Indicates surgery or trauma, liver disease, or stretching of skin.
11. Assess shape and symmetry, masses, or bulges of abdomen.	Allows detection of underlying tumors, fluid, and gaseous distention.
12. Assess for movement or pulsations of abdomen by looking across from side to side.	Indicates possible presence of aortic pulsation, peristaltic movements, and muscular contraction.
13. Measure size of abdominal girth using measing tape.	Enables nurse to determine increase or decrease in abdominal size.
14. Place diaphragm of stethoscope and auscultate over each quadrant of abdomen (Fig. 12-20).	Determines presence of peristalsis.
15. Auscultate for vascular sounds; notify physician of bruit.	Allows identification of bruits or damage.
16. Palpate each abdominal quadrant by gently pressing down approximately ½ inch (Figs. 12-21 and 12-22). Assess for masses and areas of tenderness.	Determines peristalsis. Allows detection of soft, nontender abdomen; discomfort; fluid or flatus build-up; and bladder distention.
17. Remove gloves and wash hands.	Helps prevent cross-contamination.
18. Document.	Documents procedure and patient's response.

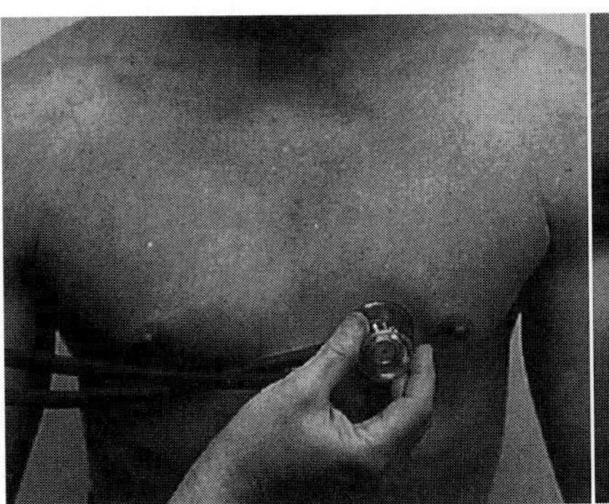

A

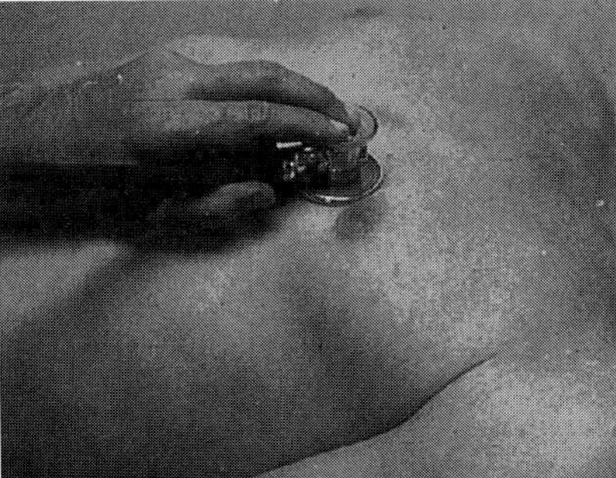

B

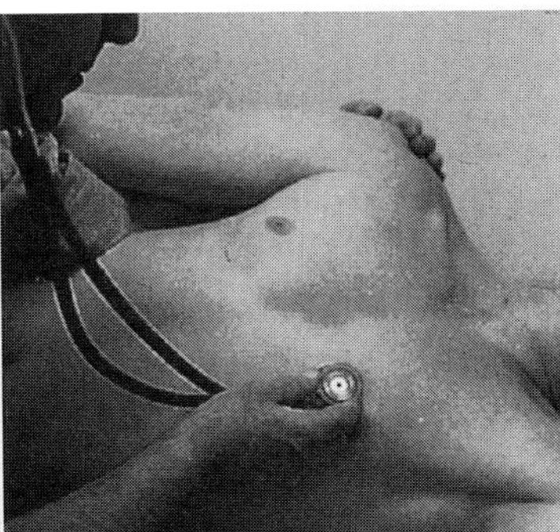

C

Fig. 12-20 Sequence of patient positions for auscultation. **A,** Sitting up, leaning slightly forward. **B,** Supine. **C,** Left lateral recumbent. (From Perry AG, Potter PA: *Clinical nursing skills and techniques,* ed 3, St Louis, 1994, Mosby.)

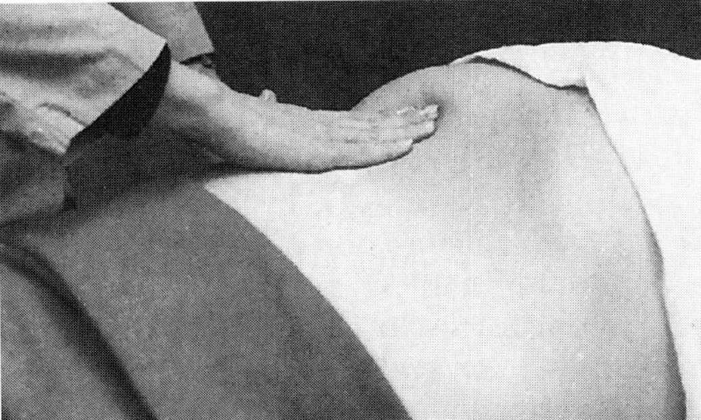

Fig. 12-21 Palpating each abdominal quadrant. (From Christensen BL, Kockrow EO: *Foundations of nursing,* ed 2, St Louis, 1995, Mosby.)

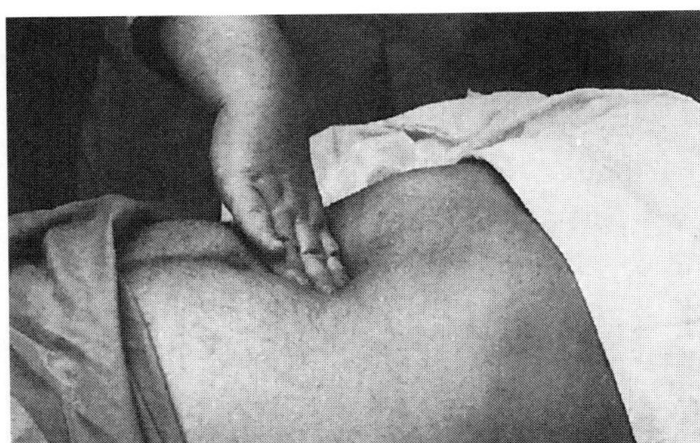

Fig. 12-22 Palpating for masses or areas of tenderness. (From Christensen BL, Kockrow EO: *Foundations of nursing*, ed 2, St. Louis, 1995, Mosby.)

SKILL 12-13 ASSESSING THE BREASTS AND AXILLAE

Steps	Rationale
1. Obtain equipment: ▪ Clean gloves	Helps organize procedure.
2. Refer to medical record, care plan, or Kardex for special interventions.	Provides basis for care.
3. Introduce self.	Decreases patient's anxiety level.
4. Identify patient by identification band.	Identifies correct patient for procedure.
5. Explain procedure to patient.	Seeks cooperation and decreases anxiety.
6. Wash hands and don clean gloves according to agency policy and guidelines from Centers for Disease Control and Prevention and Occupational Safety and Health Administration.	Helps prevent cross-contamination.
7. Prepare patient for intervention:	
a. Close door to room or pull curtain.	Provides privacy.
b. Drape for procedure if necessary.	Prevents exposure of patient.
8. Raise bed to comfortable working level.	Provides safety for nurse.
9. Arrange patient privacy.	Shows respect for patient.
FEMALE PATIENT	
10. Inspect breasts for size, symmetry, shape, change in tissue, lumps, and contour.	Allows identification of changes, which may indicate mass or inflammation.
11. Ask patient to place hands behind head or on hips and inspect breasts for flattening or unevenness.	Contracts pectoral muscles and accentuates abnormalities.
12. Inspect skin for color, vascular markings, or dimpling (puckering).	Allows detection of growth or tumor.
13. Inspect nipples and surrounding areola for shape, size, color, and discharge.	Allows identification of changes that may indicate tumor, cyst, pregnancy, lesion, discharge, or infection.
14. Examine right breast:	
a. Place patient in supine position with right hand under head. Palpate right breast, pressing tissue against chest wall, one quadrant at a time. Then move in clockwise direction, examining each quadrant (Figs. 12-23 and 12-24).	Allows detection of mass.
b. Compress nipple gently between thumb and finger to assess for discharge.	Allows identification of discharge.
c. Palpate axillae gently and along inner aspect of upper arm to examine lymph nodes (Fig. 12-25).	Allows detection of problems.
15. Repeat step 14a-4c for left breast.	Allows assessment of both breasts.

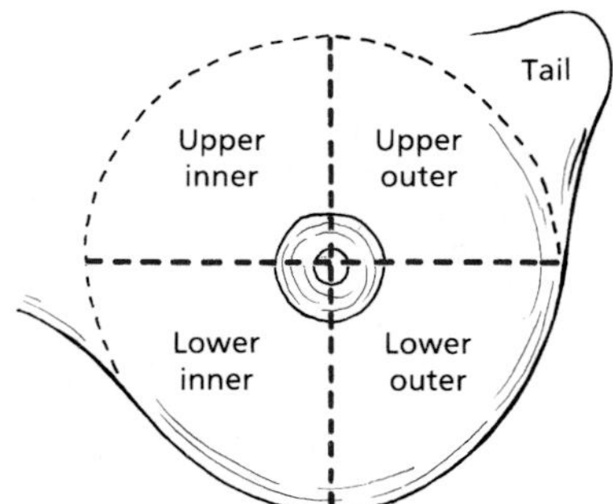

Fig. 12-23 Quadrants of the breast. (From Perry AG, Potter PA: *Clinical nursing skills and techniques,* ed 3, St Louis, 1994, Mosby.)

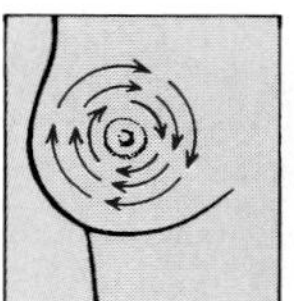
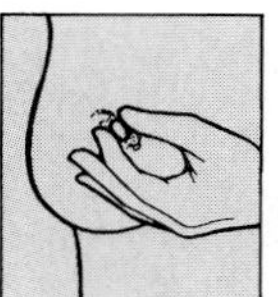
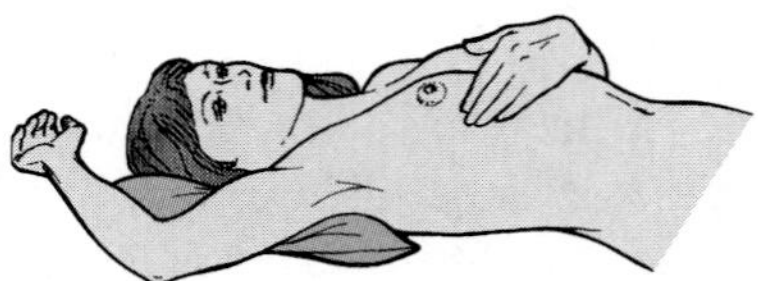

Fig. 12-24 Moving in clockwise direction, examining each quadrant. (From Perry AG, Potter PA: *Clinical nursing skills and techniques,* ed 3, St. Louis, 1994, Mosby.)

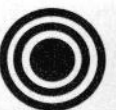

SKILL 12-13 ASSESSING THE BREASTS AND AXILLAE—cont'd

Steps	Rationale
MALE PATIENT	
16. Assess nipples, areolae, and breast tissue for swelling, discharge, lumps, or lesions.	Allows identification of changes, which may indicate mass or edema caused by obesity.
17. Remove gloves and wash hands.	Helps prevent cross-contamination.
18. Document.	Documents procedure and patient's response.

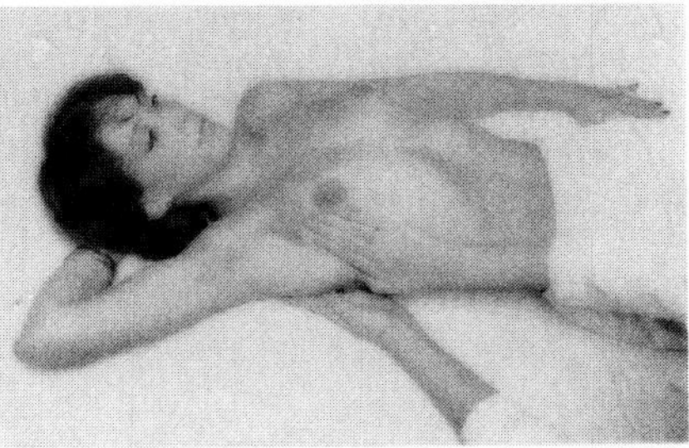

Fig. 12-25 Palpating axillae and along inner aspect of upper arm to examine lymph nodes. (From Perry AG, Potter PA: *Clinical nursing skills and techniques*, ed 3, St. Louis, 1994, Mosby.)

SKILL 12-14 ASSESSING THE FEMALE GENITALIA AND RECTUM

Steps	Rationale
1. Obtain equipment: ▪ Clean gloves ▪ Penlight ▪ Vaginal speculum ▪ Lubricant (water-soluble) ▪ Slides ▪ Specimen container	Helps organize procedure.
2. Refer to medical record, care plan, or Kardex for special interventions.	Provides basis for care.
3. Introduce self.	Decreases patient's anxiety level.
4. Identify patient by identification band.	Identifies correct patient for procedure.
5. Explain procedure to patient.	Seeks cooperation and decreases anxiety.
6. Wash hands and don clean gloves according to agency policy and guidelines from Centers for Disease Control and Prevention and Occupational Safety and Health Administration.	Helps prevent cross-contamination.
7. Prepare patient for intervention:	
a. Close door to room or pull curtain.	Provides privacy.
b. Drape for procedure if necessary.	Prevents exposure of patient.
8. Raise bed to comfortable working level.	Provides safety for nurse.
9. Arrange for patient privacy.	Shows respect for patient.
VAGINAL EXAMINATION	
10. Inspect external genitalia for distribution of pubic hair, color of skin, size and shape of labia, edema, or signs of infection.	Allows identification of normal female characteristics.
11. Separate labia and inspect clitoris and urinary meatus. Assess for inflammation, edema, drainage, lesions, and masses.	Permits better visualization of structures and assessment for problems.

Continued.

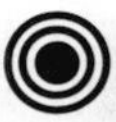

SKILL 12-14 ASSESSING THE FEMALE GENITALIA AND RECTUM—cont'd

Steps	Rationale
12. Examine vaginal opening. Ask patient to bear down as if urinating and assess for bulging or protrusion through vaginal opening.	Allows nurse to identify protrusion of bladder or rectum through vaginal opening.
13. Select appropriate size of speculum and warm blades.	Allows nurse to obtain specimens for tests and examine internal structures.
14. Sit facing patient's perineum. Insert speculum into vagina at 45-degree angle, and lock speculum in open position once cervical os (opening) is visualized.	Allows nurse to visualize cervix and vaginal walls.
15. Collect specimen for Papanicolaou smear and other smears if necessary.	Allows laboratory to test for cancer and other conditions.
16. Inspect vaginal wall for color, lesions, masses, drainage, or odor as speculum is closed and withdrawn.	Determines condition of structures.
RECTAL EXAMINATION	
17. Inspect rectum for external hemorrhoids, fissures, or other lesions.	Allows detection of anal problems.
18. Remove gloves, wash hands, and don clean gloves. Lubricate index finger.	Helps prevent cross-contamination.
19. Ask patient to bear down as if trying to have bowel movement.	Relaxes sphincter and enables examiner to insert finger into rectum.
20. Insert index finger gently into rectum and angle finger toward patient's umbiculus.	Allows finger to follow shape and direction of rectum.
21. Palpate walls of rectum for masses or nodules. Ask if patient has pain or tenderness and ask patient again to bear down and tighten sphincter muscle. Remove finger from rectum.	Allows detection of rectal problems.
22. Remove gloves and wash hands.	Helps prevent cross-contamination.
23. Document.	Documents procedure and patient's response.

SKILL 12-15 ASSESSING THE MALE GENITALIA AND RECTUM

Steps	Rationale
1. Obtain equipment: ▪ Clean gloves ▪ Penlight ▪ Lubricant (water-soluble)	Helps organize procedure.
2. Refer to medical record, care plan, or Kardex for special interventions.	Provides basis for care.
3. Introduce self.	Decreases patient's anxiety level.
4. Identify patient by identification band.	Identifies correct patient for procedure.
5. Explain procedure to patient.	Seeks cooperation and decreases anxiety.
6. Wash hands and don clean gloves according to agency policy and guidelines from Centers for Disease Control and Prevention and Occupational Safety and Health Administration.	Helps prevent cross-contamination.
7. Prepare patient for intervention:	
a. Close door to room or pull curtain.	Provides privacy.
b. Drape for procedure if necessary.	Prevents exposure of patient.
8. Raise bed to comfortable working level.	Provides safety for nurse.
9. Arrange for patient privacy.	Shows respect for patient.

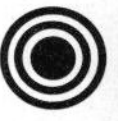

SKILL 12-15 ASSESSING THE MALE GENITALIA AND RECTUM—cont'd

Steps	Rationale
GENITAL EXAMINATION	
10. Inspect penis, assessing position of urethral opening; presence or absence of foreskin; color of skin; and presence of lesions, inflammation, or drainage.	May indicate abnormalities.
11. Inspect scrotum for symmetry, shape, skin color, and lesions.	May indicate abnormalities.
12. Assess inguinal area, palpating for lymph nodes, bulges, or hernias.	May indicate inguinal hernia.
RECTUM	
13. Ask patient to lean forward and rest body on bed.	Allows visualization of anus.
14. Spread cheeks of buttocks and inspect anus for hemorrhoids or breaks in skin.	May indicate hemorrhoids or other abnormalities.
15. Insert index finger gently into rectum and angle finger toward patient's umbilicus.	Allows finger to follow shape and direction of rectum.
16. Palpate walls of rectum for masses or nodules. Ask if patient has pain or tenderness and ask patient again to bear down and tighten sphincter muscle. Remove finger from rectum.	Allows detection of rectal problems.
17. Remove gloves and wash hands.	Helps prevent cross-contamination.
18. Document.	Documents procedure and patient's response.

SKILL 12-16 ASSESSING THE MUSCULOSKELETAL SYSTEM

Steps	Rationale
1. Obtain equipment: ▪ Tape measure ▪ Clean gloves	Helps organize procedure.
2. Refer to medical record, care plan, or Kardex for special interventions.	Provides basis for care.
3. Introduce self.	Decreases patient's anxiety level.
4. Identify patient by identification band.	Identifies correct patient for procedure.
5. Explain procedure to patient.	Seeks cooperation and decreases anxiety.
6. Wash hands and don clean gloves according to agency policy and guidelines from Centers for Disease Control and Prevention and Occupational Safety and Health Administration.	Helps prevent cross-contamination.
7. Prepare patient for intervention:	
a. Close door to room or pull curtain.	Provides privacy.
b. Drape for procedure if necessary.	Prevents exposure of patient.
8. Raise bed to comfortable working level.	Provides safety for nurse.
9. Arrange for patient privacy.	Shows respect for patient.
10. Assess patient's gait for limping, deformity, or abnormalities of balance.	Allows detection of abnormalities (Fig. 12-26).
11. Assess patient's posture.	Allows identification of deformities of joints, muscles, or bones of spine or back.

Continued.

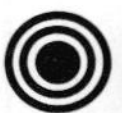

SKILL 12-16 ASSESSING THE MUSCULOSKELETAL SYSTEM—cont'd

Steps	Rationale
12. Ask patient to move each joint through full range of motion, measuring each with tape measure.	Determines need for range-of-joint-motion exercises.
13. Assess patient's muscle strength.	Determines condition of structures and possible need for intervention.
14. Examine joints of upper and lower body, assessing for edema or inflammation. Palpate for tenderness, malformation, nodules, or pain.	Allows detection of edema, inflammation, and pain.
15. Remove gloves and wash hands.	Helps prevent cross-contamination.
16. Document.	Documents procedure and patient's response.

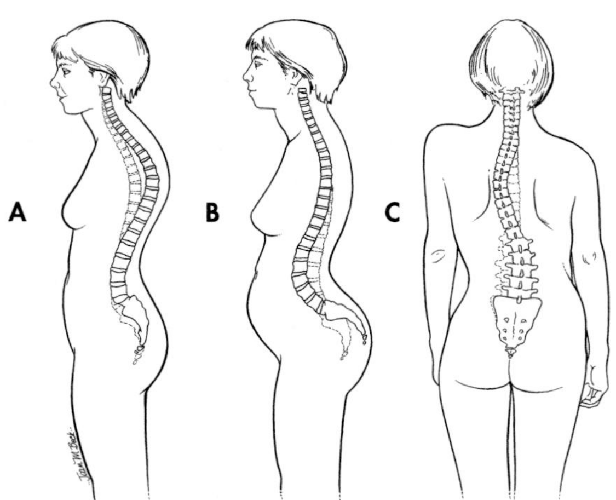

Fig. 12-26 Abnormal spine curvatures. **A**, Kyphosis. **B**, Lordosis. **C**, Scoliosis. (From Christensen BL, Kockrow EO: *Foundations of nursing,* ed 2, St. Louis, 1995, Mosby.)

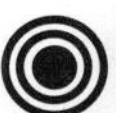

SKILL 12-17 ASSESSING THE NEUROLOGIC SYSTEM

Steps	Rationale
1. Obtain equipment: ▪ Clean gloves ▪ Reflex hammer ▪ Penlight ▪ Tongue depressor	Helps organize procedure.
2. Refer to medical record, care plan, or Kardex for special interventions.	Provides basis for care.
3. Introduce self.	Decreases patient's anxiety level.
4. Identify patient by identification band.	Identifies correct patient for procedure.
5. Explain procedure to patient.	Seeks cooperation and decreases anxiety.
6. Wash hands and don clean gloves according to agency policy and guidelines from Centers for Disease Control and Prevention and Occupational Safety and Health Administration.	Helps prevent cross-contamination.
7. Prepare patient for intervention:	
a. Close door to room or pull curtain.	Provides privacy.
b. Drape for procedure if necessary.	Prevents exposure of patient.
8. Raise bed to comfortable working level.	Provides safety for nurse.
9. Arrange for patient privacy.	Shows respect for patient.
10. Assess patient's level of consciousness by asking questions. Make certain patient is awake and paying attention and there is no language barrier.	Allows detection of disturbances of cerebral functioning that may result from brain disorders, drugs, metabolic changes, or electrolyte imbalance.
11. Asking questions such as "What is your name?" "Where are you?" and "What day is this?"	Enables measurement of patient's orientation.
12. Give commands for communication if patient is unable to speak.	Determines a method for communicating with patient.
13. Test patient's response to painful stimuli.	Allows identification of lack of feeling of painful stimuli.
14. Assess intellectual status and memory of past events.	Allows detection of memory loss, which may indicate brain disorder.
15. Assess abstract ideas by asking meaning of phrases.	Allows identification of brain disorder.
16. Remove gloves and wash hands.	Helps prevent cross-contamination.
17. Document.	Documents procedure and patient's response.

SUMMARY

When performing a physical assessment the nurse is aware of its importance: It helps the nurse chose nursing diagnoses, formulate the plan of care, and develop the care plan, which in turn help the nurse to administer quality nursing care. The nurse prepares the patient for the assessment, ensuring privacy and comfort. The patient is encouraged to be an active participant and is given the opportunity to ask questions. Each body system is assessed, and the nurse should be aware of findings that need to be reported as well as possible interventions. The nurse should perform assessment in an assertive manner to earn the patient's trust.

Key Concepts

- Findings during the first physical assessment provide a baseline for future assessments.
- The collection of accurate data helps in defining appropriate nursing diagnoses.
- Patient teaching helps prevent anxiety and helps understanding of the role of the patient to prevent disease and promote optimal health.
- Techniques of physical assessment—palpation, percussion, auscultation, and inspection—are used throughout assessment, and the nurse should be skilled in their use.
- The nurse should remember the affects of the aging process on findings while examining older adults.
- An excellent time to perform physical assessment is during the morning bath.

Critical Thinking Questions

1. The nurse palpates a mass while examining a patient's neck. Describe any additional assessments the nurse would make.
2. The nurse is assigned to work in a well-baby clinic. He is assessing 8-month-old John Henry. His weight is 12 pounds. His mother states that he "mostly drinks milk." What additional assessment data does the nurse need to determine the presence of a nutritional deficit in this patient?
3. Mrs. Tice, a 40-year-old mother of two, is entering the outpatient surgery clinic for a breast biopsy. She has never had surgery. She is a smoker and takes medication for high blood pressure. What factors will the nurse assess before surgery in developing a plan for surgical care?

REFERENCES AND SUGGESTED READINGS

Christensen BL, Kockrow EO: *Foundations of nursing,* ed 2, St Louis, 1995, Mosby.

McFarland GR, McFarlane EA: *Nursing diagnosis and intervention: planning for patient care,* ed 2, St Louis, 1993, Mosby.

Potter PA, Perry AG: *Basic nursing: theory and practice,* ed 3, St Louis, 1995, Mosby.

Potter PA, Perry AG: *Fundamentals of nursing: concepts, process, and practice,* ed 3, St Louis, 1993, Mosby.

Seidel HM et al: *Mosby's guide to physical examination,* ed 3, St Louis, 1995, Mosby.

■ CHAPTER 13 ■

Laboratory and Diagnostic Tests

Learning Objectives

After studying this chapter, the student should be able to . . .

- Define the key terms.
- State general nursing responsibilities before, during, and after a diagnostic test.
- Describe basic x-ray procedure.
- Discuss why four different types of x-ray studies might be ordered for a patient.
- Discuss three common tests that assess electrical impulses.
- Identify three types of endoscopic examination.
- Identify five laboratory studies that assess bodily fluids.
- List and explain nursing actions required for collecting specimens.
- Identify the role of the nurse when performing procedures for specimen collection.
- Provide patient teaching for a specimen collection.
- Recognize normal and abnormal laboratory values of various specimens.
- Appropriately label a collected specimen.
- Demonstrate appropriate collection of assigned specimens.
- Prepare a patient for a specimen collection.
- Collect urine, stool, and sputum specimens.
- Obtain a sterile culture.
- Measure capillary glucose levels.

Key Terms

Amniocentesis
Angiogram
Barium enema
Bone marrow aspiration
Bronchography
Bronchoscopy
Cholecystogram
Computerized axial tomography
Contrast medium
Culture
Cystoscopy
Electrocardiography
Electroencephalography
Electromyography
Endoscope
Esophagogastroduodenoscopy
Hemoccult test
Intravenous pyelogram
Lumbar puncture
Magnetic resonance imaging
Myelogram
Occult
Papanicolaou test
Paracentesis
Proctoscopy
Radiography
Radiopaque
Sensitivity
Sigmoidoscopy
Small bowel x-ray series
Thoracentesis
Ultrasonography
Upper gastrointestinal series
Urinalysis

Skills

13-1 Measuring capillary blood glucose levels
13-2 Collecting a midstream urine specimen
13-3 Collecting a sterile urine specimen
13-4 Collecting a stool specimen
13-5 Measuring occult blood in stool
13-6 Collecting sputum
13-7 Obtaining a throat culture
13-8 Assisting with a Papanicolaou test

Laboratory and diagnostic tests provide valuable information and assist the physician in making a medical diagnosis. If the specimen is not collected appropriately, labeled accurately, and taken to the laboratory at the appropriate time, the patient may suffer another day of hospitalization and extra expense as well as a possible delay in diagnosis and treatment. The patient may be taken to a special area for a test to be performed or may stay in the room where the physician performs the test at the bedside and where the laboratory technologist draws blood and then performs the test in the laboratory.

The responsibilities of the nurse include teaching the patient about the upcoming test, preparing the patient for the test, assisting the physician with the test, caring for the patient after the procedure, providing follow-up care of supplies and equipment, and documenting all teaching and care. The nurse must also know how the procedure is performed, since the nurse often assists the physician with the procedure. The nurse is also responsible for seeing that informed consent is obtained.

Many members of the health care team play integral roles in performing laboratory and diagnostic tests. These tests are frequently done to determine how the body is functioning and to pinpoint different disease processes. Recent advances allow visualization of internal areas without surgery. The result is that diseases can be detected earlier and treatment initiated. The nurse's role can be quite diverse. The nurse frequently is responsible for collecting the body fluid necessary to complete the test. However, many diagnostic tests are completed by other members of the health care team. In these situations the nurse plays a primary role in teaching and preparing the patient and equipment and providing follow-up nursing care.

Most important, the nurse needs to recognize abnormal laboratory values. It is the nurse's responsibility to notify the physician when laboratory and diagnostic studies deviate from the norm and patient intervention is necessary. Each health care facility usually has its own policy and procedure manuals. These manuals contain routine orders for each diagnostic test. The manuals are a valuable resource that prevent the nurse from overlooking critical patient preparation information. This chapter highlights basic care necessary for several commonly prescribed tests.

Remembering the meaning of root words, prefixes, and suffixes can assist the new nurse in identifying many confusing test names. The following suffixes in combination with already learned root words for body structures can be helpful and include:

-ography	Procedure in which an image is produced
-ogram	Actual image or results of a test
-oscopy	Visualization of body structures
-centesis	Puncture of a body cavity

NURSING CARE

Diagnostic tests are often ordered to assist the health care team in determining the best plan of care. Nursing care depends on the specific test ordered. However, general nursing responsibilities exist before, during, and after the procedure. Frequently ordered diagnostic tests and their accompanying nursing actions are outlined in Table 13-1.

Providing complete information regarding the test should decrease a patient's anxiety and ensure cooperation. It is important for the nurse to consider the patient's growth and developmental status. The use of medical terminology should be avoided. Special considerations of the older adult should be made (see gerontologic box).

Assessment by Radiography

X-rays produce electromagnetic energy that passes throughout the body and produces an image on a film. This is **radiography.** A plain-film x-ray study uses no other media to produce the image. These types of x-ray studies can be performed on almost any part of the body such as the chest, hand, foot, and abdomen. No special preparation or follow-up care is necessary.

If a plain x-ray film does not define the image clearly, contrast media can be used. **Contrast media** are radiopaque materials that fill a body cavity or area, increasing the density. **Radiopaque** materials do not permit the passage of x-rays. Thus the shape of the object is more clearly visualized on the film. Examples of some contrast studies include cholecystogram, myelogram, intravenous pyelogram, and angiogram. Special preparation and follow-up care are necessary for these examinations. The nurse is responsible for this care and corresponding patient teaching. The nurse also checks for allergies. Many of the contrast media are iodine based,

Text continued on p. 203.

GERONTOLOGIC CONSIDERATIONS

- If multiple procedures are necessary, adequate rest time should be scheduled.
- Sputum collection is often difficult because of poor cough. Respiratory-induced sputum collection may be necessary.
- The older adult may experience a decrease in the agility needed to collect a midstream urinalysis. Catheterization may be necessary.

Table 13-1 NURSE'S ROLE IN PREPARATION OF PATIENT FOR TESTS

Test	Preparation	Reference Values	Nurse's Duties	Follow-Up
Laboratory				
Urinalysis, routine	None			Report results.
Color	Laboratory slip	Amber yellow	Collect and label specimen.	
Clarity		clear	Know reference values.	
pH		4.6-8.0 (average—6.0)		
Specific gravity		1.003-1.035		
Protein		0-8 mg/dl		
Sugar		0		
Ketone		0		
RBCs		0-4		
		0-5		
WBCs		0		
Complete blood count (CBC)	None	See below	Know reference values.	Report results.
RBCs		3.8-5.3		
WBCs		4.1-10.0.		
Hematocrit		Male: 45%-52% Female: 37%-48%		
Hemoglobin		Male: 13-18 g/dl Female: 12-16 g/dl		
Leukocyte count (WBC)		4300-10,800 mm^3		
Erythrocyte count (RBC)		4.2-5.9 million mm^3		
Mean corpuscular volume		80-94 mm^3		
Mean corpuscular hemoglobin platelet count		27-32 pg 150,000-350,000 mm^3		
Blood Chemistry Level				
Fasting blood glucose	NPO or hold sign Laboratory slip	70-110 mg/dl	Place NPO or "hold" sign on door.	Report results.
Blood urea nitrogen		5-20 mg/dl		
Uric acid		3.0-7.0 mg/dl		
Serum glutamic-oxaloacetic transaminase (SGOT)		10-40 U/ml	Inform patient not to eat or drink until blood is drawn.	
Creatine phosphokinase (CPK)		Female: 5-35 mU/ml Male: 5-55 mU/ml	Inform patient of test.	Report results.
Calcium (Ca)		8.5-10.5 mg/dl		
Lactate dehydrogenase (LDH)	Alkaline	60-120 U/ml		
Phosphates	Phosphatase-SMA	3-5 mg/dl		
Cholesterol		102-287 mg/dl		
Triglycerides		20-200 mg/dl		
Alkaline phosphatase		32-139 IU/L		
SMA 12, 16, 24, 36, 60				
Glucose tolerance test	NPO Laboratory slip	Normal: 60-125 mg/dl Urine negative for glucose	Inform patient of test and place sign on door.	Report results.

RBCs, Red blood cells; *WBCs,* white blood cells, *NPO,* nothing by mouth, *SMA,* sequential multiple analysis.

Continued.

Table 13-1 NURSE'S ROLE IN PREPARATION OF PATIENT FOR TESTS—cont'd

Test	Preparation	Reference Values	Nurse's Duties	Follow-Up
Glucose given to patient orally or intravenously, blood samples drawn, and blood glucose amount determined				
Lumbar puncture Spinal needle inserted into subarachnoid space of spine to examine spinal fluid	NPO	Negative findings	Inform patient of test and place sign on door.	Report results.
Radiology				
Chest x-ray Lungs examined to show lungs and surrounding structures	None Requisition	Negative findings	Inform patient of test.	Report results.
Myelogram Spinal needle inserted into spinal column to determine disease or disorder	Consent form Requisition	Negative findings	Inform patient of test and answer questions.	Report results.
Mammography X-ray study given to reveal deeper structures of breasts	Requisition	Negative findings	Inform patient of test and answer questions.	Read results.
Scans				
Computerized tomography (see Fig. 13-1) Analysis of tomographic x-ray films of specific body organs and tissues	Consent form Requisition	Negative findings	Inform patient of test and answer questions.	Read results.
Brain scan	Consent form Requisition	Negative findings	Inform patient of test and answer questions.	Read results.
Body scan	Consent form Requisition	Negative findings	Inform patient of test and answer questions.	Read results.
Lung scan	Consent form Requisition	Negative findings	Inform patient of test and answer questions.	Read results.
Ultrasound/Sonogram Ultrasound used to produce image or photograph of organ or tissue; performed on major organs such as liver, gallbladder, pancreas	Consent form Requisition	Negative findings	Inform patient of test and answer questions.	Read results.

Table 13-1 NURSE'S ROLE IN PREPARATION OF PATIENT FOR TESTS—cont'd

Test	Preparation	Reference Values	Nurse's Duties	Follow-Up
Gastrointestinal Laboratory Tests				
Bronchoscopy Examination of tracheobronchial tree (see Fig. 13-2)	Consent form Requisition	Negative findings	Prepare supplies and assist physician with procedure.	Assess patient's responses and monitor postoperative vital signs.
Endoscopy Visualization of upper and lower gastrointestinal tract (see Fig. 13-3)	Requisition	Density differences examined	Inform patient of test and answer questions.	None.
Gastroscopy Visualization of stomach and adjacent structures	Requisition	Negative findings	Inform patient of test and answer questions.	None.
Colonoscopy Visualization of colon	Requisition Administration of electrolyte solution	Negative findings	Inform patient of test and answer questions.	If polypectomy performed, monitor vital signs and assess bleeding.
Proctoscopy Examination of rectum with proctoscope (see Fig. 13-4)	Requisition	Negative findings	Inform patient of test and answer questions.	If polypectomy performed, monitor vital signs and assess bleeding.
Sigmoidoscopy Examination of anus, rectum, and sigmoid colon with sigmoidoscope	Requisition	Negative findings	Inform patient of test and answer questions.	If polypectomy performed, monitor vital signs and assess bleeding.
Urinary Studies				
Cystoscopy Examination of bladder with light	Consent form Requisition	Negative findings	Inform patient of test and assess for complications.	Read results. Monitor postoperative vital signs. Provide comfort measures.
Retrograde cystoscopy	Consent form Requisition	Negative findings	Inform patient of test and answer questions.	Monitor postoperative vital signs and administer preoperative medication.
Intravenous pyelogram Examination of urinary system after injection of dye	NPO Consent form Requisition	Negative findings	Inform patient of test and answer questions.	Monitor postoperative vital signs.
Heart				
Electrocardiogram Graphic records of electrical impulses of heart	Requisition	Within normal limits	Inform patient of test and answer questions.	None.

Continued.

Table 13-1 **NURSE'S ROLE IN PREPARATION OF PATIENT FOR TESTS—cont'd**

Test	Preparation	Reference Values	Nurse's Duties	Follow-Up
Arteriogram X-ray study of arteries after injecting radiopaque dye	Consent form Requisition	Negative findings	Inform patient of test and answer questions.	Monitor postoperative vital signs. Assess patient's response.
Echocardiogram Use of ultrasound to visualize internal cardiac structures	Consent form	Negative findings	Inform patient of test and answer questions.	Assess patient's response.
Electroencephalogram Tracing of brain waves on electrocephalograph	Consent form Requisition	Normal brain waves	Keep patient awake before examination and shampoo hair night before. Inform patient of test and answer questions.	None.
Renal angiography Serial x-ray study of blood vessel taken in rapid sequence after dye injection (in this case, kidney)	Consent form Requisition	Negative findings	Inform patient of test and answer questions, administer cathartic or enema and shave injection sites, and palpate peripheral pulses and assess color and temperature.	Read results and monitor vital signs.
Amniocentesis Examination of amniotic fluid after insertion of long scope into abdomen of pregnant woman	Consent form Requisition	Fetal maturity and well-being	Inform patient of test and answer questions.	Read results.
Thoracentesis Needle placed in pleural cavity to remove excess fluid (see Fig. 13-5)	Consent form Requisition	Negative findings	Prepare supplies and assist physician.	Monitor vital signs every 15 min for 1 hr. Place patient on bedrest.
Paracentesis, abdominal Removal of peritoneal fluid for observation or testing	Consent form Requisition	Negative findings	Prepare supplies and assist physician.	Monitor vital signs. Read results.
Fluoroscopy Use of fluoroscope for medical diagnosis by x-ray study	Consent form Requisition	Negative findings	Inform patient of test and answer questions.	None.
Gastrointestinal series X-ray of upper gastrointestinal tract	Requisition NPO	Negative findings	Inform patient of test, place NPO sign on door, and answer questions.	Monitor patient's response.
Gallbladder series X-ray study of gallbladder after taking drug to make gallbladder opaque	Requisition NPO	Negative findings	Inform patient of test, place NPO sign on door, and answer questions.	None.

Table 13-1 NURSE'S ROLE IN PREPARATION OF PATIENT FOR TESTS—cont'd

Test	Preparation	Reference Values	Nurse's Duties	Follow-Up
Cardiac catheterization Very small tube passed into heart through blood vessel and samples taken for testing	Consent form Requisition	Negative findings	Inform patient of test and answer questions.	Monitor vital signs.
Bone marrow aspiration Removal of small amount of bone marrow for testing (see Fig. 13-6)	Consent form Requisition	Negative findings	Prepare supplies and assist physician.	Assess patient's response.

and a significant portion of the population has this allergy. The allergy can range from a mild reaction of a slight rash to a severe, life-threatening reaction requiring immediate emergency treatment.

An **upper gastrointestinal series** (UGI series) studies the structures of the esophagus, stomach, duodenum, and upper jejunum as the patient swallows a contrast medium (barium). The use of fluoroscopy enables the examiner to visualize the motion of the organs. This study is frequently ordered to diagnose tumors, ulcers, hiatal hernias, narrowing of structures, and gastritis.

A **small bowel x-ray series** can be ordered with a UGI. It is performed in the same manner as a UGI, but the entire small bowel is visualized. This includes all of the jejunum and ileum. It can take 2 to 6 hours to perform this examination. In contrast, an UGI alone requires 45 minutes. This study is frequently ordered to diagnose tumors, obstruction, diverticulitis, and ulcerative colitis.

A **barium enema** involves distention of the colon and rectum through the use of air and barium administered through the anus. This radioactive material allows visualization of the lower intestine. Fluoroscopy aids in the visualization process. This study is frequently ordered to diagnose lesions and inflammatory disorders of the colon. It can also identify obstructions.

A **cholecystogram** is an x-ray study of the gallbladder and its ducts. A dye is usually used as a contrast medium. This study can assess the function and abnormalities of the gallbladder and related ducts. This study is frequently ordered to diagnose gallbladder disease such as tumors, gall stones, and obstructions.

An **intravenous pyelogram** (IVP) is an x-ray examination of the urinary tract. An iodine-based contrast medium is injected into a vein to assist the technician in visualization of urinary structures. This study is frequently ordered to diagnose abnormal functioning of the urinary system, including abnormalities of the kidneys and ureters.

An **angiogram** is an x-ray examination of the vascular system. The blood vessels that supply the heart are frequently studied. However, blood vessels in the brain, lungs, and kidneys can also be examined. A radiopaque dye is used. There is a risk of allergic reactions, which is assessed before the test is begun. This is an invasive test generally performed in a specialized area. This study is frequently ordered to determine the location and degree of vessel narrowing.

A **myelogram** is a radiographic study using contrast material to study the spinal cord, nerve roots, and vertebrae. Fluoroscopy enables the spinal cord to be visualized on a screen, assisting diagnosis. This study is frequently ordered to diagnose ruptured disks, tumors, and compression of the spinal cord.

A **bronchography** is a radiographic study using contrast media to study the bronchial tree. It is often performed during bronchoscopy. This test is frequently ordered to diagnose bronchiectasis or bronchial obstructions.

The **computerized axial tomography** (CAT or CT) uses special narrow x-ray beams to provide a cross-sectional view of a body part (Fig. 13-1). The CAT machine rotates around the motionless patient. Whole-body CAT scan machines are now available. CAT scans can sometimes be used in lieu of a more invasive test such as an angiogram. An agitated or claustrophobic patient could inhibit the test procedure. Sedation may be necessary. The test can be

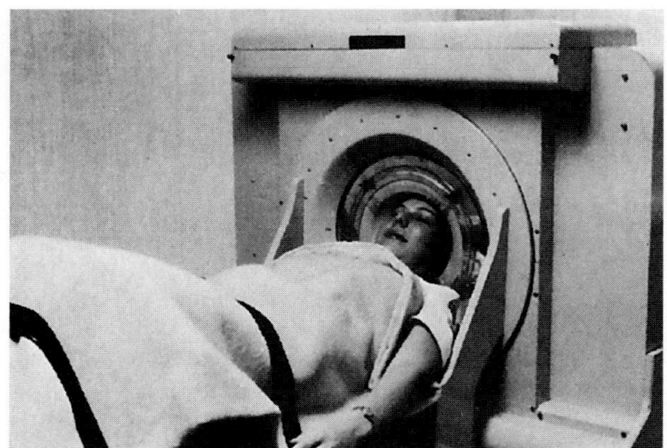

Fig. 13-1 Patient receiving computerized axial tomographic scanning. (From Christensen BL, Kockrow EO: *Foundations of nursing,* ed 2, St Louis, 1995, Mosby.)

performed with contrast dye. Again, allergies are an important consideration.

In **magnetic resonance imaging** (MRI) a powerful magnetic field produces detailed images of internal organs that are translated into visual images by a computer. Radiographic dyes or x-rays are not necessary for the test. Therefore MRI is a safe diagnostic tool. Three-dimensional imaging enhances the physician's ability to make diagnoses. MRI is contraindicated for patients who have metallic implants, gold fillings, pacemakers or heart valve prostheses, metal intravenous intracatheters, and claustrophobia. It is also contraindicated for metal workers and those who cannot lie still on the back for 45 minutes. Objects that contain iron are affected by the magnet and may cause injury to the patient. Objects made of steel such as dental braces do not injure the patient but may result in a less sharp image. All jewelry must be removed before MRIs.

Assessment of Electrical Impulses

Electrical impulses may also be tested. Nerve activity throughout the body produces these impulses. Wires, called *electrodes,* are attached to various portions of the body, depending on what area is being observed. A clear gel is used to aid in transmitting the impulses to the machine. The machine provides a visual image, usually in the form of a graph, to interpret the data. The patient feels no particular sensation during the procedure. No preparation is necessary for the test.

Electrocardiography (EKG or ECG) is an examination that records the electrical impulses of heart muscle activity. A total of 3 to 12 leads are placed on the person's chest and peripheral limbs. Heart rhythms may be monitored for 24 hours through the use of a Holter monitor. This test is frequently ordered to determine the heart rate, the rhythm, and possible heart damage.

Electroencephalography (EEG) examines the electrical activity of the brain. The technician attaches 19 to 25 gold electrodes to the patient's scalp using a conducting gel. The patient is encouraged to sleep while brain waves are measured. The patient may need medication to induce sleep. This test is frequently ordered to diagnose the absence of brain activity and a multitude of neurologic disorders.

The **electromyography** is an examination of nerve impulses in skeletal muscles. Electrodes are placed over the muscles, and needle electrodes are inserted into muscles. This test is frequently ordered to diagnose neurologic disorders with signs of paralysis, paresis (partial paralysis), and paresthesia (numbness or tingling of a part).

Assessment by Ultrasonography

Ultrasonography is a noninvasive test using sound waves to produce images of internal structures. These images are viewed on a screen. This test can detect pathologic changes in muscles and joints. It plays a critical role in obstetric medicine by assessing the development of the fetus.

Assessment by Endoscopy

An **endoscope** is a flexible, lighted scope that can be inserted into any orifice of the body, thus permitting direct visualization, examination, and biopsy of a body part. A biopsy is the removal of a small piece of tissue for microscopic examination.

A **bronchoscopy** is a direct examination of the larynx, trachea, and bronchi. The throat is anesthetized to prevent gagging as the scope is inserted (Fig. 13-2). This test is frequently ordered to diagnose and remove obstructions and thick secretions, obtain specimens, and identify tumors.

Esophagogastroduodenoscopy is an examination of the esophagus, stomach (Fig. 13-3), and duodenum. A gastroscope is used to perform this test. This study can be ordered to biopsy or remove polyps or tumors, identify ulcers, stretch strictured areas, and assist with feeding tube placement. The patient is frequently sedated but remains conscious.

During assessment by **proctoscopy** and **sigmoidoscopy,** a scope is passed into the gastrointestinal tract through the anus (Fig. 13-4) to examine the rectum and sigmoid colon. These tests are frequently ordered to diagnose tumors and inflammatory disorders of the colon.

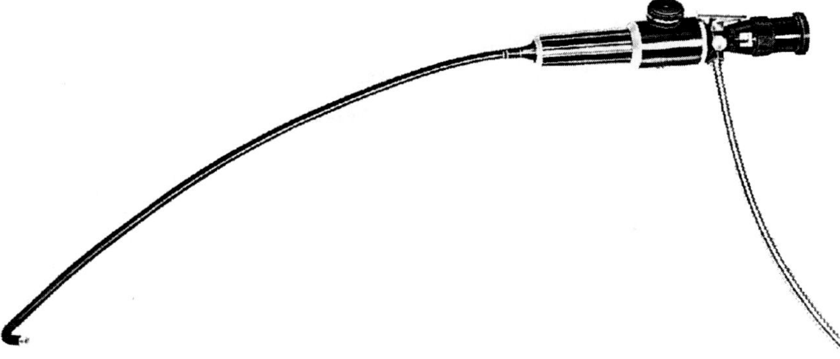

Fig. 13-2 Flexible fiberoptic bronchoscope. (Courtesy American Cystoscope Makers, Inc, Pelham, NY; from Christensen BL, Kockrow EO: *Foundations of nursing,* ed 2, St Louis, 1995, Mosby.)

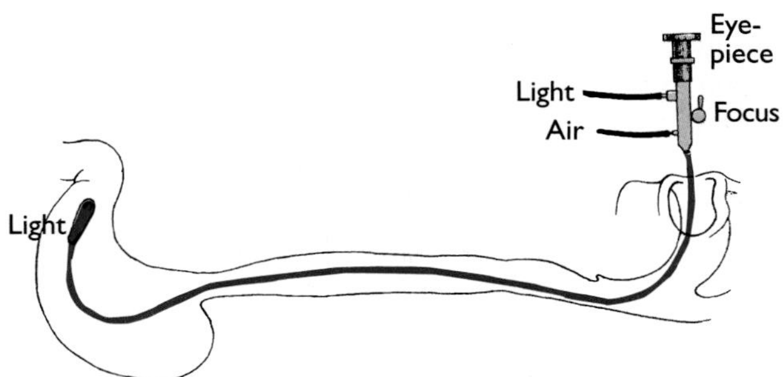

Fig. 13-3 Fiberoptic endoscope. (From Christensen BL, Kockrow EO: *Foundations of nursing,* ed 2, St Louis, 1995, Mosby.)

In **cystoscopy** an instrument called a *cystoscope* is inserted through the urethra to allow visualization of the urethra, bladder, and openings of the ureters. This procedure is frequently ordered to diagnose urinary tract abnormalities and infections, identify tumors, and remove a calculus (a stone).

Assessment of Body Fluids

Examination of body fluids is a key component of confirming a diagnosis and implementing a plan of care. The specific assessment required determines whether the nurse assists the physician or the nurse obtains the specimen. After the specimen is obtained, it is usually necessary to send it to the laboratory for analysis. Some analyses of urine, stool, and capillary blood can be completed at the bedside by the nurse. The policy and procedure of the institution may dictate when this is permissible. The universal precautions of the Centers for Disease Control and Prevention must be used at all times when coming in contact with body secretions. Several types of frequently ordered tests will be examined in more detail.

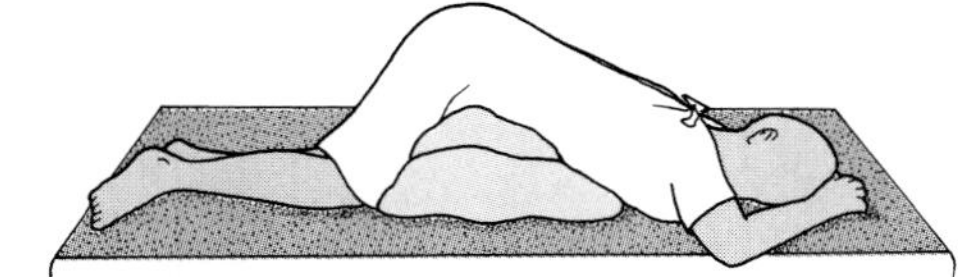

Fig. 13-4 Position for proctoscopy. (From Christensen BL, Kockrow EO: *Foundations of nursing,* ed 2, St Louis, 1995, Mosby.)

Gastric analysis

A gastric analysis is performed to examine stomach contents. A nasogastric tube is inserted, and a 50- or 60-ml syringe is attached to the tube for aspiration. A drug may be administered during the test to stimulate the production of gastric acid and observe the stomach's response. The specimen is usually sent to the laboratory for analysis. The pH level (acidity vs. alkalinity) can be immediately tested at the bedside using a test strip. A number below 7 indicates acidity, and a number above 7 indicates alkalinity. A normal value is 1 to 4. An absence of hydrochloric acid in the stomach can signify pathologic conditions. The secretions can also be tested to determine the presence of blood. This test is generally performed to evaluate gastritis, ulcers, or pathologic conditions.

Lumbar puncture

A **lumbar puncture,** or spinal tap, is performed to obtain a sample of cerebrospinal fluid. The needle is placed into the subarachnoid space, usually between the third and fourth or fourth and fifth lumbar vertebrae. The area of the needle insertion is critical to avoid hitting the spinal cord, which ends at the second lumbar vertebra. A lumbar puncture may be ordered for a variety of reasons. The specimen is usually sent to the laboratory for analysis. The results may assist in diagnosing a variety of neurologic disorders, including neoplasms, cerebral

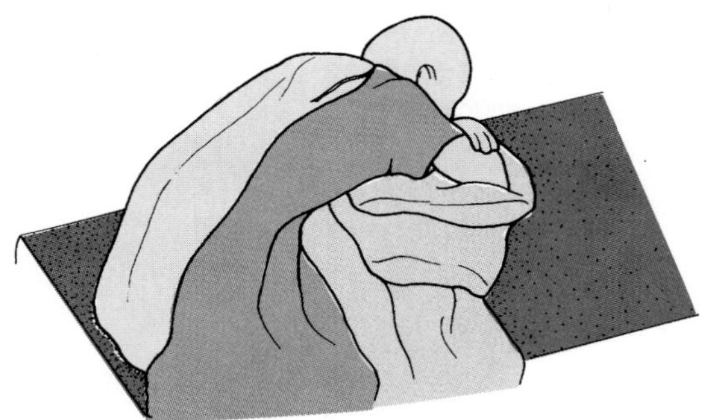

Fig. 13-5 Position for thoracentesis. (From Perry AG, Potter PA: *Clinical nursing skills and techniques,* ed 3, St Louis, 1994, Mosby.)

hemorrhage, meningitis, and encephalitis. The procedure may also be performed to instill medications and to withdraw a volume of fluid to decrease intracranial pressure.

Abdominal paracentesis

A **paracentesis** is a procedure involving puncturing the abdominal cavity to withdraw fluid. The puncture is made with a needle called a *trocar.* A cannula (flexible tube) surrounds the trocar and is left in the abdomen while the needle is withdrawn. Fluid drains through the cannula into a container until the procedure is completed. The procedure is most frequently ordered to relieve pressure and dyspnea caused by the accumulation of fluid in the abdominal cavity. This condition of fluid accumulation is called *ascites.* A sample of the fluid may be sent to the laboratory for examination.

Thoracentesis

A **thoracentesis** is a procedure involving the sterile puncture of the chest wall for removal of fluid from the pleural cavity (Fig. 13-5). The test is usually performed to remove accumulated fluid or air and thus relieve pressure, pain, or dyspnea. The fluid may be sent to the laboratory and examined for signs of infection or cancer.

Liver biopsy

A liver biopsy is a sterile procedure involving the removal of liver tissue for examination by the laboratory. It is usually ordered to determine the progress of liver disease. The procedure is contraindicated if blood clotting studies are abnormal.

Bone marrow aspiration

A **bone marrow aspiration** is a sterile procedure involving the insertion of a needle into the upper portion of the sternum or iliac crest (Fig. 13-6) to obtain a specimen, which is sent to the laboratory for examination. It is frequently ordered to diagnose a wide range of blood disorders, infections, and malignancies, such as leukemia, infectious diseases, and tumors. Bone marrow biopsy is also performed when necessary to make definitive diagnoses.

Amniocentesis

An **amniocentesis** is the puncturing of the amniotic sac to remove amniotic fluid for laboratory examination. This procedure is performed with an ultrasound to assist correct placement of the needle. This procedure is usually ordered for high-risk pregnancies. It may assist in diagnosing congenital disorders and lung maturity. The gender of the fetus can be determined during this test.

Blood studies

A wide variety of tests may be completed on a sample of blood. Most diagnostic workups require several different components of blood. Some commonly ordered tests include a complete blood count, blood chemistries, and clotting factors. Laboratory personnel usually draw blood from veins or by fingerstick. However, this may be a nursing role. The state nurse practice act and institutional policy determine this responsibility.

Measurement of capillary blood glucose is a frequently ordered blood test that is usually performed at the bedside by the nurse. Through the use of a glucometer or a similar device the nurse obtains a fairly accurate blood glucose level within a minute. This test is significantly more accurate than a dipstick urine test. Frequently the patient receives regular insulin to cover elevated blood glucose readings. This test may also easily be performed by the patient at home.

Urine studies

A laboratory examination of urine may help diagnose many different conditions. The study ordered dictates how the specimen is to be collected. A commonly ordered study is a **urinalysis**, which requires a clean specimen collection. The patient may simply void into a clean receptacle. It is best to obtain an early morning specimen. It is important to note whether a woman is menstruating and to delay urine specimen collection until the urine contains no blood.

There are several methods for collecting a urine specimen for urinalysis, one of the most widely ordered diagnostic tests. A urinalysis can include measurement of pH; protein, glucose, and ketone levels; blood; and specific gravity. The nurse collects a urine sample, labels and takes the specimen to the laboratory, and assesses the results of a urinalysis. The nurse also explains test collection to the patient.

The patient must be made aware of the upcoming test and told to contact the nurse before the next voiding. The nurse should instruct the patient to

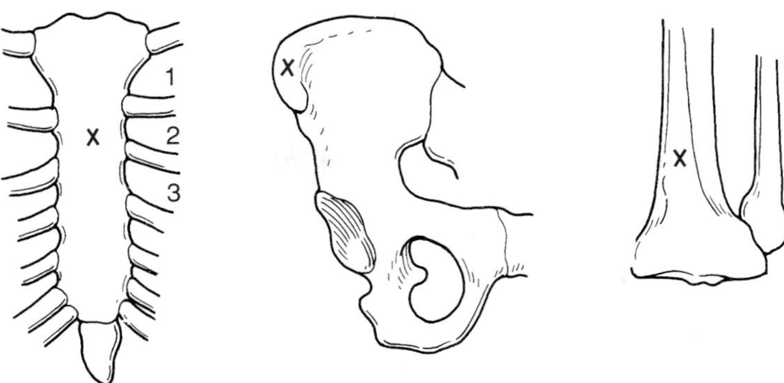

Fig. 13-6 Sites for bone marrow aspiration: sternum, iliac crest (most common), and tibia. (From Perry AG, Potter PA: *Clinical nursing skills and techniques,* ed 3, St Louis, 1994, Mosby.)

drink extra water to assist voiding, not to put toilet tissue in the container, and not to allow feces to come in contact with the urine specimen.

A midstream urine specimen may be obtained for a urinalysis or a urine culture and sensitivity. If the patient is incontinent or unable to cooperate, a sterile urine specimen is obtained by inserting a straight French catheter and collecting the specimen of urine. If a Foley catheter is already in place, the specimen can be obtained through the catheter port using sterile technique. Urine from the Foley drainage bag should not be used for a specimen, since it is old, stagnant urine and will not give accurate test results.

Residual urine (urine left in the bladder after voiding) can be measured by catheterization. The patient voids, and the catheterization is performed within 10 minutes.

The nurse must prepare the patient for the procedure by explaining what type of urine specimen will be collected. It is important that the patient's anxiety be relieved. The nurse should assure the patient that there will be no discomfort during the procedure if the patient remains relaxed. The only thing the patient should feel is pressure from the catheter when it is inserted. The patient experiences no discomfort when urine is collected from the catheter port. The urine test for glucose and acetone is not used as frequently as it once was because of the glucometer blood glucose test. The presence of all of the following abnormal components may be determined by the use of a single dipstick test performed at the bedside: albumin (albuminuria), ketone bodies (ketonuria), and glucose (glycosuria). Instructions are given on the bottle for each test.

Stool specimen

Stool specimens are collected and examined for a variety of reasons: to check for infection, bleeding, or hemorrhage; to analyze the amount, color, and consistency of the stool; and to identify parasites, fat, ova, and bacteria. The nurse collects the feces,

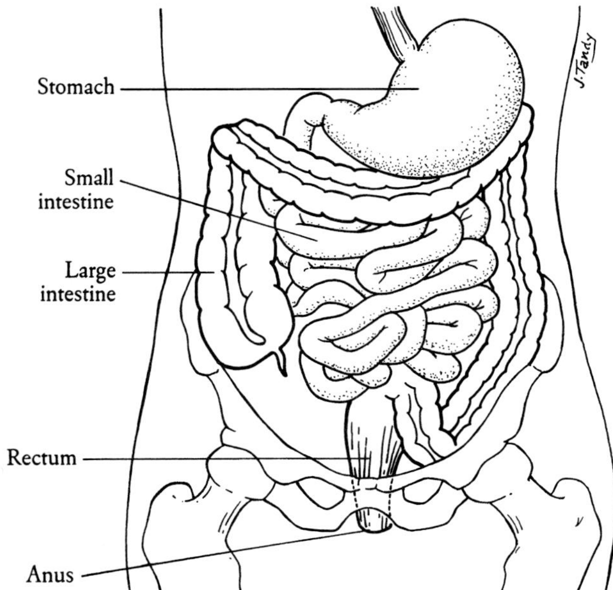

Fig. 13-7 Gastrointestinal system.

labels the specimen appropriately, and takes the specimen and laboratory request to the laboratory. Stool to be examined for parasites must be taken immediately to the laboratory so that the parasites can be examined under the microscope while alive. A stool specimen may also be collected from a colostomy or ileostomy (Fig. 13-7).

The nurse should inform the patient that a stool specimen is needed and collects the stool in such a manner that will not cause stress or make the patient feel hurried. The nurse is responsible for arranging supplies if the patient is to collect the stool.

Blood in any body waste is abnormal. Blood in the stool may be bright red. Black tarry feces indicates that old blood is present higher in the gastrointestinal tract. When blood is present in the stool but cannot be seen, it is called ***occult,*** or *hidden.* It may be seen only with the use of a microscope. A **hemoccult test** is used to detect occult blood in the feces

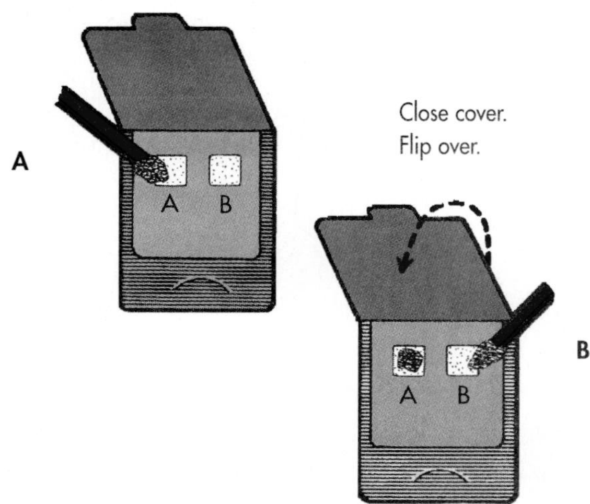

Fig. 13-8 Equipment for measuring occult blood in stool. **A,** The nurse smears a very small amount of stool in the first box. **B,** The nurse smears a very small amount of stool from another part of stool in the second box. (From Perry AG, Potter PA: *Clinical nursing skills and techniques,* ed 3, St Louis, 1994, Mosby.)

(Fig. 13-8). The hemoccult test or guaiac test may be performed on the unit. If the test is performed on the nursing unit, instructions are provided. The nurse indicates that the stools have been obtained by erasing or crossing them off of the list on the Kardex. A meat-free diet may be ordered for the 3 days before the test.

Sputum specimen

A sputum specimen is frequently obtained to diagnose respiratory conditions. Sputum (mucus from the lung) is collected to determine whether pathogenic microorganisms, cancer cells, or tubercle bacilli are present in the sputum. A culture and sensitivity test may also determine to what drugs the organism is sensitive and indicate appropriate antibiotics. A **culture** is a laboratory test involving the cultivation of microorganisms or cells in a special growth medium. **Sensitivity** is a laboratory method of determining the effectiveness of antibiotics.

A sputum specimen must come from deep within the respiratory tree. Expectoration from throat and mouth secretions cannot be used as a sputum specimen. Early morning is the best time to collect a sputum specimen because the patient has not had time to clear the respiratory passages. Many tests can be performed on sputum (for example, culture and sensitivity, cytology [study of cells], and acid-fast bacillus test). Some patients cannot cough up a specimen, so pharyngeal suctioning must be performed to obtain sputum. Collection containers that use a closed method for collection protect the nurse from contamination from body fluids. The nurse explains the

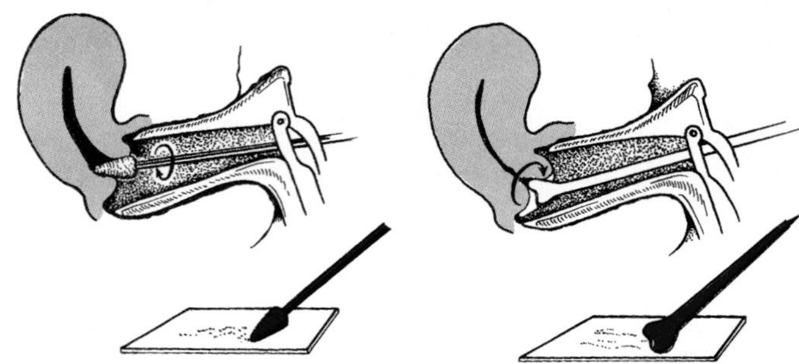

Fig. 13-9 Collection of specimen for a Papanicolaou smear. (From Perry AG, Potter PA: *Clinical nursing skills and techniques,* ed 3, St Louis, 1994, Mosby.)

procedure and prepares the patient for the test.

The nurse instructs the patient to drink extra fluids the night before the test, since this will loosen secretions and make them easier to cough up for the specimen. Saliva cannot be used as a specimen, and the patient must understand this.

Throat culture

A throat culture is used to determine whether the patient has an infection and whether the infection is viral or bacterial in nature. Antibacterials and antibiotics are administered for bacterial infections. A small part of the specimen from the throat is placed on a culture medium and allowed to grow. Readings are taken usually at 48 and 72 hours, and the organisms are identified. If a sensitivity test is ordered with the culture, the results of the test determine what organisms are present and what antibiotics will help to clear the infection.

The nurse must assess the patient's ability to understand and cooperate during the collection of a throat specimen. Patients often gag during this procedure, and the nurse should provide an emesis basin and tissues.

Papanicolaou test

The **Papanicolaou test,** or Pap smear, is performed for early detection of cancer cells. The cells are taken from the cervix and vagina and are microscopically examined (Table 13-2). There has been a success rate of almost 100% for treating cervical cancer since the Pap smear has been in use. Young women who are sexually active and women 20 years of age or older who are free of disease should have regular Pap smears. Women at risk for cancer should have annual Pap smears. Methods for obtaining a Pap smear are seen in Fig. 13-9.

The nurse often assists the physician in performing a Pap smear by preparing the supplies and the patient for the procedure. The nurse also performs patient teaching when applicable.

Table 13-2 METHODS FOR OBTAINING PAP SMEARS

Location	Technique	Location	Technique
Outer cervix	Use plastic spatula. Place tip of longer arm in os. Rotate spatula, scraping outer surface of cervix. Apply cells to glass slide. Apply fixative solution and label slide.	Endocervical	Use cervical brush (cytobrush). Gently insert brush through os. Rotate brush 180-360 degrees. Apply cells by rolling and twisting brush on glass slide. Apply fixative solution and label slide. WARNING: Do *not* use on pregnant clients.

From Potter PA, Perry AG: *Basic nursing: theory and practice,* ed 3, St Louis, 1995, Mosby.

SKILL 13-1 MEASURING CAPILLARY BLOOD GLUCOSE LEVELS

Steps	Rationale
1. Obtain equipment: ▪ Clean gloves ▪ Lancet ▪ Automatic lancing device ▪ Alcohol swab ▪ Watch with second hand ▪ Vial of test strips ▪ Glucometer	Helps organize procedure.
2. Refer to medical record, care plan, or Kardex for special interventions.	Provides basis for care.
3. Introduce self.	Decreases patient's anxiety level.
4. Identify patient by identification band.	Identifies correct patient for procedure.
5. Explain procedure to patient.	Seeks cooperation and decreases anxiety.
6. Wash hands and don clean gloves according to agency policy and guidelines from Centers for Disease Control and Prevention and Occupational Safety and Health Administration.	Helps prevent cross-contamination.
7. Prepare patient for intervention:	
a. Close door to room or pull curtain.	Provides privacy.
b. Drape for procedure if necessary.	Prevents exposure of patient.
8. Raise bed to comfortable working level.	Provides safety for nurse.
9. Arrange for patient privacy.	Shows respect for patient.
10. Remove cap from lancet using sterile technique.	Maintains sterility of point.
11. Place lancet into automatic lancing device according to instructions in operating manual.	Maintains appropriate procedure.
12. Select site on side of any fingertip. (Use heel for infant.)	Allows blood to be drawn from side of finger, which is less responsive to pain from puncture.
13. Wipe selected site with alcohol swab and discard.	Prepares site.

Continued.

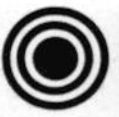

SKILL 13-1 MEASURING CAPILLARY BLOOD GLUCOSE LEVELS—cont'd

Steps	Rationale
14. Ask patient to hold arm at side for 30 sec.	Increases blood flow to site and allows site to dry.
15. Gently squeeze fingertip with thumb of same hand.	Increases blood supply to site.
16. Hold lancing device.	Provides easy access to device.
17. Place trigger platform of lancing device on side of finger and press (Fig. 13-10).	Activates lancing mechanism.
18. Squeeze finger in downward motion (wipe off first drop of blood).	Obtains enough blood to cover test pad on test strip. Removes surface contamination.
19. While holding strip level, touch drop of blood to test strip (Fig. 13-11).	Enables covering of test pad without smearing.
20. Begin recommended timing. Place reagent strip into meter. After 60 sec, blot blood off test strip in appropriate site on glucometer and wait for numeric readout (Figs. 13-12 through 13-14).	Ensures test accuracy.

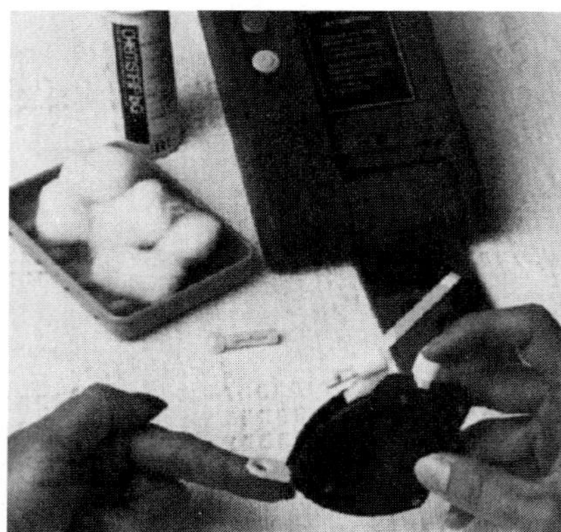

Fig. 13-10 The nurse places a trigger platform of the lancing device on the side of finger and presses.

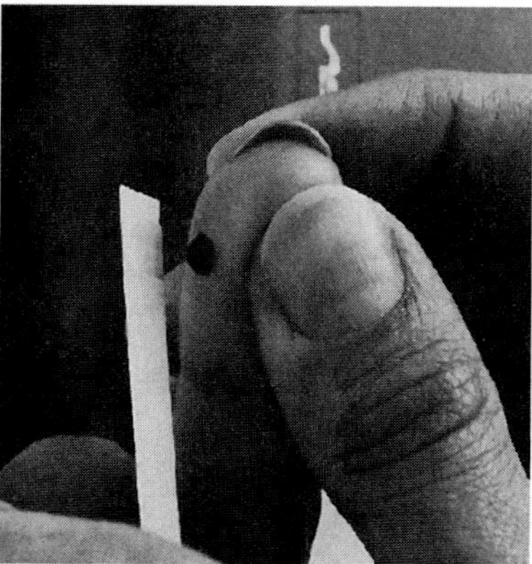

Fig. 13-11 While holding strip level, the nurse obtains a large, hanging drop and touches a drop of blood to the test strip.

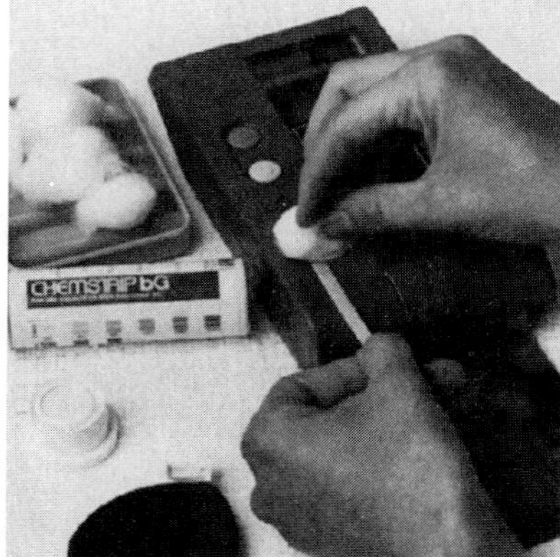

Fig. 13-12 The nurse begins recommended timing and places the reagent strip into the glucometer.

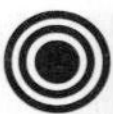

SKILL 13-1 MEASURING CAPILLARY BLOOD GLUCOSE LEVELS—cont'd

Steps	Rationale
21. **Remove lancet from device and discard.**	Prevents needle puncture of nurse.
22. **Remove gloves and wash hands.**	Helps prevent cross-contamination.
23. **Document.**	Documents procedure and patient's response.

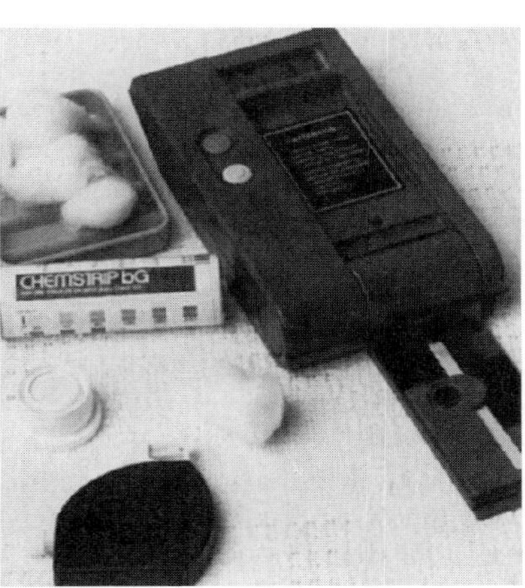

Fig. 13-13 The nurse waits 60 seconds before blotting the test strip.

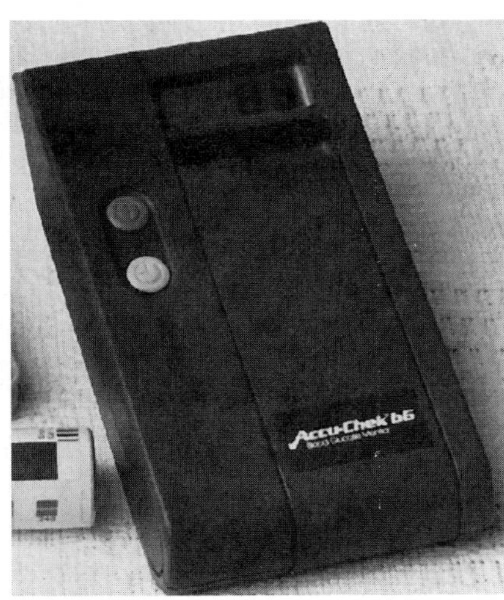

Fig. 13-14 After 60 seconds, the nurse blots blood off the test strip in an appropriate site on meter and waits for the numeric readout.

SKILL 13-2 COLLECTING A MIDSTREAM URINE SPECIMEN

Steps	Rationale
1. **Obtain equipment:** ▪ Clean gloves ▪ Midstream kit ▪ Urine specimen container ▪ Toilet seat collector (Fig. 13-15) ▪ Label ▪ Laboratory requisition and computer control number ▪ Biohazard bag	Helps organize procedure.
2. **Refer to medical record, care plan, or Kardex for special interventions.**	Provides basis for care.

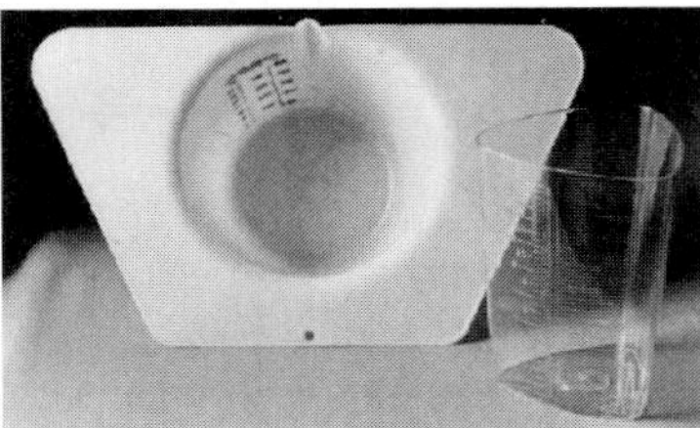

Fig. 13-15 Specimen hat container. (From Perry AG, Potter PA: *Clinical nursing skills and techniques,* ed 3, St Louis, 1994, Mosby.)

Continued.

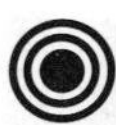

SKILL 13-2 COLLECTING A MIDSTREAM URINE SPECIMEN—cont'd

Steps	Rationale
3. Introduce self.	Decreases patient's anxiety level.
4. Identify patient by identification band.	Identifies correct patient for procedure.
5. Explain procedure to patient.	Seeks cooperation and decreases anxiety.
6. Wash hands and don clean gloves according to agency policy and guidelines from Centers for Disease Control and Prevention and Occupational Safety and Health Administration.	Helps prevent cross-contamination.
7. Prepare patient for intervention:	
a. Close door to room or pull curtain.	Provides privacy.
b. Drape for procedure if necessary.	Prevents exposure of patient.
8. Raise bed to comfortable working level.	Provides safety for nurse.
9. Arrange for patient privacy.	Shows respect for patient.
10. Instruct female patient to open midstream kit and prepare to cleanse perineum by separating labia minora with thumb and forefinger and cleansing as follows:	
a. Wipe downward from above clitoris to below anus and discard wipe.	Cleanses area for obtaining specimen. Prevents contamination.
b. Cleanse left labium and discard wipe.	Cleanses to prevent contamination of specimen.
c. Cleanse right labium and discard wipe.	Cleanses to prevent contamination of specimen.
d. Cleanse down center once again and discard wipe.	Provides a final cleansing of area.
11. Request that patient begin to void into toilet seat collector and then, without stopping flow, to void small amount into sterile specimen cup. Then instruct patient to finish voiding into toilet seat collector without stopping flow.	Collects specimen appropriately.
12. Secure lid on container.	Prevents spillage.
13. Cleanse and return toilet seat collector, if applicable.	Prepares collector for next use.
14. Label specimen appropriately.	Ensures accuracy.
15. Take specimen to laboratory with requisition using biohazard bag.	Ensures fresh specimen for testing and helps prevent contamination of nurse and laboratory personnel who handle specimens.
16. Remove gloves and wash hands.	Helps prevent cross-contamination.
17. Document.	Documents procedure and patient's response.

SKILL 13-3 COLLECTING A STERILE URINE SPECIMEN

Steps	Rationale
1. Obtain equipment: *Catheter port collection:* ▪ Sterile specimen cup with lid ▪ 20-ml syringe ▪ 21- or 22-inch needle ▪ Tube clamp ▪ Alcohol swab *Straight catheter collection:* ▪ Straight French catheter tray: female 14-16 Fr; male 16-20 Fr; children 8-10 Fr ▪ Sterile drape	Helps organize procedure.

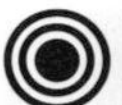

SKILL 13-3 COLLECTING A STERILE URINE SPECIMEN—cont'd

Steps	Rationale
Both: ▪ Sterile specimen cup with lid ▪ Label ▪ Double specimen bag ▪ Requisition slip and computer control number ▪ Biohazard bag for each specimen	
2. Refer to medical record, care plan, or Kardex for special interventions.	Provides basis for care.
3. Introduce self.	Decreases patient's anxiety level.
4. Identify patient by identification band.	Identifies correct patient for procedure.
5. Explain procedure to patient.	Seeks cooperation and decreases anxiety.
6. Wash hands and don clean gloves according to agency policy, and guidelines from Centers for Disease Control and Prevention and Occupational Safety and Health Administration.	Helps prevent cross-contamination.
7. Prepare patient for intervention:	
a. Close door to room or pull curtain.	Provides privacy.
b. Drape for procedure if necessary.	Prevents exposure of patient.
8. Raise bed to comfortable working level.	Provides safety for nurse.
9. Arrange for patient privacy.	Shows respect for patient.
CATHETER PORT COLLECTION	
10. Clamp just below catheter port for 30 min (Fig. 13-16).	Allows urine to collect for removal.
11. Return in 30 mins and clean port with alcohol wipe.	Cleanses port for needle puncture. Prevents urine from backing up in ureters and kidneys, causing damage.
12. Insert needle into port at 30-degree angle and withdraw enough urine for specimen (Fig. 13-17).	Provides urine for testing.
13. Place urine in sterile specimen cup and unclamp catheter.	Keeps specimen sterile and allows urine to flow.
14. Label specimen and take to laboratory with requisition using biohazard bag.	Provides accuracy of specimen and helps prevent contamination of nurse and laboratory personnel who handle specimens.
STRAIGHT CATHETER COLLECTION	
15. Open catheter tray and prepare supplies using sterile technique.	Begins sterile procedure.
16. Place sterile drape under patient's hips.	Prepares sterile field.

Fig. 13-16 The nurse clamps just below the catheter port for about 30 minutes. (From Christensen BL, Kockrow EO: *Foundations of nursing,* ed 2, St Louis, 1995, Mosby.)

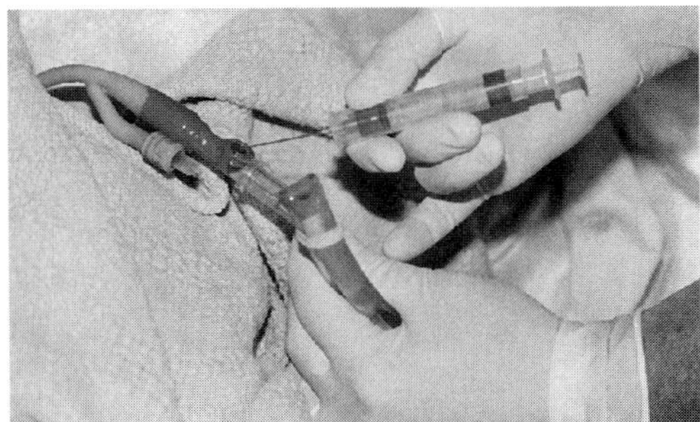

Fig. 13-17 The nurse inserts a needle into the port at a 30-degree angle and withdraws enough urine for a specimen. (From Christensen BL, Kockrow EO: *Foundations of nursing,* ed 2, St Louis, 1995, Mosby.)

Continued.

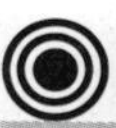

SKILL 13-3 COLLECTING A STERILE URINE SPECIMEN—cont'd

Steps	Rationale
17. Don sterile gloves.	Promotes sterile procedure.
18. For female patient, separate labia with thumb and index finger. Using cotton ball, cleanse from above clitoris to below anus and discard wipe.	Cleanses area for obtaining specimen.
a. Cleanse left labium and discard wipe.	Cleanses to prevent contamination of specimen.
b. Cleanse right labium and discard wipe.	Cleanses to prevent contamination of specimen.
c. Cleanse down center once more.	Provides a final cleansing of area.
19. Lubricate catheter and insert through urinary meatus.	Provides easy insertion.
20. When urine flows, place end of catheter in specimen cup.	Collects urine specimen.
21. Place lid on urine cup and label. Clean up supplies.	Prevents spillage and appropriately labels specimen.
22. Take specimen to laboratory with requisition using a biohazard bag.	Provides accuracy of specimen and helps prevent contamination of nurse and laboratory personnel who handle specimens.
23. Remove gloves and wash hands.	Helps prevent cross-contamination.
24. Document.	Documents procedure and patient's response.

SKILL 13-4 COLLECTING A STOOL SPECIMEN

Steps	Rationale
1. Obtain equipment: ▪ Clean gloves ▪ Stool specimen cup ▪ Tongue depressor ▪ Clean bedpan and specimen device for commode ▪ Label ▪ Laboratory requisition and computer control number ▪ Biohazard bag	Helps organize procedure.
2. Refer to medical record, care plan, or Kardex for special interventions.	Provides basis for care.
3. Introduce self.	Decreases patient's anxiety level.
4. Identify patient by identification band.	Identifies correct patient for procedure.
5. Explain procedure to patient.	Seeks cooperation and decreases anxiety.
6. Wash hands and don clean gloves according to agency policy and guidelines from Centers for Disease Control and Prevention and Occupational Safety and Health Administration.	Helps prevent cross-contamination.
7. Prepare patient for intervention:	
a. Close door to room or pull curtain.	Provides privacy.
b. Drape for procedure if necessary.	Prevents exposure of patient.
8. Raise bed to comfortable working level.	Provides safety for nurse.
9. Arrange for patient privacy.	Shows respect for patient.
10. Assist patient to bathroom when necessary.	Provides for patient safety.
11. Request that patient defecate into commode specimen device (Fig. 13-18) and to prevent urine from entering specimen.	Prevents contamination of specimen.
12. Transfer stool to specimen cup with tongue depressor and close lid (Fig. 13-19).	Protects specimen from dirt.

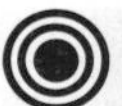

SKILL 13-4 COLLECTING A STOOL SPECIMEN—cont'd

Steps	Rationale
13. **Attach laboratory request and take specimen to laboratory using a biohazard bag.**	Identifies specimen for laboratory and helps prevent contamination of nurse and laboratory personnel who handle specimens.
14. **Remove gloves and wash hands.**	Helps prevent cross-contamination.
15. **Document.**	Documents procedure and patient's response.

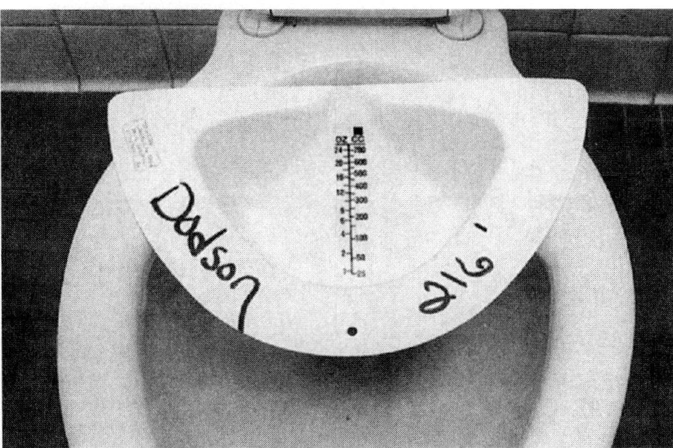

Fig. 13-18 The nurse asks the patient to defecate into the commode specimen device. (From Christensen BL, Kockrow EO: *Foundations of nursing,* ed 2, St Louis, 1995, Mosby.)

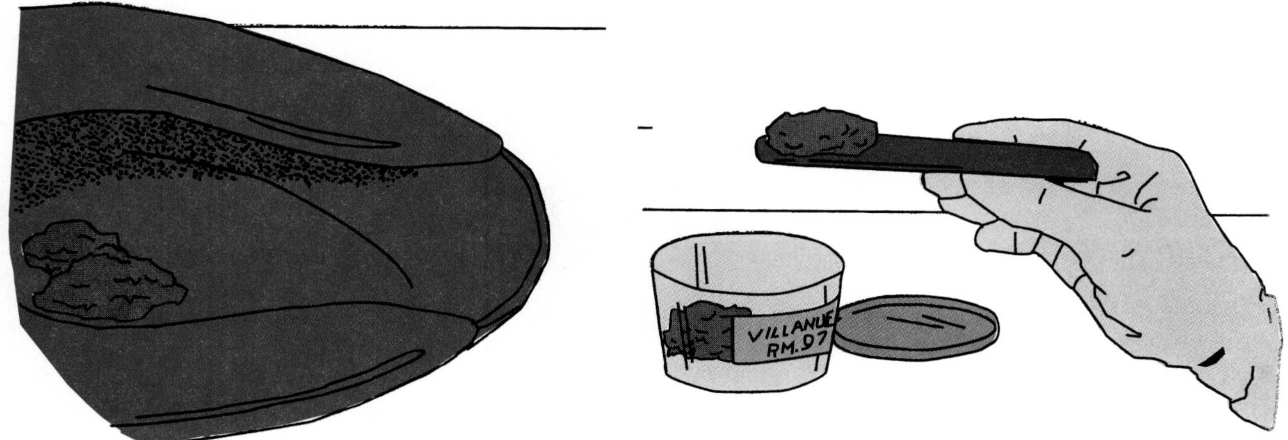

Fig. 13-19 The nurse transfers stool to the specimen cup and closes the lid. (From Christensen BL, Kockrow EO: *Foundations of nursing,* ed 2, St Louis, 1995, Mosby.)

SKILL 13-5 MEASURING OCCULT BLOOD IN STOOL

Steps	Rationale
1. Obtain equipment: ▪ Clean gloves ▪ Hemoccult card ▪ Wooden applicator ▪ Biohazard bag	Helps organize procedure.
2. Refer to medical record, care plan, or Kardex for special interventions.	Provides basis for care.
3. Introduce self.	Decreases patient's anxiety level.
4. Identify patient by identification band.	Identifies correct patient for procedure.
5. Explain procedure to patient.	Seeks cooperation and decreases anxiety.
6. Wash hands and don clean gloves according to agency policy and guidelines from Centers for Disease Control and Prevention and Occupational Safety and Health Administration.	Helps prevent cross-contamination.
7. Prepare patient for intervention:	
a. Close door to room or pull curtain.	Provides privacy.
b. Drape for procedure if necessary.	Prevents exposure of patient.
8. Raise bed to comfortable working level.	Provides safety for nurse.
9. Arrange for patient privacy.	Shows respect for patient.
10. Collect stool specimen (see Skill 13-4).	Provides stool for hemoccult test.
11. Follow steps on hemoccult slide test.	
12. Open flap.	Begins test.
13. Smear very small amount of stool in box A.	Prepares slide.
14. Smear very small amount from another part of stool in box B.	
15. Close card and label.	Ensures accuracy of specimen.
16. Take specimen to laboratory using a biohazard bag.	Provides fresh specimen for testing and helps prevent contamination of nurse and laboratory personnel who handle specimens.
17. Remove gloves and wash hands.	Helps prevent cross-contamination.
18. Document.	Documents procedure and patient's response.

SKILL 13-6 COLLECTING SPUTUM

Steps	Rationale
1. Obtain equipment: ▪ Clean gloves ▪ Sputum collector ▪ Tissues ▪ Label ▪ Laboratory requisition and computer control number ▪ Biohazard bag	Helps organize procedure.
2. Refer to medical record, care plan, or Kardex for special interventions.	Provides basis for care.
3. Introduce self.	Decreases patient's anxiety level.
4. Identify patient by identification band.	Identifies correct patient for procedure.
5. Explain procedure to patient.	Seeks cooperation and decreases anxiety.
6. Wash hands and don clean gloves according to agency policy and guidelines from Centers for Disease Control and Prevention and Occupational Safety and Health Administration.	Helps prevent cross-contamination.

SKILL 13-6 COLLECTING SPUTUM—cont'd

Steps	Rationale
7. Prepare patient for intervention:	
a. Close door to room or pull curtain.	Provides privacy.
b. Drape for procedure if necessary.	Prevents exposure of patient.
8. Raise bed to comfortable working level.	Provides safety for nurse.
9. Arrange for patient privacy.	Shows respect for patient.
10. Place patient in Fowler's position.	Assists coughing.
11. Instruct patient to take three breaths and force cough into container (Fig. 13-20).	Helps patient cough up mucus.
12. Label specimen container.	Ensures that appropriate specimen reaches laboratory.
13. Attach laboratory requisition and immediately take specimen to laboratory using biohazard bag.	Ensures that specimen reaches laboratory and helps prevent contamination of nurse and laboratory personnel who handle specimens.
14. Remove gloves and wash hands.	Helps prevent cross-contamination.
15. Document.	Documents procedure and patient's response.

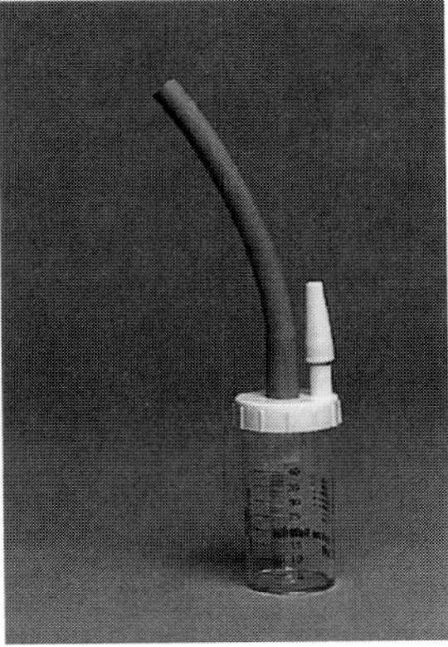

Fig. 13-20 The nurse instructs patient to take three breaths and force a cough into container. (From Perry AG, Potter PA: *Clinical nursing skills and techniques,* ed 3, St Louis, 1994, Mosby.)

SKILL 13-7 OBTAINING A THROAT CULTURE

Steps	Rationale
1. Obtain equipment: ▪ Clean gloves ▪ Culture tube and sterile swab ▪ Tongue depressor ▪ Light for examining patient's throat ▪ Laboratory requisition and computer control number ▪ Biohazard bag	Helps organize procedure.
2. Refer to medical record, care plan, or Kardex for special interventions.	Provides basis for care.
3. Introduce self.	Decreases patient's anxiety level.
4. Identify patient by identification band.	Identifies correct patient for procedure.
5. Explain procedure to patient.	Seeks cooperation and decreases anxiety.

Continued.

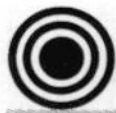

SKILL 13-7 OBTAINING A THROAT CULTURE—cont'd

Steps	Rationale
6. Wash hands and don clean gloves according to agency policy and guidelines from Centers for Disease Control and Prevention and Occupational Safety and Health Administration.	Helps prevent cross-contamination.
7. Prepare patient for intervention:	
a. Close door to room or pull curtain.	Provides privacy.
b. Drape for procedure if necessary.	Prevents exposure of patient.
8. Raise bed to comfortable working level.	Provides safety for nurse.
9. Arrange for patient privacy.	Shows respect for patient.
10. Place patient in sitting position unless contraindicated.	Positions patient for easy access to perform procedure.
11. Open sterile swab.	Prepares for procedure.
12. Request that patient lean head back and open mouth wide.	Allows nurse to see area for taking specimen.
13. Gently but completely swab tonsillar region only from side to side and collect appropriate exudate or drainage (Fig. 13-21). Use tongue depressor if necessary, since some patients cannot open mouth wide enough.	Ensures appropriate collection of specimen.
14. Place swab in culture tube, crush ampule at bottom of tube, and push tip of swab with exudate into culture medium.	Ensures that contaminated exudate will remain alive for growth.
15. Replace top on culture tube.	Prevents contamination of personnel.
16. Discard swab or tongue depressor.	Helps prevent cross-contamination.
17. Label specimen container.	Ensures that specimen reaches laboratory.
18. Attach laboratory requisition and immediately take specimen to laboratory using a biohazard bag.	Ensures that specimen reaches laboratory and helps prevent contamination of the nurse and laboratory personnel who handle specimens.
19. Remove gloves and wash hands.	Helps prevent cross-contamination.
20. Document.	Documents procedure and patient's response.

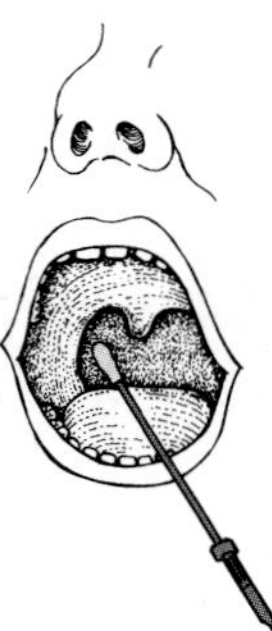

Fig. 13-21 The nurse gently, but completely, swabs tonsillar region only from side to side and collects appropriate exudate or drainage. (From Perry AG, Potter PA: *Clinical nursing skills and techniques,* ed 3, St Louis, 1994, Mosby.)

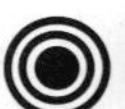

SKILL 13-8 ASSISTING WITH A PAPANICOLAOU TEST

Steps	Rationale
1. **Obtain equipment:** ▪ Clean gloves ▪ Sterile vaginal speculum ▪ Adjustable light ▪ Water soluble lubricant ▪ Glass slides ▪ Sponge forceps or swabs ▪ Specimen bottles ▪ Biohazard bag ▪ Laboratory requisition and computer control number	Helps organize procedure.
2. **Refer to medical record, care plan, or Kardex for special interventions.**	Provides basis for care.
3. **Introduce self.**	Decreases patient's anxiety level.
4. **Identify patient by identification band.**	Identifies correct patient for procedure.
5. **Explain procedure to patient.**	Seeks cooperation and decreases anxiety.
6. **Wash hands and don clean gloves according to agency policy and guidelines from Centers for Disease Control and Prevention and Occupational Safety and Health Administration.**	Helps prevent cross-contamination.
7. **Prepare patient for intervention:**	
a. Close door to room or pull curtain.	Provides privacy.
b. Drape for procedure if necessary.	Prevents exposure of patient.
8. **Raise bed to comfortable working level.**	Provides safety for nurse.
9. **Arrange for patient privacy.**	Shows respect for patient.
10. **Arrange for patient to empty bladder.**	Empty bladder needed for examination.
11. **Place patient in lithotomy position.**	Provides access for examination.
12. **Drape patient.**	Provides privacy.
13. **After physician completes test, cleanse equipment.**	Provides a clean work area.
14. **Remove gloves and wash hands.**	Helps prevent cross-contamination.
15. **Document.**	Documents procedure and patient's response.

SUMMARY

Many diagnostic procedures are available to assist the health care team in confirming diagnoses. Nursing responsibilities vary according to the test ordered. The nurse may be responsible for care before, during, or after the procedure.

Key Concepts

- Universal precautions must be maintained at all times when collecting body fluid specimens.
- Nursing care before a diagnostic procedure may include scheduling the test, administering prescribed medication or procedures, educating the patient regarding the test, preparing equipment, and transporting the patient to the test area.
- Nursing care during a diagnostic procedure may include obtaining a baseline assessment, obtaining the specimen, assisting another member of the health care team, and continuing evaluation and support of the patient.
- Nursing care after a diagnostic procedure may include ongoing assessment of the patient, preparation and delivery of the specimen to the laboratory, cleaning and disposal of equipment, notification of significant others regarding the completion of the procedure, and documentation.
- X-rays produce electromagnetic energy that passes through the body and produces an image on a film.
- A computerized axial tomographic scan uses special narrow x-ray beams to provide a cross-sectional view of a orifice.
- In magnetic resonance imaging, a powerful magnetic field produces detailed images of internal organs, which are translated into visual images by a computer.
- Electrical impulses can also be examined. Electrocardiography, electroencephalography, and electromyography are examples of this type of examination.
- An endoscope is a lighted scope that can be inserted into any orifice.
- A variety of body fluids can be obtained and analyzed in the laboratory.

Critical Thinking Questions

1. Mrs. G must provide a sputum specimen for culture and sensitivity. Her diagnosis is pneumonia. She is in a very weakened state and is unable to cough out sputum. What other option is available to the nurse to obtain the specimen?
2. A 16-year-old girl is scheduled for a follow-up x-ray study of the right femur. She states that she is sexually active and uses inconsistent birth control measures. She states that she is sure she is not pregnant. Her period is due in 5 days. How should the nurse proceed?
3. Mr. P, age 72, is admitted for an arteriogram. During the nursing admission interview, Mr. P states that his arthritis has been acting up and that he has been taking 12 to 15 aspirin per day, along with his prescribed ibuprofen (Motrin). What should the nurse do to correct this problem?

REFERENCES AND SUGGESTED READINGS

Brunner LS, Suddarth DS: *Textbook of medical-surgical nursing,* ed 7, Philadelphia, 1992, Lippincott.

Centers for Disease Control: Update: universal precautions for prevention of transmission of human immunodeficiency virus, hepatitis B virus, and other blood borne pathogens in health-care settings, *MMWR* 37:377, 1988.

Doenges M, Moorhouse MF, Geissler A: *Nursing care plans guidelines for planning and documenting patient care,* ed 3, Philadelphia, 1993, Davis.

Earnst V: *Clinical skills in nursing practice,* ed 2, Philadelphia, 1993, Lippincott.

Perry AG, Potter PA: *Clinical nursing skills and techniques,* ed 3, St Louis, 1994, Mosby.

Potter PA, Perry AG: *Fundamentals of nursing: concepts, process, and practice,* ed 3, St Louis, 1993, Mosby.

CHAPTER 14

Medical Asepsis

Learning Objectives

After studying this chapter, the student should be able to . . .

- Define the key terms.
- State the growth needs of microorganisms.
- Differentiate between medical and surgical asepsis.
- Describe the characteristics of the five elements of the infectious process.
- Describe the rationale for immunizations.
- Describe nursing interventions used as barrier techniques to interrupt the infectious process.
- Describe circumstances under which nosocomial infections are most likely to occur.
- Demonstrate the appropriate procedure for a 2-minute handwashing.
- Describe and perform methods used to follow universal precautions.
- List situations when specific isolation techniques should be used.
- Demonstrate appropriate gowning, gloving, masking, and the use of goggles for isolation or universal precautions.
- Perform the appropriate method for double bagging contaminated articles.
- Differentiate among disinfection, antisepsis, and sterilization methods.
- Perform the accepted techniques of preparation for disinfection and sterilization.
- Identify the body's first line of defense against microorganisms.
- Describe the antigen-antibody response.
- Describe the inflammatory process.

Key Terms

Agar
Antibody
Antigen
Antiseptic
Asepsis
Culture
Disinfection
Fomite
Gram staining
Host
Immunization
Immunoglobulin
Inflammation
Isolation techniques
Medical asepsis
Microorganism
Nosocomial infection
Parasite
Pathogen
Portal of entry
Portal of exit
Reservoir
Reverse isolation
Sensitivity
Serum
Spore
Sterilization
Surgical asepsis
Susceptible host
Transmission
Universal precautions
Vaccine
Vector

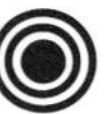

Skills

14-1 Performing a 2-minute handwashing
14-2 Gloving
14-3 Gowning for isolation
14-4 Donning a mask
14-5 Performing double bagging
14-6 Performing isolation technique
14-7 Preparing for antisepsis, disinfection, and sterilization

HISTORY OF MICROBIOLOGY

Microbiology is an important part of medical science because it has led to the discovery of the causes and cures of many diseases. Microorganisms have existed since early man and possibly before. This has been determined by research using the bones of mummies and early man. The study of microbiology is nearly as old as the mummies. For example, the early Egyptians and Chinese knew to bathe to decrease the incidence of disease. They isolated the sick from the well. Warriors from both cultures used contaminated materials to pollute the water supply of their enemies.

Leviticus, a book in the Bible, is called the "First Book on Public Health." This book contains descriptions of appropriate hygiene, the necessity of burying waste, and isolation of the sick. This book prohibited the eating of animals that had died of natural causes. The processes of koshering, as well as strictures about what parts of animals to eat, are outlined in this book.

In the Middle Ages, epidemics caused physicians to look for causes of disease. Some of the theories led to rather bizarre treatments such as leeches with which to bleed the patient, drilling holes in the head to let out the demons, and methods used to drive the devil away. In 1590, the microscope was developed by Zacharias Janssen, but it was not until 1667 that the three shapes of bacteria were described by Antoni van Leeuwenhoek.

Developments in Microbiology

Louis Pasteur

Developments in microbiology occurred slowly at first. It was not until the mid-1800s that the man now called the "Father of Microbiology" began making his discoveries. Louis Pasteur developed five major advances in microbiology:

1. The fact that life comes only from preexisting life
2. The germ theory of disease: A specific disease is caused only by a specific organism
3. The germ theory of fermentation: A specific microorganism causes a specific change in the substance in which it grows
4. Methods of sterilization and the process of pasteurization
5. The development of vaccines from a dead or weakened rabies virus

Robert Koch

Robert Koch, credited with discovering the causes of cholera and tuberculosis, used Pasteur's germ theory of disease in his research. He developed methods to prove the theory. His methods were not valid for every disease or under every circumstance, but he did advance the study of microbiology.

During his efforts to prove the theory he and his assistant (Julius Petri) developed the petri dish. This is a flat dish with a jellylike media made from agar. **Agar** is made from seaweed and is capable of sustaining bacterial and viral life. It is used to grow bacteria and viruses even today.

Ignaz Semmelweis

Around the same time, a man named Ignaz Semmelweis proved that infection developing after childbirth was caused by the organisms present either in the mother or on the hands of the doctors or midwives. He taught that handwashing would greatly reduce the incidence of the infection. Semmelweis' theory was not readily accepted during this time.

Joseph Lister

In 1864, Joseph Lister discovered the antiseptic called *carbolic acid.* He made the discovery from seeing farmers throw it on sick cows that subsequently recuperated. He then began using it in surgery by spraying it in the air with a perfume bottle.

Florence Nightingale

Modern nursing techniques have closely followed the discoveries and developments in microbiology. Florence Nightingale is credited with developing the principles of nursing, methods for training nurses, and procedures for organizing hospitals to reduce the spread of disease. Much of what Nightingale wrote and developed is still in practice today.

MICROBIOLOGY AND NURSING PRACTICE

Microbiology is a branch of biology. *Micro-* means "very small, visible only through a microscope." *Bio-* is the root word for "living organism," and *-ology* is the suffix for "the study of." Thus microbiology is the study of very small living organisms that are visible only through a microscope.

Microorganisms, sometimes called *microbes,* are what the layperson refers to as *germs.* They are generally single-celled living organisms. Microorganisms that produce disease are called ***pathogens.*** Only about 3% of all microorganisms are pathogenic. Normal flora are generally harmless microorganisms that live in or on the human body. They may live on the skin, in the colon, in the mouth, or in other areas without causing harm. They become harmful only if they get into the wrong place at the right time or if the balance of one microorganism to another becomes upset. For example, *Escherichia coli* normally lives in the large intestine of humans without causing harm. If it somehow travels to the mouth and upper gastrointestinal tract, illness can occur. If some of the other bacteria of the large bowel are killed by antibiotics, *E. coli* overgrows and causes illness. Some 97% of all normal flora are capable of causing disease in one of these ways. For that reason, they are called *opportunists.*

Man's Use of Microorganisms

Mankind has learned to use microorganisms. Some microorganisms are effective in fighting disease. For example, penicillin is grown from a type of mold. Other microorganisms are used in the decomposition of waste products. Saprophytes are microorganisms that break down organic material, including plants, animals, and sewage. Still other microorganisms are used to ferment foods. Yogurt is cultured from milk. Microorganisms are used in the curing of cheeses, wine, beer, gin, and bourbon. Yeast is used in the baking of bread.

Classification of Microorganisms

All microorganisms are classified as Protista (see box). This means they are generally unicellular and capable of rapid growth. They are then subdivided as plant or animal.

Animal kingdom

Protozoa Protozoa are a group of microorganisms that live in water. Some are found in swamps, oceans, streams, and even puddles. They are larger than bacteria, and only a few cause disease. The protozoans most likely to cause disease include amoebae, ciliates, flagellates, and sporozoa. Each is distinguished by how it moves. Amoebae propel themselves with a "false foot." This is simply part of the animal's protoplasm that flows outward and pushes the animal in the opposite direction. One type of ameba can cause amebic dysentary.

Ciliates propel themselves with tiny hairs all over their bodies. These hairs, or cilia, move in a wavelike motion. A ciliate may contribute to the development of a colon ulcer.

Flagellates propel themselves with the use of long, whiplike filaments. Two diseases caused by flagellates are vaginal infection *(Trichomonas vaginalis)* and African sleeping sickness (*Trypanosoma* organisms, which are carried by the tsetse fly.)

Sporozoa have no method of propulsion and thus must live inside another animal. One type of sporozoa, carried by the mosquito, can cause malaria.

Parasitic worms Parasitic worms are another Protista of the Animal Kingdom. A disease caused by a worm is termed an *infestation.* There are several types of parasitic worms. The roundworm looks like an earthworm. It lays its eggs, which are ingested by a person. Often the transmission is related to raw sewage in dirt. The dirt gets onto human hands or on food. The roundworm affects the digestive system as well as other areas of the body.

The pinworm is much smaller than a roundworm. It is commonly transmitted by contact with contaminated inanimate objects. The infested person touches an item with contaminated hands. The next person that touches the item becomes contaminated. Hands travel to the mouth or food. Sometimes people reinfest themselves by scratching the anal region and then touching their mouths. The pinworm also affects the digestive system.

The hookworm has a mouth shaped like a hook. This allows the worm to "hook" onto the body (generally the inside of the intestine) and suck the host's blood. This can lead to anemia. Most hookworm infections in the Western Hemisphere are caused by the species *Necator americanus.*

Trichina is a worm that can be found in pork muscle. It is encapsulated, meaning that it has a capsule around it. When a human eats pork, the gastrointestinal tract breaks down the capsule and releases the worm. It then travels to the muscles and reencapsulates. The larvae mature in the intestines of the host, with mature worms depositing their larvae in the intestinal wall.

The flatworm or tapeworm can grow to be 5 to 50 feet long. A person can acquire it from eating undercooked pork, beef, or fish. If the head is not destroyed, the worm will simply rejuvenate the rest of

CLASSIFICATION OF PROTISTA

Animal Kingdom

- Protozoa (protozoon)*
  - Amoebae (amoeba)
  - Ciliates
  - Flagellates
  - Sporozoa (sporozoan)
- Parasitic worms

Plant Kingdom

- Algae (alga)
- Fungi (fungus)
- Bacteria (bacterium)
  - Bacilli (bacillum)
  - Cocci (coccus)
  - Spirilla (spirillum)
- Rickettsiae (rickettsia)
- Viruses

*The singular forms are in parentheses.

its body. Tapeworms grow to adulthood in the intestine of humans. Diagnosis is made when eggs or portions of the adult worm are passed in the stool.

Plant kingdom

Algae Many types of microorganisms are in the plant kingdom. Most do not move on their own. An example is algae, one-celled plants that contain chlorophyll. Because they contain this substance, they need sun to grow. Algae do not cause disease. Many species are found worldwide in fresh water, in salt water, and on land.

Fungi Another member of the plant kingdom is fungus. Usually, fungi have more than one cell. These plants have no chlorophyll, so they prefer to grow in dark, damp places. Examples include molds, yeast, puffballs, and mushrooms. A few fungi are pathogenic. When a disease is caused by a fungi, it is called a *mycotic infection.* Two examples are athlete's foot and ringworm.

Bacteria Bacteria are microscopic one-celled plants accounting for the largest group of pathogens. Bacteria can be cultured and grown in a laboratory. The nature, severity, and outcome of any infection vary from bacterium to bacterium.

Bacteria are classified according to shape and arrangement (see box). Bacilli can be short or long, pointed or blunt. They may be alone, in pairs (diplobacilli), or in chains (streptobacilli). Bacilli are capable of forming spores. A **spore** is a hard-shelled, seedlike structure that contains the genetic material of the bacilli. If conditions become harsh, the bacillus forms a spore and lays dormant (inactive). When conditions become favorable again, the bacillus once again develops from the spore. Spores are very hard to kill and can lay dormant for years. Tuberculosis, a disease caused by a spore-forming bacillus, has been known to redevelop as much as 50 years later. Another type of bacillus was cultured and grown from the frozen bodies of seamen who had been buried in Arctic ice over 140 years. Two other examples of diseases caused by a bacillus are tetanus and diphtheria.

Cocci can be arranged in pairs (diplococci), in chains (streptococci), and in clusters (staphylococci). One type of diplococci can cause meningitis. Streptococci can cause "strept throat," scarlet fever, or rheumatic fever. Staphylococci cause boils, soft tissue infections, and nephritis (kidney disease).

Spirilla come in two shapes. Vibrio has a slight curve, like a fat comma. One type of vibrio causes cholera. Spirillum is shaped like a spiral or a corkscrew. Syphilis is caused by a spirillum.

Another method of classifying bacteria and rickettsiae is by **gram staining,** named for Hans Gram, the man who developed the method. A microorganism may be called *gram-positive* or *gram-negative.* A gram-positive microorganism will stain violet with Gram's stain, but a gram-negative microorganism will not change color with this stain. To see and study gram-negative microorganisms, researchers commonly counterstain them red. Two examples of gram-positive microorganisms are *Streptococcus* and *Staphylococcus.* Two examples of gram-negative microorganisms are *E. coli* and *Pseudomonas aeruginosa,* sometimes nicknamed the "water bug" because it lives in water. An infection caused by this bacteria can produce a blue-green discharge (pus).

Bacteria may also be classified as acid-fast. These bacteria are neither gram positive nor gram negative. They have a waxy outer coating that is very hard to penetrate. The most important example of an acid-fast microorganism is *Mycobacterium tuberculosis.* For this reason, it is referred to as the *acid-fast bacilli.*

CLASSIFICATION OF BACTERIA

Shape
- Bacillus (pl: *bacilli*): rod shaped
- Coccus (pl: *cocci*): round

Arrangement
- Spirillum (pl: *spirilla*): curved rods
- Diplo: arranged in pairs
- Strepto: arranged in chains
- Staphylo: arranged in clusters

Rickettsiae Rickettsiae are plants that are smaller than bacteria. They also cannot live outside a host. In other words, they are **parasites.** They are a genus that combines aspects of both bacteria and viruses. They can be transmitted by bites from fleas, lice, or ticks. Two diseases caused by a rickettsiae are Rocky Mountain spotted fever and typhus.

Viruses The last division of microorganisms in the plant kingdom are viruses. These are the smallest known microorganisms. A special microscope, called an *electron microscope,* is needed to see these microorganisms. Viruses grow only in living tissue, making them parasites. They are not susceptible to antibiotics, as are bacteria, and they are not stopped by most isolation techniques, except latex gloves. Examples of diseases caused by viruses are plentiful and include chickenpox, the common cold, polio, and acquired immunodeficiency syndrome (AIDS).

Sizes of Microorganisms

Pathogenic bacteria can cause damage in one of two ways: by entering the body and producing a poison or toxin and by entering the body and multiplying. As bacteria grow and obtain a certain size, they

Table 14-1 MICROORGANISM GROWTH

Hours	Number of Microorganisms	Hours	Number of Microorganisms
—	1	6½	8192
½	2	7	16,284
1	4	7½	32,568
1½	8	8	65,136
2	16	8½	130,272
2½	32	9	260,544
3	64	9½	521,088
3½	128	10	1,042,176
4	256	10½	2,084,352
4½	512	11	4,168,704
5	1024	11½	8,337,408
5½	2048	12	16,674,816
6	4096		

divide about every half hour. For an estimate on how quickly the number of bacteria can increase, see Table 14-1.

The unit of measure used with microorganisms is the micron (μ), which is 1/1000 of a millimeter. The average microorganism is approximately 1 μ long. Approximately 1000 bacteria this size fit onto the head of a pin. In comparison, the largest virus is only 0.4 μ long. Polio is caused by three strains of the smallest known virus, which is only 0.027 μ long.

Growth Needs of Microorganisms

All pathogenic microorganisms have four basic needs: water, darkness, food, and warmth. Water can be simply moisture or dampness. It can be the liquid in blood and other body fluids. Their food is usually body tissue or blood. Warmth is provided by the natural temperature of the human body. Although freezing may not kill bacteria, it will keep them from growing or multiplying. Some microorganisms have one additional need—oxygen—providing another way to classify microorganisms. Those requiring oxygen are called *aerobes* or *aerobic*. Those that can survive only with a lack of oxygen are called *anaerobes* or *anaerobic*. Most bacteria are aerobic. Only a few pathogens are anaerobic.

Body Defenses

The defenses of the body acting against an invading organism may be looked at as a war. The body has certain strategies of defense. The first line of defense is the skin. Unbroken skin and mucous membranes are physical barriers to microorganisms. The perspiration on the skin is slightly acidic to help repel microorganisms. The sticky secretions of mucous membranes help the body trap and remove microorganisms. The tears contain lysozyme, an enzyme that kills certain microorganisms. If a microorganism makes it to the stomach, it may be killed by the acidic digestive juices. The hairs in the nose and ears act as filters to keep microorganisms out. Cilia, the small hairlike projections of the respiratory tract, propel foreign material up and out of the body. Coughing, sneezing, vomiting, and diarrhea are all actions meant to rid the body of microorganisms.

The secondary line of defense activates if the microorganism manages to enter the body systems. One such defense is the antigen-antibody response. An **antigen** is a foreign protein that invades the body and stimulates the body to make antibodies. An **antibody** is a protein formed by the body to fight against an antigen. It is formed by the bone marrow, spleen, and other parts of the immune system. Antibodies are specific for specific antigens. This means that the antibody for pertussis (whooping cough) helps fight off pertussis but will not help fight off any other disease.

Another secondary defense is the inflammatory process. **Inflammation** is a protective vascular reaction that delivers fluid, blood products, and nutrients to interstitial tissues in an area of injury. This process is regulated by the reticuloendothelial system (a system of cells throughout the body that can phagocytize [engulf and destroy] foreign matter). This occurs during an antigen-antibody response. There are five classic signs of inflammation (see box). The nurse should assess for the inflammatory

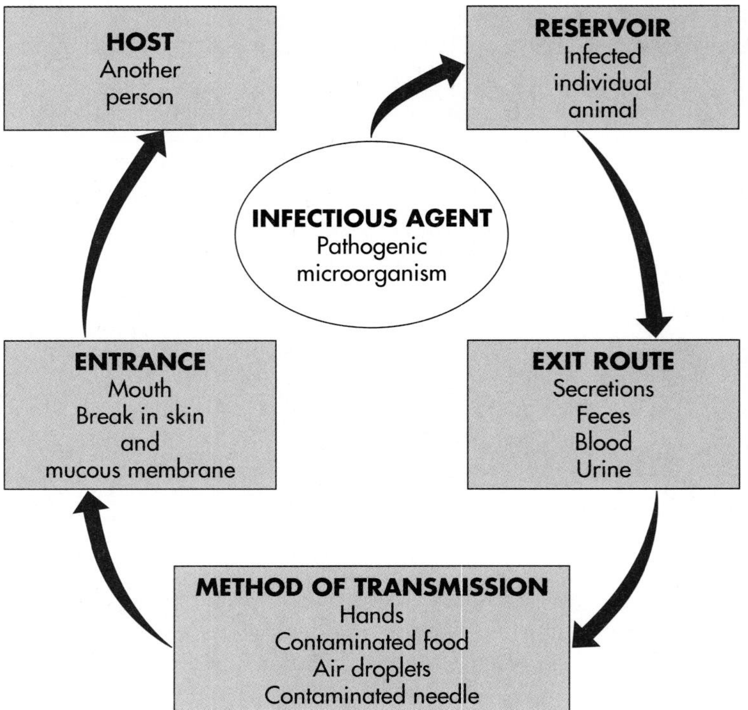

Fig. 14-1 Infectious cycle.

CLASSIC SIGNS OF INFLAMMATION

- Redness
- Swelling (edema)
- Warmth (heat)
- Pain
- Limitation of motion

process and remember the five factors of the infectious cycle.

Inflammatory process

1. Tissue injury occurs.
2. Histamine and other chemicals are released at the site.
3. Blood vessels dilate and increase blood flow to the area. This causes redness, swelling, and warmth.
4. Capillary permeability increases. (A permeable structure allows substances to pass through it.)

Infectious cycle

For infection from a microorganism to occur, five elements must be present. The microorganism is transported through the elements in the following step-by-step cycle (Fig. 14-1):

1. The pathogen may grow and multiply in a **host** or another **reservoir.** This is usually in a person or an animal, but the environment, water, or even food may also be reservoirs.
2. The **portal of exit** is the microorganism's means of escape from the body. This may be through secretions of the nose, mouth, ears, eyes, gastrointestinal tract, genitourinary tract, or wounds.
3. The microorganism must also have a means of transmission. **Transmission** is the carrying of a microorganism from one place or person to another. There are two types of transmission:
   a. With *direct contact*, there is human-to-human transmission. This contact may be through touch or the passage of contaminated blood or body fluids into a cut or another open area of the skin or onto the mucous membranes of another person. Microscopic droplets that become airborne when an infected person speaks, sings, coughs, or sneezes are breathed into the respiratory passages of the next host.
   b. With *indirect contact*, transmission is via a fomite or a vector:
      (1) A **fomite** is a nonliving carrier. It may be referred to as a *vehicle of transmission* or *contaminated article.* For example, a stethoscope, thermometer, bandage scissors, tissue, drinking glass, needle, bedpan, dish, linen, dressing, or food may all act as fomites for certain diseases.

(2) A **vector** is a living carrier. For example, insects, such as fleas, mosquitos, or flies, and animals, such as bats, cows, dogs, and raccoons, may all be vectors for certain diseases.

4. The **portal of entry** is the way that a microorganism enters another body. The skin; mucous membranes of the mouth, nose, or respiratory tract; genitourinary tract; gastrointestinal tract; or the eyes may all be portals of entry.
5. A **susceptible host** is any person whose body cannot fight off organisms. This person's resistance is low because of poor nutrition, lack of rest, lack of exercise, or a coexisting illness such as chronic obstructive pulmonary disease, diabetes, or even a cold. Once an infection develops in a susceptible host, that person then becomes a reservoir, and the cycle repeats.

NURSING PROCESS FOR MEDICAL ASEPSIS

Assessment

By evaluating signs and symptoms revealed during assessment, the nurse can determine whether a patient's clinical condition indicates the onset or extension of an infection. Early recognition of infection assists the nurse in making the correct nursing diagnosis and establishing a treatment plan.

The nurse must assess ways in which an infection affects the patient and family. The nurse should also assess the patient's ability to adjust to a disease and the need for resources to manage health problems.

Nursing Diagnosis

The selection of a nursing diagnosis is based on data collected during assessment. Possible nursing diagnoses for patients susceptible to or affected by infection include the following:

Body-image disturbance
Impaired tissue integrity
Risk for impaired skin integrity
Risk for infection
Social isolation

Planning

Nursing interventions are chosen with the patient, family, physician, and other members of the health care team. During discharge planning, it is important to determine the extent to which the family will be involved in caring for the patient at home. The care plan on p. 235 details care for a specific patient.

The plan of care focuses on achieving specific goals and outcomes related to the nursing diagnoses identified. These may include the following:

Goal #1: Transmission of infectious organisms is controlled.

Outcome

Patient does not experience onset of nosocomial infection.

Goal #2: Progression of infection is controlled or decreased.

Outcome

Inflammation over an involved site decreases in 5 days.

Implementation

The nurse prevents the onset and spread of infection and promotes measures for treatment. Eliminating reservoirs of infection, controlling portals of exit and entry, and avoiding actions that transmit microorganisms prevent bacteria and viruses from finding a site to grow. Getting adequate nutrition, resting, maintaining physiologic protective mechanisms, and obtaining immunizations protect a patient from invasion by pathogens.

When a patient develops an infection, the nurse continues preventive care so that health care personnel and other patients do not acquire the infection. Good handwashing minimizes exposure of the staff and patients. Patients with communicable diseases and infections that are easily transmitted to others require special precautions. It is important that the patient and family understand the precautions that should be observed (see teaching box). Interventions for the older adult should also be considered (see gerontologic box).

Evaluation

Because a patient's condition can change at any time, evaluation is ongoing. The nurse must use assessment skills to determine the patient's progress. It is important to evaluate the results of interventions so that the nurse can continue nursing care therapies, revise them as needed, or determine that the problem has been resolved.

The nurse refers to the goals and outcomes identified when planning care and uses evaluative measures to determine the status of each goal.

Goal #1: Transmission of infectious organisms is controlled.

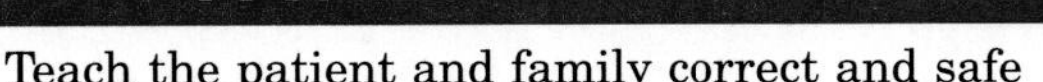

PATIENT TEACHING

- Teach the patient and family correct and safe methods of storing and preparing food.
- Teach patient and family about the dangers of sharing items such as drinking glasses and toothbrushes.
- Emphasize the importance of adequate exercise, a well-balanced diet, and current immunizations.
- Instruct patient about signs and symptoms of wound infection.
- Stress how and when handwashing should be performed to be effective in preventing infection.
- Teach the patient and family about the need for wearing gloves, gowns, and masks, if necessary, and should ensure that the family understands how to perform these procedures.
- Teach the patient and family proper cleaning and sterilization techniques.

Evaluative measures

Assess patient's temperature.

Observe wound sites for redness, swelling, tenderness, or discharge.

Inspect character of any body fluids such as urine or sputum.

Goal #2: Progression of infection is controlled or decreased.

Evaluative measures

Inspect size of inflamed area over consecutive intervals.

Palpate involved site to note reduction in tenderness.

BARRIER TECHNIQUES

Barrier techniques are methods used to break the infectious cycle. The cycle may be broken at each point on the cycle. Often, these barrier techniques are called ***asepsis.*** **Medical asepsis,** also called *clean technique,* includes practices that *reduce* the number and spread of microorganisms. **Surgical asepsis,** also called *sterile technique,* includes practices that *kill* all microorganisms. This type of asepsis is used in surgery, during urinary catheterization, in the care of wounds, or in other situations in which the body or a body cavity has been opened or invaded.

Infectious Agent

To begin the infectious cycle, there must be an infectious agent. Microorganisms capable of causing infection are known as *infectious agents.* These may include bacteria, viruses, yeasts, or fungi. The strength of the microorganism, the number of microorganisms present, the effectiveness of a person's immune system, and the length of exposure to a microorganism determine the pathogen's ability to produce disease. The nurse helps identify the microorganism by accurately documenting signs and symptoms and appropriately collecting specimens.

GERONTOLOGIC CONSIDERATIONS

- The dermal and epidermal skin layers of the older adult become thinner, and elasticity is decreased. The nurse should frequently turn the patient who is on bedrest and carefully observe the skin for breakdown.
- The older adult experiences an alteration in the integrity of the oral mucosa. The nurse should promote careful oral hygiene and regular dental care.
- Some older adults may not be able to see adequately to perform all aspects of self-care. The nurse should include in all teaching those who will be assisting with care of the older adult.

Reservoir

A reservoir is a nonhuman host that serves as a means of sustaining an infectious organism as a potential source of human infection. The cycle may be broken if a reservoir is discovered quickly. This may be accomplished by regular health checkups and early treatment. A microorganism must be cultured to appropriately identify it. A **culture** is a test involving the growth of microorganisms outside the body. Once a microorganism has been cultured, it may then be tested for **sensitivity** to specific antibiotics. In this way the physician will know what medication works best for this infection. The treatment is more likely to be effective, thus eliminating a reservoir.

Environmental sanitation measures also aim at reservoirs by ensuring that contaminated materials are not allowed to accumulate. The sanitarian division of the local health department enforces regulations that ensure fresh, clean food and water. This includes mandating the pasteurization of milk, inspecting and licensing food handlers and restaurants, providing appropriate garbage disposal, and educating the public. The nurse can stop the infectious cycle by quickly identifying reservoirs with accurate and timely nursing assessment and evaluation so that medical treatment can begin. Techniques that isolate a normal flora in its own body area, such as washing the genital and rectal areas last, also help stop the cycle.

Portal of Exit

Measures that help maintain the integrity of the skin or mucous membranes help prevent a portal of exit. These measures may include turning the patient frequently, applying skin lotion, giving a backrub with warmed lotion, providing mouth care, lubricating the lips, or covering an infected wound. Other portals of exit may be prevented by cleaning away drainage as it occurs; having the patient wear a mask when around other persons; and appropriately disposing of urine, feces, emesis, and blood according to agency policy and guidelines from the Centers for Disease Control and Prevention (CDC) and Occupational Safety and Health Administration (OSHA).

Means of Transmission

Measures that prevent transmission include washing the hands (Skill 14-1), wearing gloves (Skill 14-2), wearing gowns (Skill 14-3), wearing a mask (Skill 14-4), double bagging contaminated trash or linens (Skill 14-5), performing isolation techniques (Skill 14-6), and using a disinfectant or sterilizing fomites (Skill 14-7). Transmission is also prevented when a person covers the mouth to cough or sneeze, throws away tissues appropriately, or flushes urine and stool promptly. The patient and family should be taught to never use "community property" such as a drinking glass. Some families even share toothbrushes and should be taught the danger in this practice. A patient should receive a personal set of care articles, such as a bedpan (urinal), bath basin, water pitcher, drinking glass (preferably disposable), and hand and bath soap, to prevent cross-contamination. Linens and supplies are kept away from the uniform. To avoid scattering microorganism-laden dust, the nurse should learn to lean over slightly when handling soiled linen. The nurse should also discard disposable equipment immediately after use, as well as discard or clean anything that falls to the floor because the floor is considered the most contaminated area of the room. The least soiled area of an item or body part is always cleaned first, or the item is cleaned from "clean to dirty." For example, a bedside table would be wiped clean before the floor. The nurse should be sure to wrap a contaminated wet dressing in a water-proof bag. Contaminated equipment and soiled linen should be placed in special waste containers or laundry bags. Negative-airflow units are used in some isolation rooms. These units maintain a negative air flow to keep microorganisms from traveling into the hallway. Sanitarian divisions of the local health department also help control insects, rodents, and animals that may carry disease; regulate waste and refuse disposal; and monitor food services and animal health.

With the increased awareness of contamination from blood-borne pathogens (for example, the hepatitis B virus [HBV] and the human immunodeficiency virus [HIV] that causes AIDS) came the realization that precautions need to be taken even more carefully than in the past to prevent infection. CDC is conducting continuing studies on health care workers with documented skin or mucous-membrane exposures to blood or body fluids of infected patients. CDC statistics confirm the infection of many health care workers who did not use protective measures. The nurse must carefully use protective measures. Today's nurse simply cannot fail to protect the self, patient, and family.

It is difficult to accurately identify all patients infected with blood-borne pathogens. Major concerns were raised about protective practices because they were at one time instituted only after a person was diagnosed, thus causing the health care team to be exposed before the diagnosis. This system also missed many people who harbor microorganisms (that is, carriers) or those who did not reveal a known illness to their health care workers. Some diseases require a certain length of time before diagnostic tests become positive. For example, during the 6 to 8 weeks between exposure to HIV and positive test results, the patient may spread the virus to others.

The CDC, American Hospital Association, and the Association for Practitioners of Infection Control all recommend that universal blood and body-fluid precautions or **universal precautions** be used by health care workers when caring for all patients to prevent exposure to blood-borne pathogens such as HBV and HIV. All blood and body substances are capable of spreading disease and should be handled as if they are infectious. This includes feces, urine, wound drainage, oral secretions, sputum, vaginal and penile drainage and secretions, and emesis. These recommendations include the following precautions:

1. Gloves should be worn during any procedure that could result in contact with blood or body fluid, open skin lesions, or mucous membranes. Goggles, masks, or face shields should be worn if there is a risk of droplets spraying. Aprons or gowns should be worn to protect uniforms.
2. The handwashing procedure should be performed immediately after removal of gloves and if known contamination with blood or body fluid has occurred.
3. The health care worker should prevent injury from needles, scalpels, and other sharp instruments. Disposable sharp instruments should be

dated advice from the CDC (1987) on wearing gloves includes the following:

1. Gloves are worn once for the care of a single patient and then placed into infectious-waste containers for safe disposal.
2. If the nurse has not completed the patient's care but has come into contact with infectious material, the gloves should be changed before continuing the patient's care.
3. There is a chance that gloves could be perforated during use, so handwashing is highly recommended after gloves have been removed.

Some facilities are advocating the use of "double-gloving": wearing two gloves on each hand to decrease the risk of exposure. The nurse should use appropriate judgment regarding the need for wearing gloves.

Family members should understand the importance of the use of gloves. The nurse should explain that gloves become contaminated if they touch infected material or a contaminated object.

Wearing Gowns

The use of gowns in protective asepsis is important primarily to keep clothing from getting soiled during administration of patient care. The gown also blocks contact with infectious microorganisms from the patient. It is recommended that gowns not be reused but be discarded in the appropriate recepticle when the nurse leaves the patient's room. This practice aids in preventing the spread of pathogens to other patients or personnel. This procedure also applies to visitors. Another rationale for use of gowns is protection of a patient in reverse isolation. In this case, the gown is worn to prevent the transfer of pathogens from health care personnel and visitors to the patient. The nurse should carefully teach and demonstrate the gowning technique and ask for return demonstrations from the family and other visitors to ensure that they have mastered the skill.

Isolation gowns are open at the back but have ties at the neck and the waist that keep the gown securely closed, protecting the back of the uniform as well as the front. The gown should be long enough to cover the uniform and have long sleeves with cuffs for added protection. Waterproof aprons may also be used to protect the clothing from soiling in special circumstances. The apron would not be adequate to provide protection to a patient with lowered immune response or an airborne infection. Donning an isolation gown is indicated when the nurse deals with diseases or conditions characterized by heavy drainage, infectious and acute diarrhea, gastrointestinal problems, respiratory problems, skin problems or burns, and urinary problems.

Wearing Masks and Goggles

When a mask is appropriately applied, it fits snugly over the nose and mouth, and the top edge fits below eyeglasses to prevent fogging of the lenses. A mask should be changed at least every 20 to 30 minutes or if it becomes moist. Masks should not be reused or dangled around the neck and then reused. The patient and family members should be instructed on the appropriate use of the mask. The nurse may need to use specialized masks in the case of certain diseases such as tuberculosis.

Goggles are worn to protect the eyes when the nurse handles blood and body fluids.

Double Bagging Waste Materials

Items that may need to be double bagged include trash, dirty linen, reusable food trays, equipment, and specimens. A single bag is adequate if the contaminated articles can be placed in the bag without contaminating the outside of the bag. Double bagging is recommended by the CDC when it is impossible to keep the outer surface of a single bag free from contamination. The second bag should be labeled or color coded to alert nursing personnel and to prevent contamination of housekeeping personnel when handling contaminated material.

Isolation

Isolation techniques are used to separate or segregate persons with communicable diseases. Universal precautions are used for every person, based on the hypothesis that any identified or, as yet, unidentified pathogen can be present in that person. Isolation techniques begin after a definitive diagnosis is made and are used in addition to those of universal precautions. Isolation techniques may also be called *protective asepsis.*

General isolation techniques used include a private room, a segregated room (all persons in the room have the same diagnosis), or a special isolation room; closed door; private bath; exclusive use of equipment such as the blood pressure cuff or thermometer; washing of the hands before entering and exiting the room, and the use of a protective gown, mask, gloves, and goggles or eye shields. Not all of these techniques are used in each situation.

The CDC has issued specific guidelines for isolation techniques in a controlled environment. There are two systems for implementing these guidelines: the disease-specific system, in which certain procedures are performed for each type of in fectious disease, and the category-specific system.

The category-specific system recognizes seven ways by which a microorganism is transmitted (Table 14-2). In this category, similar isolation precautions are used for different diseases because the microorganism is transmitted in the same manner. Although the disease-specific system has proved to be less time consuming and less costly because some diseases need only minimal precautions added to universal precautions, the category-specific system is still commonly used in some health care agencies.

BASIC ISOLATION PRINCIPLES

1. Thorough handwashing should be performed before entering and before leaving a patient's room.
2. An understanding of the disease process and method of transmission of the infectious microorganism helps determine the use of protective barriers.
3. Contaminated equipment and articles are to be disposed of in a safe and effective manner to prevent transmission of pathogens to other individuals.
4. If the patient is to be transported to other areas in the agency (away from the isolation room), necessary measures should be taken to protect those who may be exposed. This is accomplished by having the patient wear a gown and mask.

The patient with an infectious disease should be placed in a private or isolation room equipped with the appropriate handwashing and toilet facilities. The routine care of a patient in isolation is the same hygienic care given to all patients. The health care

Table 14-2 CATEGORY-SPECIFIC ISOLATION PRECAUTIONS

Type of Isolation	Description	Examples of Conditions
Strict	Diseases transmitted by air or contact require full-isolation technique.	Diphtheria
Direct contact precautions	Nurse should wear gown, mask, and gloves only when coming into contact with infectious substance.	Impetigo, herpes simplex, acute respiratory infections in infants and small children
Respiratory isolation	Health care personnel must wear masks when in room with patient because pathogen is transmitted by air droplets over short distances.	Pneumonia, measles, bacterial meningitis
Enteric precautions	Disease is spread through fecal material. Nurse should wear gown and gloves for protection against feces.	Viral hepatitis, infectious diarrhea
Tuberculosis isolation	Pathogen is transmitted by air droplet and sputum. Nurse may need to wear gown and mask if patient is coughing without covering mouth, but gloves are not indicated.	Tuberculosis
Drainage and secretion precautions	Pathogen is transmitted by direct or indirect contact with drainage from infected body site. Nurse should wear gown and gloves to prevent contact with infectious material. Mask is not needed.	Infected burns or wounds
Blood and body fluid precautions	Direct or indirect contact or risk of contact with infected body fluids or blood requires use of gown or gloves and goggles.	
Care of immunosuppressed patient	This is known as *reverse isolation.* Health care personnel caring for immunosuppressed patient should wear gowns, masks, and gloves to prevent transmission of pathogens by contact or air droplet.	Leukemia, burns, or organ transplantation

worker should remember that all articles that come into contact with the patient are contaminated and should be handled in the appropriate manner to maintain protective asepsis.

Equipment used for assessing vital signs remains in the room if possible. Otherwise, the equipment must be disinfected safely when removed from the room. The nurse's watch may be placed on a clean paper towel or sealed in a plastic bag and placed on the bedside unit stand before touching any article in the room.

It is important to consider the psychologic implications of isolation. The patient is forced into solitude and is deprived of normal social contacts. The nurse should make the patient feel wanted and cared for, like all other patients. To do this, the nurse should spend extra time with the patient, keep the room clean and pleasant, and teach the patient the rationale for use of this technique. The emotional state of the patient may interfere with recovery unless the nurse minimizes the feeling of psychologic and physical isolation. The patient and family should have an understanding of the patient's disease and know the importance of following protective asepsis. Family and visitors are taught how to wear isolation garb, and the nurse must ensure that the procedure is followed each visit.

Antiseptics, Disinfection, and Sterilization

Pathogenic microorganisms are believed to be present on most articles in the home and in public areas, including health care agencies. By following basic clean or aseptic technique, the nurse can interrupt the infection process to prevent and control the spread of infection. **Antiseptics** are used to inhibit the growth of microorganisms but do not kill them. Antiseptics may also be referred to as *bacteriostatic solutions. Bacterio-* means "microorganism," and *-static* means "referring to that which cannot move or grow." Antiseptics may be used on human tissue and therefore may be used before surgery, during wound care, for mouth care, and for washing hands.

Disinfection is used to destroy microorganisms. However, it does not destroy spores. The solutions used are called *disinfectants* or possibly *bacteriocidal solutions.* (*-cidal* means "to die.") These solutions are too strong for the human skin and are used only on inanimate objects. If a disinfectant solution comes in contact with human tissue, the tissue feels "slippery." This is the first step of tissue breakdown. When using a disinfectant solution, the nurse should use clean gloves to protect the skin.

Sterilization refers to methods used to kill all microorganisms, including spores. There are two types of sterilization methods: physical and chemical (see box).

Before equipment can be sterilized, it must be appropriately prepared. This is the responsibility of the nurse. First, the equipment must be washed in warm water and detergent. If the item has blood, drainage, sputum, mucus, or another body fluid on it, it is rinsed in cold water before cleansing to decoagulate the protein of the fluid. The equipment is then dried. Many organisms live in water. Each nurse is responsible for the equipment used and must decide what method of destroying microorganisms to use for each situation. The method used depends on the following factors:

1. The type of microorganism present, since spore-forming bacteria are resistant to destruction
2. The number of microorganisms present, since it takes longer to kill a large number
3. The type of article in need of cleansing, since heat or certain chemicals can destroy some materials

Other factors determining the sterilization method are the intended use of the article (for example, surgical asepsis requires all organisms to be

PRINCIPLES OF DISINFECTION AND STERILIZATION

Physical Method

- *Steam under pressure* or moist heat is most practical and dependable method for destruction of all microorganisms. This technique is called *sterilization.* Examples of sterilization equipment are autoclave, which is used in hospitals and other agencies, and pressure cooker, which is used in the home.
- *Boiling water* is best method for home use and is least expensive. However, this technique will not destroy bacterial spores and some viruses. Article should be boiled for minimum of 20 minutes for disinfection.
- *Radiation* sterilizes pharmaceutical goods, foods, and heat-sensitive items. It is extremely effective on articles difficult to sterilize.
- *Dry heat* is used for disinfecting articles destroyed by moisture. Health agencies seldom use this method, but in home, article can be disinfected by placing it in the oven for 2 hours at 320° F or 45 minutes at 350° F.

Chemical Process

- *Gas* (ethylene oxide) is used for sterilization. It destroys spores formed by bacteria.
- *Chemical solutions* are often used to disinfect instruments because they are effective in destroying microorganisms. Clinical thermometers can be stored in chemical solution, and some articles are soaked in solution to prepare them for another method of disinfection or sterilization.

destroyed, whereas medical asepsis requires only removal of pathogens) and the methods of sterilization available.

In most health care agencies, a central supply department sterilizes some supplies and disinfects reusable equipment and supplies. Although most supplies used today for patient care are disposable, some situations still require the use of sterilization and disinfection techniques. The patient and family may also be taught cleansing and disinfecting principles for the home.

Effective chemicals used in disinfection are carbolic acid, phenylphenol, LPH, and chlorine compounds such as bleach. A 10% solution of chlorine is effective in killing the virus that causes AIDS. Chlorine is useful for disinfection in the household and of water but should never be mixed with ammonia because of the resulting toxic fumes. Chlorine has a tendency to corrode some metals.

Chemical sterilization with solutions has limited uses, usually only if another method is not available. The method will be effective only if the appropriate strength of solution is used, the solution is newly made or was kept covered, and the item is in the solution for the appropriate length of time. Chemical sterilization may also be accomplished with the use of gas, usually ethylene oxide. This gas is normally used if sterilization is necessary for cloth items, such as linen packs or stuffed animals.

Solutions that may be used as antiseptics include iodine or its relatives such as povidine-iodine, alcohol, hydrogen peroxide, and potassium permanganate. Iodine may also be an appropriate bactericidal agent under certain circumstances (that is, it kills bacteria but not spores). However, because iodine stains articles and many patients are allergic to it, its use is as common as it was in the past. Alcohol stings when it comes into contact with open areas of the skin. Potassium permanganate may also stain. It is an oxidizing agent, meaning that it performs its function by releasing free oxygen. It is a bluish purple color before use but turns dark brown after it has lost an oxygen molecule. Hydrogen peroxide is also an oxidizing agent. It foams as it loses its oxygen on coming into contact with the protein of body fluids.

■ NURSING CARE PLAN ■

RISK FOR INFECTION

Mrs. L, age 61, has chronic obstructive pulmonary disease. She is susceptible to infection, but infections worsen her condition.

NURSING DIAGNOSIS

Risk for infection related to chronic pulmonary disease as evidenced by symptoms of inflammation, increased cough, worsened breath sounds, fever, and increased pain

GOAL

- Patient will be free of infection in 72 hours.

EXPECTED OUTCOMES

- Patient will be free of symptoms of inflammation.
- Cough will be decreased, and breath sounds will be more clear.
- Body temperature will be normal.
- Patient will state relief of pain by discharge date.

NURSING INTERVENTIONS

- Assess body temperature, breath sounds, level of cough, and pain every 4 hours.
- Wash hands before and after care of patient.
- Encourage activity to improve lung expansion.
- Keep any member of health care team from entering room if that person has symptoms of infection.
- Teach patient and family symptoms of infection.
- Teach patient and family methods of avoiding infection.
- Institute protective isolation techniques if white blood cell count is low.

EVALUATION

- Patient states that cough, pain, and other symptoms relating to inflammation have decreased since admission.

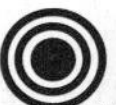

SKILL 14-1 PERFORMING A 2-MINUTE HANDWASHING

Steps	Rationale
1. **Obtain equipment:** ▪ Warm, running water ▪ Paper towels ▪ Liquid soap (if possible) ▪ Orange stick ▪ Hand lotion (unless contraindicated)	Helps organize procedure. (Procedure is usually performed in utility area.)
2. **Assess hands, observing for visible dirt, breaks, or cuts in skin and cuticles.**	Permits identification of dirt and open areas of skin, which provide places where microorganisms grow.
3. **Determine contaminant on hands (for example, dirt).**	Helps determine need for 2-minute handwashing.
4. **Assess areas around sink that are contaminated or clean.**	Prevents contamination of hands during and after procedure.
5. **Remove jewelry (except plain wedding band and watch) and push long sleeves above elbow.**	Removes source of microorganisms, which can collect in jewelry and watchbands. Makes it easier to wash all areas of hands and wrists.
6. **Adjust water to right temperature and force.**	Prevents chapping from hot water. Allows appropriate lathering, which is inhibited by water. Prevents spread of microorganisms to other areas from splashing.
7. **Wet hands and wrists thoroughly under warm, running water, always keeping hands lower than elbows (Fig. 14-2).**	Allows water to flow from least contaminated area to most contaminated area of arm.

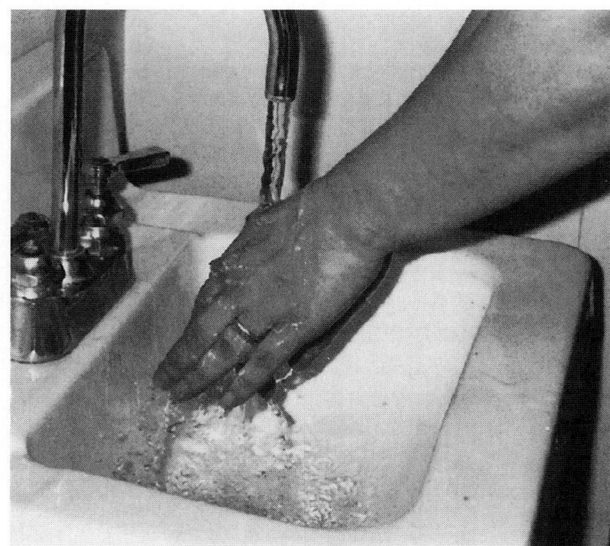

Fig. 14-2 Wetting hands.

Steps	Rationale
8. **Lather hands with liquid soap (about 1 teaspoon).**	Emulsifies fat and aids in cleansing.
9. **If bar soap must be used, rinse bar and rub hands on bar to produce enough lather to wash entire area. Then rinse bar off under running water.**	Removes dirt and microorganisms from use.
10. **Wash hands thoroughly using firm, circular motion and friction on back of hands, palms, and wrists. Wash each finger individually. Pay special attention to areas between fingers and knuckles by interlacing fingers and thumbs and moving hands back and forth (Fig. 14-3).**	Helps loosen dirt and microorganisms, both transient (acquired from contamination) and resident (normally present).

SKILL 14-1 PERFORMING A 2-MINUTE HANDWASHING—cont'd

Steps	Rationale

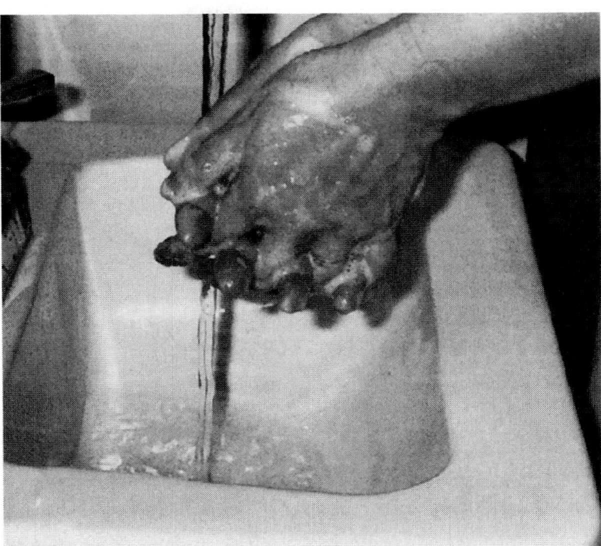

Fig. 14-3 Washing hands.

Steps	Rationale
11. **Wash 1 minute, rinse thoroughly, relather, and wash another minute, using continuous amount of friction.**	Removes loosened microorganisms and ensures thorough cleaning. (The greater the contamination, the more need for longer washing.)
12. **Rinse wrists and hands completely, keeping hands lower than elbows (Fig. 14-4).**	Allows water to run from cleaner area (wrists) to area that is less clean.

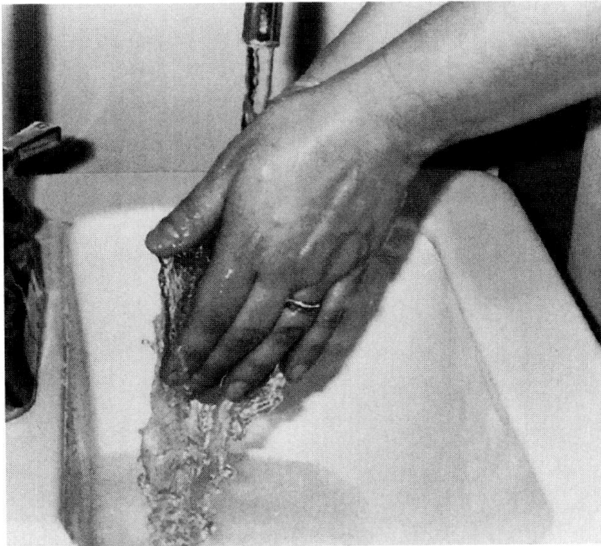

Fig. 14-4 Rinsing hands.

Steps	Rationale
13. **Clean fingernails carefully under running water using fingernails of other hand or blunt end of orange stick.**	Reduces chance of microorganisms remaining under nails.
14. **Dry hands thoroughly with paper towels. Pat fingertips, hands, and then wrists and forearms.**	Prevents chapping. Allows drying from cleanest areas (fingers and hands) to areas that are less clean.
15. **Turn off faucets with dry paper towel (Fig. 14-5).**	Prevents clean hands from touching contaminated handles.

Continued.

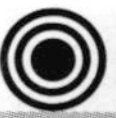

SKILL 14-1 PERFORMING A 2-MINUTE HANDWASHING—cont'd

Steps	Rationale
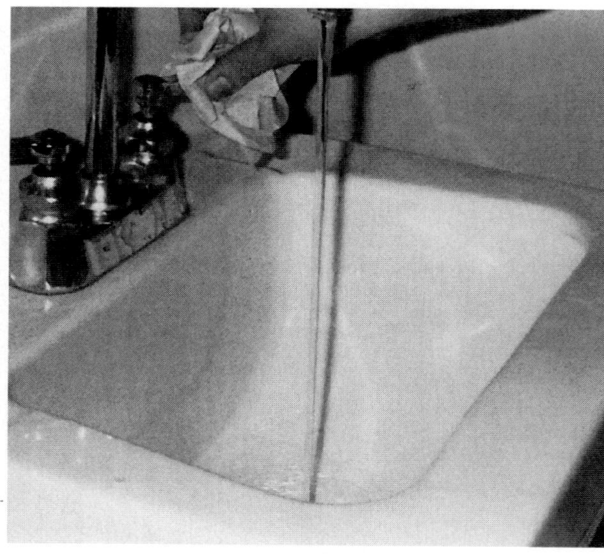 Fig. 14-5 Turning off faucet.	
16. Use hand lotion if desired, unless contraindicated.	Keeps skin soft and lubricates skin so that it will not crack easily, possibly causing infection.
17. Dispose of waste materials.	Helps prevent spread of microorganisms.

SKILL 14-2 GLOVING

Steps	Rationale
1. Obtain equipment: ▪ Pair of gloves ▪ Soap ▪ Warm, running water	Helps organize procedure.
2. Wash hands (see Skill 14-1).	Helps prevent cross-contamination.
3. Assess for need for gloves.	Determines whether wearing gloves is necessary.
DONNING GLOVES	
4. Remove gloves from dispenser.	Keeps gloves handy and ready for use.
5. Inspect gloves for perforation.	Prevents pathogenic microorganisms from entering through perforation in gloves.
6. Don gloves when ready to begin patient care (Fig. 14-6). If gloves are to be worn with gown, wear them pulled over cuffs of gown.	Provides protection for patient and nurse. Ensures full coverage of nurse's skin.
7. Change gloves after direct handling of infectious drainage. Do not touch side rails, tables, or bedstands with contaminated gloves.	Prevents contamination of patient. Prevents spread of microorganisms throughout environment.

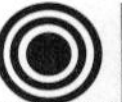

SKILL 14-2 GLOVING—cont'd

Steps	Rationale

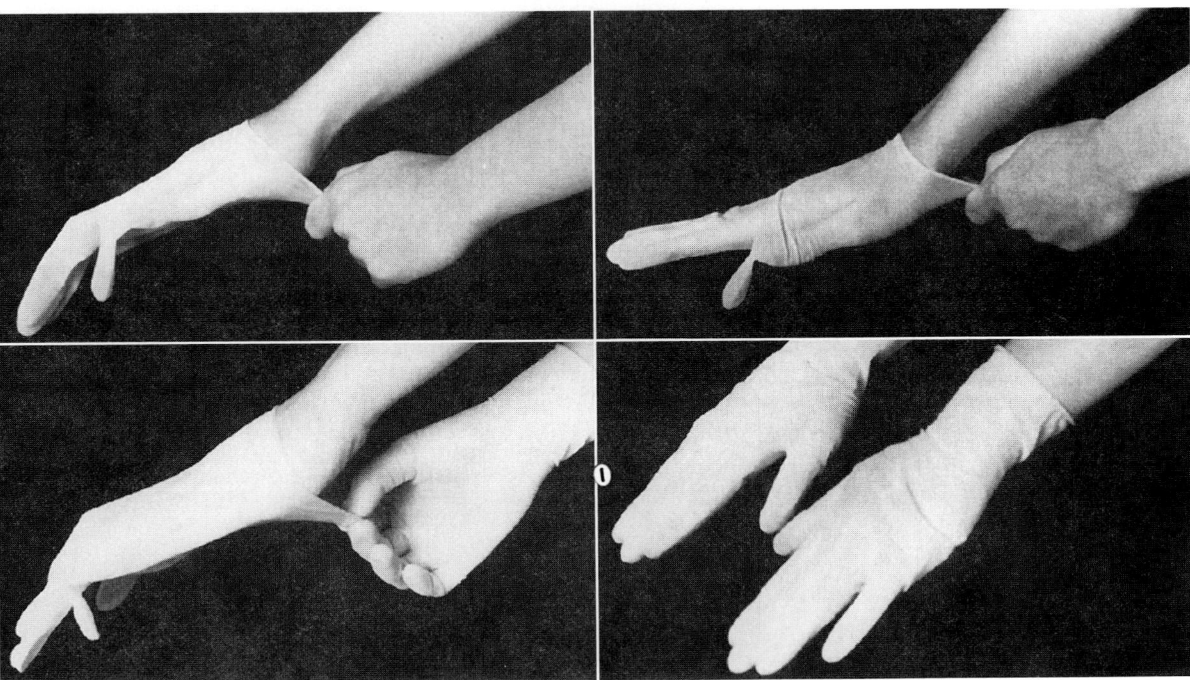

Fig. 14-6 Donning gloves.

REMOVING GLOVES

Steps	Rationale
8. Remove first glove by grasping at palm with other gloved hand and pulling glove off and inside out (Fig. 14-7). Place this glove in other hand.	Prevents nurse from touching own skin with contaminated glove.

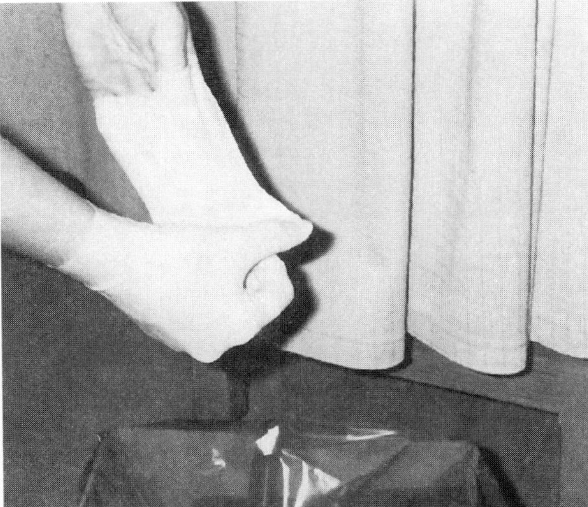

Fig. 14-7 Removing gloves.

Steps	Rationale
9. Remove second glove by placing finger under cuff edge and turning glove inside out and over other glove. Drop gloves into waste container.	Prevents nurse from touching contaminated glove. Wraps contamination inside gloves to help protect others.
10. Wash hands.	Helps prevent cross-contamination.

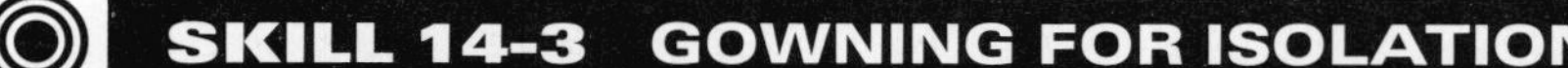

SKILL 14-3 GOWNING FOR ISOLATION

Steps	Rationale
1. Obtain equipment: ▪ Paper towel or plastic bag ▪ Isolation gown	Helps organize procedure.
2. Determine need for use of isolation gown.	Ensures use of universal precautions and isolation techniques when necessary.
3. Explain need for procedure to patient.	Decreases patient's anxiety.
4. Make certain patient is informed that isolation procedure is to help protect patient and nursing staff.	Prevents patient from feeling dirty. Prevents patient from feeling nurses fear patient.
5. Remove watch and push up long sleeves.	Ensures that uniform sleeve is under gown sleeve for protection.
6. Place watch on paper towel or place it in plastic bag and close bag before taking vital signs.	Prevents contamination of watch.
7. Wash hands.	Helps prevent cross-contamination.
DONNING ISOLATION GOWN	
8. Open gown by placing hands on inside of gown sleeves (Fig. 14-8, *A*).	Prevents touching outside of gown (cleanest part to protect patient).
9. Pull gown on and securely tie it at neck and then waist (Fig. 14-8, *B* and *C*).	Provides protective covering of entire uniform.

A

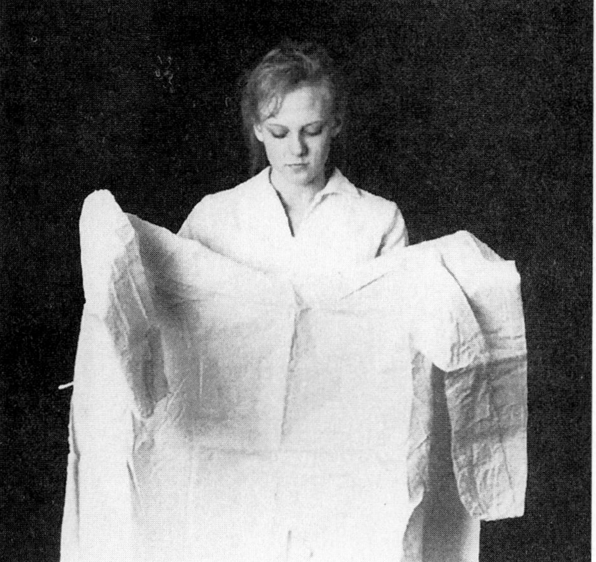

B

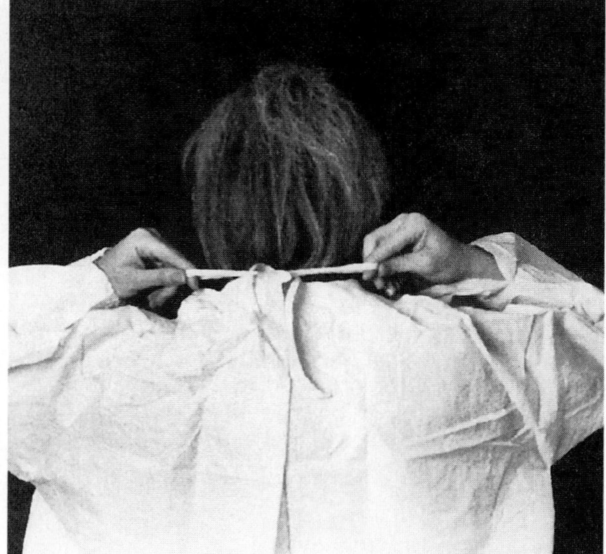

C

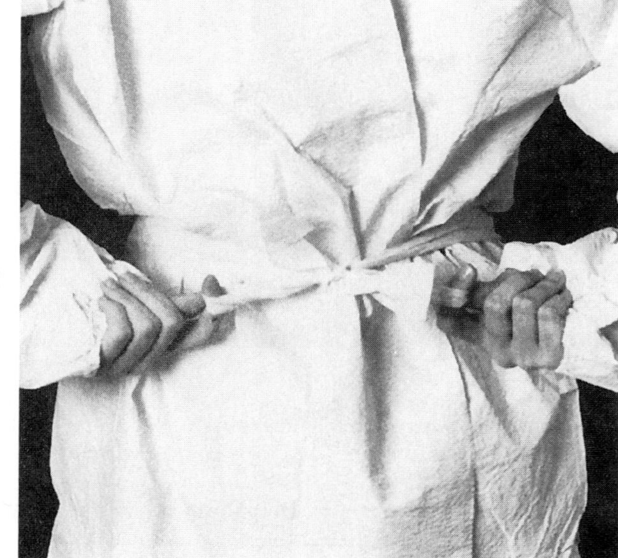

Fig. 14-8 Donning isolation gown. **A,** Opening gown. **B,** Pulling on gown. **C,** Tying gown.

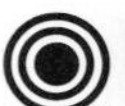

SKILL 14-3 GOWNING FOR ISOLATION—cont'd

Steps	Rationale
10. Don gloves and mask as necessary.	Protects nurse's hands and face.
REMOVING ISOLATION GOWN	
11. Untie waist.	Prevents contamination from waist ties.
12. Remove gloves.	Prevents contamination from gloves, which should not touch nurse's neck.
13. Untie neck ties (Fig. 14-9, *A*).	Allows removal of neck ties, which are considered clean.
14. Remove hands carefully from gown sleeves (Fig. 14-9, *B*).	Prevents contamination from outside of gown.
15. Do not allow sleeves to be turned inside out to avoid touching outside of gown (Fig. 14-9, *C*).	Prevents contamination.
16. Fold gown with outside surfaces touching (Fig. 14-9, *D*).	Prevents contamination of nurse.

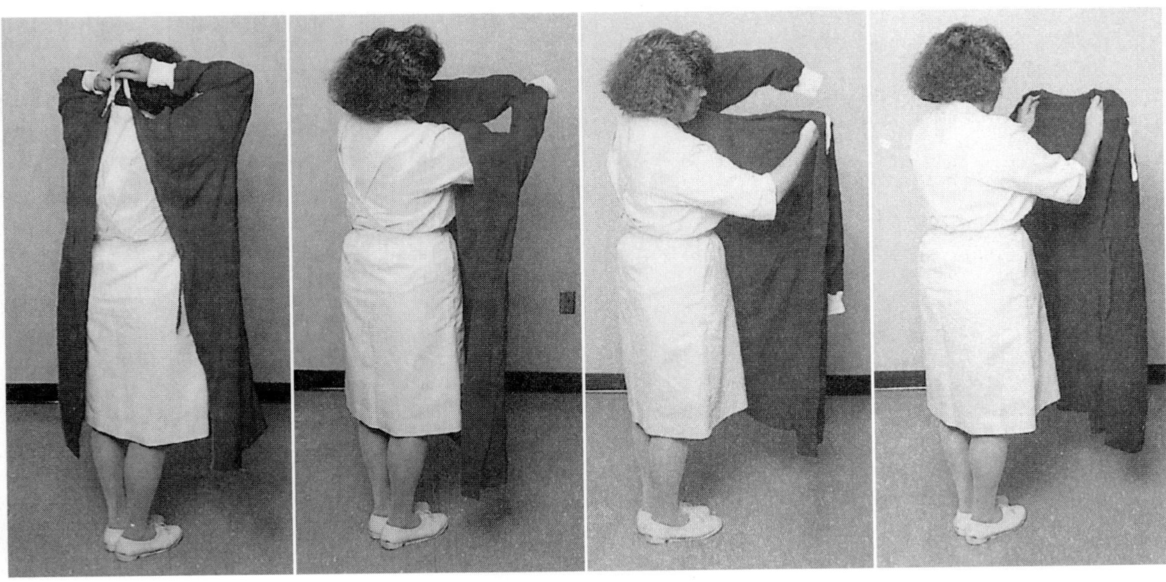

A B C D

Fig. 14-9 Removing isolation gown. **A,** Nurse loosens neck ties. **B,** Hands are carefully removed from sleeves. **C,** Sleeves are not allowed to be turned inside out. **D,** Gown is folded with outside surfaces touching. (From Potter PA, Perry AG: *Basic nursing: theory and practice,* ed 3, St Louis, 1995, Mosby.)

Steps	Rationale
17. Dispose of gown in appropriate receptacle in room.	Helps prevent spread of microorganisms.
18. Wash hands.	Helps prevent cross-contamination.
19. Remove mask by untying.	Ensures prevention of contamination of nurse's face.
20. Dispose of any waste in room.	Helps prevent spread of microorganisms.

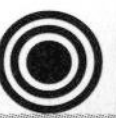

SKILL 14-4 DONNING A MASK

Steps	Rationale
1. Obtain equipment: ▪ Isolation mask	Helps organize procedure.
2. Wash hands.	Helps prevent cross-contamination.
3. Remove mask from container.	Keeps masks handy and ready for use.
4. Choose appropriate mask for task.	Helps ensure optimal protection for nurse.
DONNING MASK	
5. Don mask when ready to begin patient care by covering nose and mouth with mask (Fig. 14-10, *A*).	Provides protection from microorganisms.
6. Secure mask with elastic band. If strings are used, string on top is tied in back of head. String on bottom is tied on top of head (Fig. 14-10, *B*).	Secures mask for maximum protection.

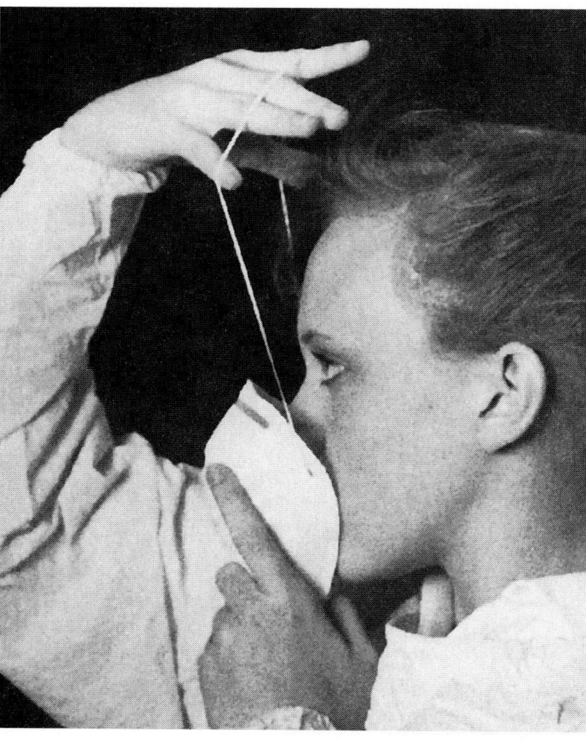

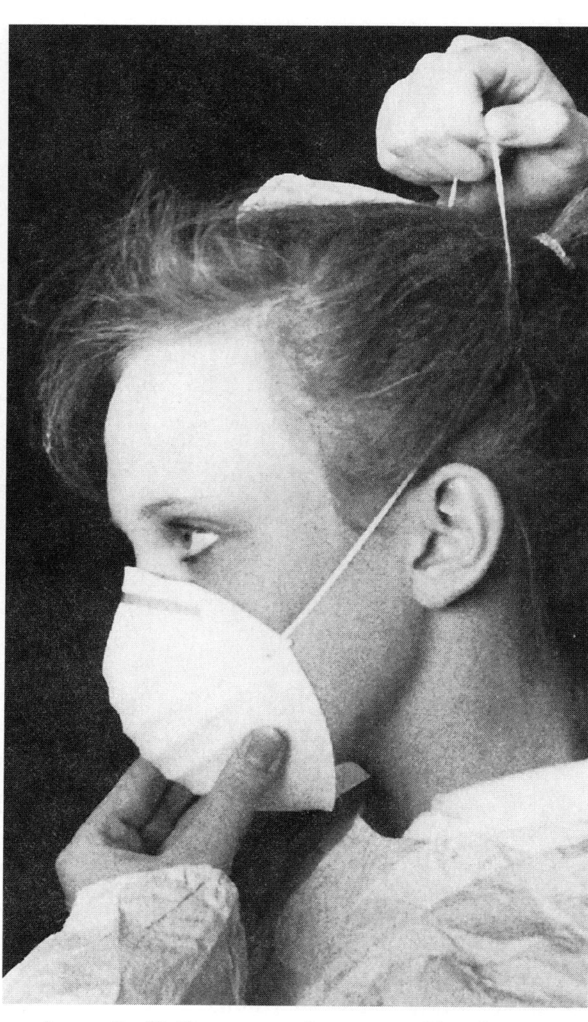

Fig. 14-10 Donning a mask. **A,** Place mask over nose and mouth. **B,** Secure mask on top of head.

Steps	Rationale
7. Wear mask until it becomes moist but not longer than 20-30 min.	Keeps moisture from rendering mask ineffective. Prevents growth of microorganisms.
REMOVING MASK	
8. Remove mask by untying strings or moving elastic, making certain not to touch contaminated area.	Protects nurse from coming into contact with contaminated mask.
9. Dispose of contaminated mask.	Protects nurse and other health care workers.
10. Wash hands.	Helps prevent cross-contamination.

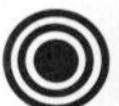

SKILL 14-5 PERFORMING DOUBLE BAGGING

Steps	Rationale
1. **Obtain equipment:** ▪ Single isolation bag ▪ Special color-coded double bag ▪ Holder for isolation bag ▪ Isolation gown ▪ Isolation mask ▪ Clean gloves ▪ Holder for laundry bag	Helps organize procedure.
2. **Wash hands.**	Helps prevent cross-contamination.
3. **Don gown, mask, and gloves before entering patient's room or perform double bagging before removing isolation garb after nursing care.**	Prevents contact with contaminated articles.
4. **Collect all contaminated disposable articles in isolation bag and tie securely without excess air.**	Prepares for double bagging.
5. **Summon second health care worker to remain outside patient area.**	Prevents risk of contamination of personnel.
6. **Have second person hold double bag with top edge of bag folded over to make clean edge and to cover hands (Fig. 14-11).**	Prevents risk of contamination of personnel.

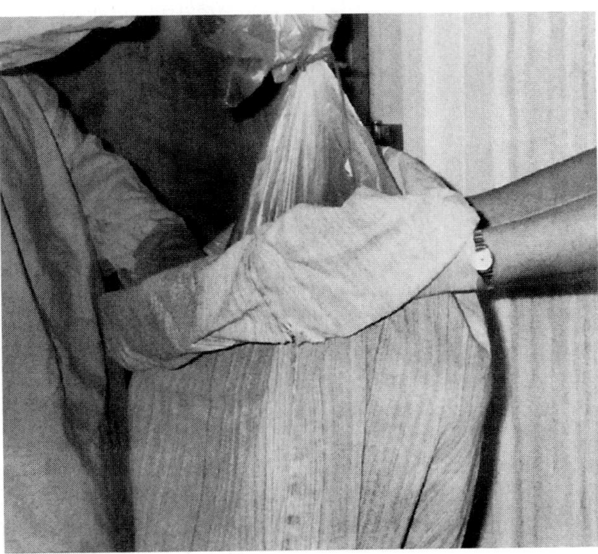

Fig. 14-11 Double bagging.

Steps	Rationale
7. **Drop contaminated bag in double bag without touching edges of bag. Hold outside bag open by touching only inside of bag.**	Keeps outside of double bag clean.
8. **Have second person seal or tie and label bag.**	Prevents spread of infectious microorganisms.
9. **Place new bags in holder.**	Keeps articles ready for use.
10. **Remove gown, gloves, and mask without contamination.**	Prevents spread of pathogens.
11. **Dispose of waste materials.**	Helps prevent spread of microorganisms.
12. **Wash hands.**	Helps prevent cross-contamination.

SKILL 14-6 PERFORMING ISOLATION TECHNIQUE

Steps	Rationale
1. **Obtain equipment:** *Outside patient's room or in anteroom:* ▪ Isolation gowns ▪ Isolation masks ▪ Isolation gloves ▪ Clean linens ▪ Single isolation bags ▪ Double isolation bags ▪ Paper towels ▪ Running water ▪ Soap with dispenser *Inside patient's room or in anteroom:* ▪ Holder for isolation bag ▪ Holder for laundry bag	Helps organize procedure.
2. **Determine causative microorganism or determine whether patient's immune system is deficient.**	Helps nurse know virulence of causative pathogen.
3. **Refer to medical record, care plan, or Kardex for special interventions.**	Provides basis for care.
4. **Introduce self.**	Decreases patient's anxiety level.
5. **Identify patient by identification band.**	Identifies correct patient for procedure.
6. **Explain procedure to patient.**	Seeks patient's cooperation and decreases anxiety.
7. **Prepare patient for intervention:**	
a. Close door to room or pull curtain.	Provides privacy.
b. Drape for procedure if necessary.	Prevents exposure of patient.
8. **Raise bed to comfortable working level.**	Provides safety for nurse.
9. **Arrange for patient privacy.**	Shows respect for patient.
10. **Follow agency policy for type of isolation used.**	Increase awareness of isolation methods available in agency.
11. **Post isolation category instruction on door to room.**	Alerts personnel, patient, family, and visitors to need for special precautions.
12. **Plan time to explain isolation to patient and family.**	Promotes cooperation for using isolation and reduces patient's anxiety.
13. **Wash hands and don isolation garb according to agency policy and guidelines from OSHA and CDC.**	Prepares for administration of patient care.
14. **Provide required nursing care.**	Meets patient's needs.
15. **Dispose of waste materials in isolation container.**	Helps prevent spread of microorganisms.
16. **Remove isolation garb and place in isolation container.**	Prevents contamination.
17. **Document.**	Documents procedure and patient's response.

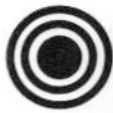

SKILL 14-7 PREPARING FOR ANTISEPSIS, DISINFECTION, AND STERILIZATION

Steps	Rationale
1. **Obtain equipment:**	Helps organize procedure.
▪ Appropriate disinfectant for cleansing	Aids in appropriate care of equipment and reusable supplies.
▪ Clean gloves	Protects nurse from contamination.
▪ Running water	Aids in cleansing and rinsing of articles.
▪ Scrub brush	Aids in cleansing grooves.
▪ Cloth wrappers	Provides means for wrapping articles requiring sterilization in autoclave.
2. **Assess contamination of article and need for cleansing, disinfection, or sterilization.**	Ensures continuity of universal precautions to protect all personnel and patients.
3. **Wash hands and don clean gloves according to agency policy and OSHA and CDC guidelines.**	Helps prevent cross-contamination.
4. **Rinse article under cold, running water.**	Decoagulates protein for easier removal.
5. **Wash article with detergent and warm water.**	Emulsifies or softens dirt for removal.
6. **Use scrub brush to remove material in grooves.**	Loosens material in corners and grooves.
7. **Dry article thoroughly.**	Helps prevent growth of microorganisms.
8. **Prepare article for autoclave by wrapping in appropriate cloth wrappers.**	Ensures appropriate sterilization and ease of opening package without contaminating articles.
9. **Dispose of waste materials.**	Helps prevent spread of microorganisms.
10. **Remove gloves and wash hands.**	Helps prevent cross-contamination.

SUMMARY

Isolation protects the patient, health care team, family members, and friends of the patient. Appropriate handwashing techniques are imperative to prevent cross-contamination. Nurses should consider preventing infection of their own family members by performing appropriate handwashing. Wearing gloves at appropriate times helps prevent nosocomial infection and protects the nurse.

Key Concepts

- Normal body flora resist infection by releasing antibacterial substances and inhibiting multiplication of pathogenic microorganisms.
- Immunity to infection is measured by the capacity to produce antibodies in response to exposure to an antigen.
- An infection cannot develop as long as the elements composing the infection chain are interrupted.
- Microorganisms are transmitted by direct and indirect contact, by airborne spread, and by vectors and contaminated vehicles.
- Masks with eye-protection devices such as goggles or glasses with solid side shields are worn when splashes or spray of blood or potentially infectious material may be generated.
- The Centers for Disease Control and Prevention recommends that health care workers consider all patients as potentially infected with the human immunodeficiency virus and other bloodborne pathogens and to reduce the risk of exposure to blood and body fluids.
- Following aseptic principles is the key to a nurse's success in preventing patients from acquiring infections.
- Poor handwashing is the main cause of nosocomial infections.

Critical Thinking Questions

1. Identify the six elements of the chain of infection. Identify those elements of the chain that are broken when the nurse does not wash hands between contact with patients.
2. Each year health care facilities spend millions of dollars for isolation barrier protection (for example, gowns, gloves, goggles, masks). For this reason, nurses must carefully choose personal protective equipment (PPE) to establish barriers without creating additional costs for their facility. In the following patient care situations, select the appropriate PPE and give rationale.
   a. Initiating venipuncture
   b. Blood pressure checks on a patient with hepatitis B
   c. Changing the bed linen for an incontinent patient
   d. Entering the room of a patient with meningococcal meningitis
   e. Emptying a suction bottle containing bloody fluid
   f. Bathing a baby born to a mother who is HIV positive
3. The nurse has admitted Mr. Cobbs to a general medical unit with a diagnosis of tuberculosis. The physician has not ordered isolation precautions. Should the patient be isolated? If so, what kind of isolation?

REFERENCES AND SUGGESTED READINGS

Anderson KN, Anderson LE, Glanze WD, editors: *Mosby's medical, nursing, and allied health dictionary,* ed 4, St Louis, 1994, Mosby.

Brunner LS, Suddarth DS: *The Lippincott manual of nursing practice,* ed 6, Philadelphia, 1994, Lippincott.

Lewis SM, Collier IC, Heitkemper MM: *Medical-surgical nursing: assessment and management of clinical problems,* ed 4, St Louis, 1996, Mosby.

McFarland GK, McFarlane EA: *Nursing diagnosis and intervention: planning for patient care,* ed 2, St Louis, 1993, Mosby.

Phipps WJ et al, editors: *Medical-surgical nursing: concepts and clinical practice,* ed 5, St Louis, 1995, Mosby.

Potter PA, Perry AG: *Basic nursing: theory and practice,* ed 3, St Louis, 1995, Mosby.

Scanlon VC, Sanders T: *Essentials of anatomy and physiology,* Philadelphia, 1995, Davis.

CHAPTER 15

Medication Administration

Learning Objectives

After studying this chapter, the student should be able to . . .

- Define the key terms.
- Identify personal skills in basic mathematics that may need improvement and work to improve the skills.
- Calculate doses of medications using appropriate formulas.
- Convert systems of measurement to calculate doses of medication.
- Implement concepts for the administration of medication.
- Explain the legal aspects of the administration of medication.
- Implement the five rights.
- Describe four primary routes for administration of medication.
- Describe five types of medication preparation and name at least three nursing responsibilities associated with each.
- Demonstrate the appropriate procedures for the preparation and administration of oral, topical, rectal, eye, ear, parenteral, transdermal, intravenous, and inhalation medications.

Key Terms

Ampule
Buccal
Controlled substance
Diluent
Enteric coated
Gauge
Infusion
Infusion pump
Inhalant
Injection
Instillation
Intradermal
Intramuscular
Intravenous
Irrigation
Narcotic
Parenteral
Patent
Patient-controlled analgesia (PCA)
Piggyback
Precipitate
Subcutaneous
Sublingual
Topical
Vial
Z-track method

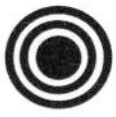

Skills

15-1 Administering oral medications
15-2 Applying a transdermal medication patch
15-3 Administering eye medications
15-4 Administering ear medications
15-5 Administering rectal medications
15-6 Administering injections

The administration of medication places great responsibility on the nurse. Before administering medication, the nurse should know (1) drug classification (brand and generic names), (2) usual dosage, (3) route, (4) nursing implications, (5) actions (uses), (6) therapeutic effects, (7) adverse effects, and (8) side effects. Knowledge of specific drug classifications and guidelines is important. The nurse must learn legal guidelines to meet expected standards of law when administering medication.

The beginning of this chapter offers a review of mathematical processes to assist the student in solving basic math problems. The purpose for accurately calculating a *dosage* is to ensure the correct amount of medication is administered to the patient.

The nurse should have knowledge in the following areas before administering medication to a patient:

1. Basic math skills for the calculation of correct dosages of medication
2. Guidelines for administering medication, medication abbreviations and symbols, and legal aspects to meet the standards of accountability and responsibility
3. Various routes of administration and nursing measures to consider for each *route of administration*
4. Injection sites and variations that meet the needs of adults, children, and infants
5. Reporting of medication errors
6. Medication preparations and appropriate administration techniques
7. Principles of administering medication, including the five rights

Because of the variety of medications available today, the nurse faces an enormous task in learning information about each one. This task may be facilitated by using drug cards. A drug card is usually an index-type card used to write information about a specific medication and includes medication classification, brand and generic names, actions, adverse reactions, route, usual dosage, contraindications, and nursing implications. The individual card system may be used each time the nurse needs information about medication. A nursing drug reference book is another useful tool.

NURSING PROCESS

Assessment

The nurse assesses many factors to determine the need for and potential response to drug therapy. These factors include the patient's medical history, diet, and allergy history. The nurse also assesses the patient's current physical and mental status. Coordination limitations may interfere with the patient's ability to prepare doses and take medications correctly. The patient's knowledge and understanding of drug therapy should also be considered. It is important for the nurse to know as much as possible about each drug given, including normal dosages, purpose, action, routes, side effects, and interaction with other drugs.

Nursing Diagnosis

Assessment findings are used to determine actual or potential problems with drug therapy. Certain data reveal nursing diagnoses. These may include the following:

Anxiety
Impaired physical mobility
Impaired swallowing
Knowledge deficit (specify)
Noncompliance: drug regimen
Sensory/perceptual alterations (specify) (auditory, gustatory, kinesthetic, olfactory, tactile, visual)

PATIENT TEACHING

- Instruct patient to keep each drug in its original labeled container.
- Instruct patient to discard outdated medications.
- Advise patient to notify physician of side effects.

Planning

The plan of care should focus on the safe administration of drugs (see care plan on p. 282). The nurse can use time during drug administration to teach patients about their medications (see teaching box). The nurse should collaborate with the patient's family and friends about drug regimens after discharge.

The plan of care may include the following goal and outcome:

Goal: Patient and family understand drug therapy.

Outcome

Patient and family describe information about the drug, dosage, schedule, purpose, and adverse effects.

Implementation

The nurse identifies factors that may improve or diminish a patient's health and well-being. Physical limitations, beliefs, values, and habits may influence a patient's compliance with medication schedules. The nurse is responsible for knowing about medications and their potential adverse effects on the patient, especially if there are multiple prescriptions. The capabilities and limitations of the older adult are especially important considerations (see gerontologic box).

Evaluation

The nurse uses evaluative measures to determine whether patient outcomes were met. The nurse must always be prepared to revise the care plan based on the evaluation.

GERONTOLOGIC CONSIDERATIONS

- The older adult may have difficulty swallowing because of dry mouth. Sipping water before swallowing the medication may facilitate swallowing.
- Visual alterations in the older adult may make it difficult to read prescriptions.
- Hospitalized older adults often have one or more chronic illnesses for which they are taking multiple medications.

Goal: Patient and family understand drug therapy.

Evaluative measure

Ask patient to describe purpose, dosage, and adverse effects of each prescribed medication.

MATH REVIEW

Many errors in medication dosages are caused by carelessness in failing to add, subtract, multiply, or move a decimal point appropriately. For this reason a review of basic mathematical processes is presented.

Adding Fractions

For adding of fractions, a common denominator (bottom number) is first obtained. For example, in the equation $1/5 + 1/2$, 10 is the common denominator because it is the smallest number into which 2 and 5 divide evenly.

The numerator (top number) and denominator then should be multiplied by the same number to create the common denominator. For example,

$$\frac{1 \times 2}{5 \times 2} = \frac{2}{10} \text{ and } \frac{1 \times 5}{2 \times 5} = \frac{5}{10}$$

The fractions now can be added by determining the sum of the numerators; the denominator remains the same. For example, $2/10 + 5/10 = 7/10$. Therefore $1/5 + 1/2 = 7/10$.

For practice, the student should add the following fractions:

1. $\frac{1}{6} + \frac{1}{7} =$
2. $\frac{1}{6} + \frac{1}{2} =$
3. $\frac{2}{3} + \frac{5}{6} + \frac{7}{20} =$
4. $\frac{2}{4} + \frac{2}{4} =$
5. $\frac{1}{2} + \frac{3}{6} =$

Subtracting Fractions

For subtraction of fractions, a common denominator is first obtained. For example, in the equation $1/2 - 1/5$, 10 is the common denominator because it is the smallest number into which 2 and 5 divide evenly. The numerator and denominator then should be multiplied by the same number to create the common denominator. For example,

$$\frac{1 \times 5}{2 \times 5} = \frac{5}{10} \text{ and } \frac{1 \times 2}{5 \times 2} = \frac{2}{10}$$

The fractions now can be subtracted by determining the difference of the numerators; the denominator remains the same. For example, $5/10 - 2/10 = 3/10$. Therefore $1/2 - 1/5 = 3/10$.

For practice, the student should subtract the following fractions:

1. $\frac{3}{16} - \frac{5}{42} =$
2. $\frac{5}{11} - \frac{1}{11} =$
3. $\frac{1}{6} - \frac{1}{7} =$
4. $\frac{3}{4} - \frac{2}{4} =$
5. $\frac{2}{3} - \frac{5}{6} =$

Changing Mixed Numbers to Improper Fractions

For changing mixed numbers to improper fractions, the whole number is multiplied by the denominator, and the answer is added to the numerator. For example, $6\frac{2}{3} = 6 \times 3 + 2$ or 20. The total of this equation is the numerator of the improper fraction. The denominator remains the same. Therefore $6\frac{2}{3} = 20/3$.

For practice, the student should change the following mixed numbers to improper fractions:

1. $5\frac{3}{8} =$
2. $3\frac{1}{5} =$
3. $3\frac{3}{8} =$
4. $2\frac{1}{3} =$
5. $7\frac{1}{5} =$

Changing Improper Fractions to Mixed Numbers

For changing improper fractions to mixed numbers, the denominator is divided into the numerator. For example, $^{28}/_{5}$ would be changed to 28 ÷ 5, which equals 5 with 3 left over. The remainder becomes the numerator; the old denominator remains the same. Therefore $^{28}/_{5} = 5^{3}/_{5}$.

For practice, the student should change the following improper fractions to mixed numbers:

1. $\frac{9}{3} =$
2. $\frac{22}{5} =$
3. $\frac{17}{4} =$
4. $\frac{36}{8} =$
5. $\frac{100}{75} =$

Multiplying Fractions

Before fractions are multiplied, they should always be reduced to the lowest form. For example, $^{16}/_{20} \times ^{2}/_{8} = ^{4}/_{5} \times ^{1}/_{4}$. The numerators *and* denominators then should be multiplied. For example, $^{4}/_{5} \times ^{1}/_{4} = ^{4}/_{20}$. The answer should be reduced to lowest form (that is, $^{4}/_{20} = ^{1}/_{5}$). If the numbers diagonal from one another in the equation can be divided into one another, the answer will be in the lowest form.

For practice, the student should multiply the following fractions:

1. $\frac{2}{4} \times \frac{4}{6} =$
2. $\frac{6}{8} \times \frac{1}{4} =$
3. $\frac{2}{3} \times \frac{3}{6} =$
4. $\frac{1}{3} \times \frac{1}{4} =$
5. $\frac{3}{5} \times \frac{1}{5} =$

Dividing Fractions

Before fractions are divided, they should be reduced to their lowest form. For example, $^{5}/_{21} \div ^{8}/_{12} = ^{5}/_{21} \div ^{2}/_{3}$. For dividing one fraction by another, the second fraction should be inverted and the two fractions multiplied. For example, $^{5}/_{21} \div ^{2}/_{3} = ^{5}/_{21} \times ^{3}/_{2} = ^{15}/_{42} = ^{5}/_{14}$. (See the section on multiplying fractions.)

For practice, the student should divide the following fractions:

1. $\frac{4}{10} \div \frac{2}{5} =$
2. $\frac{1}{2} \div \frac{1}{4} =$
3. $\frac{1}{2} \div \frac{1}{6} =$
4. $\frac{3}{3} \div \frac{3}{9} =$
5. $\frac{1}{3} \div \frac{2}{3} =$

Changing Fractions to Decimals

For changing a fraction into a decimal, the numerator should be divided by the denominator. For example, $^{2}/_{5}$ = 2.0 ÷ 5 = .4. A zero should be added before the decimal point to denote a fraction of a part and to help prevent a dosage error. For example, 2.0 ÷ 5 = 0.4.

For practice, the student should change the following fractions to decimals:

1. $\frac{1}{100}$
2. $\frac{2}{5}$
3. $\frac{3}{4}$
4. $2\frac{1}{2}$
5. $\frac{50}{35}$

Adding Decimals

For adding decimals, the decimal points are vertically aligned, and the two numbers added. For example,

$$\begin{array}{r} 0.57 \\ 2.98 \\ \underline{32.90} \\ 36.45 \end{array}$$

Therefore 0.57 + 2.98 + 32.9 = 36.45.

For practice, the student should add the following decimals:

1. 3.5 + 0.2 =
2. 50 + 0.7 + 3.049 =
3. 2.003 + 12.8 =
4. 14 + 0.007 + 8.40 =
5. 123.45 + 678.90 + 11.12 =

Subtracting Decimals

For subtracting decimals, the decimal points should be vertically aligned and the two numbers subtracted. For example,

$$\begin{array}{r} 62.40 \\ \underline{-\ 6.98} \\ 55.42 \end{array}$$

Therefore 62.40 − 6.98 = 55.42.

For practice, the student should subtract the following decimals:

1. 6.25 − 0.22 =
2. 65 − 0.8 =
3. 0.17 − 0.06 =
4. 127.20 − 67.40 =
5. 575.04 − 323.90 =

Multiplying Decimals

Decimals are multiplied just as whole numbers are multiplied. The decimal points must be vertically aligned but should be disregarded during multiplication. For example,

$$\begin{array}{r} 29.87 \\ \times \quad 6.42 \\ \hline 59\ 74 \\ 1194\ 80 \\ 17922\ 00 \\ \hline 191.76\ 54 \end{array}$$

However, a decimal point must be added to the answer. To determine where the decimal point should be placed, one should count the total number of spaces after the decimal point to the right in the numbers multiplied. For example, in the equation 29.87 × 6.42, there are a total of four spaces after the decimal points. Therefore there should be four spaces after the decimal point in the answer (four spaces from the right): 29.87 × 6.42 = 191.7654.

For practice, the student should multiply the following decimals:

1. 2.57 × 0.2 =
2. 15.07 × 2.57 =
3. 1000 × 15.10 =
4. 0.0073 × 9 =
5. 123.45 × 0.06 =

Dividing Decimals

For dividing decimals, the dividing number (the divisor) should be made a whole number by moving the decimal point to the right until it is a whole number. For example, 0.63 = 063.0. The decimal point is moved two spaces to the right to create the whole number 63. Next, the decimal point in the number into which the divisor is being divided (the dividend) must be moved the same number of places to the right as the decimal point in the divisor. For example, 29.90 = 2990.0. Now the decimals can be divided:

$$\begin{array}{r} 47.460 \\ 63.\overline{)2990.000} \\ \underline{252} \\ 470 \\ \underline{441} \\ 290 \\ \underline{252} \\ 380 \\ \underline{378} \\ 20 \end{array}$$

The decimal point in the quotient (answer) must align with the decimal point in the dividend.

For practice, the student should divide the following decimals:

1. 0.63 ÷ 3 =
2. 3 ÷ 0.63 =
3. 0.9 ÷ 3.3 =
4. 40.20 ÷ 8 =
5. 0.063 ÷ 0.3 =

Changing Ratios to Percentages

For changing a ratio to a percentage, the ratio should be changed to a fraction. For example:

$$1{:}3 = \frac{1}{3}$$

Next, the fraction is multiplied by 100. For example:

$$1{:}3 = \frac{1}{3} \times \frac{100}{1} = \frac{100}{3}$$

Then the fraction is reduced to the lowest form and the numerator is divided by the denominator. For example:

$$1{:}3 = \frac{1}{3} \times \frac{100}{1} = \frac{100}{3}$$

$$\begin{array}{r} 33.3\% \\ 3\overline{)100.0} \\ \underline{9} \\ 10 \\ \underline{9} \\ 10 \\ \underline{9} \\ 1 \end{array}$$

Therefore the ratio 1:3 = 33.3%.

For practice, the student should change the following ratios to percentages:

1. 1:2
2. 1:1000
3. 1:4
4. 1:100
5. 1:15

Changing Percentages to Ratios

For changing percentages to ratios, the percent (%) sign is omitted. For example:

$$75\% = 75$$

Second, the whole or mixed number is placed as the numerator. For example:

$$\frac{75}{}$$

Third, 100 is placed as the denominator. For example:

$$\frac{75}{100}$$

Next, the fraction is reduced to the lowest terms. For example:

$$\frac{75}{100} = \frac{3}{4}$$

Then the fraction is written as a ratio. For example:

$$3:4$$

Therefore 75% = 3:4.

For practice, the student should change the following percentages to ratios:

1. 25%
2. 1%
3. 45%
4. 50%
5. 20%

Converting a Percentage to a Decimal

For converting a percentage to a decimal, the percent sign is removed, and the decimal point is moved 2 places to the left. For example, for 75%, the percent sign is removed (that is, 75). Then the decimal point is moved 2 places to the left to create a decimal. For example:

$$0.75$$

For practice, the student should convert the following percentages to decimals:

1. 15%
2. 60%
3. 40%
4. 35%
5. 100%

Converting a Decimal to a Percentage

For converting a decimal to a percentage, the decimal point is moved 2 places to the right, and a percent sign is added. For example, for 0.45, the decimal point is moved 2 places to the right (that is, 45.0).

A percent sign is added to create a percentage. For example:

$$0.45 = 45\%$$

For practice, the student should convert the following to percentages:

1. 0.65
2. 75
3. 25
4. 50
5. 90

SYSTEMS OF MEASUREMENT

Three systems of measurement are used when drug dosages are calculated: metric, apothecary, and household.

Metric System

The metric system is a decimal system based on ratios of tens. The system can be converted easily through multiplication and division.

The basic units of measurement in the metric system are:

meter (m)	length
liter (L or l)	volume
gram (g or gm)	weight

Each basic unit has a numerical value of 1 and is organized into units of ten. The following Latin and

Greek prefixes are used to designate subdivisions and multiples of the basic unit when written with the unit of measurement:

deci = 0.1 of the unit
centi = 0.01 of the unit
milli = 0.001 of the unit
deka = 10 times the unit
hecto = 100 times the unit
kilo = 1000 times the unit

Multiplying or dividing the basic unit changes the metric value of the unit. A simple rule to remember is as follows: For *multiplication,* the decimal point of the unit being converted is moved as many places to the *right* as there are zeros. For *division,* the decimal point of the unit being converted is moved as many places to the *left* as there are zeros. When converting larger units to smaller units, one should always multiply, and when converting smaller units to larger units, one should always divide.

For example, to change the basic unit gram to a milligram, one must multiply by 1000 (that is, move the decimal point 3 places to the right). *Milli-* has three zeros, and the basic unit gram is 1.0. Moving the decimal 3 places to the right converts the gram to a milligram. Therefore 1 gram equals 1000 milligrams.

To change the basic unit gram to a kilogram, one should divide by 1000 (that is, move the decimal point 3 places to the left). *Kilo-* has three zeros, and the unit gram is 1.0. Moving the decimal 3 places to the left converts the gram to a kilogram. Therefore 1 g equals 0.001 kg.

To appropriately write drug dosages using the metric unit measurement, the nurse should remember the following rules:

1. The dosage is written in a decimal form instead of a fraction. A zero is *always* placed in front of the decimal to prevent a medication error (for example, 0.25).
2. The form of measurement is placed after the dose (for example, 0.25 milligram).
3. Lowercase letters are appropriate abbreviations for the subdivisions (for example, milligram = mg; milliliter = ml).

For practice, the student should convert liters to milliliters:

1. 2.75 l =
2. 3.46 l =
3. 0.45 l =
4. 1 l =
5. 0.005 l =

! REMEMBER

- To change grams to milligrams, one should multiply by 1000.
- To change milligrams to grams, one should divide by 1000.
- To change liters to milliliters, one should multiply by 1000.
- To change milliliters to liters, one should divide by 1000.

For practice, the student should convert milliliters to liters:

1. 2752 ml =
2. 9735 ml =
3. 1500 ml =
4. 1000 ml =
5. 5 ml =

For practice, the student should convert grams to milligrams:

1. 0.250 g =
2. 0.0025 g =
3. 0.030 g =
4. 0.001 g =
5. 0.0003 g =

For practice, the student should convert milligrams to grams:

1. 30 mg =
2. 500 mg =
3. 0.3 mg =
4. 0.04 mg =
5. 2 mg =

The nurse should learn the metric and apothecary systems of measurement. Equivalents for these systems are given in Table 15-1. Weight equivalent measurements are given in Table 15-2.

Apothecary System

The apothecary system can be used as a measurement of weight or volume. The grain is the basic unit of weight.

Abbreviations used in the apothecary system of measurement are as follows:

ʒ = dram	iii = 3
℥ = ounce	iv = 4
fʒ = fluidram	v = 5
f℥ = fluidounce	vi = 6
ss = one half	vii = 7
i = 1	viii = 8
ii = 2	ix = 9
	x = 10

Table 15-1 VOLUME EQUIVALENTS OF MEASUREMENT

Metric	Apothecary	Household
1 ml	15 minims (m)	15 drops (gtt)
15 ml	4 fluidrams (f3)	1 tablespoon (tbsp)
30 ml	1 fluid ounce (f3)	2 tablespoons (tbsp)
240 ml	8 fluid ounces (f3)	1 cup (c)
480 ml (approximately 500 ml)	1 pint (pt)	1 pint (pt)
960 ml (approximately 1 L)	1 quart (qt)	1 quart (qt)
3840 ml (approximately 4000 ml)	1 gallon (gal)	1 gallon (gal)

From Perry AB, Potter PA: *Clinical nursing skills and techniques,* ed 3, St Louis, 1994, Mosby.

Table 15-2 WEIGHT EQUIVALENTS OF MEASUREMENT

Metric	Apothecary	Household
1 mg	1/60 gr	—
60 mg	1 gr	—
1 g	15 gr	—
4 g	1 ʒ	—
30 g	1 oz (℥)	1 oz
500 g	1.1 lb	1 lb
1000 g (1 kg)	2.2 lb	2 lb

From Perry AB, Potter PA: *Clinical nursing skills and techniques,* ed 3, St Louis, 1994, Mosby.

The following list of equivalents should be learned by the nurse:

Volume

60 minims (m) = 1 fluidram (fʒ)
8 fluidrams (fʒ) = 1 fluidounce (f℥)
16 fluidounces (f℥) = 1 pint (pt or O)
2 pints (pt or O) = 1 quart (qt)
4 quarts (qt) = 1 gallon (gal or C)

Weight

60 grains (gr) = 1 dram (ʒ)
8 drams (ʒ) = 1 ounce (℥)
12 ounces (℥) = 1 pound (lb)

To appropriately write drug dosages using the apothecary system, the nurse should remember the following rules:

1. Small letters or symbols are used to designate the units of measurement (for example, grain = gr; minim = m, min, or mx; dram = dr or ʒ; ounce = oz or ℥).
2. Because the dram and ounce may be a unit of weight or volume, volume is always designated with f or fl and the symbol (for example, fʒ, f℥).
3. Roman numerals are still used by many physicians for ordering drugs and writing prescriptions. Lowercase Roman numerals designate the amount or dose and always follow the unit of measurement (for example, 3 grains = gr iii; 10 grains = gr x).
4. Fractions and whole numbers may also be used with the apothecary unit but only when it is appropriate (for example, grains 1/60 = 1/60 gr; grain 1 = 1 gr).
5. The fraction ½ is designated with the symbol $\overline{ss}$ (for example, 3½ ounces = ℥iii$\overline{ss}$).

HOUSEHOLD MEASUREMENTS

- Drop (gtt)
- Teaspoon (tsp)
- Tablespoon (tbsp)
- Cup (c)
- Glass (gl)
- Ounce (oz)
- Pint (pt)
- Quart (qt)
- Gallon (gal)
- Pound (lb)

Household System

Most people are familiar with the household system of measurement (see box). The system applies only to measurement of volume.

The nurse must know approximate equivalents in all systems of measurement to convert desired dosages when necessary (see Tables 15-1 and 15-2).

For practice, the student should answer the following:

1. Write the prescription symbol for 2 fluidrams:
2. Write the prescription symbol for 6 fluidounces:
3. Write the symbol for grain 10:
4. 3ii = gr =
5. 3i = drams =

CALCULATING DRUG DOSAGE

In the administration of some *medications,* the nurse must calculate an accurate *dosage* of *medication.* There are five points to remember when calculating dosages:

1. If the systems of measurement are different, the nurse should convert to the same system.
2. The appropriate *formula* is worked as a fraction problem.
3. Scored tablets or those with a line or indentation across the center can be used in calculating less than a one tablet dose because the tablet can be broken evenly in half.
4. An unscored tablet should not be cut because the dose will not be accurate.
5. When the formula is used for liquid or injection calculation, one should convert to minims if the amount is less than 1 ml.

There are several formulas to assist the nurse in calculating an accurate dosage of medication.

Formula I

This formula is used for dosage calculation of solid forms of medication, such as tablets:

$$\frac{\text{Dose ordered (dose the physician orders)}}{\text{Dose on hand (dose available)}} = \text{Amount (dose to be given)}$$

The formula is shortened to:

$$\frac{DO}{DH} = A$$

For example, the physician orders 60 mg of a medication; the nurse has available 1 gr of tablets. How many tablets would the nurse administer?

$$\frac{DO = 60\text{ mg}}{DH = 1\text{ gr}} = A$$

1. Convert to the same system.

$$D = 60\text{ mg}$$

$$H = 1\text{ gr} = 60\text{ mg}$$

2. Work the problem as a fraction.

$$\begin{array}{r} 1.0\text{ tab.} \\ 60\text{ mg})\overline{60\text{ mg}} \\ \underline{60} \\ 0 \end{array}$$

$$\frac{DO}{DH} = \frac{60\text{ mg}}{60\text{ mg}} = 1\text{ tablet}$$

If the systems are the same, the formula is used and worked as a fraction. For example, the physician orders 75 mg of a medication; the nurse has 50 mg on hand. How much would the nurse give?

$$\begin{array}{r} 1.5\text{ tabs.} \\ 50)\overline{75.0} \\ \underline{50} \\ 250 \\ \underline{250} \\ 0 \end{array}$$

$$\frac{D}{H} = \frac{75\text{ mg}}{50\text{ mg}} = 1.5\text{ tablets}$$

Formula II

This formula is used for dosage calculation of liquid and injectable forms of medication:

$$\frac{DO}{DH} \times \frac{\text{Quantity (Volume)}}{1} = A$$

For example, the physician orders 75 mg of Demerol intramuscularly; the nurse has a ampule that holds 50 mg/ml. How much would the nurse give?

$$\frac{DO}{DH} = \frac{75\text{ mg}}{50\text{ mg}} \times \frac{1\text{ ml}}{1} = 1.5\text{ ml}$$

Ratio Proportion Formula

Formula #1:

A ratio expresses a relationship between two items. Ratios are used in everyday life. For example, if a recipe calls for 2 cups of milk to make 4 servings of pudding, how many cups of milk is needed to make 8 servings of pudding? The following is an example of how the process works:

2 cups = the known (fact)	x = the unknown (what nurse needs to know)
4 servings = known	8 servings = unknown

The known (fact) goes to the *left* in the formula. The unknown (what the nurse needs to know) goes to the *right* in the formula.

For example, the colon (:) means "is to," and the equal sign (=) means "as." In other words, 4 servings "is to" 2 cups "as" 8 servings "is to" x (unknown). Written as a formula, this information gives the following information:

$$4\text{ servings}:2\text{ cups} = 8\text{ servings}:x\text{ cups}$$

Next, the *extremes* (outer numbers) are multiplied:

4 servings : 2 cups = 8 servings : x cups

OR

4x = 8 servings : 2 cups

Then the *means* are multiplied:

4 servings : 2 cups = 8 servings : x cups

OR

4x = 16

Putting the problem all together completes the problem as shown:

$$4:2 = 8:x$$
$$4x = 16$$
$$x = 4 \text{ cups}$$

The same formula applies for finding the correct medication dose. The medication order is for 62 mg of a medication. The bottle of medication available is labeled 40 mg per 1 ml. How many milliliters contain 62 mg?

Known: 40 mg per 1 ml
Unknown: 62 mg or x

$$40 \text{ mg} : 1 \text{ ml} = 62 \text{ mg} : x$$
$$40x = 62 \text{ mg}$$
$$x = 1.5 \text{ ml}$$

Formula #2

Using a different ratio formula:

$$(\textit{known ratio})\ \frac{1 \text{ ml}}{40 \text{ mg}} \quad \frac{x \text{ ml (unknown)}}{62 \text{ mg (what nurse needs to know)}}$$

$$40 \times x = 40x$$

$$1 \times 62 = 62$$

$$62 = 40x \qquad 62 \div 40 = 1.5$$

$$x = 1.5 \text{ ml}$$

The ratio formula will work only when the same systems of measurement are used. To convert from grains to milligrams, the nurse must convert into the same system. For example, the order is for morphine ¼ gr, and the morphine is in 30-mg tablets. The nurse must first convert to a common system. Consulting a table the nurse finds that 1 gr = 60 mg.

$$\frac{60 \text{ mg}}{1 \text{ gr}} \text{(known ratio)} \qquad \frac{x \text{ mg (unknown)}}{1/4 \text{ gr (wanted amount)}}$$

$$60 \times 1/4 \text{ (or 0.25)} = 15$$

$$1 \times x = 1x$$

$$1/4 \text{ gr} = 15 \text{ mg}$$

Now the problem can be solved:

$$\frac{1 \text{ tablet}}{30 \text{ mg}} \text{(known ratio)} \quad \frac{x \text{ tablet (unknown)}}{15 \text{ mg (wanted amount)}}$$

$$1 \times 15 = 15$$

$$30 \times x = 30x$$

$$15 \div 30 = 0.5 \text{ or } 1/2 \text{ tablet}$$

For further assistance in mathematical conversions, the student should consult a pharmacology text.

Formula #3:

In another example, the physician orders 50 mg of Demerol intramuscularly. The nurse has an ampule that holds 75 mg/ml. How many millimeters would the nurse give to equal 50 mg?

$$\frac{DO}{DH} = \frac{50 \text{ mg}}{75 \text{ mg}} \times \frac{1 \text{ ml}}{1} = 0.6 \text{ ml}$$

Pediatric Dosage Calculation

Milligram per kilogram formula

First, the nurse determines the child's weight in kilograms: 1 kg = 2.2 lb

To go from pounds to kilograms:	Divide by 2.2
To go from kilograms to pounds:	Multiply by 2.2

A 1-year-old child weighs 25 lb. How many kilograms?

$$25/2.2 = 11.3 \text{ kg.}$$

The medical order for this child is aminophylline 65 mg by mouth every 6 hours. To recheck the dosage, the nurse checks the drug source book, which indicates children from 1-9 yr: 24 mg/kg daily. An example using the child's calculated weight is follows:

$$11 \text{ kg} \times 24 \text{ mg} = 264 \text{ mg/daily}$$

Every 6 hours = 4 times daily

$$264 \div 4 = 66 \text{ mg}$$

What would be the appropriate dosage of aminophylline for a 6-year-old weighing 74 lb?

$$74/2.2 = 33.6 = 34 \text{ kg}$$

$$34 \text{ kg} \times 24 \text{ mg} = 816 \text{ mg/daily}$$

$$816 \div 4 = 204 \text{ mg every 6 hours}$$

Body-surface formula

The body-surface formula is based on the ratio of a child's body surface area (BSA) compared with the BSA of an average adult, which is 1.7 square meters (1.7 m^2). Many standard nomograms, representations by graphs or charts, show the relationship between a child's BSA by weight and approximate age. These are used for reference when determining a child's BSA. To use the nomogram (Fig. 15-1), the nurse draws a line from the child's height (in the left column) to the child's weight (in the right column). The place where the line intersects, the SA line, is the BSA of the child. This number is placed into the formula, and the child's dosage is calculated. The formula to apply with this rule is:

$$\frac{\text{BSA of child}}{1.7 \text{ m}^2} \times \frac{\text{Normal adult dose}}{1} = \text{Child's dose}$$

For example, if a normal single adult dose of ampicillin is 250 mg, how much would a child who weighs 12 kg need? The standard nomogram list shows that a child who weighs 12 kg and is 24 inches tall has a BSA of 0.54 m^2. Therefore:

$$\frac{0.54 \text{ m}^2}{1.7 \text{ m}^2} \times 250 = \text{Child's dose}$$

Since the units (m^2) are constant, they can be ignored.

$$\frac{0.54}{1.7} = 0.3; 0.3 \times 250 \text{ mg} = 75 \text{ mg}$$

Dosage determined according to the BSA should be calculated accurately, and comparisons should be made to a standard nomogram.

For practice, the student should calculate the following drug dosages and show the work:

1. The physician prescribes 250 mg of a medication. The nurse has 100-mg scored tablets on hand. How many tablets would the nurse give?

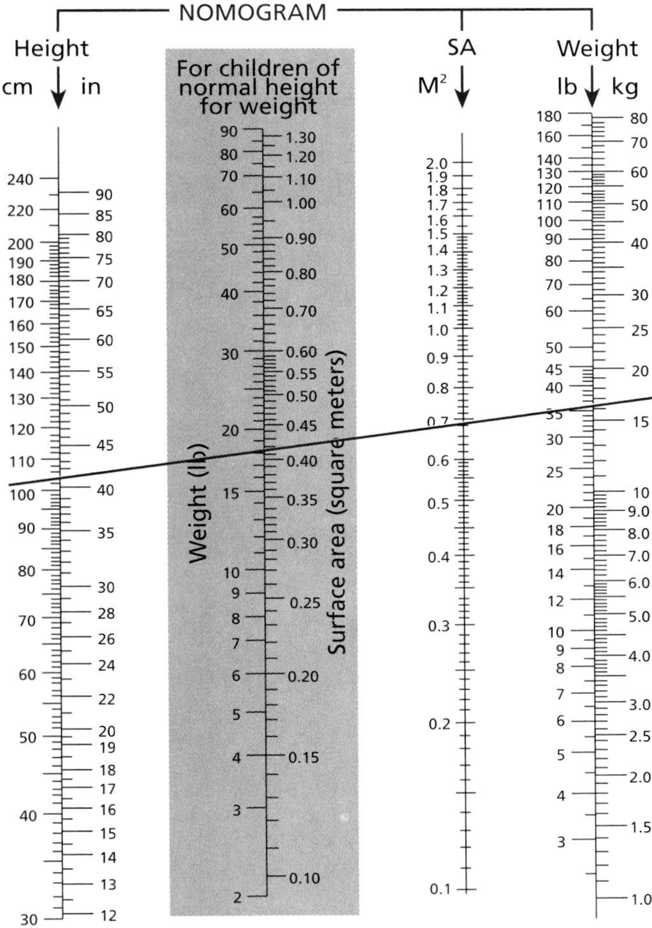

Fig. 15-1 West nomogram for the estimation of surface areas of children. A straight line is drawn between the height and weight. The point where the line crosses the surface area column is the estimated body surface area. (From Behrman RE, Vaughan VC, editors: *Nelson textbook of pediatrics*, ed 15, Philadelphia, 1996, Saunders; modified from data of Boyd E by West CD.)

2. The nurse has gr ½ tablets. The physician orders gr ¼ tablets. How many tablets would the nurse give?
3. The physician orders grain xv of a liquid medication. The label on the bottle reads 7½ gr/5 ml. How many milliliters would the nurse give?
4. The physician orders the nurse to give a patient 35 mg of Demerol. The ampule label reads 50 mg/ml. How many minims would the nurse administer?
5. A child weighing 30 lb is to be given Tylenol. The normal adult dose is 325 mg. What would be the correct dose for a child?

6. The physician orders Duricef 30 mg/kg for a child weighing 52 lb. The dose is to be divided and given every 12 hours. How many milligrams will the nurse give at each dose?

LEGAL ASPECTS

Federal and state legislation set forth standards of control for producing, distributing, prescribing, and administering drugs. Acts have been established in the United States to provide a safe, controlled, and effective means of using drugs by use of written standards.

The Food and Drug Act (FDA), enacted in 1906, was the first federal law to establish standards of purity for food distribution. It includes standards for safe and effective drugs and requires manufacturers to label all drugs accurately, including the contents, strength, and purity.

Amendments have been made to the FDA that provide governmental control of the distribution and sale of drugs, drug naming and labeling, drug testing, and regulation of controlled substances, such as narcotics. An amendment in 1912 prohibited false claims of a drug providing certain health benefits.

Drug Legislation

The Drug Enforcement Agency (DEA) is an agency of the Drug Enforcement Administration of the federal government. This agency enforces regulations regarding the import or export of narcotic drugs and certain other substances and the traffic of these substances across state lines.

Each state and local governing body has additional policies and standards for administering medication. The nurse should be knowledgeable about the laws and expectations of the state and institution where employed.

Controlled Substances and Narcotics

Controlled substances (psychoactive drugs) and **narcotics** (drug that alters perception of pain) are kept in special double-locked cabinets, drawers, boxes, or rooms on nursing units. Because of the high risk for abuse of these medications, federal law governs the dispensing of them. According to the law, records for dispensing controlled substances or narcotics must include the following:

1. Name of the patient receiving the drug
2. Dosage administered (dosage wasted with two signatures affirming the waste)
3. Date and time administered
4. Prescribing physician's name
5. Name of nurse administering the narcotic

When a dose of a controlled substance or narcotic must be wasted or a partial dose wasted, another person must witness its disposal and must cosign as witness that it was indeed wasted. The need to waste a controlled substance or narcotic may occur when a patient refuses medication that has been prepared, when the required dosage is less than the supplied amount, when the medication is accidentally dropped or contaminated, or when the packaging appears to have been damaged. In most agencies, a count is done at change of shift. A nurse from both shifts verify that the number of each controlled substance or narcotic agrees with the number of original supply, less those administered during the shift. An inaccurate count is verified and recorded. Precautions in accounting for controlled substances or narcotics help control drug abuse and meet the requirements of the law (see box).

GUIDELINES FOR SAFE ADMINISTRATION AND CONTROL OF CONTROLLED SUBSTANCES AND NARCOTICS

- All controlled substances and narcotics must be stored in locked, secure cabinet or container.
- Nurses in charge carry sets of keys for controlled substances and narcotics cabinet.
- During institution's change-of-shift, nurse going off duty counts all controlled substances and narcotics with nurse coming on duty. Both nurses sign record to indicate that count is correct.
- Discrepancies in counts are reported immediately.
- Special inventory record is used each time that controlled substance or narcotic is dispensed. (Some agencies have computerized narcotic dispensing with automatic record printouts.)
- Record is used to document patient's name, date, time of drug administration, name of drug, dosage, and signature of nurse dispensing drug.
- Form provides an accurate, ongoing count of medications used and remaining.
- If only one part of premeasured dose of controlled substance or narcotic is given, second nurse witnesses disposal of unused portion and documents such on record form.

From Potter PA, Perry AG: *Basic nursing: theory and practice,* ed 3, St Louis, 1995, Mosby.

NURSING RESPONSIBILITIES

Administering medications is one of the nurse's responsibilities. Guidelines should be carefully followed (see box). Knowledge of the medication classifications, normal doses, routes of administration, therapeutic effects, adverse and side effects, and legal standards and laws governing the ordering, dispensing, and administration of drugs helps the nurse provide safe and legal nursing care. The nurse is expected to interpret the abbreviations used in many drug prescriptions and medical orders. Some common abbreviations are listed in Table 15-3. The nurse should read the specific agency abbreviation list, which is usually located in the policy manual.

Five Rights

The five rights for administering medications should be used each time that a nurse gives medication to a patient. These guidelines are referred to as the *five rights:*

1. The right patient
2. The right drug
3. The right dose
4. The right route
5. The right time

Right patient

The nurse should identify the patient to make certain that the prescribed medication is being administered to the right patient. The appropriate procedure for identification is:

1. Compare the name on the patient's identification band with the medication profile. If a band is not available, another means of identification should be established, or an identification band must be placed on the patient's wrist.
2. Ask the patient to state the full name.
3. Compare photographs if available. In some facilities, especially nursing homes and long-term care facilities, photographs are used to appropriately identify patients.

Right drug

The nurse should compare the label on the medicine container with the medication profile. Spelling should be checked because many drugs have nearly the same spelling but different effects thus the wrong drug may be ordered.

Right dose

The nurse should compare the dosage on the medicine container with the specified dosage on the medication profile. This is the step to calculate the dosage, if necessary. The nurse should then recheck steps before administration.

Right route

The route of medication is designated by the physician. If there is a question about the appropriate

GUIDELINES FOR ADMINISTERING MEDICATIONS

- Read medication profile or medication record with medical order.
- Read medication label 3 times: when taking from drawer, when placing in container, and when unwrapping.
- Administer only medications nurse prepares.
- Reassess medication before administering if patient questions anything about drug.
- Send unlabeled or illegible label of medication to pharmacy for correction before administration.
- Have another nurse check dosage of anticoagulants, insulin, or other drugs of like nature before administration.
- Use appropriate measurement for medication dosages (that is, teaspoon for teaspoon, dram for dram, ounce for ounce) on liquid medication cup.
- Break scored tablet straight across center line after washing hands.
- Clean mortar and pestle appropriately, removing all medication residue after each use.
- Use common generic name as well as trade names.
- Assess patient's ability to swallow medications.
- Remain with patient until patient swallows medication.
- Never leave medication at bedside without medical order.
- Look up unfamiliar medications before administration, noting classification, action or uses, side effects, adverse reactions, usual dosage, route, contraindications, and nursing implications.
- Cease pouring medications when someone interrupts to talk. Talk and then return to pouring medication to avoid making errors.
- Read liquid plastic medication cup at eye level for accuracy.
- Open unit dose medications in patient's room, not in medication room. If patient refuses medication, place it back in medication cart drawer.
- Pour tablet into lid of medication container from multidose container and transfer medication to medication cup without touching medication.
- Pour liquids away from medication label.
- Assess expiration date on all medications.
- Keep medication cart locked when not in use.

Table 15-3 ABBREVIATIONS FOR MEDICATION ADMINISTRATION

Abbreviation	Definition	Abbreviation	Definition
ac	Before meals	po	By mouth
ad lib	As desired	PO	Postoperatively
AD	Right ear	prn	As needed
AS	Left ear	pt	Pint
AU	Each ear	qam	Each morning
bid	Twice a day	qd	Every day
cap	Capsule	qh	Every hour
cc	Cubic centimeter	q2h	Every 2 hours
dr	Dram	q3h	Every 3 hours
DS	Double strength	q4h	Every 4 hours, etc.
elix	Elixir	qid	Four times a day
gm, g	Gram	qn	Every night
gal	Gallon	qod	Every other day
gr	Grain	qt	Quart
gtt	Drop or drops	R	Rectally or by rectum
hs	At bedtime or hours of sleep	Ⓡ	Right
IM	Intramuscular	SA	Sustained action
IV	Intravenous	SQ	Subcutaneous
IVPB	Intravenous piggyback	SL	Sublingual
kg	Kilogram	sol	Solution
L	Liter	sp	Spirits
Ⓛ	Left	$\overline{ss}$	One half
LA	Long-acting	STAT	Immediately
liq	Liquid	supp	Suppository
mcg	Microgram	susp	Suspension
mEq	Milliequivalent	syr	Syrup
mg	Milligram	tab	Tablet
ml	Milliliter	tbs	Tablespoon
m	Minim	tid	Three times a day
NGT	Nasogastric tube	tr	Tincture
OD	Right eye (oculus dexter)	tsp	Teaspoon
OS	Left eye (oculus sinister)	U	Unit
OU	Both eyes (oculus unitus)	ung	Ointment
pc	After meals	ʒ	Dram
		℥	Ounce

route of medication, the nurse should notify the physician.

Some medications come in powder form and are to be mixed with solution before being administered. The nurse should read the instructions carefully on the label for mixing such medications and use the appropriate solution for mixing. If it is an injectable medication, the solution should be specific for injections to avoid error. For example, some drugs may be administered intramuscularly but not intravenously. Some drugs may be administered both intramuscularly and intravenously but must state so on the instructions.

Right time

It is important to administer the medication on a regular schedule for maximal results. The medication should be given as close to the prescribed time as possible. A medication administered 30 minutes before or after the hour due is considered on time.

Medication Order

Since the nurse is responsible for assessing and carrying out the medication order, it is important to determine whether the order includes seven essential components. A medication order cannot be followed if it lacks any of the following parts:

1. Patient's full legal name
2. Medication name (generic or trade name)
3. Dose to be administered
4. Route by which medication is to be administered
5. Time or frequency of administration

6. Date and time the medical order was written
7. Signature of person writing the order

If the medical order is not valid, does not contain all seven parts, or is illegible, questionable, or unclear, the nurse has a legal obligation to clarify it. When there is a question about a medication order, it is best to communicate with the person who has written it.

Storing and Dispensing Drugs

The nurse is responsible for receiving and safeguarding medications on the nursing unit. In many agencies, pharmacy personnel deliver medications to the nursing unit. The medications may be delivered as stock supply, larger quantities of frequently used medications, individual containers for specific patients, or unit-dose system in which each dose is individually packaged for specific patients (Fig 15-2). Each health care agency has a system for receiving, safeguarding, and dispensing medications, which the nurse is expected to learn and follow.

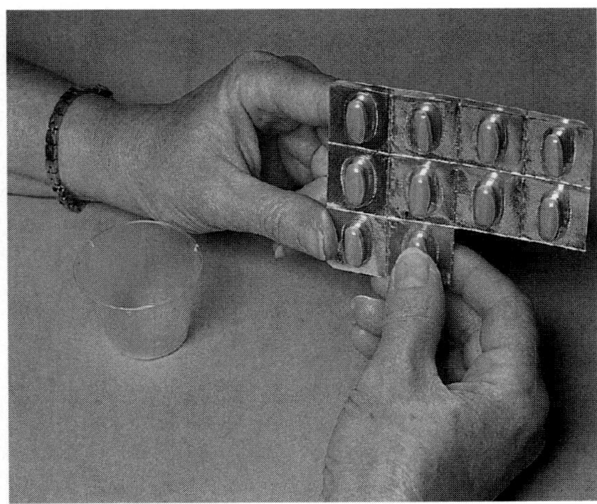

Fig. 15-2 Unit-dose package. (From Christensen BL, Kockrow EO: *Foundations of nursing,* ed 2, St Louis, 1995, Mosby.)

Patient's Health History

Another nursing responsibility in administering medications is reviewing information in the patient's health history. Information concerning the patient's nonprescription medications; allergies; daily habits; mobility; body size; ability to understand, follow directions, and care for the self; and support system is helpful in planning care.

Nonprescription drugs may alter the action of prescribed drugs or cause an adverse reaction. Knowledge of allergies to various foods and medications helps determine appropriate alternatives to medical treatment and helps avoid reactions that could prove life threatening. Drug therapy may be influenced by the consumption of alcohol, caffeine, and herbal teas or by dietary restrictions or excesses. Evaluation of the patient's mobility and body size enables the nurse to select appropriate equipment for administering parenteral medications. Recognition of the patient's support system and ability for self-care gives the nurse additional resources for ensuring that the patient receives medications in a safe and appropriate manner.

When preparing to administer medications, the nurse evaluates the ability of the patient to take medication by the prescribed route. If the patient is unable to receive medication by this route, the nurse communicates with the medical provider to see whether the route can be changed.

Incident Report

When an error is made in medication administration, it is the nurse's ethical and professional responsibility to notify the supervisor and the physician. An error in medication may be a serious matter and must be brought to the attention of the physician as soon as it is recognized. The only person who knows an error has been made is the nurse who makes the error.

A medication error form is completed by the nurse as soon as the error is discovered. The incident is described accurately. The form is used to help correct errors by correcting the problem relating to a medication error. Most facilities have a review committee that reviews medication error reports and offers suggestions to help resolve existing problems.

Most medication errors are a result of deviations from appropriate procedure. Investigations have shown that one or more of the five rights were violated and led to the medication error.

MEDICATION ROUTES

There are several routes or means by which medication may be administered (see Table 15-4). Each method is chosen because of the type of medicine to be administered and the desired effect. There are four routes for administering medications:

1. Oral
2. Topical
3. Inhalation
4. Parenteral

Table 15-4 ROUTES OF MEDICATION ADMINISTRATION

Route	Advantages	Disadvantages
Oral		
Given by mouth or nasogastric tube—tablets, capsules, caplets, time-release capsules	Convenient, noninvasive, economical route Preferred route of patients	Possible stomach irritation Slower onset of action Contraindication in patients unable to swallow Destruction of some drugs by stomach acid
Buccal		
Placed between gums and inner cheek	Slow absorption into mucosa	Possible mucosal irritation Patient swallowing medication and not receiving expected effect
Sublingual		
Placed under tongue for slow absorption	Noninvasive route Absorption while dissolving under tongue	Inability of patient to eat or drink while medication is dissolving Contraindication in unconscious or confused patient
Topical		
Placed on skin or mucous membranes (rectum, vagina, ear, nose, eye)	Usually painless application to local area for local effect Limited side effects	Possible systemic effects Possible local irritation or patient embarrassment Lack of control over rate of absorption
Inhalation		
Given into respiratory tract	Rapid relief Easy access Ability to be delivered to unconscious patient Local or systemic effects	Possible systemic effects Potentially dangerous side effects of oxygen and anesthetics
Parenteral		
Subcutaneous, intramuscular, intradermal, intravenous	Lack of irritation of gastrointestinal system Lack of alteration by stomach acid or loss through vomiting Ability to be given to unconscious patients or those unable to swallow Ability to prescribe precise dose Rapid, direct, effective absorption	Possible allergic reaction Possible injury to tissues, nerves, and blood vessels Possible local irritation, pain, swelling, and abscess Possible injection into wrong tissue and resulting improper absorption Patient refusal of injectable medications

The nurse may choose several appropriate sites for an injection but allows the patient to make the final choice. In this way the nurse encourages cooperation, gives the patient some control over the situation, and enhances self-esteem. The nurse selects the appropriate needle and syringe based on the type of medication to be given, explains the procedure, and answers any questions. Instructing the patient and family on the desired and adverse effects of the medication helps ensure patient cooperation and safety.

Preparations

Solid preparations

A tablet is a powder that has been compressed or molded into a hard, disklike form of various shapes and sizes. Some have special markings that designate the manufacturer, and some are scored so that they can be broken into smaller doses, if needed.

Some tablets are **enteric coated.** That is, they have a thin shell covering and do not dissolve in the stomach. An enteric coating is used if the drug causes irritation to the delicate lining of the stomach. The coating does not dissolve until the medication reaches the intestines, where it dissolves and releases the medication for absorption into the bloodstream.

A capsule is a thin gelatin covering that contains powder, liquid, oil, or time-release pellets. After a capsule is swallowed, the gelatin cover dissolves, and the medication is released through the digestive system. The time-release beads allow sustained medication action because they release at different rates in the gastrointestinal tract.

A troche (lozenge) is a hard, candylike form that comes in a variety of shapes. This preparation contains the medication as well as ingredients to enhance the taste. It should be dissolved in the mouth.

A suppository is a hard form of a drug mixed in a special substance that melts at body temperature. The shape and size differ according to its use. Suppositories are inserted into the rectum or vagina, and the drug is released through the mucous membranes when the suppository melts.

Liquid preparations

An elixir is a clear solution that contains the medication, water, and a small percentage of alcohol. It usually has a sweetener added to make it more palatable for oral ingestion.

A tincture is also a solution composed of the drug, alcohol, and/or water. The drug is usually of a plant origin or synthetic chemical.

A fluid extract is a drug made into a solution from a vegetable source.

A suspension is drug particles that are dispersed or suspended in a solution and do not dissolve. If a suspension is left standing, the particles settle to the bottom. The solution appears clear on top and opaque on the bottom. Suspensions should be shaken well to disperse the particles evenly before they are administered to a patient.

A syrup is a thick, heavy sugar solution with dissolved particles of medication. A variety of flavors, such as orange or cherry, helps to make the drug more palatable.

A liniment is a preparation made of a medication contained in an oil, alcohol, or soap base. It is rubbed onto the skin for local effects and is used only externally.

A lotion is a liquid suspension containing a drug and is used only externally. It is applied to the skin and used as a coolant, for soothing and protection, or as a lubricant.

Ointments are semisolids that contain a drug in a jellylike substance, such as petroleum. An ointment is applied to the skin for local effects. Ointments can be used for the eye and ear. They are labeled specifically for ophthalmic use when used in the eyes and must be sterile.

ADMINISTERING ORAL MEDICATIONS

Medications administered by the oral route are given by mouth. **Sublingual** drugs are placed under the tongue and dissolved. A solid medication given the **buccal** route is placed inside the cheek. The drug is absorbed into the bloodstream through the digestive system. Therefore the onset of the *drug action* is slower than most other routes, but the effects of the medicine are prolonged. Oral medications are less expensive and are the preferred route of administration.

Oral medications include tablets, capsules, caplets, time-release capsules, and sublingual preparations. Skill 15-1 is the procedure for these forms of medication.

Specific guidelines to remember when preparing oral medications follow:

1. Encourage adequate fluid intake.
2. If a patient has a nasogastric tube, assess placement of the tube before instilling liquid. Crush tablets and mix with at least 20 to 30 ml of tepid water, and administer them through the tube. Follow the medication with 30 to 60 ml of tepid water to rinse tubing (see box).
3. If a nasogastric tube is connected to suction, clamp the tube for 30 minutes to 1 hour after administration of medication, or the medicine will be suctioned out, preventing absorption.
4. Do not attempt to break unscored tablets or crush enteric-coated tablets. Contact the pharmacist for questions or assistance (see box).
5. Administer effervescent tablets immediately after they are dissolved in water or juice according to package instructions and patient preference.
6. Position the patient in a sitting or side-lying position and offer medications as preferred by the patient.
7. Know that some oral medications require special procedures for administration. For example, digoxin (Lanoxin) should be placed in a medicine cup by itself to remind the nurse to assess the apical pulse before administration. Sublingual drugs (that is, tablets placed under the tongue) should also be placed in a separate medicine cup to remind the nurse to teach the patient not to swallow this type of medication.
8. Do not follow medications that have a syrup base, such as cough medicines, with liquids. Certain

GUIDELINES FOR GIVING DRUGS THROUGH NASOGASTRIC TUBE, J-TUBE, G-TUBE, OR SMALL-BORE FEEDING TUBE

- Determine placement of tube before administering medications.
- Administer medications in liquid form (suspension, elixir, or solution) when possible to prevent tube obstruction.
- Read medication labels carefully before crushing tablet or opening capsule.
- Do *not* administer buccal, sublingual, or enteric-coated tablets or sustained-action medications through enteral feeding tube.
- Dissolve crushed tablets, powders, and soft gelatin capsules in warm water.
- Irrigate tube before and after each medication with 50 to 100 ml of water.
- Avoid giving syrups or medications with a pH of less than 4.
- Do not attempt to give whole or undissolved medications.

From Potter PA, Perry AG: *Basic nursing: theory and practice,* ed 3, St Louis, 1995, Mosby; modified from Petrosin BM et al: *Critical Care Nursing Quarterly* 12:1, 1989.

cough medications will be washed away and the intended effect prevented.

9. Remember that dietary factors can be important. Some nutrients can interfere with the absorption of certain oral medications. For example, ampicillin, an antibiotic, should not be given with fruit juices or other foods containing acid because such nutrients inactivate the drug.

DRUGS THAT SHOULD NOT BE CRUSHED OR CHEWED

- Enteric-coated tablets.
- Sustained-release forms. These often have the following suffixes attached to the drug name:
  - Dur (*dur*ation)
  - SR (*s*ustained *r*elease)
  - CR (*c*ontrolled or *c*ontinuous *r*elease)
  - SA (*s*ustained *a*ction)
  - Contin (*contin*uous)
  - LA (*l*ong *a*cting
- Trade names that imply sustained release such as spansules, extentabs, extencaps.
- Trade names with twice-a-day abbreviation in the name, such as Theobid, Lithobid, Cardabid.
- Liquid-containing capsules, although occasionally it may be acceptable to puncture capsule and squeeze out contents; consult pharmacist or manufacturer.

The name alone may not provide enough information. Consult the pharmacist if in doubt. Some forms that look like sustained forms are not, and vice versa. Some capsules containing small, slow-release pellets may be opened and pellets sprinkled on applesauce or gently mixed into liquid or food, but they should not be crushed or dissolved.

Scored tablets may be broken along scored line but should not be chewed or crushed.

From Clark JB et al: *Pharmacologic basis of nursing practice,* ed 4, St Louis, 1993, Mosby.

ADMINISTERING TOPICAL MEDICATIONS

Lotions, liniments, ointments, pastes, medicated dressings, plasters, and transdermal patches, which are applied to the skin or mucous membranes, are designed to coat, protect, soothe, or penetrate the skin or relieve symptoms of inflammation or infection. Other medications considered **topical** are applied locally to areas of the body by irrigation, instillation, or insertion into body cavities. Examples of **irrigation** (flushing the membranes with a solution to remove secretions or soothe tissues) include eye and ear irrigations and vaginal douches. Nose sprays and drops and eye and ear drops are examples of **instillations** (introduction of a solution into a body cavity). Suppositories and creams are inserted into the rectum or vagina. Transdermal patches are designed to provide a systemic effect by absorption through the skin. Drugs administered by transdermal patch include nitroglycerin, scopolamine, estrogen, nicotine, clonidine, and fentanyl.

Lotions are usually swabbed or soothed onto the skin for their soothing effects, relieving irritation, itching, and dryness. Calamine and tolnaftate are examples of lotions. Liniments are meant to be rubbed into the skin to relieve joint and muscle soreness. An important aspect of applying liniment is the psychologic and muscle-relaxing effect of the massage. Mentholated agents are examples of liniments.

Ointments, pastes, plasters, and medicated dressings are applied to the skin to provide various systemic and local effects. The nurse applies a fine, even coating of the ointment or paste to the designated area. Overly thick application may alter the action of the medication and is wasteful. Zinc or silver oxide are examples. Plasters and medicated dressings are cotton or gauze materials saturated with a medication and placed on the area to be treated. Examples of this include corn and mustard plasters and potassium permanganate or dilute iodine solutions.

Several precautions should be observed when applying topical medication because of the chemical composition and concentration of certain drugs as well as the condition of the patient's skin and mucous membranes:

1. The nurse should use gloves to avoid direct contact with these drugs.
2. In the case of open wounds, sterile technique is indicated.
3. Appropriate cleansing or debridement of the area is required before medication is applied.
4. Old medication, skin crusts, and dead tissues are removed before new medication is applied.
5. Using a sterile tongue depressor to remove medications from containers avoids cross-contamination of the medication left in the container.
6. Gloved hands or applicators may be used to spread the medication evenly over the area.
7. Sometimes, dressings are ordered to prevent removal of the medication or soiling of clothing.
8. Each medication should be applied according to its specific indications and order.

Applying a Transdermal Patch

Transdermal patches have the advantage in that they do not interfere with the daily activities of the patient and give a sustained dose of the needed medication. When properly applied, these patches do not interfere with bathing, showering, or swimming because their outer layer is a water barrier material. Skill 15-2 lists the steps in applying a transdermal patch.

Applying Ointments

Ointments (for example, nitroglycerin) come in tubes and are usually ordered by the linear inch. The same precautions that apply to the transdermal patch apply. The nurse cleans the old site, properly prepares the new site, wears gloves, and properly disposes of soiled materials. The ointment is squeezed out for the prescribed length and placed against the patient's skin. The ointment is evenly distributed under the paper guide and then covered with clear plastic wrap and taped to the skin. Documentation follows regular medication administration guidelines.

Administering Eye Medications

The eye is a sensitive organ of the body–it has multiple pain fibers—and requires careful administration of medication to avoid discomfort or pain. Because of the sensitive and delicate tissue structure of the eye, it is imperative that the nurse use sterile equipment and technique during the application of eye medication (Skill 15-3). Eye medications are usually used to treat eye inflammation or infection, prepare for eye examinations, or soothe and lubricate the eyes. There are general precautions to follow when administering eye medications.

Administering Ear Medications

The delicate structures within the internal ear are sensitive to temperature changes. The nurse must make certain that the medicated solution being instilled into the ear is at body temperature to prevent severe dizziness and nausea (Skill 15-4). The external ear canal should be free of cerumen (earwax) before the medication can penetrate beyond the external canal.

Another delicate structure that requires protection when introducing medication into the ear is the tympanic membrane. The tympanic membrane can be perforated or ruptured if the solution is introduced directly onto the tympanic membrane with force. Ear medications are usually administered to treat infection, soften impacted cerumen, irrigate the external ear to remove obstruction, and prevent microorganisms from entering middle or inner ear.

Administering Nasal Medications

Nasal medications are usually sprays or drops. Nose drops are administered in the same manner as ear drops (Fig. 15-3). Most nasal medications are saline based, and those with oil bases must be used with caution to prevent aspiration into the lungs as well as irritation and inflammation. Many people self-medicate with nose drops and sprays and forget to consider them as medications. The nurse should alert the patient about side effects of long-term use of nasal preparations.

Administering Rectal Medications

Rectal medications are administered for a variety of reasons. These medications help to relieve fever, pain, and vomiting; help relieve rectal irritation; and stimulate peristalsis or defecation. Many medications usually given via the oral route can be given rectally when the patient is unable to tolerate or re-

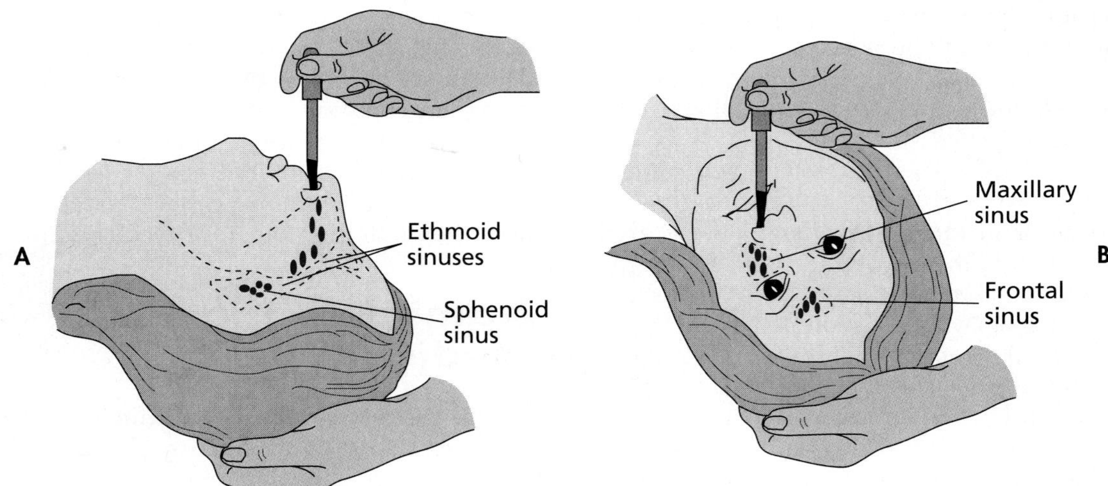

Fig. 15-3 **A,** Ethmoid or sphenoid sinus: Tilt head back over the edge of the bed or place a pillow under the shoulder and tilt the head back. **B,** Frontal and maxillary sinus: tilt the head back over the edge of the bed or pillow with the head turned toward the side treated. (From Potter PA, Perry AG: *Basic nursing: theory and practice,* ed 3, St Louis, 1995, Mosby.)

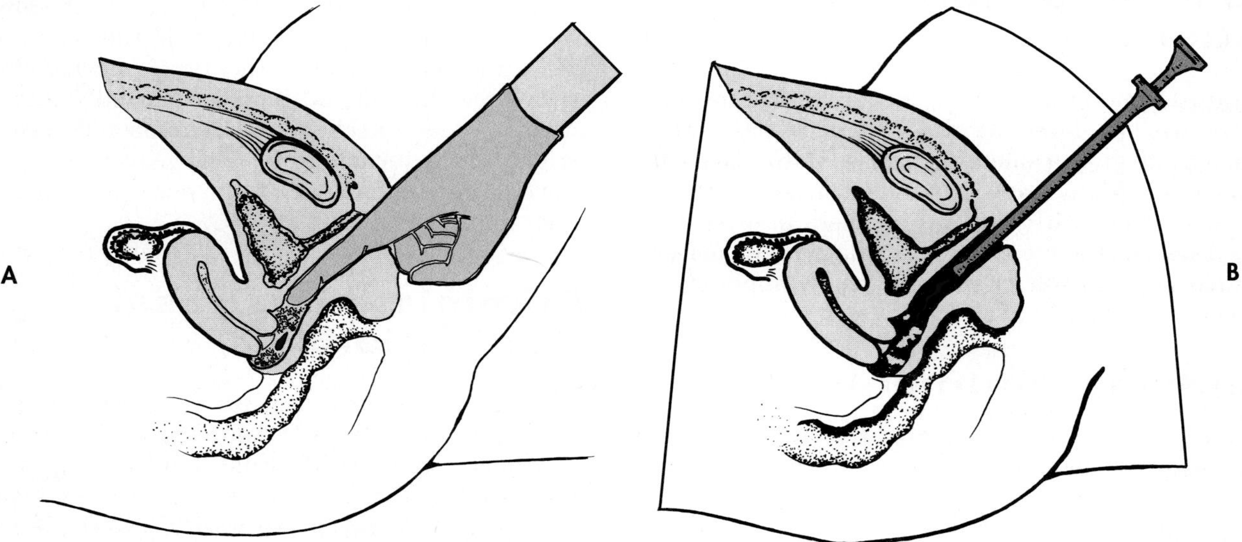

Fig. 15-4 **A,** Insert the rounded end of the suppository along the posterior wall of the vaginal canal using entire length of finger (7.5 to 10 cm [3 to 4 in]). **B,** With dominant gloved hand, insert the applicator approximately 5 to 7.5 cm (2 to 3 in). Push the applicator plunger to deposit medication into the vagina. (From Potter PA, Perry AG: *Basic nursing: theory and practice,* ed 3, St Louis, 1995, Mosby.)

tain oral medications. The steps for administering rectal medications are listed in Skill 15-5.

One type of rectal medication is a suppository. The medication in a rectal suppository is suspended in a glycerin or cocoa-butter base that melts at body temperature, allowing the medication to be absorbed slowly through the rectal mucosa. This type of medication is usually refrigerated until needed. Suppositories should be left in their wrappers until insertion. If a suppository becomes softened, it is placed under cold running water until it is solid enough to insert. Rectal suppositories are contraindicated for patients who have had recent surgery or trauma to the rectum, prostate, or perineum. Suppositories are also contraindicated for patients with

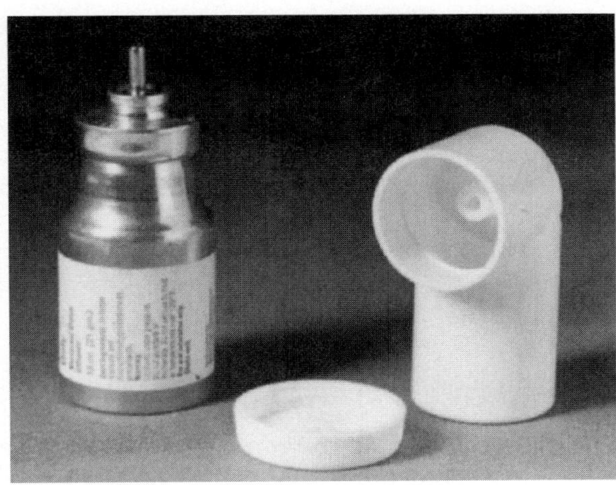

Fig. 15-5 Metered-dose inhaler with medication canister. (From Perry AG, Potter PA: *Clinical nursing skills and techniques,* ed 3, St Louis, 1994, Mosby.)

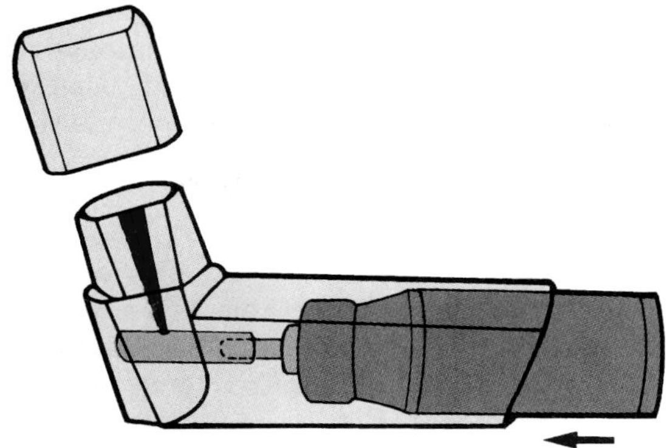

Fig. 15-6 Metered-dose inhaler is inserted into the end of the aerochamber. (From Perry AG, Potter PA: *Clinical nursing skills and techniques,* ed 3, St Louis, 1994, Mosby.)

cardiac dysarhythmias because of vagal nerve stimulation.

Administering Vaginal Medications

Medications placed within the vagina include creams and suppositories (Fig. 15-4). Medical asepsis is used because the vagina is not sterile. Vaginal medications are usually administered at bedtime, when the woman will be able to remain lying flat for several hours to retain the medication. Clean perineal pads should be available, especially when the woman is upright because gravity causes the medication to drain from the body, soiling clothing and bedding. Multiuse applicators used to insert the medication should be washed and dried thoroughly to prevent recontamination. Some newer vaginal medications come in prefilled, disposable applicators.

ADMINISTERING INHALED MEDICATIONS

Inhalants are medications designed to be inhaled. Types of inhalants include aerosol spray, mist, and fine powder. The medication may be quickly absorbed into the bloodstream in much the same manner as oxygen and carbon dioxide are exchanged through the alveolar-capillary network. Therefore adverse systemic effects can occur from some forms of medication if they are not appropriately prepared. Medications frequently administered by inhalation include antibiotics, bronchodialators, steroids, and expectorants.

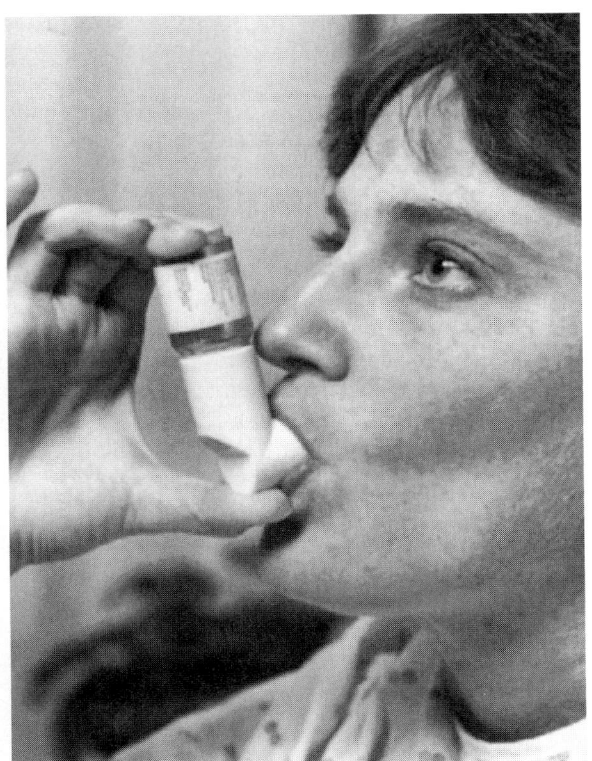

Fig. 15-7 Instruct patient to exhale fully and then grasp the mouthpiece with the teeth and lips while holding the inhaler with the thumb at the mouthpiece and the index finger and middle finger at the top. (From Perry AG, Potter PA: *Clinical nursing skills and techniques,* ed 3, St Louis, 1994, Mosby.)

Inhalant drugs are vaporized into fine particles when they are passed through a narrow channel under pressure. The finer the mist, the deeper the droplets pass into the respiratory system. Most hand-held inhalers provide relief in the upper respiratory tract (Fig. 15-5). Larger machines used by respiratory therapists mix oxygen or compressed air with medications and are used for reaching and treating the deeper structures of the respiratory tract.

Nursing care includes an evaluation of the patient's ability to manipulate and assemble an inhaler (Fig. 15-6). The patient must understand the appropriate use of the inhaler, frequency of use, and care of the equipment (Fig. 15-7). Assessment of the patient's knowledge and understanding of the respiratory problem is essential before the nurse develops a plan to instruct or reinforce teaching. The patient and the family should be involved in learning about the patient's care. Encouraging patient and family participation can increase self-confidence and self-esteem as well as prepare the family for home care.

ADMINISTERING PARENTERAL MEDICATIONS

Parenteral administration involves giving a medication by a route other than the gastrointestinal tract. The nurse should understand and use appropriate technique in preparing to administer parenteral medication (Skill 15-6). Parenteral medication includes all types of injections and intravenous infusions. When medication is administered by injection, the medicine reaches the bloodstream more quickly and is faster acting than with other methods.

Injections involve forcing a liquid into the body via a syringe. They are invasive procedures that cause more risk to the patient than oral medication administration. Risks include infection, allergic reaction, inflammation, abscess, and skin and nerve damage. The nurse must inject a needle at the required angle to administer medication into the appropriate tissue.

Parenteral Routes

The physician orders the route of administration, and the nurse determines the appropriate site of *injection.* The routes of parenteral administration are **intradermal** (into the dermis), **subcutaneous** (into the subcutaneous layer of skin), **intravenous** (into a vein), **intramuscular** (into a muscle). The nurse must assess the patient's general body build, such as thinness, obesity, and muscular structure, for signs of atrophy, flaccidity, or firmness to determine the site of injection. The age of the patient is also a determining factor.

Sites for intradermal injections

The most common site for intradermal (ID) injection is the inner surface of the forearm. When determining the site for ID injections, the nurse should avoid skin areas that are lightly pigmented or discolored and areas with lesions or hair.

Since the injection is given just below the epidermis with the needle bevel up, a small bleb (raised

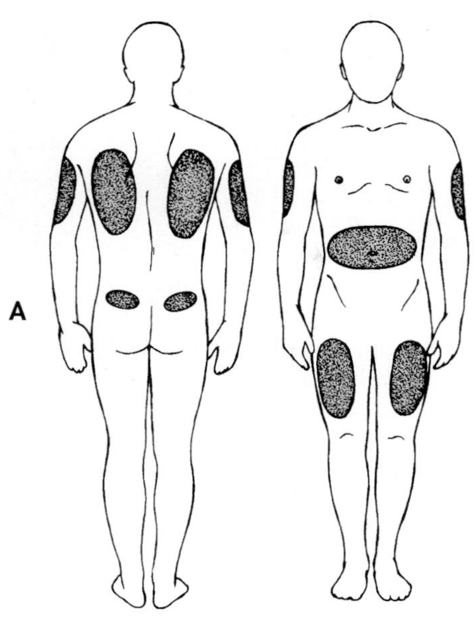

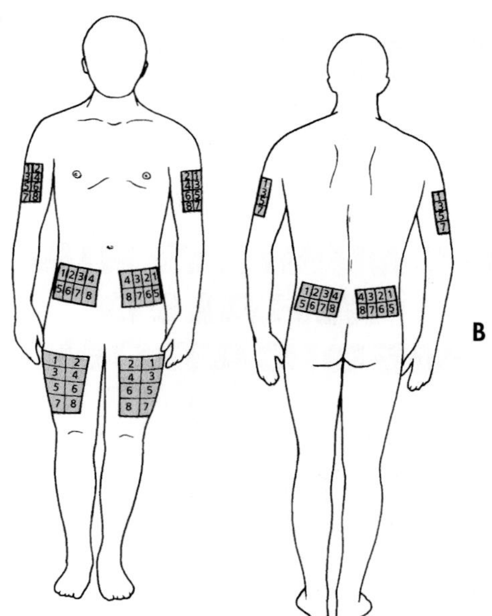

Fig. 15-8 **A,** Common sites for SQ injections. **B,** SQ injection site diagram. (From Perry AG, Potter PA: *Clinical nursing skills and techniques,* ed 3, St Louis, 1994, Mosby.)

area similar to a mosquito bite) should appear. If a bleb does not appear, the injection will be given too deep and result in an invalid test result. For special skin tests, such as allergy tests, the ID injection may be given on the upper chest or upper back. Using the inner aspect of the forearm provides easy access for the nurse to observe and record results at specific time intervals. Information such as location, time, and date is recorded and read at designated times.

Sites for subcutaneous injections

Subcutaneous (SQ) injections are given below the dermis. Common injection sites include the upper, outer surface of either arm; area below the costal margins to the iliac crest; anterior surface of either thigh; upper back; and umbilicus (Fig. 15-8). The nurse must not inject within 2 inches of the umbilicus, large areas of scar tissue, moles, or warts.

Most patients receiving regular SQ injections, such as diabetics, must have injection sites rotated. The sites are rotated to the arms, legs, buttocks, or other areas. Multiple sites in one area an inch apart are recommended because of the different rates of absorption of insulin.

Sites for intramuscular injections

The dorsogluteal muscle is the muscle most commonly used for intramuscular (IM) injections in the adult. As with all IM injections, special precautions are necessary to avoid damage to underlying structures, such as nerves and major blood vessels. With this particular location, the sciatic nerve must be avoided. Damage to the sciatic nerve can be painful and cause temporary or permanent paralysis of the affected leg.

To locate the dorsogluteal site, the nurse locates the postero superior iliac spine and the greater trochanter, draws an imaginary line between the two landmarks, and finds the site above and to the side of the line (upper outer quadrant) (Fig. 15-9).

A

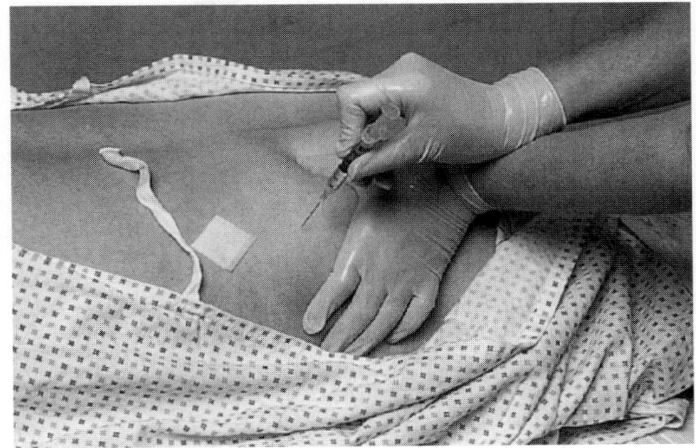

B

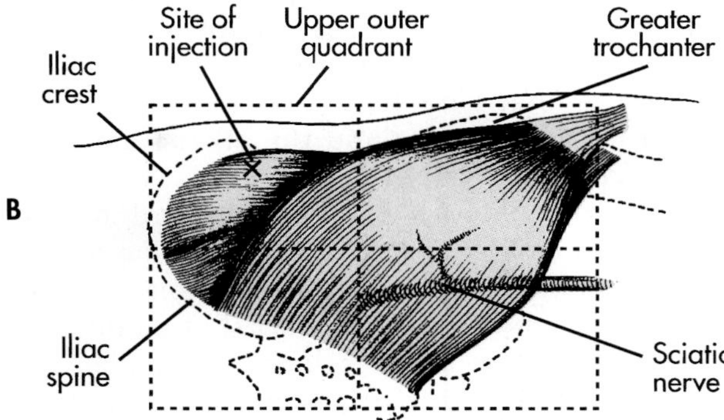

Fig. 15-9 **A,** Site of injection into the left dorsogluteal muscle. **B,** Imaginary diagonal line extending from the posterosuperior iliac spine to the greater trochanter is the landmark for selecting the dorsogluteal injection site. (From Perry AG, Potter PA: *Clinical nursing skills and techniques,* ed 3, St Louis, 1994, Mosby.)

A

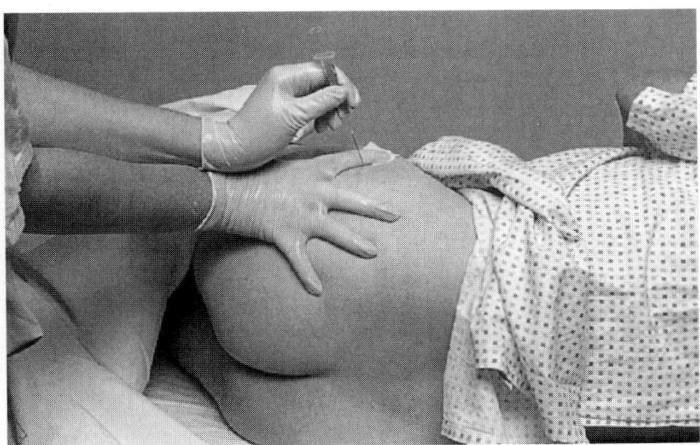

B

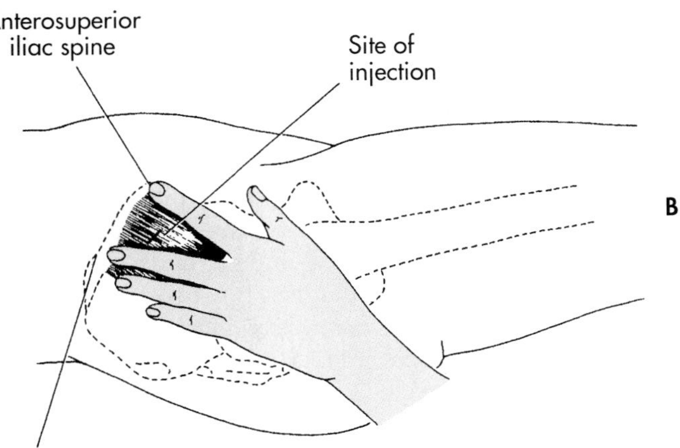

Fig. 15-10 **A,** Injection site for ventrogluteal muscle avoids major nerves and blood vessels. **B,** Anatomic view of the ventrogluteal muscle injection site. (From Perry AG, Potter PA: *Clinical nursing skills and techniques,* ed 3, St Louis, 1994, Mosby.)

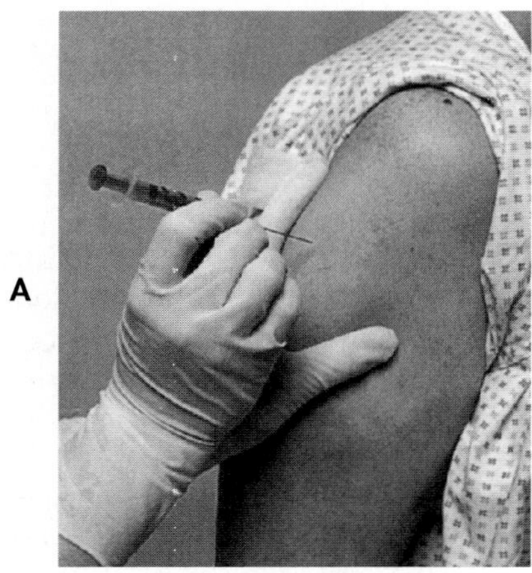

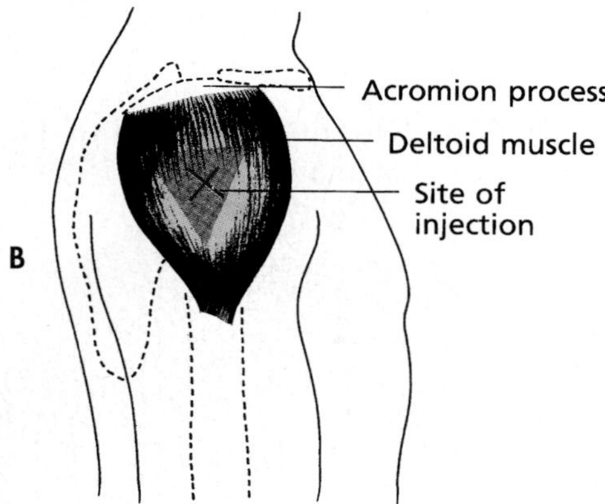

Fig. 15-11 **A,** Site of IM injection into the deltoid muscle. **B,** Site of deltoid muscle injection below the acromion process. (From Perry AG, Potter PA: *Clinical nursing skills and techniques,* ed 3, St Louis, 1994, Mosby.)

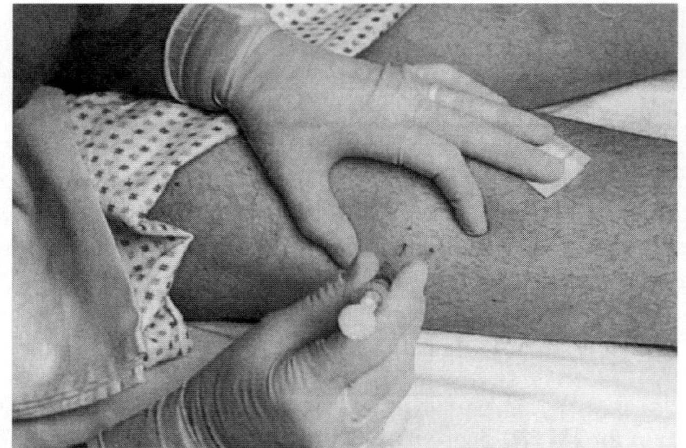

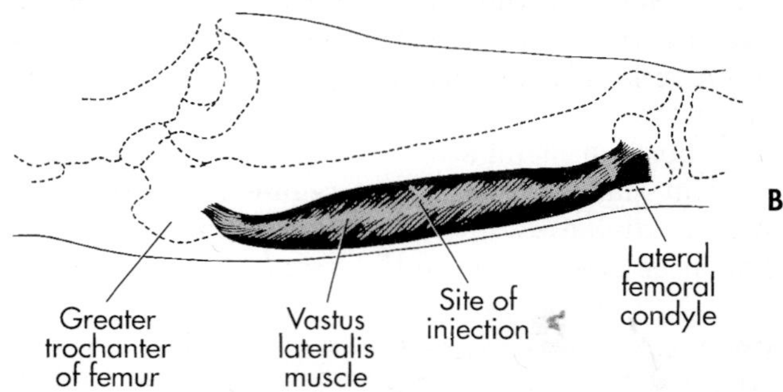

Fig. 15-12 **A,** Injection site for the vastus lateralis muscle. **B,** Anatomic view of the site for IM injection into vastus lateralis muscle. (From Perry AG, Potter PA: *Clinical nursing skills and techniques,* ed 3, St Louis, 1994, Mosby.)

The ventrogluteal muscle is located near the dorsogluteal muscle and involves the gluteus medius and minimus (Fig. 15-10).

To find the ventrogluteal muscle, the nurse places the palm of the hand over the patient's greater trochanter with the fingers toward the iliac crest, uses the right hand for the left hip and the left hand for the right hip, and places the index finger over the antero superior iliac spine and spreads the middle finger backward along the iliac crest toward the buttock. The index and middle fingers form a V. The ventrogluteal muscle is inside the V.

The deltoid muscle is located in the upper arm beginning approximately two fingers below the shoulder joint (acromion process) and forming a triangle with the point toward the elbow (Fig. 15-11). The injection should be given in the thickest part of the muscle. To locate the thickest part of the deltoid muscle, the nurse should locate the *acromion process,* visualize a triangle with the point toward the elbow, and place two fingers just below the acromion process. The injection site is in the bulk of the deltoid muscle.

The deltoid is small in many patients. It is recommended for injections of 1 ml or less.

The vastus lateralis muscle is located on the lateral anterior aspect of the thigh and extends a handbreadth above the knee and a handbreadth below the greater trochanter of the femur (Fig. 15-12).

To find the injection site, the nurse should place one hand above the knee and the other hand just below the greater trochanter.

The injection site is the middle third of the muscle. This is the preferred site of injection for infants and small children and is often specified by physicians. This is based on the fact that an infant's gluteal muscles are not developed until about 3 years of age for the dorsogluteal injection and that there is less danger of injury to the muscle.

Syringes and Needles

Syringes and needles are needed to administer SQ, IM, ID, and intravenous (IV) therapy. The

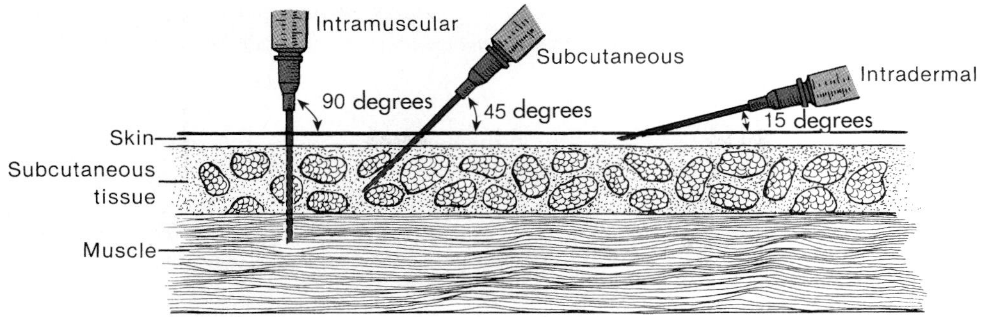

Fig. 15-13 Comparison of angles of insertion for injections: IM (90 degrees), SQ (45 degrees), and ID (15 degrees). (From Perry AG, Potter PA: *Clinical nursing skills and techniques,* ed 3, St Louis, 1994, Mosby.)

angles for injections are shown in (Fig. 15-13). A Z-track injection is a widely used method of administering an intramuscular injection.

Syringes

The parts of a syringe are a plastic or glass cylindrical barrel with a tip designed to fit snugly in the hub of a hypodermic needle. A close-fitting plunger is contained in the barrel of the syringe. Syringes are individually prepackaged in a sterile paper or rigid plastic container and may have a sterile needle attached.

To prevent contamination the nurse should touch only the outside of the syringe barrel and the protruding round disk end of the plunger. The inside of the barrel, shaft of the plunger, tip of the syringe, and needle should remain sterile.

Needles

Most needles are made of stainless steel. However, some are plastic, such as intravenous catheters. A needle has three parts: (1) the *hub,* which connects snugly onto the tip of the syringe; (2) the *shaft,* which is connected to the hub; and (3) the *bevel,* which is the slanted tip of the needle.

The only part of the needle that may be handled by the nurse without using sterile technique is the hub. The hub is usually held to support the needle while the injection is being administered. The shaft and the bevel of the needle should remain sterile. The term ***gauge*** is used to designate the diameter of a needle. The viscosity, or thickness, of the solution to be injected determines the selection of an appropriate gauge for an injection. A small needle gauge designates a large needle diameter.

The length of the needle varies from ¼ to 5 inches, with 1½ inches being the preferred length for IM injections to ensure injection into deep muscle mass (Fig. 15-14). The length of the needle to be used is determined by the nurse, who assesses the size and weight of the patient and the site and type of tissue to be injected. A site that is emaciated and contains little or no muscle mass or a site that is paralyzed may not be able to take a 1½ inch needle. A 1-inch needle may be used in this situation.

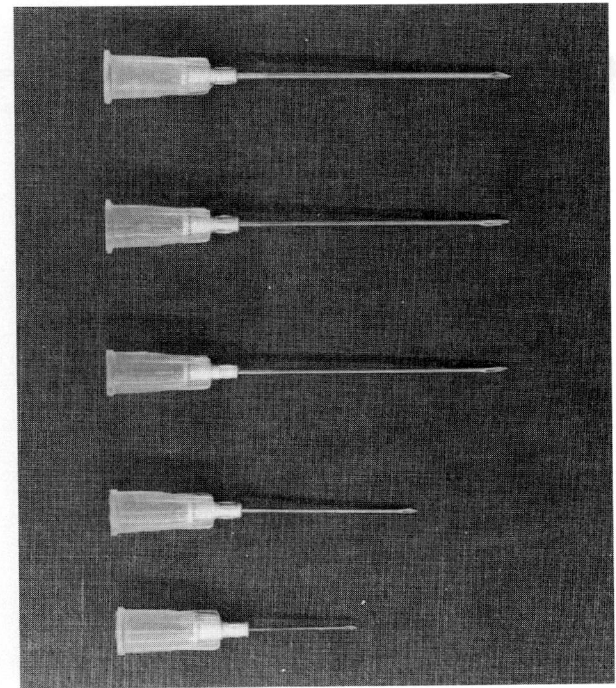

Fig. 15-14 Hypodermic needles arranged in order of gauge. *Top to bottom:* 16 gauge, 19 gauge, 20 gauge, 23 gauge, and 25 gauge. (From Perry AG, Potter PA: *Clinical nursing skills and techniques,* ed 3, St Louis, 1994, Mosby.)

Steps to follow in selecting the appropriate needle and syringe (Table 15-5):

1. Review the medical medication order
2. Determine route
3. Determine quantity of medication to be administered

Table 15-5 SELECTING APPROPRIATE EQUIPMENT

Type of Injection	Syringe Size	Needle Size
Insulin (SQ)	Specially provided 1-ml syringe with insulin unit calibrations: U50, U100 (sometimes correct needle is permanently fused to syringe)	½- to ⅝-inch length; 25, 26, 27 gauge
SQ	1, 2, or 3 ml with 0.1- or 0.2-ml calibrations	½- to ⅝-inch length; 23, 25, 26 gauge
ID	1 ml with 0.1- or 0.01-ml or minim calibrations	½- to ⅝-inch length; 25, 26, 27 gauge
IM	1, 2, 3, or 5 ml with 0.1- or 0.2-ml calibrations	1-, 1½-, or 2-inch length; 20, 21, 22, 23 gauge

Table 15-6 STEPS FOR FILLING A SYRINGE

Using Medication from a Vial	Using Medication from an Ampule
Assess medication and dose.	Assess medication and dose.
Remove metal cap from vial to expose rubber stopper.	Tap or shake any liquid from area above neck into bottom of ampule.
Clean rubber stopper with antiseptic swab.	Cover ampule neck with gauze or cotton square to protect fingers when glass neck breaks.
Fill syringe with air equal to amount of medicine to be withdrawn from vial.	Briskly snap glass top from ampule and discard it in sharps container.
Insert needle into center of rubber stopper.	Stabilize ampule and carefully insert needle into fluid without touching outside surface or rim of ampule.
Inject air into air space in vial to avoid injecting air bubbles into solution.	Maintaining needle tip in solution, draw back on plunger to withdraw medication into syringe.
Invert vial, and keeping needle tip in solution, draw back plunger to draw medication into syringe.	Remove filled syringe and hold with needle pointing up and syringe at eye level.
Without removing needle from vial, tap syringe to cause any air bubbles to rise to needle hub.	Tap syringe to cause any air bubbles to rise to needle hub.
Press gently on plunger to expel any air or excess medication back into vial.	Press gently on plunger to expel any air or excess medication from syringe.
Remove needle from vial and reassess medication label on vial before discarding.	Reassess medication label printed on ampule before discarding in puncture-resistant sharps container.
Replace protective sheath over needle carefully to prevent contamination.	Carefully replace protective sheath over needle to prevent contamination.

4. Determine the thickness (viscosity) of the solution
5. Assess the body size and build of the patient
6. Select injection site

After selecting the appropriate syringe and needle, the nurse needs to follow the appropriate steps to safely fill the syringe with the required medication (Table 15-6). Medications are supplied in ampules, single and multidose vials, and prefilled cartridges. Prefilled cartridges may be available with a permanently attached sterile needle. Some medications are available prefilled in their own self-contained syringe. The syringe is prepared for use by following the directions on the package label. Although these medications save time and are convenient, the nurse is the person responsible for ensuring that the patient receives the correct medication and dose. By always following standard nursing procedure and assessing the medication label *3 times* for medication name, dose, and recommended route, the nurse minimizes the possibility of a medication error (Table 15-7).

Needles are discarded in an appropriate "sharps" container, and syringes are not recapped after use. These measures help protect the nurse from needle punctures.

Table 15-7 WAYS TO PREVENT DRUG ADMINISTRATION ERRORS

Precaution	Rationale	Precaution	Rationale
Read drug labels carefully.	Many products come in similar containers, colors, and shapes.	When new or unfamiliar drug is ordered, consult resource.	If physician is also unfamiliar with drug, there is greater risk of inaccurate dosages being ordered.
Question administration of multiple tablets or vials for single dose. Be aware of drugs with similar names. Check decimal point. Question abrupt and excessive increases in dosages.	Most doses are one or two tablets or capsules or one single-dose vial. Incorrect interpretation of order may result in excessively high dose. Many drug names sound alike (for example, digoxin and digitoxin, Keflex and Keflin, Orinase and Ornade). Some drugs come in quantities that are multiples of one another (for example, Coumadin in 2.5- and 25-mg tablets, Thorazine in 30 and 300 mg spansules). Most dosages are increased gradually so that physician can monitor therapeutic effect and response.	Do not administer drug ordered by nickname or unofficial abbreviation. Do not attempt to decipher illegible writing. Know patients with same last names. Also have patients state their full names. Check name bands carefully. Do not confuse equivalents.	Many physicians refer to commonly ordered medications by nicknames or unofficial abbreviations. If nurse or pharmacist is unfamiliar with name, wrong drug may be dispensed and administered. When in doubt, ask physician. Unless nurse questions order that is difficult to read, chance of misinterpretation is great. It is common to have two or more patients with same or similar last names. Special labels on Kardex or medication book can warn of potential problem. When in hurry, it may be easy to misread equivalents (for example, milligram instead of milliliter).

From Potter PA, Perry AG: *Fundamentals of nursing: concept, process, and practice,* ed 3, St Louis, 1993, Mosby.

Injection Containers

Two types of containers are used in withdrawing solutions for injections. Each requires special technique to withdraw medication with a needle and syringe. The two common types of containers are ampules and vials (Fig. 15-15).

Ampule

An **ampule** is a glass container with a narrow neck. It usually contains a single dose of medication. It may contain from 1 to 10 ml of medication. The top of an ampule must be broken off so that the medication can be withdrawn. The nurse must use caution to avoid cutting the fingers when working with an ampule. When the sharp-edged pieces of an ampule are discarded, they should be placed in a puncture-resistant sharps container and not in the trash container in the patient's room. The sharps

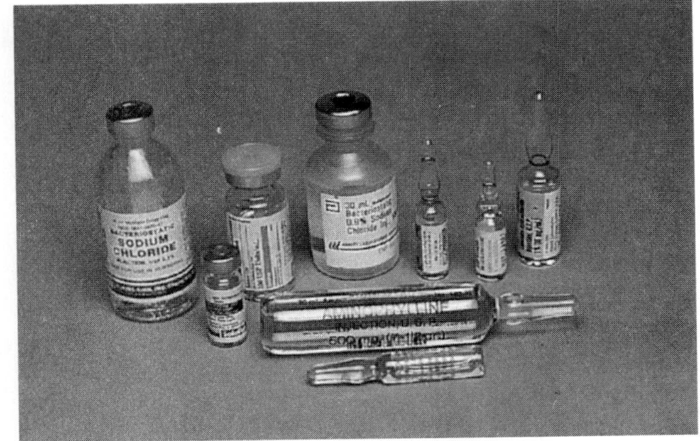

Fig. 15-15 Ampules and vials. (From Perry AG, Potter PA: *Clinical nursing skills and techniques,* ed 3, St Louis, 1994, Mosby.)

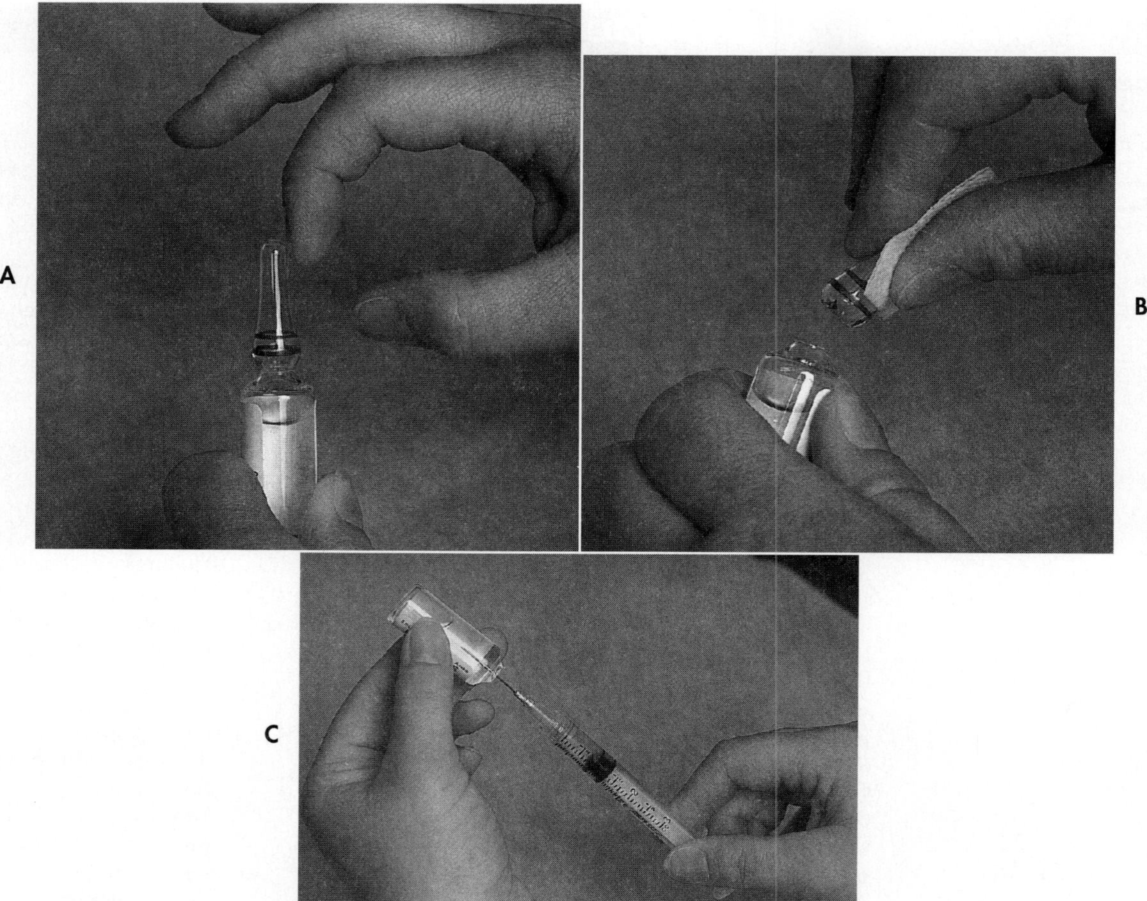

Fig. 15-16 **A,** Tap the top of the ampule to move the solution from the top of the ampule to the bottom of the ampule. **B,** Cover the neck of the ampule with an alcohol sponge. Break off the top of the ampule. Deposit the top of the glass ampule in the sharps container. **C,** Inject diluent into the vial of powdered drug. Gently shake and tap the vial to dissolve the powder into the solution. (From Christensen BL, Kockrow EO: *Foundations of nursing,* ed 2, St Louis, 1995, Mosby.)

container is usually conveniently located on the wall in the room.

Vial

A **vial** is a glass or plastic container that contains single doses or multidoses of medication. It may contain 1 to 50 ml of medication. The top of the vial is sealed with a metal cap that must be removed for use. Under the metal cap is a rubber stopper that must be cleaned with an alcohol swab before the medication is withdrawn. A needle is inserted into the center of the rubber stopper to withdraw medication.

Withdrawal of medications from ampules and vials

There is a difference between withdrawing medication from an ampule and doing so from a vial. The nurse should remember the following points:

1. When medication is withdrawn from an ampule, there is no need to inject air into the ampule. There is no vacuum in the ampule (Fig. 15-16).
2. When medication is withdrawn from a vial, air is injected into the vial to draw out its contents because there is a vacuum. The nurse should inject the same amount of air into the vial as the amount of medication to be withdrawn from the vial (Fig. 15-17).

Reconstituting a Powdered Medication

Although many injectable medications come in liquid form, some are supplied as a powder in a sterile vial and must be reconstituted before administering. It is important for the nurse to read the label to know what **diluent** (liquid used to dissolve a powder) is required. Common diluents are sterile normal saline or sterile water, which are

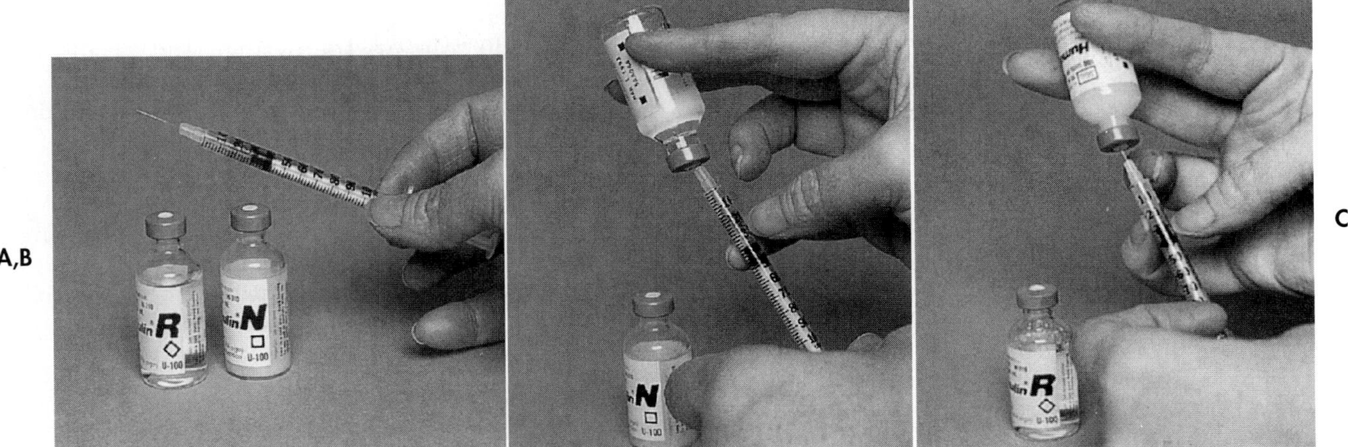

Fig. 15-17 **A,** Take the insulin syringe and aspirate the volume of air equivalent to the dose to be withdrawn from the modified insulin (cloudy vial). **B,** Insert the needle into the vial of the unmodified regular insulin (clear vial), inject air, and then fill the syringe with the proper regular insulin dose. **C,** Insert the needle into the vial of modified insulin (cloudy vial). Be careful not to push the plunger and expel the medication into the vial. Invert the vial and carefully withdraw the desired amount of insulin into the syringe. (From Perry AG, Potter PA: *Clinical nursing skills and techniques,* ed 3, St Louis, 1994, Mosby.)

usually available with unit stock medications. Sometimes the pharmacy dispenses the appropriate diluent along with the medication vial containing the powdered medication. The nurse must read the label carefully to determine the amount and type of diluent to use. If the reconstituted medication vial holds more than one dose, the nurse is required to waste the rest of the medication unless administered in a given time. The information on the label helps the nurse avoid medication errors caused by using a medication past its expiration date.

When drawing up the diluent, the nurse follows the steps for filling a syringe and then removes the metal cap from the vial containing the powder, cleans the rubber cap with an antiseptic swab, inserts the needle through the rubber stopper, and injects the diluent into the vial. The vial is gently rotated or rolled between the nurse's hands to help the powder become completely dissolved. The vial should not be shaken vigorously because this produces air bubbles within the medication that may alter the volume of medication when it is drawn into a syringe. The warmth of the nurse's hands and the gentle rotation of the vial should produce a transparent liquid with no observable particles in the vial. Medication should not be used if it is not clear. The liquid volume of reconstituted medication in the vial is greater than the amount of injected diluent but is still considered the required dose. The medication may then be prepared for administration to the patient.

Mixing Compatible Medications

An important aspect of mixing two medications in one syringe is to ensure that the drugs are compatible. A drug compatibility chart may be available in the nursing unit, but if in doubt, the nurse may always consult the pharmacist. Some medications form a precipitate when mixed together and must not be used for parenteral administration. A **precipitate** is a substance that has separated from or settled out of a solution. Expensive medications may be wasted and time lost when questions of compatability are not assessed before mixing.

The method for mixing compatible medications varies depending on the containers in which they are packaged. The same principles and aseptic techniques are followed as in filling a syringe from a vial or an ampule. The sequencing (timing of air injection into containers and container to withdraw from first) varies. By adhering to the following sequencing guidelines, the nurse prevents contamination of medications and helps prevent medication errors:

Sequence for mixing from a single-dose vial and an ampule:

1. Following the steps for filling a syringe from a vial, withdraw the desired volume of medication from the vial first.
2. Following the steps for filling a syringe from an ampule, carefully withdraw the required volume of medication from the ampule.

Sequence for mixing from a multidose vial and an ampule:

1. Following the steps for filling a syringe from a vial, withdraw the desired volume of medication from the vial first.
2. Following the steps for filling a syringe from an ampule, carefully withdraw the required volume of medication from the ampule.

Sequence for mixing from a single-dose vial and a multidose vial (Fig. 15-18).

1. Fill the syringe with air equal to the amount of medication required from vial A.
2. Inject vial A with air, being careful not to let the needle touch the solution.
3. Withdraw the empty syringe and fill it with air equal to the amount of medication to be withdrawn from vial B.
4. Inject the air into vial B and withdraw the required medication from vial B into the syringe.
5. Remove the needle from vial B.
6. Apply a new sterile needle onto the syringe and carefully insert it into vial A, being careful not to expel any medicine from the syringe into vial A.
7. Carefully withdraw the desired amount of medicine from vial A.
8. Carefully remove the syringe and needle from vial A.
9. Apply a new sterile needle and reassess all doses and vial labels.

Sequence for mixing from two multidose vials:

1. Follow the sequencing for mixing from a single-dose vial and a multidose vial.
2. Mentally label the vials "A" and "B" and follow the previous steps.

Changing a Needle

Sometimes it is necessary to change the needle on a syringe. If the needle becomes contaminated, it must be changed before another injection is administered to the patient. Accidentally dropping a filled syringe or inadvertantly allowing the needle to touch anything causes it to become contaminated. If the nurse has the slightest suspicion that the needle may have brushed against something, no matter how lightly, it is considered contaminated and must be changed. Needles also need to be changed when

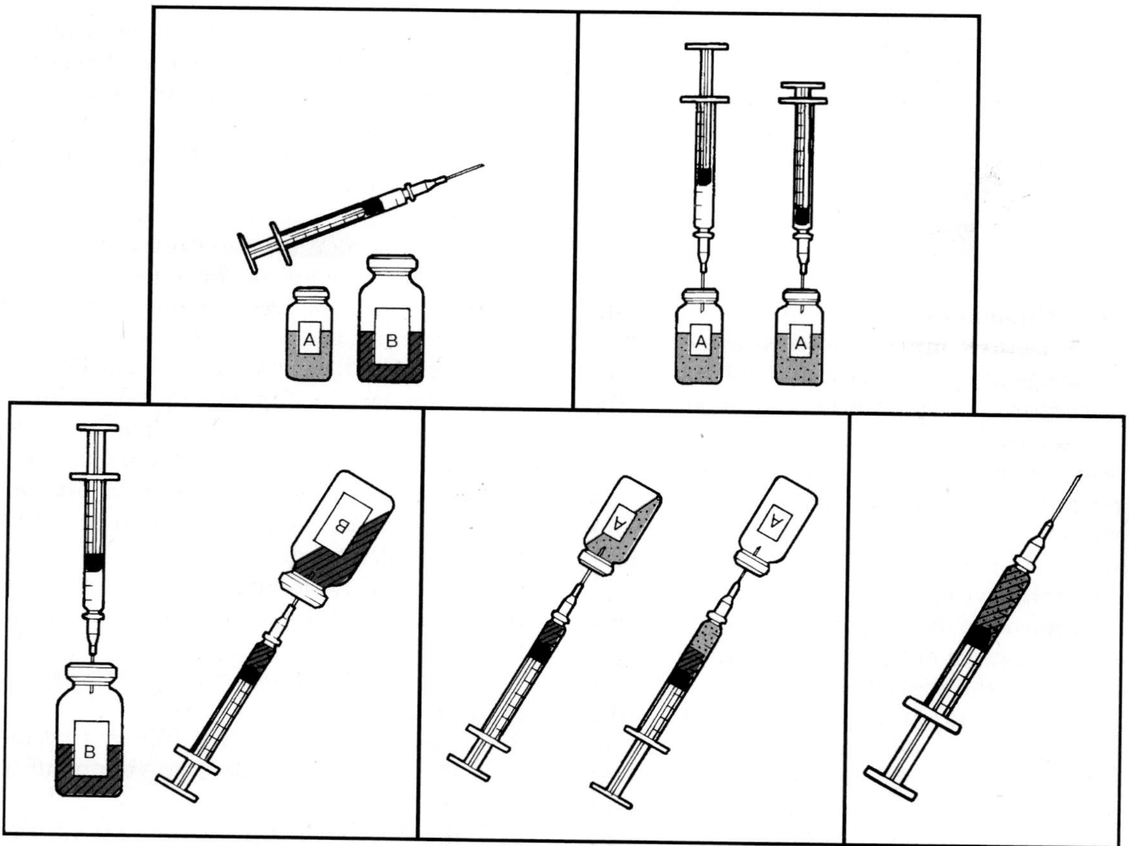

Fig. 15-18 Steps in mixing medications from two vials. (From Perry AG, Potter PA: *Clinical nursing skills and techniques,* ed 3, St Louis, 1994, Mosby.)

mixing various medications to avoid cross-contamination of the medication within the container. When drawing up medications that may be irritating to the tissues (for example, injectable iron medications), the nurse changes the needle to prevent the medication on the outside of the needle from irritating the patient at the injection site or from staining tissues. The steps for changing a needle follow:

1. Select another appropriate aseptic needle of the same size and gauge.
2. Break the seal to ensure sterility of the contents.
3. Hold syringe carefully by the barrel in the non-dominant hand.
4. Remove the contaminated needle, place it in the sharps container, and hold medication to prevent spillage.
5. Handle new sterile needle by the needle sheath and place it on the syringe.
6. Push and twist the needle and syringe together at the hub.

Administration Techniques

Preparation for giving parenteral medications includes comparison of the medical medication order, washing of the hands, aseptic filling of the syringe according to procedure, explanation of the procedure to the patient, assistance of the patient to a position of comfort, selection of the injection site, and appropriate cleansing of the site. It is also expected that appropriate disposal of contaminated equipment, handwashing, and prompt and accurate documentation follow injection administration.

Z-track injection method

Another technique used to administer IM medication is the **Z-track method.** This method works well with drugs that are irritating to the tissues such as iron preparations or hydroxyzine (Vistaril). A Z-track injection seals the medication within the muscle and prevents it from escaping out of the needle-insertion track. Larger, deeper muscles such as the dorsogluteal or ventrogluteal muscles are the sites of choice for Z-track administration. Because of the extremely irritating nature of these medications, it is best to replace the needle used to fill the syringe with a new, sterile needle for injecting the medication. After checking the dosage in the filled syringe for accuracy, the nurse draws 0.2 to 0.5 ml of air into the tip of the syringe, depending on the amount of air needed. This "airlock" ensures that all the medication passes through the shaft of the needle into the muscle. After appropriate cleansing of the site, the nurse, using the nondominant hand, pulls the skin and subcutaneous tissues laterally (to the side) about 1 to 1½ inches (2.5 to 3.5 cm). Maintaining the skin taut (pulled tight) with the nondominant hand, the nurse quickly darts the needle into the muscle at a 90-degree angle. By holding the syringe like a dart, the barrel held by the fingers of the hand with the thumb at the plunger, the nurse can "walk up" the syringe, place the index and middle finger around the barrel, and aspirate and administer the medication. The nondominant hand must maintain the lateral pull on the tissue. After ensuring that the needle is not in a blood vessel, the nurse uses the thumb to slowly inject the medication into the muscle. Allowing the needle to remain in the muscle for 10 seconds before removal allows the medicine to be dispersed within the muscle. After withdrawing the needle quickly, the nurse releases the skin and applies pressure for 30 seconds with an antiseptic wipe. The skin springs back to its normal position, leaving a zig-zag path that seals the needle track, effectively preventing the escape of the medication from the muscle tissue.

Intravenous medications

Medications that are administered directly into the circulatory system are effective immediately. Because there is little time to counteract any dangerous effects of these drugs, nurses who are permitted to administer them have had special training. Not all nurses are expected or required to administer IV medications. State nurse practice acts determine the legal guidelines, and agency policies further define the qualifications of nurses allowed to give medications through the IV route. The nurse must know and practice within the legal and agency guidelines.

An existing IV access must be available for the administration of IV medication. This may be activated through a port on a primary IV infusion (also called *piggyback*), the primary IV infusion itself, or a heparin or saline lock. Medications are administered intermittently or continuously according to the medical order. The rate of both the IV solution and the medication administration are usually regulated through an infusion pump (Fig. 15-19) to ensure that the correct, prescribed amount is delivered accurately. Newer connection equipment is available to provide greater safety to both patients and nurses.

Diluting medications in large volumes of IV solutions (500 to 1000 ml) is safest and easiest because of the low concentration of medication infused over a longer time. Potassium chloride and vitamins are examples of medications frequently added to IV solutions. The medical order specifies which type of IV solution is to be used, and the person adding any

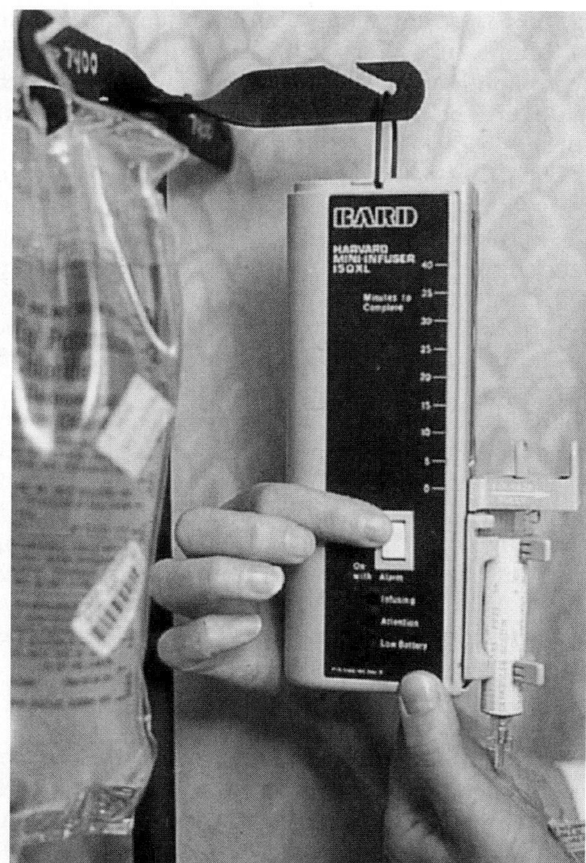

Fig. 15-19 Hang the infusion pump with the syringe on the IV pole along the main IV bag. Press the button on the pump to begin infusion. (From Perry AG, Potter PA: *Clinical nursing skills and techniques,* ed 3, St Louis, 1994, Mosby.)

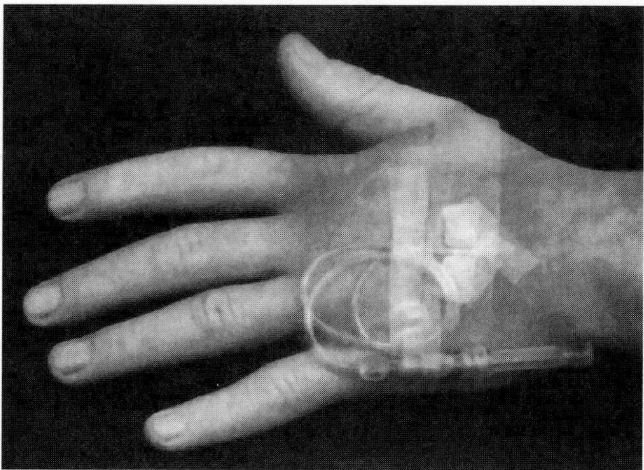

Fig. 15-20 Butterfly, scalp, or wing-tipped needle in place as a heparin lock. (From Christensen BL, Kockrow EO: *Foundations of nursing,* ed 2, St Louis, 1995, Mosby.)

medication must assess for any possible incompatabilities between the solution and the medication. The nurse may be required to add medication to an IV fluid container. However, in many institutions, the primary responsibility for mixing IV medications belongs to the pharmacist. The solution container is then labeled with the name of the medication, the dose added to the container, the time and date the medication was added, the initials of the person who added the medication, the patient's name, and the name of the person who wrote the medical medication order. The nurse who administers the medicated IV solution has the responsibility to follow the five rights of medication administration. If there is any question about the medicated solution, the nurse has the right and responsibility to clarify the medical order or resolve questions concerning the solution before administration.

A **piggyback** infusion involves the administration of medication that has been diluted in a 50- or 100-ml bag of a compatible solution attached to a short tubing line and joined to the primary IV infusion through an IV tubing port (hence the term *piggyback*). The medication bag is hung higher than the primary IV line so that gravity enables the medication to run through the primary tubing into the patient. Medications administered by the piggyback method are regulated by an infusion pump to ensure accurate infusion. An advantage of administering medication by the piggyback method is that the medication can be discontinued without affecting the primary IV infusion, therefore maintaining access to the patient's circulatory system for administration of an antidote or emergency medication.

Volume-control infusion devices can be used to piggyback medications or accurately control the volume administration during IV therapy. Both piggyback and volume-control devices allow the control of fluid volume intake and administration of medications over a limited or specific time frame. The nurse must be familiar with different types of equipment and their setup, maintenance, and disposal to provide accurate, safe IV medication administration.

A third method of administering IV medications is through a heparin lock device (Fig. 15-20). For patients who do not require the continuous administration of IV fluids, this device provides the needed access for administration of IV medications at regular intervals. The heparin lock eliminates the need to repeatedly puncture the patient, and the patient has more freedom of movement than when attached to a continuous IV administration setup. The procedure is now referred to in many areas as a *saline lock.* The nurse may use a syringe to inject medica-

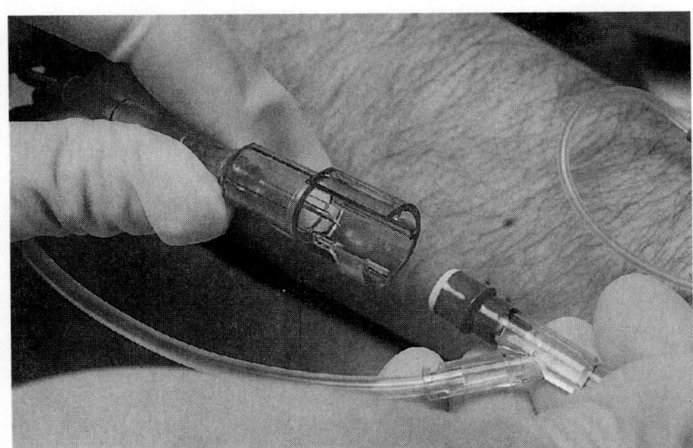

Fig. 15-21 Use needle-lock device to secure the needle of a secondary piggyback line through the injection port of the main line. (From Potter PA, Perry AG: *Basic nursing: theory and practice,* ed 3, St Louis, 1995, Mosby.)

tions directly into the heparin lock. Medication "pushed" should never be injected too fast. The necessary time allowed for administering medication by this method depends on the type and amount of medication being injected. The nurse should carefully read the medication container insert for directions for use. A standard rule is not to exceed 1 ml/min. A watch with a second hand should be used to time the administration of "push" medications.

A needleless device may also be used to administer medication (Fig. 15-21). The use of this device reduces the risk of needlestick injury to the nurse.

Because certain medications are irritating to the blood vessels, they must be diluted before infusing. In this case a small bag (50, 100, or 250 ml) of fluid in which the ordered medication has been diluted is piggybacked into the heparin lock for a short time while the medication is infused. After infusion of the medication, the tubing is unattached from the heparin lock and appropriately guarded for the next medication dose or discarded according to agency policy.

Care of a heparin lock device usually involves periodic flushing to ensure that it is **patent** (open and unblocked) and free of clots. Agency policy dictates the appropriate interval and solution for flushing. There are also agency guidelines for the periodic changing of IV access equipment and sites. Nurses who are qualified and approved to work with IV lines are required to know and observe agency policies concerning these procedures.

Certain general guidelines are to be followed by those administering IV medications. Before administering any IV medication, the nurse should compare the medical order with the medication to be administered. If there is any question of compatibility, a compatibility chart or the pharmacist should be consulted. The medication should be prepared using aseptic technique and the syringe filled with the appropriate dose.

The nurse should be able to perform the following procedures:

Adding medication to a bag of solution:
1. Cleanse the port site of the bag with an antiseptic wipe.
2. Carefully insert the needle into the middle of the cleansed port.
3. Inject the medication into the bag.
4. Remove the needle and discard it immediately in a sharps container.
5. Gently rotate the bag of medicated solution to mix well. (Do not shake the bag because this causes small air bubbles to be trapped within the solution.)
6. Hang the bag at the appropriate time and adjust the flow pump to administer the medication at the appropriate rate.

Adding medication to a volume-flow regulator:
1. Allow the correct volume of solution to flow into the volume-control chamber from the primary solution bag.
2. Cleanse the port on the top of the volume control chamber with an alcohol swab.
3. Carefully insert the needle of the medication-filled syringe into the center of the port.
4. Inject the medication into the volume-container fluid.
5. Remove the needle from the port and discard it in the sharps container.
6. Adjust the flow control to administer the medication at the appropriate rate.

Hanging a piggyback medication bag:
1. Assess whether the patient has a primary IV line or a heparin lock.
2. Assess whether there is appropriate tubing at the patient's bedside. (If not, issue appropriate tubing to the patient.)
3. Attach the tubing to the piggyback bag and slowly open the flow valve to flush the tubing to remove any air bubbles.
4. Close the flow valve of the piggyback tubing.

With a primary IV line:
1. Assess the site for infiltration, irritation, and patency.
2. Select the port on the primary tubing and cleanse it with an alcohol swab.
3. Hang the piggyback bag higher than the primary

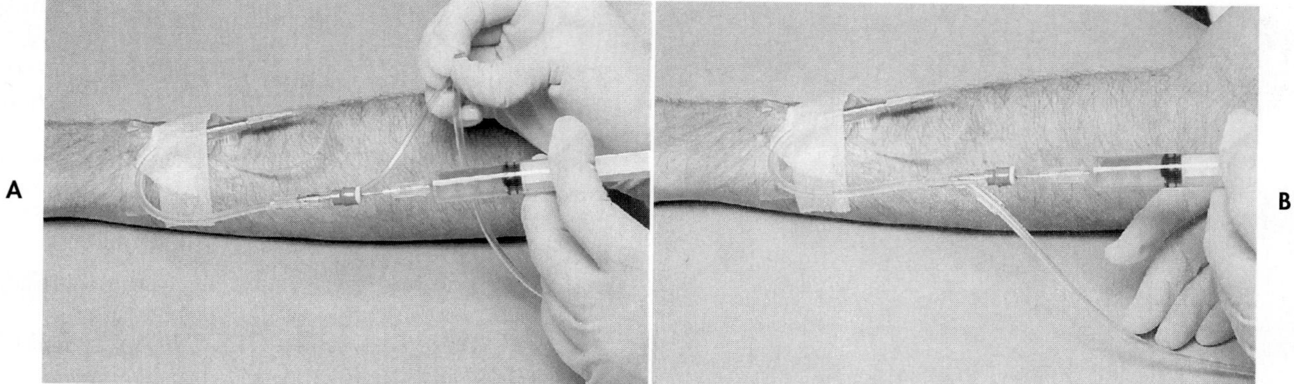

Fig. 15-22 **A,** Occlude the IV line by pinching the tubing just above the injection port. Pull back gently on the syringe's plunger to aspirate for blood return. **B,** After noting blood return, inject the medication slowly over several minutes. (Read directions on drug package.) Use a watch to time administrations. (From Potter PA, Perry AG: *Fundamentals of nursing: concepts, process, and practice,* ed 3, St Louis, 1993, Mosby.)

IV bag to allow gravity to assist the flow through the tubing.

4. Insert the needle, or nonneedle end of the piggyback tubing, into the port and secure it using agency guidelines.
5. Open the flow valve of the piggyback bag and adjust the flow control to administer the appropriate dose.

With a heparin lock:

1. Assess the site for swelling, bruising, and redness.
2. Cleanse the port with an alcohol swab.
3. Insert a sterile needle and syringe into the port.
4. Aspirate for a blood return into the heparin lock tubing to ensure that the device remains in the vein.
5. Remove the syringe and needle and discard them immediately in the sharps container.
6. Recleanse the port with another alcohol swab, attach the needle or nonneedle end of the piggyback tubing into the port, and secure it following agency guidelines.
7. Open the flow valve of the piggyback bag and adjust the flow control to administer the appropriate dose.
8. After the piggyback medication has infused, follow agency guidelines for guarding or discarding the piggyback bag, tubing, and needle.
9. Follow agency guidelines for flushing a heparin lock after medication administration.

Flushing a heparin or saline lock

There is controversy concerning whether sterile saline solution or a dilute heparin flush solution is best for assessing placement and patency of heparin lock devices. Some agencies use a combination of both solutions. Using a heparin solution was thought to prevent blood clotting, but recent research has indicated that a saline solution may provide the same effect. Broad guidelines follow, but nurses who are qualified to flush a heparin lock must follow agency policy for the frequency, solution, and procedure guidelines:

1. Wash hands.
2. Assemble equipment.
3. Explain procedure to patient.
4. Assess site for redness and swelling.
5. Cleanse the port and insert the needle containing the flush solution.
6. Aspirate for blood return.
7. Flush per agency policy.
8. If a second syringe must be used, cleanse the port each time.
9. Discard equipment into appropriate containers.
10. Document promptly and accurately.

IV push

The qualified nurse may be required to give medications directly into the vein through an existing IV or heparin lock device. This procedure is not without risk because a concentrated dose of a drug immediately enters the circulatory system, leaving no time to correct for adverse effects. Most agency policies specifically indicate which drugs and what doses may be administered by the nurse. Sometimes during emergencies, a nurse is asked to give medications in dosages and by routes that exceed legal parameters. The nurse should not practice beyond the law. A safe alternative is to provide the correct medication and syringe to someone who has the legal qualifications to administer the medication. Guidelines for push medications follow:

1. Follow the five rights of medication administration.

2. Use aseptic technique.
3. Cleanse the port of the IV tubing or heparin lock.
4. Insert the needle into the center of the port. (Occlude or pinch off the primary IV tubing to ensure that the medication is delivered into the vein and is not backing up into the IV tubing [Fig. 15-22].)
5. Aspirate to determine the patency and placement of medication into bloodstream.
6. Inject medication slowly (according to drug package directions), not exceeding 1 ml/min.
7. Use a watch with a second hand to time the injection.
8. Inject all the medication.
9. Release the pinched IV tubing before withdrawing the syringe.
10. Withdraw the syringe and needle and discard them immediately in the sharps container (Fig. 15-23).
11. Reassess IV infusion rate or flush heparin lock if indicated per agency policy.
12. Wash hands.
13. Document promptly and accurately.

Infusion pumps

An **infusion** is the introduction of a substance directly into a vein or insterstitially (between tissues) by means of gravity flow.

Infusion pumps are mechanical devices that regulate the flow of fluids. Usually used to control IV fluid infusion rates, these pumps may also control tube feeding infusions. Each manufacturer's pump may vary slightly, but the basic function is to provide a programmed rate of infusion. Some pumps have an electronic eye that monitors and counts the number of drops, whereas others provide a pulsating mechanism against the tubing to propel the fluid forward through the tubing at appropriate intervals. Each agency provides instruction for using their pumps.

Patient-controlled analgesia

Special mechanical devices allow patients to administer pain medication to themselves. This is **patient-controlled analgesia (PCA).** The nurse or pharmacist is responsible for preparing the medication. However, the nurse is responsible for assessing the medication and programming the PCA pump to deliver the accurate amount into the patient's IV line according to the medical order. Since most medications administered by PCA pumps are controlled substances, they are accounted for according to strict procedures.

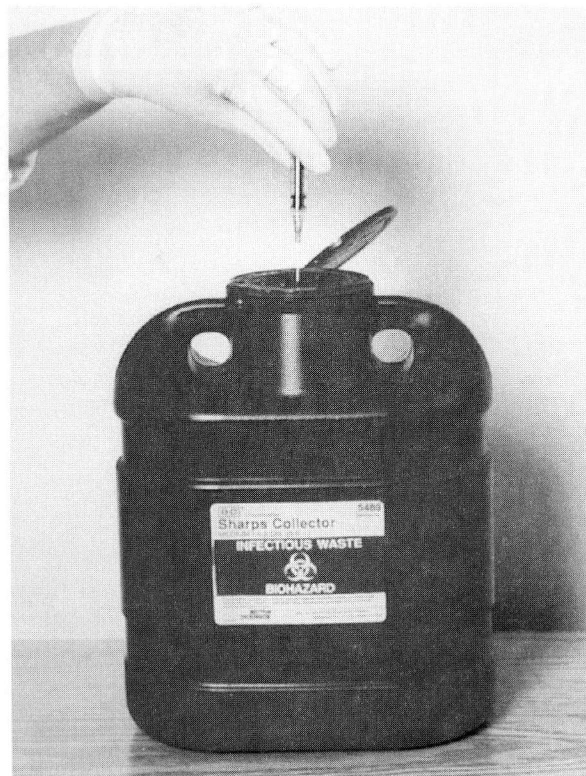

Fig. 15-23 Special sharps containers are available in nursing units for disposal of contaminated syringes. (From Potter PA, Perry AG: *Basic nursing: theory and practice,* ed 3, St Louis, 1995, Mosby.)

The frequency rate, designated by the medical order, is programmed to prevent the disoriented patient from causing an overdose. The programming functions of the pump are protected by a locked door to prevent unauthorized persons from changing the dose or interval. Keys to these PCA pumps are guarded per agency policy. Any unused portion of medication must be discarded following legal guidelines.

The patient may receive small frequent doses of medication by pushing a button. The medication is released at a programmed dose and time. Small, frequent doses help the patient avoid some of the negative side effects that may be caused by infrequently administered, larger doses. The button releases the programmed dose into the patient's IV line, ensuring adequate, prompt pain control. Because the patient is able to control pain before it becomes severe, anxiety decreases, and many patients require less medication.

■ NURSING CARE PLAN ■

IMPAIRED SWALLOWING

Mrs. R, age 76, has been admitted with difficulty swallowing.

NURSING DIAGNOSIS

Impaired swallowing related to neuromuscular impairment as evidenced by difficulty swallowing food and medications, choking, and aspiration

GOAL

- Patient will swallow liquid medication or powdered medication in soft foods in 48 hr.

EXPECTED OUTCOMES

- Patient complies with treatment regimen.
- Patient can swallow powdered medication in soft foods.

NURSING INTERVENTIONS

- Elevate head of bed 90 degrees for meals and for taking medications to decrease risk of aspiration.
- Crush medications with mortar and pestle to help patient swallow medications.
- Assure patient someone will remain in attendance during meals and while taking medications to reduce fear of choking.

EVALUATION

- Patient does not aspirate.
- Patient takes medications in compliance with treatment regimen.
- Patient is no longer fearful about taking medications.

SKILL 15-1 ADMINISTERING ORAL MEDICATIONS

Steps	Rationale
1. Obtain equipment: ▪ Medication profile ▪ Portion cup ▪ Liquid medication cup ▪ Unit-dose medications ▪ Bottles of medication	Helps organize procedure.
2. Compare medical order with medication profile for all medications for accuracy.	Determines medication, dose, route, and times to be administered.
3. Wash hands before preparing medications.	Helps prevent cross-contamination.
4. Prepare medications for one patient at a time while comparing medical order with medication profile:	Helps prevent medication errors.
a. Take one unit-dose medication or one tablet out of medication bottle at a time from patient's drawer and compare label with medication profile. Place dose in portion cup without opening package until in patient's room.	Decreases risk for making medication error. Allows medication to be placed back in system if not contaminated by being opened.
b. Pour tablets and capsules from multidose container into portion cup without touching medication.	Avoids contamination from touching medications.
c. Hold liquid medication bottle with palm against label to pour into appropriate liquid medication cup. Read dose at eye level. Read amount of liquid at bottom of meniscus (curved upper surface of a liquid column) (Fig. 15-24).	Prevents label from being obscured from damage caused by spilled liquid medication, which may result in medication error. Prevents dosage error.

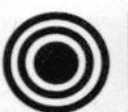

SKILL 15-1 ADMINISTERING ORAL MEDICATIONS—cont'd

Steps	Rationale
5. Assess by reading container a third time when returning medication bottle to storage.	Concludes checking medication 3 times. If error was made, nurse has last chance to catch and correct it.
6. Take patient's medications to correct room.	Prevents administration to wrong patient in wrong room.
7. Introduce self.	Decreases patient's anxiety level.
8. Identify patient by identification band.	Identifies correct patient for procedure.
9. Explain procedure to patient.	Seeks cooperation and decreases anxiety.
10. Wash hands.	Helps prevent cross-contamination.
11. Raise bed to comfortable working level.	Provides safety for nurse.
12. Arrange for patient privacy.	Shows respect for patient.
13. Assist patient to sit up in bed to take medications, unless contraindicated.	Prevents choking when patient is attempting to swallow medications.
14. Assist patient to take medications, allowing patient preference as much as possible. Encourage patient to drink plenty of water.	Allows patient some control over taking medications.
15. Remain at bedside until all medications are swallowed.	Prevents patient from removing medication from mouth or storing medications.
16. Wash hands.	Helps prevent cross-contamination.
17. Document.	Documents procedure and patient's response.

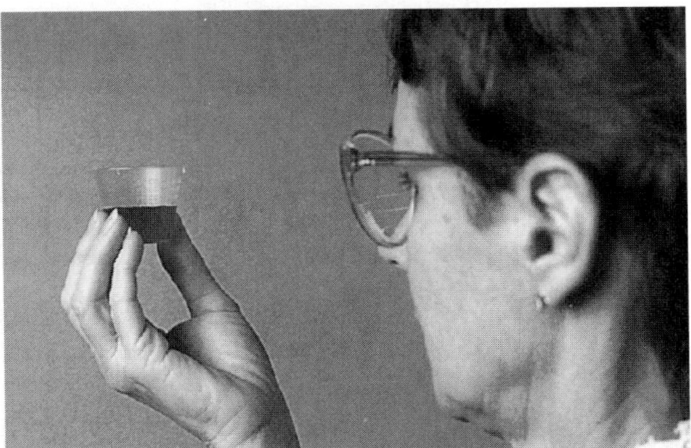

Fig. 15-24 Hold the medication cup at eye level or place it on counter and fill it to the desired level on the scale. (From Perry AG, Potter PA: *Clinical nursing skills and techniques,* ed 3, St Louis, 1994, Mosby.)

SKILL 15-2 APPLYING A TRANSDERMAL MEDICATION PATCH

Steps	Rationale
1. Obtain equipment: ▪ Medication profile ▪ Transdermal patch ▪ Clean gloves	Helps organize procedure.
2. Refer to medical record, care plan, or Kardex for special interventions.	Provides basis for care.
3. Introduce self.	Decreases patient's anxiety level.
4. Identify patient by identification band.	Identifies correct patient for procedure.
5. Explain procedure to patient.	Seeks cooperation and decreases anxiety.

Continued.

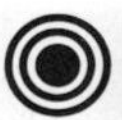

SKILL 15-2 APPLYING A TRANSDERMAL MEDICATION PATCH—cont'd

Steps	Rationale
6. Wash hands and don clean gloves according to agency policy and guidelines from Centers for Disease Control and Prevention and Occupational Safety and Health Administration.	Helps prevent cross-contamination.
7. Prepare patient for intervention:	
a. Close door to room or pull curtain.	Provides privacy.
b. Drape for procedure if necessary.	Prevents exposure of patient.
8. Raise bed to comfortable working level.	Provides safety for nurse.
9. Arrange for patient privacy.	Shows respect for patient.
10. Compare medical order with medication profile for accuracy.	Helps prevent medication error.
11. Remove old patch, place it in appropriate container, and cleanse and dry site. Assess for irritation, redness, or broken skin.	Avoids medicating patient with residual medication.
12. Select and cleanse new site.	Clean, dry skin ensures therapeutic absorption of medication.
13. Peel off patch backing, avoiding contact with drug.	Prevents touching patch, which will contaminate medication and possibly change dose of medication.
14. Dispose of soiled supplies.	Prevents cross-contamination.
15. Remove gloves and wash hands.	Helps prevent cross-contamination.
16. Document.	Documents procedure and patient's response.

SKILL 15-3 ADMINISTERING EYE MEDICATIONS

Steps	Rationale
1. Obtain equipment: ▪ Medication profile ▪ Eye medication ▪ Clean gloves	Helps organize procedure.
2. Compare medical order with medication profile for medications for accuracy.	Determines medication, dose, route, and times to be administered.
3. Refer to medical record, care plan, or Kardex for special interventions.	Provides basis for care.
4. Introduce self.	Decreases patient's anxiety level.
5. Identify patient by identification band.	Identifies correct patient for procedure.
6. Explain procedure to patient.	Seeks cooperation and decreases anxiety.
7. Wash hands and don clean gloves according to agency policy and guidelines from Centers for Disease Control and Prevention and Occupational Safety and Health Administration.	Helps prevent cross-contamination.
8. Prepare patient for intervention:	
a. Close door to room or pull curtain.	Provides privacy.
b. Drape for procedure if necessary.	Prevents exposure of patient.
9. Raise bed to comfortable working level.	Provides safety for nurse.
10. Arrange for patient privacy.	Shows respect for patient.
11. Assess condition of eyes.	Determines need to cleanse eyes before administering medication.
12. Assist patient to supine position with head tilted back.	Provides access to eyes and promotes comfort and cooperation.
13. Press gently and pull eyelid downward.	Prevents eye trauma.
14. Ask patient to look up and back toward ceiling.	Retracts cornea away from conjunctival sac and reduces blinking reflex.

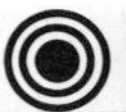

SKILL 15-3 ADMINISTERING EYE MEDICATIONS—cont'd

Steps	Rationale
15. Drop prescribed number of drops into conjunctival sac of lower eyelid or apply thin stream of ointment across lower eyelid from inner to outer canthus (Fig. 15-25).	Provides even distribution of dose of medication in eyes.
16. Have patient gently close eyes and gently move eyes from side to side and up and down. Encourage patient not to squeeze eyes since this forces medication out.	Distributes medication evenly in eyes.
17. Apply gentle pressure to nasolacrimal duct for 30 to 60 sec.	Prohibits medication from flowing into nose and throat and being absorbed by mucous membranes, producing systemic effect.
18. Wipe away excess medication gently from inner to outer canthus.	Promotes patient comfort.
19. Remove gloves and wash hands.	Helps prevent cross-contamination.
20. Document.	Documents procedure and patient's response.

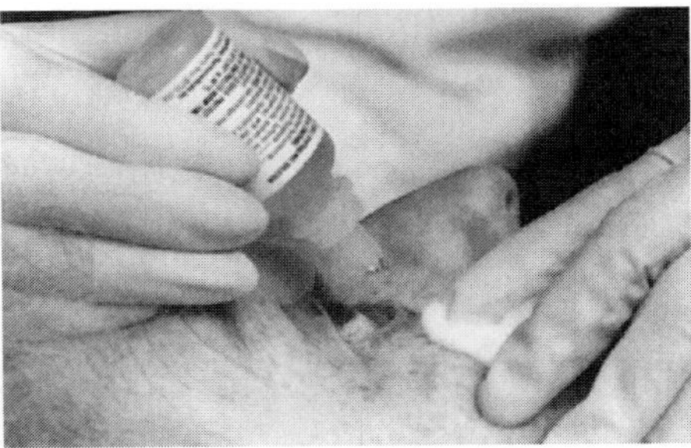

Fig. 15-25 To apply drops, expose the lower conjunctival sac by having the patient look upward while applying gentle traction to the lower eyelid. (From Christensen BL, Kockrow EO: *Foundations of nursing,* ed 2, St Louis, 1995, Mosby.)

SKILL 15-4 ADMINISTERING EAR MEDICATIONS

Steps	Rationale
1. Obtain equipment: ▪ Medication profile ▪ Ear medication ▪ Clean gloves	Helps organize procedure.
2. Compare medical order with medication profile for all medications for accuracy.	Determines medication, dose, route, and times to be administered.
3. Warm medication to body temperature.	Prevents discomfort, vertigo (dizziness), and nausea.
4. Refer to medical record, care plan, or Kardex for special interventions.	Provides basis for care.
5. Introduce self.	Decreases patient's anxiety level.
6. Identify patient by identification band.	Identifies correct patient for procedure.
7. Explain procedure to patient.	Seeks cooperation and decreases anxiety.
8. Wash hands and don clean gloves according to agency policy and guidelines from Centers for Disease Control and Prevention and Occupational Safety and Health Administration.	Helps prevent cross-contamination.

Continued.

SKILL 15-4 ADMINISTERING EAR MEDICATIONS—cont'd

Steps	Rationale
9. Prepare patient for intervention:	
a. Close door to room or pull curtain.	Provides privacy.
b. Drape for procedure if necessary.	Prevents exposure of patient.
10. Raise bed to comfortable working level.	Provides safety for nurse.
11. Arrange for patient privacy.	Shows respect for patient.
12. Cleanse outer ear if necessary.	Prevents interference from cerumen and drainage and helps absorption of medication.
13. Assist patient to supine position.	Provides access to ears.
14. Straighten ear canal by pulling up and backward for adult (Fig. 15-26) or downward and backward for a young child.	Allows medication to reach structures in ear canal.
15. Hold ear dropper ½ inch above ear canal.	Prevents contamination of dropper.
16. Gently drop prescribed number of drops onto side of ear canal.	Provides accurate dose. Prevents unpleasant sensation of drops falling directly on eardrum.
17. Encourage patient to remain in position for 3 to 5 min.	Allows time for medication to reach deeper structures and to absorb.
18. Allow medication to absorb for few minutes before treating opposite ear.	Prevents medication from leaking out.
19. Treat opposite ear in same manner as previous ear.	Ensures that medication is instilled in both ears.
20. Allow opposite ear to absorb medication.	Prevents medication from leaking out.
21. Remove gloves and wash hands.	Helps prevent cross-contamination.
22. Document.	Documents procedure and patient's response.

A 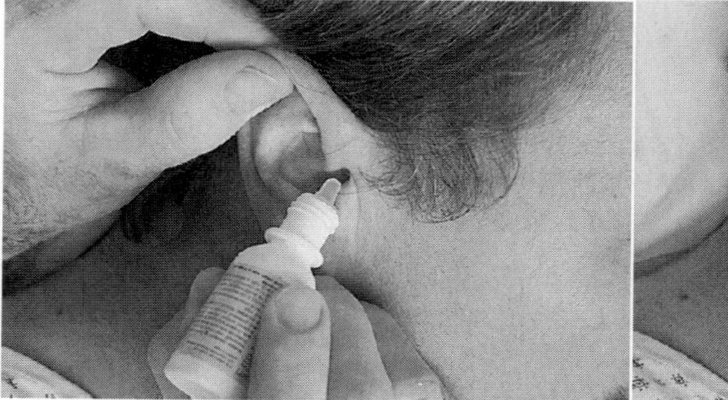

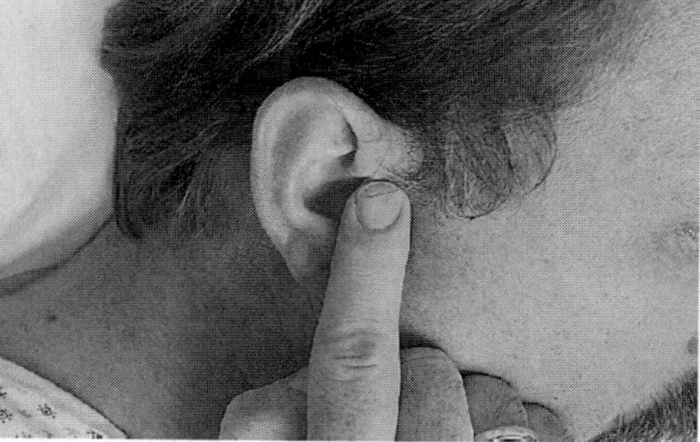 B

Fig. 15-26 **A,** Instill prescribed drops holding the dropper 1 cm (½ inch) above the ear canal. **B,** Ask the patient to remain in a side-lying position 2 to 3 minutes. Apply gentle massage to the tragus of the ear with the finger. (From Potter PA, Perry AG: *Basic nursing: theory and practice,* ed 3, St Louis, 1995, Mosby.)

SKILL 15-5 ADMINISTERING RECTAL MEDICATIONS

Steps	Rationale
1. Obtain equipment: ▪ Medication profile ▪ Rectal medication ▪ Lubricant (water soluble) ▪ Ink pen ▪ Clean gloves	Helps organize procedure.
2. Compare medical order with medication profile for all medications for accuracy.	Determines medication, dose, route, and times to be administered.

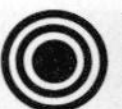

SKILL 15-5 ADMINISTERING RECTAL MEDICATIONS—cont'd

Steps	Rationale
3. Refer to medical record, care plan, or Kardex for special interventions.	Provides basis for care.
4. Introduce self.	Decreases patient's anxiety level.
5. Identify patient by identification band.	Identifies correct patient for procedure.
6. Explain procedure to patient.	Seeks cooperation and decreases anxiety.
7. Wash hands and don clean gloves according to agency policy and guidelines from Centers for Disease Control and Prevention and Occupational Safety and Health Administration.	Helps prevent cross-contamination.
8. Prepare patient for intervention:	
a. Close door to room or pull curtain.	Provides privacy.
b. Drape for procedure if necessary.	Prevents exposure of patient.
9. Raise bed to comfortable working level.	Provides safety for nurse.
10. Arrange for patient privacy.	Shows respect for patient.
11. Assist patient to left Sims' position and expose buttocks.	Provides access to rectum.
12. Examine anus for hemorrhoids or variations at site.	Determines access and prevents trauma to rectum and hemorrhoids.
13. Open lubricant package to ready lubrication of suppository.	Reduces friction on insertion of suppository.
14. Remove suppository from package and lubricate tip.	Reduces friction for easy insertion.
15. Gently insert suppository past sphincter muscle by placing it between index, middle, and ring fingers of dominant hand. Insert it approximately 4 in, allowing index finger to push suppository away from finger and upward. (Nurse should feel suppository push itself away and upward, or it will lodge in rectum and will not provide expected action.) For child, insert suppository approximately 1 to 2 in.	Ensures that peristalsis takes suppository up for absorption.
16. Withdraw finger. Hold cheeks of buttocks together for few seconds and wipe lubricant and drainage, if necessary, from anal area.	Provides hygiene and comfort. Prevents suppository from slipping out.
17. When necessary, place call light within patient's reach.	Provides help from nurse.
18. Remove gloves and wash hands.	Helps prevent cross-contamination.
19. Document.	Documents procedure and patient's response.

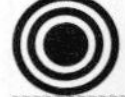

SKILL 15-6 ADMINISTERING INJECTIONS

Steps	Rationale
1. Obtain equipment: ▪ Medication profile ▪ Correct syringe ▪ Needle (if not attached to syringe) ▪ Alcohol swab ▪ Clean gloves	Helps organize procedure.
2. Refer to medical record, care plan, or Kardex for special interventions.	Provides basis for care.

Continued.

SKILL 15-6 ADMINISTERING INJECTIONS—cont'd

Steps	Rationale
3. Introduce self.	Decreases patient's anxiety level.
4. Identify patient by identification band.	Identifies correct patient for procedure.
5. Explain procedure to patient.	Seeks cooperation and decreases anxiety.
6. Wash hands and don clean gloves according to agency policy and guidelines from Centers for Disease Control and Prevention and Occupational Safety and Health Administration.	Helps prevent cross-contamination.
7. Prepare patient for intervention:	
a. Close door to room or pull curtain.	Provides privacy.
b. Drape for procedure if necessary.	Prevents exposure of patient.
8. Raise bed to comfortable working level.	Provides safety for nurse.
9. Arrange for patient privacy.	Shows respect for patient.
INTRADERMAL (ID) INJECTION	
10. Choose appropriate site. Pull skin taut over site with thumb and index finger of nondominant hand.	Protects tissues, facilitates accurate entry into tissue, and allows needle to enter skin smoothly when skin is pulled taut.
11. Insert needle at 10- to 25-degree angle to inside of forearm and slide needle tip under skin where approximately 3 mm of tip will be visible through skin. Do not aspirate.	Facilitates needle entering dermis and ensures that medication is injected between skin layers and will not leak. Prevents tissue trauma from aspiration.
12. Inject medication slowly, assessing formation of a bleb (Fig. 15-27).	Confirms that medication is deposited into dermis.
13. Remove needle quickly at 10- to 15-degree angle and do not massage site. Mark site with skin marker with date, time, and nurse's initials. Circle site away from insertion of medication.	Minimizes discomfort and tissue trauma and prevents alteration of results. Facilitates reading of skin test in 48 to 72 hr.
INTRAMUSCULAR (IM) INJECTION	
14. Spread skin taut using nondominant hand. With dominant hand, quickly dart needle into muscle at 90-degree angle.	Compresses subcutaneous tissue to ensure that medication enters muscle. Minimizes discomfort from injection.

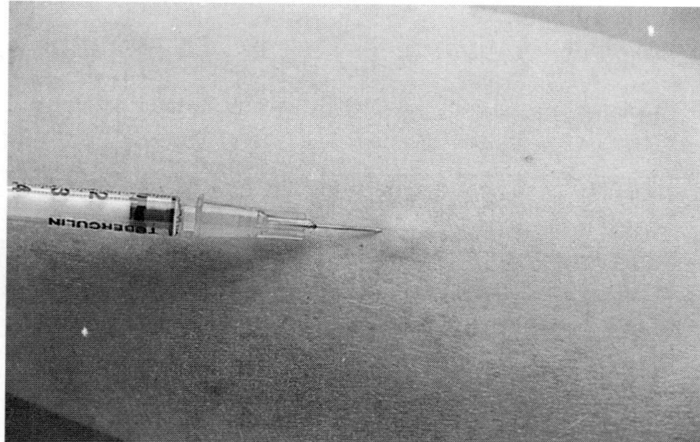

Fig. 15-27 During ID injection, note formation of small bleb on skin's surface. (From Potter PA, Perry AG: *Basic nursing: theory and practice,* ed 3, St Louis, 1995, Mosby.)

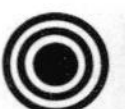

SKILL 15-6 ADMINISTERING INJECTIONS—cont'd

Steps	Rationale
15. Move nondominant hand to stabilize syringe barrel near needle hub. Aspirate by gently drawing back on plunger. If blood appears in syringe, quickly withdraw needle, change needle (if agency policy), and choose another site for injection. Repeat.	Stabilizes needle placement during aspiration. Assesses whether blood enters syringe, which indicates that needle is in vessel.
16. Inject medication slowly if no blood appears. Quickly remove needle, placing alcohol swab along needle hub. Apply pressure and massage site unless contraindicated.	Minimizes feeling of pressure and pain and prevents pain when needle is removed. Prevents medication from leaking and helps clotting. Disperses medication and promotes absorption.
SUBCUTANEOUS (SQ) INJECTION	
17. Choose site and pinch skin between thumb and forefinger. With dominant hand, quickly dart needle into tissue at 45- to 90-degree angle, depending on medication being administered and syringe being used.	Elevates subcutaneous tissue and tightens skin over site for easy penetration and entrance of medication into subcutaneous tissue. Reduces pain of injecting needle through skin.
18. Stabilize syringe by holding hub and lower part of syringe barrel. Aspirate unless contraindicated. If blood appears in syringe, quickly withdraw needle, change needle (if agency policy), and choose another site for injection. Repeat.	Prevents movement of needle and tissue trauma and relaxes tissue. Assesses whether blood entered syringe, which indicates needle is in vessel.
19. Inject medication slowly. Remove needle quickly and apply pressure with alcohol swab against site. Massage site.	Allows medication to enter tissue slowly and minimizes tissue trauma. Helps absorption of medication.
20. Remove gloves and wash hands.	Helps prevent cross-contamination.
21. Document.	Documents procedure and patient's response.

SUMMARY

The safety and well-being of the patient depends on the nurse's knowledge and application of principles of medication administration. The nurse must be able to accurately calculate dosages, follow aseptic principles, and use clinical judgment in providing drug therapy. Physical assessment of the patient and knowledge of the medical history, allergies, and diet assist the nurse in planning and providing safe, effective nursing care.

Key Concepts

- Nurse practice acts legally define the nurse's qualifications and scope of practice in administering medications.
- Controlled substances are regulated according to federal law. The nurse follows strict procedures to safeguard and account for these medications.
- The five rights are followed for every medication administration.
- Prompt and accurate documentation should follow every drug administration.
- The nurse has the right and responsibility to question incomplete or illegible medical medication orders.
- Medication should not be left unattended.
- The nurse is responsible for knowing drug classifications, routes, actions, side effects, and nursing implications when administering medications.
- The nurse is expected to perform accurate medication calculations.
- Safety precautions are observed when preparing, administering, and disposing of medications and equipment used to administer medications.
- The nurse immediately reports any medication errors, reactions, or discrepancies.
- The nurse uses clinical judgment in assessing

the patient's ability to receive the medication by the ordered route and in selecting equipment and injection sites.

- Patient and family education and patient safety are nursing responsibilities.
- Handwashing is the most important means to control infection and cross-contamination for both patients and health care providers.
- The nurse is required to use universal precautions when indicated.

Critical Thinking Questions

1. Your 84-year-old patient is having visual difficulties. What specific interventions should you use to promote compliance and safety in administering medications?
2. In preparing a medication, you discover that the physician's order is illegible and that you are unsure of the drug dosage. The primary nurse informs you she wrote it correctly on the medication record. What should you do?
3. Mrs. Calhoun has heart failure and is taking Lanoxin and Lasix to treat the heart failure. The nurse practitioner managing Mrs. Calhoun's care noted that her serum potassium level in March was 3.6 mEq/L and, in consultation with the physician, ordered a potassium supplement to be given. Now, in September, Mrs. Calhoun is admitted to the hospital because she has fractured her right hip and has a total hip replacement. Three days after surgery, she begins taking oral medications and the Lanoxin, Lasix, and potassium supplement are again ordered. At this time, the nurse notes that Mrs. Calhoun's heart rate is irregular, that her previous 24 hour input and output showed intake of 2050 ml and output of 800 ml, and that her urine is now very dark amber. What serum electrolyte level should the nurse immediately check? What other assessment data should the nurse gather? Which medications should be held until the staff nurse consults with Mrs. Calhoun's health care provider?
4. Mrs. Kline is a 42-year-old woman admitted with pneumonia. She is placed on IV antibiotics every 6 hours at 0600, 1200, 1800, and 2400 hours. At 0900 on the second day of treatment, the nurse notes a skin rash and notifies the physician, who changes her antibiotic. The medication nurse gives the 1200 dose of the original antibiotic, and the patient has a severe allergic reaction. Identify the elements of neglect. Establish how such negligence can be avoided.

REFERENCES AND SUGGESTED READINGS

Asperheim MK: *Pharmacology, an introductory text,* ed 7, Philadelphia, 1992, Saunders.

Avey MA: TB skin testing: how to do it right, *American Journal of Nursing* 93(9):42, 1993.

Bohony J: 9 common IV implications and what to do about them, *American Journal of Nursing* 93(10):45, 1993.

Bowles K, Lynch M: These products and procedures prevent needlesticks, *RN* 55(7):42, 1992.

Clark JB, Queener SF, Karb VB: *Pharmacologic basis of nursing practice,* St Louis, 1993, Mosby.

Drass J: What you need to know about insulin injections, *Nursing 92* 22(11):40, 1992.

McConnell EA: How to administer a Z track injection, *Nursing 93* 23(4):18, 1993.

Millam DA: IV technology helps you stay out of harm's way, *Nursing 93* 23(10):62, 1993.

Nicholson SH: Infusion therapy program requires nursing skill and knowledge, *Provider* 19(4):38, 1993.

Nursing procedures, student version, Springhouse, Penn, 1993, Springhouse.

Perry AG, Potter PA: *Clinical nursing skills and techniques,* ed 3, St Louis, 1994, Mosby.

Potter PA, Perry AG: *Fundamentals of nursing concepts, process, and practice,* ed 3, St Louis, 1993, Mosby.

Rice JB, Skelley EG: *Medications and math for the nurse,* ed 7, Albany, NY, 1993, Delmar.

Shoaf J, Oliver S: Efficacy of normal saline injection with and without heparin for maintaining intermittent intravenous site, *Applied Nursing Research* 5(1):9, 1992.

Spencer RT et al: *Clinical pharmacology and nursing management,* ed 4, Philadelphia, 1993, Lippincott.

Taylor HJ: Patients deserve painless injections: Z-track technique, *RN* 55(3):25, 1992.

Weakland BS: Administering insulin through an indwelling catheter, *Nursing 93* 23(11):58, 1993.

Wilson JA: Preventing infection during IV therapy, *Professional Nurse* 9(6):388, 1994.

CHAPTER 16

Parenteral Therapy

Learning Objectives

After studying this chapter, the student should be able to . . .

- Define the key terms.
- Identify the nurse's responsibility in administering intravenous therapy.
- Identify the nurse's responsibility in administering blood therapy.
- Identify the nurse's responsibility in administering chemotherapy.
- Implement appropriate nursing measures to help alleviate the side effects of chemotherapy.
- Distinguish the types of blood reactions that may occur during a blood transfusion.
- Discuss complications of intravenous therapy.
- List the equipment and steps necessary for initiating an intravenous infusion.
- Discuss guidelines for patient education about parenteral therapy.

Key Terms

Air embolus
Alopecia
Angiocatheter
Anorexia
Antibody
Antigen
Antineoplastic
Autotransfusion
Blood transfusion
Bone marrow depression
Chemotherapy
Crossmatching
Drop factor
Erythroblastosis fetalis
Hemolysis
Infiltration
Parenteral therapy
Phlebitis
Rh factor
Stomatitis
Transfusion reaction
Typing
Venipuncture

Skills

16-1 Initiating venipuncture
16-2 Administering blood
16-3 Administering chemotherapy

Parenteral therapy is treatment administered by a route other than the digestive tract. Chemotherapy, blood and blood product administration, and intravenous fluid and medication administration are special parenteral therapies. *Chemotherapy* describes any drug therapy, but the term usually refers to the administration of antineoplastic medications specifically related to treatment of the patient who has cancer. Blood and blood products are replaced because these elements are "lost" through trauma or diseases. Intravenous therapy is used to correct or prevent imbalances of fluids and electrolytes. The fluid to be administered is medically determined depending on the individual's needs.

State nurse practice acts determine the legal guidelines and agency policies further define the qualifications of nurses allowed to administer intravenous medications, blood and blood products, and chemotherapy. Only nurses who have been specially trained and who meet the legal qualifications and agency guidelines are involved in intravenous administration. Not all nurses are expected or required to administer intravenous therapy.

Nurses qualified to administer intravenous therapy are expected to initiate, regulate, maintain, and discontinue intravenous therapy according to medical orders and agency policies and to identify complications of such therapy. Solutions, tubings, and other equipment may vary from agency to agency. However, there are some principles.

Universal precautions should be followed when exposure to blood or body fluids is possible. Gloves are also required when certain antineoplastic agents are handled because of their toxic nature. Therefore

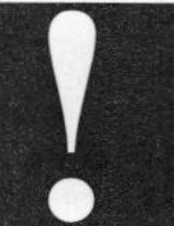

REMEMBER

- The nurse should know and practice within legal guidelines.
- The nurse should use universal precautions when exposure to blood or body fluids is possible.
- Very young and very old patients are at greater risk for intravenous infusion complications.
- Older adult and pediatric veins may be fragile.
- The nurse must calculate and monitor intravenous infusion therapy very carefully and frequently.
- Intravenous infusion complications include infiltration, infection, phlebitis, allergic reactions, circulatory overload, and air embolus.

when equipment is prepared for the administration of nonblood, nontoxic products, gloves are not required, since no risk of exposure exists. However, when initiating venipuncture, handling any blood or blood products and toxic antineoplastics, changing an intravenous infusion to a heparin or saline lock, and discontinuing intravenous therapy and handling soiled supplies from these procedures, the nurse must wear gloves.

ASSESSING INTRAVENOUS COMPLICATIONS

When assessing for complications from an intravenous infusion the nurse should observe for infiltration, phlebitis, allergic reactions, circulatory problems, and vein and skin trauma. **Infiltration** occurs when intravenous fluids enter the subcutaneous space around the venipuncture site. Signs of infiltration include a feeling and appearance of tightness and edema of the extremity or at the point of entry of the needle or intracatheter. Other signs are pallor, pain, coolness, burning, and stinging. Often, the rate of the infusion slows.

Phlebitis is inflammation of a vein. Signs of inflammation are redness, swelling, pain, local heat, and red streaks that spread away from the site. Allergic reactions to medications may cause rash, shortness of breath, and temperature elevation. Blood reactions, always considered life threatening, are common and include chills, fever, and hematuria (blood in the urine). Circulatory problems are produced by excess fluid volume or particles circulating through the bloodstream. Circulatory overload may lead to pulmonary edema, and particles in the circulatory system may produce pulmonary embolism. These complications are life threatening and must receive prompt attention.

PATIENT TEACHING

- Teach patient and family signs and symptoms of infiltration.
- Encourage the patient and family to promptly report signs of infiltration to the nurse.
- Discuss the importance of not changing the flow rate, lying on the tubing, or kinking the tubing.
- Demonstrate the care of intravenous site while performing hygiene measures.
- Discuss the need for intravenous fluid container to be above the insertion site.
- Teach performance of allowed activities to prevent dislodging of the equipment.

Burning, redness, or warmth at the intravenous insertion site may indicate an infection. Certain medications may irritate the vein and, if infiltration occurs, may cause necrosis (tissue death) and sloughing. A generally acceptable nursing measure is to stop the infusion; notify the physician; and apply warm, moist compresses to the area. Agency policy, however, dictates the specific steps nurses should take to control these complications and the interventions to be initiated. Prompt and accurate documentation of assessments, observations, and nursing interventions is expected.

Nursing care includes discussing the side effects of medications and complications of parenteral therapy with the patient and family (see teaching box), suggesting strategies to minimize side effects, allowing the patient and family to ask questions and ventilate frustrations, promoting nutrition and hygiene, recognizing the significance of laboratory reports, and providing comfort and safety measures. The evaluation of the patient's physical and emotional response to the illness and treatment is an important nursing responsibility. Monitoring the patient for adverse effects, complaints, and objective findings, the nurse provides information that the physician needs to determine the continued course of treatment.

PERFORMING VENIPUNCTURE

It may be necessary to initiate intravenous therapy, or venipuncture. **Venipuncture** is the technique by which a vein is punctured by a stylet, a cannula, a needle, or a needle attached to a syringe. If such therapy is necessary, the nurse assembles equipment to perform the venipuncture and prepares the solution and tubing to deliver the infusion (Skill 16-1). In addition to the solution, tubing, and infusion pump, the nurse will need gloves, a tourniquet, antiseptic wipes, adhesive tape and dressing, and an **angiocatheter** (see Fig. 16-3, *A*), a hollow, flexible tube inserted into a blood vessel to withdraw or instill fluids. Some agencies have all the necessary equipment assembled in an intravenous tray that the nurse carries to the bedside.

Selecting Veins

The veins of the hands and arms are preferred to allow easy access and patient mobility (see Fig. 16-5). A patient usually prefers an intravenous infusion in the nondominant hand when possible. The nurse should avoid the wrist and elbow veins whenever possible. Straight veins are more easily entered. Those that feel hard, lumpy, or bumpy should be avoided. The venipuncture should be initiated at distal sites to allow for future sites when an intravenous infusion is needed. An infusion should not be started over bruises, scar tissue, joints, or areas of compromised circulation.

Calculating an Infusion Rate

The medical order for an intravenous infusion should identify the type of fluid, the amount of fluid, and the frequency of administration. If the order is for different solutions, the sequencing of the solutions must be specified. An example of an intravenous infusion order follows:

1000 ml Ringer's lactate solution Q8hr

The nurse must calculate the number of milliliters per minute to program the infusion pump to administer the correct amount of fluid over the prescribed time. The formula for this calculation follows:

Number of total milliliters ÷ Number of hours to be infused = Number of milliliters per hour

1000 ml ÷ 8 hr = 125 ml/hr

To then determine the number of milliliters per minute the nurse divides the number of milliliters per hour by 60, since there are 60 minutes in each hour:

125 ml ÷ 60 = 2.08 ml/min

Many pumps require programming by drops per minute. The nurse must recognize that not all intravenous tubing is the same size and therefore the number of drops per minute **(drop factor)** varies. The drop factor is printed on the tubing package. Some common drop factors follow:

1 ml equals 15 drops
1 ml equals 20 drops
1 ml equals 60 drops (also called *microdrops*)

The drop factor for most blood administration tubing is 10 drops = 1 ml

The nurse should carefully assess the drop factor and continue the calculations to determine the correct infusion rate in drops per minute. Using the previous example of 2.08 ml/min and a tubing set that delivers 15 drops/ml, the nurse multiplies 2.08 by 15, which equals 31.2 drops per minute. By rounding off to 31 drops/min, the nurse programs the infusion pump to accurately deliver the prescribed volume of fluid over the prescribed time.

Another example follows:

1000 ml dextrose q6hr Tubing drop factor 1 ml = 20 drops

1000 ml ÷ 6 hr = 166.6 ml/hr

166.6 ml ÷ 60 min = 2.77 ml/min (rounded to 2.8 ml/min)

2.8 ml × 20 drops = 56 drops/min

Preparing the Solution

Sterile, prepackaged solutions are available in plastic bags of varying volumes. Bags holding 1000, 500, 250, 100, and 50 ml are usually available. The nurse follows aseptic technique and the five rights of medication administration when providing intravenous therapy.

After reviewing the medical order and calculating the correct number of drops per minute, the nurse selects the appropriate intravenous solution bag (Table 16-1). If the solution is ordered to follow therapy already in progress, the nurse assesses the intravenous site, tubing patency, and infusing fluid to ensure safety and continuity. The used bag of fluid is removed and the new bag hung using aseptic technique (see Chapter 14). The fluid level in the bag in use is almost allowed to empty. When there is 30 to 50 ml left in the bag, the new bag is readied. The new bag is removed from the sterile packaging and inverted, and the insertion port cover is removed. The used bag is taken from its hanger and inverted, and the tubing is grasped firmly above the tubing spike. A sharp tug removes the spike from the insertion port of the used bag. Using aseptic technique, the nurse inserts the spike into the fresh bag's port, pressing until the port diaphragm has been pierced by the spike (Fig. 16-1). The new bag is then turned upright and hung on the hanger. The

Table 16-1 COMMON NAMES FOR INTRAVENOUS SOLUTIONS

Solution	Other Names
0.9% sodium chloride	Normal saline 0.9% NaCl 0.9% NS NS
0.45% sodium chloride	One-half–strength normal saline 0.45% NaCl 0.45% NS ½ NaCl ½ NS
Dextrose 5% in 0.9% sodium chloride	D5 normal saline D5 0.9% NaCl D5 0.9% NS D5 NS
Dextrose 5% in 0.45% sodium chloride	D5 One-half–strength normal saline D5 0.45% NaCl D5 0.45% NS D5 ½ NaCl D5 ½ NS
Ringer's lactate	RL
Dextrose 5% in Ringer's lactate	D5 RL

drip chamber should remain about one third full of fluid. If the drip chamber is too full, the tubing below the drip chamber is pinched off, the container is inverted, the drip chamber is squeezed, the bag is hung, and the tubing is released (Fig. 16-2, *A*). The tubing is assessed for air bubbles.

Displacing Air Bubbles

Air bubbles must be displaced so that they do not enter the patient's circulatory system, causing an **air embolus,** the abnormal presence of air in the cardiovascular system, resulting in obstruction of blood flow through the vessel. To move the bubbles up the tubing into the drip chamber, the nurse firmly grasps the tubing to straighten it and, using a finger, pencil, or pen, briskly taps the tubing below the bubbles, thumping until they rise (Fig. 16-2, *B*). This action is continued until the bubbles disperse into the drip chamber. Another method to diplace air bubbles is to wrap the tubing around a pencil, pen, or syringe barrel. Slowly moving the object upward should propel the bubbles up and into the drip chamber. A third method is to locate a port below the bubbles. The nurse cleanses the port and then inserts a sterile needle into it to allow the fluid and bubbles to slowly move toward it. In this way, the air is released through the needle. The needle must be removed and discarded into the sharps container and the port recleansed.

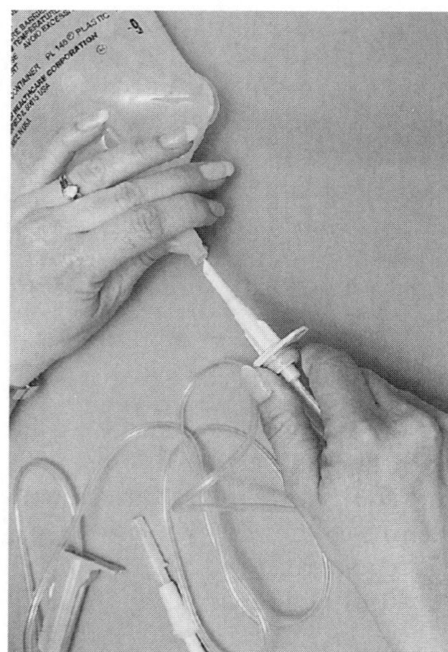

Fig. 16-1 Insert spike in fresh solution port. (From Potter PA, Perry AG: *Basic nursing: theory and practice,* ed 3, St Louis, 1995, Mosby.)

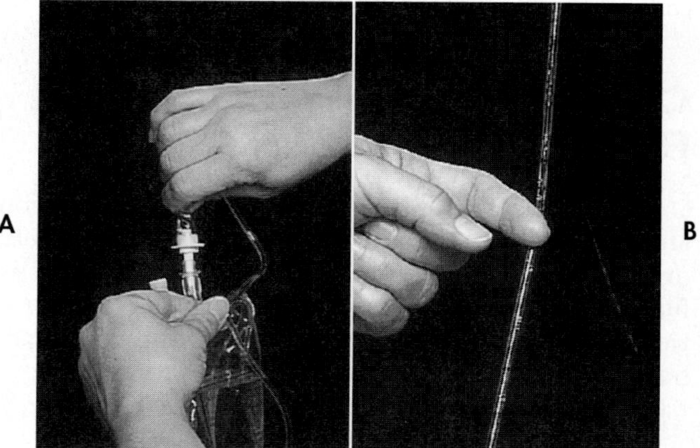

Fig. 16-2 **A,** Make adjustments if drip chamber is too full. **B,** Thump tubing to move air bubbles. (From Perry AG, Potter PA: *Clinical nursing skills and techniques,* ed 3, St Louis, 1994, Mosby.)

Initiating Therapy

There are several steps to performing a venipuncture (Skill 16-1). Before the procedure, the nurse must assemble and ready the equipment. The patient's veins must be assessed, a puncture site selected and cleansed, the venipuncture performed, and the infusion begun and secured. The nurse teaches the patient about the signs and symptoms

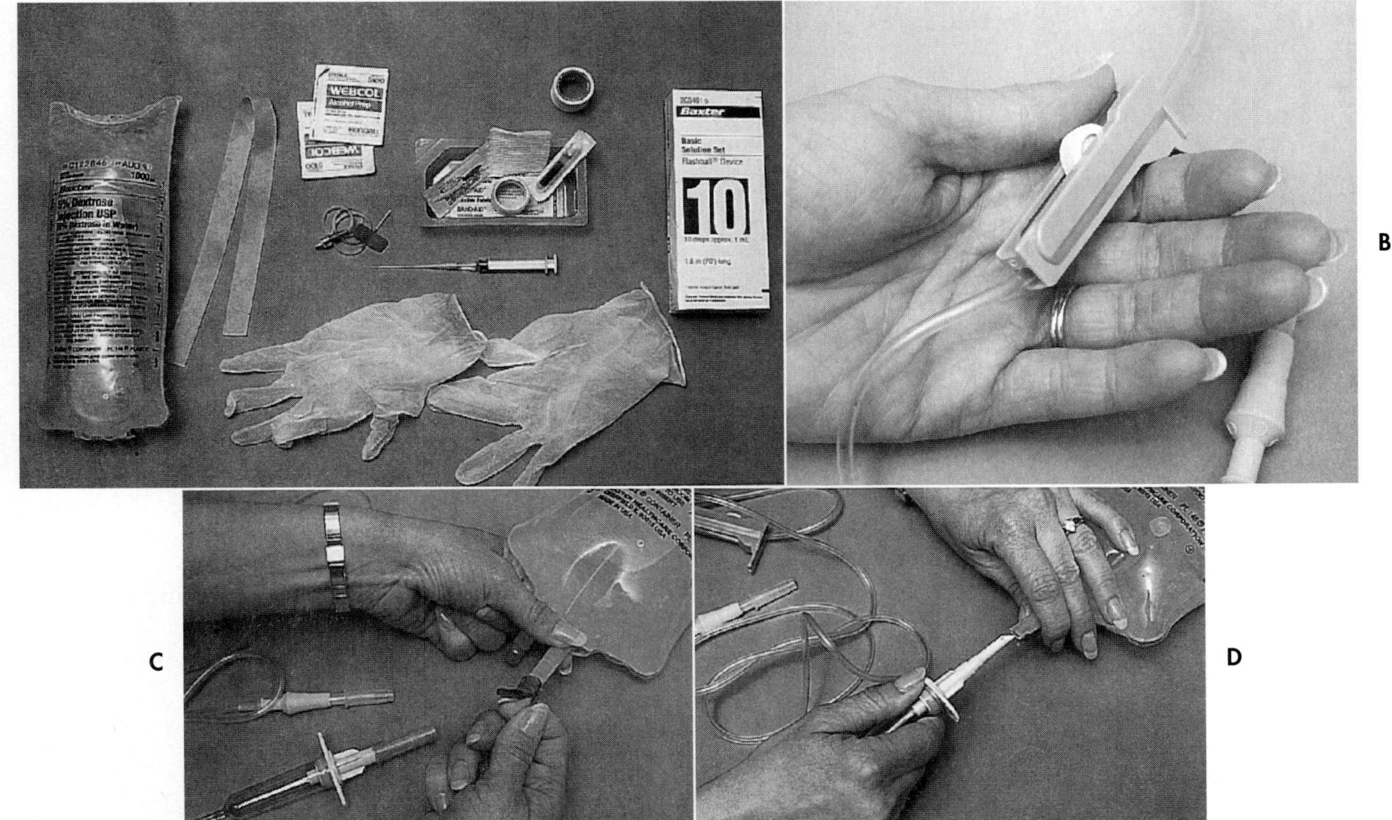

Fig. 16-3 **A,** Supplies for venipuncture. **B,** Close valve. **C,** Remove insertion port cover. **D,** Insert spike into port. (From Potter PA, Perry AG: *Fundamentals of nursing: concepts, process, and practice,* ed 3, St Louis, 1993, Mosby.)

of problems and ways to perform activities while on venipuncture (see teaching box). Because venipuncture is invasive and the pierced skin is no longer a barrier to microorganisms, this procedure must be performed following strict aseptic principles. Equipment packaging should be inspected for breakage of sterile seals and used before the dates marked on the packaging barriers. Equipment with damaged outer packaging should not be used.

The nurse selects the new tubing based on the needs of the patient and the type of infusion to be initiated. The tubing's sterile packaging is removed and the tubing inspected for kinks. The nurse also ensures that the flow valve is functional. The valve is closed, and the tubing is placed within easy reach (Fig. 16-3, *B*). The correct fluid bag is removed from its sterile packaging and inverted to allow easy access to the tubing insertion port. The insertion port cover is removed (Fig. 16-3, *C*), the tubing spike end cover is removed, and the spike is inserted into the port until the plastic diaphragm covering the port is pierced (Fig. 16-3, *D*). The fluid bag is then held upright and the tubing drip chamber gently squeezed to partially fill it with fluid. The flow valve is slowly opened to permit the flow of the solution down the tubing. This priming (filling of the tubing with solution) prevents air from being forced through the tubing into the patient's circulatory system, creating an air embolus.

Changing the Tubing

Changing intravenous tubing is most easily accomplished when a new bag of fluid is added. The nurse connects and primes the new solution container and tubing, takes it to the patient's bedside, and hangs it on the pole hanger. After donning gloves, the nurse carefully removes the tape securing the old tubing to the intravenous catheter hub while gently stabilizing the catheter and site. Working carefully but quickly, the nurse turns off the flow valve of the old tubing, removes the old tubing from the intravenous catheter hub and, using aseptic technique, inserts the new tubing into the catheter hub and opens the flow valve (Fig. 16-4). The connection and site are then secured with tape and/or dressing per agency policy. The new tubing is labeled with the time and date, and the old tubing, intrave-

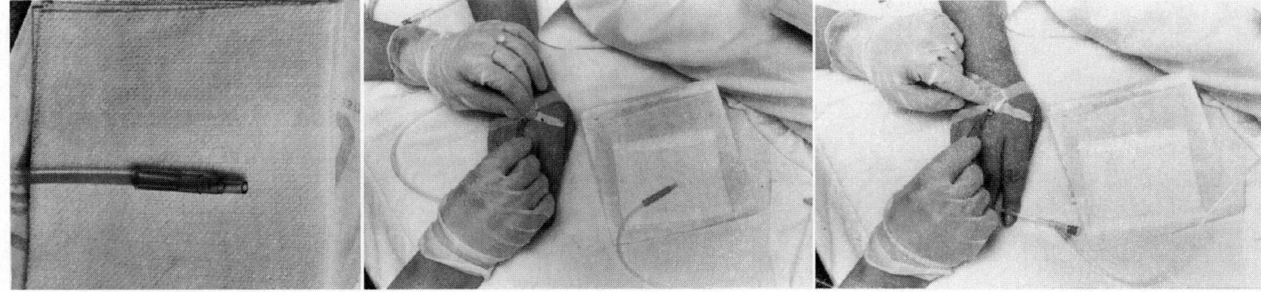

Fig. 16-4 Insert new tubing into catheter hub and open flow valve. (From Perry AG, Potter PA: *Clinical nursing skills and techniques,* ed 3, St Louis, 1994, Mosby.)

nous bag, and soiled supplies are discarded according to the guidelines of the Centers for Disease Control and Prevention, Occupational Safety and Health Administration, and agency policy.

The venipuncture needle and catheter should be selected according to the solution to be infused and the size and condition of the patient's veins. The catheter should be smaller than the vein, yet large enough for the solution to flow through it without clogging. Normally, a 20, 21, or 22 gauge is acceptable for an adult. However, if blood is to be administered, a larger lumen (18 or 19 gauge) should be used. Plastic intravenous catheters are flexible and have blunt tips that reduce infiltration and allow the patient to move more than the metal needles used several years ago. These plastic catheters have a metal needle inside them that pierces the skin and guides them into the vein. The catheter is then threaded over the needle and into the vein, and the metal guide needle is removed.

Discontinuing Therapy

Intravenous infusions are discontinued when the prescribed amount of solution has infused, when there are signs of infiltration, or if the patient has developed phlebitis or other complications. Steps for discontinuing an intravenous infusion include the following:

1. Collect supplies.
2. Wash hands.
3. Explain the procedure to the patient.
4. Don gloves.
5. Turn intravenous flow regulator to the "off" position.
6. Gently remove tape and any dressing from the site while carefully stabilizing the needle or catheter to keep it from from pulling on the insertion site.
7. Place dry gauze pad over needle insertion site.
8. Swiftly withdraw needle or catheter from the site while applying gentle pressure over the site.
9. Hold site above level of the heart while continuing to apply direct pressure for 45 seconds to 1 minute.
10. Assess for bleeding from the site. If bleeding continues, maintain pressure for another minute, then reassess.
11. Apply a bandage or sterile dressing according to agency policy.
12. Discard soiled supplies and gloves in appropriate containers.
13. Remove gloves.
14. Wash hands.
15. Document promptly and accurately.
16. Reevaluate site in 10 to 15 minutes.

ADMINISTERING BLOOD

A **blood transfusion** is an introduction of blood or blood products into the bloodstream. Patients may require only red blood cells, serum, platelets, or albumin. Any one of these components may be given, or whole blood may be transfused. Blood transfusions replace blood or blood components to increase the number of red blood cells in patients with anemia, to increase blood volume after hemorrhage, and to provide blood clotting factors to control bleeding.

Strict guidelines are established for typing, receiving, storing, issuing, and transfusing blood and blood products. Qualified personnel responsible for the administration of blood and blood products must be familiar with the strict procedures and extensive documentation that must accompany this responsibility. Life-threatening reactions may occur during blood administration, so the nurse must take every precaution to recognize signs of a reaction and intervene immediately according to established protocol.

A **transfusion reaction** occurs when the donor blood is incompatible with the patient's blood. This incompatibility could be an allergic, hemolytic, or febrile reaction (Table 16-2). Even after **typing** (a test

Table 16-2 BLOOD TRANSFUSION REACTIONS

Type of Reaction	Cause	Symptoms
Allergic	Hypersensitivity to antibodies in donor's blood	Urticaria (hives), pruritus (itching), fever, anaphylactic shock
Hemolytic	Incompatibility	Nausea, vomiting, pain in lower back, hypotension, increase in pulse rate, decrease in urinary output, hematuria
Pyogenic febrile (most common)	Antibodies to donor platelets or leukocytes or contamination of blood	Fever, chills, nausea, headache, flushing, tachycardia, palpitations

From Harkness-Hood G, Dincher JR: *Total patient care,* ed 8, St Louis, 1992, Mosby.

performed to determine the blood group to which an individual belongs) and **crossmatching** (a test performed to determine the compatibility of a donor's blood to a recipient's blood before transfusion), blood reactions may occur.

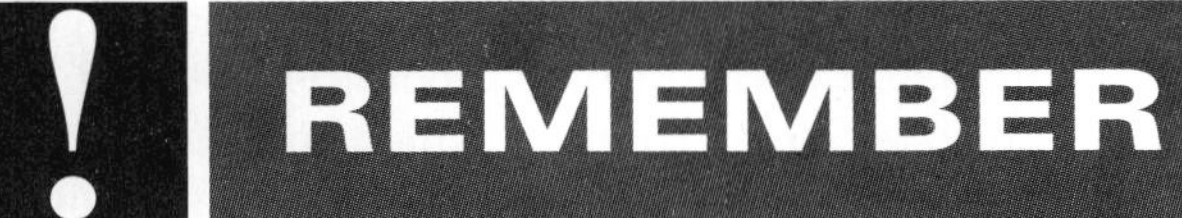

- The nurse should use only 0.9% normal saline with blood administration.
- Many blood reactions occur within the first 15 minutes of a transfusion.
- Whole blood and packed red blood cells should not hang at room temperature longer than 2 hours.
- Only legally qualified nurses administer blood and blood products.

Blood Types

There are four major blood groups—A, B, AB, and O. Therefore they are named the *ABO blood groups.* The groups are distinguished by the presence or absence of A or B **antigens** (substances that induce antibody formation) on the surface of the red blood cells. Type A blood has A antigens, type B has B antigens, type AB contains both A and B antigens, and type O contains no antigens.

Various **antibodies** (substances providing immunity) circulate in the plasma of the different blood types. Type A blood contains anti-B antibodies, type B contains anti-A antibodies, type AB contains no antibodies, and type O contains antibodies in the plasma.

Since antibodies destroy antigens, compatibility is vital. If a person has type A blood and receives type B blood, the anti-A antibodies react and destroy the recipient's red blood cells. Therefore type O blood, which has no antigens, can be donated to people with all blood types, so people with this blood type are called *universal donors.* People with AB blood, which has no antibodies, can receive all types of blood and are thus known as *universal recipients.* Today, patients are given their own types to prevent blood reactions.

Rh Factor

Another consideration before initiation of a blood transfusion is the **Rh factor,** which is the presence or absence of the Rh-factor antigen on the red blood cell. Persons whose blood contains the antigen are considered Rh positive (Rh^+), and those whose blood lacks the antigen are considered Rh negative (Rh^-). Antibodies destroy antigens, so if a person with Rh^- blood receives Rh^+ blood, the antibodies in the Rh^+ blood eventually destroy the recipient's own Rh^- red blood cells.

During pregnancy, the Rh factor is of major concern. If the mother is Rh^+, there is no need for concern: The growing fetus may have Rh^- or Rh^+ blood, so the mother's body does not develop antibodies. However, if the mother is Rh^- and the baby has inherited the Rh factor antigen (that is, has Rh^+ blood) from the father, problems may develop. If the fetal and maternal blood intermingle because of a microscopic leak caused by trauma or delivery, the mother's body recognizes the Rh^+ antigen in the infant's blood and produces antibodies against it. During a subsequent pregnancy with an Rh^+ fetus, the antibodies cross the placenta and begin **hemolysis** (destruction of the infant's red blood cells). This is a life-threatening fetal condition called **erythroblastosis fetalis.** The incidence of this condition has decreased considerably since the introduction of RhoGAM, a blood product that can be given to Rh^- pregnant women to prevent the development of antibodies against the fetus.

Autotransfusion

A newer method for administering blood is **autotransfusion,** a technique in which individuals who

BENEFITS OF AUTOTRANSFUSION

- Blood is immediately available.
- The need for typing and cross-matching is eliminated.
- The technique can be used when religious beliefs prevent administration of blood.
- The risk of adverse reaction is negligible.
- The technique is cost effective.
- The procedure may be useful in elective surgery.

are in good health and who have scheduled elective surgery may donate their own blood to be stored and then administered to them at the time of surgery. This technique is used to eliminate transfusion of incompatible blood or blood infected with serum hepatitis or HIV antibodies. Although all donated blood is screened and tested before being released for transfusions, fears exist that blood transfusions may transmit blood-borne diseases or cause severe reactions. This method eliminates the problems of incompatability and cross-contamination (see box). Blood can be stored 3 to 5 weeks, giving the body time to build up blood volume before surgery. Except in cases of elective surgery, it is difficult to predict when a person may need a transfusion, and blood cannot be kept for long periods. However, blood may now be frozen for a certain time, making it last longer.

Initiating Transfusion

The nurse is responsible for assessing and monitoring the patient before, during, and after the transfusion. After an informed consent has been signed, a primary intravenous infusion of 0.9% normal saline is initiated, and the established protocol is followed for obtaining the blood, double-checking the compatibility of the blood with the patient's blood, and the identity of the patient (Skill 16-2). Baseline vital signs are taken and recorded. Then the nurse primes the special blood administration tubing and piggybacks it into the primary infusion line. Remaining with the patient while slowly infusing the first 50 ml of blood allows the nurse to assess the patient's response and monitor vital signs. Transfusion reactions may occur at any time during or even after a blood transfusion. However, many reactions occur within the first 15 minutes. The nurse must know the symptoms of a blood transfusion reaction (see box) and the nursing interventions to initiate for them.

SYMPTOMS OF TRANSFUSION REACTIONS

- Flushing
- Itching
- Urticaria
- Wheezing
- Headache
- Sudden chills and fever
- Cough
- Chest pain
- Dyspnea
- Low back pain
- Abdominal pain
- Nausea
- Vomiting
- Cyanosis
- Jaundice
- Tachycardia
- Anxiety
- Laryngeal edema
- Anaphylaxis
- Acute renal failure
- Circulatory collapse
- Death

The medical order specifies the rate of infusion. Ideally each unit of blood should infuse within 2 hours. The risk of blood cell damage and infection increase after that time. The protocol regarding discarding or returning of container to the blood bank must be followed when one unit of blood is infused. In addition, the primary tubing should be flushed with normal saline before another unit is infused so that the blood from both units is not mixed within the tubing. Each new unit of blood should be administered through new tubing and piggybacked into the primary intravenous line. This prevents clotting within the tubing and keeps blood from mixing from unit to unit.

CHEMOTHERAPY

The term **chemotherapy** describes any type of drug therapy. However, it usually means the administration of **antineoplastic** medications (those used to prevent the proliferation of malignant [cancer] cells). These chemicals are effective in controlling cellular metabolism or the physical and chemical processes that occur within the cell. The drugs are classified by their mechanism of action. Table 16-3 lists selected chemotherapeutic drugs. Steroid and hormonal therapy is occasionally used to treat certain cancers.

Antineoplastic chemicals destroy cancer cells or prevent them from reproducing, but healthy cells

Table 16-3 AGENTS USED IN CANCER CHEMOTHERAPY

Agent	Mechanism of Action	Major Toxic Manifestations
Alkylating		
Busulfan (Myleran) Carmustine (BCNU) Chlorambucil (Leukeran) Cisplatin (Platinol) Cyclophosphamide (Cytoxan) Lomustine (CCNU) Melphalan (Alkeran) Streptozocin (Zanosar)	Interfere with DNA replication by attacking DNA synthesis throughout cell cycle (cell cycle nonspecific)	Bone marrow depression with thrombocytopenia and bleeding, pulmonary fibrosis possible, renal failure
Antimetabolites		
Cytarabine (ara-C, Cytosar) 5-Fluorouracil (5-FU) Mercaptopurine/6-MP (Purinethol) Methotrexate (Mexate)	Interfere with synthesis of essential metabolites (cell cycle specific)	Bone marrow depression, oral and gastrointestinal ulceration
Antibiotics		
Bleomycin (Blenoxane) Dactinomycin (Cosmegan) Daunorubicin (Cerubidine) Doxorubicin (Adriamycin) Mitomycin (Mutamycin) Plicamycin (Mithracin)	Interfere with DNA or RNA synthesis, varying with the drug (cell cycle nonspecific)	Bone marrow depression (except for bleomycin), pulmonary fibrosis with bleomycin or mitomycin, renal failure with mitomycin, cardiac toxicity with doxorubicin
Plant alkaloids		
Vinblastine (Velban) Vincristine (Oncovin)	Interfere with mitosis	Bone marrow depression, areflexia Neurotoxicity with ataxia and impaired fine motor skills, paralytic ileus
Steroid hormones		
Adrenocorticosteroids (prednisone) Androgens (testosterone proprionate) Antiestrogens (tamoxifen citrate [Nolvadex]) Estrogens (diethylstilbestrol) Progestins (Medroxyprogesterone [Depoprovera])	Alter host environment for cell growth (cell cycle nonspecific)	Specific for action of hormone

From Long BC, Phipps WJ, Cassmeyer VL: *Medical-surgical nursing: a nursing process approach,* ed 3, St Louis, 1993, Mosby.

are often destroyed as well. This adverse (unintended) effect is unavoidable and certainly not a goal of therapy. These chemicals can also adversely affect professionals who handle them. Chemotherapeutic medications can be absorbed through inhalation or by direct contact with the skin or mucous membranes. Exposure can damage fast-growing cells such as ova and sperm and fetal tissue.

Chemotherapy is commonly used to enhance surgery and radiation. Patients may receive chemotherapy in the hospital, at outpatient clinics, or in their home. Although this chapter focuses on the intravenous administration of chemotherapy (Skill 16-3), these drugs may also be administered orally, into arteries, between the pleurae, into the peritoneum, and intrathecally (into the cerebrospinal fluid). Only nurses specially trained and qualified by law may administer chemotherapeutic agents.

Adverse Reactions

When chemotherapy is administered in the hospital, outpatient settings, or the home, emergency drugs and equipment should be available in case of an emergency. Nurses who administer chemotherapy in the home must have access to telephone and emergency medical services.

Nurses involved in the care of patients receiving chemotherapy must be aware of medication reactions. Nausea, vomiting, diarrhea, **stomatitis** (inflammatory condition of the mouth), and **anorexia** (lack or loss of appetite, resulting in the inability to eat) are common with most chemotherapeutic agents. The intensity of the side effects may be dose related, with severity increasing as doses and frequency of administration increase.

Hair loss and bone marrow supression are other common reactions to chemotherapeutic agents. Loss of hair **(alopecia)** is usually of great concern to the patient and may threaten self-esteem. **Bone marrow supression** decreases the number of blood cells produced. The number of red blood cells and their oxygen-carrying capabilities are decreased, so the patient may feel fatigued and short of breath. A low platelet count increases the likelihood of bruising and bleeding, and an increased susceptibility to infection results from the low white blood cell count. The daily tasks of shaving, brushing teeth, and clipping nails may cause bleeding and infection. Venipuncture and injections may need to be halted until the patient's clotting time is improved. Knowledge of these adverse effects help the nurse to reduce or prevent many symptoms and complications caused by these toxic chemicals (see box).

Safety Measures

When preparing chemotherapeutic medications, the pharmacist and nurse wear protective clothing, including gowns, masks, goggles, caps, and gloves. Preparation is done under strict aseptic technique within a safety cabinet or air-flow hood. All supplies and equipment are disposed of in clearly labeled, leak-proof, puncture-resistant containers to warn others of the potential hazard. Strict protocols are followed in the preparation, handling, and administration of these drugs (see box). These severely toxic chemicals can cause necrosis and sloughing of tissue if they are infused into the tissues rather than the vein.

Although family members are encouraged to accompany the patient, young children, pregnant women, older adults, and patients with chronic illnesses are prohibited from being in the room with the patient during administration of the drugs. The patient and family are instructed on the appropriate disposal of waste and supplies to prevent exposure of others at home. The patient is instructed to avoid exposure to persons who are ill because of the compromised immune system resulting from chemotherapy.

CARE FOR PATIENTS RECEIVING CHEMOTHERAPY

Bone Marrow Suppression or Infection

- Check blood counts.
- Assess infection-prone areas daily to identify early signs of infection.
- Maintain medical asepsis through careful handwashing.
- Maintain intact skin and mucous membranes:
  - Teach avoidance of bumping and breaking skin.
  - Maintain aseptic technique during intravenous infusion and dressing changes.
  - Keep fingernails short.
  - Teach good perineal hygiene.
  - Teach avoidance of excessive friction and importance of vaginal lubrication.
  - Teach avoidance of anal intercourse.
  - Teach avoidance of enemas, rectal medications, or rectal thermometers.
  - Encourage fastidious orgal hygiene with soft toothbrush.
  - Inspect mouth daily for ulcers and white patches.
  - Use lubricants to prevent drying and cracking of lips.
- Maintain optimal respiratory function:
- Assess for early signs of respiratory infection.
- Auscultate lung sounds.
- Instruct family and friends not to visit if they have colds.
- Maintain reverse isolation if ordered.

Gastrointestinal Effects: Stomatitis, Nausea, Vomiting

- Administer oral nystatin, as ordered.
- Use rinse and lidocaine before meals to lubricate and provide analgesic effect.
- Use cleansing rinse of plain water or normal saline after meals.
- Administer antiemetic as ordered.
- Determine from patient best time for food and fluid intake in relation to treatment.
- Teach relaxation techniques and imagery, if appropriate.

CARE FOR PATIENTS RECEIVING CHEMOTHERAPY—cont'd

Alopecia
- Explain that drug-induced alopecia is not permanent.
- Allow expression of feelings about hair loss.
- Apply scalp tourniquets or scalp hypothermia via ice pack (if ordered) for patients with solid tumors to minimize hair loss with some agents (for example, vincristine, doxorubicin).
- Encourage use of wigs, hats, and scarves.

Effects on Skin
- Inspect administration site for signs of infiltration or extravasation.

Organ Toxicities
- Assess signs and symptoms of liver dysfunction.
- Monitor cardiac status (dysrhythmias, congestive heart failure).
- Assess signs and symptoms of pulmonary toxicity.

Urinary Effects: Hemorrhagic Cystitis, Renal Toxicity
- Maintain hydration by encouraging drinking of large amounts of fluid (if receiving cyclophosphamide).
- Monitor renal function: Check serum creatinine level or creatinine clearance (with cisplatin or streptozocin).

Sterility
- Assess knowledge of known and possible effects on fertility.
- Provide birth control and reproductive counseling, as appropriate.

From Long BC, Phipps WJ, Cassmeyer VL: *Medical-surgical nursing: a nursing process approach,* ed 3, St Louis, 1993, Mosby.

PRECAUTIONS FOR HANDLING ANTINEOPLASTIC AGENTS

All persons handling cytotoxic (hazardous) drugs, such as antineoplastic agents, should be properly trained in safety procedures and have access to policies and procedures that follow current government and professional practice standards.

Drug Preparation and Administration
Wash hands thoroughly then wear a disposable gown, surgical latex gloves, and eye protection when preparing or administering cytotoxic drugs.

Whenever possible, it is highly recommended that preparation of injectable antineoplastic agents be performed in the clean-air work station (Hepa filter in BSC or biohazard cabinet).

Use areas for the preparation of drugs only for that purpose. Limit access to that area.

Remove only the required amount of the drug into the syringe. If more is withdrawn accidently, inject the excess back into the vial and dispose of it properly.

Vent vials with a 20-gauge needle to avoid the creation of aerosol particles.

Nurses should not prepare or administer intravenous chemotherapy if they are pregnant because of suspected risk to the fetus from these agents.

Disposal of Antineoplastic Drugs and Equipment
All antineoplastic drugs and all vials, needles, syringes, tubing, and equipment used in their administration need to be discarded with caution. Special leak-proof, puncture-proof, double-bagged containers should be used and labeled BIOHAZARD for disposal by incineration.

Needles and syringes should not be broken and/or separated before disposal because leakage of the medication may occur.

Spillage or Antineoplastic Drug Contact with Nurse or Client
Spillage
Wear two pairs of gloves when cleaning up an antineoplastic drug spill. Wash hands before and after.

Wear a mask and eye protection if the medication is powdered.

Place the spilled substance in a plastic bag. Wipe up the remainder with a damp cloth and also place the cloth in the plastic bag.

Seal the bag and place it inside of a second bag, and seal the second bag. Label it BIOHAZARD and send it for disposal by incineration.

Drug contact with nurse or client
Thoroughly wash the affected area with soap and water. If clothing was contaminated, remove clothing immediately.

If eye contact was made, flush the eyes with copious amounts of water, holding the eyelids open during flushing.

Disposal of Client Excreta
Urine, vomitus, and other body fluids from clients receiving antineoplastic drugs should be handled with caution. Flush excreta down the toilet. Wear gloves to avoid contact. Wash containers thoroughly.

From McKenry LM, Salerno E: *Mosby's pharmacology in nursing,* ed 19, St Louis, 1995, Mosby.

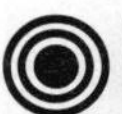

SKILL 16-1 INITIATING VENIPUNCTURE

Steps	Rationale
1. Obtain equipment: ▪ Intravenous infusion tray, including tourniquet, alcohol wipe, angiocatheter, tubing, adhesive tape and dressing ▪ Clean gloves ▪ Solution to be infused	Helps organize procedure.
2. Refer to medical record, care plan, or Kardex for special interventions.	Provides basis for care.
3. Introduce self.	Decreases patient's anxiety level.
4. Identify patient by identification band.	Identifies correct patient for procedure.
5. Explain procedure to patient.	Seeks patient's cooperation and decreases anxiety.
6. Wash hands and don clean gloves according to agency policy and guidelines from Centers for Disease Control and Prevention and Occupational Safety and Health Administration.	Helps prevent cross-contamination.
7. Prepare patient for intervention:	
a. Close door to room or pull curtain.	Provides privacy.
b. Drape for procedure if necessary.	Prevents exposure of patient.
8. Raise bed to comfortable working level.	Provides for safety for nurse.
9. Arrange for patient privacy.	Shows respect for patient.
10. Identify venipuncture sites (Fig. 16-5).	Promotes patient movement and comfort and adequate vein for infusion.
11. Apply tourniquet (Fig. 16-6, *A*).	Facilitates observation and puncture of distended veins.
12. Select venipuncture site (Fig. 16-6, *B*).	
13. Cleanse site with alcohol swab or special agent using friction (Fig. 16-6, *C*).	Helps remove organisms from puncture site.

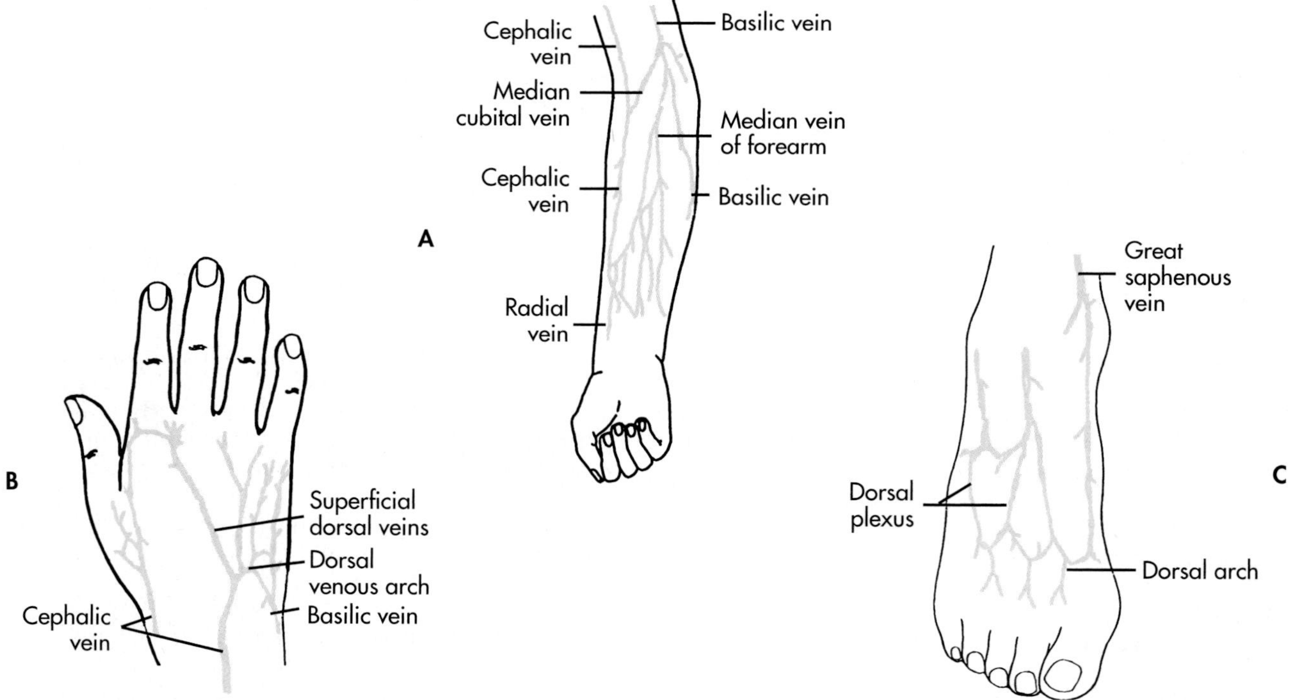

Fig. 16-5 Common intravenous sites. **A,** Dorsal surface of the hand. **B,** Inner arm. **C,** Dorsal surface of the foot. (From Potter PA, Perry AG: *Fundamentals of nursing: concepts, process, and practice,* ed 3, St Louis, 1993, Mosby.)

SKILL 16-1 INITIATING VENIPUNCTURE—cont'd

Steps	Rationale
14. Stretch skin taut and stabilize vein with nondominant hand (Fig. 16-6, *C*).	Prevents vein from moving during process.
15. Holding angiocatheter bevel up, pierce skin above and slightly to side of vein at 45-degree angle.	Allows needle to enter smoothly through skin and approach vein wall.
16. Lower angle to 10 degrees and enter vein wall. Slight resistance and "pop" accompany entry into vein.	Reduces risk of going completely through vein and ensures placement within vein.
17. Follow vein lumen with tip of needle to ensure placement within vein, watching for blood return through angiocatheter backflow chamber (Fig. 16-6, *D*).	Confirms placement within vein.
18. Release tourniquet.	Decreases potential for vein rupture.
19. Holding guide needle in place, gently thread plastic catheter off needle and into vein.	Prevents needle going through catheter and vein. Prevents catheter from being dislodged by slight movement.
20. Applying gentle pressure over catheter in vein, remove guide needle, and attach sterile connection end of primed tubing into catheter hub.	Avoids backflow, connects fluid source to venous access, and maintains sterility of system.
21. Stabilizing insertion site, slowly open flow valve to begin intravenous infusion.	Maintains catheter in place, prompts infusion, and avoids clotting of blood in catheter.
22. Following agency policy, secure and dress site with tape, medications, and dressings.	Prevents unintentional dislodging of catheter from vein and helps prevent infection.
23. Label site and tubing according to agency policy.	Serves as reminder to change site and tubing.
24. Adjust fluid flow rate according to accurate drop-rate calculations.	Provides fluid therapy according to medical order.
25. Remove gloves and wash hands.	Helps prevent cross-contamination.
26. Document.	Documents procedure and patient's response.

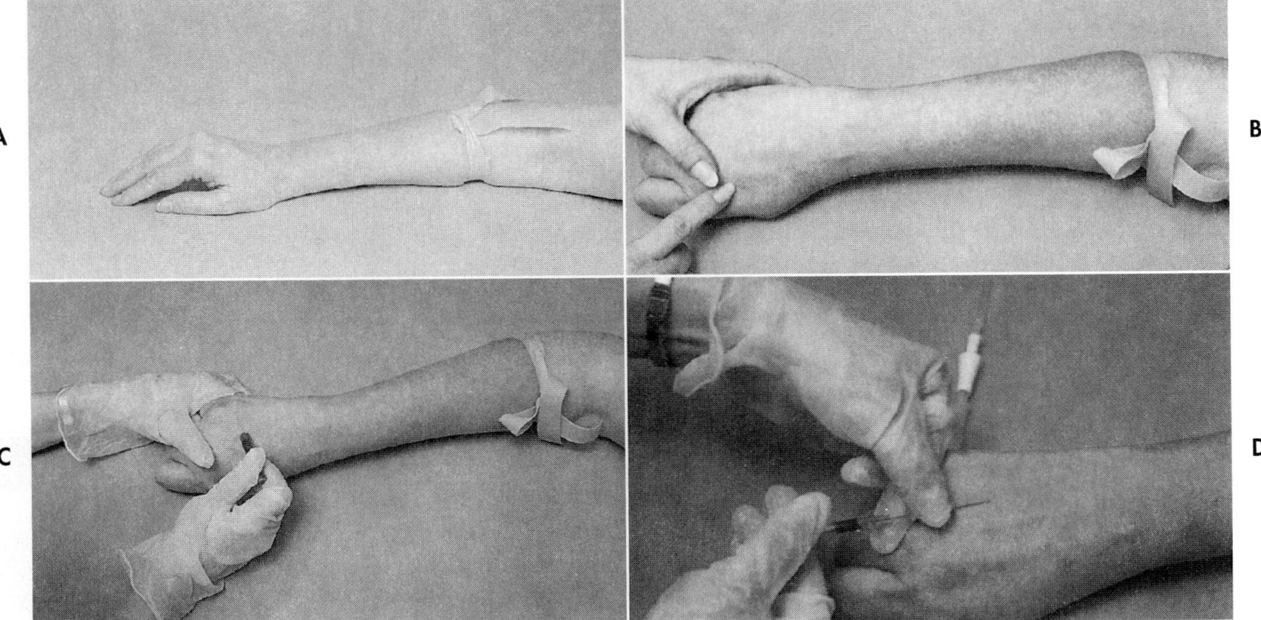

Fig. 16-6 **A,** Apply tourniquet. **B,** Select intravenous site. **C,** Cleanse site for venipuncture. **D,** Watch for blood return through angiocatheter. (From Potter PA, Perry AG: *Fundamentals of nursing: concepts, process, and practice,* ed 3, St Louis, 1993, Mosby.)

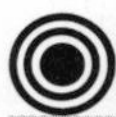

SKILL 16-2 ADMINISTERING BLOOD

Steps	Rationale
1. Assess for informed consent form.	Indicates legal approval for procedure.
2. Obtain equipment: ▪ Intravenous tray ▪ Clean gloves	Helps organize procedure.
3. Refer to medical record, care plan, or Kardex for special interventions.	Provides basis for care.
4. Introduce self.	Decreases patient's anxiety level.
5. Identify patient by identification band.	Identifies correct patient for procedure.
6. Explain procedure to patient.	Seeks patient's cooperation and decreases anxiety.
7. Wash hands and don clean gloves according to agency policy and guidelines from Centers for Disease Control and Prevention and Occupational Safety and Health Administration.	Helps prevent cross-contamination.
8. Prepare patient for intervention:	
a. Close door to room or pull curtains.	Provides privacy.
b. Drape for procedure if necessary.	Prevents exposure of patient.
9. Raise bed to comfortable working level.	Provides for safety of nurse.
10. Arrange for patient privacy.	Shows respect for patient.
11. Initiate primary intravenous infusion or hang 0.9% normal saline container and flush tubing into existing intravenous infusion.	Prevents hemolysis.
12. Obtain blood immediately before infusion.	Decreases potential for clotting and contamination.
13. Verify patient identity and blood compatibility per agency protocol.	Helps prevent blood transfusion error.
14. Attach filtered blood administration tubing to blood unit container and prime it.	Prevents air embolus and clots.
15. Piggyback blood-filled tubing to Y-connector closest to patient.	Prevents additional blood from infusing if a reaction occurs, and maintains primary intravenous infusion.
16. Obtain baseline vital signs.	Identifies pretransfusion norms.
17. Begin transfusion slowly.	Helps avoid blood reaction.
18. Take vital signs every 5 minutes for 15 minutes.	Assesses for early signs of reaction.
19. If reaction symptoms occur, stop transfusion and follow steps of nursing interventions for transfusion reactions (see box).	Prevents complications and severe adverse reactions to transfusion.
20. Instruct patient to immediately report any rash, itching, chills, or headache.	Helps prevent severe reactions.
21. Adjust flow rate using infusion pump.	Provides safe blood administration at prescribed rate.
22. Observe and assess patient frequently per protocol.	Ensures stability of patient's condition.
23. Discontinue blood transfusion when blood is infused and maintain primary intravenous infusion of 0.9% normal saline.	Allows time for patient to respond to infusion and maintains venous access.
24. Remove gloves and wash hands.	Helps prevent cross-contamination.
25. Document.	Documents procedure and patient's response.

NURSING INTERVENTIONS FOR TRANSFUSION REACTIONS

If a blood reaction occurs the nurse should:

- Stop the blood transfusion immediately.
- Maintain the primary intravenous infusion with 0.9% normal saline.
- Stay with the patient, monitoring vital signs every 3 to 5 minutes.
- Call or ring for assistance.
- Notify the physician and blood bank.
- Prepare to administer emergency care (cardiopulmonary resuscitation, emergency medications).
- Obtain urine specimen and send it to the laboratory.
- Complete reports, forms, and other necessary documentation.
- Save the blood container, remaining blood, and tubing for laboratory or blood bank follow-up.

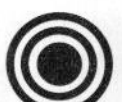

SKILL 16-3 ADMINISTERING CHEMOTHERAPY

Steps	Rationale
1. **Obtain equipment:** ▪ Drug ▪ Intravenous tray ▪ Clean gloves	Helps organize procedure.
2. **Refer to medical record, care plan, or Kardex for special interventions.**	Provides basis for care.
3. **Introduce self.**	Decreases patient's anxiety level.
4. **Identify patient by identification band.**	Identifies correct patient for procedure.
5. **Explain procedure to patient.**	Seeks patient's cooperation and decreases anxiety.
6. **Wash hands and don clean gloves according to agency policy and guidelines from Centers for Disease Control and Prevention and Occupational Safety and Health Administration.**	Helps prevent cross-contamination.
7. **Prepare patient for intervention:**	
a. Close door to room or pull curtain.	Provides privacy.
b. Drape for procedure if necessary.	Prevents exposure of patient.
8. **Raise bed to comfortable working level.**	Provides for safety of nurse.
9. **Arrange for patient privacy.**	Shows respect for patient.
10. **Verify that informed consent has been granted.**	Indicates legal approval for procedure.
11. **Review laboratory reports, record current patient history and vital signs, and provide opportunity for patient to discuss feelings.**	Verifies patient's physical and emotional state to receive medication.
12. **Read medical order and medication label 3 times and verify dosage, medication, and patient.**	Helps prevent medication errors.
13. **Administer preventive measures as ordered (for example, antiemetic, ice chips, ice cap to scalp, cool cloth to forehead or neck).**	Maintains patient stability.
14. **Don protective gear.**	Helps prevent contamination and hazard.
15. **Place emergency equipment and medications nearby.**	Prevents delay if emergency occurs.
16. **Perform venipuncture or verify placement of intravenous infusion or heparin lock by assessing for blood return.**	Verifies that tissue damage has not occurred.
17. **Cleanse injection port and insert stopcock device.**	Avoids puncture of tubing and leakage of medication.
18. **Insert syringe or piggyback tubing connection into stopcock device (Fig. 16-7).**	Provides medication into intravenous infusion.

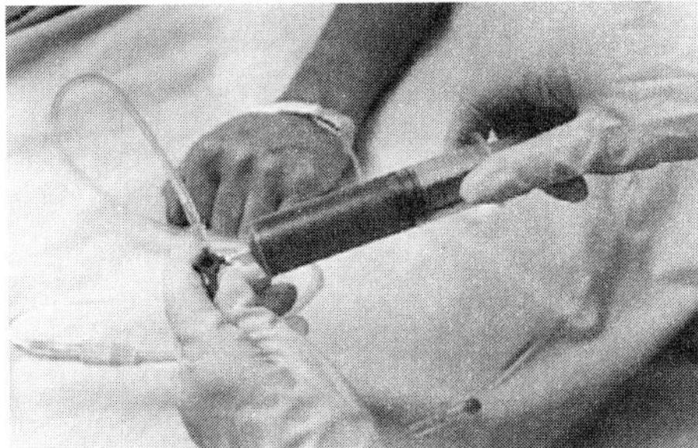

Fig. 16-7 Insert syringe to piggyback tubing into stopcock. (From Perry AG, Potter PA: *Clinical nursing skills and techniques,* ed 3, St Louis, 1994, Mosby.)

Continued.

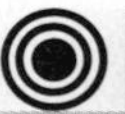

SKILL 16-3 ADMINISTERING CHEMOTHERAPY—cont'd

Steps	Rationale
19. Slowly begin medication infusion.	Prevents onset of side effects.
20. Administer medication by pump or volume-control device, aspirating and frequently assessing patient's response.	Provides accurate, controlled dosage; verifies that route remains intravenous; determines patient's response; and prevents complications.
21. Stop chemotherapy immediately if severe reaction or infiltration occurs.	Promotes patient's safety.
22. Flush intravenous infusion lines between multiple medication administration.	Prevents mixing of medications.
23. Frequently observe and assess infusion and patient (Fig. 16-8).	Prevents complications.
24. When completely infused, remove piggyback tubing and container or syringe and dispose in biohazardous containers according to agency policy (Fig. 16-9).	Avoids contamination and protects others from biohazardous material.
25. Remove protective gear and dispose of it according to agency policy.	Provides protection for nurse and others.
26. Instruct patient on disposal of body fluids for next 48 hr.	Promotes patient's safety.
27. Remove gloves and wash hands.	Helps prevent cross-contamination.
28. Document.	Documents procedure and patient's response.

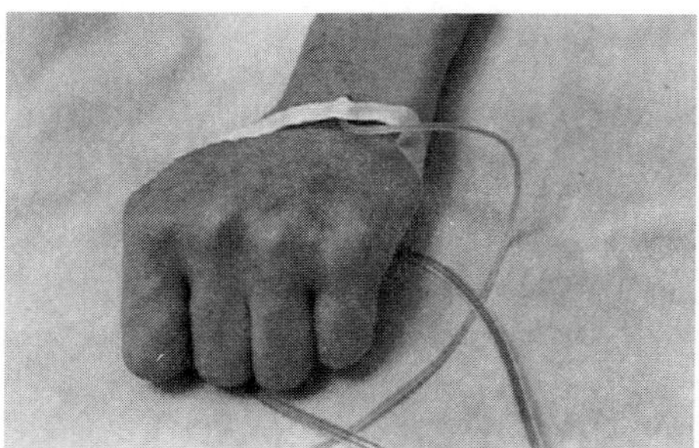

Fig. 16-8 Observe and assess intravenous infusion and patient. (From Perry AG, Potter PA: *Clinical nursing skills and techniques,* ed 3, St Louis, 1994, Mosby.)

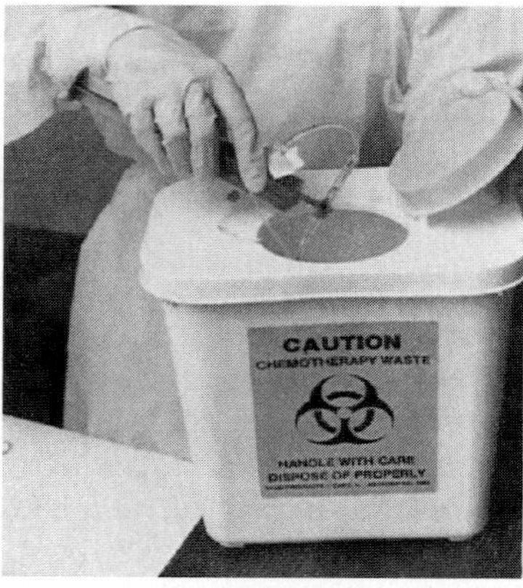

Fig. 16-9 Disposal into biohazard container. (From Perry AG, Potter PA: *Clinical nursing skills and techniques,* ed 3, St Louis, 1994, Mosby.)

SUMMARY

Special parenteral therapies are administered only by specially trained and legally qualified nurses. These therapies are medically ordered to meet individual needs for specific reasons. Fluid and electrolyte imbalances, hemorrhage, blood diseases, and cancer may be life threatening. Safe and accurate administration and regulation of fluids, blood, and antineoplastic agents are the responsibility of the nurse. Another important responsibility of the nurse is patient and family education. Taking the time to answer questions and give guidance for home follow-up encourages patient cooperation and enhances patient self-esteem.

Key Concepts

- Aseptic technique is used for all intravenous therapy.
- Knowledge of various complications of intravenous therapies and nursing interventions is required of any nurse involved in administering these therapies.
- Nurse practice acts legally define the nurse's qualifications and scope of practice in administering parenteral therapy.
- Universal precautions are indicated in the administration of intravenous therapy.
- Patient and family education and safety are important nursing responsibilities.
- Specially marked biohazardous containers are used for the disposal of supplies and equipment used to administer intravenous therapy.
- Intravenous solution tubings must be primed before solutions are administered through them.
- Blood must be refrigerated until it is used.
- Blood reactions may occur immediately after administration is begun or may occur several days later.
- Protective gear is used in the handling of chemotherapeutic agents.
- Reactions to chemotherapy may increase with increased dosage or frequency.
- Alopecia from chemotherapy is not permanent.

Critical Thinking Questions

1. Mr. Jones is receiving intravenous fluids because he is to have nothing by mouth after surgery earlier today. His fluid order is 1000 ml of lactated Ringer's solution with 20 mEq/L KCl to run over 6 hours. What tubing should be used to administer these fluids in terms of drop size? The nurse hangs a new bag of fluids at 5 PM. At 8 PM, the nurse notes that 300 ml have infused from the bag. Are these fluids on time? If not, what assessments should be done to determine the reason?
2. While starting an intravenous infusion the nurse begins to advance the ONC and notes that the area immediately around the insertion site is swelling. What should the nurse do?

REFERENCES AND SUGGESTED READINGS

Bohony J: 9 common IV implications and what to do about them, *American Journal of Nursing 93*(10):45, 1993.

Clark JB, Queener SF, Karb VB: *Pharmacologic basis of nursing practice,* St Louis, 1993, Mosby.

Edmunds MW: *Introduction to clinical pharmacology,* ed 2, St Louis, 1995, Mosby.

Harovas J, Anthony HH: Managing transfusion reactions, *RN* 56(12):32, 1993.

Jagger J, Blackwell B: Needless needles remain in hospital invironment: needles used to connect IV lines are strictly unnecessary needles, *Today's OR Nurse 16*(3):3, 1994.

Long et al: *Medical-surgical nursing: a nursing process approach,* ed 3, St Louis, 1993, Mosby.

McKenry LM, Salerno E: *Mosby's pharmacology in nursing,* ed 19, St Louis, 1995, Mosby.

Millam DA: How to teach good venipuncture technique, *American Journal of Nursing* 93(7):38, 1993.

Perry AG, Potter PA: *Clinical nursing skills and techniques,* ed 3, St Louis, 1994, Mosby.

Perucca R, Micek J: Treatment of infusion related phlebitis: review and nursing protocol, *Journal of Intravenous Nursing* 16(5):277, 1993.

Potter PA, Perry AG: *Basic nursing: theory and practice,* ed 3, St Louis, 1995, Mosby.

Potter PA, Perry AG: *Fundamentals of nursing: concepts, process, and practice,* ed 3, St Louis, 1993, Mosby.

Querin JJ, Stahl LD: 12 simple, sensible steps for successful blood transfusions, *Nursing 1990* 20(10):68, 1990.

Rice JB, Shelley EG: *Medications & math for the nurse,* ed 7, Albany, NY, 1993, Delmar.

Robinson S: Principles of chemotherapy, *European Journal of Cancer Care* 2(2):55, 1993.

Sheldon JE: What you should know about IV dressings, *Nursing 1994* 24(8):32, 1994.

Thurkauf GE: Understanding the beliefs of Jehovah's Witnesses, *Focus on Critical Care* 16(3):199, 1989.

Wilson JA: Preventing infection during IV therapy, *Professional Nurse* 9(6):388, 1994.

CHAPTER 17

Perioperative Nursing

Learning Objectives

After studying this chapter, the student should be able to. . .

- Define the key terms.
- List the steps in preoperative preparation.
- Identify the high-risk surgical patient.
- Differentiate among the preoperative preparation of the child, older adult, and high-risk patient.
- Complete a preoperative checklist.
- Teach controlled coughing, breathing techniques, and leg exercises.
- Describe the major assessment skills needed in the preoperative, intraoperative, and postoperative stages.
- Explain the steps necessary to perform a surgical shave.
- Make a surgical bed.
- Explain the purpose of informed consent.
- Perform general postoperative measures such as obtaining vital signs; assessing the level of consciousness; detecting and caring for postoperative complications; assessing surgical pain; and assessing dressings, drains, and tubes.
- Report and document common postoperative complications.
- Explain the procedure for receiving the patient from the postanesthesia care unit (recovery room).
- Assess for a patent airway.
- Apply antiembolism stockings when needed.
- Apply heat and cold applications.
- Clean and care for a surgical drain.
- Apply bandages and binders.

Key Terms

Ambulatory surgery
Antiembolism stockings
Autologous transfusion
Bandaging
Binder
Cardiac arrest
Dehiscence
Distention
Drainage
Elective surgery
Evisceration
Flatulence
Hemorrhage
Hypovolemia
Incentive spirometry
Ischemia
Normovolemic hemodilution
Perioperative blood salvage
Perioperative nursing
Postanesthesia care unit (PACU)
Rebound effect
Respiratory arrest
Sequential compression device (SCD)
Splinting
Thrombophlebitis
Thrombus
T-tube

Skills

17-1 Teaching postoperative breathing techniques and leg exercises
17-2 Teaching controlled coughing
17-3 Performing a surgical shave
17-4 Making a surgical bed
17-5 Receiving the patient from the postanesthesia care unit
17-6 Applying antiembolism stockings
17-7 Applying heat
17-8 Applying cold
17-9 Caring for surgical drains
17-10 Applying a bandage
17-11 Applying a binder, arm sling, or T-binder

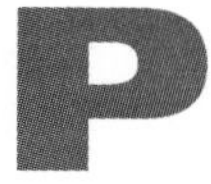

Perioperative nursing refers to the nursing care administered to a patient for the entire surgical experience. It begins when the patient is admitted to the hospital and concludes when the patient is discharged from the physician's care. Included in this experience for the patient are preoperative preparation and teaching, the intraoperative or surgical experience, and postoperative care and follow-up teaching. The family patient needs to be involved in each step of this experience.

Even though one nurse seldom follows the patient through all of the phases, each nurse is responsible for providing competent and safe nursing care. The goal for all nurses is to assist the patient to return to as healthy a state as possible.

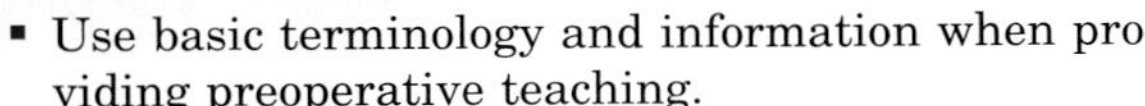

- Use basic terminology and information when providing preoperative teaching.
- Give the patient and family a tour of the new unit if the patient will be transferred after surgery.
- Reassure the patient and family that pain will be controlled.
- Teach the patient measures to lessen the effects of anesthesia and surgery, such as taking only the amount of pain medication needed to fully relieve pain and increasing ambulation early in the postoperative period.

NURSING PROCESS

Assessment

General assessment of the preoperative patient includes obtaining a nursing history. This consists of any prior surgery, allergies, current medications, use of other drugs or alcohol, and smoking status. The nurse also assesses the patient's physical condition, high-risk data, emotional status of the patient and family members, and preoperative diagnostic data. It is important for the patient and family to understand the surgical procedure and the expected outcomes. In the intraoperative stage, the nurse completes any procedures such as shaving or catheterization. During surgery and recovery, the nurse continually assesses the patient's condition. The nurse also provides postoperative care to prevent and detect complications and return the patient to wellness.

Nursing Diagnosis

Nursing diagnoses establish direction for care that will be provided during one or all surgical phases. Nursing diagnoses may focus on intraoperative and postoperative risks. Preventive care is essential for effective management of the surgical patient. Nursing diagnoses related to this patient may include the following:

Altered role performance
Anxiety
Body-image disturbance
Fear
Impaired physical mobility
Impaired skin integrity
Ineffective airway clearance
Ineffective breathing pattern
Ineffective individual coping
Knowledge deficit (specify)
Pain
Powerlessness
Risk for infection

Planning

The plan of care begins before surgery and follows through the postoperative period to provide the best nursing care possible. It is important for the nurse to include the patient in health care planning (see care plan on p. 330). A patient informed about the surgical experience is less likely to be fearful and is able to prepare for expected outcomes (see teaching box).

Goals and expected outcomes for the surgical patient may include the following:

Goal #1: Patient achieves physical and psychologic comfort.

Outcome
Patient verbalizes relief of pain.

Goal #2: Patient returns to functional health state within limitations posed by surgery.

Outcome
Patient independently participates in self-care activities.

Implementation

Nursing interventions before surgery physically and psychologically prepare the patient for the surgical procedure. The nurse acts as an advocate for the patient during and after surgery to ensure that the patient's dignity and rights are protected at all times. The nurse provides interventions for the older patient according to the individual's capabilities (see gerontologic box).

Evaluation

The effectiveness of the plan of care is evaluated by the nurse. The plan is revised as needed. Ex-

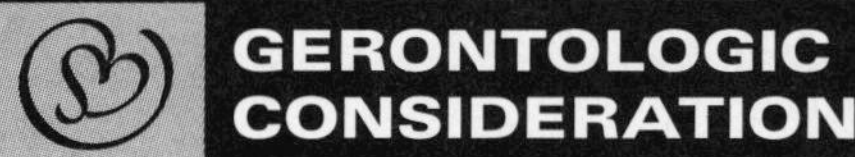

GERONTOLOGIC CONSIDERATIONS

- Older patients tend to recover more slowly from surgery. Recovery may be affected by the level of mental functioning, individual ability to cope, and availability of a support system.
- Preoperative and postoperative teaching may require extra time. Directions should be repeated and reinforced.
- Risks of aspiration, pneumonia, and infection are increased in the older adult.
- Disorientation can occur after anesthetics or sedatives have been administered. This condition may last days after initial administration.

amples of goals and evaluative measures include the following:

Goal #1: Patient achieves physical and psychologic comfort.

Evaluative measure

Observe patient for nonverbal signs of discomfort.

Goal #2: Patient returns to functional health state within limitations posed by surgery.

Evaluative measure

Observe patient perform hygiene activities and exercise.

PREOPERATIVE EXPERIENCE

Surgical patients enter the hospital in different states of health. A patient may be admitted for **elective surgery** to correct a condition that is not currently life threatening, or a patient may be admitted for emergency surgery that must be performed immediately to save a life or preserve a body part. Regardless of the type of surgery a patient is to undergo, it is preferable for the patient to be appropriately prepared both physically and psychologically.

Ambulatory Surgery

Many surgical patients now have the option to enter the hospital early in the morning, have the surgery, and return home the same day. Other terms for **ambulatory surgery** are *outpatient surgery, one-day surgery,* and *same-day surgery.* This type of surgery is generally reserved for patients who need "minor" surgical procedures, who are in excellent health, and whose surgical outcome is expected to be uneventful. Although much of the surgery continues to be performed in the regular hospital surgical unit, ambulatory surgical centers have been designed to meet the needs of the ambulatory surgical patient.

The advantages of ambulatory surgery are many. The patient is generally more rested and relaxed before surgery. The cost of surgery is greatly reduced when a longer hospital stay is not required. The patient spends less time away from work, home, or school, and daily routines are not completely disrupted.

One of the main disadvantages of ambulatory surgery is the difficulty of appropriately preparing a patient before surgery. Patient preparation and teaching are usually completed in a much shorter time in the surgeon's office or the outpatient unit before surgery. The nurse continues to administer competent nursing care physically and emotionally.

23-Hour or Short-Term Stay

A short-term stay involves the admission of a patient after surgery for a short period, which usually does not exceed 23 hours. This type of stay is recommended for the patient who needs to have some follow-up but is not expected to have complications or require close assessment after the first day. If complications occur or the patient needs to be closely assessed for a longer time, the patient is admitted as an acute care patient.

Inpatient Surgery

The patient requiring inpatient surgery is admitted to the hospital for surgery and remains in the hospital until released by the surgeon. An inpatient stay may last from 2 to 10 days or longer if complications occur. This type of admission continues to be essential for the high-risk surgical patient or for more complicated surgeries.

Autologous Transfusion

Because of the increase in infectious blood-borne pathogens (for example, acquired immunodeficiency syndrome [AIDS], hepatitis B), a greater number of patients are choosing **autologous transfusion,** the collection and reinfusion of a patient's own blood or blood components. This can be done in one of three ways. The most commonly used method is preoperative autologous blood donation. Two methods used somewhat less commonly are perioperative blood salvage and acute normovolemic hemodilution.

The preoperative autologous blood donation involves the patient donating blood 4 to 6 weeks before surgery. This method can be used only for patients undergoing planned surgery. Blood cannot be donated any later than 72 hours before surgery. Because of their size and blood volume, children are not good candidates for preoperative donation. Patients with cardiac conditions and geriatric patients are also not considered candidates for autologous transfusion. The American Red Cross has specific guidelines describing who is eligible. One disadvantage is the cost for processing, tracking, and storing the blood, which is considerably greater than that of a regular transfusion.

Perioperative blood salvage involves collecting blood during surgery or up to 12 hours after surgery. This is accomplished by collecting the blood under sterile conditions using suction at the operative site or collecting the blood from chest drains after surgery. The salvaged blood may be transfused directly after collection or processed (washed) before infusion. The salvaged blood cannot be stored. This method of transfusion is contraindicated in surgeries involving spilled intestional contents, bacterial peritonitis, intraabdominal abscesses, osteomyelitis, or malignancies.

Acute **normovolemic hemodilution** involves the removal of the patient's blood immediately before or after administration of the anesthesia. At the same time a colloid solution is given intraveniously to the patient to help replace the volume of blood and maintain normovolemia (normal volume). During surgery or immediately after, the removed blood can be reinfused to provide the patient with additional volume and blood components. This option is used only for the patient who can tolerate the rapid withdrawal of blood before surgery.

High-Risk Surgical Patient

Children, older adults, and other high-risk patients present a real challenge for the nurse. Assessment must be thorough, and baseline data must be well documented for postoperative comparison. The nurse must be aware of the possible complications and assess the patient for any signs that may indicate a problem. Any person who is undergoing surgery should be evaluated for possible risks.

Obesity Obese patients are considered to be at high risk for many reasons. Surgical procedures are difficult because of the amount of fatty tissue, sutures are difficult to tie, and wound dehiscence is more likely (see Chapter 18). After surgery, the obese patient is harder to turn, and the lungs are harder to ventilate, which may lead to respiratory complications. The healing process may be slower, and resistance is usually lower, causing the possibility for infection.

Dehydration Patients who are dehydrated, have a fluid and electrolyte imbalance, or are malnourished are at greater risk for postoperative shock, poor healing, and impaired skin integrity.

Chronic diseases The presence of chronic diseases increases the risk for surgical patients. Alcoholism, pulmonary and upper respiratory diseases, diabetes, and cardiovascular diseases are a few conditions that should alert the nurse to the possibility of potential complications.

Medications Patients taking certain prescription medications are considered to be at high risk for surgery. Anticoagulants interfere with the clotting process. Steroids alter the ability to heal and fight infections because of their antiinflammatory action. Oral contraceptives increase the possibility of blood clots. Diuretics increase the possibility of electrolyte imbalances.

Elevated temperature A patient with an elevated temperature is at greater risk when undergoing anesthesia, and the need for fluids and calories is increased for these patients.

Children Children who are admitted to the hospital for surgery require special consideration. Physically the child presents different problems than the adult. The younger the age, the more closely the child needs to be assessed (see box).

Psychologically, the child and family need emotional support; adequate explanation of all procedures, including the surgical procedure; and preparation for any postoperative changes, such as new or different equipment. The family needs to know how the child will feel after surgery and, especially, if the child will be located in a different room or unit when returned from surgery. Questions from the child or family should be answered honestly to help alleviate fear and anxiety. A doll is frequently used to explain procedures to the small child. A painful procedure is not explained to the child until the time

NEEDS OF THE HOSPITALIZED CHILD

- Infants and young children have faster metabolic rates, which require that they be fed more often. Because of their faster metabolism, children usually heal more rapidly than adults.
- Abnormal fluid loss in infants or young children is more serious than in adults, requiring that their intake and output be measured accurately.
- Unlike adults, children lack physical body reserves, so their conditions are more unpredictable. Their general condition may quickly worsen without warning.
- Children usually require proportionally less analgesia or pain medication than adults.

for the procedure so that the child will not overreact.

Older adults Many patients undergoing surgery are older adults. Because of the deterioration of the body systems, an older adult's ability to adapt to the stress of surgery may be hampered. Many older adults have other physical problems that must be considered when the nurse prepares them for surgery. Factors to be taken into consideration are listed in the box.

Nursing Intervention

The responsibilities of the nurse before surgery include the following:

1. Explaining and maintaining nothing-by-mouth (NPO) status because the patient needs an empty gastrointestinal tract to prevent the possibility of vomitus aspiration during or immediately after surgery
2. Examining the chart for appropriate physical examination, laboratory tests, special examination reports, history, and patient allergies
3. Obtaining a signed informed consent or surgical consent form
4. Taking and assessing the patient's vital signs
5. Providing personal hygiene, including bathing, oral care, donning of a clean gown, and preparation of a surgical bed
6. Preparing the surgical site according to orders
7. Removing or securing the patient's jewelry (It is best if the patient allows the nurse to place the jewelry and other valuables in the hospital safe, but when the patient objects, a ring may be taped in place or secured with gauze, or valuables are given to appropriate family member.)
8. Removing glasses, contact lenses, prostheses, wigs, false eyelashes, dentures, hairpins, clips, combs, nail polish, and make-up; placing a surgical cap over the patient's hair in some institutions.
9. Assessing the patient's identification band and allergy band for correct information and correct placement on the patient's arm
10. Providing for elimination or insertion of a Foley catheter
11. Administering preoperative medication as ordered at the designated time; raising the side rails, placing the call light or bell within reach, and informing the patient of possible drowsiness; emphasizing the need to remain in bed; ensuring that all forms are signed before the administration of any preoperative medications
12. Documenting and completing the preoperative checklist

In most instances, the surgeon orders an enema to cleanse the bowel before surgery. This is performed to prevent an involuntary bowel movement during anesthesia and to reduce the possibility of postoperative abdominal distention. It also helps prevent postoperative straining or constipation. If bowel surgery is to be performed, enemas may be ordered "until clear," meaning that no fecal material is present in the returning solution.

The surgeon may order a vaginal douche for female patients before vaginal surgery or for surgery involving the reproductive organs. The douche cleanses the vagina and adjacent parts and lessens the possibility of infection.

Preoperative medications are ordered to help the patient relax, relieve apprehension, lower the metabolic rate, reduce secretions, minimize spasm, produce a sedative effect, and reduce the possibility of vomiting. It is important that the nurse administer the medication at the time ordered by the physician. Most of the medications should be administered 45 to 75 minutes before the administration of the anesthetic to provide the maximal effect. If it is not possible to administer the medication as ordered, the anesthesiologist should be made aware of the situation so that appropriate changes in anesthesia can be made for patient safety.

PHYSIOLOGIC CHANGES WITH AGING

- Sensory losses can occur with increased age. Diminished hearing and eyesight can make communication more difficult. Reduced sensitivity to touch and increased pain tolerance may delay the discovery of injury or complications from the surgery.
- Loss of skin elasticity, subcutaneous fat, and mobility may create an environment for skin breakdown over bony prominences, causing pressure ulcers (see Chapter 21).
- Reduced kidney functioning—particularly the ability to remove wastes or drugs—provides an opportunity for an undesirable cumulative effect of drugs. Some medications (barbiturates) in usual dosages may cause confusion and disorientation in the older adult.
- Lower metabolic rates and a reduced blood supply from decreased cardiac output and increased deposits of minerals and plaque in the blood vessels cause slower healing.
- Loss of mobility may make it more difficult to move the patient and to change the patient's position frequently.
- Reduced size and mobility of the rib cage may make deep respirations more difficult, increasing the chances for respiratory complications.
- Reduced functioning of the gastrointestinal system may result in dehydration, malnutrition, and constipation.

Preoperative checklist

The preoperative essential checklist may be used for completing the aspects of preoperative care. Also, having all of the appropriate information on one sheet eliminates the need to look through the entire chart. Preoperative checklists vary from institution to institution; however, most preoperative checklists include the items in the box.

The checklist is completed and signed by the unit nurse. The surgical nurse receiving the patient is also asked to assess the checklist, verify that the patient has been appropriately prepared, and sign the checklist.

Psychologic preparation

Anticipation of surgery frequently leads to fear and anxiety. The patient may associate surgery with pain, disfigurement, a potential change in body image, dependence on others, disruption of lifestyle, cancer, or even death. It is therefore vital that the patient be given an opportunity to voice these fears. The nurse listens to the patient and/or family member and determines the type of nursing action needed. Appropriate explanations should be provided to the patient and family members. A spiritual leader may be called to provide spiritual support. If a patient or family member requires further explanation to alleviate fear regarding the surgery, the physician should be notified.

Preoperative teaching

The nurse is responsible for preoperative teaching. The extent of teaching is determined on an individual basis and takes into account the patient's previous knowledge or experience, desire to learn, emotional and physical condition, and amount of time available. Appropriate preoperative teaching should result in a more positive attitude, which in turn will ensure a more rapid recovery. The need for medications for pain may be lessened, and the possibility of complications may be reduced, resulting in a shorter hospital stay.

Hospital procedures and policies also should be explained to the patient and family. The location of the surgical suites and the surgical waiting room should be pointed out. When the patient and family are familiar with hospital routine, the patient is more cooperative and comfortable.

In some instances when extensive surgery is performed, the patient may be transferred to the intensive care unit. If this is a possibility, the family needs to be aware of the location of the unit. If any equipment is required after surgery, it should be adequately explained to the family to alleviate anxiety or fears.

Teaching deep-breathing and leg exercises Teaching is most effective if performed before surgery when the patient is alert and more receptive and willing to cooperate (Skill 17-1). The nurse should emphasize the importance of performing deep-breathing and leg exercises after surgery to counteract the effects of anesthesia and inactivity during surgery. If the patient seems to be reluctant to perform these exercises, the nurse should explain that pain medication may be ordered and ad-

PREOPERATIVE CHECKLIST

- Ensure that patient's name is correct.
- Write date.
- Obtain patient's height and weight.
- Ensure that identification or allergy band is placed on patient's wrist.
- Ensure that patient has had nothing by mouth after midnight or as ordered.
- Administer preoperative medication. List medication and amount.
- Perform preoperative teaching.
- Remove patient's bobby pins, combs, and hairpieces.
- Remove patient's nail polish.
- Remove patient's make-up.
- Ensure that allergies are noted on front of chart.
- Remove dentures or partial plates.
- Ensure that informed consent or surgical permit has been obtained according to agency policy (Fig. 17-1).
- Prepare operative site.
- Ensure that results of history and physical examination are in chart.
- Remove glasses or contact lenses.
- Remove prosthesis.
- Remove or secure jewelry.
- Ensure that complete blood count or other laboratory work is reported on chart.
- Ensure that urinalysis report is in chart.
- Ensure that blood has been typed and crossmatched.
- Ensure that chest x-ray report is in chart.
- Ensure that electrocardiographic report is in chart.
- Bathe patient.
- Place surgical gown on patient.
- Obtain vital signs.
- Remove hearing aid, or ensure that it goes to surgery with patient.
- Ensure that Foley catheter is in place.
- Record amount of urine voided and time.
- Know location of family members.
- Ensure that x-ray films are sent to surgery.
- Ensure that surgical team knows about presence of any loose teeth (especially in children).
- Write any special comments on instructions.

Wilson N. Jones Memorial Hospital
500 North Highland • Sherman, Texas 75090

DISCLOSURE AND CONSENT
MEDICAL AND SURGICAL PROCEDURES

TO THE PATIENT: *You have the right, as a patient, to be informed about your condition and the recommended surgical, medical, or diagnostic procedure to be used so that you may make the decision whether or not to undergo the procedure after knowing the risks and hazards involved. This disclosure is not meant to scare or alarm you; it is simply an effort to make you better informed so you may give or withhold your consent to the procedure.*

I (we) voluntarily request Dr. Blankenship as my physician and such associates, technical assistants and other health care providers as they may deem necessary, to treat my condition which has been explained to me as:

Remove my uterus, tubes, and ovaries

I (we) understand that the following surgical, medical and/or diagnostic procedures are planned for me and I (we) voluntarily consent and authorize these procedures:

Remove my uterus, tubes, and ovaries

I (we) understand that my physician may discover other or different conditions which require additional or different procedures than those planned. I (we) authorize my physician, and such associates, technical assistants and other health care providers to perform such other procedures which are advisable in their professional judgement.
I (we) understand that no warranty or guarantee has been made to me as to result or cure.
Just as there may be risks and hazards in continuing my present condition without treatment, there are also risks and hazards related to the performance of the surgical, medical, and/or diagnostic procedures planned for me. I (we) realize that common to surgical, medical, and/or diagnostic procedures is the potential for infection, blood clots in veins and lungs, hemorrhage, allergic reactions, and even death. I (we) also realize that the following risks and hazards may occur in connection with this particular procedure:

1. Abdominal hysterectomy (total).
1. Uncontrollable leakage of urine.
2. Injury to bladder.
3. Sterility.
4. Injury to the tube (ureter) between the kidney and the bladder.
5. Injury to the bowel and/or intestinal obstruction.

3. All fallopian tube and ovarian surgery with or without hysterectomy, including removal and lysis of adhesions.
1. Injury to the bowel and/or bladder.
2. Sterility.
3. Failure to obtain fertility (if applicable).
4. Failure to obtain sterility (if applicable).
5. Loss of ovarian functions or hormone production from ovary(ies).

8. Removal of the cervix.
1. Uncontrolled leakage of urine.
2. Injury to bladder.
3. Sterility.
4. Injury to the tube (ureter) between the kidney and the bladder.
5. Injury to the bowel and/or intestinal obstruction.
6. Completion of operation by abdominal incision.

I (we) understand that anesthesia involves additional risks and hazards but I (we) request the use of anesthetics for the relief and protection from pain during the planned and additional procedures. I (we) realize the anesthesia may have to be changed, possibly without explanation to me (us).
I (we) understand that certain complications may result from the use of any anesthetic including respiratory problems, drug reactions, paralysis, brain damage or even death. Other risks and hazards which may result from the use of general anesthetics range from minor discomfort to injury to vocal cords, teeth or eyes. I (we) understand that other risks and hazards resulting from spinal or epidural anesthetics include headache and chronic pain.
I (we) have been given an opportunity to ask questions about my condition, alternative forms of anesthesia and treatment, risks of nontreatment, the procedures to be used, and the risks and hazards involved, and I (we) believe that I (we) have sufficient information to give this informed consent.
I (we) certify this form has been fully explained to me, that I (we) have read it or have had it read to me, that the blank spaces have been filled in, and that I (we) understand its contents.
I (we) hereby authorize the hospital pathologist to dispose of any tissue that may be removed.

DATE: 1-26-96 TIME: 10:30 A.M. / P.M.

Judith Cameron
PATIENT/OTHER LEGALLY RESPONSIBLE PERSON SIGN

WITNESS:
Name Jo Jones, LPN
1930 Scott Ave.
Address (Street or P.O. Box)
Creekwater, Tx 70251
City, State, Zip Code

Fig. 17-1 Informed consent form. (Courtesy Wilson N. Jones Memorial Hospital, Sherman, Texas.)

ministered before the exercises to help relax and permit more comfortable compliance. Often, patients require only a minimal reminder to perform the exercises after they are awake and somewhat alert.

Patients who are healthy and active before surgery may develop respiratory problems after surgery. Many factors increase this possibility. Adequate ventilation may be inhibited by inactivity. Patients are often reluctant to move because they fear pain or opening the incision. The body relies on an intake of food and fluid to produce body secretions. When none is taken, secretions, especially respiratory secretions, become thick and difficult to expectorate. The entire respiratory tract is lined with mucous membranes. Anesthetics and oxygen have a drying effect on the respiratory mucous membranes, creating a more susceptible environment for infection. Alveoli have a tendency to fill with this sticky mucus, preventing full inflation.

Deep-breathing exercises may help prevent an accumulation of thick secretions in the respiratory tract by getting air to the alveoli to assist with reinflating these tiny air sacs. When combined with coughing exercises, deep-breathing exercises can rid the respiratory passages of the thick secretions.

In addition, the immobility of the patient and the slowing of bodily processes cause the blood return from the legs to slow, which could initiate the formation of a **thrombus** (blood clot). A thrombus may become dislodged, travel through the bloodstream, and become lodged in an artery of a vital organ (for example, brain, lung, heart), shutting off the blood supply to that area and causing serious damage or death. For this reason, it is also very important that the legs not be massaged or rubbed by the patient or family. Leg exercises increase circulation through the contraction and flexion of muscles, which pushes blood through the blood vessels. Leg exercises are most effective when they are performed as soon after surgery as possible and repeated every 1 to 2 hours. The nurse should emphasize to the patient the importance of performing deep-breathing and leg exercises to counteract the effects of the surgery.

Older adults. Older patients may need to be reminded and encouraged to practice the deep-breathing and leg exercises because they may not fully understand the importance of the procedure. If there is a diminished physical capacity for deep breathing or exercising the legs, it may be necessary for the nurse or family members to assist with the exercises.

Children. Teaching children to do deep-breathing and leg exercises might be difficult and depends on their age. The child may be afraid of new people and situations and must be approached slowly and carefully. Other family members are included in teaching and performing the exercises. It will be challenging to the nurse to create ways for the child to cooperate. Developing games using the exercises is one method of getting the child to perform.

Patients in home care. For the patient entering the hospital for ambulatory surgery, the teaching of deep-breathing and leg exercises may be performed in the physician's office, in the preoperative area, or after surgery before the patient is discharged. The home health nurse may need to reinforce the importance of performing the exercises for 2 to 3 days after surgery.

Patients with chronic obstructive pulmonary disease. Patients who have chronic respiratory conditions may need assistance and encouragement to carry out the breathing exercises. Smokers and patients with chronic respiratory diseases who are at higher risk for developing respiratory complications may need to use incentive spirometry to ensure adequate inflation of the lungs.

Teaching controlled coughing Coughing is the natural automatic method for clearing the airways of secretions. Cilia, which are hairlike structures that line the mucous membranes of the respiratory tract, move the secretions in an upward motion. Each cough moves the secretions closer to expectoration. Deep breathing is sometimes enough of a stimulus to produce a cough. A deep, productive cough is more beneficial than a shallow cough or a mere clearing of the throat.

Preoperative medications, NPO status, anesthesia, and oxygen produce a drying effect on mucous membranes, causing the secretions to become thick and more difficult to expectorate. Adequate amounts of postoperative fluids should be encouraged to prevent thick secretions.

Coughing may be dangerous for patients undergoing surgery for hernias or certain types of surgery on the brain and eyes. Coughing increases pressure in the operative area and may even cause damage. For these patients, coughing should not be encouraged unless the physician specifically orders it.

After surgery, the nurse should listen to the patient's lungs to assess for the presence of secretions before and after the patient coughs. Normal breath sounds are smooth and should resemble the sound of air moving in and out of a passageway. When secretions have accumulated, the nurse may hear no sounds in an area or sounds such as wheezing, gurgling, or crackling (rales) as the patient inhales and exhales.

In most instances, unless moist secretions are heard in the lungs, coughing should not be forced. Forced coughing has a tendency to collapse the alveoli and can cause more harm than good. For patients who have moist-sounding respirations, coughing should be encouraged to raise the accumulated secretions for expectoration (Skill 17-2).

The patient with an abdominal or thoracic incision may fear coughing because of pain. **Splinting** the incision with both hands or with a towel, pillow, or folded bath blanket provides light pressure or support to the surgical area to help minimize pain and to make the patient feel more secure.

When deep breathing is performed before coughing, the cough reflex may be stimulated. Frequently, deep-breathing exercises and coughing are performed together. If possible, the exercises should not be performed close to mealtime because expectoration of secretions may greatly diminish the appetite. If expectoration follows the mealtime too closely, the gag reflex may be triggered, and vomiting may occur.

Patients should be taught appropriate disposal of secretions. It is best if the secretions are expectorated into a tissue or emesis basin. The tissue is disposed of in a plastic bag, and the emesis basin is rinsed in cold water and the contents disposed of in the toilet and flushed. The secretions may be contaminated with microorganisms or pathogens. Appropriate handwashing is a must for both the patient and the nurse to avoid contaminating others (see Chapter 14).

If a patient chooses not to perform the controlled coughing, hypostatic pneumonia and other lung complications may occur.

Surgical shaving

The skin harbors microorganisms in great numbers. Microorganisms normally grow and multiply on the skin of all persons. Body hair, which covers the majority of the body externally, also harbors large numbers of microorganisms. For this reason, many surgeons order preoperative shaving of the surgical site (Skill 17-3).

Current controversy exists as to whether the operative area of a patient being prepared for surgery should be shaved. The wound infection rate for patients shaved before surgery is higher than for those not shaved before surgery. Because of this, shaving of the surgical site is not performed as commonly as it once was. The Centers for Disease Control and Prevention recommends using clippers or a depilatory to remove hair from the site and cleansing the site with antimicrobial agents just before surgery.

Some surgeons may order a surgical shave the night before surgery, but ideally this is best performed immediately before surgery in the holding area of the surgical suite. Minor abrasions or cuts caused by shaving are prime areas for the growth of bacteria, and the longer the period between the shave and surgery, the greater the potential for an infection or increase in bacterial growth. Because skin is a natural barrier against pathogens, when a break in the skin occurs, pathogens may enter and multiply quickly.

If surgical shave is ordered, the nurse shaves an area much larger than the incisional site. This reduces the number of microorganisms on the surrounding or adjacent skin areas. Hospital policies differ regarding the description of areas to shave. Therefore it is best to review the hospital or agency policy to determine the area to be surgically shaved (Fig. 17-2). The surgeon may give specific orders concerning the area to be surgically shaved.

Before shaving the patient, the nurse should closely assess the surgical site for infection, breaks in the skin, moles, irritations or rashes, bruises, growths, or exudate. Anything unusual should be recorded and reported to the surgeon.

Surgical shaving of the operative site must be completed with care. The nurse must prevent nicking or impairment of skin integrity. The goal is to remove the hair without causing injury to the skin.

Making of a surgical bed

After the patient has been taken to surgery, the nurse prepares the room for the patient's return. This includes making the bed to receive the patient (Skill 17-4). The surgical bed is also called the *anesthetic bed, postoperative bed,* or *recovery bed.* Transfer of the patient to the bed should be completed as easily as possible and with minimal exertion required from the patient or nurses. Therefore the bed should be placed even with height of the stretcher from recovery.

Room for a stretcher should be provided. The stretcher will be placed next to the bed for easy transfer of the patient.

The principles for bedmaking also apply to making the surgical bed (see Chapter 23). The bed should be neat, tight, and free of wrinkles to promote the physical comfort for the surgical patient. The bed should be made with clean linens to provide a clean environment. Sometimes, a bath blanket is placed over the bottom sheet to provide extra warmth. Hospital procedures differ, but all surgical beds are prepared with the top sheet and spread fanfolded to the side or foot of the bed so that the sheet can be easily pulled over the patient after transfer from the stretcher to the bed.

In addition to making of the surgical bed, the patient's room is straightened, and the emesis basin and tissues are placed on the bedside table because the patient may become nauseated and may vomit. The nurse must check medical orders for preparing

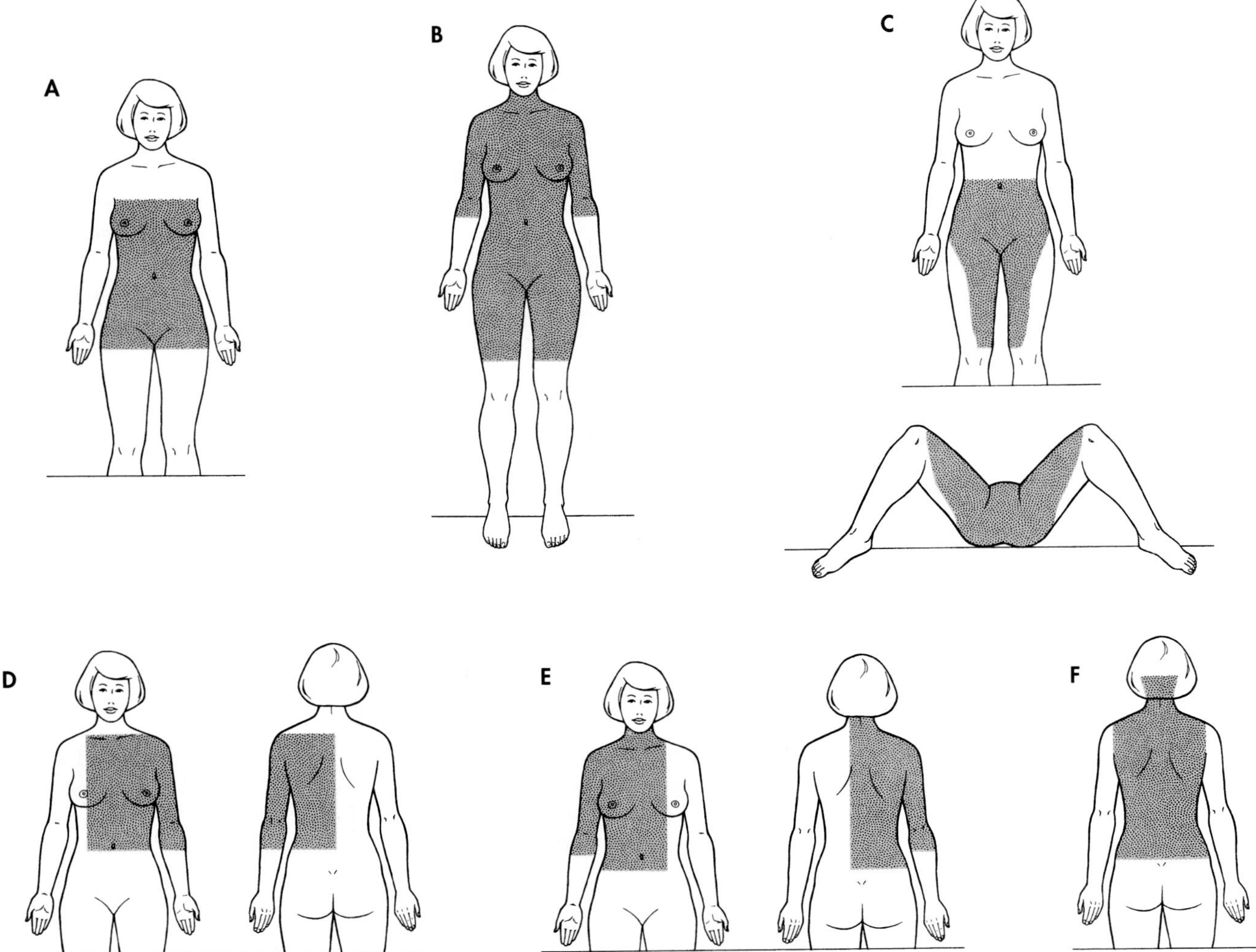

Fig. 17-2 Skin preparation sites for surgery on various body areas. The shaded area indicates the area that should be shaved. **A,** Abdominal surgery. **B,** Open-heart surgery. **C,** Perineal surgery. **D,** Chest or thoracic surgery. **E,** Breast surgery. **F,** Cervical spine surgery.

other special equipment for use, such as an intravenous pole, traction device, or infusion pump.

INTRAOPERATIVE CARE

Intraoperative nursing care involves intense focus and assessment of the patient during surgery and recovery from the anesthetic. The surgical patient is transported to a "holding" area or preanesthesia room to be prepared for surgery. Admission to the surgical unit and assessment of the patient are completed by a licensed person. Often, the surgical shave and skin scrub are completed in this area. A catheter may be inserted, and an intravenous infusion is sometimes started in the preanesthesia area before the patient's entrance to the operating room (OR).

The surgical team consists of the surgeon and an assistant surgeon, the anesthesiologist or nurse anesthetist, the circulating nurse, and the surgical technician. Many hospitals train the licensed practical/vocational nurse to function as the surgical technician. This surgical technician is responsible for continually assessing the patient and ensuring that all instruments and supplies are on hand or obtained as needed. The surgical technician and circulating nurse are responsible for completing all counts (for example, instruments, needles, sponges). Responsibilities and functions for surgical nurse may be different for each institution.

Since both the surgical procedure and anesthesia pose potential threats, after surgery, patients are taken to the **postanesthesia care unit (PACU)** or recovery room until they are awake and stable enough to be returned to the surgical nursing unit. Nurses who are educated to care for the postoperative patient continuously assess the patient, including closely monitoring for blood loss and fluid and electrolyte balance. The surgery itself causes trauma to the body and decreases resistance to infection. The anesthetic impairs the ability of patients to respond to environmental stimuli and to help themselves in any way. Therefore constant attention is required during the postanesthesia waking period. Frequent assessment is vital for patient safety. The length of time the patient remains in the PACU is determined by the type of surgery, type of anesthesia, and condition of the patient. Patients who have had extensive surgery or whose conditions are serious and unstable usually spend more time in recovery and may be transferred to the intensive care unit (ICU) instead of the surgical nursing unit.

Once a patient has regained consciousness and is considered stable (that is, the patient is awake, vital signs are consistently within normal range for the patient, ventilation is adequate, and patient knows where he or she is), the transfer from PACU to the surgical nursing unit for continued postoperative care is performed. In most institutions, a licensed person must transfer the patient from the PACU to the nursing unit. The transporter may be a licensed practical/vocational or registered nurse, who is responsible for providing a patient condition report to the receiving nurse on the unit.

For the patient who has been admitted for outpatient surgery, the follow-up to the PACU is usually completed in an outpatient room designed for the complete recovery of the patient. Patients are usually discharged when they are alert and stable. Postoperative teaching is completed, and instructions are sent home with the patient.

POSTOPERATIVE CARE

Postoperative nursing care is designed to prevent and detect complications, assist the patient to safely recover from anesthesia, relieve pain or discomfort, and help the patient return to a level of self-care, independence, and improved physiologic functioning.

Receiving the Patient From the Postanesthesia Care Unit

The patient is returned to the surgical nursing unit when the condition is stable. This is indicated by stable vital signs; appropriate respiratory functioning; orientation to surroundings or return of the reflexes such as blinking, gagging, and swallowing; controlled wound drainage; and minimal pain and nausea.

When receiving the patient on the surgical nursing unit (Skill 17-5), the nurse must be aware that the patient's safety depends on the nurse's ability to assess and provide immediate care. Since the patient may still be drowsy, the nurse continues to orient the patient to the environment. Explanation that the surgery is over and that the patient is back in the room may help reduce anxiety. The presence of tubes or drains may need to be explained immediately if the patient is aware of them or pulling or rubbing them. The nurse frequently repeats and clarifies information for the patient.

Family members are notified of the patient's location and condition. The nurse should be aware of the information given to the family by the surgeon so that reinforcement of information or answers to questions can be provided. The family also needs the nurse's support, especially when the patient's condition is serious or the prognosis is not positive. The patient's unit must be ready for the patient's return. The surgical bed should be ready for easy transfer of the patient, and any necessary or special equipment should be on hand (Fig. 17-3). Assessment should begin immediately on return of the patient and performed at frequent, regular intervals according to hospital procedure or medical orders.

Documentation should be thorough, and the initial assessment should be used as a baseline for comparison of patient status as the postoperative period progresses. After the first assessment is performed

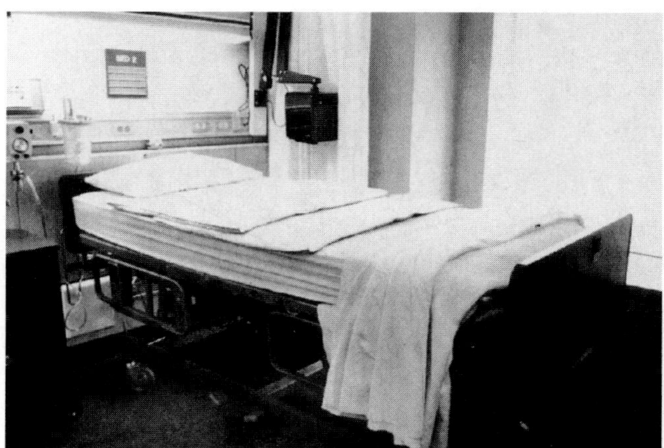

Fig. 17-3 Bed in the high position for the easy transfer of the patient from a stretcher to an unoccupied surgical bed. (From Perry AG, Potter PA: *Clinical nursing skills and techniques,* ed 3, St Louis, 1994, Mosby.)

and the patient is made as comfortable as possible, the family is allowed to visit. The nurse should be prepared to explain procedures and equipment. The family needs to know that the patient will sleep most of the first day because of the effects of the anesthesia. The nurse explains the necessity for frequent assessments by the nurse to prevent anxiety and worry. Preoperative medical orders are automatically canceled when the patient leaves for surgery. New medical orders are issued for the postoperative patient.

Children The child who has been well prepared preoperatively should be more cooperative after surgery. Anxiety in the child and parents is common and may be lessened if the parents are allowed to assist the nurse in caring for the child. Parents who are taught procedures will be better prepared to care for the child after discharge. It is best to explain a procedure to a child immediately before implementing it so that there is no chance for fear to build. Children should be allowed to handle equipment that will be used, if possible.

Older adults Pneumonia is the most frequent respiratory complication of the older adult, and chances for developing it may be reduced with early ambulation. Older adults may require extra blankets for warmth, since their body temperatures are labile (unstable). Nighttime confusion is more common and may be reduced by frequent visits from the nursing personnel. Healing may be slower in the older adult and the poorly nourished individual.

Patients in home care Patients undergoing ambulatory surgery are discharged as soon as they are stabilized and alert. Instructions are given to the patient and family that include cautioning the patient not to drive a vehicle or operate equipment for 24 to 36 hours after surgery. The family and patient are taught the signs and symptoms of potential complications. The nurse gives the surgeon's phone number to the patient in case of an emergency. Special instructions are given to the family and patient before discharge (Fig. 17-4).

Nursing Care

Assessment

The nurse who receives the patient on the surgical nursing unit completes an initial assessment. Procedures may vary somewhat for each institution or facility, but most require initial assessment of the patient's airway patency; vital signs; level of consciousness; condition of dressings, drains, and tubes; intravenous fluids; comfort level; and skin color, temperature, and condition. Because a patient's condition may change rapidly, ongoing assessment and nursing care are vital. Vital signs (see Chapter 11) are assessed according to hospital procedure or medical orders. Typically, vital signs are taken every 15 minutes for 1 hour. If the vital signs are stable, the nurse then monitors them every 1 hour for 4 hours, and if they are still stable, they are monitored every 4 hours for 48 hours. A sudden variation in the vital signs requires closer assessment (for example, every 5 to 15 minutes). All vital signs will need to be documented on the patient's medical record.

Safety and comfort

The nurse should assess safety measures, such as the side rails placed in the raised position. It is common for the older adult to become confused and for a patient continuing to recover from anesthesia to attempt to get out of bed. The nurse contacts the confused patient frequently. The call light must always be within the patient's reach.

The nurse should also thoroughly assess the patient's level of pain or discomfort. Consideration should be given to the location, type, and duration of pain; amount of relief from pain medication; and time the last dose of pain medication was given.

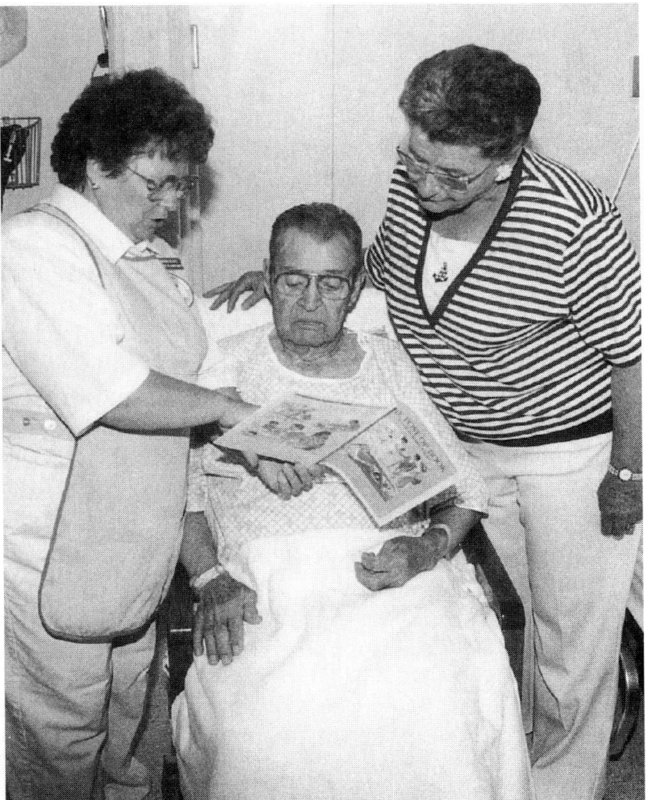

Fig. 17-4 Reviewing discharge planning instructions. (From Christensen BL, Kockrow EO: *Foundations of nursing,* ed 2, St Louis, 1995, Mosby.)

Some patients complain, and others only display nonverbal signs (see Chapter 27). Pain from surgery should diminish after the first 24 to 48 hours. Providing other comfort measures in addition to the pain medication often relieves pain or discomfort. These measures include changing the patient's position, assisting the patient to void, rubbing the patient's back, and sometimes just spending a extra time with the patient to listen and talk.

Coughing and deep breathing

Coughing and deep breathing help remove secretions from the respiratory tract. Coughing, if indicated, should be performed with deep breathing every 2 hours during the patient's waking hours. These exercises are most effective when started as soon as possible after surgery. Since both exercises may be uncomfortable for the patient, the operative site may be splinted. Incentive spirometry may also be ordered to assist the patient to reexpand the lungs after surgery. **Incentive spirometry** is a method of encouraging voluntary deep breathing by providing visual feedback of the inspiratory volume that patients have achieved. The postoperative patient restricted to bed also needs to be encouraged to turn every 1 to 2 hours while awake and to sit up as soon as possible to allow for greater chest expansion.

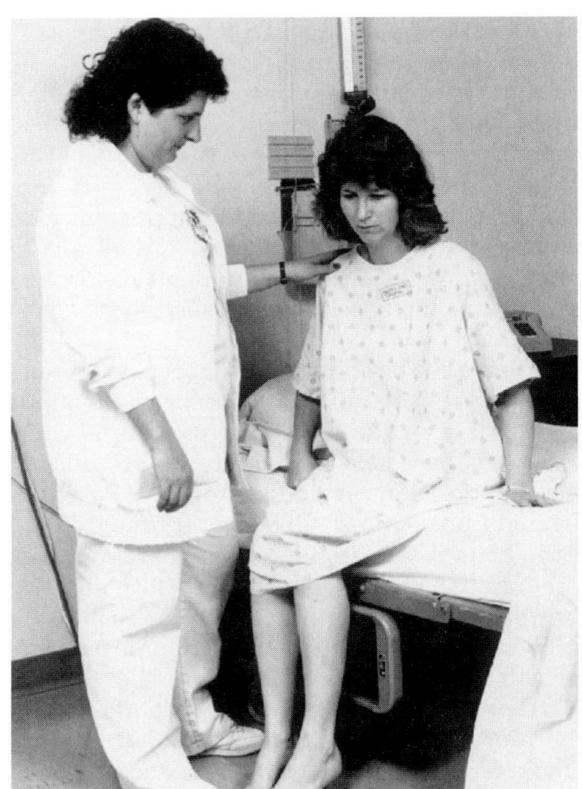

Fig. 17-5 The nurse assists the patient to ambulate for the first time after surgery.

Early ambulation

Early ambulation facilitates normal functioning of all body systems and should be encouraged as soon as the surgeon allows. The first time that the patient ambulates the nurse should assist the patient to a sitting position, allowing the patient time to adjust to the change in position. The bed should be in a low position and the patient's feet (in slippers) should rest on the floor, a stool, or chair (Fig. 17-5). The patient's legs should not be allowed to dangle from the edge of the bed. If the patient becomes dizzy or light-headed, the nurse should encourage the patient to take slow deep breaths, hold the head erect, and avoid looking down. If the dizziness persists, the patient should be returned to bed. Two persons should accompany the patient on the first attempt to ambulate, since this is frequently ordered to be initiated later the day of surgery or the day after surgery. The patient is usually still somewhat weak and unsteady. Early ambulation helps provide a more rapid recovery for the patient and helps prevent complications that could otherwise occur.

Intake and nutrition

Patients returning from surgery are usually NPO until they are fully awake. Typically, surgeons order clear liquids as tolerated and increase the diet as the patient tolerates it until the patient is receiving solid foods. The nurse should begin by offering the patient only small sips of water. Ice chips often relieve the thirst and dry mouth and are refreshing to the patient. Usually, within a few days, peristalsis has fully returned, and the patient can tolerate a full diet. Peristalsis is the coordinated, rhythmic, and serial contractions that force food through the digestive tract. Too much ice given to a patient who has a nasogastric tube causes electrolytes to be washed out of the stomach (see Chapter 19). Intravenous fluids are usually continued to balance the loss of fluids during the perioperative period when fluids are withheld. The nurse is responsible for maintaining the appropriate intravenous drip rate and assessing the infusion site at regular intervals. Intake and output are carefully measured and documented for 48 hours after surgery unless medical orders say otherwise.

Voiding

Patients who have had rectal, pelvic, vaginal, or lower abdominal surgery are more likely to have difficulty voiding after surgery. The nurse assesses the patient for urinary retention (see Chapter 30). A distended bladder may cause discomfort. A patient should not be allowed to go longer than 8 hours without voiding if fluid intake has been adequate. The nurse should use measures designed to help the patient void, such as assisting the patient to a sitting position (which is a normal voiding position), running water for the sound, or pouring premeasured, warm water slowly over the perineum. Catheterization should be performed only as a last resort and may be performed only with a medical order. If catheterization is ordered, it should be performed using strict surgical asepsis to help prevent infection.

Skin care

Skin care is important for the postoperative patient. The antiseptic solutions used to cleanse the operative site and the wound drainage on the patient's skin serve as irritants. A complete bed bath given the first day after surgery makes the patient more comfortable and removes these irritants. To prevent skin breakdown, a wound with a large amount of drainage should be cleansed and dressed frequently (see Chapter 18). Care is taken to prevent contamination of the surgical site.

Postoperative complications

Abdominal distention Abdominal **distention** (swelling) is fairly common after surgery and should not be taken lightly. The problem is frequently uncomfortable for the patient, and measures should be taken to relieve it. Abdominal distention is usually caused by an accumulation of **flatulence** (gas) in the intestines related to the loss of peristalsis during surgery, but it may also indicate hemorrhage. The nurse should assess the patient thoroughly. In addition to assessing vital signs, the nurse should also listen for bowel sounds. If the blood pressure suddenly drops, internal hemorrhage should be suspected and the surgeon notified immediately. To determine whether the abdomen is continuing to enlarge, the nurse should measure the abdominal girth at the line of the umbilicus. A measurement should be performed every few hours for comparison. The surgeon may order a carminative to relieve the flatulence or the insertion of a rectal tube to help stimulate the bowel and relieve the flatulence. X-ray studies may be ordered to decide whether there is an organic problem.

Evisceration and dehiscence The nurse will need to assess the incision for **dehiscence** (the separation of a surgical incision or rupture of a wound closure), **evisceration** (the protrusion of an internal organ through a wound or surgical incision, especially in the abdominal wall) (Fig. 17-6), and wound infection. If evisceration occurs, the nurse should cover the wound with sterile dressings. The surgeon should be notified immediately. If the bowel or abdominal contents are outside the abdomen, the surgeon may order that they be kept moist with sterile normal saline, sterile abdominal pads, or sterile towels until surgery can be performed to resuture the incision. If dehiscence occurs, care should be taken to prevent infection in the open wound. The nurse should always be alert for signs of a pressure ulcer and provide extra nursing measures to prevent impaired skin integrity (see Chapter 21).

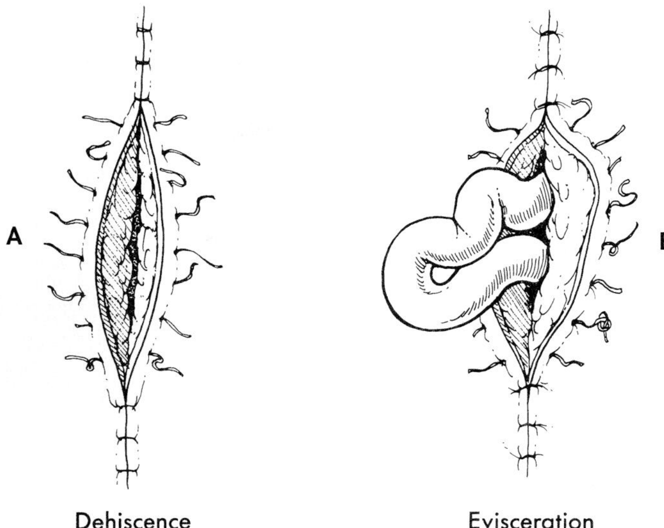

Fig. 17-6 **A,** Wound dehiscence. **B,** Evisceration. (From Christensen BL, Kockrow EO: *Foundations of nursing,* ed 2, St Louis, 1995, Mosby.)

Thrombophlebitis The surgeon may order the application of elastic antiembolism stockings as a measure to help prevent **thrombophlebitis** (inflammation of a vein, often accompanied by formation of a clot) (Fig. 17-7). The stockings are usually donned in the morning before the patient arises and are removed for personal hygiene and reapplied.

Shock Shock, or **hypovolemia,** is one of the most serious and common postoperative complications. Shock is the body's reaction to inadequate circulation and is usually caused by hemorrhage. The loss of fluids and electrolytes and the trauma of surgery, anesthetics, and preoperative medications may be precipitating factors. Types of shock includes hypovolemic, which is caused by decreased fluid volume such as fluid or blood loss; cardiogenic, which results from cardiac failure or interference with heart functioning; neurogenic, which occurs because of peripheral vascular dilation that may be caused by spinal anesthetic; and septic, which results from severe infection. Symptoms of shock include a rapid, thready pulse; a drop in blood pressure at 90 systolic or below; pallor (paleness) or cyanosis (bluish discoloration); cold, clammy skin; restlessness; and low body temperature. Respirations are usually

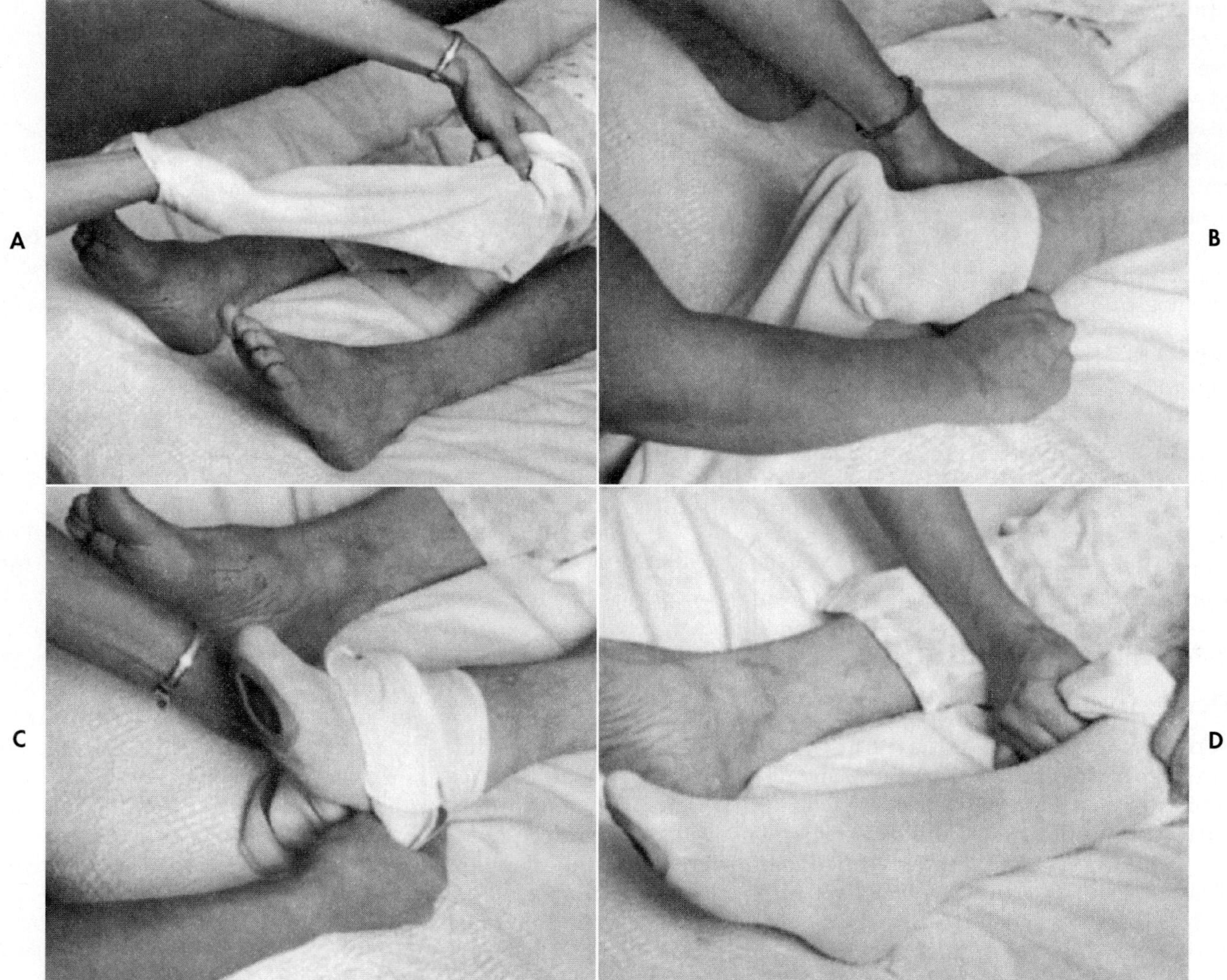

Fig. 17-7 Applying antiembolism stockings. **A,** Turn the elastic stocking inside out by placing one hand into the sock, holding the toe of the sock with the other hand, and pulling. **B,** Place the patient's toes into the foot of the elastic stocking, making sure that the sock is smooth. **C,** Slide remaining portion of the sock over the patient's foot, making sure that the toes are covered. Sock will now be right-side out. **D,** Slide the sock up over the patient's calf until the sock is completely extended. Be sure that the sock is smooth and that no ridges are present. (From Perry AG, Potter PA: *Clinical nursing skills and techniques,* ed 3, St Louis, 1994, Mosby.)

rapid and deep, and as shock becomes more severe, they become rapid and shallow. Shock is an emergency and needs to be detected early and treated. The patient will die if remedial action is not taken.

Vital signs should be taken frequently, recorded, and reported. Dressings should be assessed frequently for excessive bleeding. The nurse should remember to assess for a pooling of blood under the patient. Unless ordered by the physician, the patient should be kept flat. Some physicians may order the feet and legs to be elevated to encourage blood flow away from the extremities toward the vital organs. The patient may need an extra blanket for warmth, but the nurse must not allow the patient to become overheated, since this causes blood to be diverted away from the vital organs to the body's superficial surfaces. The nurse should be prepared to monitor an intravenous infusion, administer blood transfusions or blood components, and administer medications or oxygen as ordered by the physician (see Chapters 16 and 29). The approach to the treatment of shock is to determine the cause and correct it. The nurse provides accurate documentation of continual assessment of the patient.

Hemorrhage **Hemorrhage** is the loss of a large amount of blood in a short time. It may occur at the time of surgery (primary hemorrhage), within the first few hours after surgery (intermediary hemorrhage), or some time after surgery (secondary hemorrhage). Bleeding may be external and considered evident or may be internal and classified as concealed hemorrhage. Symptoms include apprehension; restlessness (constant movement); thirst; cold, moist, and pale skin; increased pulse; low body temperature; and respirations that are rapid and deep (air hunger). These symptoms also indicate that the patient is in shock.

The treatment for hemorrhage is to discover the source, stop the bleeding, and replace fluids. If bleeding is external, diagnosis is easily made, but if the hemorrhage is concealed, documentation of it is vital. Surgery is usually required to expose the source of bleeding and to correct the defect. The nurse should continually monitor vital signs, inspect and reinforce dressings, and document the color and amount of drainage.

Respiratory arrest **Respiratory arrest** is inadequate ventilation from cessation of respirations. Respiratory arrest may occur after surgery for several reasons. One of the primary causes is upper airway obstruction. Arrest may occur as a result of the tongue relaxing and falling back into the pharynx, blocking the airway. It may also be caused by the accumulation of secretions that block the airway. Another possible cause for respiratory arrest in the postoperative patient is central nervous system depression, which may be caused by drug overdose or anesthesia. Respiratory failure may also occur in the immediate postoperative period as a result of inadequate ventilation, especially after major chest or abdominal surgery. Anesthetic drugs have long-lasting effects, depressing respirations and enhancing the effects of narcotics, which also depress respirations. If muscle relaxants are also administered during anesthesia, the effect may be cumulative for some patients, causing the patient to become very weak.

To treat the patient, the cause for the respiratory arrest must be determined. If an obstruction is present, it should be cleared so that a patent (open) airway can be maintained. The nurse should assess the patient for an obstruction and relieve it, if possible. Suctioning may be indicated. The nurse often initiates cardiopulmonary resuscitation (CPR). Assessment and documentation are important to help the physician make a correct diagnosis. If the arrest is related to central nervous system depression or a cumulative effect of drugs, the patient may be placed on a mechanical ventilator until the effect of the drugs is diminished and the patient can resume breathing without mechanical aid.

Cardiac arrest **Cardiac arrest** is the sudden, unexpected cessation of the heartbeat and circulation. All of the action of the heart may stop, or fibrillation (muscular twitching) may occur. After surgery, the patient may immediately lose consciousness, and no pulse can be felt or heart sounds heard. The pupils begin to dilate within 45 seconds. Convulsions may occur. If circulation is not restored 4 to 5 minutes from the cessation of circulation, permanent brain damage results.

The most reliable symptom of cardiac arrest is an absence of the carotid pulse. Valuable time should not be wasted taking the blood pressure if the pulse is absent and other symptoms are present. CPR is initiated immediately. Accurate documentation of assessment and actions should be made.

If successful resuscitation results, the nurse carefully monitors the patient. The patient may be transferred to the intensive care unit for closer monitoring because the risk for another cardiac arrest is increased. The decision to terminate unsuccessful resuscitation is made by the physician based on the assessment reported by the nurse and the physician's own observations.

Application of antiembolism stockings

Thrombophlebitis may occur when patients lie still for long periods without moving the legs. The problem occurs because venous circulation may be impaired and the blood flows slowly through the veins, predisposing the patient to inflammation and consequent clot formation. Usually, symptoms of thrombophlebitis develop within 7 to 10 days after surgery. The nurse and patient should assess for pain or cramping in the calf of the leg, painful swelling in the calf, an increase in body temperature, redness, and tenderness. The use of elastic stockings, or **antiembolism stockings,** helps compress the veins in the legs and facilitates venous blood return to the heart.

Several types of antiembolism stockings are available, and the surgeon orders the type preferred. One type extends from the foot to the knee and another extends from the foot to midthigh. Another type extends from the foot to the waist. The heel or toe of the stocking is open so that assessment of the foot may be carried out. The stockings usually come in small, medium, and large sizes. Accurate measurement should be completed by the nurse to determine the appropriate size. The stockings are ineffective if the fit is incorrect.

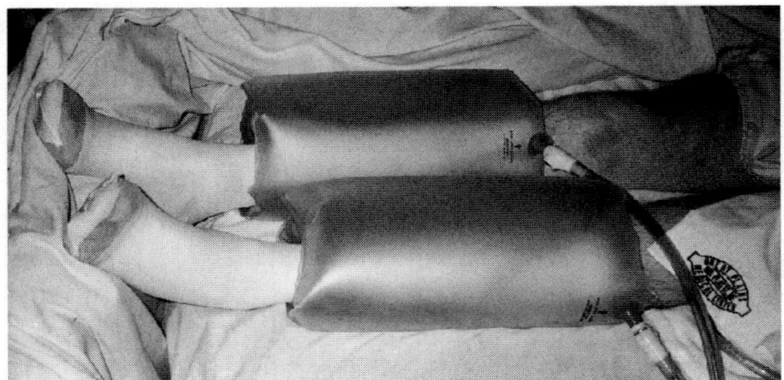

Fig. 17-8 Intermittent external pneumatic compression system. (From Christensen BL, Kockrow EO: *Foundations of nursing,* ed 2, St Louis, 1995, Mosby.)

Hospital procedures vary, but antiembolism stockings usually are donned before patients get out of bed in the morning and may be removed at night, when they return to bed (Skill 17-6). They are removed for personal hygiene and then reapplied. Some agencies require the stockings to be worn except for removal once each shift.

Recently, surgeons have been ordering graduated or **sequential compression devices (SCDs)** for surgical patients to help prevent deep vein thrombosis. These stockings are applied after surgery (usually in the PACU) and are taken to the unit with the patient. They are usually made of plastic with several different chambers that fill with air delivered by a pump (Fig. 17-8). The action of the sequential stocking is to apply varying degrees of external compression by exerting the greatest compression at the ankle (100%) and a lesser compression at the midcalf (70%) and the midthigh (40%). Physiologically, the pressure on the vein walls causes the valves to contract and increase blood flow. Patients who have massive edema of the legs; extreme leg deformities; arterial ischemia; inflammation or phlebitis; trauma; severe arteriosclerosis; congestive heart failure with leg or pulmonary edema; skin conditions such as infections, lesions or ulcers; or very large thighs are not candidates for use of the sequential pneumatic or graduated compression stockings.

Application of heat

The body can adapt to a wide range in temperatures. Therapeutically, heat may be applied to the body in different forms and for a variety of reasons. Heat is used to promote vasodilation (widening of blood vessels) and improve blood flow to a body part, to reduce joint stiffness by decreasing the viscosity (thickness) of synovial fluid, and to relieve pain by increasing circulation to ischemic areas. **Ischemia** is a decreased supply of oxygenated blood to a body organ or part. Application of heat may be in dry or moist form (Skill 17-7). Moist heat applications are provided through conduction (a transfer from one surface to another surface) by means of sitz baths, soaks, and compresses. Sterile technique is used in treating open wounds with heat. Dry heat may be applied locally for heat conduction by means of an aquathermia pad, electric pad, hot water bottle, or disposable chemical pack. Chemical packs are commercially prepared packs that, when activated, produce a specific amount of heat for a specific amount of time. Dry heat by radiation (sent out in rays) may be applied by means of a heat lamp.

The body has the ability to adapt to temperature changes. This creates a problem in protecting patients from becoming injured from temperatures that are too hot or too cold. An extreme temperature change is felt at first, but within a short time the patient adapts and hardly notices the temperature. This causes a patient who is insensitive to heat and cold to have tissue damage, which further compromises the patient's health.

Heat is therapeutic and produces maximal vasodilation in 20 to 30 minutes. Continuing heat therapy beyond that time provides a **rebound effect** (opposite effect). After 30 to 40 minutes, the blood vessels constrict, and the patient is at greater risk for burns. Heat treatments must be discontinued before this rebound effect begins. The temperatures that the body can tolerate vary according to body part. Areas where the skin is thinner (for example, the forearm, neck, wrist, and abdomen) tend to be more sensitive. The larger the size of the exposed area, the lower the tolerance. Damaged or injured areas create a more sensitive environment, and the length of exposure affects sensitivity. Tolerance is increased with time.

In some situations, the use of heat is contraindicated. These include the first 24 hours after traumatic injury, which increases hemorrhage; noninflammatory edema from heat, a skin condition in which redness and blisters are present; areas where metallic implants are present; and areas of acute inflammation.

A medical order is required for the application of heat. To prevent injury, the nurse should adhere to time frames for the application of heat and should frequently perform assessments. Special care should be taken with the patient who is not mentally alert or mentally able to warn the nurse about discomfort or symptoms of complications. The nurse should remain with the patient who is not cooperative or who has a mental impairment. Persons with neurosensory impairment are unable to feel heat and are at risk for tissue damage. Persons who are known to have delicate or sensitive skin may burn more easily and will need to be assessed closely.

Children Young children have a greater sensitivity to heat and should be assessed frequently. Teaching parents to watch for signs and symptoms of complications is important.

Older adults The older adult has a greater sensitivity to heat and should be assessed frequently. Because of the possibility of compromised circulation, the older adult might not feel the adverse effects of heat or signs and symptoms of complications. Stroke victims who have some neurosensory impairment may not be able to determine when symptoms of complications occur.

Patients in home care Patients or family should be taught appropriate techniques for heat application, especially safety precautions. Patients or family should be aware of heat tolerance and the rebound effect. A timer should be used to ensure appropriate timing of treatments.

Application of cold

The adaptation of the body to cold is the same as it is with heat. After the first few seconds of treatment, the skin receptors begin to adapt to the change in temperature. This adaptation continues throughout the treatment. The patient may feel the cold when it is first applied but gradually gets used to it. This may create a problem in protecting the patient from very cold temperatures. Also, the rebound effect occurs with cold applications. This means that after the maximal therapeutic effect has been reached and maximal vasoconstriction (narrowing of the blood vessels) has occurred, the blood vessels start to dilate. This usually occurs after the skin has been cooled to keep the body tissue from freezing. Therefore cold applications can cause harm if left in place too long.

Cold may be applied to the body in different forms and for a variety of reasons (Skill 17-8). It is usually ordered to decrease inflammation by causing vasoconstriction; to prevent edema; to decrease bleeding by constricting blood vessels; to reduce body temperature and the body's metabolic rate; to relieve pain, especially after an injury; and to produce an anesthetic affect for certain surgical procedures. Cold application is usually recommended after an injury to help control swelling and pain. Cold is especially effective for injured eyes, headaches, tooth extractions, and hemorrhoids. Prolonged exposure to cold and vasoconstriction may increase the blood pressure by increasing the blood supply to the internal organs. It may also cause tissue ischemia, which is evident in the appearance of the skin (purplish or blue and mottled, with numbness and burning pain), or shivering, which is the body's attempt to create warmth.

SITUATIONS CONTRAINDICATING THE USE OF COLD APPLICATIONS

- Edema
- Impaired circulation
- Shivering
- Open wounds
- Allergy or hypersensitivity to cold
- Neurosensory impairment

The tolerance of the body to cold varies depending on length of exposure, body part exposed, condition of skin and tissue treated, size of exposed body part, and patient's age and general physical condition. Dry cold may be tolerated better than moist cold. Also the maximal safe limits for cold temperatures can be tolerated by small areas of skin for shorter periods. A situation using maximal cold requires constant monitoring for patient safety.

A medical order is required for the application of cold. To prevent injury, the nurse should adhere to time frames for applying cold and frequently perform assessments. There are contraindications to the use of cold (see box). The unconscious patient should never be left alone during cold application. Cold should not be applied to an open wound. Cold should not be applied to patients who are allergic or hypersensitive to cold. Diabetics have a greater sensitivity to cold.

Children Young children have a greater sensitivity to cold and should be assessed frequently. Children should never be left alone while cold is being applied. It is important that parents be taught to watch for signs and symptoms of complications.

Older adults The older adult has a greater sensitivity to cold and should be assessed frequently. Because of the possibility of poor circulation, the older adult might not feel the adverse effects or signs and symptoms of complications. Stroke victims who have some neurosensory impairment may not be able to determine when symptoms of complications occur.

Patients in home care The patient and family need to be taught the proper techniques and principles of cold application. They also need to know about the rebound effect. Timing is important, and a timer should be used. The patient and family should also know the symptoms of overexposure.

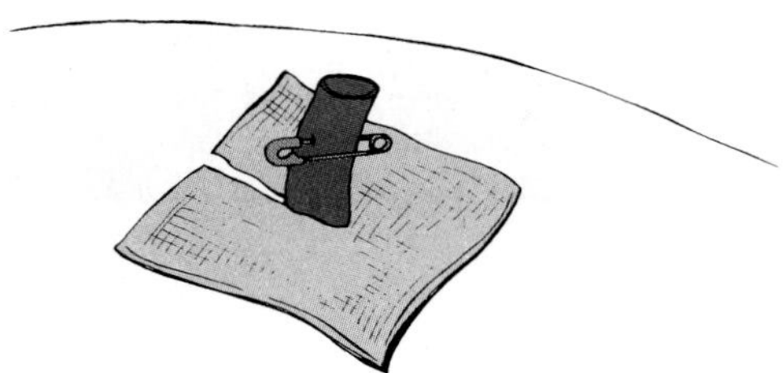

Fig. 17-9 Commercial drain dressing around the tube-insertion site.

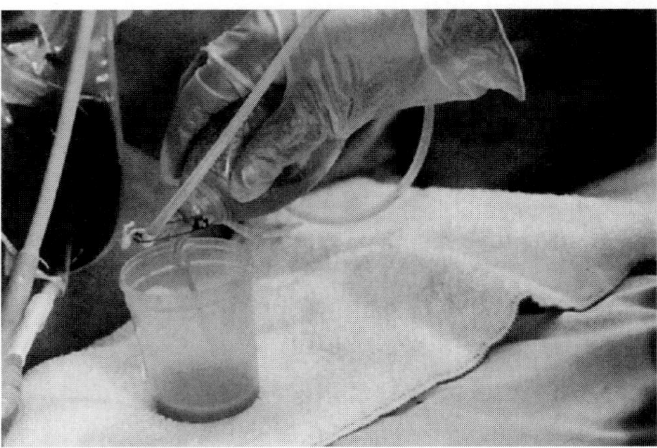

Fig. 17-10 Graduated container receptacle is placed under the outlet of collection system. Remove cap and drain the contents.

Care of the surgical drain site and drainage

Drains are used for surgeries in which a large amount of drainage is expected. Most **drainage** contains an accumulation of blood, body fluids, pus, and necrotic material and provides a good medium for the growth of microorganisms. Adequate drainage of a wound helps reduce the risk of infection (see Chapter 18). Open drainage may be provided with a Penrose drain, a flexible rubber drain, or a silicone or plastic drain (Fig. 17-9). A Penrose drain is inserted during surgery to promote drainage and healing. The drain is inserted through a stab wound a few centimeters from the incision to prevent irritation of the incision. To keep the drain from being suctioned or retracted into the wound, it is sutured in place, or a safety pin or clip is placed on the end of the drain or where the physician prefers (Skill 17-9). Drains may vary from 10 to 14 inches in length and ½ to 1½ inches in width. As the wound heals, the Penrose drain may be shortened a little each day to promote healing from the inside out. The open drain allows drainage to accumulate on the dressing and requires that the dressing be changed often.

Closed drains are preferred because they decrease the chance for infection even further. The drain is connected to a receptacle for the drainage. The receptacle may be a part of a suction machine, which provides a continuous, gentle suctioning action to remove the drainage, or a part of a portable wound-suction device. The portable suction apparatus operates from the creation of a vacuum suction inside the receptacle when it is manually depressed and plugged. It should be emptied using sterile technique to prevent wound contamination and is referred to as a *Jackson-Pratt drain* (Fig. 17-10).

The drainage is included in the output for the patient. Portable wound devices are preferred because they are lightweight, inexpensive, disposable, and quiet and allow for easy ambulation.

After surgical removal of the gallbladder, the bile duct is often inflamed and edematous. A drainage tube is frequently inserted into the duct to maintain a free flow of bile until the swelling subsides. This tube is called a ***T-tube*** (Fig. 17-11). The long end of the T-tube exits through the abdominal incision or through a separate surgical wound. The tube drains by gravity into a closed drainage system. The collection bag is emptied and measured every shift or as necessary.

Nursing care considerations for bile drainage include the following:

1. Include specific interventions or techniques for dressing change in the nursing care plan to provide continuity of care.
2. Assess the patency of drainage tube frequently, avoiding twists or kinks to ensure appropriate, open drainage.
3. Keep the receptacle for vacuum drainage collection below the level of the wound to ensure appropriate drainage.
4. Keep the collection receptacle compressed and frequently monitor it to maintain a vacuum.
5. Protect the skin surrounding the wound from bile drainage to prevent tissue breakdown.
6. Assess excessive bile leakage from the wound, since it may indicate a blocked drainage tube.
7. Assess for normal bile drainage: amount varying from 500 to 1000 ml per 24 hours and color normally thick and greenish-brown and slightly blood tinged in the first 24 hours.
8. Consider the use of Montgomery straps (Fig. 17-12) when the dressing requires frequent changing.
9. Assess the need for patient teaching during the dressing change and wound care.
10. Secure the vacuum unit to the patient's gown, avoiding tension on the tubing.
11. Record the amount of drainage on the intake and

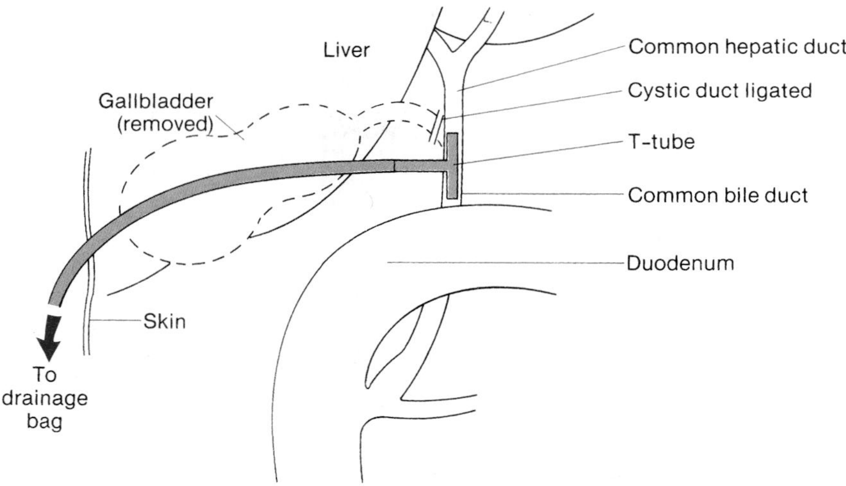

Fig. 17-11 T-tube in the common bile duct. (From Christensen BL, Kockrow EO: *Foundations of nursing,* ed 2, St. Louis, 1995, Mosby.)

output sheet to provide an accurate intake and output record.

Children Children must be assessed carefully so that the drain will not be pulled out. Parents should be taught sterile technique and the appropriate procedure for caring for the drainage site and equipment.

Older adults Healing may be somewhat slower in the older patient. The older patient, diabetics, and patients with chronic conditions are more susceptible to infection.

Patients in home care The patient should be taught appropriate care of the drain and dressing change before going home. The patient should be given instructions as to what to do if the drain accidently comes out. The drain should be protected from the confused patient who may pull it out.

Application of a bandage

Bandaging involves applying a continuous strip of woven material to a part of the body. Bandages are available in rolls of various sizes and materials. Elastic woven materials, such as Ace bandages, provide support and are frequently used to exert pressure to prevent bleeding or swelling. Gauze bandages are made of soft, woven, lightweight cotton, which is easily molded to body parts. Stockinet (tubular) bandages are made of stretchable material and are used to encircle body parts, such as the extremities or head. Other bandage materials include muslin, flannel, or synthetic fabrics.

There are several principles involved in bandaging (Skill 17-10). During application of a roller bandage, the outer surface of the material is placed against the patient's skin. Bandages should be ap-

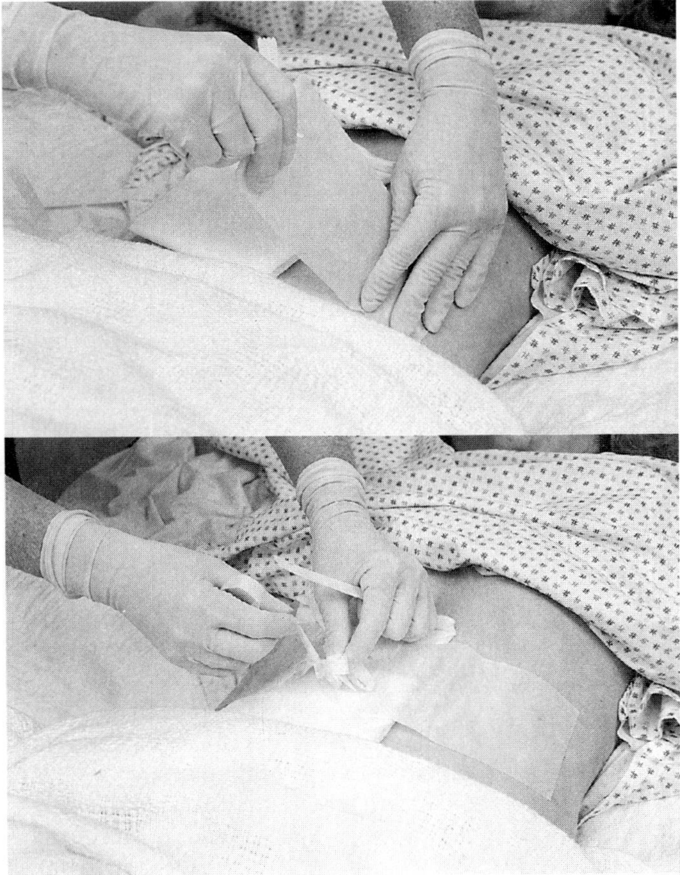

Fig. 17-12 Montgomery ties. (From Potter PA, Perry AG: *Basic nursing: theory and practice,* ed 3, St Louis, 1995, Mosby.)

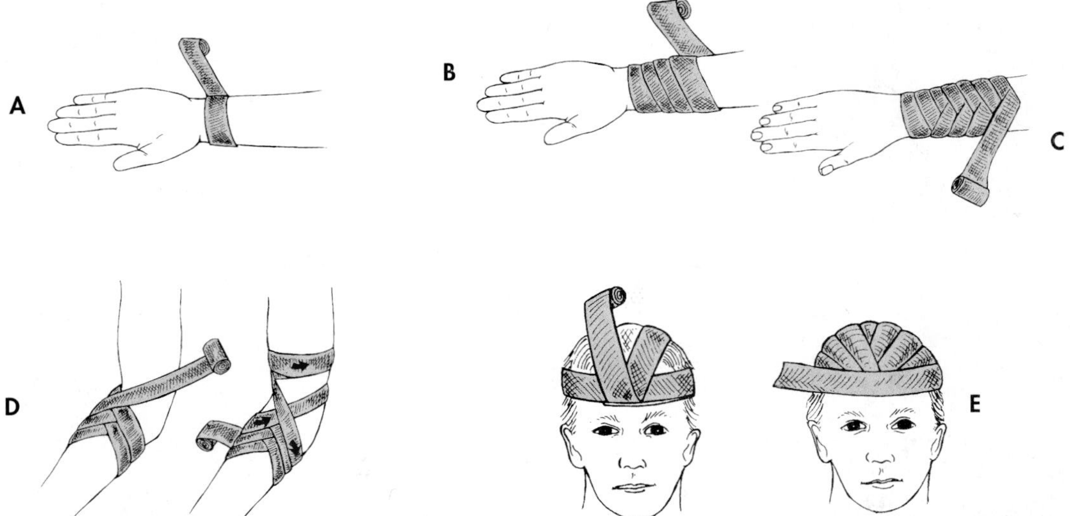

Fig. 17-13 Types of bandage turns. **A,** Circular. **B,** Spiral. **C,** Spiral-reverse. **D,** Figure-eight. **E,** Recurrent.

plied securely to prevent slipping when the patient moves. The body part to be bandaged should be positioned in a comfortable position in alignment to reduce the risk of deformity or injury. When bandaging extremities, the bandage should be applied to the distal end and wrapped toward the body trunk to aid the flow of venous blood. Bandages should be applied firmly and with equal tension exerted with each turn or layer. Excess overlapping of bandages should be avoided. Skin surfaces should not be bandaged together. For example, toes and fingers should have cotton or gauzes placed between them before they are bandaged. If possible, the end of the body part should be left exposed so that assessment of circulation and condition can be performed. The heel should be left exposed when wrapping the foot.

The five basic bandaging turns used for the various parts of the body are seen in Fig. 17-13. They are as follows:

1. Circular turns, which are used to anchor bandages and to terminate them
2. Spiral turns, which are used on parts of the body that are fairly uniform in circumference, such as the fingers, arms, and legs
3. Spiral-reverse turns, which are used on cylindrical parts of the body that are not uniform in circumference, such as the lower leg or lower arm
4. Figure-eight turns, which permit some movement and are usually used on the elbows, knees, or ankles
5. Recurrent turns, which are used to cover distal parts of the body, such as the skull or stump of an amputation (Fig. 17-14)

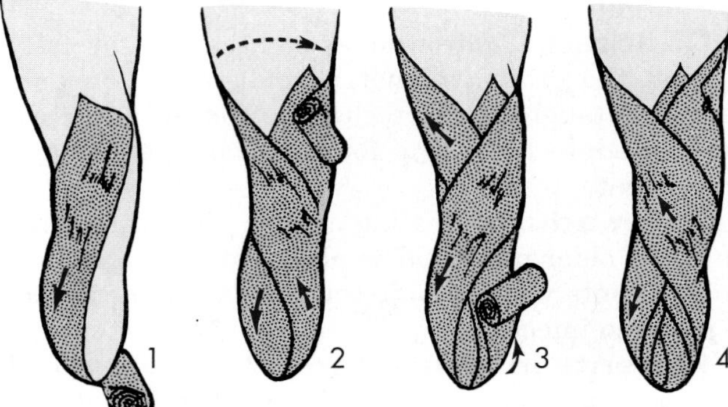

Fig. 17-14 Applying a stump bandage. Pass the bandage roll back and forth over the end of the body part to be covered, covering first one side from the center out and then the other side.

Nursing care considerations for bandages include the following:

1. Assist the patient who has an amputation in maintaining a positive self-image.
2. Ask the patient to inform the nurse if the bandage feels too tight. Assess bandages at least every hour when they are first applied.
3. Loosen the bandage if the patient complains of tingling, burning, numbness, or pain to prevent compressed circulation.

Children Bandages are difficult to keep on the small child. Parents should be taught the appropri-

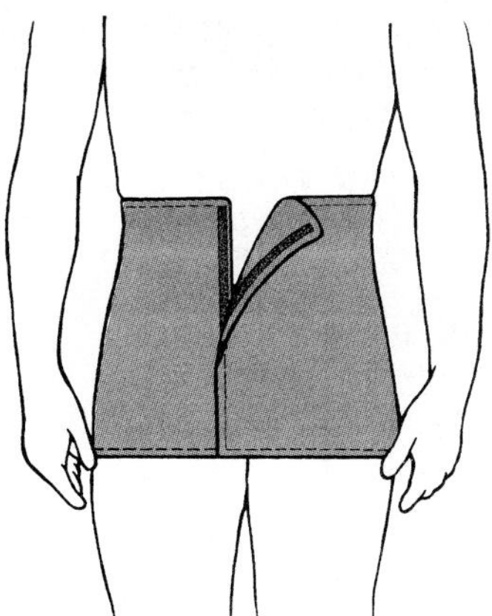

Fig. 17-15 Straight abdominal binder. (From Perry AG, Potter PA: *Clinical nursing skills and techniques,* ed 3, St Louis, 1994, Mosby.)

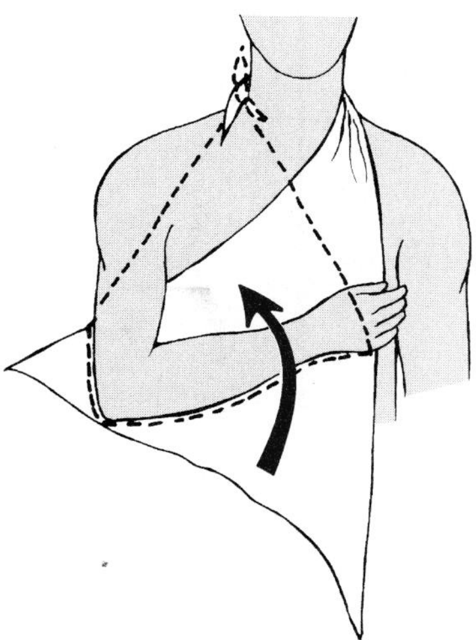

Fig. 17-16 Triangular sling. (From Perry AG, Potter PA: *Clinical nursing skills and techniques,* ed 3, St Louis, 1994, Mosby.)

ate technique for applying bandages and the signs of complications.

Older adult The older patient must be reassessed more often than other patients because circulatory problems are common. The older adult is more prone to impaired skin integrity and possible infection.

Patients in home care The patient and family should be taught the technique for applying the bandage as well as caring for a bandage. The patient and family should be taught to report changes to the physician. Signs and symptoms of complications should be explained to the family.

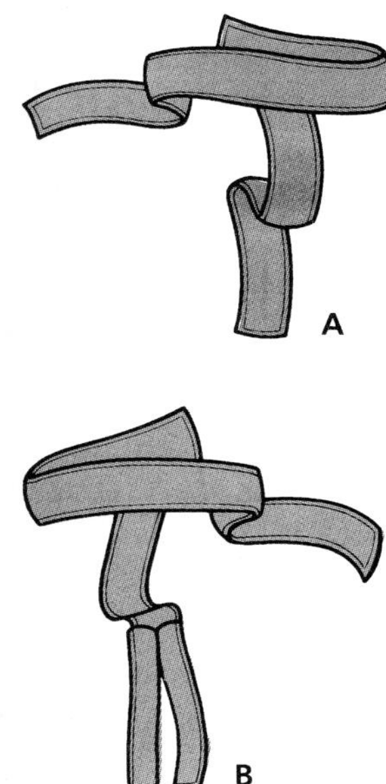

Fig. 17-17 **A,** T-binder (female). **B,** Double T-binder (male). (From Perry AG, Potter PA: *Clinical nursing skills and techniques,* ed 3, St Louis, 1994, Mosby.)

Application of a binder

Binders are bandages made of large pieces of material designed for various parts of the body. They may be made of material such as flannel, muslin, or elasticized material, which fastens with hooks and eyes or Velcro.

There are several types of binders. An abdominal binder is used to provide pressure on the abdomen after surgery to help prevent evisceration. This binder has a Velcro closing (Fig. 17-15).

Another type of binder is a triangular arm binder, which is also called a *sling.* The binder is used to support the arm, elbow, and forearm in the treatment of muscular sprains or fractures (Fig. 17-16). It may be commercially made or homemade from a large, triangular piece of cloth. It is made of various fabrics.

A T-binder is so named because it is shaped like the letter T (Fig. 17-17). The binder helps secure rectal or perineal dressings. Because of the location, a T-binder is easily soiled and requires frequent changing (Skill 17-11).

A nursing care consideration for binders follows:

1. Patients with tubes or drains with binders should be assessed frequently to ensure patency of the tubes and drains.

Patients in home care The patient should be taught appropriate application if the binder will be applied at home. The patient should also know appropriate care of the binder.

■ NURSING CARE PLAN ■

BODY-IMAGE DISTURBANCE

Mrs. R, age 48, discovered a lump 3 days before while performing her monthly breast self-examination. This was confirmed by her gynecologist, and she was referred to the surgeon for a breast biopsy and possible right modified radical mastectomy. Surgery was performed, the lump found to be malignant, and the mastectomy was performed. Mrs. R is having emotional difficulty accepting the diagnosis and resulting surgery.

NURSING DIAGNOSIS

Body-image disturbance related to loss of breast as evidenced by refusal to look at surgical site, crying, and verbalization of fear of rejection by husband

GOAL

- Patient will accept diagnosis and treatment.

EXPECTED OUTCOMES

- Patient will be able to look at surgical site.
- Patient will be able to discuss the diagnosis with her husband.

NURSING INTERVENTIONS

- Encourage patient to express grief related to the loss of her breast.
- Discuss the "Reach to Recovery" program and encourage the patient to allow a member to visit.
- Encourage patient to look at the surgical site.
- Provide patient with information regarding reconstructive surgery and breast forms.
- Encourage patient to use a temporary breast form as soon as permitted by the physician.
- Encourage patient to verbalize fears and feelings regarding diagnosis and surgery.

EVALUATION

- Patient has discussed fears related to diagnosis, body-image disturbance, and rejection from husband.
- Patient has looked at surgical site.
- Patient has visited with a member of "Reach to Recovery."

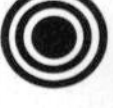

SKILL 17-1 TEACHING POSTOPERATIVE BREATHING TECHNIQUES AND LEG EXERCISES

Steps	Rationale
1. **Obtain equipment:** ▪ Support pillow, towel, or folded bath blanket ▪ Gloves ▪ Emesis basin ▪ Facial tissues ▪ Chair ▪ Pain medication, if indicated	Helps organize procedure.
2. **Refer to medical record, care plan, or Kardex for special interventions.**	Provides basis for care.
3. **Introduce self.**	Decreases anxiety level.
4. **Identify patient by identification band.**	Identifies correct patient for procedure.
5. **Explain procedure to patient.**	Seeks cooperation and decreases anxiety.
6. **Wash hands and don clean gloves according to agency policy and guidelines from Centers for Disease Control and Prevention and Occupational Safety and Health Administration.**	Helps prevent cross-contamination.

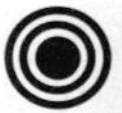

SKILL 17-1 TEACHING POSTOPERATIVE BREATHING TECHNIQUES AND LEG EXERCISES—cont'd

Steps	Rationale
7. Prepare patient for intervention:	
a. Close door to room or pull curtain.	Provides privacy.
b. Drape for procedure if necessary.	Prevents exposure of patient.
8. Raise bed to comfortable working level.	Provides safety for nurse.
9. Arrange for patient privacy.	Shows respect for patient.
10. Premedicate with pain medication, if indicated.	Helps elicit patient compliance.
DEEP BREATHING	
11. Place pillow between patient and bed or chair.	Allows for fuller chest expansion. (Bed or chair itself is too firm to provide expansion.)
12. Sit or stand facing patient.	Allows patient to observe nurse.
13. Demonstrate taking slow, deep breaths. Avoid using shoulder and chest while inhaling. Inhale through nose.	Prevents panting and hyperventilation. Prevents unnecessary expenditure of energy. Moistens, filters, and warms inhaled air.
14. Hold breath for count of 3 and slowly exhale through pursed lips.	Allows for gradual expulsion of all air.
15. Repeat exercise 3 to 5 times. Have patient practice exercise.	Allows patient to observe appropriate technique. Allows nurse to assess patient's technique and correct errors.
16. Instruct patient to take 10 slow deep breaths every 2 hours after surgery during waking hours until ambulatory.	Helps prevent postoperative complications.
17. If patient has abdominal or chest incision, instruct patient to splint incisional area using pillow or bath blanket, if desired, during breathing exercises.	Provides support and additional security for patient.
LEG EXERCISES	
18. Lifting one leg at time and supporting joints, gently flex and extend leg 5 to 10 times (Fig. 17-18).	Stimulates circulation and helps prevent formation of thrombi.

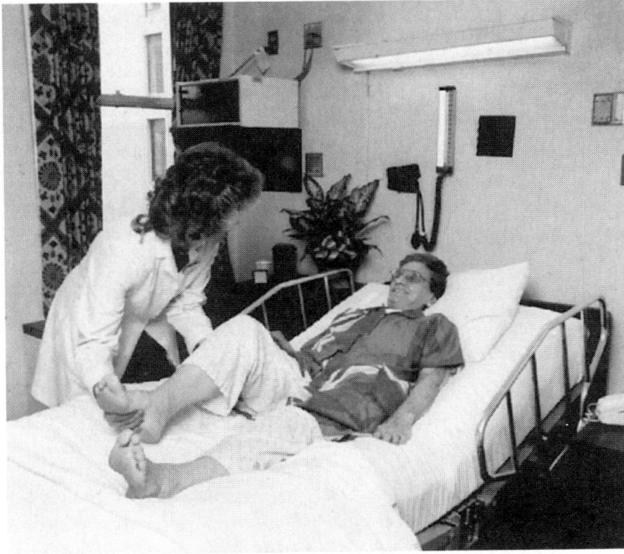

Fig. 17-18 The nurse lifts one leg at a time, supporting the joints, and extends the leg 5 to 10 times.

Continued.

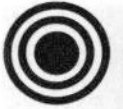

SKILL 17-1 TEACHING POSTOPERATIVE BREATHING TECHNIQUES AND LEG EXERCISES—cont'd

Steps	Rationale
19. Repeat exercise with opposite leg. Lifting leg while supporting joints, gently flex leg 5 to 10 times.	Stimulates circulation and helps prevent formation of blood clots.
20. Alternately point toes toward chin and toward foot of bed 4 to 5 times.	Uses additional muscle flexion and contraction to stimulate circulation.
21. Make circles with ankles of both feet 4 to 5 times to left and 4 to 5 times to right (Fig. 17-19).	Further stimulates circulation through muscle contraction and flexion.
22. Assess pulse, respiration, and blood pressure.	Helps determine complications from exercise.
23. Remove gloves and wash hands.	Helps prevent cross-contamination.
24. Document.	Documents procedure and patient's response.

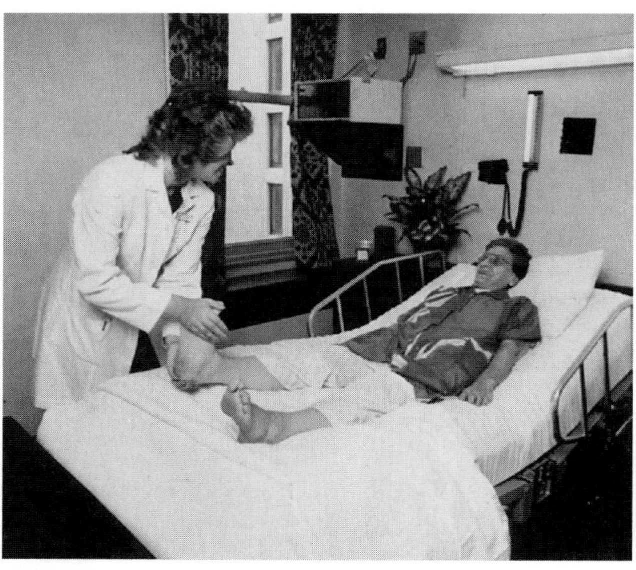

Fig. 17-19 The nurse gently flexes the leg.

SKILL 17-2 TEACHING CONTROLLED COUGHING

Steps	Rationale
1. Obtain equipment: ▪ Support pillow, towel, or bath blanket ▪ Gloves ▪ Emesis basin ▪ Facial tissues ▪ Chair ▪ Pain medication, if indicated	Helps organize procedure.
2. Refer to medical record, care plan, or Kardex for special interventions.	Provides basis for care.
3. Introduce self.	Decreases anxiety level.
4. Identify patient by identification band.	Identifies correct patient for procedure.
5. Explain procedure to patient.	Seeks cooperation and decreases anxiety.
6. Wash hands and don clean gloves according to agency policy and guidelines from Centers for Disease Control and Prevention and Occupational Safety and Health Administration.	Helps prevent cross-contamination.

SKILL 17-2 TEACHING CONTROLLED COUGHING—cont'd

Steps	Rationale
7. Prepare patient for intervention:	
a. Close door to room or pull curtain.	Provides privacy.
b. Drape for procedure if necessary.	Prevents exposure of patient.
8. Raise bed to comfortable working level.	Provides safety for nurse.
9. Arrange for patient privacy.	Shows respect for patient.
10. Premedicate with pain medication, if indicated.	Helps elicit patient compliance.
11. Assist patient to an upright position. Place pillow between bed or chair and patient.	Enhances expansion of lungs. Helps provide soft, pliable surface to further allow complete expansion of lungs.
12. Explain importance of maintaining upright position.	Facilitates appropriate movement of diaphragm and chest expansion.
13. Demonstrate coughing exercise for patient:	
a. Take several deep breaths.	Expands lungs fully so that mucus can be loosened.
b. Inhale through nose.	Warms, filters, and moistens inhaled air.
c. Exhale through mouth with pursed lips.	Helps provide more forceful and complete exhalation.
d. Inhale deeply again and hold breath for count of 3.	Helps air move behind mucus.
e. Cough two or three consecutive coughs without inhaling between coughs.	Gets all air out of lungs. Helps move mucus more effectively than forceful coughing.
14. Splint abdominal or thoracic incision with hands, pillow, towel, or bath blanket before coughing (Figs. 17-20 and 17-21).	Minimizes pain and discomfort and provides support and sense of security.
15. Encourage patient to practice coughing while splinting incisional area once or twice per hour during waking hours.	Discourages patient from coughing hard and forcefully, since this can damage respiratory tract and patient should not experience severe pain.
16. Provide facial tissues and emesis basin for any phlegm or secretions expectorated.	Prevents contamination of nurse.
17. Provide washcloth and warm water for washing hands and face and return patient to comfortable position.	Makes patient more comfortable.
18. Clean emesis basin and appropriately dispose of tissues.	Prevents spread of microorganisms.
19. Remove gloves and wash hands.	Helps prevent cross-contamination.
20. Document.	Documents procedure and patient's response.

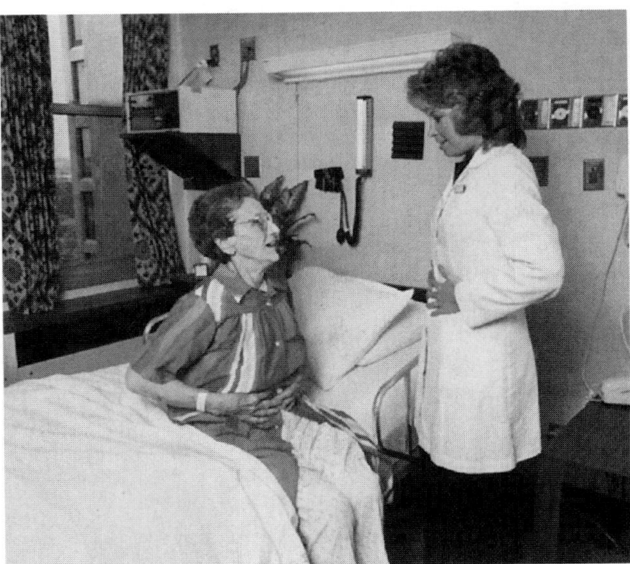

Fig. 17-20 Splinting the surgical incision with the hands.

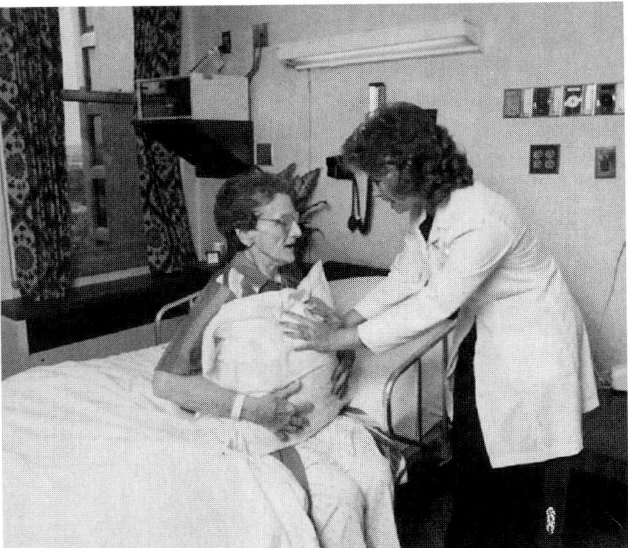

Fig. 17-21 Splinting the surgical incision with a pillow.

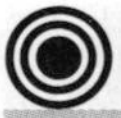

SKILL 17-3 PERFORMING A SURGICAL SHAVE

Steps	Rationale
1. Obtain equipment: ▪ Appropriate light ▪ Razor and new blades or disposable razors ▪ Basin ▪ Antiseptic or antimicrobial soap ▪ Gauze squares ▪ Bath blanket ▪ Towels and washcloth ▪ Waterproof pad ▪ Clean gloves ▪ OR prep kit ▪ Warm water	Helps organize procedure.
2. Refer to medical record, care plan, or Kardex for special interventions.	Provides basis for care.
3. Introduce self.	Decreases anxiety level.
4. Identify patient by identification band.	Identifies correct patient for procedure.
5. Explain procedure to patient.	Seeks cooperation and decreases anxiety.
6. Wash hands and don clean gloves according to agency policy and guidelines from Centers for Disease Control and Prevention and Occupational Safety and Health Administration.	Helps prevent cross-contamination.
7. Prepare patient for intervention:	
a. Close door to room or pull curtain.	Provides privacy.
b. Drape for procedure if necessary.	Prevents exposure of patient.
8. Raise bed to comfortable working level.	Provides safety for nurse.
9. Arrange for patient privacy.	Shows respect for patient.
10. Position patient.	Maintains appropriate body mechanics for patient.
11. Place towel or waterproof pad under area to be shaved.	Protects bed and linens from soiling.
12. Fill basin with warm water.	Allows nurse to lather soap and rinse skin.
13. Place bath blanket over patient.	Exposes only area to be shaved.
14. Adjust lighting.	Allows thorough assessment of skin and helps decrease chance of injuring skin.
15. Lather skin with antiseptic soap or lather and warm water using gauze squares (Fig. 17-22).	Cleanses skin, softens hair, and reduces friction from razor.
16. Hold razor at a 30- to 45-degree angle to skin:	Minimizes chances of cutting or nicking skin.
a. Shave small areas while holding skin taut.	
b. Use short, smooth strokes.	Prevents pulling of skin.
c. Shave hair in same direction it grows (Fig. 17-23).	Removes hair close to skin surface.
17. Rinse razor frequently:	Removes accumulation of hair from razor.
a. Change blade as needed.	Sharp blade minimizes chance of injuring skin.
b. Replace razor if disposable razor is used.	
c. Change water as needed.	Prevents contamination from dirty water.
18. When entire area is shaved, use washcloth and clean, warm water to cleanse area. Dry skin.	Removes excess shaved hair, body oils, and dirt on skin. Reduces number of microorganisms. Promotes comfort of patient.
19. Reassess skin for cuts, nicks, or hair.	Prevents growth of microorganisms and possible infection from disruption of skin integrity.
20. Return patient to appropriate position.	Provides patient comfort and safety.
21. Clean and dispose of equipment.	Minimizes chances for spreading microorganisms.
22. Remove gloves and wash hands.	Helps prevent cross-contamination.
23. Document.	Documents procedure and patient's response.

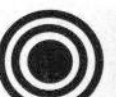

SKILL 17-3 PERFORMING A SURGICAL SHAVE—cont'd

Steps | **Rationale**

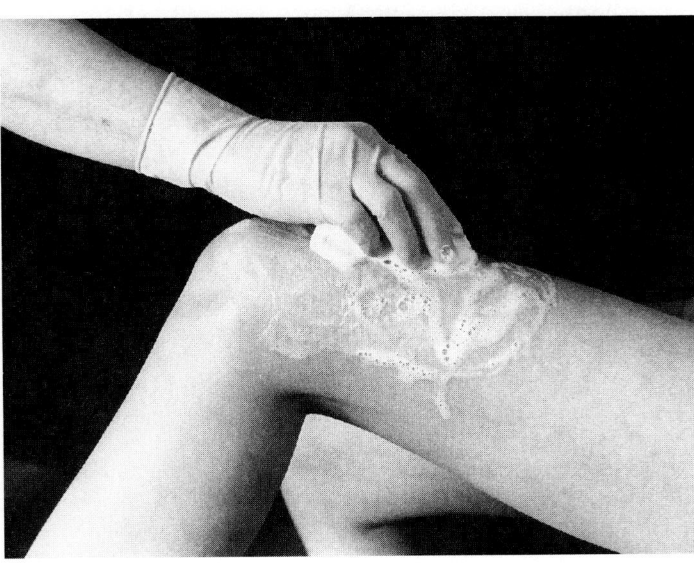

Fig. 17-22 The nurse lathers the skin well with an antiseptic soap or lather and warm water using gauze squares.

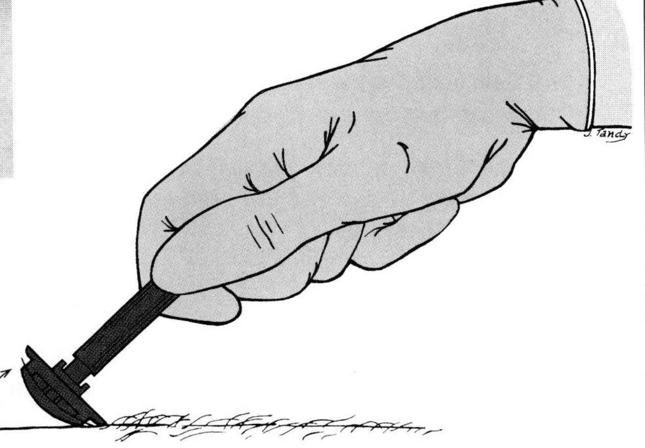

Fig. 17-23 The razor is held at a 30- to 45-degree angle to the skin. (From Perry AG, Potter PA: *Clinical nursing skills and techniques,* ed 3, St Louis, 1994, Mosby.)

SKILL 17-4 MAKING A SURGICAL BED

Steps	Rationale
1. **Obtain equipment:** ▪ Two clean sheets ▪ One clean drawsheet, if used ▪ One clean bath blanket ▪ One clean bedspread ▪ Disposable pad or towel ▪ Emesis basin ▪ Facial tissues ▪ Clean gloves	Helps organize procedure and saves time for the nurse. Provide clean environment for patient.
2. **Refer to medical record, care plan, or Kardex for special interventions.**	Provides basis for care.
3. **Wash hands and don clean gloves according to agency policy and guidelines from Centers for Disease Control and Prevention and Occupational Safety and Health Administration.**	Helps prevent cross-contamination.
4. **Raise bed to comfortable working level.**	Provides safety for nurse.
5. **Examine room to determine which side of bed patient will be returned.**	Facilities patient safety when patient is returned to bed.
6. **Place linens within easy reach.**	Saves time and energy and reduces chance of dropping linens.

Continued.

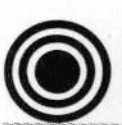

SKILL 17-4 MAKING A SURGICAL BED—cont'd

Steps	Rationale
7. Strip bed according to procedure in Chapter 23.	Helps prevent cross-contamination.
8. Make the foundation of bed according to procedure in Chapter 23.	Protects patient's skin integrity.
9. Place bath blanket or flannel sheet on foundation bed, if called for in agency procedure.	Supplies extra warmth for patient returning from surgery.
10. Place disposable pad or towel for patient's head (optional).	Protects bed linens if patient vomits.
11. Place top sheet and spread on bed, leaving both untucked.	Facilitates fanfolding of linens for easy return of patient to bed.
12. Fold top covers down about 6 in from top of bed and 6 in from bottom of bed.	Prepares linens for fanfolding.
13. Fanfold top sheets according to agency policy (usually to foot of bed).	Allows sheets to be easily pulled over patient after returning to bed. (Sheets will be tucked in at foot of bed with corners mitered and room allowed for patient's feet to be loose, preventing pressure.)
14. Change pillow case and place pillow on bedside chair.	Keeps pillow out of way of returning patient.
15. Lock wheels of bed (see p. 318).	Prevents bed from moving while transferring patient from stretcher.
16. Leave bed in high position.	Facilitates transfer of patient from stretcher to bed.
17. Place emesis basin and tissues at bedside.	Prepares for patient who may vomit.
18. Provide any other equipment ordered by surgeon.	Prepares for patient's needs after surgery.
19. Discard dirty linen and tidy room.	Provides clean and neat environment for returning patient.
20. Wash hands and remove gloves.	Helps prevent cross-contamination.
21. Document.	Documents procedure.

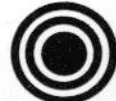

SKILL 17-5 RECEIVING THE PATIENT FROM THE POSTANESTHESIA CARE UNIT

Steps	Rationale
1. Obtain equipment: ▪ Sphygmomanometer ▪ Stethoscope ▪ Thermometer ▪ Watch with a second hand ▪ Emesis basin ▪ Tissues ▪ Bath blanket ▪ Side rails ▪ Intravenous pole or stand ▪ Clean gloves	Helps organize procedure.
2. Refer to medical record, care plan, or Kardex for special interventions.	Provides basis for care.
3. Introduce self to patient if awake.	Decreases anxiety level.
4. Identify patient by identification band.	Identifies correct patient for procedure.
5. Explain procedure to patient as level of consciousness allows.	Seeks cooperation and decreases anxiety.
6. Wash hands and don clean gloves according to agency policy and guidelines from Centers for Disease Control and Prevention and Occupational Safety and Health Administration.	Helps prevent cross-contamination.
7. Prepare patient for intervention:	
a. Close door to room or pull curtain.	Provides privacy.
b. Drape for procedure if necessary.	Prevents exposure of patient.

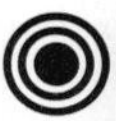

SKILL 17-5 RECEIVING THE PATIENT FROM THE POSTANESTHESIA CARE UNIT—cont'd

Steps	Rationale
8. Raise bed to comfortable working level.	Provides safety for nurse.
9. Arrange for patient privacy.	Shows respect for patient.
10. Determine time of arrival on unit.	Documents return to unit.
11. Transfer patient to surgical bed.	Provides safe return of patient.
12. Place patient on side unless contraindicated or turn head to one side.	Prevents secretions from draining into lungs or aspiration of vomitus. Helps keep tongue from obstructing airway.
13. Assess level of consciousness.	Determines patient's need for more frequent assessment.
14. Assess airway for patency.	Ensures that patient is receiving adequate oxygen.
15. Obtain vital signs (see Chapter 11).	Provides baseline for comparison.
16. Assess skin for color, diaphoresis; coolness, clamminess, pallor, or cyanosis.	Assists in assessing for surgical shock and respiratory problems.
17. Assess dressings for bleeding or drainage (see Chapter 18).	Provides baseline for comparison or detects hemorrhage.
18. Assess intravenous infusion and assess site (see Chapter 16).	Assesses for infiltration and ensures that solution is infusing.
19. Read medical orders for further instructions: ▪ Diet or fluids per mouth ▪ Additional intravenous fluids ▪ Medications ▪ Specific positioning ▪ Intake and output ▪ Laboratory tests ▪ Activity ▪ Special orders, such as oxygen, suctioning, dressing changes, and wound care	Provides means for administering postoperative nursing care.
20. Assess tubes or drains for patency.	Ensures appropriate drainage.
21. Assess patient for pain or discomfort.	Determines need for pain medication.
22. Raise side rails, lower bed, and place call light within reach of patient.	Helps provide patient safety while continuing to recover from anesthesia.
23. Remove gloves and wash hands.	Helps prevent cross-contamination.
24. Communicate with family.	Answers questions for family.
25. Document.	Documents procedure and patient's response.

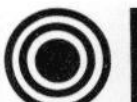

SKILL 17-6 APPLYING ANTIEMBOLISM STOCKINGS

Steps	Rationale
1. Obtain equipment: ▪ Antiembolism stockings or SCD ▪ Clean gloves ▪ Tape measure	Helps organize procedure.
2. Refer to medical record, care plan, or Kardex for special interventions.	Provides basis for care.
3. Introduce self.	Decreases anxiety level.
4. Identify patient by identification band.	Identifies correct patient for procedure.
5. Explain procedure to patient.	Seeks cooperation and decreases anxiety.
6. Wash hands and don clean gloves according to agency policy and guidelines from Centers for Disease Control and Prevention and Occupational Safety and Health Administration.	Helps prevent cross-contamination.
7. Prepare patient for intervention: a. Close door to room or pull curtain. b. Drape for procedure if necessary.	 Provides privacy. Prevents exposure of patient.

Continued.

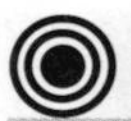

SKILL 17-6 APPLYING ANTIEMBOLISM STOCKINGS—cont'd

Steps	Rationale
8. Raise bed to comfortable working level.	Provides safety for nurse.
9. Arrange for patient privacy.	Shows respect for patient.
10. Examine legs and assess for high-risk conditions.	Helps nurse determine presence of pigmentation around ankles, pitting edema, peripheral cyanosis, which may indicate poor circulation.
11. Assess patient for calf pain or positive Homan's sign (pain in calf with dorsiflexion of foot).	May indicate presence of thrombophlebitis.
12. Measure legs for stockings according to agency policy and order stockings.	Allows nurse to apply correct size to accomplish purpose of stockings.
ANTIEMBOLISM ELASTIC STOCKINGS	
13. Assist patient to supine position to apply stockings before patient rises.	Prevents veins from becoming distended or edema from occurring.
14. Turn stocking inside out as far as heel. Place thumbs inside foot part, and slip stocking on until heel is correctly aligned.	Positions stocking for appropriate application.
15. Gather fabric and ease it over ankle and up leg (see p. 322).	Prevents bunching of stocking, which can cause local pooling of blood.
16. Pull leg portion of stocking over foot and up as far as it will go, making certain that gusset lies over femoral artery. Adjust stocking to fit evenly and smoothly with no wrinkles.	Allows appropriate fit and application, which are vital for maintaining even pressure. Prevents irritation and impediments to circulation.
17. Repeat Steps 13-16 for opposite leg.	Ensures appropriate application.
SEQUENTIAL COMPRESSION DEVICES	
18. Place sleeve under patient's leg with fuller portion at top of thigh.	Ensures that fuller portion is placed under larger part of leg.
19. Apply sleeve with opening at front of knee and closed portion behind knee.	Ensures appropriate placement and desired effect.
20. When in place, make sure there are no wrinkles or creases in stockings and fold Velcro strips over to secure stockings.	Allows proper functioning of stockings and prevents irritation.
21. Attach tubing to SCD after both sleeves are applied. Align arrows for correct connection and appropriate effect. Plug in unit.	Allows air to inflate stockings in sequential order.
22. Assess patient periodically.	Helps determine presence of swelling or cyanosis.
23. Assess stocking at regular intervals.	Ensures that top has not rolled down or loosened and that no wrinkles are present.
24. Remove gloves and wash hands.	Helps prevent cross-contamination.
25. Document.	Documents procedure and patient's response.

SKILL 17-7 APPLYING HEAT

Steps	Rationale
1. Obtain equipment: *Dry heat:* ▪ Hot water bag with cover ▪ Aquathermia pad ▪ Distilled water for aquathermia pad ▪ Heat lamp with 60-watt bulb ▪ Chemical pack with cover *Moist heat:* ▪ Gauze squares or washcloth ▪ Container	Helps organize procedure.

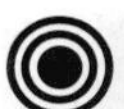

SKILL 17-7 APPLYING HEAT—cont'd

Steps	Rationale
▪ Solution ▪ Waterproof pad ▪ Towel	
2. Refer to medical record, care plan, or Kardex for special interventions.	Provides basis for care.
3. Introduce self.	Decreases anxiety level.
4. Identify patient by identification band.	Identifies correct patient for procedure.
5. Explain procedure to patient.	Seeks cooperation and decreases anxiety.
6. Wash hands and don clean gloves according to agency policy and guidelines from Centers for Disease Control and Prevention and Occupational Safety and Health Administration.	Helps prevent cross-contamination.
7. Prepare patient for intervention:	
a. Close door to room or pull curtain.	Provides privacy.
b. Drape for procedure if necessary.	Prevents exposure of patient.
8. Raise bed to comfortable working level.	Provides safety for nurse.
9. Arrange for patient privacy.	Shows respect for patient.
10. Expose only area to be treated.	Provides for modesty of patient.
HOT WATER BOTTLE	
11. Measure temperature of water: adult, 120° F; debilitated or unconscious patient, 110° F; and small child, 105° F. Monitor temperature closely.	Keeps temperature from exceeding recommendations and prevents burns.
12. Fill bottle one-third to one-half full.	Ensures that bottle will mold to body part and not fall off site.
13. Expel air from bottle (Fig. 17-24, *A*).	Allows for flexibility of bottle. Allows better conduction of heat.
14. Secure stopper.	Prevents leaking on bedclothes or sheets.
15. Assess for leaks by holding bottle upside down over sink.	Prevents leaking on bedclothes or sheets.
16. Dry bottle and apply cover.	Maintains dry equipment and prevents burns from application of hot water bottle directly to skin.
17. Apply to treatment area and assess for skin reactions such as pain, redness, and burning.	Helps prevents problems.
18. Assess treatment area every 10 min or according to agency policy.	Helps prevent burns.
19. Allow patient to remain on affected area for approximately 30 min or as ordered by physician.	Allows heat to produce maximal effect, which occurs in 20-30 min, and prevents rebound effect, which begins after 30-45 min.
HEAT LAMP	
20. Assess patient's skin to make sure that it is clean and dry.	Prevents burning of skin, which is less likely if the skin is dry.
21. Position lamp at appropriate angle and 18-24 in from area to be treated (by measurement), with bulb no greater than 60 watts (Fig. 17-24, *B*).	Prevents lamp from falling on site if it is knocked over. Produces adequate heat without burning.
22. Do not cover lamp.	Prevents heat from causing material to catch on fire.
23. Assess patient at least every 10 min.	Helps prevent burns.
24. Remove lamp at appropriate time or according to agency policy.	Allows heat to produce maximal effect, which occurs in 20-30 min, and prevents rebound effect, which begins after 30-45 min.
WARM COMPRESSES	
25. Position patient in comfortable position.	Ensures appropriate body alignment.
26. Prepare appropriate solution.	Ensures correct treatment of site.

Continued.

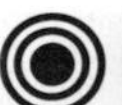

SKILL 17-7 APPLYING HEAT—cont'd

Steps	Rationale
27. Saturate gauze or clean washcloth in solution and wring excess solution from gauze or washcloth.	Prevents gown and bed linens from getting wet.
28. Place gauze or washcloth slowly over area to be treated.	Helps determine appropriate temperature and prevents burns.
29. Cover gauze or washcloth with dry towel and piece of plastic.	Prevents cooling of device.
30. Secure compress with tape or ties.	Holds in heat.
31. Apply aquathermia pad to outer cover if required (Fig. 17-24, *C*).	Helps hold in heat.
32. Assess skin frequently, at least every 10 min.	Helps prevent burns.
33. Remoisten gauze as needed to keep it warm.	Ensures treatment to provide expected outcomes.
34. After appropriate time, remove gauze or washcloth and dispose appropriately.	Helps prevent spread of microorganisms.
35. Remove gloves and wash hands.	Helps prevent cross-contamination.
36. Document.	Documents procedure and patient's response.

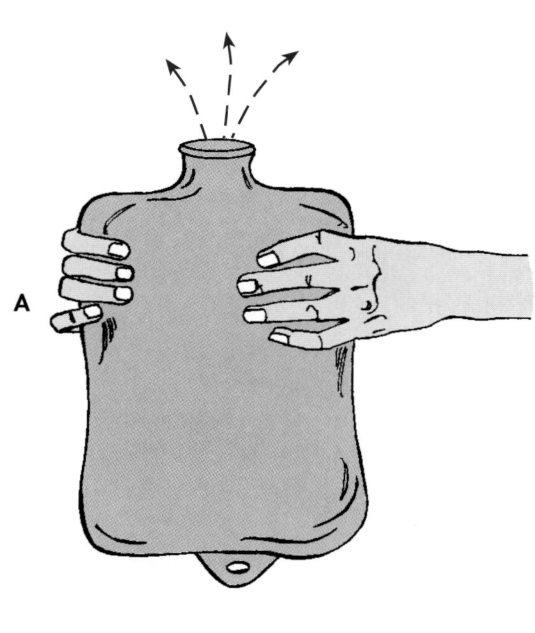

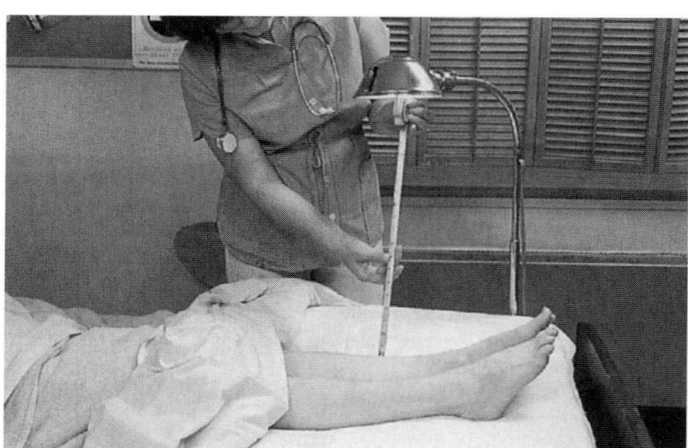

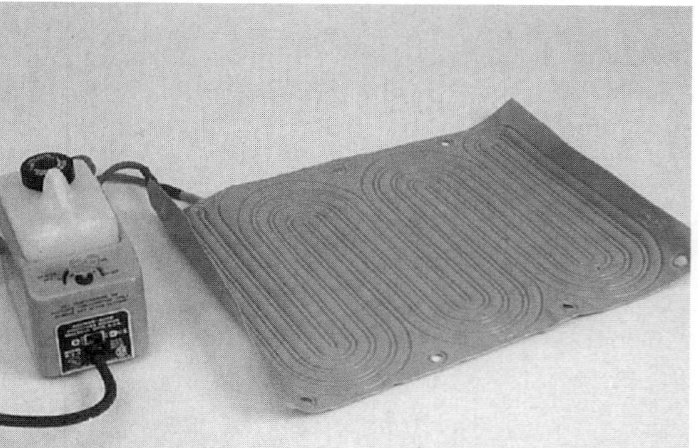

Fig. 17-24 **A,** Hot water bottle is squeezed to remove air. **B,** Gooseneck lamp. **C,** The aquamic pad and heating unit.

SKILL 17-8 APPLYING COLD

Steps	Rationale
1. **Obtain equipment:** *Dry Cold:* ▪ Ice bag or collar ▪ Mattress or hypothermia blanket pad ▪ Chemical Pack *Moist Cold:* ▪ Container for solution ▪ Solution ▪ Thermometer ▪ Gauze squares or washcloth ▪ Towel for insulation ▪ Plastic or waterproof pad ▪ Ties or tape	Helps organize procedure.
2. **Refer to medical record, care plan, or Kardex for special interventions.**	Provides basis for care.
3. **Introduce self.**	Decreases anxiety level.
4. **Identify patient by identification band.**	Identifies correct patient for procedure.
5. **Explain procedure to patient.**	Seeks cooperation and decreases anxiety.
6. **Wash hands and don clean gloves according to agency policy and guidelines from Centers for Disease Control and Prevention and Occupational Safety and Health Administration.**	Helps prevent cross-contamination.
7. **Prepare patient for intervention:**	
a. Close door to room or pull curtain.	Provides privacy.
b. Drape for procedure if necessary.	Prevents exposure of patient.
8. **Raise bed to comfortable working level.**	Provides safety for nurse.
9. **Arrange for patient privacy.**	Shows respect for patient.
10. **Position patient in comfortable position with only treatment area exposed.**	Protects privacy and modesty of patient.
ICE BAG	
11. **Fill bag one-third to one-half full of crushed ice (Fig. 17-25).**	Allows molding of ice bag to area.

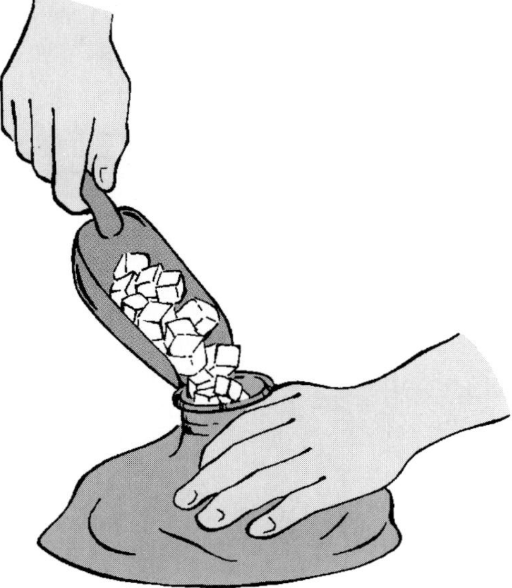

Fig. 17-25 Ice bag is filled with ice.

Continued.

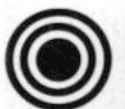

SKILL 17-8 APPLYING COLD—cont'd

Steps	Rationale
12. Expel excess air.	Allows bag to mold to site.
13. Secure stopper.	Prevents leaking on bedclothes and sheets.
14. Assess for leaks by holding bottle upside down over sink.	Prevents leaking on bedclothes and sheets.
15. Dry bottle and apply cover.	Maintains dry application.
16. Apply to treatment area.	Supports as necessary to keep in place.
17. Assess treatment area every 5-10 min.	Helps prevent mottling.
18. Allow to remain in place for appropriate time (usually 20 to 30 min) or as ordered by physician.	Allows coldness to produce maximal effect.
ICE COLLAR	
19. If ice collar needs to be filled, follow Steps 11-15.	Allows application of collar to body part.
20. If prefilled ice bag is used, remove from freezer and apply cover.	Prevents plastic or rubber from being placed directly against skin.
21. Position ice collar on patient.	Allows application of treatment.
22. Secure with roller gauze or binder, tape, or safety pins. Avoid puncturing collar with safety pin.	Prevents leakage.
23. Assess patient for comfort and skin reaction every 5-10 min. Assess temperature of ice collar.	Allows nurse to note relief of discomfort or mottling.
24. Remove ice collar at appropriate time (usually 20-30 min).	Allows coldness to produce maximal effect.
COLD COMPRESSES	
25. Prepare appropriate solution.	Ensures accuracy.
26. Saturate gauze or clean washcloth in solution.	Absorbs moisture and cold.
27. Wring excess solution from gauze or washcloth.	Prevents solution from dripping on bed linens and patient.
28. Place gauze or washcloth over area to be treated.	Allows patient time to adjust to temperature change.
29. Cover gauze or washcloth with dry towel or waterproof pad.	Insulates area, maintains temperature, and protects bedclothes.
30. Secure in place with ties or tape.	Holds in place close to skin.
31. Apply bag to the outside surface of the compress.	Maintains temperature.
32. Assess skin frequently, at least every 10 min.	Helps prevent mottling.
33. Remoisten compress as needed.	Maintains temperature and moisture.
34. Remove gauze or washcloth at appropriate time (usually 20-30 min) and dispose of according to agency policy.	Allows coldness to produce maximal effect.
ICE MATTRESS (HYPOTHERMIC BLANKET)	
35. Prepare pad or blanket.	Ensures that thermostatically controlled solution is for cooling effect.
36. Take patient's temperature.	Determines base temperature.
37. Place one bath blanket beneath patient and over cooling pad and one bath blanket over patient.	Protects patient and prevents overcooling.
38. Connect pad or blanket to cooling unit.	Starts cooling action.
39. Plug in unit.	Begins treatment.
40. Take patient's temperature frequently.	Keeps nurse aware of patient status.

SKILL 17-8 APPLYING COLD—cont'd

Steps	Rationale
41. Remove blanket when desired body temperature (usually within 2° F of desired temperature) is reached or according to agency policy.	Allows body to continue to cool after blanket is removed.
CHEMICAL PACK	
42. Read all instructions before use. Squeeze or knead pack.	Allows nurse to follow specific instructions. Activates chemical reaction.
43. Cover with cloth, if needed. (Some packs are covered with soft outer covering and do not need additional cover.)	Protects patients.
44. Assess skin and temperature of pack every 5-10 min.	Helps prevent mottling.
45. Remove after treatment is completed (usually 15-20 min).	Allows coldness to produce maximal effect.
46. Place patient in comfortable position after treatment.	Meets patient's needs.
47. Dispose of or clean and return equipment to appropriate storage or cleaning area.	Helps prevent spread of microorganisms.
48. Remove gloves and wash hands.	Helps prevent cross-contamination.
49. Document.	Documents procedure and patient's response.

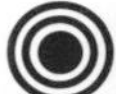

SKILL 17-9 CARING FOR SURGICAL DRAINS

Steps	Rationale
1. Obtain equipment: ▪ Sterile gloves ▪ Clean gloves ▪ Antiseptic solution ▪ Gauze squares ▪ Moisture-proof padding ▪ Sterile dressing ▪ Pain medication, if indicated	Helps organize procedure.
2. Refer to medical record, care plan, or Kardex for special interventions.	Provides basis for care.
3. Introduce self.	Decreases anxiety level.
4. Identify patient by identification band.	Identifies correct patient for procedure.
5. Explain procedure to patient.	Seeks cooperation and decreases anxiety.
6. Wash hands and don clean gloves according to agency policy and guidelines from Centers for Disease Control and Prevention and Occupational Safety and Health Administration.	Helps prevent cross-contamination.
7. Prepare patient for intervention:	
a. Close door to room or pull curtain.	Provides privacy.
b. Drape for procedure if necessary.	Prevents exposure of patient.
8. Raise bed to comfortable working level.	Provides safety for nurse.
9. Arrange for patient privacy.	Shows respect for patient.
10. Premedicate patient with pain medication, if indicated.	Helps elicit compliance.
11. Ask patient to not touch drain site.	Prevents contamination of drain site.
12. Place soiled dressing in moisture-proof bag. Remove gloves and discard.	Provides for safe disposal. Prevents contamination from microorganisms.
13. Wash hands and don clean gloves.	Helps reduce number of microorganisms.
14. Pour antiseptic solution into sterile container.	Provides means for cleaning site.

Continued.

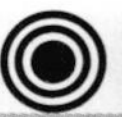

SKILL 17-9 CARING FOR SURGICAL DRAINS—cont'd

Steps	Rationale
15. Place sterile gauze squares in solution and remove contaminated gloves.	Maintains sterile technique.
16. Don sterile gloves.	Prevents contamination of drain site.
17. Squeeze excess solution out of gauze square and clean drain site. Work in full circles, starting at drain site and moving outward. Use new gauze square for each wipe. Continue cleaning until all drainage has been removed.	Prevents dripping solution on bed. Prevents contamination from use of one wipe.
18. Place sterile, precut 4 × 4 drain gauze around drain.	Helps with absorption of drainage to reduce excoriation of skin.
19. Apply sterile dressing, if appropriate. Avoid kinking tubing.	Absorbs drainage. Prevents obstruction of drainage.
20. Place graduated container under outlet of closed drainage collection container (Hemovac, Jackson-Pratt, T-tube, Penrose. Remove cap or clamp and pour contents into container. Assess drainage, note measurement, and discard (Fig. 17-26).	Accurately records output.
21. Remove gloves and wash hands.	Helps prevent cross-contamination.
22. Document.	Documents procedure and patient's response.

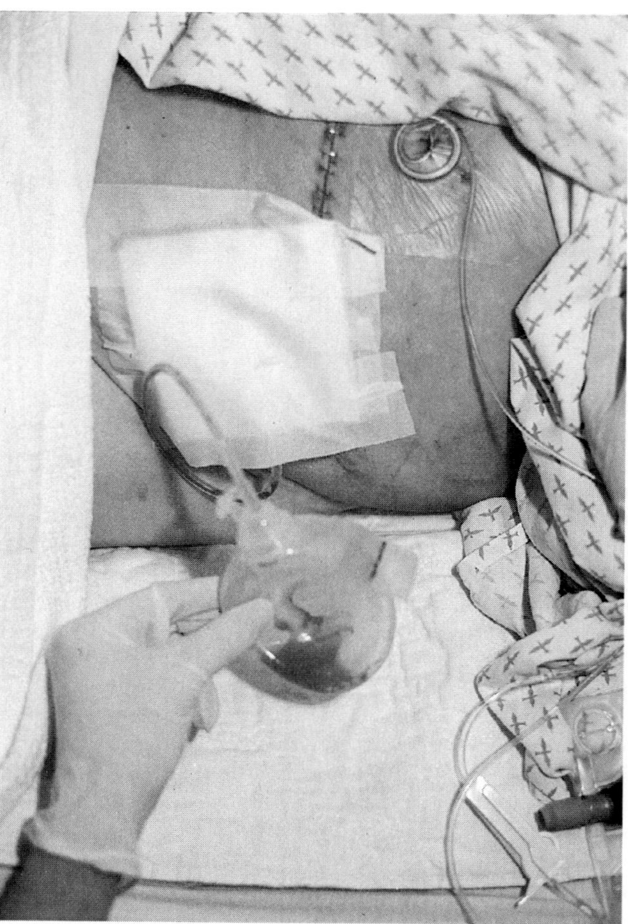

Fig. 17-26 Jackson-Pratt drainage tubes and reservoir. (From Potter PA, Perry AG: *Basic nursing: theory and practice,* ed 3, St Louis, 1995, Mosby.)

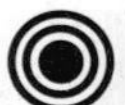

SKILL 17-10 APPLYING A BANDAGE

Steps	Rationale
1. Obtain equipment: ▪ Clean dressing ▪ Bandage ▪ Cotton padding ▪ Tape ▪ Clips or safety pins to secure bandage ▪ Pain medication, if indicated	Helps organize procedure.
2. Refer to medical record, care plan, or Kardex for special interventions.	Provides basis for care.
3. Introduce self.	Decreases anxiety level.
4. Identify patient by identification band.	Identifies correct patient for procedure.
5. Explain procedure to patient.	Seeks cooperation and decreases anxiety.
6. Wash hands and don clean gloves according to agency policy and guidelines from Centers for Disease Control and Prevention and Occupational Safety and Health Administration.	Helps prevent cross-contamination.
7. Prepare patient for intervention:	
a. Close door to room or pull curtain.	Provides privacy.
b. Drape for procedure if necessary.	Prevents exposure of patient.
8. Raise bed to comfortable working level.	Provides safety for nurse.
9. Arrange for patient privacy.	Shows respect for patient.
10. Premedicate patient with pain medication, if indicated.	Helps elicit patient compliance.
11. Position patient in comfortable position, arranging support for area to be bandaged.	Ensures easier application of bandage and provides patient comfort.
12. Ensure that skin and/or dressing is clean and dry.	Allows bandages to be applied to clean, dry areas to prevent further impaired skin integrity.
13. Separate any adjacent skin surfaces.	Prevents irritation and impaired skin integrity.
14. Align part to be bandaged, providing slight flexion if appropriate and not contraindicated.	Promotes comfort and functional use.
15. Apply bandage from distal to proximal part.	Encourages return of venous blood flow to heart.
16. Apply bandage with even distribution of pressure.	Prevents interference with circulation and slowing of healing process.
CIRCULAR BANDAGE (SEE FIG. 17-13, *A*)	
17. Apply bandage so that each round overlaps previous turn.	Allows for anchoring bandage where it begins and ends for even, equal pressure.
18. Secure bandage in place, if appropriate.	Anchors bandage.
SPIRAL BANDAGE (SEE FIG. 17-13, *B*)	
19. Make two circular turns.	Anchors bandage.
20. Continue so that each round of bandage slightly overlaps previous round by about two thirds, progressing up limb.	Allows application of equal pressure. Encourages return of venous blood flow to heart.
21. End with two circular turns and secure with pins, tape, or clips. Do not clip or pin over injured area.	Anchors bandage.
SPIRAL-REVERSE BANDAGE (SEE FIG. 17-13, *C*)	
22. Make two circular turns.	Anchors bandage.
23. Bring bandage upward at 30-degree angle.	Guides bandage in correct direction.
24. Place thumb of free hand on upper edge of bandage.	Holds fold of bandage in place.
25. Fold bandage back on itself.	Reverses direction.
26. Continue to bandage limb, overlapping previous turn by two-thirds width of bandage.	Helps equalize pressure.

Continued.

SKILL 17-10 APPLYING A BANDAGE—cont'd

Steps	Rationale
27. Perform reversal of bandage at same spot on each turn.	Aligns turns.
28. End with two circular turns and secure with safety pins, tape, or clips.	Anchors bandage and holds it in place.
RECURRENT (STUMP) BANDAGE (SEE FIG. 17-13, *E*)	
29. Holding dressings in place, anchor bandage proximal to wound with two circular turns.	Begins recurrent type bandage.
30. Hold roller bandage with roll facing upward. Hold initial part of bandage in opposite hand.	Facilitates turning and maintains even tension.
31. Pass bandage roll back and forth over end of body part to be covered, covering first one side from center out, then other side.	Anchors dressing.
32. Recircle around bandage area, using figure-eight turns.	Secures and supports bandage.
33. Secure bandage with tape or clips.	Secures bandage.
FIGURE-EIGHT BANDAGE (SEE FIG. 17-13, *D*)	
34. Make two circular turns.	Anchors bandage.
35. Carry bandage above joint and around it and then below joint and around it.	Makes figure-eight style bandage.
36. Continue above and below joint, overlapping previous turn by about two-thirds width of bandage.	Equalizes pressure.
37. End bandage above joint making two circular turns.	Anchors bandage.
38. Assess tension of bandage and circulation of extremity.	Ensures that bandage is applied appropriately.
39. Position patient for comfort.	Meets patient's needs.
40. Remove gloves and wash hands.	Helps prevent cross-contamination.
41. Document.	Documents procedure and patient's response.

SKILL 17-11 APPLYING A BINDER, ARM SLING, OR T-BINDER

Steps	Rationale
1. Obtain equipment: ▪ Binder ▪ Safety pins ▪ Washcloth ▪ Towel ▪ Soap ▪ Water ▪ Cotton or gauze pad ▪ Pain medication, if indicated	Helps organize procedure.
2. Refer to medical record, care plan, or Kardex for special interventions.	Provides basis for care.
3. Introduce self.	Decreases anxiety level.
4. Identify patient by identification band.	Identifies correct patient for procedure.
5. Explain procedure to patient.	Seeks cooperation and decreases anxiety.
6. Wash hands and don clean gloves according to agency policy and guidelines from Centers for Disease Control and Prevention and Occupational Safety and Health Administration.	Helps prevent cross-contamination.

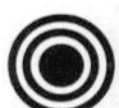

SKILL 17-11 APPLYING A BINDER, ARM SLING, OR T-BINDER—cont'd

Steps	Rationale
7. Prepare patient for intervention:	
a. Close door to room or pull curtain.	Provides privacy.
b. Drape for procedure if necessary.	Prevents exposure of patient.
8. Raise bed to comfortable working level.	Provides safety for nurse.
9. Arrange for patient privacy.	Shows respect for patient.
10. Premedicate patient with pain medication, if indicated.	Helps elicit patient compliance.
11. Assist patient to comfortable position.	Meets patient's needs.
12. Change dressing if appropriate and wash skin if needed.	Binders will need to be applied over clean dressings or skin to prevent impaired skin integrity, infection, and soiling of binder.
ABDOMINAL BINDER (SEE FIG. 17-15)	
13. Separate skin surfaces or pad bony prominences.	Preserves skin integrity.
14. Apply Velcro binder by placing it under patient's waist and hips and pulling it tight but not allowing it to become constrictive.	Prevents pressure on surgical wound on abdomen.
TRIANGULAR BINDER (SLING) (SEE FIG. 17-16)	
15. Have patient flex arm at approximately 80-degree angle, depending on purpose. (If swelling is present, angle may be more acute.)	Allows proper angle for application.
16. Place end of triangular binder over shoulder of injured side (front to back). (Binder should now be located at front of chest.)	Places point of triangle under patient's elbow of injured arm.
17. Pick up other end of binder and bring it up and over injured arm to shoulder of injured arm.	Supports arm.
18. Use square knot to tie two ends together at side of neck on injured side (not over bony prominences, especially at back of neck over vertebrae).	Prevents slippage of knot and wear on bony prominences.
19. Support wrist well with binder. Do not allow it to hang down over end of binder.	Maintains body alignment and appropriate circulation.
20. Fold third triangle end neatly around elbow and secure with safety pins.	Secures binder and ensures that arm will not slip out.
T-BINDER (SEE FIG. 17-17)	
21. Using appropriate binder, place waistband smoothly under patient's waist. Place tails under patient.	Allows use of appropriate binder: single tail for female patients and two tails for male patients.
22. Secure two ends of waistband horizontally with safety pin.	Allows bending at waist.
23. For single tail, bring tail between legs to secure dressing.	Secures dressing, pad, or other item.
24. For two tails, bring tails up one on each side of penis or large dressing.	Secures dressing without causing pressure on penis.
25. Bring tails under and over waistband and secure horizontally with safety pins.	Allows for more comfortable movement.
26. Remove gloves and wash hands.	Helps prevent cross-contamination.
27. Document.	Documents procedure and patient's response.

SUMMARY

The patient must be assessed in all phases of the surgical experience. Children, older adults, and persons with chronic medical conditions who are undergoing surgery are more difficult to manage perioperatively. The nurse caring for the patient in each of the phases (preoperative, intraoperative, and postoperative) must be aware of the need for explaining each procedure and providing continuous patient teaching.

Key Concepts

- Perioperative nursing care involves providing competent, caring nursing intervention to patients and families.
- Teaching is important in providing for patient comfort and cooperation during the preoperative and postoperative periods.
- Assessment is important during each phase of the perioperative period.
- A patient may enter the hospital or ambulatory surgery center in a variety of ways, including ambulatory surgery, 23-hour surgery, and inpatient surgery.
- The child and gerontologic patient have special needs during the surgical experience and must be frequently assessed.
- Patients and family members should be given explanations in terms that they can understand.
- The family and other caregivers should be included in caring for the postoperative patient.
- Autologous transfusions may be obtained for the patient who wants to ensure that the blood received in a transfusion is safe.
- Obesity, dehydration, chronic diseases, certain medications, and elevated temperatures are situations that may increase the risk for the surgical patient.
- A preoperative checklist is completed to help ensure that the patient will be appropriately prepared for surgery.
- Surgeons may order specific procedures to be completed to further prepare the patient for surgery.
- Deep breathing and coughing should help to reexpand the lungs after the administration of an anesthetic.
- Constant attention is essential for the patient in the PACU.
- The transporter should supply a detailed report to the nurse on the surgical unit when returning the patient from the PACU.
- The patient and family should be made aware of the signs and symptoms of postoperative complications, such as shock and hemorrhage.
- Sterile technique must be used when providing care to the drain or incisional area.

Critical Thinking Questions

1. Mr. Wilson is a 76-year-old patient admitted for a fractured hip. He has a history of emphysema. What risk does Mr. Wilson face as a result of surgery and why?
2. Mr. Joseph is the nurse working in the third floor PACU. Mr. Sennett is admitted after abdominal surgery for removal of a colonic tumor. What should Mr. Joseph assess first when the patient enters the PACU?
3. Ms. Lyons is recovering from surgery on the first postoperative day. The nurse finds that the patient's abdomen is distended. What might this indicate?

REFERENCES AND SUGGESTED READINGS

Harkness G, Dincher JR: *Medical-surgical nursing: total patient care,* ed 9, St Louis, 1996, Mosby.

Kozier B, Erb G: *Techniques in clinical nursing,* ed 4, Menlo Park, Calif, 1993, Addison-Wesley.

Long BC, Phipps WJ, Cassmeyer VL: *Medical-surgical nursing: a nursing process approach,* ed 3, St Louis, 1993, Mosby.

National Blood Resource Education Program's Nursing Education Working Group: Autologous transfusion, *American Journal of Nursing* 91(6):47, 1991.

Postop effects of OR positioning, *RN* 56(2):50, 1993.

Potter PA, Perry AG: *Basic nursing: theory and practice,* ed 3, 1995, Mosby.

Surgical update '95, *Nursing 95* 25(2):52, 1995.

The use of sequential compression devices in the prevention of deep vein thrombosis, *Journal of Practical Nursing* 43(4):38, 1993.

What to do when the diabetic patient faces surgery, *Journal of Practical Nursing* 41(4):36, 1991.

CHAPTER 18

Wound Care

Learning Objectives

After studying this chapter, the student should be able to . . .

- Define the key terms.
- Give examples of open and closed wounds.
- Explain each stage of healing.
- Differentiate between healing by primary and secondary intention.
- Use sterile technique in providing wound care.
- Don and remove sterile gloves using open technique.
- Apply a dry sterile dressing.
- Apply a wet-to-dry dressing.
- Apply a sterile compress to a wound.
- Obtain a sterile wound culture.
- Demonstrate the ability to perform a wound irrigation.
- Remove sutures or staples from a surgical wound.

Key Terms

Cellular debris
Compress
Debridement
Dehiscence
Dressing
Evisceration
Exudate
Granulation tissue
Hematoma
Inflammation
Irrigation
Maturation
Necrosis
Primary intention
Proliferation
Purulent
Sanguineous
Secondary intention
Serosanguineous
Serous
Staple
Suture
Wound

Skills

18-1 Performing sterile glove technique (open gloving)
18-2 Performing sterile dressing change
18-3 Obtaining a sterile wound culture
18-4 Applying a wet-to-dry dressing
18-5 Applying a sterile compress
18-6 Performing sterile irrigation
18-7 Removing sutures or staples

A **wound** is any physical injury involving a break in the skin, usually caused by an act or accident rather than by a disease. Wounds are classified as closed wounds (contusions) or open wounds (incisions or breaks in the skin). Open wounds may be the result of a laceration, burn, pressure ulcer, surgical incision, or puncture of the skin, mucous membrane, or underlying tissue. When a wound is open, the risk for infection is greater.

All wounds heal by primary or secondary intention. Healing by **primary intention** is the simplest form of healing. Little tissue damage or reaction occurs in healing by primary intention because there has been little or no tissue loss and the edges of the wound are held together by sutures, staples, or clips. This healing process is short, with little or no visible **granulation tissue,** or scar tissue. When the edges of the wound cannot be brought together because of the size or nature of the wound and the loss of tissue, the open wound must heal by **secondary intention,** or from inside out. This process takes longer, results in more granulation tissue, and leaves a larger, more noticeable scar.

WOUND HEALING

Normal wound healing occurs in stages (see box). The first stage, the inflammatory stage, is charac-

STAGES OF WOUND HEALING

Inflammatory Stage

- Lasts about 3 days
- Is characterized by redness, warmth, and throbbing

Internal activity

- Blood vessels constrict.
- Platelets increase to stop bleeding.
- Fibrin is formed to provide framework for repair.
- Histamine is released by cells, which causes vasodilation.
- Serum and white blood cells are released into the traumatized tissue, causing symptoms.
- White blood cells engulf bacteria or debris to help clean wound.
- Epithelial cells migrate from wound edges under base of scab or clot.

Proliferative Stage

- Lasts 3 to 24 days
- Is characterized by formation of new tissue

Internal activity

- New blood vessels form as part of reconstruction.
- New tissue is formed.
- Risk of wound separation decreases.

Maturation Stage

- Lasts up to 1 year
- Is final stage of healing
- Is characterized by formation of scar tissue

Internal activity

- Collagen fibers increase.
- Scar tissue is strengthened.

terized by **inflammation** (protective response of body tissues to irritation or injury). The signs and symptoms of inflammation are localized redness, warmth, edema, and throbbing pain near the wound. These symptoms gradually decrease and usually disappear by the end of the third day. The second stage, **proliferation,** results in tissue regeneration and lasts up to 3 weeks. During this stage, the wound is usually deep pink and may be tender or bleed easily if irritated or traumatized. The third stage of healing, **maturation,** usually lasts about a year, and tissue is strengthened during this time. The scar resulting from the wound is usually lighter in color than the surrounding tissue. Factors affecting wound healing are found in the box.

After an accident that causes an open wound, foreign material (for example, dirt, rocks, glass, and damaged tissue) may be lodged in the wound. This material creates a more complicated situation, and like **necrosis** (localized tissue death), **dehiscence** (separation of wound edges), and **evisceration** (organs protruding through an incision), it delays wound healing (Table 18-1). Any open wound should be well cleansed before a dressing is applied. The removal of foreign material or dead tissue is called ***debridement.*** Often pain medication is administered 30 to 45 minutes before a scheduled debridement to alleviate or prevent pain. If foreign material is lodged deep in the wound, the patient may need to have surgery to complete the debridement.

The surgeon or physician usually uses **sutures** to sew the edges of the wound together so that healing will take place with less chance of infection. Sutures are made of silk, cotton, sheep intestine (catgut), or synthetic materials. Sutures used to sew deeper layers of tissue together are catgut and are usually absorbable, whereas those used to close the dermis and epidermis usually need to be removed. Steel **staples** are often used to close the outer layers of skin after surgery because they are less traumatic to the wound and provide extra strength for the incision. The physician usually orders that the sutures or staples be removed by the nurse. Steri-strips or butterfly closure strips may be used to close a small wound when the edges are well approximated.

Over 2000 commercial products are available to aid wound healing. Many of these have been developed to incorporate the use of moisture in wound healing. A dressing should be suited to a specific wound's characteristics to promote healing. A **dressing** is a clean or sterile covering applied directly to wounded or diseased tissue for absorbing secretions, protecting the wound from trauma, administering medication, keeping the wound clean, and stopping bleeding. An understanding of the variety and purpose of dressings is essential for the nurse (Table 18-2).

NURSING PROCESS

Assessment

The nurse performs a thorough assessment of the wound, which should be clean and dry. The edges should be well approximated. The nurse should note the presence of drains, tubes, sutures, staples, signs of increased inflammation, **hematoma** (blood trapped in skin tissue or an organ), purulent drainage, dehiscence, or evisceration.

Drainage from a wound site or drainage system, such as a Hemovac or T-tube (see Chapter 17), should be assessed for amount, color, odor, and consistency. Wound drainage, also called ***exudate,*** is fluid that is deposited on the skin or dressing cover-

FACTORS INFLUENCING WOUND HEALING

Age
- Blood circulation and oxygen delivery to wound, clotting, inflammatory response, and phagocytosis may be impaired in very young and older adults. Risk of infection is greater.
- Cell growth and differentiation in reconstruction are slower with advancing age.
- Scar tissue is more taut and less pliable, increasing risk of altered body part function in older adults.

Nutrition
- Tissue repair and infection resistance depend on balanced diet. Surgery, severe wounds, serious infections, and preoperative nutritional deficits increase nutritional requirements.

Obesity
- Less abundant supply of blood vessels in fatty tissue impairs delivery of nutrients and cellular elements needed for healing.
- Suturing of adipose tissue is more difficult. If wound heals by secondary intention, dehiscence or evisceration and subsequent infection are greater.

Extent of Wound
- Deeper wounds with more tissue loss heal more slowly and by secondary intention and thus are more vulnerable to complications.

Oxygenation
- Reduced oxygen delivery to wound inhibits repair.
- Low arterial oxygen tension alters synthesis of collagen and formation of epithelial cells.
- Wound heals more slowly when local blood flow is reduced and wound is not exposed to oxygen.
- Low hemoglobin levels exhibited in severe anemia reduce oxygenation and impede tissue repair.

Smoking
- Functional hemoglobin levels decrease. Oxygen release in tissues is impaired.

Immunosuppression
- Reduced immune response contributes to poor healing.
- Cortisone depresses fibroblast activity and capillary growth and thereby impairs wound closure.
- Because steroids mask inflammatory response, nurse may not be able to detect early signs of inflammation or infection.
- Chemotherapeutic drugs and certain cancerous diseases interfere with leukocyte production and immune response.

Diabetes Mellitus
- Diabetic patient has small vessel disease that impairs tissue perfusion. Thus oxygen delivery may be poor.
- Elevated blood glucose level impairs macrophage function.
- Risk of infection is increased because of poor wound healing.

Radiation
- Radiotherapy, which eventually results in fibrosis and vascular scarring, interferes with postoperative wound healing when surgery is delayed more than 4 to 6 weeks and irradiated tissues have become fragile and poorly perfused.

Wound Stress
- Sustained stress (for example, vomiting, abdominal distention, and coughing) disrupts wound layers and tissue repair.

From Potter PA, Perry AG: *Basic nursing: theory and practice,* ed 3, St Louis, 1995, Mosby.

ing a wound. Exudate is made up of tissue fluid, fluid from blood, and various types of cells. **Serous** fluid or drainage is the clear portion of blood without cells. **Sanguineous** drainage contains mostly red blood cells and is red. **Serosanguineous** drainage is a combination of serous fluid and sanguineous drainage and is reddish or pinkish tinged. **Purulent** drainage contains pus, is thicker, and is usually whitish, yellowish, or greenish. Pus consists of dead tissue, cells, leukocytes, and living and dead microorganisms.

The skin surfaces around the wound should be assessed for redness, blisters, or tape residue, which may indicate an allergic reaction to the dressing or tape. All dressings should be frequently assessed for bleeding in the first hours following surgery. The wound should be assessed at least daily or more often.

Nursing Diagnosis

The nurse reviews data gathered during assessment and establishes nursing diagnoses. The diagnoses help the nurse anticipate the need for preventive or supportive care. Possible nursing diagnoses related to wound care include the following:

Altered tissue perfusion (peripheral)
Body-image disturbance
Impaired skin integrity
Pain
Risk for infection
Risk for impaired skin integrity

Table 18-1 COMPLICATIONS OF WOUND HEALING

Symptom	Nursing Action
Bright bleeding from wound	Bright bleeding from wound is never normal and may indicate hemorrhage. Nurse should monitor and report.
Continued or increased redness	Although inflammatory stage is normal part of healing and lasts up to 3 days, persistent redness accompanied by pain may indicate infection. Nurse should report and document.
Yellow drainage	Yellow drainage indicates pus caused by infection. This drainage must be cleaned from the wound before healing can occur. Nurse should report to physician because wound cultures and other medical interventions may be ordered. Risk factors for infection include altered immune response, anemia, traumatized tissue, advancing age, and metabolic disorders, such as diabetes.
Black tissue in a wound	Black tissue in wound indicates necrotic tissue that must be removed before wound can heal. Nurse should notify physician.
Severe or increased pain	Nurse should inspect wound. Complications, such as infection or hematoma, may be developing.
Dehiscence	This indicates that wound is not healing properly. It most commonly occurs in abdominal wounds 3 to 11 days after surgery but may occur at any time. Dehiscence may occur in patients who are obese, medically compromised, or malnourished. Straining from severe coughing or vomiting may be cause. Nurse should report immediately because reclosure may be indicated.
Evisceration	This is emergency that requires immediate surgical intervention. Nurse should report immediately and cover area with sterile saline dressings to keep it moist.

Table 18-2 DRESSING MATERIALS

Dressing	Description
Gauze	Gauze is most commonly used dressing. It is placed directly on wound to collect exudate and debris. Sizes used most frequently include 2×2s, 4×4s, 4×8s, or rolls. It is used for wet and dry dressings.
Fluff	Large absorbent section of loosely folded gauze is used to absorb drainage or pack wounds.
Petroleum gauze	Petroleum gauze is nonadherent. Gauze impregnated with petroleum jelly will not cause tissue damage when removed.
Telfa	Telfa is nonadherent. Exudate will collect in middle layers, but dressing will not adhere to wound when removed. It is not used when debridement is desired and is used over clean wounds.
Abdominal pad	Larger, thick dressing is used over smaller gauze dressings. It is very absorbent and is used when drainage is present.
Transparent	It is adhesive and nonabsorbent. Most are semipermeable and allow gases and oxygen to pass through material. It promotes tissue healing by providing moist environment and is used for small wounds.
Hydrocolloid	Hydrocolloid is occlusive. It is small wafer that can be cut to desired shape or size and placed over open wound. It is useful in absorbing drainage, providing moisture for healing, and liquifying necrotic tissue. It is usually used over open ulcers or wounds.
Hydrogel	Hydrogel adds moisture to dry wounds. It works better on shallow crater wounds than on deep wounds. It may macerate surrounding skin, so it must be cut to fit within wound edges.

PATIENT TEACHING

- Teach importance of keeping dressings, sutures, and staples dry and clean.
- Explain importance of washing hands before and after dressing changes.
- Teach signs and symptoms of infection.
- Instruct patient to notify physician if signs of wound infection appear.

GERONTOLOGIC CONSIDERATIONS

- The nurse should assess the ability of the older adult to perform self-care: to reach the wound and to manipulate the wound dressings.
- The skin of older adults is fragile and may not tolerate adhesives. Frequent dressing changes should be avoided.

Planning

The nurse establishes a plan of care based on the patient's health care needs. The patient's plan for discharge should be considered, since patients are discharged earlier than in the past. The nurse should teach the patient and family appropriate wound-management and healing-promotion techniques for use after discharge (see teaching box). The special needs of the older adult should be considered when performing wound care (see gerontologic box).

The plan of care may be based on one or more of the following goals:

Goal #1: Patient's wound is free of infection.

Outcome

There is no purulent drainage or separation during healing.

Goal #2: Patient achieves comfort.

Outcome

Patient uses less pain medication as wound heals.

Implementation

While implementing these goals during wound care, the nurse should observe the wound for signs of infection. The nurse ensures sterile technique is used when gloving, handling sterile equipment and dressings, and performing procedures that involve care of the open wound (see care plan on p. 358). Documentation of wound care should include the appearance of the wound, presence of drainage, medications or solutions used in wound care, type of dressing applied, and patient response to the procedure. Any deviation from normal healing should be reported.

Evaluation

The nurse evaluates wound healing with each dressing change, after application of heat and cold therapies, after wound irrigations, and after stress to the wound site. The nurse determines whether expected outcomes have been met. Examples of goals and evaluative measures used in identifying outcomes include the following:

Goal #1: Patient's wound is free of infection.

Evaluative measure

Inspect the wound bed or dressings for odor, drainage, and separation.

Goal #2: Patient achieves comfort.

Evaluative measure

Compare dosage and frequency of pain medication delivered over recovery period.

GUIDELINES FOR WOUND CARE

1. Follow the medical orders or agency policy for wound care.
2. Read previous documentation of wound care to assess progress of healing and be aware of special interventions.
3. Obtain supplies before approaching the patient.
4. Use cost-effective measures without compromising asepsis.
5. Maintain aseptic technique during all wound-care procedures.
6. Assess the wound's condition, including the presence of sutures, staples, or drains.
7. Evaluate the patient's physical and psychologic response to wound care.
8. Include family members in wound care as appropriate.
9. Teach the patient regarding wound care, including principles of asepsis and signs of infection.
10. Evaluate the presence of factors that may interfere with or delay the healing process (that is, older adulthood, obesity, diabetes, inadequate nutrition, chronic illness).
11. Document findings and report deviations.

Sterile (Open) Gloving

The use of sterile gloves permits the nurse to handle sterile equipment without contamination

Table 18-3 PRINCIPLES OF STERILE TECHNIQUE

Principle	Rationale
Sterile objects become contaminated when touched by unsterile objects.	Microorganisms are present on almost all surfaces, and even clean surfaces are considered contaminated.
If in doubt about sterility of object, the nurse should consider it unsterile.	When unsure, it is best to assume that article is not sterile rather than risk contaminating other objects and risk spreading microorganisms.
The nurse should consider item unsterile if expiration date has passed.	Expiration dates indicate time that object is no longer considered sterile.
Sterile wrapper should always be opened away from nurse. Last fold to be opened should be the fold toward nurse.	This prevents reaching over sterile field, thus rendering it contaminated.
Wet object is considered contaminated.	Water is vehicle for microorganisms and can travel through wet surface.
Sterile field is contaminated if nurse reaches across it.	Dust, lint, or clothing particles can fall onto sterile field and carry microorganisms, causing contamination.
All sterile objects must be kept above waist level.	Viewing of objects lower than waist level is difficult, and when object is not in visual field, it is considered unsterile.
Outer inch of sterile field is considered contaminated and must not be touched with sterile gloves or equipment.	Outer edges of any sterile object are most likely to be touched or come in contact with unsterile areas.
Talking, sneezing, or coughing over sterile field causes contamination.	Droplets and spray containing microorganisms can fall onto sterile field by gravity.
Sterile field left unattended is considered unsterile.	Sterility cannot be guaranteed if it is not observed at all times.
Sterile field becomes more contaminated the longer it is open.	Microorganisms are transported by dust and air currents.

(Table 18-3). Sterile gloves also protect a wound, body cavity, or opening from microorganisms residing on a nurse's hands.

Gloves should fit snugly but should not constrict. To maintain asepsis, the sterile package and the gloves should be dry and free from tears, holes, or other defects (Skill 18-1).

Sterile Dressing Changes

The majority of wounds are covered with dressings and bandages. The dressing fits against the wound and protects it from injury and contamination, absorbs drainage, helps promote wound healing, and provides physical and psychologic comfort. The bandage fits over the dressing and provides more absorption and protects the dressing.

The location and size of the wound determines the type and amount of dressing needed. Some dressing materials absorb drainage but will not adhere to the wound when removed. Gauze dressings may also be used to cover the wound. Dressings are commercially packaged in various sizes. Large abdominal dressings may also be used for larger or draining wounds. Dressings are secured with adhesive, silk, or paper tape. If frequent dressing changes are required, Montgomery straps may be used to prevent skin irritation from frequent tape removal. If the dressing change is likely to be painful, the patient should be medicated 30 to 60 minutes before the procedure (Skill 18-2).

Sterile Wound Cultures

If assessment of a wound or drainage indicates an infection, a wound culture may be ordered. Some institutions have a policy requiring a culture of any open or draining wound. The culture determines whether a pathogen is present and growing and assists in identifying the bacteria causing the infection. Identifying the causative microorganism allows for specific medical intervention. Physicians order a culture and sensitivity (C&S) test. The culture identifies the microorganism and determines the sensitivity of the microorganism to specific medications. The best specimen for a culture is obtained from fresh drainage or from within the wound itself (Skill 18-3).

Wet-to-Dry Dressings

Wet-to-dry dressings are frequently indicated for infected or draining wounds to debride the wound. Debridement removes damaged tissue and **cellular debris** (dead, diseased, or damaged tissue in a wound). As the wet dressing dries, the damaged tissue clings to the dressing and is removed when the dressing is changed (Skill 18-4).

The dressing should be just wet enough to dry between dressing changes. A saturated dressing promotes tissue breakdown and bacterial growth. Various solutions, such as povidine-iodine (Betadine), acetic acid, hydrogen peroxide, or normal saline, may be ordered for wet-to-dry dressings. The type of solution used is determined by the nature of the wound. For example, povidine-iodine or acetic acid is used for infected wounds, whereas normal saline is used for noninfected, draining wounds.

Sterile Compresses

Sterile **compresses** are used to improve circulation, localize infection, promote drainage of purulent material, and increase patient comfort. Compresses are made of sterile gauze soaked in warmed, prescribed solutions (Skill 18-5). They are usually covered with a layer of waterproof material. A hot water bag or another aquathermic device is applied over the compress to maintain the heat for a prescribed length of time. Care must be taken not to burn the patient. Commercially packaged compresses are used in some agencies, and manufacturers' directions should be followed.

Sterile Irrigation

A wound **irrigation** aids in the removal of wound drainage and infectious debris. Irrigations are commonly ordered for deep, open wounds (Skill 18-6). The removal of exudate and debris helps the wound to heal from deep within the wound out toward the skin surface. This process of healing avoids the formation of a pus pocket or other infectious tracts beneath a closed surface. Although normal saline solution can be used for irrigating a wound, antiseptic or antibiotic solutions may also be used. Irrigations should be performed slowly and gently to avoid discomfort, tissue damage, and the spread of bacteria to other areas.

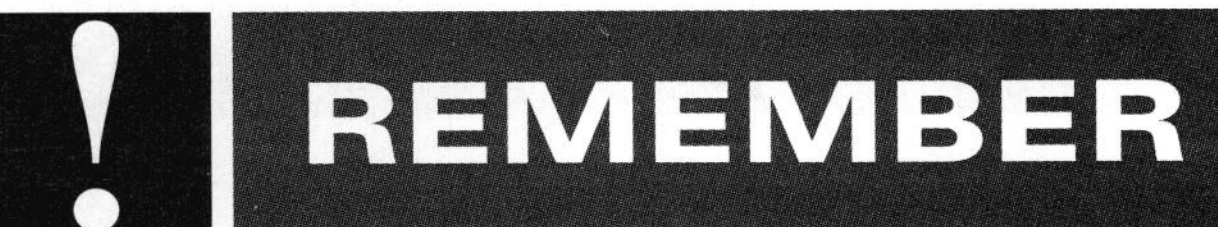

- If there is any doubt as to whether gloves are sterile, consider them contaminated and use another pair.
- When removing surgical staples, carefully count and document the number of staples removed.
- It is sometimes helpful to work the skin off the staple rather than pull on the staple itself.

Removal of Sutures or Staples

Agency policy determines who may remove sutures or staples. The progress of wound healing determines when wound-closure materials are removed. A medical order is required and should be followed specifically (Skill 18-7). Usually, closure materials are removed from the fourth to the twelfth postoperative day, depending on their location and the progress of healing. Staples or sutures that remain longer than necessary may be a source of infection.

■ NURSING CARE PLAN ■

RISK FOR INFECTION

Mr. S, a 43-year-old male, experienced a deep laceration on his forehead as a result of a fall on a gravel driveway. He was taken to the emergency room by a family member. The physician repaired the wound and sent the patient home with instructions to change the dressing for the next 5 days.

NURSING DIAGNOSIS

Risk for infection related to contamination of the wound as evidenced by the presence of foreign materials in the wound

GOAL

- Patient will use sterile technique while caring for wound.

EXPECTED OUTCOMES

- Patient will remain free of infection.
- Wound will heal without complications.

NURSING INTERVENTIONS

- Teach patient and other family members the principles of sterile technique to use while changing the dressing.
- Change dressing daily.
- Teach patient to recognize symptoms of an impending infection.
- Encourage patient to have a well-balanced diet and maintain an adequate health regimen.
- Encourage patient to ask questions about wound or care.

EVALUATION

- Patient's wound exhibits no symptoms of infection.
- Patient has a clean, dry wound with appropriate healing.

SKILL 18-1 PERFORMING STERILE GLOVE TECHNIQUE (OPEN GLOVING)

Steps	Rationale
1. **Obtain equipment:** ▪ Sterile gloves	Helps organize procedure. Must be appropriate size.
2. **Place package of sterile gloves on a clean, dry surface at waist level or above.**	Moist surfaces will contaminate gloves.
3. **Carefully peel back outer wrapper of glove package.**	Maintains sterility of gloves.
4. **Open inner package (wrapper) with cuff ends of gloves facing self. Do not touch inside of wrapper.**	Allows for ease in application and prevents contamination of gloves.
5. **With thumb and index finger of nondominant hand, pick up folded cuff of glove of dominant hand (Fig. 18-1).**	Allows unsterile hand to touch only inside of glove while outside of glove remains sterile.
6. **Hold gloves with fingers facing slightly upward and lift up and away from wrapper.**	Avoids risk of contaminating sterile glove on surface or wrapper.
7. **Carefully insert dominant hand into glove without touching outside of glove (Fig. 18-2).**	Helps prevent cuff from rolling and contaminating outside of glove.
8. **Insert fingers of gloved hand under cuff of second glove, keeping thumb away from hand (Fig. 18-3). Pick glove up and away from sterile wrapper.**	Maintains sterile-to-sterile contact. Avoids touching skin of other hand with thumb. Lessens chance for contaminating glove on wrapper.
9. **Insert nondominant hand into glove, being careful not to touch gloved hand with ungloved hand (Fig. 18-4).**	Prevents contamination of gloved hand.

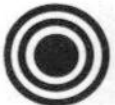

SKILL 18-1 PERFORMING STERILE GLOVE TECHNIQUE (OPEN GLOVING)—cont'd

Steps	Rationale
10. Adjust fit of both gloves, especially smoothing fingers, touching only outer surfaces of both gloves and not touching above the wrist (Fig. 18-5).	Prevents contamination from inner surface of glove, which is unsterile. Ensures smooth fit by removing wrinkles and air pockets. Prevents contamination from area above wrist, which is unsterile.
11. To remove gloves, grasp glove of nondominant hand near cuff and remove by inverting glove. Collect contaminated glove in gloved hand and wad into fist (Fig. 18-6).	Avoids contact of skin surface with contaminated glove. Ensures that microorganisms remain inside contaminated glove.
12. Slide fingers of ungloved hand inside opposite glove and remove by turning inside out and pulling over both gloves.	Avoids contact of skin surface with contaminated glove. Ensures that all contaminated areas are enclosed in second glove.
13. Remove gloves and wash hands.	Helps prevent cross-contamination.
14. Document.	Documents procedure and patient's response.

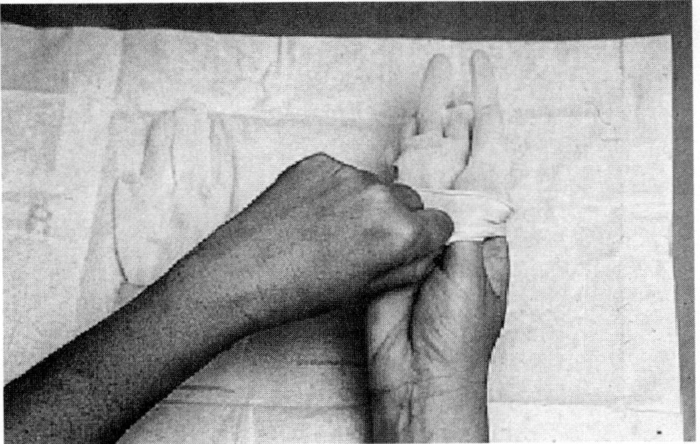

Fig. 18-1 Pick up the folded cuff of the glove for the dominant hand. (From Perry AG, Potter PA: *Clinical nursing skills and techniques,* ed 3, St Louis, 1994, Mosby.)

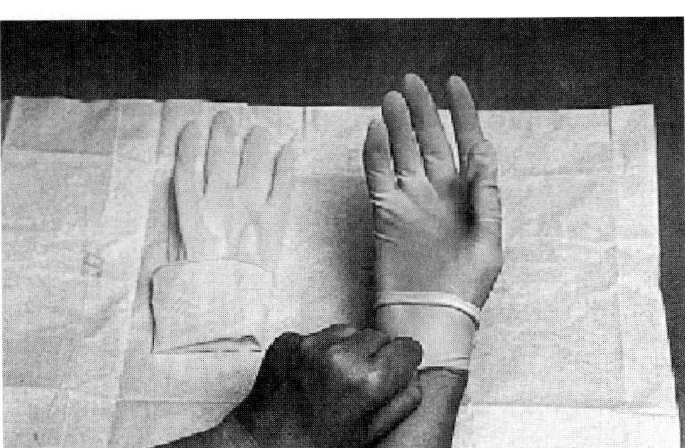

Fig. 18-2 Insert the dominant hand into the glove. (From Perry AG, Potter PA: *Clinical nursing skills and techniques,* ed 3, St Louis, 1994, Mosby.)

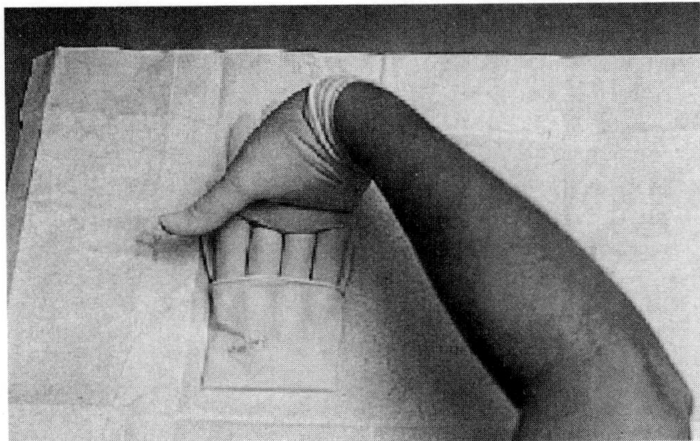

Fig. 18-3 Insert the fingers of the gloved hand under the cuff of the second glove. (From Perry AG, Potter PA: *Clinical nursing skills and techniques,* ed 3, St Louis, 1994, Mosby.)

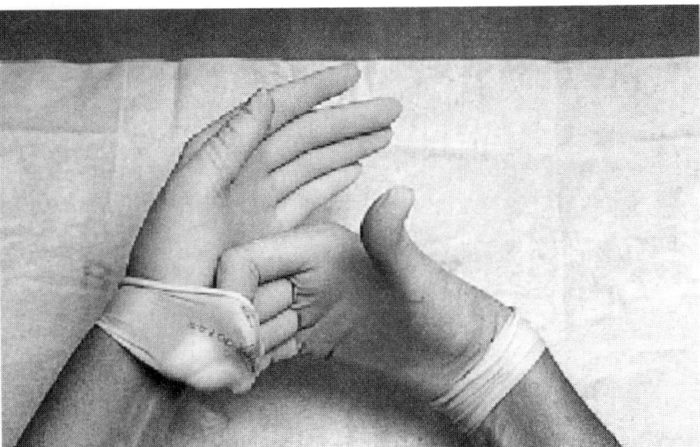

Fig. 18-4 Insert the nondominant hand. (From Perry AG, Potter PA: *Clinical nursing skills and techniques,* ed 3, St Louis, 1994, Mosby.)

Continued.

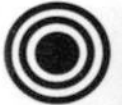

SKILL 18-1 PERFORMING STERILE GLOVE TECHNIQUE (OPEN GLOVING)—cont'd

Steps	Rationale

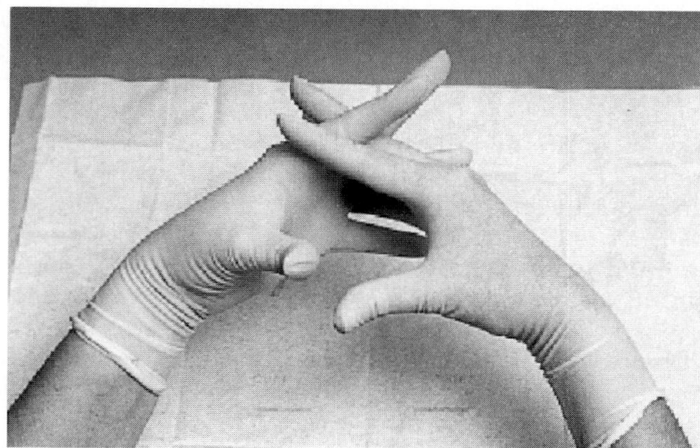

Fig. 18-5 Adjust the fit of the gloves. (From Perry AG, Potter PA: *Clinical nursing skills and techniques,* ed 3, St Louis, 1994, Mosby.)

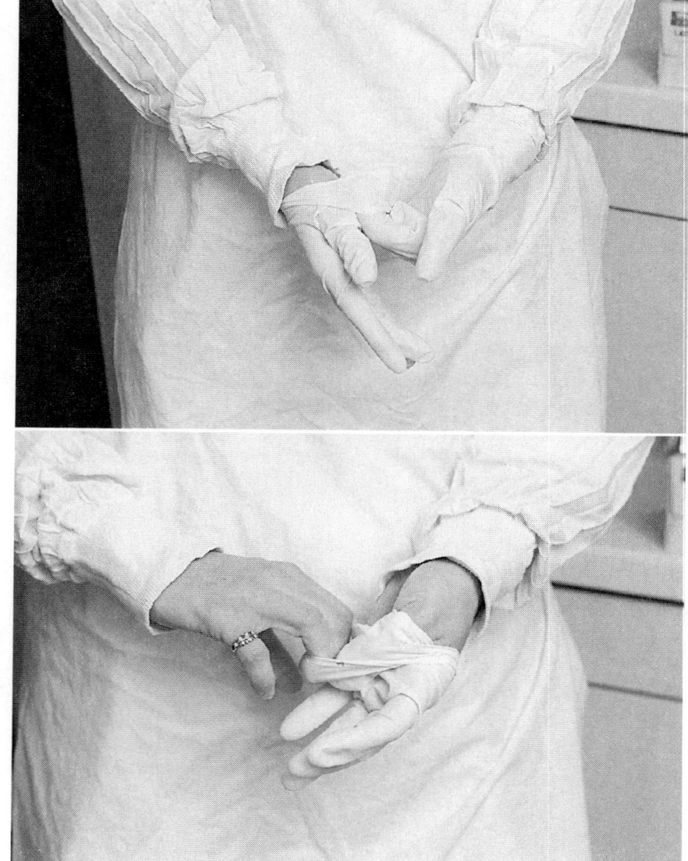

Fig. 18-6 Removing gloves. **A,** Nurse places gloved finger inside cuff to pull first glove off hand. **B,** Second glove is removed as nurse slides finger inside glove cuff and pulls.

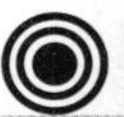

SKILL 18-2 PERFORMING STERILE DRESSING CHANGE

Steps	Rationale
1. Obtain equipment: ▪ Clean gloves ▪ Sterile gloves ▪ Refuse container ▪ Dressing set ▪ Antiseptic swabs ▪ Ointment, if ordered ▪ 4×4 gauze squares ▪ Nonadherent dressing ▪ Fluff or loose gauze ▪ Abdominal pads ▪ Barrier drape (optional) ▪ Sterile waterproof drape ▪ Tape, Montgomery straps, or binder ▪ Biohazard bag	Helps organize procedure.
2. Refer to medical record, care plan or Kardex for special interventions.	Provides basis for care.
3. Introduce self.	Decreases anxiety level.
4. Identify patient by identification band.	Identifies correct patient for procedure.
5. Explain procedure to patient.	Seeks cooperation and decreases anxiety.
6. Wash hands and don clean gloves according to agency policy and guidelines from Centers for Disease Control and Prevention and Occupational Safety and Health Administration.	Helps prevent cross-contamination.
7. Prepare patient for intervention:	
a. Close door to room or pull curtain.	Provides privacy.
b. Drape for procedure if necessary.	Prevents exposure of patient.
8. Raise bed to comfortable working level.	Provides safety for nurse.
9. Arrange for patient privacy.	Shows respect for patient.
10. Place refuse container in convenient location away from sterile field.	Avoids reaching across sterile field to prevent contamination.
11. Set up sterile field (Fig. 18-7): a. Open sterile dressing. b. Use barrier drape if needed. c. Open sterile gloves. d. Open dressing set, if needed. e. Provide antiseptic swabs.	Maintains asepsis during procedure and organizes approach to procedure.
12. Loosen tape by pulling toward incision and gently pulling skin away from tape.	Minimizes tissue trauma and decreases patient discomfort.
13. Remove dressing and discard. (Biohazard refuse bag should be used for additional soiled material.)	Protects nurse from contamination.
14. Assess status of wound and wound drainage on dressing.	Evaluates healing process and collects data for accurate documentation.
15. Wash hands and don sterile gloves.	Maintains surgical asepsis.

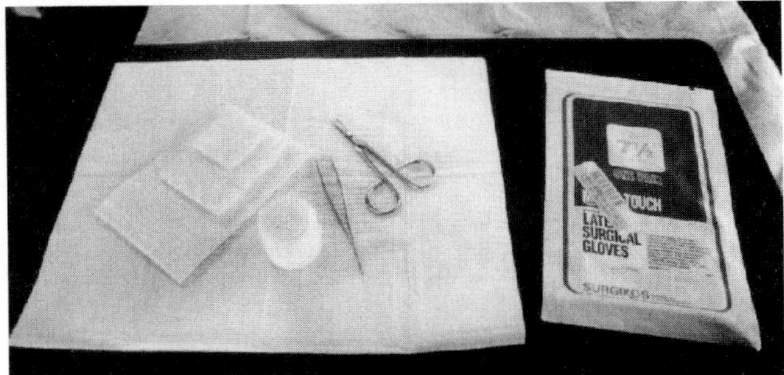

Fig. 18-7 Supplies for a sterile dressing change. (From Perry AG, Potter PA: *Clinical nursing skills and techniques,* ed 3, St Louis, 1994, Mosby.)

Continued.

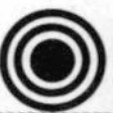

SKILL 18-2 PERFORMING STERILE DRESSING CHANGE—cont'd

Steps	Rationale
16. Cleanse wound and surrounding area with antiseptic swab, starting from incision outward, one stroke per swab (Fig. 18-8).	Removes bacteria from wound area.
17. Cleanse drain site if applicable (Fig. 18-9).	
18. Apply ointment (for example, antibiotic, debridement granules) if applicable.	Reduces infection or debrides wound.
19. Cover wound with appropriately sized dry sterile dressing and use drain dressing if applicable.	Protects wound and skin around drain site.
20. Secure dressing with tape, Montgomery straps, or binder (Fig. 18-10).	Keeps dressing secure.
21. Remove sterile gloves appropriately and don clean gloves.	Decreases possibility of cross-contamination.
22. Discard refuse in biohazard bag.	Avoids spread of microorganisms.
23. Reposition patient.	Provides patient comfort.
24. Remove gloves and wash hands.	Helps prevent cross-contamination.
25. Document.	Documents procedure and patient's response.

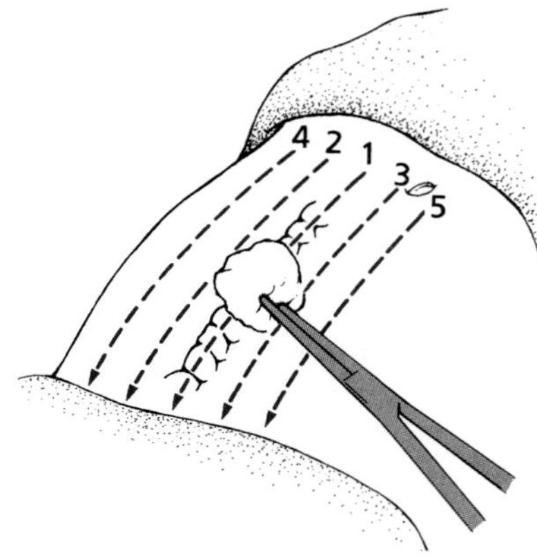

Fig. 18-8 Cleansing the wound and the surrounding area. (From Perry AG, Potter PA: *Clinical nursing skills and techniques,* ed 3, St Louis, 1994, Mosby.)

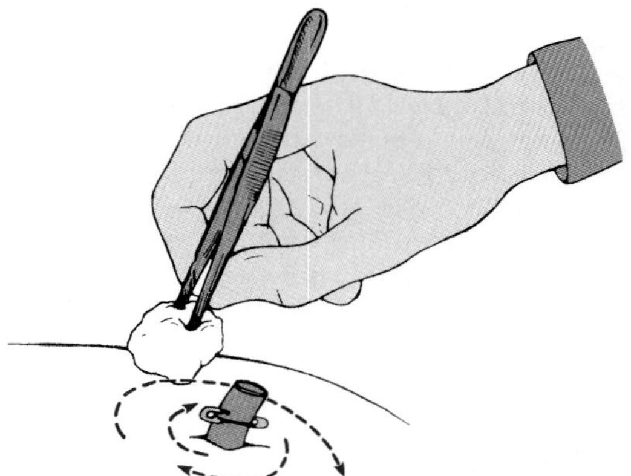

Fig. 18-9 Cleansing the drain site. (From Perry AG, Potter PA: *Clinical nursing skills and techniques,* ed 3, St Louis, 1994, Mosby.)

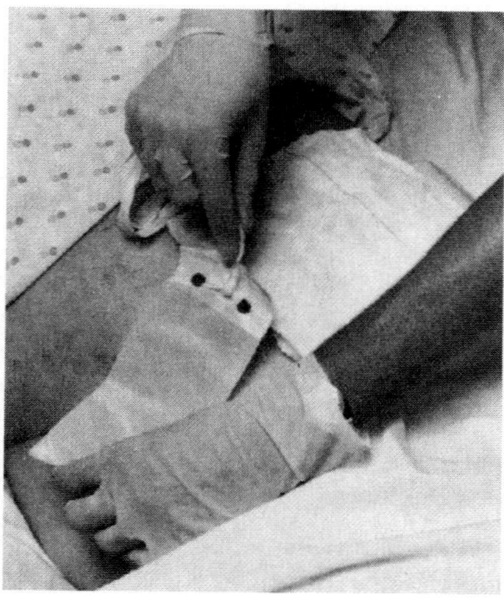

Fig. 18-10 Applying Montgomery straps. (From Perry AG, Potter PA: *Clinical nursing skills and techniques,* ed 3, St Louis, 1994, Mosby.)

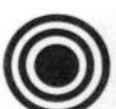

SKILL 18-3 OBTAINING A STERILE WOUND CULTURE

Steps	Rationale
1. Obtain equipment: ▪ Culture tube and kit ▪ Refuse container ▪ Clean gloves ▪ Sterile gloves ▪ Dressing set (optional) ▪ Antiseptic swabs ▪ 4×4 gauze squares ▪ Telfa ▪ Fluff or loose gauze ▪ Abdominal pads ▪ Barrier drape (optional) ▪ Tape or roller gauze ▪ Elastic bandage	Helps organize procedure.
2. Refer to medical record, care plan, or Kardex for special interventions.	Provides basis for care.
3. Introduce self.	Decreases patient's anxiety level.
4. Identify patient by identification band.	Identifies correct patient for procedure.
5. Explain procedure to patient.	Seeks cooperation and decreases anxiety.
6. Wash hands and don clean gloves according to agency policy and guidelines from Centers for Disease Control and Prevention and Occupational Safety and Health Administration.	Helps prevent cross-contamination.
7. Prepare patient for intervention:	
a. Close door to room or pull curtain.	Provides privacy.
b. Drape for procedure if necessary.	Prevents exposure of patient.
8. Raise bed to comfortable working level.	Provides safety for nurse.
9. Arrange for patient privacy.	Shows respect for patient.
10. Position patient.	Ensures patient comfort and provides exposure of wound.
11. Place refuse container in convenient location away from sterile field.	Avoids reaching across sterile field and prevents contamination.
12. Set up sterile field: ▪ Open sterile dressing ▪ Use barrier drape, if needed ▪ Open sterile gloves ▪ Place antiseptic swabs ▪ Prepare wound culture tube and kit	Maintains asepsis during procedure and organizes approach to procedure.
13. Loosen dressing tape by pulling toward incision and, using thumb, gently pulling skin away from tape (using counter traction).	Minimizes tissue trauma and decreases patient discomfort.
14. Using clean gloves, remove dressing, and discard into refuse bag. (Refuse bag may be used for additional soiled material.)	Protects nurse from microorganisms and prevents contamination from soiled dressing.
15. Assess status of wound and wound drainage on dressing.	Determines healing status of wound and collects data for accurate documentation.
16. Wash hands and don sterile gloves.	Maintains surgical asepsis.
17. Cleanse wound and surrounding area with antiseptic swab and discard.	Removes old drainage and reduces risk of contaminating specimen with skin bacteria.
18. Remove sterile culture swab from culture tube and gently insert into drainage or into wound itself.	Culture specimen should be taken from fresh drainage.
19. Remove swab from wound and insert into sterile culture tube.	Prevents specimen contamination.
20. Crush ampule of culture medium at bottom of tube and push swab into fluid (Fig. 18-11).	Allows bacteria to thrive during transport to laboratory.
21. Put cap or lid on culture tube tightly.	Ensures that culture is not contaminated.

Continued.

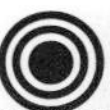

SKILL 18-3 OBTAINING A STERILE WOUND CULTURE—cont'd

Steps	Rationale
22. Cleanse wound with antiseptic swab and apply sterile dressing.	Protects wound and absorbs drainage.
23. Remove sterile gloves appropriately and don clean gloves.	Decreases possibility of cross-contamination.
24. Discard refuse appropriately.	Avoids spread of microorganisms.
25. Label culture specimen with exact location of culture source and send promptly to laboratory with requisition.	Helps laboratory to determine type of media to use for growth of microorganisms.
26. Remove gloves and wash hands.	Helps prevent cross-contamination.
27. Document.	Documents procedure and patient's response.

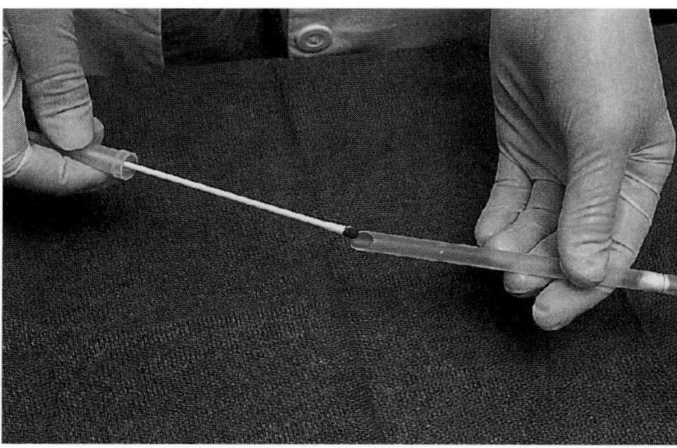

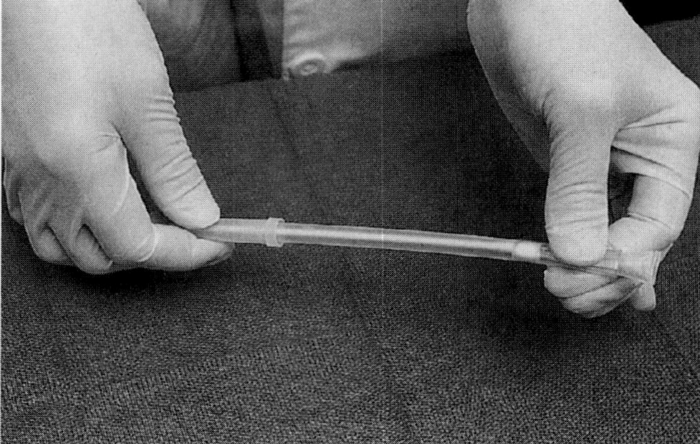

Fig. 18-11 Crush the ampule in a sterile culture tube. (From Perry AG, Potter PA: *Clinical nursing skills and techniques,* ed 3, St Louis, 1993, Mosby.)

SKILL 18-4 APPLYING A WET-TO-DRY DRESSING

Steps	Rationale
1. Obtain equipment: ▪ Open barrier drape ▪ Sterile dressing ▪ Gauze ▪ Sterile basin ▪ Sterile solution ▪ Antiseptic swabs ▪ Instrument set, if needed ▪ Clean gloves ▪ Sterile gloves ▪ Refuse container ▪ Tape or Montgomery straps ▪ Waterproof pad	Helps organize procedure.
2. Refer to medical record, care plan, or Kardex for special interventions.	Provides basis for care.
3. Introduce self.	Decreases patient's anxiety level.
4. Identify patient by identification band.	Identifies correct patient for procedure.
5. Explain procedure to patient.	Seeks cooperation and decreases anxiety.

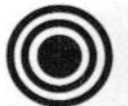

SKILL 18-4 APPLYING A WET-TO-DRY DRESSING—cont'd

Steps	Rationale
6. Wash hands and don clean gloves according to agency policy and guidelines from Centers for Disease Control and Prevention and Occupational Safety and Health Administration.	Helps prevent cross-contamination.
7. Prepare patient for intervention:	
a. Close door to room or pull curtain.	Provides privacy.
b. Drape for procedure if necessary.	Prevents exposure of patient.
8. Raise bed to comfortable working level.	Provides safety for nurse.
9. Arrange for patient privacy.	Shows respect for patient.
10. Position patient.	Ensures patient comfort and provides exposure of wound.
11. Place waterproof pad appropriately.	Prevents soiling of clothes or linens.
12. Place refuse container appropriately.	Avoids reaching across sterile field and thus prevents contamination.
13. Set up sterile field: a. Open barrier drape. b. Add sterile dressing and gauze. c. Add sterile basin. d. Pour sterile solution into basin. e. Add instrument set, if needed. f. Add antiseptic swabs.	Maintains asepsis during procedure and organizes approach to procedure.
14. Loosen tape by pulling toward incision and, using thumb, gently pulling skin away from tape (countertraction).	Minimizes tissue trauma and decreases patient discomfort.
15. Don clean gloves. Remove dressing and discard it into refuse bag. (Refuse bag may be used for additional soiled material.)	Protects nurse from microorganisms and prevents contamination from soiled dressing.
16. Assess status of wound and wound drainage on dressing.	Evaluates healing process and collects data for accurate documentation.
17. Wash hands and don sterile gloves.	Maintains surgical asepsis.
18. Cleanse wound from incision outward, one stroke per swab, and discard.	Removes old drainage and bacteria from skin area.
19. Place gauze into basin.	Wets gauze with solution.
20. Wring excess solution from dressing, leaving it slightly moist.	Prevents growth of bacteria from dressing that is too wet.
21. Place gauze over open wound surfaces and press into depressed areas (Fig. 18-12).	Allows solution to come into contact with wound, which makes it effective.

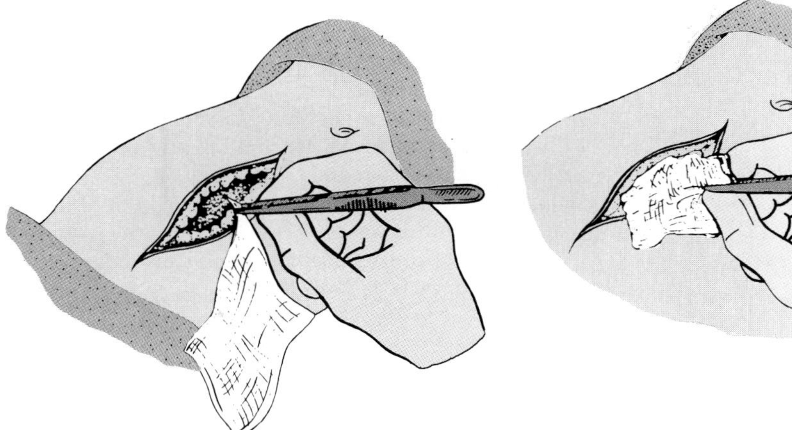

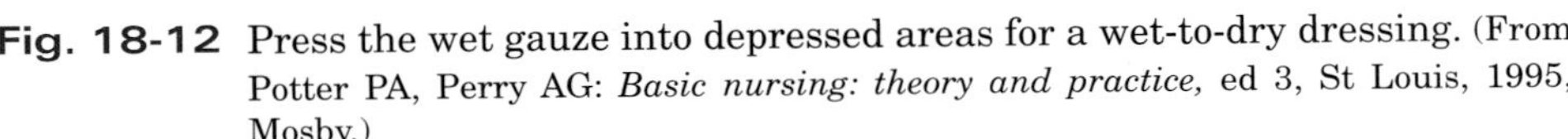

Fig. 18-12 Press the wet gauze into depressed areas for a wet-to-dry dressing. (From Potter PA, Perry AG: *Basic nursing: theory and practice,* ed 3, St Louis, 1995, Mosby.)

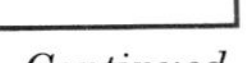

Continued.

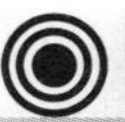

SKILL 18-4 APPLYING A WET-TO-DRY DRESSING—cont'd

Steps	Rationale
22. Apply dry dressing over wet gauze.	Allows for absorption of excess moisture.
23. Cover with additional dressing as needed.	Protects wound from bacteria.
24. Secure with tape or Montgomery straps.	Holds dressings in place.
25. Remove sterile gloves and don clean gloves.	Decreases contamination.
26. Reposition patient.	Provides patient comfort.
27. Discard refuse appropriately.	Avoids spread of microorganisms.
28. Remove gloves and wash hands.	Helps prevent cross-contamination.
29. Document.	Documents procedure and patient's response.

SKILL 18-5 APPLYING A STERILE COMPRESS

Steps	Rationale
1. Obtain equipment: ▪ Refuse container ▪ Clean gloves (2 pairs) ▪ Sterile gloves (2 pairs) ▪ Dressing set ▪ Antiseptic swabs ▪ Sterile basin ▪ Warmed sterile solution (100° to 115° F) ▪ Barrier drape ▪ Sterile gauze ▪ Appropriate dressings ▪ Appropriate tape/gauze	Helps organize procedure.
2. Refer to medical record, care plan, or Kardex for special interventions.	Provides basis for care.
3. Introduce self.	Decreases patient's anxiety level.
4. Identify patient by identification band.	Identifies correct patient for procedure.
5. Explain procedure to patient.	Seeks cooperation and decreases anxiety.
6. Wash hands and don clean gloves according to agency policy and guidelines from Centers for Disease Control and Prevention and Occupational Safety and Health Administration.	Helps prevent cross-contamination.
7. Prepare patient for intervention:	
a. Close door to room or pull curtain.	Provides privacy.
b. Drape for procedure if necessary.	Prevents exposure of patient.
8. Raise bed to comfortable working level.	Provides safety for nurse.
9. Arrange for patient privacy.	Shows respect for patient.
10. Position patient.	Ensures patient comfort and provides adequate exposure of wound.
11. Place refuse container in convenient location away from sterile field.	Avoids reaching across sterile field and prevents contamination.
12. Set up sterile field: ▪ Add sterile basin. ▪ Add sterile warmed solution to basin. ▪ Add gauze for compresses to solution in basin. ▪ Open sterile gloves. ▪ Open dressing set (optional). ▪ Place antiseptic swabs.	Maintains asepsis during procedure and organizes approach to procedure.
13. Remove outer tape gently.	Minimizes tissue trauma.
14. Remove dressing and discard in refuse container.	Protects nurse from microorganisms and prevents contamination from soiled dressing.

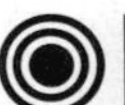

SKILL 18-5 APPLYING A STERILE COMPRESS—cont'd

Steps	Rationale
15. Assess status of wound and wound drainage on dressing.	Evaluates healing process and collects data for accurate documentation.
16. Wash hands and don sterile gloves.	Maintains surgical asepsis.
17. Cleanse wound and surrounding area with antiseptic swab following principles of asepsis.	Removes old drainage and bacteria from wound area.
18. Wring out solution-soaked gauze and apply to total wound area.	Prevents excess moisture from altering tissue integrity and allows all wound surfaces to be exposed to compress.
19. Cover compress with sterile drape.	Retains heat and moisture and prevents transfer of microorganisms into wound.
20. Apply aquathermic device (for example, waterproof heating pad or hot water bag) over drape for 20 to 30 min.	Maintains desired warmth during treatment.
21. Monitor patient frequently during procedure and inspect site.	Avoids burns and tissue trauma.
22. Remove gloves and discard soiled dressings.	Decreases contamination.
23. Reposition patient.	Provides patient comfort.
24. Remove compress in 30 min, or as ordered, using clean gloves. Discard appropriately.	Maintains therapeutic effect of heat application.
25. Assess wound and surrounding skin.	Notes effects of compress application.
26. Don sterile gloves.	Maintains asepsis.
27. Redress wound, if applicable, following sterile dressing-change procedure.	Protects wound from injury and microorganisms, promotes wound healing, and provides for patient comfort.
28. Remove gloves and wash hands.	Helps prevent cross-contamination.
29. Document.	Documents procedure and patient's response.

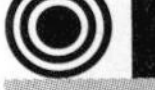

SKILL 18-6 PERFORMING STERILE IRRIGATION

Steps	Rationale
1. Obtain equipment: ▪ Refuse container ▪ Clean gloves ▪ Sterile gloves ▪ Dressing set ▪ Antiseptic swabs ▪ Sterile basin ▪ Warmed sterile irrigation solution (200-1000 ml) ▪ Irrigation syringe or soft catheter for deep wounds ▪ Clean basin ▪ Waterproof pad ▪ Sterile dressings ▪ Gown and goggles, if needed ▪ Tape, gauze, and elastic bandage, if appropriate ▪ Mask, if needed	Helps organize procedure.
2. Refer to medical record, care plan, or Kardex for special interventions.	Provides basis for care.
3. Introduce self.	Decreases anxiety level.
4. Identify patient by identification band.	Identifies correct patient for procedure.
5. Explain procedure to patient.	Seeks cooperation and decreases anxiety.

Continued.

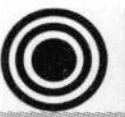

SKILL 18-6 PERFORMING STERILE IRRIGATION—cont'd

Steps	Rationale
6. Wash hands and don clean gloves according to agency policy and guidelines from Centers for Disease Control and Prevention and Occupational Safety and Health Administration.	Helps prevent cross-contamination.
7. Prepare patient for intervention:	
a. Close door to room or pull curtain.	Provides privacy.
b. Drape for procedure if necessary.	Prevents exposure of patient.
8. Raise bed to comfortable working level.	Provides safety for nurse.
9. Arrange patient privacy.	Shows respect for patient.
10. Position patient and waterproof pad appropriately (Fig. 18-13).	Ensures patient comfort and provides adequate exposure of wound. Protects patient and bed linens from contaminated fluid.
11. Place refuse container in convenient location away from sterile field.	Prevents reaching across sterile field and prevents contamination.
12. Set up sterile field: ▪ Set up sterile basin. ▪ Add sterile warmed irrigation solution to basin. ▪ Add antiseptic swabs. ▪ Open sterile gloves. ▪ Add dressing set (optional). ▪ Add sterile syringe and catheter if necessary.	Maintains asepsis during procedure and organizes approach to procedure.
13. Don gown and goggles if appropriate.	Protects nurse if splashing is anticipated.
14. Don clean gloves and remove dressing. Discard dressing in refuse container.	Protects nurse from pathogens and prevents contamination from soiled dressing.
15. Remove gloves and wash hands.	Helps prevent cross-contamination.
16. Assess status of wound and wound drainage on dressing.	Evaluates healing process and collects data for accurate documentation.
17. Place collection basin appropriately.	Collects contaminated solution.
18. Wash hands and don sterile gloves.	Maintains asepsis.
19. Cleanse area around wound with antiseptic swabs.	Removes bacteria and drainage.
20. Fill irrigating syringe with solution. Attach soft catheter if irrigating a deep wound with small opening.	Allows for direct flow of solution into wound.
21. Instill solution gently into wound, holding syringe approximately 1 inch above wound. If using catheter, gently insert into wound opening until slight resistance is met, pull back, and gently instill solution.	Minimizes tissue trauma, irritation, and bleeding.

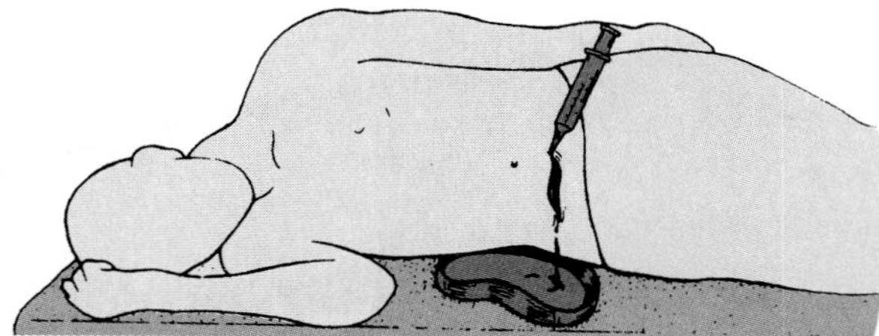

Fig. 18-13 Position the patient and waterproof pad. The solution for sterile irrigation from the syringe flows from a clean to a dirty area. (From Perry AG, Potter PA: *Clinical nursing skills and techniques,* ed 3, St Louis, 1994, Mosby.)

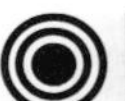

SKILL 18-6 PERFORMING STERILE IRRIGATION—cont'd

Steps	Rationale
22. Allow solution to flow from clean area of wound to dirty area.	Prevents contamination of clean tissue by drainage.
23. Pinch off catheter during withdrawal from wound.	Avoids aspiration of contaminating fluid into syringe.
24. Refill syringe and continue irrigation until solution returns clear.	Thoroughly cleanses wound.
25. Blot wound edges with sterile gauze.	Prevents tissue breakdown from excess moisture.
26. Redress wound, if applicable.	Protects wound from injury and microorganisms and provides for patient comfort.
27. Remove sterile gloves and don clean gloves.	Decreases possibility of cross-contamination.
28. Discard soiled material and contaminated solution appropriately.	Avoids spread of bacteria.
29. Reposition patient.	Provides patient comfort.
30. Remove gloves and wash hands.	Helps prevent cross-contamination.
31. Document.	Documents procedure and patient's response.

SKILL 18-7 REMOVING SUTURES OR STAPLES

Steps	Rationale
1. Obtain equipment: ▪ Refuse container ▪ Clean gloves ▪ Sterile gloves ▪ Sterile suture and staple-removal set ▪ Antiseptic swabs ▪ Appropriate sterile dressings	Helps organize procedure.
2. Refer to medical record, care plan, or Kardex for special interventions.	Provides basis for care.
3. Introduce self.	Decreases patient's anxiety level.
4. Identify patient by identification band.	Identifies correct patient for procedure.
5. Explain procedure to patient.	Seeks cooperation and decreases anxiety.
6. Wash hands and don clean gloves according to agency policy and guidelines from Centers for Disease Control and Prevention and Occupational Safety and Health Administration.	Helps prevent cross-contamination.
7. Prepare patient for intervention:	
a. Close door to room or pull curtain.	Provides privacy.
b. Drape for procedure if necessary.	Prevents exposure of patient.
8. Raise bed to comfortable working level.	Provides safety for nurse.
9. Arrange for patient privacy.	Shows respect for patient.
10. Position patient.	Ensures patient comfort and provides exposure of wound.
11. Place refuse container in convenient location away from sterile field.	Avoids reaching across sterile field and prevents contamination.
12. Set up sterile field: a. Open suture and staple set. b. Open sterile dressings (use sterile barrier if necessary for sterile field).	Maintains asepsis during procedure and organizes approach to procedure.
13. Remove dressing. Discard into plastic refuse bag. (Bag may then be used for additional refuse.)	Protects nurse from microorganisms and prevents contamination from soiled dressing.
14. Assess status of wound and drainage on dressing.	Determines alterations in healing process and collects data for accurate documentation.

Continued.

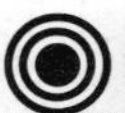

SKILL 18-7 REMOVING SUTURES OR STAPLES—cont'd

Steps	Rationale
15. Wash hands and don sterile gloves.	Maintains surgical asepsis.
16. Cleanse area with antiseptic swab, starting from incision outward, one stroke per swab.	Removes bacteria from wound area.
REMOVAL OF INTERRUPTED SUTURES (Fig. 18-14)	
17. Grasp and elevate knotted end of suture with hemostat or forceps (Fig. 18-15).	Ensures correct suture removal and maintains skin integrity.
18. Cut suture at skin level on opposite side, distal to knot.	Avoids pulling exposed contaminated suture through skin.
19. Gently remove entire suture with forceps and discard on sterile gauze (Fig. 18-16).	Reduces tension on suture line, reduces patient discomfort, and maintains asepsis.
20. Repeat steps 17-19 until all sutures have been removed.	Ensures removal of all sutures.
REMOVAL OF CONTINUOUS SUTURES (see Fig. 18-14)	
21. Cut first suture close to skin on side away from knot.	Ensures correct suture removal and maintains skin integrity.
22. Remove gently from knotted side with forceps and discard on sterile gauze.	Begins count of sutures.
23. Cut second suture on same side (away from knot).	Ensures correct suture removal.
24. Repeat steps 21-23 until all sutures have been removed.	Ensures removal of all sutures to prevent abscess from suture left.
STAPLE REMOVAL	
25. Place staple remover under both sides of staple; squeeze handles together and gently remove staple from skin (Fig. 18-17).	Ensures correct staple removal and maintains skin integrity.
26. Release handles and discard staple in refuse container.	Avoids wound contamination.
27. Repeat steps 25-26 until all staples have been removed.	Ensures complete removal of all staples.
28. Count number of staples removed.	Ensures count for documentation.
29. Assess healing status of wound.	Determines need for butterfly or Steri-strip skin closures.
30. Cleanse area with antiseptic swabs.	Decreases possibility for infection.

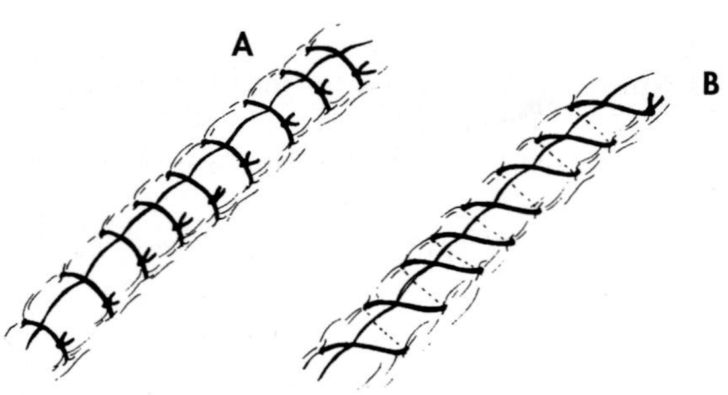

Fig. 18-14 Examples of suturing methods. **A,** Interrupted. **B,** Continuous. (From Perry AG, Potter PA: *Clinical nursing skills and techniques,* ed 3, St Louis, 1994, Mosby.)

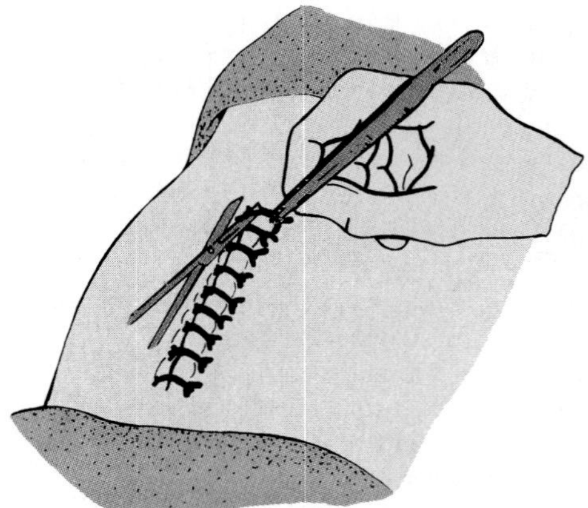

Fig. 18-15 Grasp knot of suture. (From Potter PA, Perry AG: *Basic nursing: theory and practice,* ed 3, St Louis, 1995, Mosby.)

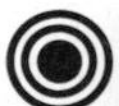

SKILL 18-7 REMOVING SUTURES OR STAPLES—cont'd

Steps	Rationale
31. Apply sterile dressing or leave open to air as applicable. (Dressing may not be needed unless patient's clothing will irritate wound area.)	Protects wound and facilitates healing process.
32. Remove gloves and wash hands.	Helps prevent cross-contamination.
33. Document.	Documents procedure and patient's response.

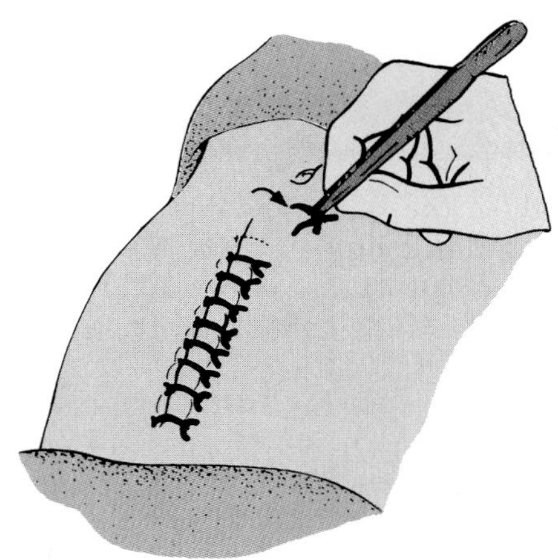

Fig. 18-16 Remove entire suture. (From Potter PA, Perry AG: *Basic nursing: theory and practice,* ed 3, St Louis, 1995, Mosby.)

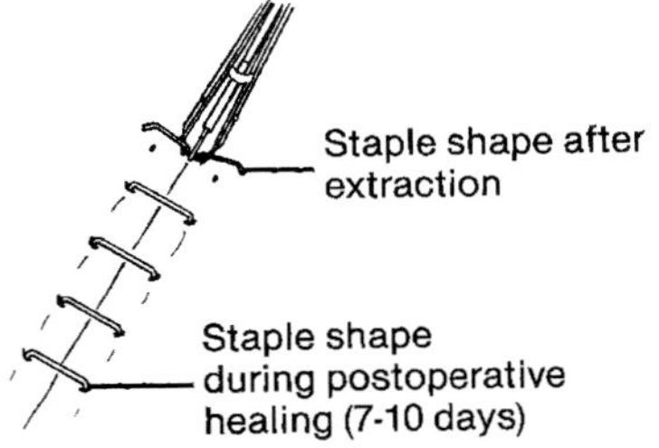

Fig. 18-17 Remove staple. (From Perry AG, Potter PA: *Clinical nursing skills and techniques,* ed 3, St Louis, 1994, Mosby.)

SUMMARY

The nurse should be aware of the stages of the healing process to effectively assess wounds. Wound care involves providing care for the clean surgical wound and the contaminated wound. Prevention of infection is the key to wound care. Wound healing is dependent upon many factors, including nutritional status, age, and circulation. The nurse should recognize the patient who is at risk for complications of wound healing and assess the patient's wound frequently. The nurse should also know the principles of sterile technique and apply them when caring for a patient with an open wound.

Key Concepts

- Wounds are described as open or closed. Care of the open wound is determined by the extent of the wound.
- Wounds heal by primary or secondary intention. The greater the size of the wound, the longer and more extensive the healing process.
- It is essential to maintain sterile technique when providing care for an open wound. Any item coming in contact with an open wound should be sterile.
- Signs of wound infection include redness; tenderness; pain; swelling; yellow, green, or white thick drainage; and heat to touch.
- When a wound contains foreign matter, the surgeon usually debrides it. The chance for infection is greater if the wound is contaminated or contains rocks, glass, dirt, or other foreign matter.
- Dressings are applied to wounds to medicate or protect the wound, absorb drainage, apply pressure, or help debride or provide a better medium to encourage healing.
- Careful assessment of wounds is essential to

evaluate wound healing and the presence of infection or other complications, such as dehiscence or evisceration.

- Dressings should be removed gently to prevent further injury to the wound. Used dressings need to be discarded appropriately to prevent cross-contamination.
- Cultures are obtained to determine whether the wound is infected and, if so, what type of microorganism it is. A sensitivity test may also be performed to determine which antibacterial medication to administer.
- Wound care involves assessment of the wound and surrounding area, cleansing of the wound, and changing of the dressing. Care may also include irrigating the wound or removing sutures or staples.

Critical Thinking Questions

1. You have just admitted a patient from a nursing home to the nurse's division. On initial assessment, the nurse assesses a stage II pressure ulcer. How does the nurse determine the type of care and dressing to use with this particular pressure ulcer?
2. Explain the correct first aid procedures for an abrasion, laceration, and puncture wound. Include application of dressing, if appropriate.
3. The nurse's patient has a 3-cm left trochanteric ulcer, full thickness, as evidenced by necrotic slough in the base. The edges of the ulcer are smooth and rounded with the necrotic tissue lifting. What method of wound cleansing would be best suited to this situation with a bedfast patient?
4. There is an order to cleanse a lower abdominal wound with normal saline with each dressing change. On inspection, the nurse identifies a 1-cm wound with a depth of 4.5 cm. The nurse is unable to visualize the base. What steps should you take in caring for this patient?

REFERENCES AND SUGGESTED READINGS

Bryant RA: *Acute and chronic wounds: nursing management,* St Louis, 1992, Mosby.

Harkness GH, Dincher JR: *Medical-surgical nursing: total patient care,* ed 9, St Louis, 1996, Mosby.

Lewis LW, Timby BK: *Fundamental skills and concepts in patient care,* ed 5, New York, 1992, Lippincott.

Moncada GA: The healing wound: clinical management, *Plastic Surgical Nursing* 12(2):56, 1992.

Potter PA, Perry AG: *Fundamentals of nursing: concepts, process, and practice,* ed 3, St Louis, 1993, Mosby.

Ryan TJ: Wound dressing, *Dermatologic Clinics* 11(1): 207, 1993.

CHAPTER 19

Gastrointestinal Intubation

Learning Objectives

After studying this chapter, the student should be able to . . .

- Define the key terms.
- Identify the guidelines used in gastrointestinal intubation.
- Explain the importance of assessing a patient's knowledge of intubation.
- Explain the purposes of intubation.
- Insert and remove a nasogastric tube.
- Perform a gastric gavage.
- Perform irrigation of the stomach.
- Monitor and maintain gastrointestinal suctioning.
- Explain nursing care for a patient with a gastrostomy tube.

Key Terms

Aspiration	Gastrostomy
Bolus	Gavage
Compression	Jejunostomy
Decompression	Lavage
Distention	Nasogastric (NG) intubation
Dysphagia	Peristalsis
Enteral feeding	
French (Fr)	

Skills

19-1 Performing nasogastric tube insertion and tube feeding
19-2 Performing gastrostomy and jejunostomy tube care
19-3 Performing gastric lavage or irrigation
19-4 Performing gastric suctioning
19-5 Removing a nasogastric tube

Frequently, patients who are acutely ill may require alternative ways of feeding to maintain appropriate nutrition or may require removal of the contents of the stomach or intestine. Many conditions may affect the function of the gastrointestinal (GI) tract. Some cerebral disorders, inadequate food intake, impaired or loss of motility of the intestinal tract, and impaired mucosal integrity may indicate use for intubation of the GI system. **Nasogastric (NG) intubation** is the insertion of a tube into the stomach or intestine. Intubation is accomplished with various types of tubes. The type of tube chosen depends on the purpose of intubation (Table 19-1).

Intubation is performed for many reasons such as **gavage** (feedings through an NG tube), **lavage** (washing out or irrigation), gastric analysis (analyzing the stomach's contents), **compression** (applying internal pressure), **decompression** (removal of liquid or gas), and administration of medication. Single-lumen tubes such as the Levin tube (Fig. 19-1, *A*) or the small-bore feeding tube (approximately 3 feet long) are often chosen for gavage. A double-lumen tube such as the Salem sump (Fig. 19-1, *B*) may be chosen for continuous gastric suctioning. The Salem tube's blue secondary tube acts as a vent to prevent adherence to the gastric mucosa during suction through the clear primary lumen. This enables the tube to remain patent and decreases trauma to the mucosa. The blue tail must remain open to ensure

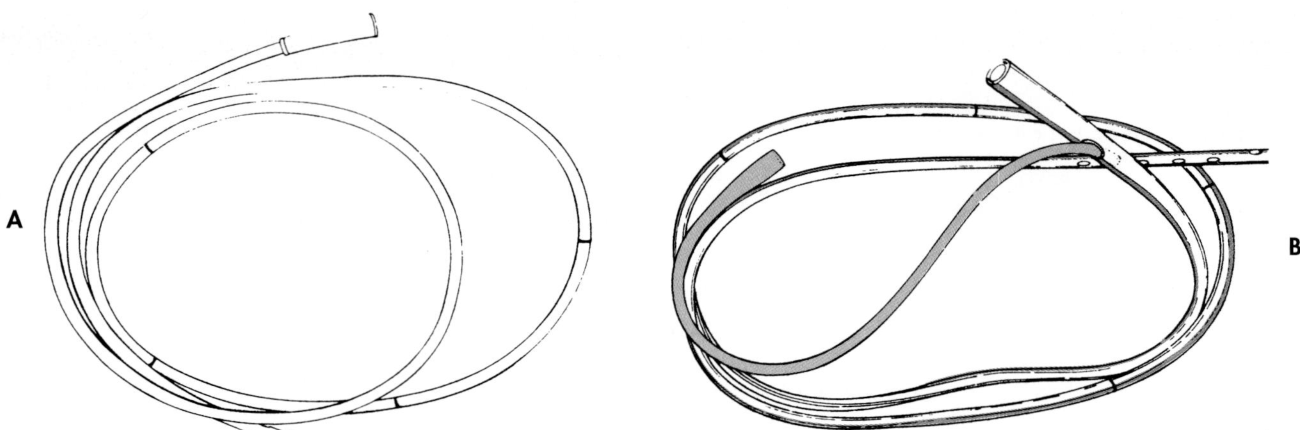

Fig. 19-1 NG tubes. **A,** Levin tubes. **B,** Salem sump tube. (From Christensen BL, Kockrow EO: *Foundations of nursing,* ed 2, St Louis, 1995, Mosby.)

Table 19-1 NASOGASTRIC AND INTESTINAL TUBES

Tube	Purpose	Characteristic	Use
Nasogastric tubes			
Levin	Removal of fluid and gas from stomach (decompression) and tube feedings	Has single lumen; is easy to maintain; may cause trauma to stomach wall	Use intermittent suction at low-pressure setting.
Salem sump	Same purpose as Levin tube (more commonly used)	Has double lumen, one to provide drainage and one to provide air vent to prevent tube adherence to stomach wall	Use low (30 mm Hg) *constant* suction. Attach larger lumen of tube only to suction.
Entron	Tube feedings for gastric feedings only	Is no. 6 Fr (small bore); has stylet for easier insertion but no weighted end	Clamp off when not in use. Do not attach to suction (collapses).
Dobbhoff enteric	Tube feedings for gastric or intestinal feedings	Is No. 8 Fr (small bore), has stylet for easier insertion and weighted end to pass into intestines	Use same techniques as for Entron tube.
Intestinal tubes			
Miller-Abbott	Removal of fluid and gas from intestines (decompression)	Has double lumen, one for balloon inflation and one for drainage	Use low-pressure, intermittent suction. Clamp off balloon tube and attach drainage tube only to suction.
Cantor	Same purposes as Miller-Abbott tube (less frequently used)	Has single lumen; allows mercury to be injected into balloon with needle and syringe before insertion	Use low-pressure, intermittent suction.

From Long BC, Phipps WJ, Cassmeyer VL: *Medical-surgical nursing: a nursing process approach,* ed 3, St Louis, 1993, Mosby.

appropriate function. The air vent is never clamped, attached to suction, or used as an irrigation lumen.

The term **French (Fr)** is used to denote the size of the lumen of the tube. A 12-Fr tube is smaller than a 14-Fr tube.

NURSING PROCESS

Assessment

Intubation is an invasive procedure that requires a medical order. The nurse should read the medical

PATIENT TEACHING

- Explain the purpose of a tube in supplementing nutrition.
- Explain how the decompression tube will prevent nausea, vomiting, and abdominal distention.
- Teach patient and family how to care for the NG tube at home.
- Discuss the need to maintain moist mucous membranes with special mouth care.

order for details of specific actions to be taken during the procedure and ways that they are to be performed. The patient's knowledge of the procedure and its purpose should be assessed. Baseline data regarding the condition of the oral mucous membrane and the patient's abdomen should be collected. Evaluation of bowel sounds and the degree of abdominal **distention** (swelling) enables the nurse to compare the patient's condition before and after insertion of the tube. Noting the baseline condition of the mucous membrane prepares the nurse for follow-up oral care during tube use. If the membrane is already impaired, it will be necessary to perform frequent mouth care to prevent further breakdown of the tissue, since the patient usually has nothing by mouth during tube use.

Nursing Diagnosis

The nurse reviews data gathered during assessment and clusters defining characteristics to reveal a diagnosis. Possible nursing diagnoses include the following:

Altered nutrition: less than body requirements
Altered oral mucous membranes
Anxiety
Fear
Fluid volume deficit
Impaired swallowing
Risk for fluid volume deficit

Planning

The plan of care should focus on the types or methods of care and on the many care measures that the nurse can perform. The nurse can assess the patient's readiness to learn and teach health promotion (see teaching box).

The following goal may be included in the plan of care:

Goal: Patient's skin around feeding tube remains clean, so integrity is maintained.

Outcome

Patient's skin is intact.

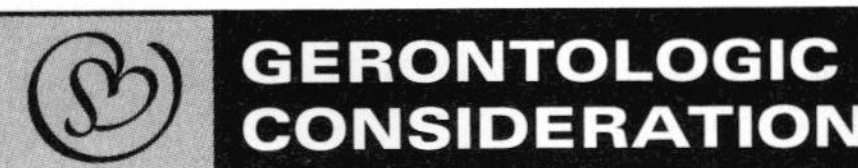

GERONTOLOGIC CONSIDERATION

- Nighttime confusion is common in older adults. The nurse should use soft restraints or ask the family to sit with the patient to remind the patient not to pull on the tube.

Implementation

Eliciting patient cooperation through explanation and education helps make implementation of the care plan easier and helps reduce patient discomfort. Explaining the role of the patient alleviates fear and allows the patient some control during tube care (see care plan on p. 380). Establishing signals for "stop" or "need time" gives the patient a feeling of control. The nurse should consider the special needs of the older adult with an intestinal tube (see gerontologic box).

Evaluation

Nursing interventions are evaluated by determining the patient's response to nursing therapies and by determining whether goals were achieved:

Goal: Patient's skin around feeding tube remains clean, so integrity is maintained.

Evaluative measure

Clean skin around feeding tube daily with warm water and mild soap.

NURSING CARE

It is important for the nurse to assess each nostril for patency. To determine which nostril is the most patent, the nurse occludes one nostril at a time while the patient breathes out through the nose. Using a pen light the nurse inspects the nostril for any deviation of the canal or polyps (small tumorlike growths) that may interfere with passage of the tube. The nurse should also determine the patient's ability to assist or cooperate in the procedure.

The tube is inserted into the nose (left or right nares) and then passed through the pharynx (posterior oronasal area) and down the esophagus into the stomach (Skill 19-1) and may be further passed into the jejunum. The tube should be measured for the length to be inserted (Fig. 19-2). The traditional method is to measure the distance from the tip of the nose to the earlobe and then down to the xiphoid process of the sternum (Fig. 19-3). The tube should then be marked with a small piece of tape. Nasogas-

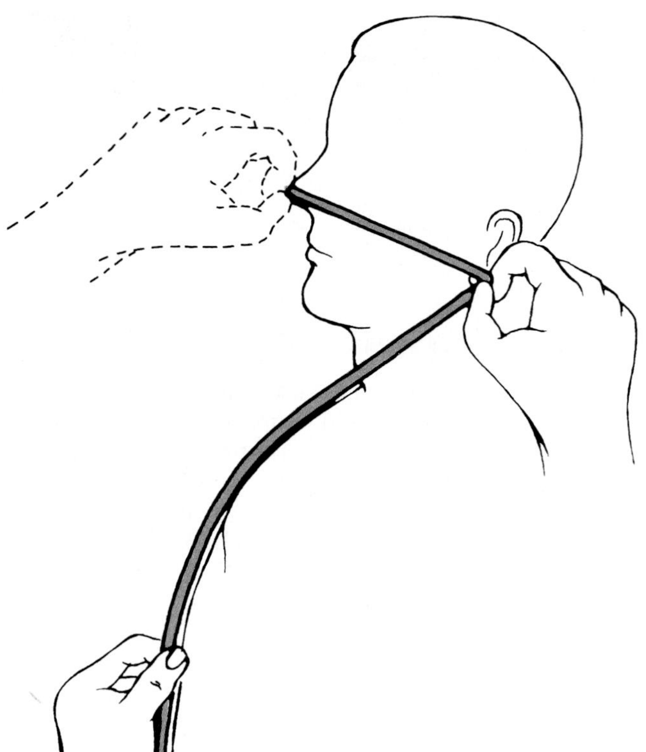

Fig. 19-2 Measuring for length of NG tube to be inserted. (From Perry AG, Potter PA: *Clinical nursing skills and techniques,* ed 3, St Louis, 1994, Mosby.)

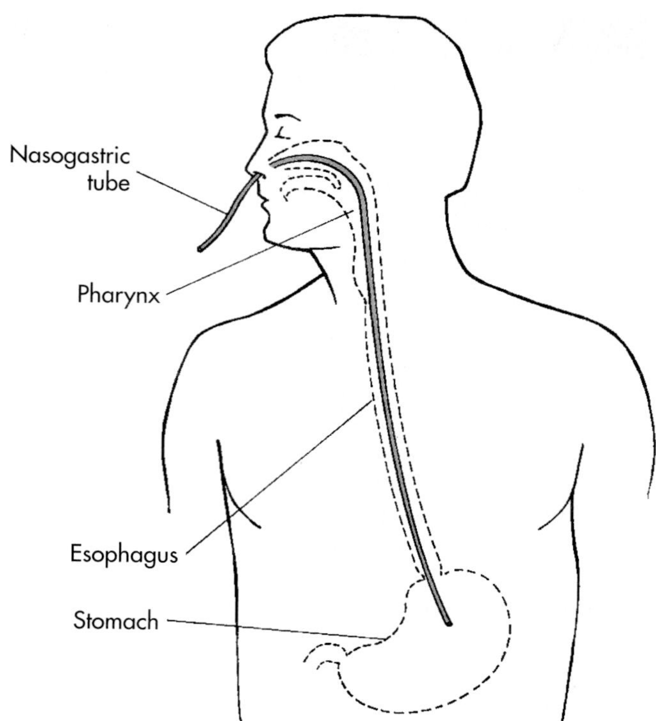

Fig. 19-3 Placement of nasogastric tube in stomach.

tric tubes can be mechanically passed into the stomach, but passing the tube farther depends on gravity and peristaltic action, which carry the tube along the GI tract. **Peristalsis** is the coordinated, rhythmic, serial contraction of smooth muscle that forces food through the digestive tract.

To ensure appropriate tube placement during intubation the nurse uses a penlight and tongue blade to examine the oral passage way for signs of a coiled tubing or movement of the tube up into the mouth. During advancement of the tube in a patient who is unconscious or has **dysphagia** (difficulty swallowing), stroking the neck encourages the swallowing reflex and passage of the tube. Sometimes during insertion, the tube enters the trachea instead of the stomach. Before instilling liquids through the tube or attaching the tube to suction, the nurse must first determine that the tube is in the stomach. The following are methods of testing for proper NG tube placement:

1. Inject 10 to 20 ml of air into the tube while auscultating over the epigastric area. Confirm a "whooshing" or gurgling sound.
2. Aspirate gastric contents. (**Aspiration** is the withdrawal of fluid from the body by a suction device.)
3. Test gastric contents for acidity (pH) with litmus paper.

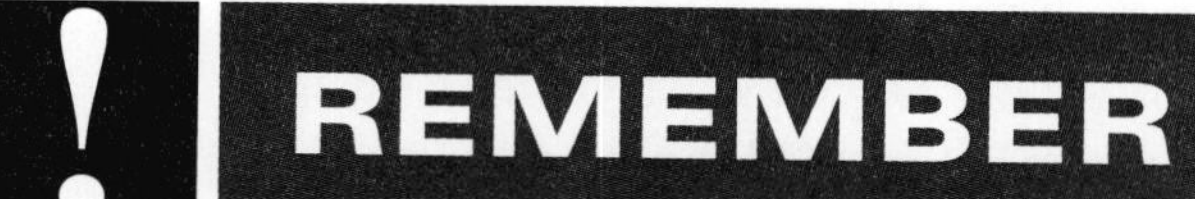

REMEMBER

- If permissible, allow the patient to suck on hard candy or ice chips to keep the mucous membranes moist.
- Place an ice bag against the patient's throat to reduce pharyngeal soreness.

The last method (litmus test) is generally considered to be the most accurate method for ensuring tube placement in the stomach. Other ways of testing for placement is to ask the patient to talk or hum. If neither is possible, it is more than likely that the tube has entered the trachea. Some agencies require x-ray verification of tube placement before instillation of any fluids or attachment of the tube to suction.

The nurse is usually responsible for inserting and caring for the NG tube once it is in place. Patient comfort and safety are the most important duties of the nurse in this procedure.

The following guidelines are useful to the nurse

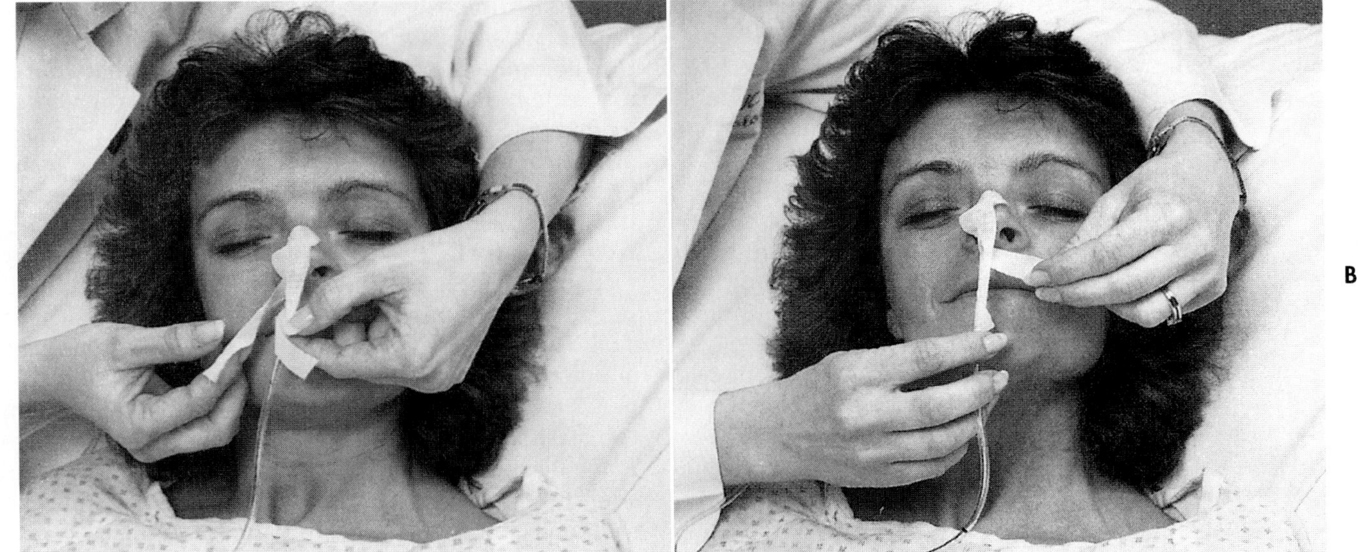

Fig. 19-4 **A,** Tape tube to nose. **B,** Carefully wrap two split ends around tube. (From Potter PA, Perry AG: *Basic nursing: theory and practice,* ed 3, St Louis, 1995, Mosby.)

when helping patients through the NG intubation:

1. For most patients, NG intubation is a new and frightening experience. The nurse may help by thoroughly explaining the procedure and the reason for its use.
2. The inability to chew, taste, and swallow food and liquids may contribute to patient anxiety during NG intubation.
3. A patient with a NG or intestinal tube is usually given nothing by mouth. Frequent oral hygiene may relieve discomfort and keep the mucous membranes moist.
4. The presence of an NG or intestinal tube is a constant irritant to the nasopharynx and requires frequent care of the nose and mouth.
5. Patients with NG tubes are often afraid that moving will dislodge the tube. Tubes are stabilized with tape to the nose (Fig. 19-4). The patient should be taught about movement with the tube. The nurse must intervene with frequent position changes to enhance tube functioning and prevent complications of immobility.

The nurse is responsible for knowing all types of GI tubes as well as their application and use (see Table 19-1).

Enteral Feedings

Enteral feedings are administered into the small intestine. The most common enteral feedings are given through small-bore NG feeding tubes. These tubes are passed through the nose or mouth and pharynx, down through the esophagus, into the stomach or farther (into the jejunum). When a larger tube is used for suctioning or decompression of the stomach or intestinal tract, it is passed in the same way. Small-bore feeding tubes are easily dislodged and should be assessed for placement before instillation of any liquids. Because the small-bore tube is soft, it easily collapses with aspiration, making it difficult to determine placement. Placement may be verified by x-ray study.

Equipment for instilling feedings is usually an Asepto bulb syringe used for bolus feedings. (A **bolus** is a round mass, specifically of chewed food ready to be swallowed.) Bolus feedings are ordered with a specific number of milliliters of formula (usually 240 to 360 ml) per intermittent feeding every 4 to 6 hours. Feedings are usually followed with instillation of 60 to 100 ml of water to clear the tubing and provide hydration. Formula may also be continuously administered with a computerized monitor set for an ordered number of milliliters per hour. Asepto syringes should be carefully cleaned and placed in a clean receptacle between feedings. Asepto syringes and monitor tubes should be changed every 24 to 48 hours, depending on agency policy and procedure.

Gastrostomy or Jejunostomy Feedings

Gavage feedings may also be performed through a gastrostomy or jejunostomy tube. A gastrostomy feeding tube is inserted through the stoma of a **gastrostomy** (surgical creation of an artificial opening through the abdominal wall and into the stomach).

A jejunostomy feeding tube is inserted through the stoma of a **jejunostomy** (surgical creation of an artificial opening through the abdominal wall into the jejunum). Patients with a functioning GI tract who are unable to swallow or to consume adequate foods and fluids must be fed in this manner. When patients are comatose, have an injury to the esophagus, or have cerebral damage that interferes with the swallowing mechanism, this alternative entry into the GI tract may be necessary. These feeding routes may be permanent or temporary, depending on the reason for them.

The patient often has difficulty accepting a gastrostomy or jejunostomy tube. The trauma is usually not as great when the tube is temporary. Explanations of the process itself should be thoroughly discussed by the patient and physician before tube placement. A gastrostomy or jejunostomy feeding tube is surgically or endoscopically placed through the wall of the abdomen either into the stomach or jejunum. The tube is sutured in place, or specific devices are used to hold the tube in place. A variety of tubes are available for use. They include large-lumen latex tubes such as Foley catheters, polyurethane tubes such as the Ross Sacks-Vine tube, and silicone tubes. Feedings may be initiated 24 to 48 hours after insertion. The nurse should assess for bowel sounds to ensure return of peristalsis before feedings are begun. Patients often are discharged with percutaneous endoscopic gastrostomy (PEG) tubes or percutaneous endoscopic jejunostomy (PEJ) tubes. Aseptic technique is performed during the care of the tube (Skill 19-2), entry wound, and enteral feedings. As early as possible after insertion, the patient and family member must be taught and encouraged to participate in the care of the tube and site of insertion and the provision of feedings to be prepared for home care after discharge. The skin should be inspected around the tube for color and breaks as well as the presence of drainage, odor, and edema. Measurement of the tube length should be performed to detect dislodgment. The skin should be cleansed with soap and water and then rinsed well and dried. A dry gauze dressing is then applied around the tube and over the wound. New dressings, called *wafer dressings,* have been specifically designed for use with PEG and PEJ tubes.

Gastric Lavage and Irrigation

An NG tube inserted to provide drainage of gastric contents or to provide enteral feedings may become obstructed by secretions or formula. The tip of the tube may rest against the wall of the stomach and may also block functioning of the tube. The nurse should assess for kinks in the tube, pressure on the tube that obstructs flow, and failure of suction equipment. After other causes of restrictive flow are ruled out, irrigation is performed to restore drainage (Skill 19-3). Lavage and irrigation require a medical order for the type and amount of solution to be used, frequency, and temperature of the solution. Normal saline is usually used to reduce electrolyte loss. Gastric lavage may be an emergency measure performed to wash out the stomach contents when a patient swallows a toxic substance such as lye, bleach, or a cleaning agent. In instances of poisoning or active bleeding, continuous lavage is performed to dilute and wash the substances from the stomach. The procedure may also be used to remove drugs from the stomach when the patient has overdosed on drugs. Lavage is usually performed in the emergency unit. The NG tube may also be irrigated after some surgeries, after feedings or suction (routine care), and for any other reasons decided by the physician.

The nurse performs lavage and irrigation for the following reasons:

1. To determine patency of the NG tube
2. To maintain patency of the NG feeding tube
3. To remove toxic substances from the stomach
4. To wash the stomach during active bleeding

Gastrointestinal Suctioning

When the NG tube is used for decompression, it is attached to suction. The rate of suction is set at low, medium, or high when ordered by the physician. Some agencies have set protocols for suction rates according to the type of tube being used. Suction piped from wall outlets is available in some agencies. This suction may be regulated for continuous or intermittent suction. Another type of portable suction is the Gomco pump, which is an intermittent suction with high and low settings. This apparatus may be a floor model or may be a model in which suction is piped from the wall by the patient's bed (Fig. 19-5).

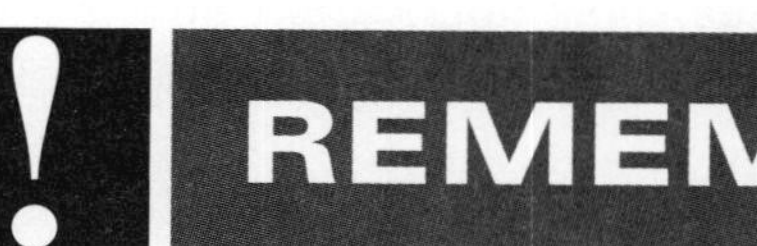

- Never use the air vent on a suction tube for irrigation or suction.
- Carefully assess tube placement in an unconscious patient.
- Give the formula at room temperature. Cold formula may cause cramping.

Two tubes used for decompression of the intestinal tract are the Miller-Abbott and the Cantor tubes (Fig. 19-6). These tubes may be passed through the entire intestinal tract. A small balloon on the tip of the tubes is filled with air, water, or mercury after the tip reaches the stomach. The filled balloon stimulates peristalsis and helps propel the tube through the pylorus and along the intestine. Intestinal tubes are attached to suction either at the time of insertion or when they reach the desired location in the intestines (Skill 19-4). These tubes are not taped to the nose until they reach the desired location. Various tubes and sizes of tubes are available, depending on the purpose of the intubation. The Sengstaken-Blakemore tube provides both compression and decompression. This tube has three lumens specifically marked: (1) inflation of the esophageal balloon for compression of esophageal bleeding, (2) inflation of the gastric balloon for stabilization of the tube, and (3) gastric suction and decompression.

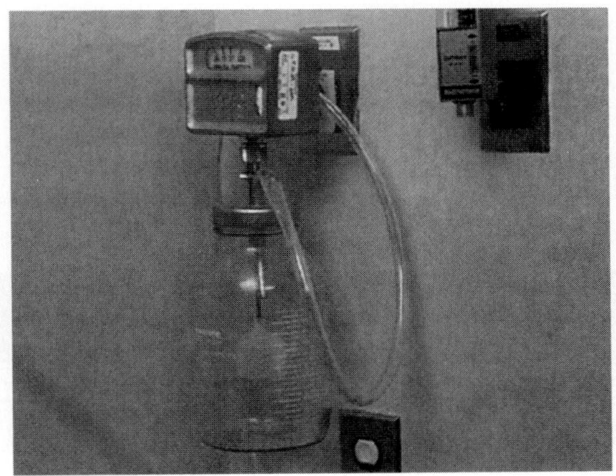

Fig. 19-5 Wall suction apparatus.

Removal of Tubes

The NG tube is removed when the treatment is no longer required or when a new tube is to be inserted. Removal requires a medical order. If the patient knows that the tube is being removed permanently, anxiety is reduced or nonexistent. If the tube was used for decompression, the patient may fear reinsertion. The patient having a new tube inserted after removal may also be anxious. Therefore it is important for the nurse to assess the patient's feelings and concerns. Time is allowed for questions and expression of fears.

There are several steps in removing an NG tube (Skill 19-5). The procedure is explained to the patient. The NG tube is clamped off to prevent backflow as the tube is removed. The patient is positioned in the high-Fowler's position, and all tube stabilizers (nose tape, rubberbands, and safety pins) are removed. The nurse should ask the patient to hold the breath and close the eyes as the tube is swiftly removed using the hand-over-hand technique. It is best to place the tube in a bath towel so that the tube is covered as it is removed. This helps reduce patient anxiety because the patient does not see the tube during removal. The nurse has facial tissues for any secretions that may follow the tube. Special mouth and nose care should follow removal. The patient should remain in a high- to medium-Fowler's position for a time to facilitate adjustment. The emesis basin and tissues should be left close to the patient, who should be told to notify the nurse if nausea or vomiting occurs.

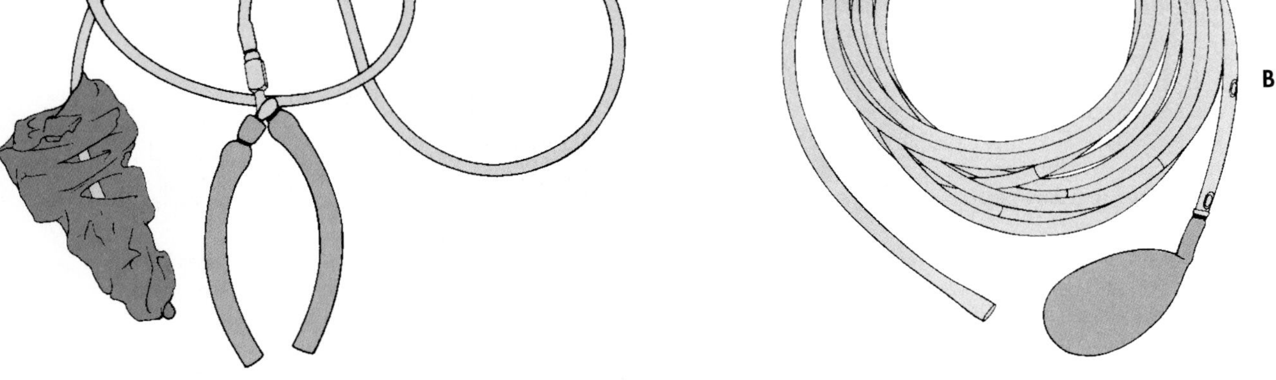
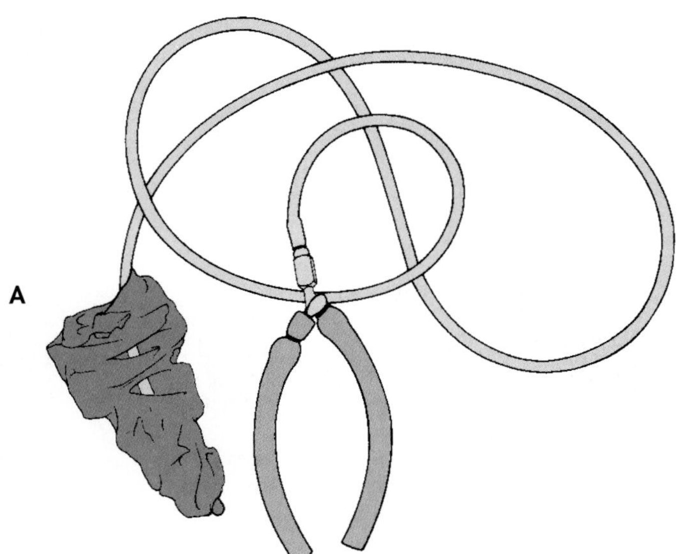

Fig. 19-6 Intestinal tubes. **A,** Miller-Abbott tube. **B,** Cantor tube.

■ NURSING CARE PLAN ■

ANXIETY

Ms. H, age 82, was diagnosed 3 days before with a cerebrovascular accident, or stroke, with resulting dysphagia and right hemiplegia (paralysis on one side of the body). She is unable to swallow but is oriented and alert. The patient is scheduled to have a small-bore NG feeding tube inserted for nutritional supplement.

NURSING DIAGNOSIS

Anxiety related to fear of the unknown as evidenced by wringing of hands and resisting the nurse's approach

GOAL

- Patient will cooperate with nurse during procedure.

EXPECTED OUTCOMES

- Patient will express understanding of what is to be performed.
- Patient will cope with need for NG tube.

NURSING INTERVENTIONS

- Teach steps of procedure to patient to help reduce anxiety.
- Encourage patient to express feelings causing anxiety to help patient relax.
- Listen to patient attentively to instill trust in nurse.

EVALUATION

- Patient demonstrates relaxation techniques.
- Patient allows procedure to be performed.

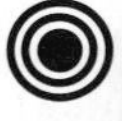

SKILL 19-1 PERFORMING NASOGASTRIC TUBE INSERTION AND TUBE FEEDING

Steps	Rationale
1. Obtain equipment: ▪ Small-bore nasogastric tube or Levin tube (8-12 Fr) ▪ Large syringe: 30 ml ▪ Luer-Lock or 30-ml Asepto syringe ▪ pH test strips ▪ Hypoallergic tape (1 inch) ▪ Glass of water and straw ▪ Tongue blade ▪ Towel or waterproof pad ▪ Penlight or flashlight ▪ Emesis basin ▪ Clean gloves ▪ Facial tissues ▪ Guidewire or stylet (if using small-bore tube) ▪ Safety pin and rubber band ▪ Prescribed formula at room temperature	Helps organize procedure.
2. Refer to medical record, care plan, or Kardex for special interventions.	Provides basis for care.
3. Introduce self.	Decreases anxiety level.
4. Identify patient by identification band.	Identifies correct patient for procedure.
5. Explain procedure to patient.	Seeks cooperation and decreases anxiety.

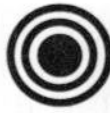

SKILL 19-1 PERFORMING NASOGASTRIC TUBE INSERTION AND TUBE FEEDING—cont'd

Steps	Rationale
6. Wash hands and don clean gloves according to agency policy and guidelines from Centers for Disease Control and Prevention and Occupational Safety and Health Administration.	Helps prevent cross-contamination.
7. Prepare patient for intervention:	
a. Close door to room or pull curtain.	Provides privacy.
b. Drape for procedure if necessary.	Prevents exposure of patient.
8. Raise bed to comfortable working level.	Provides safety for nurse.
9. Arrange for patient privacy.	Shows respect for patient.
10. Assess condition and patency of nares. Occlude one naris and have patient breathe through other to determine through which air passes more easily.	Allows easier insertion of tube and prevents meeting possible obstruction on insertion attempt.
11. Place patient in high-Fowler's position and raise bed to comfortable height for patient.	Eases insertion and enhances swallowing.
12. Stand on dominant side.	Allows easier manipulation of tube.
13. Place towel or waterproof pad over patient's chest with tissues nearby in case patient's eyes water.	Protects patient's gown and provides area for tube to rest during insertion.
14. Determine length of tube to reach stomach: Measure distance from tip of nose to tip of earlobe to tip of xiphoid process (see Fig. 19-2).	Ensures that tubing will reach patient's stomach.
15. Use tape to mark distance.	Ensures that correct length is used.
16. Cut two pieces of tape, one 3 in long and one 1½ in long. Cut or tear the 3-in strip halfway down the center.	Organizes taping procedure. Saves time.
17. Using water-soluble lubricant, lubricate first 3-4 ins (7.5-10 cm) of tube.	Eases movement of tube over mucous membrane.
18. Extend patient's head back toward pillow. Hold tube about 3 in from tip and insert it into nostril, gently guiding it straight back and down along floor of nose.	Helps tube to follow oral passageway.
19. Have patient flex head slightly forward as tube is advanced. Have patient sip water (if permitted) or swallow continuously as tube is advanced.	Enables tube to enter esophagus (in this position glottis closes over trachea). Helps advance tube toward stomach.
20. If there is excessive gagging and coughing, withdraw tube slightly:	Allows nurse to reposition tube, which may be entering larynx or may be coiled in back of pharynx.
a. Use flashlight and tongue blade to assess pharynx.	
b. If tube is curled in pharynx, pull tube back slightly, allowing patient to relax, and then begin advancing tube again.	Allows tube to continue to move toward stomach.
21. Continue advancing tube until tape mark reaches nares.	Allows NG tube to reach the stomach.
22. If patient is gasping, cyanotic, or unable to speak, stop procedure, withdraw tube, let patient relax, relubricate tube, and then reinsert.	Allows nurse to reposition tube, which may have entered trachea instead of esophagus.
23. Verify that tube is in stomach.	Ensures that tip of tube has reached stomach.

Continued.

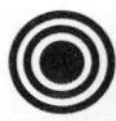

SKILL 19-1 PERFORMING NASOGASTRIC TUBE INSERTION AND TUBE FEEDING—cont'd

Steps	Rationale
24. Attach 30-ml syringe to tube. Place stethoscope over epigastric area. While auscultating, inject 10-20 ml of air into tube. Listen for "whooshing" or gurgling. Alternatively, verify placement with x-ray study.	Allows nurse to verify tube placement.
25. Aspirate gastric contents and assess acidity.	Confirms that tip of tube is in stomach. (Lung fluids are not acid.)
26. Clamp or plug tube.	Prevents gastric contents from draining onto gown or linens.
27. Have patient close eyes tightly and wipe bridge of nose carefully, avoiding eye area, with protective wipe. Allow nose to dry for 60 sec.	Helps prevent shearing of tissue when tape is removed and prevents skin damage.
28. Secure tube:	
a. Secure to gown with rubberband and safety pin.	Reduces pull on nares and permits more freedom of movement.
b. Secure to nose with tape (see Fig. 19-4): Anchors tube securely.	Supports weight of tube to prevent dislodging and damage to mucosa. Reinforces hold of tape and thus tube. Secures tube.
(1) Press wide part of 3-in tape lengthwise over bridge of nose.	
(2) Wrap ends of tape alternately around tube.	
(3) Press second piece of tape over bridge of nose and first strip of tape.	
29. Leave head of bed elevated for tube feeding and make patient comfortable.	Prevents aspiration.
ENTERAL FEEDINGS	
30. Assess placement of tube before instilling foods, fluids, or medications.	Ensures that tube is in stomach so that fluids are not instilled into lungs.
31. Aspirate gastric contents and measure for residual. If unable to aspirate contents, assess for possible abdominal distention, which may indicate retention.	Indicates gastric retention if there are more than 150 ml of contents. Prevents regurgitation and aspiration, which can occur if retention and overfilling of the gastric area is undetected.
32. Reinstill contents according to agency policy.	Prevents loss of fluids and electrolytes.
INTERMITTENT BOLUS FEEDINGS	
33. Clamp end of feeding tube.	Prevents air from entering stomach.
34. Attach syringe to end of tube.	Prepares for feeding.
35. Fill syringe with formula and raise syringe 18 in above port of entry.	Allows formula to flow slowly without exerting high pressure.
36. Unclamp tubing and allow syringe to empty gradually to just above connection and refill repeatedly until all prescribed volume has been instilled.	Reduces pressure and increased risk of diarrhea from bolus feeding.
CONTINUOUS FEEDING	
37. Fill bag and tubing with formula as prescribed and attach to clamped NG tube.	Removes air from bag and tubing, preventing air from entering stomach.
38. Connect infusion pump and set rate. Remove clamp from connection and allow formula to be delivered.	Maintains desired flow.
39. Administer additional water as prescribed or according to agency policy.	Clears tube and increases hydration for the patient.
40. Clamp or plug feeding tube when not being used.	Prevents leakage of gastric contents and air from entering the stomach between instillations.
41. Monitor gastric residuals every 6-8 hr.	Prevents complications.
42. Remove gloves and wash hands.	Helps prevent cross-contamination.
43. Document.	Documents procedure and patient's response.

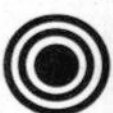

SKILL 19-2 PERFORMING GASTROSTOMY AND JEJUNOSTOMY TUBE CARE

Steps	Rational
1. Obtain equipment: ▪ Clean gloves ▪ Gauze dressing ▪ Tape ▪ Scissors or precut dressing ▪ Soap ▪ Water ▪ Ruler ▪ Stethoscope ▪ Graduated pitcher ▪ Protective ointment when ordered ▪ Plastic bag	Helps organize procedure.
2. Refer to medical record, care plan, or Kardex for special interventions.	Provides basis for care.
3. Introduce self.	Decreases anxiety level.
4. Identify patient by identification band.	Identifies correct patient for procedure.
5. Explain procedure to patient.	Seeks cooperation and decreases anxiety.
6. Wash hands and don clean gloves according to agency policy and guidelines from Centers for Disease Control and Prevention and Occupational Safety and Health Administration.	Helps prevent cross-contamination.
7. Prepare patient for intervention:	
a. Close door to room or pull curtain.	Provides privacy.
b. Drape for procedure if necessary.	Prevents exposure of patient.
8. Raise bed to comfortable working level.	Provides safety for nurse.
9. Arrange for patient privacy.	Shows respect for patient.
10. Inspect skin around tube for color; breaks; and drainage, odor, and swelling. Measure length of tube.	Provides baseline for further assessment.
11. Palpate abdomen and listen for bowel sounds.	Determines presence of peristalsis and distention.
12. Assist patient to comfortable position that allows access to dressing.	Promotes patient comfort.
13. Place open, cuffed plastic bag within easy reach.	Reduces transmission of microorganisms when disposing of soiled dressing.
14. Loosen tape by pulling toward dressing.	Reduces discomfort.
15. Remove dressing and assess drainage.	Determines healing or infection of wound.
16. Discard dressing in plastic bag.	Reduces chance of contamination.
17. Measure length of tube.	May indicate dislodgment from stomach (increased length).
18. Cleanse skin with soap and water and dry well.	Removes drainage.
19. Replace dressing and tape using sterile technique.	Prevents infection of wound.
20. Weigh patient and discuss frequency, amount, and type of feedings.	Helps determine adequacy of nourishment.
21. Provide mouth care if necessary.	Provides comfort and maintains moist mucous membrane.
22. Collect urine in graduated container and assess color, amount, consistency, and odor.	May indicate urine concentration and need for increased fluid intake (concentrated, small amount).
23. Remove gloves and wash hands.	Helps prevent cross-contamination.
24. Document.	Documents procedure and patient's response.

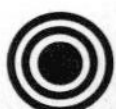

SKILL 19-3 PERFORMING GASTRIC LAVAGE OR IRRIGATION

Steps	Rationale
1. Obtain equipment: ▪ Irrigation set, including Asepto or Toomey syringe ▪ Container for irrigant (check expiration date) ▪ Clamp ▪ Towel or waterproof pad ▪ Stethoscope ▪ Clean gloves	Helps organizes procedure.
2. Refer to medical record, care plan, or Kardex for special interventions.	Provides basis for care.
3. Introduce self.	Decreases anxiety level.
4. Identify patient by identification band.	Identifies correct patient for procedure.
5. Explain procedure to patient.	Seeks cooperation and decreases anxiety.
6. Wash hands and don clean gloves according to agency policy and guidelines from Centers for Disease Control and Prevention and Occupational Safety and Health Administration.	Helps prevent cross-contamination.
7. Prepare patient for intervention:	
a. Close door to room or pull curtain.	Provides privacy.
b. Drape for procedure if necessary.	Prevents exposure of patient.
8. Raise bed to comfortable working level.	Provides safety for nurse.
9. Arrange for patient privacy.	Shows respect for patient.
10. Assess functioning of suction apparatus and suction tubing.	Prevents drainage of gastric contents caused by malfunctioning equipment.
11. Assess abdomen.	Provides baseline data for comparison.
12. Place patient in semi-Fowler's position.	Protects patient's clothing and linens.
13. Disconnect NG tubing and place suction tubing on towel or waterproof pad or towel.	Prepares for procedure.
14. Verify that tube is in stomach: Attach syringe to tube and aspirate gastric contents.	Confirms that tip of tube is in stomach.
15. If no gastric contents are aspirated, place stethoscope over epigastric area. While auscultating, inject 20-30 ml of air into tube. Listen for "whooshing" or bubbling sound.	Ensures that tube is in place.
16. Pour normal saline into container. Draw 30 ml (or amount ordered) into irrigating syringe.	Ensures that tip of irrigation syringe fits snugly into end of tube.
17. Place syringe into NG tube while pinching between index finger and thumb. Keeping syringe in upright position, gently instill solution. Do not use force, which may injure gastric mucosa.	Prevents air from being instilled into stomach.
18. If resistance is met, change patient's position and repeat step 17. Check with charge nurse or physician if there is continued resistance.	Ensures that tip of tube is not against stomach wall and that tube is not blocked with drainage.
19. Withdraw fluid into syringe and measure. Continue irrigating with appropriate amount of normal saline or until purpose of lavage or irrigation has been accomplished.	Clears tube.
20. Reclamp or plug NG tube or reconnect it to suction tubing.	Resumes purpose of tube.
21. Assess and record amount of saline instilled and withdrawn.	Helps record accurate intake and output.
22. Remove gloves and wash hands.	Helps prevent cross-contamination.
23. Document.	Documents procedure and patient's response.

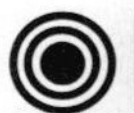

SKILL 19-4 PERFORMING GASTRIC SUCTIONING

Steps	Rationale
1. **Obtain equipment:** ▪ Asepto or Toomey syringe ▪ Towel ▪ Suction apparatus, if used ▪ Clean gloves ▪ Emesis basin ▪ Glass ▪ Straw ▪ Stethoscope	Helps organize procedure.
2. **Refer to medical record, care plan, or Kardex for special interventions.**	Provides basis for care.
3. **Introduce self.**	Decreases anxiety level.
4. **Identify patient by identification band.**	Identifies correct patient for procedure.
5. **Explain procedure to patient.**	Seeks cooperation and decreases anxiety.
6. **Wash hands and don clean gloves according to agency policy and guidelines from Centers for Disease Control and Prevention and Occupational Safety and Health Administration.**	Helps prevent cross-contamination.
7. **Prepare patient for intervention:**	
a. Close door to room or pull curtain.	Provides privacy.
b. Drape for procedure if necessary.	Prevents exposure of patient.
8. **Raise bed to comfortable working level.**	Provides safety for nurse.
9. **Arrange for patient privacy.**	Shows respect for patient.
10. **Assess patient's oral and nasal cavities.**	May indicate need for special care.
11. **Assess patient's abdomen for bowel sounds and amount of distention.**	Provides baseline for further assessments and may indicate tube malfunction.
12. **Assess nothing-by-mouth status.**	Helps maintain fluid balance.
13. **Following insertion of NG tube, assess tube placement.**	Begins maintenance of nasogastric tube and verifies that tube is in stomach.
14. **Assess NG tube drainage for amount, color, and consistency.**	Ensures that tube is functioning appropriately.
15. **Assess NG tube patency.**	Ensures patency of tube.
16. **Keep patient's lips and mouth moist by allowing sips of water or small amount of ice chips unless contraindicated.**	Helps prevent drying of mouth and lips. Prevents washing out electrolytes from stomach.
17. **Assess suction apparatus according to type:** *For Gomco:* a. Secure plugs. b. Make sure that light is blinking. c. Ensure that tubing connections are tight. d. Verify that setting is correct. *For wall suction:* e. Ensure that pressure gauge connections are tight. f. Make sure that pressure indicated on gauge is as ordered or according to agency policy. g. Verify that setting is at intermittent unless contraindicated.	Identifies whether that apparatus is functioning.
18. **Assess tubing for kinks and ensure that patient is not lying on tube.**	Verifies that weight of patient or tube itself is not causing obstruction.
19. **Ensure that tube is pinned to patient's gown with enough slack to allow movement.**	Prevents dislodging of tube and patient discomfort.
20. **Ensure that drainage is moving through tubing to drainage-collection bottle.**	Indicates that stomach or intestinal contents are being removed.

Continued.

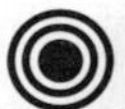

SKILL 19-4 PERFORMING GASTRIC SUCTIONING—cont'd

Steps	Rationale
21. For Salem sump tube, listen for hissing at opening of blue air vent, making certain that vent is pointing upward.	Indicates that air vent is patent and promotes drainage through vent via gravity.
22. Estimate amount of drainage in bottle and empty bottle if it is full at end of shift.	Provides baseline for further assessments, prevents overflow, and provides for accurate measurement.
23. Remove gloves and wash hands.	Helps prevent cross-contamination.
24. Document.	Documents procedure and patient's response.

SKILL 19-5 REMOVING A NASOGASTRIC TUBE

Steps	Rationale
1. Obtain equipment: ▪ Facial tissues ▪ Towel or waterproof pad ▪ Plastic bag ▪ Clean gloves ▪ Clamp (optional) ▪ Universal precautions equipment, as indicated.	Helps organize procedure.
2. Refer to medical record, care plan, or Kardex for special interventions.	Provides basis for care.
3. Introduce self.	Decreases anxiety level.
4. Identify patient by identification band.	Identifies correct patient for procedure.
5. Explain procedure to patient.	Seeks cooperation and decreases anxiety.
6. Wash hands and don clean gloves according to agency policy and guidelines from Centers for Disease Control and Prevention and Occupational Safety and Health Administration.	Helps prevent cross-contamination.
7. Prepare patient for intervention:	
a. Close door to room or pull curtain.	Provides privacy.
b. Drape for procedure if necessary.	Prevents exposure of patient.
8. Raise bed to comfortable working level.	Provides safety for nurse.
9. Arrange for patient privacy.	Shows respect for patient.
10. Assess nose and oral cavity.	Determines patient's need for oronasal care and determines the condition of oronasal cavity.
11. Assess patient's abdomen.	Provides baseline data of abdominal condition and distention for future comparison.
12. If tube is attached to suction, turn off suction and disconnect tubing.	Decreases patient discomfort.
13. Remove tape from nose and pin from gown.	Allows unrestricted removal of tube.
14. Place towel or waterproof pad across patient's chest and provide facial tissues.	Protects clothing and allows patient to wipe nose.
15. Pinch tube with fingers or clamp. Quickly and smoothly remove tube while patient holds breath.	Prevents dripping of gastric contents and minimizes discomfort.
16. Place tube in plastic bag.	Reduces transmission of microorganisms.
17. Provide oronasal care and make patient comfortable.	Provides comfort.
18. Dispose of tube and equipment and measure drainage.	Reduces transmission of microorganisms and provides for accurate measurement of output.
19. Remove gloves and wash hands.	Helps prevent cross-contamination.
20. Document.	Documents procedure and patient's response.

SUMMARY

To successfully perform care for the patient with an NG or intestinal tube, the nurse must recognize each person as an individual. The patient's emotional and physical needs must be considered. The nurse should provide careful monitoring of the function of the tube and the patient's reaction to each procedure. Considerable emotional support will be needed for patients who are embarrassed or feel trapped by the tube.

All feeding tubes must be assessed for placement before instillation of foods or fluids. Patients and families should be taught all functions and care of the tube. Aseptic technique should be maintained when handling tubes. The nursing care of each patient and each tube varies. In most cases of suction or feedings the patient depends on the nurse for successful treatment. The nurse should have a sound understanding of the tube's function and the procedures to be performed with the tube. The nurse should also attempt to relieve the discomfort and stigma associated with intubation.

Key Concepts

- Disorders of the gastrointestinal tract affect its functioning.
- The nurse should prevent trauma to oral and gastric mucosa when performing intubation.
- The rate of gastrointestinal suction should be precise and accurately maintained.
- The patient should be clear regarding the purpose of the tube to encourage cooperation.
- Tube placement should be assessed every time that a procedure is performed to prevent it from slipping into the trachea.
- Bowel sounds should be assessed as necessary.

Critical Thinking Questions

1. The nurse has received a morning report on Mr. Karl. NG tube feedings have been ordered. The night nurse stated that his abdomen was distended, and she withheld the 0500 feeding. What assessments does the nurse need to make about Mr. Karl's tolerance to the tube feeding, the placement of the tube, and the resumption of tube feedings?
2. Correctly write the following incorrect nursing interventions:
   a. Irrigate nasogastric tube with normal saline.
   b. Suction patient every 2 hours.
   c. Change patient's dressing at 0600, 1400, and 2200 hours.

REFERENCES AND SUGGESTED READINGS

DeWitt SC: *Rambo's nursing skills for clinical practice,* ed 4, Philadelphia, 1994, Saunders.

Linton AD, Matteson MA, Maebius NK: *Introductory nursing care of adults,* Philadelphia, 1995, Saunders.

Long BC, Phipps WJ, Cassmeyer VL: *Medical-surgical nursing: a nursing process approach,* St Louis, 1993, Mosby.

Potter PA, Perry AG: *Basic nursing: theory and practice,* ed 3, St Louis, 1995, Mosby.

Potter PA, Perry AG: *Fundamentals of nursing: concepts, process, and practice,* ed 3, St Louis, 1993, Mosby.

Rosdahl CB: *Textbook of basic nursing,* ed 6, Philadelphia, 1995, Lippincott.

CHAPTER 20

Body Mechanics

Learning Objectives

After studying this chapter, the student should be able to . . .

- Define the key terms.
- State the principles of appropriate body mechanics.
- Describe the purposes of appropriately positioning the patient.
- Explain appropriate technique for turning, moving, lifting, and carrying the patient.
- Demonstrate positioning the patient in the Fowler's, supine (dorsal), Sims', side-lying, prone, dorsal-recumbent, and lithotomy positions.
- Demonstrate the use of techniques when using body mechanics.
- Assess for impaired body alignment and mobility.
- Place a patient in accurate body alignment.
- Explain the role of the nurse when range-of-motion exercises are performed.
- Identify complications caused from immobility.

Key Terms

Balance
Base of support
Body alignment
Body mechanics
Contracture
Dorsal (supine)
Dorsal-recumbent
High Fowler's
Immobility
Knee-chest (genupectoral)
Lithotomy
Orthopneic
Posture
Prone
Range of motion (ROM)
Semi-Fowler's
Sims'
Trendelenburg's

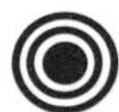

Skills

20-1 Positioning, moving, and lifting the patient
20-2 Performing passive range-of-motion exercises

Body mechanics is the field of physiology that studies muscular actions and the function of muscles in maintaining the balance and posture of the body during all the many activities necessary in daily living. In daily nursing care, body mechanics should be used to protect both the patient and the nurse from injury to the musculoskeletal and nervous systems.

PRINCIPLES OF BODY MECHANICS

To understand the principles or foundation of body mechanics the nurse should know the muscle groups and the ways that they are used. These muscle groups are used when bending, lifting, moving, and performing all other activities of daily living. **Body alignment** is the placing of the human body in appropriate anatomic position, whether standing or lying. When the body is out of alignment for extended periods, strain occurs, muscle tone is reduced, and body balance is compromised. The muscles and eventually the ligaments and tendons become permanently shortened **(contracture).** Maintaining appropriate body alignment is a key factor in the use of body mechanics.

The nurse should maintain a wide base of support when standing by keeping the feet slightly apart (Fig. 20-1). This stance provides appropriate stability and prevents the nurse from becoming overbalanced while performing an activity, such as assisting the patient in and out of bed or walking the patient in the room.

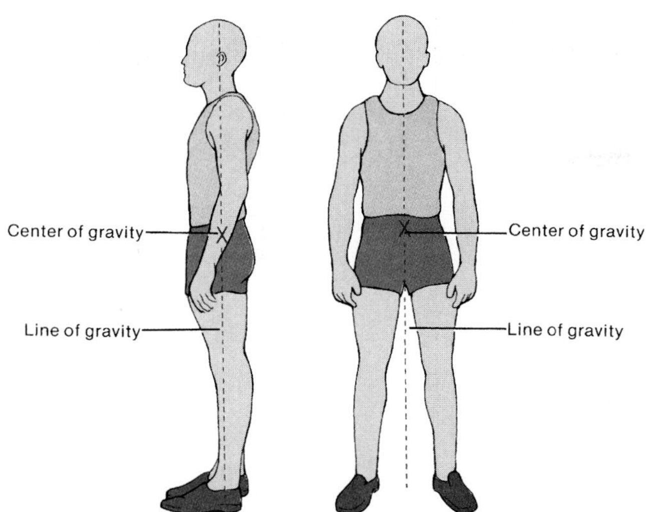

Fig. 20-1 Appropriate body alignment when standing. (From Perry AG, Potter PA: *Clinical nursing skills and techniques,* ed 3, St Louis, 1994, Mosby.)

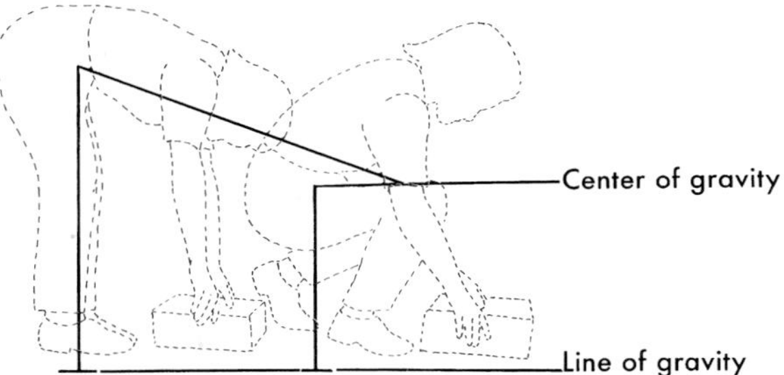

Fig. 20-2 Comparison of lifting techniques by lowering center of gravity of object to be lifted. (From Perry AG, Potter PA: *Clinical nursing skills and techniques,* ed 3, St Louis, 1994, Mosby.)

Posture

Posture is the position of the body. Posture is determined and maintained by the coordination of various muscles that move the limbs and by the sense of balance. Muscles of the lower extremities, trunk, neck, and back deal with posture. The muscles support the body's weight when standing or sitting. The nurse should be aware of common postural abnormalities and assess the patient for these types of problems (Table 20-1).

Balance

Equilibrium, or **balance,** which is maintained by muscles and the nervous system, aids appropriate body alignment when lifting, bending, moving, and performing other activities. The back is vulnerable to stress and to potential injury because of the type of physical work required in nursing. The back is protected from injury when the nurse bends the knees before performing nursing activities. Adjusting the working level to one of comfort and ease helps prevent undue stress and strain on back muscles. This may be accomplished by adjusting the position of the bed to complement the height of the nurse.

If the **base of support** is widened in the direction of movement, less effort is required to carry out an activity. A base of support is the placement of feet securely on the floor to provide protection and support to muscle groups, enabling the nurse to lift heavier objects, such as a patient. When moving an object, the nurse should stand in front of it to avoid twisting the spine. When stooping, the nurse should flex or bend the hips and maintain appropriate body alignment (Fig. 20-2). Bending from the waist should be avoided, since this activity in time, causes low back strain.

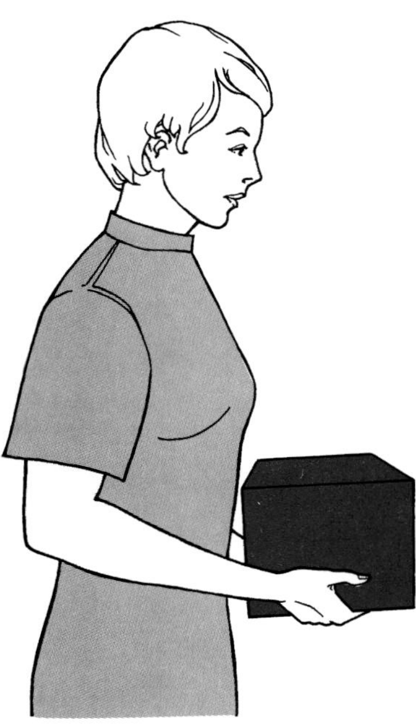

Fig. 20-3 Box being carried close to the nurse's body and base of support. (From Christensen BL, Kockrow EO: *Foundations of nursing,* ed 2, St Louis, 1995, Mosby.)

When the nurse uses large muscle groups, such as the legs, a greater workload may be performed more safely. The more muscle groups used, the better the distribution of a workload. The nurse should bend the knees when lifting and allow the leg muscles to handle most of the weight. This technique helps prevent injury to the back. The nurse may be protected further from injury by carrying objects close to the midline of the body (Fig. 20-3), avoiding reaching too far, avoiding lifting when

Table 20-1 POSTURAL ABNORMALITIES

Abnormality	Description	Cause	Treatment
Torticollis	Inclination of head to affected side, in which sternocleidomastoid muscle is contracted	Congenital or acquired	Surgery, heat, support, or immobilization, depending on cause and severity
Lordosis	Exaggeration of anterior convex curve of lumbar spine	Congenital Temporary as with pregnancy	Based on cause: frequently, spine-stretching exercises
Kyphosis	Increased convexity in curvature of thoracic spine	Congenital Rickets Tuberculosis of spine	Based on cause and severity: spine-stretching exercises, sleeping without pillows, use of bed board, bracing, and spinal fusion
Kypholordosis	Combination of kyphosis and lordosis	Congenital	Based on cause: similar to methods used in kyphosis or lordosis
Scoliosis	Lateral curvature of spine, unequal heights of hips and shoulders	Congenital Poliomyelitis Spastic paralysis Unequal leg length	Based on cause and severity: immobilization and surgery
Kyphoscoliosis	Abnormal anteroposterior and lateral curvature of spine	Congenital Poliomyelitis Cor pulmonale	Based on cause and severity: includes immobilization and surgery
Congenital hip dysplasia	Hip instability with limited abduction of hips and, occasionally, adduction contractures; head of femur does not articulate with acetabulum because of abnormal shallowness of acetabulum	Congenital; more common with breech deliveries	Maintenance of continuous abduction of thigh so that head of femur presses into center of acetabulum Abduction splints, casting, or surgery
Knock-knee (genu valgum)	Legs curved inward so that knees knock together as person walks	Congenital Rickets	Knee braces and surgery if not corrected by growth
Bowlegs (genu varum)	One or both legs bent outward at knee; normal until 2 to 3 years of age	Congenital Rickets	Slowing rate of curving if not corrected by growth With rickets, increase of vitamin D, calcium, and phosphorus intake to normal ranges
Clubfoot	95%: medial deviation and plantar flexion of foot (equinovarus) 5%: lateral deviation and dorsiflexion (calcaneovalgus)	Congenital	Based on degree and rigidity of deformity: casts, splints such as Denis Browne splint, and surgery
Footdrop	Plantar flexion, inability to invert foot because of peroneal nerve damage	Congenital Trauma Improper position of immobilized patient	Prevention through physical therapy
Pigeon-toes	Internal rotation of forefoot or entire foot, common in infants	Congenital Habitual	Growth or by wearing of reversed shoes

From Potter PA, Perry AG: *Basic nursing: theory and practice,* ed 3, St Louis, 1995, Mosby; data from McCance KL, Huether SE: *Pathophysiology: the biologic basis for disease in adults and children,* St Louis, 1990, Mosby.

other means of movement are available, and alternating periods of rest and activity.

NURSING PROCESS

Assessment

Assessment of body alignment can be performed with the patient standing, sitting, or lying. It is important for the nurse to put the patient at ease and identify the patient's learning needs for maintaining correct body alignment. The nurse should note trauma, muscle damage, or nerve dysfunction and obtain information about other factors that contribute to poor body alignment. These may include fatigue, malnutrition, and psychologic problems.

Nursing Diagnosis

The nurse reviews all data gathered during assessment. Clustering defining characteristics reveals a diagnosis. Nursing diagnoses are often related to the patient's ability to move. Possible diagnoses for improper body mechanics include the following:

Activity intolerance
Impaired gas exchange
Impaired physical mobility
Impaired skin integrity
Pain
Risk for disuse syndrome
Risk for injury
Sleep pattern disturbance

Planning

The plan of care is based on the patient's developmental stage, level of health, and lifestyle. It is important for the nurse to understand the patient's need for maintaining motor function and independence (see care plan on p. 394) Interventions should be individualized according to the level of risk to the patient. The nurse, patient, and members of the health care team should work together to determine the most effective ways to maintain optimal body alignment and mobility.

The plan of care may be based on one or more of the following goals and outcomes:

Goal #1: Patient increases activity tolerance.
Outcomes
Patient is less fatigued.
Patient's participation in self-care activities increases.

PATIENT TEACHING 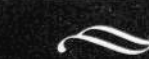

- Teach family members protective self-care when transferring a patient at home.
- Teach patients to exercise joints according to medical orders. Report complaints of discomfort immediately.

GERONTOLOGIC CONSIDERATIONS

- The older adult may experience loss of joint mobility and flexibility. Modification in normal transfer techniques may be necessary to protect the patient and the nurse.
- The older adult's skin is fragile and susceptible to injury. During transfer, the nurse should avoid pulling the older adult across the bed, which may cause tearing of the skin.

Goal #2: Patient remains free of bodily injury.
Outcome
Patient identifies factors that increase the risk of injury.

Implementation

While implementing these goals, the nurse can also assess the patient's readiness to learn and teach appropriate body mechanics (see teaching box). To maintain appropriate body alignment the nurse correctly lifts the patient, uses appropriate positioning techniques, and safely transfers the patient. Special care should be taken with the older adult (see gerontologic box).

Evaluation

The nurse evaluates the success of interventions by comparing the patient's response to the outcomes established for each nursing goal:

Goal #1: Patient increases activity tolerance.
Evaluative measures
Ask patient to rate fatigue on a scale of 1 to 10.
Ask patient about the number of activities involved in self-care.

Goal #2: Patient remains free of bodily injury.
Evaluative measure
Ask patient to list factors that increase the risk of injury.

POSITIONING, MOVING, AND LIFTING THE PATIENT

Positions

Positioning is performed often by the nurse. Many positions are used for the procedure, depending on the condition of the patient. To avoid complications the patient must be protected from injury at all times. The nurse should provide movement and comfort whenever possible. The nurse using the **dorsal (supine)** position places the patient on the back in appropriate body alignment. This position is used for comfort, position change, physical assessment, clinical assessment of the patient, changing of dressings, and talking or patient teaching.

In the **dorsal-recumbent** position, the patient is placed on the back with the legs flexed and slightly rotated outward. The position is used for pelvic examination, digital vaginal examination, female catheterization, perineal care, and douching.

The **semi-Fowler's** position supports the patient in a 45- to 60-degree (18- to 20-inch) sitting position with or without a pillow at the head. The patient's feet are elevated to prevent slipping down in the bed. The position is used for eating, enhancing breathing, reading, and talking. In the **high Fowler's** position the patient sits straight up in the bed at a 90-degree angle.

The **knee-chest (genupectoral)** position requires the patient to kneel so that the weight of the body is supported by the knees and chest, with the abdomen raised. The head is turned to one side and the arms flexed so that the upper body can be supported in part by the elbows. This position is used as an exercise to regain muscle tone for the recently delivered mother and for rectal examination.

The **lithotomy** position is assumed by the patient lying supine with the hips and knees flexed and the thighs abducted and rotated externally. The position is used for pelvic examination, vaginal hysterectomy, and other medical procedures. The patient is draped for privacy, with only the external genitalia exposed for examination.

The **orthopneic** position is used when a patient has difficulty breathing related to chronic obstructive pulmonary disease or severe heart disease. The patient is sitting up and is bent forward, with the arms supported on a table or chair arms.

When lying **prone,** the patient faces downward while lying flat on the abdomen. This may be a position for comfort or sleep. The arms are usually flexed toward the head.

In the **Sims'** position, the patient lies on the left side with the right knee and thigh drawn upward toward the chest. The chest and abdomen are allowed to fall forward. It is the position of choice for administering enemas or conducting rectal examinations.

Trendelenburg's position is one in which the head is low and the body and legs are on an inclined plane. It is sometimes used in pelvic surgery to displace the abdominal organs upward and out of the pelvis or to increase the flow of blood to the brain in hypotension and shock.

> **! REMEMBER**
>
> - Do not overtire the patient during ambulation.
> - Give the patient time to talk about ambulation needs.
> - Children on bedrest may be irritable because of restrained activity.
> - Older patients on bedrest are at risk for impaired skin integrity.

Moving and Lifting

The nurse is often required to assist in moving the patient. This includes lifting the patient up in bed, turning, dangling, and assisting the patient in and out of bed for ambulation (Skill 20-1). The nurse should assess patient mobility before moving. A patient should not be moved unless it is safe to do so. When in doubt, the nurse should request help from one or more co-workers.

Other techniques used by the nurse include using mechanical equipment for lifting the patient, such as the hydraulic lift and the Surgilift. Once the nurse knows that the patient can be moved, special devices may be used when positioning or moving the patient (Table 20-2).

These mechanical devices, such as the hydraulic lift used with a Hoyer Patient Lifter (Fig. 20-4), are used for moving patients safely, protecting the

Table 20-2 **DEVICES USED FOR APPROPRIATE POSITIONING**

Device	Uses
Pillow	Provides support of body or extremity, elevates body part, splints incisional area to reduce postoperative pain during activity or coughing and deep breathing
Foot boot	Maintains feet in dorsiflexion
Trochanter roll	Prevents external rotation of legs when patient is in supine position
Sandbag	Provides support and shape to body contours, immobilizes extremity, maintains specific body alignment
Hand roll	Maintains thumb slightly adducted and in opposition to fingers, maintains fingers in slightly flexed position
Hand-wrist splint	Is individually molded for patient to maintain appropriate alignment of thumb, is slightly adducted in opposition to fingers, maintains wrist in slight dorsiflexion
Trapeze bar	Enables patient to raise trunk from bed, enables patient to transfer from bed to wheelchair, allows patient to perform exercises that strengthen upper arms
Side rail	Allows weak patient to roll from side to side or to sit up in bed
Bed board	Provides additional support to mattress and improves vertebral alignment

From Potter PA, Perry AG: *Basic nursing: theory and practice,* ed 3, St Louis, 1995, Mosby.

nurse's back, and avoiding lifting the patient's total weight. Agency policy is followed for use of the lift. The nurse may use the lift for moving a patient to a chair, onto a stretcher, and into the bathtub.

Range-of-Motion Exercises

A joint's **range of motion (ROM)** is its range of movement. If **immobility** (inability to move about freely) occurs, complications that eventually prevent movement may occur. Every person is different in how long it takes for immobility to affect the joints, causing problems with activities of daily living. Range-of-motion exercises are used for patients confined to bed for long periods. These exercises may be performed passively by the nurse or physical therapist or actively by the patient. The process includes the range of movement of a joint, from maximum extension to maximum flexion, as measured in degrees of a circle (Skill 20-2).

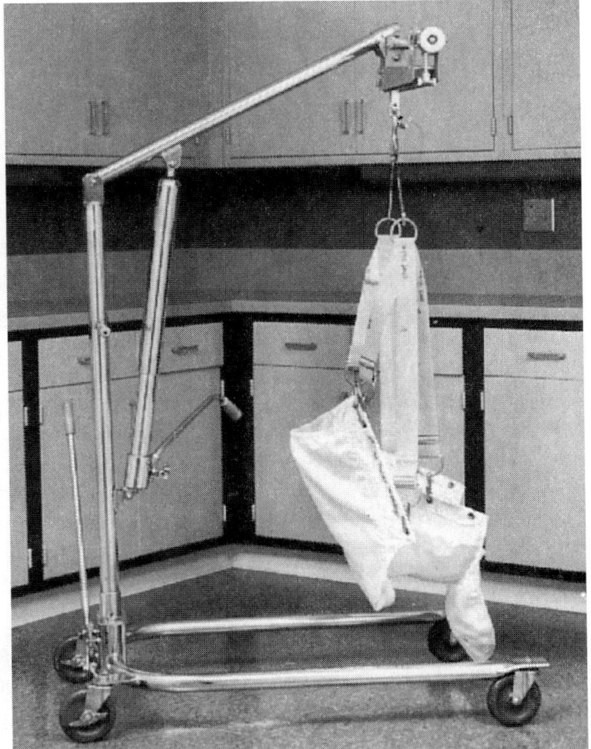

Fig. 20-4 Hoyer sling used with hydraulic lift. (From Perry AG, Potter PA: *Clinical nursing skills and techniques,* ed 3, St Louis, 1994, Mosby.)

■ NURSING CARE PLAN ■

IMPAIRED PHYSICAL MOBILITY

Mr. P, age 71, has been admitted because he is unable to care for himself because of decreased muscle strength affecting physical movement.

NURSING DIAGNOSIS

Impaired physical mobility related to neuromuscular impairment as evidenced by decreased endurance, inability to purposefully move, and limited range of motion

GOALS

- Patient will care for self.

EXPECTED OUTCOMES

- Patient will maintain muscle strength and joint range of motion.
- Patient or family members will perform mobility regimen.

NURSING INTERVENTIONS

- Perform range-of-motion exercises every 8 hr to prevent contracture of joints and muscle atrophy (wasting or diminution of size).
- Turn and place in appropriate alignment every 2 hr all three shifts to prevent impaired skin integrity.
- Encourage independence in movement by assisting when necessary to increase muscle tone.

EVALUATION

- Patient maintains muscle strength.
- Patient shows no evidence of contracture.
- Patient walks down hall and back with only arm assistance.

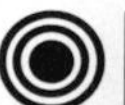

SKILL 20-1 POSITIONING, MOVING, AND LIFTING THE PATIENT

Steps	Rationale
POSITIONING THE PATIENT	
1. Obtain equipment: ▪ Gloves ▪ Pillows	Helps organize procedure.
2. Refer to medical record, care plan, or Kardex for special interventions.	Provides basis for care.
3. Introduce self.	Decreases anxiety level.
4. Identify patient by identification band.	Identifies correct patient for procedure.
5. Explain procedure to patient.	Seeks cooperation and decreases anxiety.
6. Wash hands and don clean gloves according to agency policy and guidelines from Centers for Disease Control and Prevention and Occupational Safety and Health Administration.	Helps prevent cross-contamination.
7. Prepare patient for intervention:	
a. Close door to room or pull curtain.	Provides privacy.
b. Drape for procedure if necessary.	Prevents exposure of patient.
8. Raise bed to comfortable working level.	Provides safety for nurse.
9. Arrange for patient privacy.	Shows respect for patient.
10. Place patient in dorsal (supine) position (Fig. 20-5):	
a. Move patient and mattress to head of bed and remove pillow.	Centers patient for movement.
b. Lower head of bed unless contraindicated.	Provides for patient safety.
c. Turn patient onto back.	Positions patient for moving.
d. Replace pillow.	Provides for patient comfort.

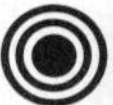

SKILL 20-1 POSITIONING, MOVING, AND LIFTING THE PATIENT—cont'd

Steps	Rationale
11. Place patient in dorsal-recumbent-position (Fig. 20-6):	
a. Move patient and mattress to head of bed and remove pillow.	Centers patient for movement.
b. Lower head of bed unless contraindicated.	Provides for patient safety.
c. Turn patient onto back.	Positions patient for moving.
d. Assist patient to raise legs, bend knees, and allow legs to relax.	Positions patient.
e. Replace pillow.	Provides for patient comfort.
12. Place patient in Fowler's position (Fig. 20-7):	
a. Move patient and mattress to head of bed and remove pillow.	Centers patient for moving.
b. Raise head of bed to 45 to 60 degrees.	Aids in appropriate positioning.
c. Replace pillow.	Provides for patient comfort.
d. Raise foot of bed no more 15 degrees.	Prevents pressure in popliteal area.

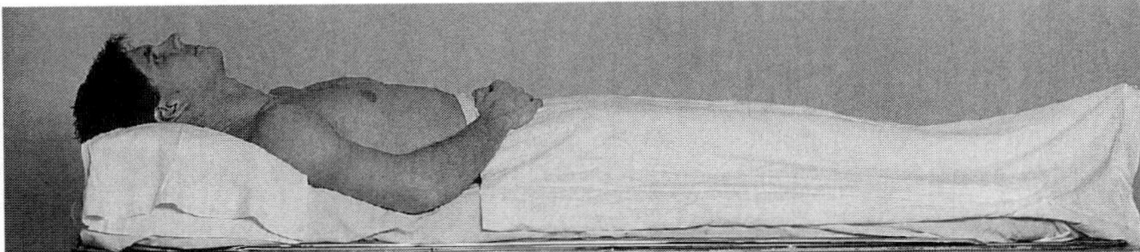

Fig. 20-5 Dorsal or supine position. (From Christensen BL, Kockrow EO: *Foundations of nursing,* ed 2, St Louis, 1995, Mosby.)

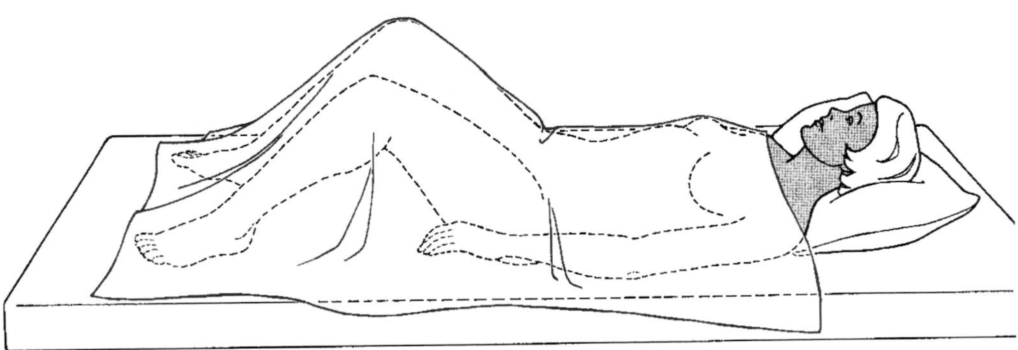

Fig. 20-6 Dorsal-recumbent position. (From Christensen BL, Kockrow EO: *Foundations of nursing,* ed 2, St Louis, 1995, Mosby.)

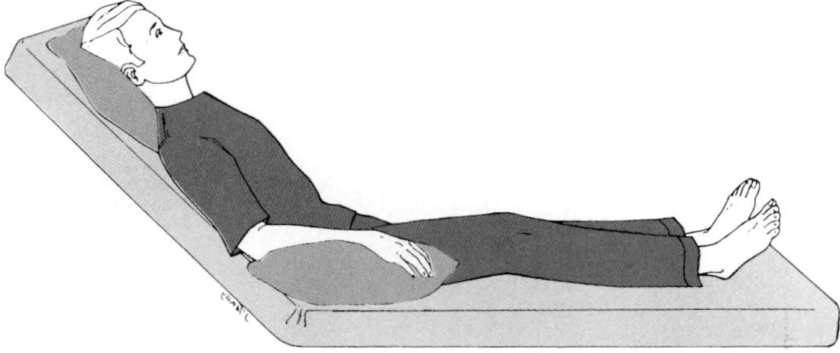

Fig. 20-7 Fowler's position. (From Christensen BL, Kockrow EO: *Foundations of nursing,* ed 2, St Louis, 1995, Mosby.)

Continued.

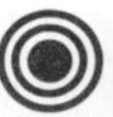

SKILL 20-1 POSITIONING, MOVING, AND LIFTING THE PATIENT—cont'd

Steps	Rationale
13. Place patient in knee-chest position (Fig. 20-8):	
a. Turn patient onto abdomen.	Facilitates positioning.
b. Assist patient to kneeling position. Position patient's arms and head on pillow while upper chest rests on bed.	Completes positioning.
14. Place patient in lithotomy position (Fig. 20-9):	
a. Request patient to move buttocks to edge of examining table.	Facilitates positioning.
b. Have patient lift both legs, bend knees, and place feet in stirrups at the same time.	Positions patient for examination.
c. Drape patient.	Provides privacy and prevents exposure.
15. Place patient in orthopneic position:	
a. Elevate head of bed to 90 degrees.	Facilitates positioning.
b. Place pillow between patient's back and mattress.	Provides back support.
c. Place pillow on overbed table and assist patient to lean over, placing head on pillow.	Eases patient's breathing.
16. Place patient in prone position (Fig. 20-10):	
a. Assist patient onto abdomen with face to one side.	Positions patient.
b. Flex arms toward head.	Provides appropriate body alignment.

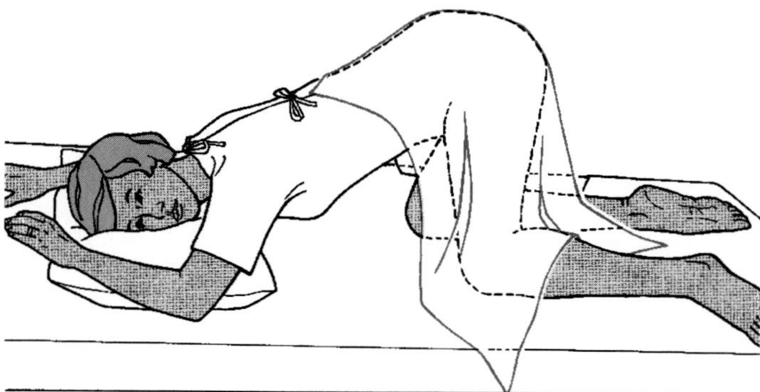

Fig. 20-8 Knee-chest (genupectoral) position. (From Christensen BL, Kockrow EO: *Foundations of nursing,* ed 2, St Louis, 1995, Mosby.)

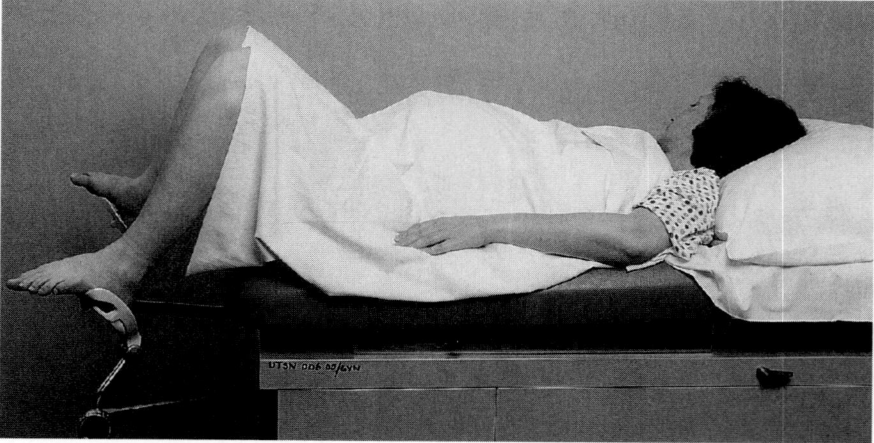

Fig. 20-9 Lithotomy position. (From Christensen BL, Kockrow EO: *Foundations of nursing,* ed 2, St Louis, 1995, Mosby.)

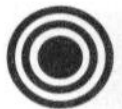

SKILL 20-1 POSITIONING, MOVING, AND LIFTING THE PATIENT—cont'd

Steps	Rationale
17. Place patient in semi-Fowler's position:	
a. Move patient and mattress to to head of bed and remove pillow.	Centers patient for movement.
b. Raise head of bed to about 30 degrees.	Provides appropriate positioning.
c. Replace pillow.	Provides for patient comfort.
d. Slightly raise foot of bed.	Helps prevent patient from slipping down in bed.
18. Place patient in Sims' position (Fig. 20-11):	
a. Move patient and mattress to head of bed and remove pillow.	Centers patient for movement.
b. Turn patient to right side.	Initiates position placement.
c. Assist patient to draw left knee and thigh up near abdomen.	Provides appropriate position for for enema.
d. Place patient's right arm along back.	Provides appropriate body alignment.
e. Allow patient to lean forward to rest on chest.	Provides for patient comfort.
19. Place patient in Trendelenburg position:	
a. Place patient's head lower than body with body and legs elevated on incline (bed may be elevated on blocks).	Indicates position for treating shock (unless head injury) and for performing some abdominal surgeries.
20. Remove gloves and wash hands.	Helps prevent cross-contamination.
MOVING THE PATIENT	
21. Obtain equipment: ▪ Hospital bed ▪ Chair ▪ Siderails ▪ Patient's slippers ▪ Cotton blanket ▪ Pillows ▪ Clean gloves ▪ Extra personnel if necessary	Helps organize procedure.
22. Lift and move patient up in bed:	
a. Place patient in supine position with head flat.	Provides less resistance on flat surface.
b. Face side of bed and provide base of support.	Protects nurse's back.
c. For one-nurse move, place one arm under patient's axilla and opposite arm under patient's shoulder and neck.	Provides for patient support and safety.
d. For two-nurse move, place one arm under patient's head and opposite shoulder and other arm under patient's thigh.	Prevents injury to patient and nurse.
e. Request that patient flex knees and push up with feet on count of 3.	Protects nurse's back and promotes patient mobility.
f. On count of 3, pull patient up to head of bed with minimum friction.	Moves patient in unison, promotes safely, and prevents shearing and friction forces.

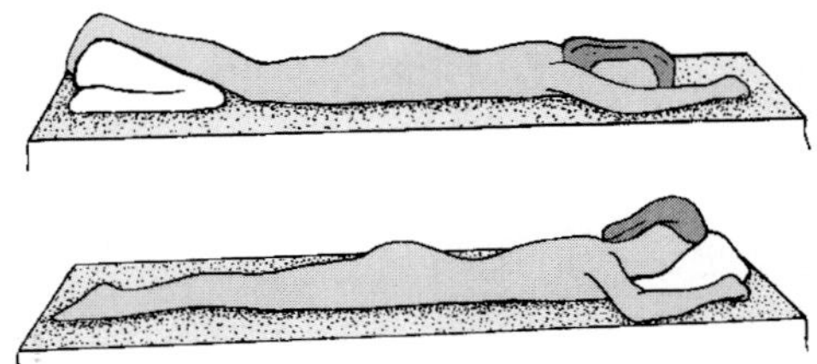

Fig. 20-10 Prone position. (From Christensen BL, Kockrow EO: *Foundations of nursing,* ed 2, St Louis, 1995, Mosby.)

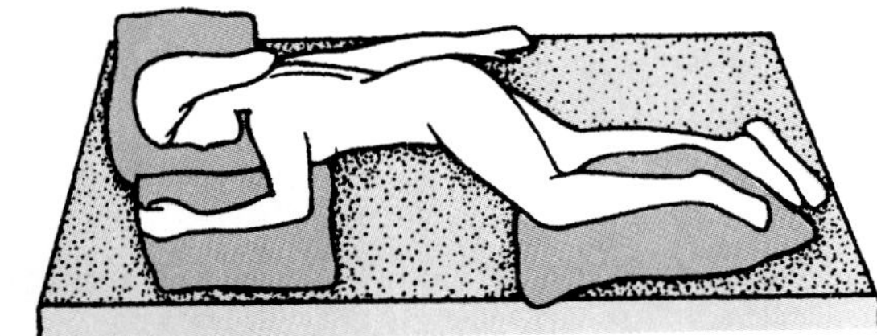

Fig. 20-11 Sims' position. (From Christensen BL, Kockrow EO: *Foundations of nursing,* ed 2, St Louis, 1995, Mosby.)

Continued.

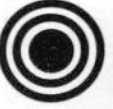

SKILL 20-1 POSITIONING, MOVING, AND LIFTING THE PATIENT—cont'd

Steps	Rationale
23. Turn patient:	
a. Stand with feet slightly apart and flex knees.	Provides patient safety and support.
b. Place arm under patient's neck and shoulders and opposite arm under patient's waist.	Provides for patient safety.
c. Pull patient *toward* nurse.	Reduces strain on patient and nurse.
d. Turn patient on side facing nurse and raise side rail.	Prevents patient fall.
e. Flex one leg over the other (Fig. 20-12).	Reduces pressure on legs.
f. Align shoulders.	Ensures appropriate body alignment.
g. Support back with pillows if necessary.	Helps keep patient in position desired.
h. Assess body alignment by standing at foot of bed and looking straight at patient.	Provides for patient safety and comfort and depicts any part of body out of alignment.
24. Logroll patient:	
a. Have three nurses stand side by side by side of bed.	Provides for patient safety.
b. Have one nurse place arms under legs, second nurse place arms under buttocks, and third nurse place arms under chest, shoulders, and neck (Fig. 20-13).	Ensures that patient is turned like a log is rolled.

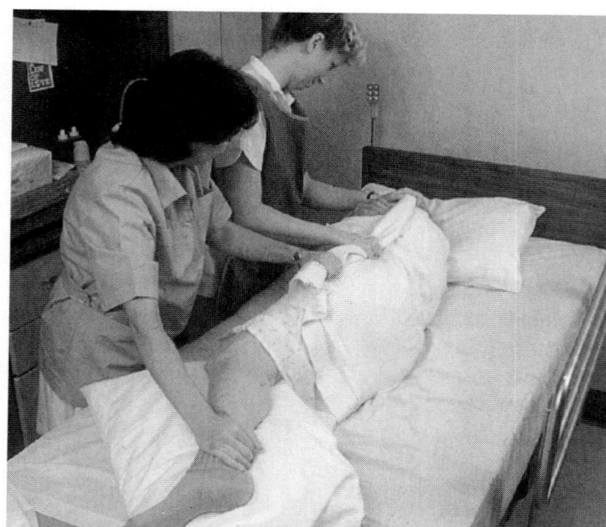

Fig. 20-12 Turning the patient and flexing one leg over the other. (From Christensen BL, Kockrow EO: *Foundations of nursing,* ed 2, St Louis, 1995, Mosby.)

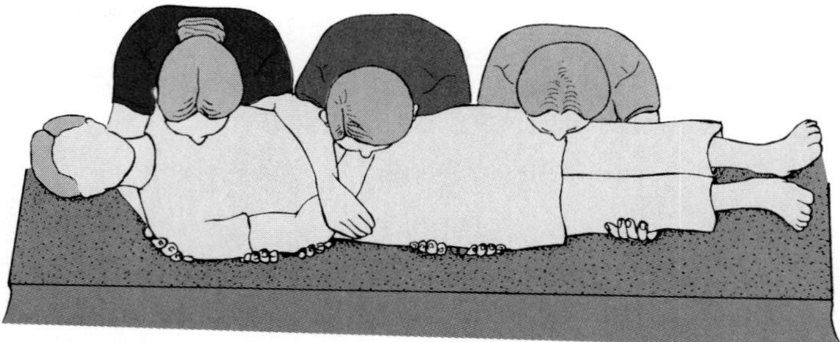

Fig. 20-13 Logrolling the patient. (From Perry AG, Potter PA: *Clinical nursing skills and techniques,* ed 3, St Louis, 1994, Mosby.)

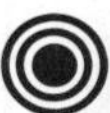

SKILL 20-1 POSITIONING, MOVING, AND LIFTING THE PATIENT—cont'd

Steps	Rationale
c. Have nurse nearest patient's head give prearranged signal to turn patient at exact time.	Ensures patient movement in unison.
d. Make patient comfortable.	Provides for patient comfort.
25. Transfer patient from bed to straight chair or wheelchair:	
a. Place chair beside bed with seat facing foot of bed.	Provides easy access to chair.
b. Lock wheelchair.	Provides patient safety.
c. Place straight chair against wall or have another nurse hold chair.	Prevents patient from falling.
d. Lower bed to lowest position.	Provides for patient safety.
e. Raise head of bed.	Helps patient to easily swing around to sit up.
f. Support patient's shoulder and help patient to swing legs around and off bed. Perform all in one motion (Fig. 20-14).	Prevents patient strain.
g. Assist patient to don robe and slippers.	Prevents chilling.
h. Stand directly in front of patient and place hands under patient's axillae.	Prepares for move to chair.
i. Assist patient to stand and swing around with back toward seat of chair.	Provides for patient safety.
j. Assist patient to sit down as nurse bends knees to assist process.	Prevents patient from slipping and falling.
k. Apply blanket to legs if needed.	Provides warmth.
26. Use lift for moving patient:	
a. Secure appropriate number of personnel to assist.	Provides for patient safety.
b. Place chair near bed (heavy chair if available).	Provides easy access to chair.
c. Raise bed to maximum height.	Assists in use of appropriate body mechanics for personnel.
d. Place canvas seat evenly under patient.	Provides support and safety of patient.
e. Slide horseshoe-shaped bar under bed on one side.	Places lift near bed.
f. Lower horizontal bar to level of sling by releasing hydraulic valve and lock valve.	Places lift near patient.
g. Fasten hooks on chain to holes in sling.	Attaches lift to sling seat.
h. Raise head of bed.	Places patient in sitting position.
i. Fold patient's arms over chest.	Prevents injury to patient's arms.
j. Pump lift-handle until patient is raised off bed.	Ensures patient safety.
k. With steering handle, pull lift off bed and down to chair.	Places patient safely in chair.
l. Release valve *slowly* to left and lower patient to chair.	Places patient in chair little at a time to prevent feeling like falling.
m. Close off valve and release straps.	Prevents patient injury.
n. Remove straps and lift.	Provides for comfort.
27. Remove gloves and wash hands.	Helps prevent cross-contamination.

Continued.

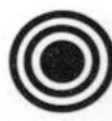

SKILL 20-1 POSITIONING, MOVING, AND LIFTING THE PATIENT—cont'd

Steps	Rationale

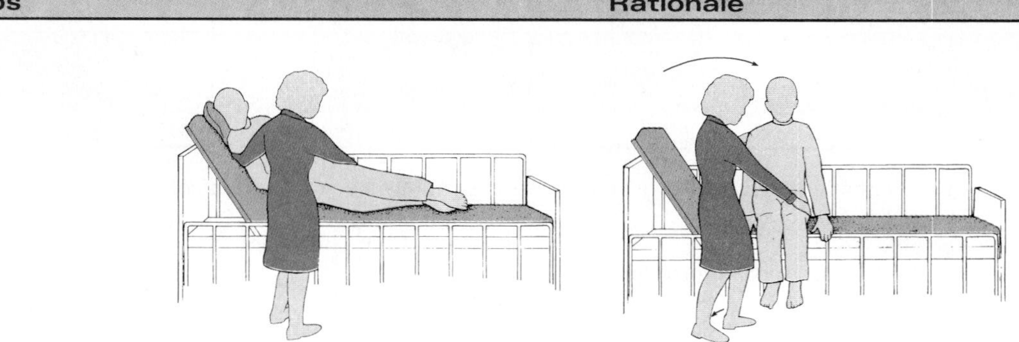

Fig. 20-14 Transferring the patient from a bed to chair or wheelchair. The nurse is supporting the patient's shoulder and helping to swing the legs around and off the bed all in one motion. (From Perry AG, Potter PA: *Clinical nursing skills and techniques,* ed 3, St Louis, 1994, Mosby.)

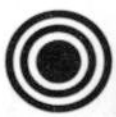

SKILL 20-2 PERFORMING PASSIVE RANGE-OF-MOTION EXERCISES

Steps	Rationale
1. Obtain equipment: ▪ Clean gloves	Helps organize procedure.
2. Refer to medical record, care plan, or Kardex for special interventions.	Provides basis for care.
3. Introduce self.	Decreases anxiety level.
4. Identify patient by identification band.	Identifies correct patient for procedure.
5. Explain procedure to patient.	Seeks cooperation and decreases anxiety.
6. Wash hands and don clean gloves according to agency policy and guidelines from Centers for Disease Control and Prevention and Occupational Safety and Health Administration.	Helps prevent cross-contamination.
7. Prepare patient for intervention:	
a. Close door to room or pull curtain.	Provides privacy.
b. Drape for procedure if necessary.	Prevents exposure of patient.
8. Raise bed to comfortable working level.	Provides safety for nurse.
9. Arrange for patient privacy.	Shows respect for patient.
10. Assist patient by putting each joint through full range of motion (Table 20-3).	Provides baseline for joint movement.
11. Adjust bed linen.	Provides comfort and privacy.
12. Remove gloves and wash hands.	Helps prevent cross-contamination.
13. Document.	Documents procedure and patient's response.

Table 20-3 RANGE OF JOINT MOTION EXERCISES

Body Part	Type of Joint	Type of Movement
Neck and cervical spine	Pivotal	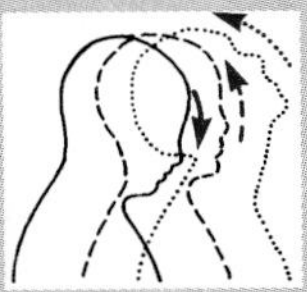 Flexion: bring chin to rest on chest Extension: return head to erect position. Hyperextension: bend head back as far as possible.
		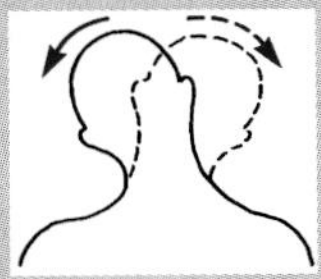 Lateral flexion: tilt head as far as possible toward each shoulder.
		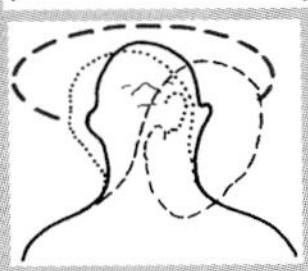 Rotation: turn head as far as possible to right and left.
Shoulder	Ball and socket	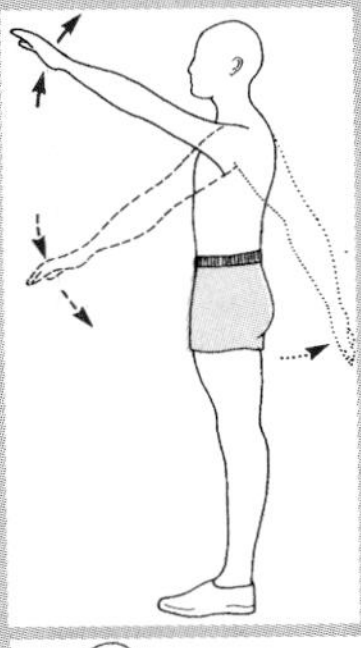 Flexion: raise arm from side position forward to position above head. Extension: return arm to position at side of body. Hyperextension: move arm behind body, keeping elbow straight.
		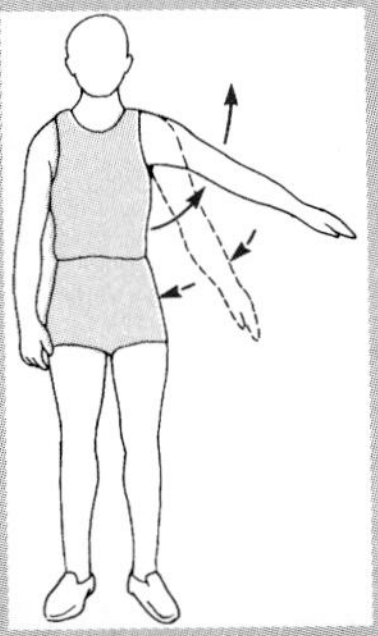 Abduction: raise arm to side to position above head with palm away from head. Adduction: lower arm sideways and across body as far as possible.
		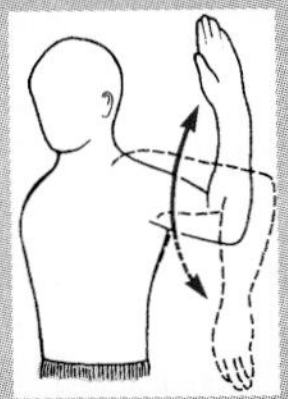 Internal rotation: with elbow flexed, rotate shoulder by moving arm until thumb is turned inward and toward back. External rotation: with elbow flexed, move arm until thumb is upward and lateral to head.
		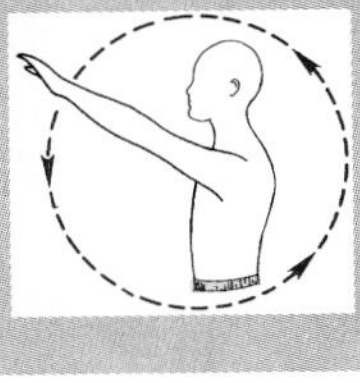 Circumduction: move arm in full circle. (Circumduction is combination of all movements of ball-and-socket joint.)
Elbow	Hinge	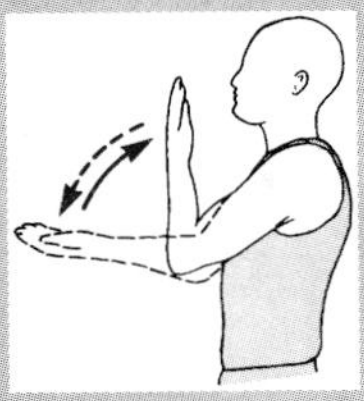 Flexion: bend elbow so that lower arm moves toward its shoulder joint and hand is level with shoulder Extension: straighten elbow by lowering hand. Hyperextension: bend lower arm back as far as possible.
Forearm	Pivotal	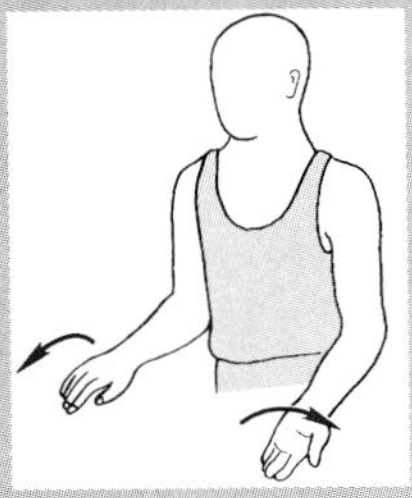 Supination: turn lower arm and hand so that palm is up. Pronation: turn lower arm so that palm is down.
Wrist	Condyloid	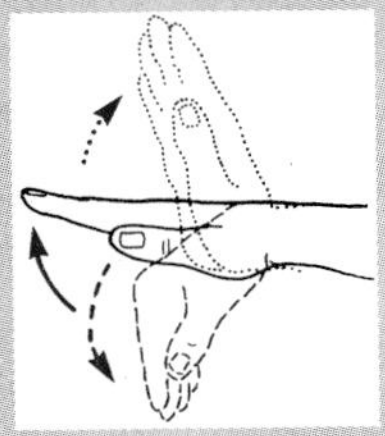 Flexion: move palm toward inner aspect of forearm. Extension: move fingers so that fingers, hands, and forearm are in same plane. Hyperextension: bring dorsal surface to hand back as far as possible.
		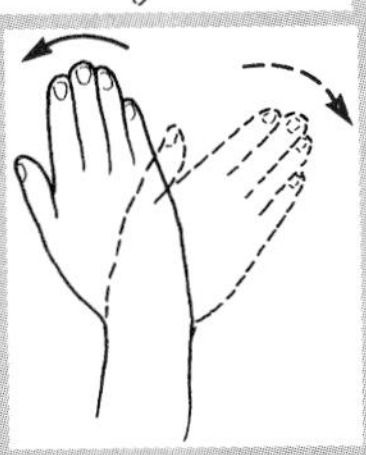 Radial flexion: bend wrist medially toward thumb. Ulnar flexion: bend wrist laterally toward fifth finger.
Fingers	Condyloid hinge	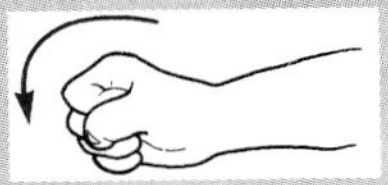 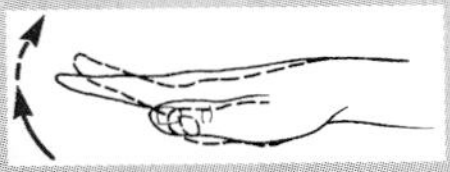 Flexion: make fist. Extension: straighten fingers. Hyperextension: bend fingers back as far as possible.
		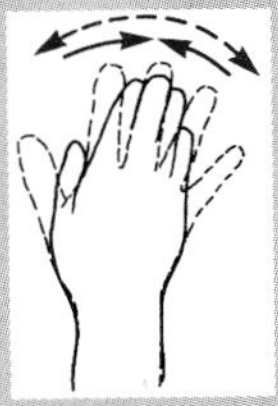 Abduction: spread fingers apart. Adduction: bring fingers together.

From Potter PA, Perry AG: *Basic nursing: theory and practice,* ed 3, St. Louis, 1995, Mosby.

Continued.

Table 20-3 RANGE OF JOINT MOTION EXERCISES—cont'd

Body Part	Type of Joint	Type of Movement
Thumb	Saddle	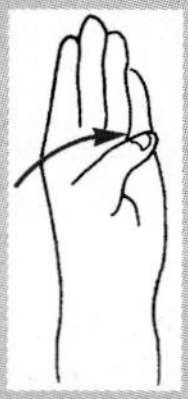 Flexion: move thumb across palmar surface of hand. Extension: move thumb straight away from hand.
		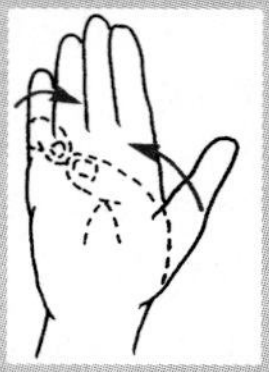 Abduction: extend thumb laterally (usually done when placing fingers in abduction and adduction). Adduction: move thumb back toward hand. Opposition: touch thumb to each finger of same hand.
Hip	Ball and socket	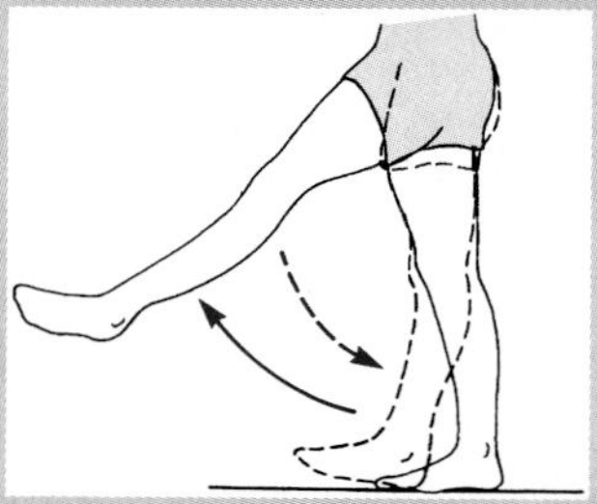 Flexion: move leg forward and up. Extension: move leg back beside other leg.
		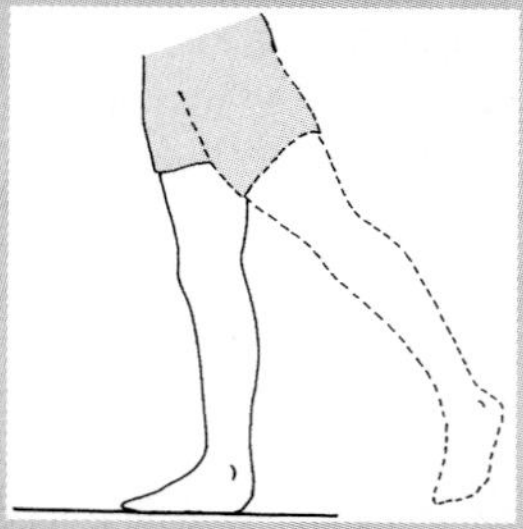 Hyperextension: move leg behind body.
		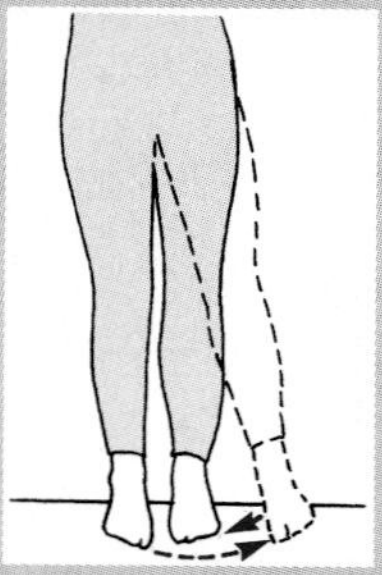 Abduction: move leg laterally away from body. Adduction: move leg back toward medial position and beyond if possible.
		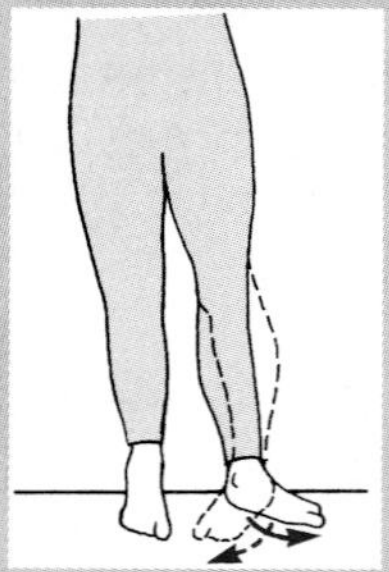 Internal rotation: turn foot and leg toward other leg. External rotation: turn foot and leg away from other leg.
		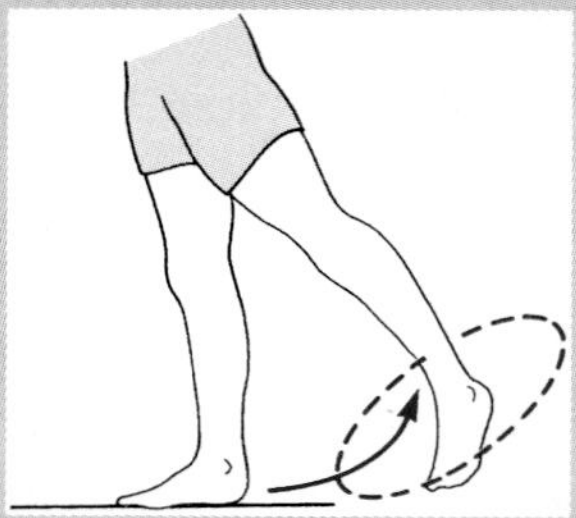 Circumduction: move leg in circle.
Knee	Hinge	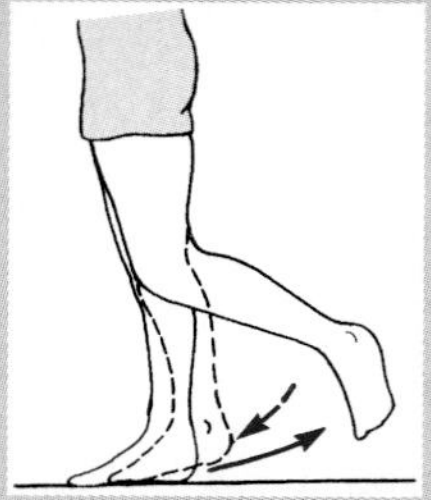 Flexion: bring heel back toward back of thigh. Extension: return heel to floor.
Ankle	Hinge	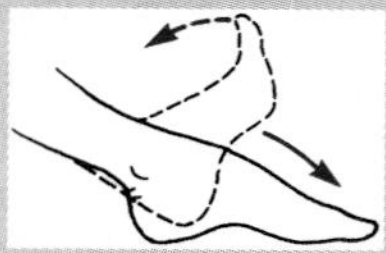 Dorsal flexion: move foot so that toes are pointed upward. Plantar flexion: move foot so that toes are pointed downward.
Foot	Gliding	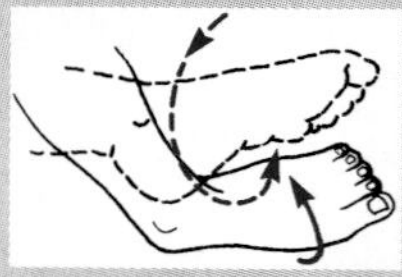 Inversion: turn sole of foot medially. Eversion: turn sole of foot laterally.
Toes	Condyloid	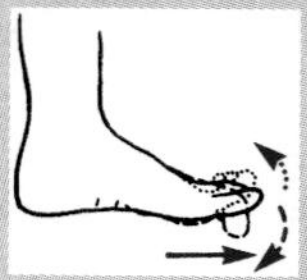 Flexion: curl toes downward. Extension: straighten toes.
		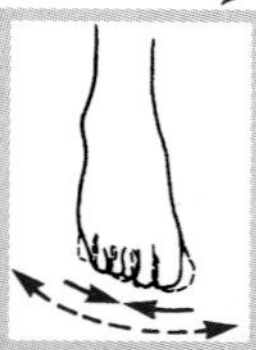 Abduction: spread toes apart. Adduction: bring toes together.

SUMMARY

The use of appropriate body mechanics protects both the patient and the nurse from injury. The nurse should learn self-protection as well as teach the patient appropriate body mechanics. Bending the knees is one of the most important aspects of protecting the back while lifting, moving, and providing nursing care. Maintaining balance and posture supports the body's weight when standing or sitting. Range-of-motion exercises for the patient should be performed by the nurse or physical therapist to prevent contractures.

Key Concepts

- The use of appropriate body mechanics helps the nurse perform nursing care.
- Body alignment of the patient should be maintained by the nurse.
- The nurse should use a wide base of support when stooping, lifting, or moving a patient.
- The more muscle groups used, the better the distribution of the workload.
- The nurse should know how all positions are used for placing patients.
- Range-of-motion exercises may be performed passively by the nurse or actively by the patient.

Critical Thinking Questions

1. Identify the appropriate placement of equipment, position of the patient, and movement of the nurse in the following situations:
   a. The nurse is helping a patient walk to the bathroom, and the patient states that he or she feels faint and starts to fall to the floor.
   b. The nurse is moving a heavy patient from a stretcher to the bed.
2. Mr. Kauffman, 69, is being released from the hospital today. He is going home with his daughter, who will be caring for him. He will be confined to bed. List and discuss the guidelines that the nurse will give to Mr. Kauffman's daughter concerning body mechanics.

REFERENCES AND SUGGESTED READINGS

Christensen BL, Kockrow EO: *Foundations of nursing,* ed 2, St Louis, 1995, Mosby.

Lewis C, Knortz KA: *Orthopedic assessment and treatment of the geriatric patient,* St Louis, 1991, Mosby.

Mosby's medical, nursing, & allied health dictionary, ed 4, St Louis, 1994, Mosby.

Mourad LM: *Orthopedic disorders: Mosby's clinical nursing series,* St Louis, 1991, Mosby.

Perry AG, Potter AG: *Clinical nursing skills and techniques,* ed 3, St Louis, 1994, Mosby.

Potter PA, Perry AG: *Basic nursing: theory and practice,* ed 3, St Louis, 1995, Mosby.

Sahrmann S: *Diagnosis and exercise management of musculoskeletal pain syndromes,* St Louis, 1995, Mosby.

UNIT IV

BASIC PATIENT NEEDS

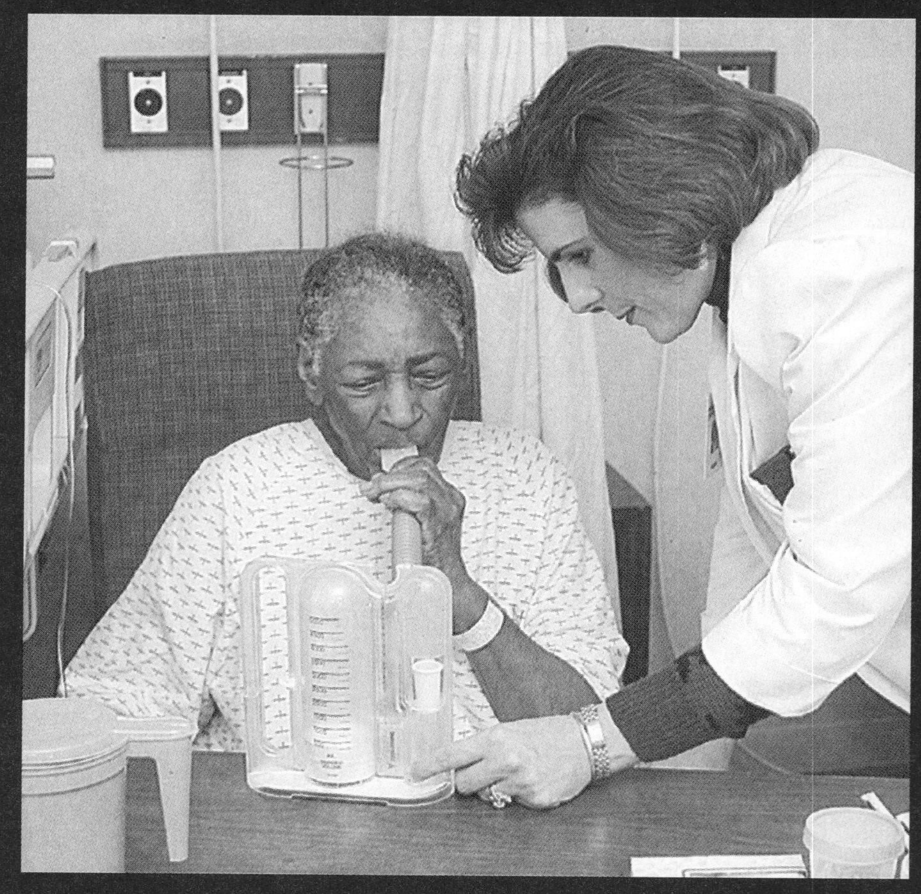

CHAPTER 21

Skin Integrity

Learning Objectives

After studying this chapter, the student should be able to . . .

- Define the key terms.
- State the impact of pressure ulcers on health care.
- Describe the pathophysiologic changes caused by a pressure ulcer.
- Discuss several factors predisposing to a pressure ulcer.
- Describe the four stages of pressure ulcer development.
- Describe nursing management of the stages of a pressure ulcer.
- Describe nursing interventions to maintain skin integrity.
- List the types of dressings used in pressure ulcer management.
- Describe the surgical management of pressure ulcers.

Key Terms

Blanching
Bony prominence
Dependent edema
Enterostomal therapist
Eschar
Friction
Granulation tissue
Hydrophilic dressing
Hydrophobic dressing
Hyperemia
Hypoxia
Ischemia
Necrosis
Negative nitrogen balance
Pressure point
Pressure ulcer
Shearing force
Skin graft

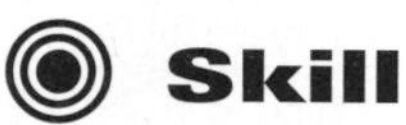

21-1 Caring for a pressure ulcer

Healthy, intact skin provides a boundary for the organs and fluids of the body and a defense against allergens, pathogens, ultraviolet radiation, and other harmful agents (Flory, 1992). An intact skin is a patient's protection against these agents and infection. The skin is the first line of defense against microorganisms. Providing nursing care that promotes the integrity of the skin is a primary focus of nursing.

PRESSURE ULCERS

As the age of the general population increases, nurses increasingly deal with patients who have multiple health problems and are immobile for longer periods. Increased immobility (bedrest) subjects a patient to prolonged periods of pressure to body areas and irritation of the skin, which may result in pressure ulcers. A **pressure ulcer** is a lesion caused by unrelieved pressure resulting in damage to the underlying tissue (National Pressure Ulcer Advisory Panel [NPUAP], 1989).

A pressure ulcer has been documented by the names *pressure sore, decubitus ulcer,* and *bedsore.* These terms describe skin that becomes red and broken in bedridden or are immobile patients. Patients particularly susceptible to pressure ulcers are stroke patients, older patients with chronic conditions, patients with casts, and patients with circulatory problems. The NPUAP recommends the term *pressure ulcer* for skin problems related to prolonged pressure (Potter, Perry, 1995).

NURSING PROCESS AND PRESSURE ULCERS

Assessment

The nurse should perform an assessment to locate problems of common pressure sites. Appropriate

PATIENT TEACHING

- Explain why patient cooperation is important for turning and positioning.
- Teach preventive care measures to reduce hazards to the patient's skin, such as staying off certain body areas for extended periods of time.
- Demonstrate appropriate skin care to the patient and family.

lighting is needed to see sites well. The environment should not be hot or cold. Each pressure area should be inspected for hyperema, abrasions, ischemia, edema, and warmth. If a pressure ulcer is discovered, the nurse should assess the lesion for location and size. The depth as well as the width should be measured. The nurse should also assess the stage of the ulcer, color of the wound bed, and presence of necrosis. Assessment should also be made for signs of infection, condition of the wound edges, amount of time the lesion has been known to exist, and any previously used treatments (Flory, 1992).

Nursing Diagnosis

The nurse reviews data gathered during assessment and clusters defining characteristics to reveal a diagnosis. Possible nursing diagnoses related to skin integrity include the following:
Altered nutrition: less than body requirements
Impaired physical mobility
Impaired skin integrity
Impaired tissue integrity
Risk for impaired skin integrity
Risk for infection
Sensory/perceptual alterations: tactile

Planning

In developing the plan of care, the nurse should focus on maintaining the patient's skin integrity and preventing complications. Goals should be aimed at reducing or preventing impaired skin integrity. The nurse must establish priorities based on the patient's activity tolerance and developmental stage (see care plan on p. 419). The patient and family should participate in planning care and setting goals. The nurse may use this opportunity to teach health-promotion practices (see teaching box).

The plan of care may be based on one or more of the following goals:

Goal #1: Skin pressure and friction are avoided.
Outcome
Patient's skin is intact.

GERONTOLOGIC CONSIDERATIONS

- Circulatory changes and decreased mobility increase the risk of pressure ulcers.
- Physiologic changes make the skin of the older adult more fragile and susceptible to impairment.
- A decrease in tissue fluid, subcutaneous fat, and sebaceous secretions in the older adult results in dryness, flaking, itching, loss of elasticity, and a wrinkled appearance.
- An older adult's perception of pain may be decreased because of a decrease in the number of cutaneous end organs responsible for the sensations of pressure and touch.

Goal #2: Patient's nutritional intake improves.
Outcome
Patient's weight returns to ideal body weight.

Implementation

Nursing interventions should focus on preventing or treating pressure ulcers. Turning schedules should be established when a patient is immobile. The skin should be promptly cleaned and dried after soiling. Special care should be taken when providing nursing care for the older adult (see gerontologic box).

Evaluation

The nurse evaluates the success of interventions and determines whether expected outcomes have been met. The nurse must always be prepared to revise to the care plan based on the evaluation. Examples of goals and evaluative measures include the following:

Goal #1: Patient avoids pressure and friction to the skin.
Evaluative measure
Observe and palpate patient's skin.

Goal #2: Patient's nutritional intake improves.
Evaluative measure
Weigh patient daily.

HEALTH CARE COSTS

The prevention of pressure ulcers is a major priority in the nursing care of patients. Studies indicate that the occurrence of pressure ulcers varies from 3% to 14% in health care settings. The incidence increases as the high-risk indicators such as age, immobility, incontinence, and chronic disease are included in the data (Ferrell et al, 1993).

Pressure ulcers have an impact on the cost of health care. According to research, pressure ulcers increase the length and thus cost of a hospital stay and also increase the cost of home nursing care. However, defining the exact cost or cost range has been difficult. The treatment of a pressure ulcer depends on the health status and commitment of each patient as well as continuity of care. Ferrell et al (1993) estimate the increased cost to be between $4000 and $40,000. For these reasons, nurses must find ways to identify and prevent rather than treat pressure ulcers.

Preventive equipment should be reviewed and the best equipment used to meet needs of each patient with pressure ulcers. The health care facility should educate the staff in the correct use of the equipment and related hygiene measures. The implementation of a prevention program can also be expensive (Bolander, 1994).

PATHOPHYSIOLOGY

Pressure ulcers usually occur over the bony prominences of the body (Fig. 21-1). **Bony prominences** are areas where bones are close to the skin's surface. These areas, called ***pressure points,*** are prone to breakdown because they are not flat or adapted for bearing weight for prolonged periods.

A person's weight when lying down is not distributed over the entire body (Bolander, 1994). The extra weight compresses the soft tissue between the body and the mattress or surface involved. The increased pressure blocks the blood flow to the pressure point, causing **ischemia** (decreased blood flow). Ischemia causes damage to the tissue at the pressure points, ultimately leading to **necrosis** (death) of the underlying tissue (Lewis, Collier, 1992).

Pressure ulcers are a direct result of ischemia. The decreased blood flow decreases cellular metabolism, which slows or stops nutrition (oxygen and glucose) to the area. Slower metabolism causes a buildup of waste products in the blood and involved tissue. As the blood flow to the area decreases, blanching results. **Blanching** is a decrease in color to the area. The involved skin looks pale in people with light complexions, but in people with dark skin, the area may take on a grayish hue, resembling ashes in a fireplace (Beare, Myers, 1994). The pressure on the skin should be removed as soon as the area is located and the blood flow reestablished. If this is not done, the tissue in the area becomes **hyperemic** (engorged with blood, causing redness and warmth). Under normal conditions, skin color returns to normal when pressure is removed. In the patient with impaired skin integrity, if the skin remains red longer than 10 minutes, the positioning schedule for the patient should be reassessed and the patient should be positioned more frequently. Skin remaining red for longer than 30 minutes usually indicates that permanent damage has occurred (Berger, Williams, 1992).

Two other factors, friction and shearing force, frequently combine with pressure to cause ulcers. **Friction** is a force acting parallel to the skin and is created when the patient pulls up in bed. The skin rubs against the sheet, creating friction. When this happens, the superficial layers of the skin may be removed, making the skin more prone to breakdown and infection (Ignatavicius, Workman, Mishler, 1995).

When a patient slides to the foot of the bed with the head of the bed elevated, a shearing force is created. The weight of the body presses down on the skin covering the sacral area, which area does not move because of the friction between the skin and sheets. As the skin and superficial vessels remain stationary in relation to the surface of the bed, the deeper tissues remain firmly attached to the skeleton and bone. This causes a **shearing force** between the superficial and the deeper tissues. The increased downward pressure constricts the flow of blood to the tissues underneath. As a result, the outward tissue may look normal, but the deep tissue is damaged and eventually becomes necrotic (Burrell, 1992).

Stages

The stages of pressure ulcers are determined by the layers of the skin affected (Fig. 21-2). Generally, pressure ulcers start in the superficial layers of the skin and can continue until the deep structures of the skin and musculoskeletal system are affected (Table 21-1).

Staging an ulcer is not always easy. Identification of a stage I pressure ulcer is difficult in patients with darkly pigmented skin. Also, when eschar is present, the staging cannot occur until the eschar has been removed. **Eschar** is a scab or crust.

RISK FACTORS

Many patients who are at high risk for developing pressure ulcers have preexisting risk factors.

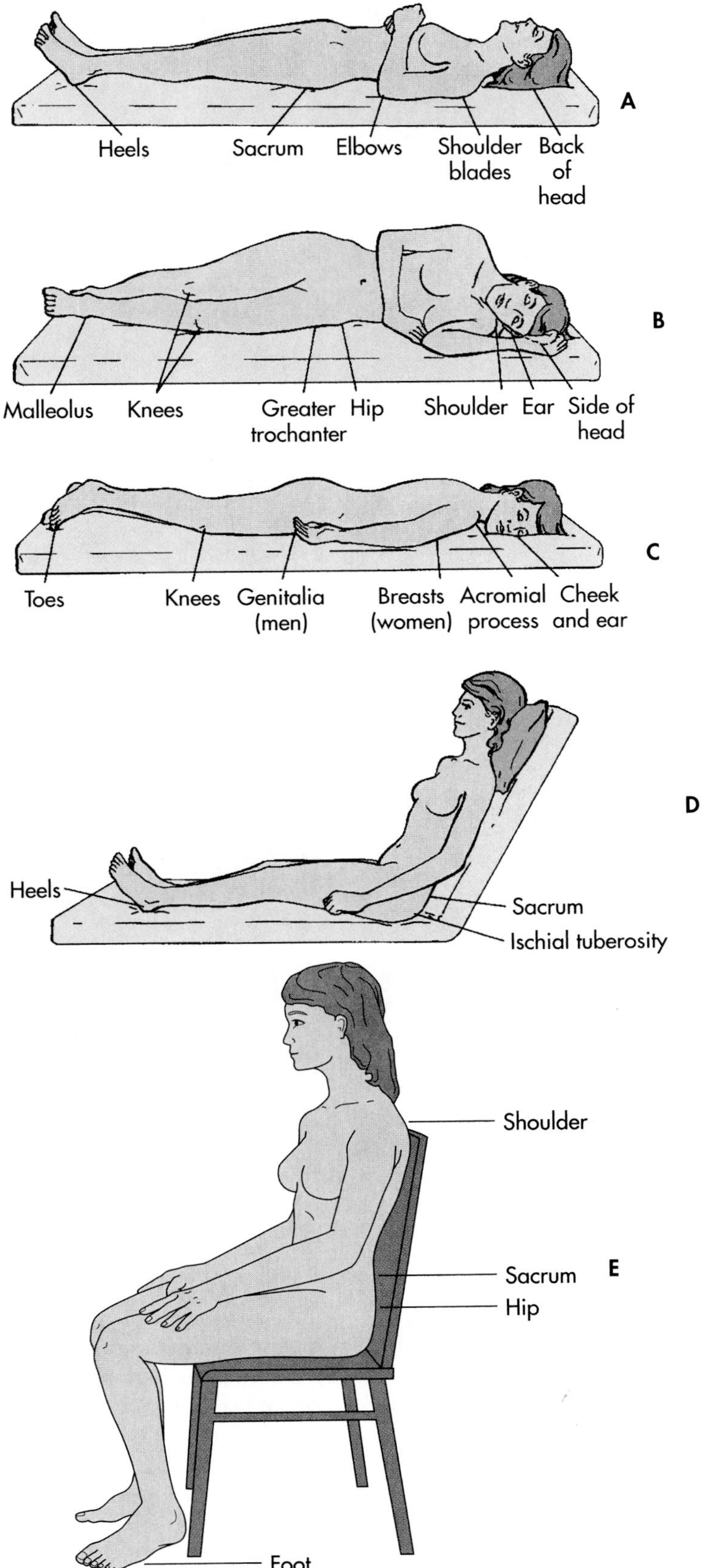

Fig. 21-1 Pressure points. **A,** Supine position. **B,** Lateral position. **C,** Prone position. **D,** Fowler's position. **E,** Sitting position.

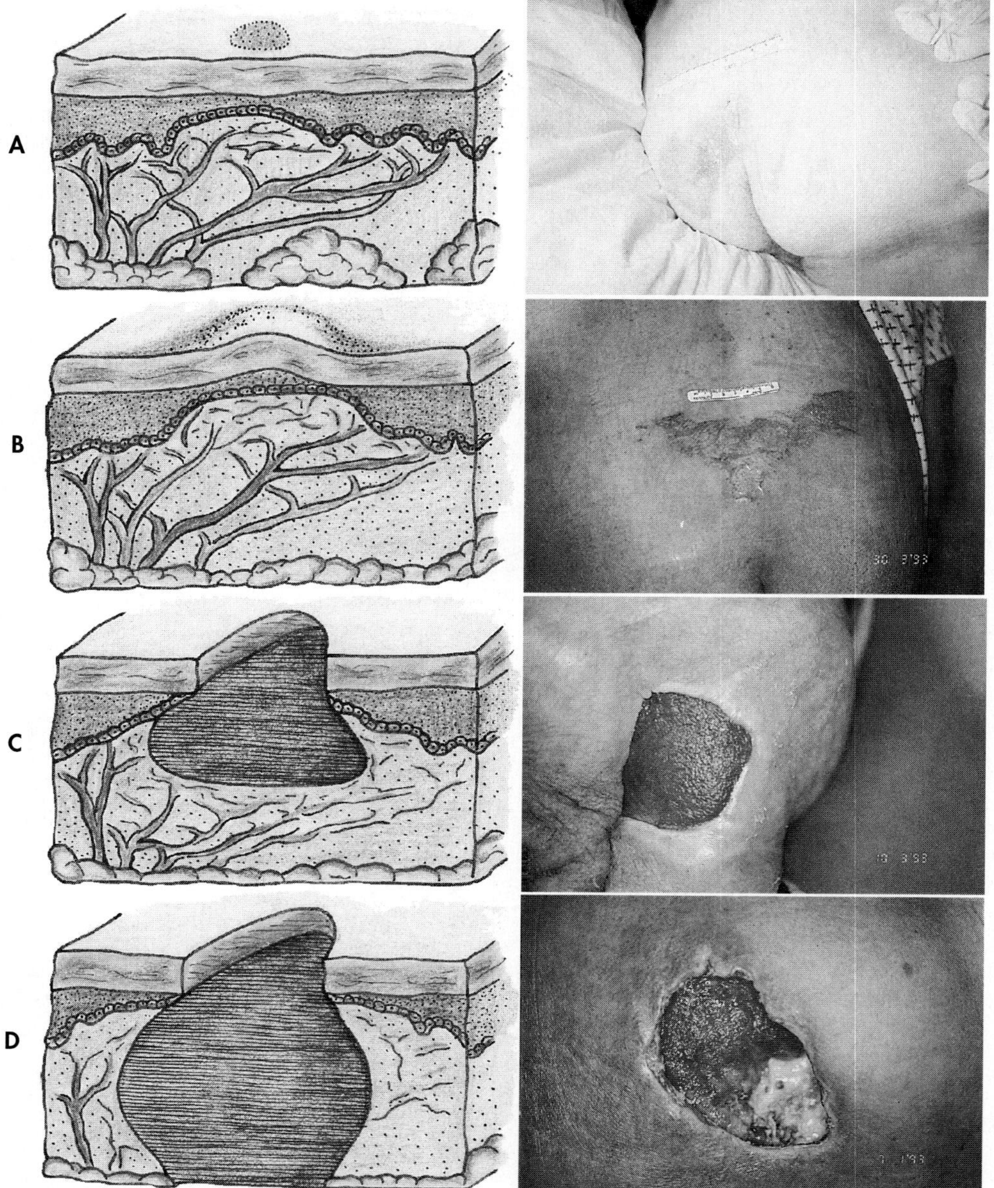

Fig. 21-2 Pressure ulcer. **A,** Stage I. **B,** Stage II. **C,** Stage III. **D,** Stage IV. (Photos from Laurel Wiersema, RN, MSN, Clinical Nurse Specialist, Barnes Hospital, St Louis; In Potter PA, Perry AG: *Basic nursing: theory and practice,* ed 3, St Louis, 1995, Mosby.)

These health conditions may relate to immobility. Examples are patients who have had strokes; who are paralyzed from injuries; who are older, undernourished, incontinent, or thin or overweight; who have circulation problems; or who have diabetes (Burrell, 1992).

Immobility Movement is natural for people. Usually a person moves when discomfort or pressure on a body part is felt. Patients who are sedated or immobile have an increased risk for developing a pressure ulcer. Compounding the problem are the patient with decreased sensation and the application of casts, safety reminder devices, or other devices that may limit movement.

Chronic disease Chronic disease may increase the chance for pressure ulcers. A condition such as emphysema places an added strain on the energy required for the body. Lack of energy, no matter what the cause, increases the risk of a pressure ulcer. Fatigue contributes to inactivity, which

STAGES OF FORMATION OF PRESSURE ULCER

- *Stage I:* This is nonblanchable erythema of intact skin, prominent sign of pressure ulcer.
- *Stage II:* This is partial-thickness loss involving epidermis or dermis. Ulcer is superficial and presents as abrasion, blister, or shallow crater.
- *Stage III:* This is full-thickness skin loss involving damage or necrosis of subcutaneous tissue, which may extend to but not through underlying fascia. Ulcer presents as deep crater with or without undermining of adjacent tissue.
- *Stage IV:* This is full-thickness skin loss with extensive destruction, tissue necrosis, or damage to muscle, bone, or supporting structures.

Data from Potter PA, Perry AG: *Basic nursing: theory and practice,* ed 3, St Louis, 1995, Mosby.

causes increased pressure on the area not being moved. For example, the risk is increased for a 70-year-old thin man with emphysema who has been admitted with a fractured femur because of the pressure related to bedrest and immobility (Kozier et al, 1995).

Aging process The normal aging process contributes to several changes in the skin and surrounding support structures. Aging causes loss of lean body mass and a generalized thinning of the epidermis. The decreased production of oil by the sebaceous glands results in decreased skin turgor, increased dryness, and scaliness. In addition, the aging process diminishes the older patient's perception of pain because the number of cutaneous end organs responsible for the sensations of pressure and touch decreases.

Alteration in nutrition Inadequate nutrition contributes to the development of pressure ulcers. A lack of nutrient reserve and inappropriate eating habits cause the undernourished patient to loose weight and develop muscle atrophy (wasting away or diminution of size or physiologic activity). As a result, the padding between the skin and bone decreases, which can affect the development of pressure ulcers. Most of these patients have diets low in protein, carbohydrates, fluids, and vitamin C (Kozier et al, 1995).

Hypoproteinemia Hypoproteinemia (a low protein content in the blood) results in a **negative nitrogen balance.** This imbalance between the nitrogen taken into the body and the nitrogen excreted from the body predisposes the patient to **dependent edema** (abnormal accumulation of fluid in the interstitial spaces of the tissues of the lowermost parts of the body). Edema further increases the risk for pressure ulcers because edematous tissue has a decreased blood supply.

SKIN ASSESSMENT

A thorough skin assessment should be performed once each shift (Table 21-1). The pressure-prone areas are inspected for color changes or other signs of pressure. High-risk patients should be assessed every 8 hours, and all hyperemic areas should be observed for blanching. Blanching of an erythemic area indicates tissue **hypoxia** (inadequate cellular oxygenation) that can be reversed (Beare, Myers, 1994).

Risk Assessment Tools

Several risk-assessment tools are available to provide a systematic, uniform method of identifying patients at risk for developing pressure ulcers. Patients are assessed by the nurse and given a score based on the available data. This score includes information such as mental state, activity, mobility, and incontinence. The assessment tool should be completed within 24 to 48 hours after the patient is admitted. Each tool assesses preexisting factors that contribute to pressure ulcer formation.

Laboratory Values

The nurse should also review the results of the patient's blood tests for a decreased protein level, which could hinder the body's ability to rebuild epidermal tissue. Results of a complete blood count may reveal anemia and signs of infection. Anemia hinders the blood's ability to carry oxygen, which decreases the body's ability to make new tissue. Both anemia and infection increase the association between nutrition deficits and the risk of pressure ulcers (Kozier et al, 1995).

ENTEROSTOMAL THERAPY

Health care agencies may use an **enterostomal therapist,** a nurse trained to provide wound-drainage services. This nurse selects and provides the primary nursing plan for pressure ulcers. The management plan selected by the nurse is approved by the physician.

In the past, nurses massaged these areas in an outward to inward fashion using massage. However,

Table 21-1 ASSESSMENT FOR RISK OF PRESSURE ULCER DEVELOPMENT

Steps	Rationale
Identify patient's risk for pressure ulcer formation:	This determines need to administer preventive care and use topical agents for existing ulcers.
Paralysis or immobilization caused by restrictive devices	Patient is unable to turn or reposition independently.
Sensory loss	Patient feels no discomfort from pressure.
Circulatory disorders	These reduce perfusion of skin's tissue layers.
Decreased level of consciousness, sedation, or anesthesia	Patient is unable to perceive pressure to turn or reposition independently.
Shearing force	This causes skin and underlying subcutaneous layers to adhere to surface of bed. Trauma occurs to underlying tissues.
Moisture: incontinence, perspiration, wound drainage, or vomitus	This reduces skin's resistance to pressure from shearing force.
Malnutrition	This can lead to weight loss, muscle atrophy, and reduced tissue mass. Less tissue is available to pad between skin and underlying bone. Poor protein, vitamin, and caloric intake limit wound-healing capabilities.
Anemia	Decreased hemoglobin level reduces oxygen-carrying capacity of blood and amount of oxygen available to tissues.
Infection	This causes increase in metabolic demands of tissues. Accompanying diaphoresis (sweating) leaves skin moist.
Obesity	Poorly vascularized excess adipose tissue is more susceptible to pressure. Body weight against bony prominences places underlying skin at risk for breakdown.
Cachexia (malnutrition associated with weakness and emaciation)	This causes loss of adipose tissue that protects bony prominences from pressure.
Hydration: edema or dehydration	Edematous tissue has decreased blood supply and thereby is less tolerant of pressure, friction, and shearing force. Dehydrated skin is less elastic, and skin turgor is poor.
Older adulthood	Skin is less elastic and drier; tissue mass is reduced.
Existing pressure ulcers	This limits surfaces available for position changes, placing available tissues at increased risk.
Assess condition of skin over regions of pressure. Look for following characteristics:	
Hyperemia	This may indicate that tissue was under pressure. Normal reactive hyperemia is normal physiologic response to hypoxemia. In dark-skinned persons, skin that was under pressure appears darker than surrounding skin and may even take on purplish hue (Pires, Muller, 1991). Normal reactive hyperemia over pressure area lasts less than 1 hour. Affected area blanches at fingertip pressure (Pires, Muller, 1991). Abnormal reactive hyperemia lasts longer than 1 hour. Surrounding tissue does not blanch (Pires, Muller, 1991).
Blanching	Blanching is normal, expected response.
Induration (hardening of tissue because of edema or inflammation)	Localized edema beneath skin surface, induration commonly occurs with abnormal reactive hyperemia (Pires, Muller, 1991).

Table 21-1 ASSESSMENT FOR RISK OF PRESSURE ULCER DEVELOPMENT—cont'd

Steps	Rationale
Pallor and mottling	Persistent hypoxia in tissues that were under pressure is abnormal physiologic response.
Absence of superficial skin layers	This represents early pressure ulcer formation.
Scabs, blisters, or pimples	There are early signs of skin damage, but damage to underlying tissue may be more progressive (Pires, Muller, 1991).
Assess client for areas of potential pressure:	Patients at high risk have multiple sites of pressure necrosis.
Nares	Pressure can occur from nasogastric tube or nasal oxygen cannula.
Tongue, lips	Oral airway and endotracheal tube are high-risk locations.
Intravenous sites (especially long-term access sites)	Stress occurs at catheter exit sites.
Drainage tubes	There is stress against tissue at exit site.
Foley catheter	There is pressure against labia, especially with edema.
Observe client for preferred positions when in bed or chair.	Weight of body will be placed on bony prominences. Contractures (flexion and fixation of joint) may result in pressure exerted in unexpected places. Phenomenon is best assessed through observation.
Observe client's mobility and ability to initiate and assist with position changes.	Potential for friction and shear increases when client is completely dependent for position changes.
Obtain risk score: Norton Scale Braden Scale	Risk score depends on instrument used and predicts client's need for preventive care (AHCPR, 1992).
Monitor length of time any area of redness persists:	Redness usually persists for half of time hypoxia occurred. For example, redness lasts 15 minutes, so hypoxia lasted approximately 30 minutes.
Determine appropriate turning interval, which should be (turning interval − hypoxia time = suggested interval)	For example, turning interval is 2 hours, hypoxia time is 30 minutes, 2 hour − 30 minutes = 1½-hour suggested turning interval.
Use pressure-relief device, if indicated	Short turning intervals (for example, 1-2 hours) may not be realistic. Therefore use of device is recommended.
Obtain nutritional assessment data, including serum albumin level, total protein level, hemoglobin level, and ideal body weight.	Poor nutritional status decreases skin's and underlying tissue's tolerance to pressure, friction, and shearing force (Hanan, Scheele, 1991).
Assess client's and family's understanding of risks for pressure ulcers.	This provides opportunity to begin prevention education.
Document assessment findings.	This provides baseline data for skin integrity and risk of pressure ulcer development.

From Potter PA, Perry AG: *Basic nursing: theory and practice,* ed 3, St Louis, 1995, Mosby.

research has documented that massaging increases the risk of damaging the capillaries in the skin. The nursing care necessary to prevent and treat pressure ulcers currently includes a combination of several components (Skill 21-1). Use of positioning schedules, therapeutic mattresses, special dressings, whirlpool treatment, and medications as well as improvement of the nutritional status of the patient are among the most important. Surgery is also used.

Positioning

Once a red area is discovered the nurse assesses for blanching. Reassessment of the area is performed an hour after the patient has been turned to determine the extent of the redness.

Positioning schedules are designed to reduce the pressure on and shearing forces of the skin. Patients should be repositioned at least every 2 hours. For

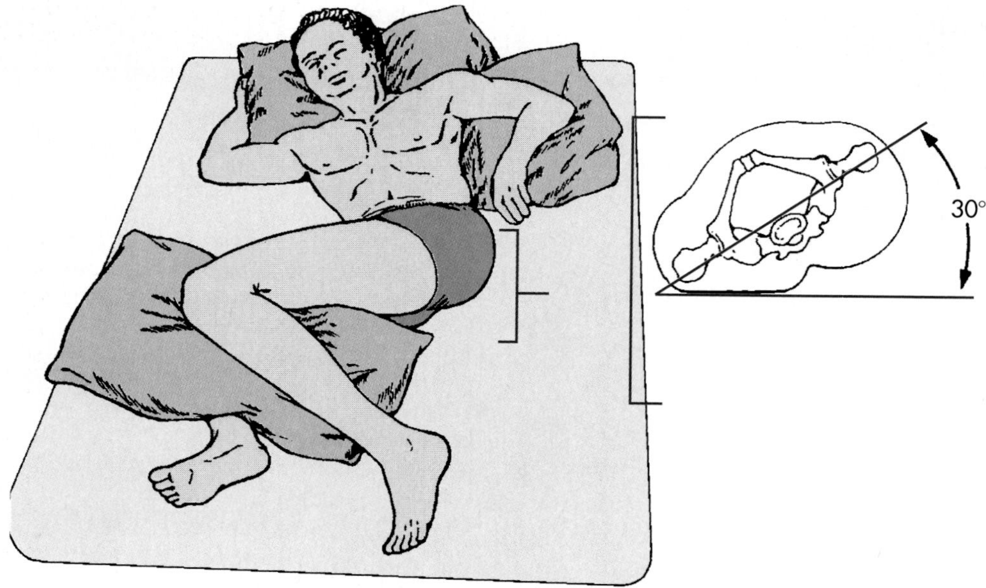

Fig. 21-3 Thirty-degree lateral position at which pressure points are avoided. (From Bryant RA: *Acute and chronic wounds: nursing management,* St Louis, 1992, Mosby.)

many, this may not be often enough to prevent skin problems. Therefore repositioning times need to be assessed and reevaluated from time to time. The exact turning schedule time may range from 1 to 2 hours. To calculate the appropriate time, the nurse uses the following formula:

Turning interval − Hypoxia time
= Suggested repositioning interval

For example, if a patient has been turned every 2 hours and the nurse finds a red area, the turning time is recalculated by subtracting the time that the involved area remains red after the removal of pressure. The suggested turning interval would be 1 hour and 15 minutes for an area that remained red 45 minutes after the patient had been turned.

A basic positioning schedule should be designed to reduce shearing force to the skin. Shearing can be reduced by keeping the head of the bed below 30 degrees, using turning sheets, and using a 30-degree lateral position to keep pressure off of the coccyx (Fig. 21-3).

Therapeutic Beds and Mattresses

Therapeutic beds and mattresses should be used for patients who are at high risk for developing pressure ulcers and who have an existing ulcer (Table 21-2). The nurse is responsible for operating the therapeutic beds and for teaching assistive staff its use.

Pressure Ulcer Dressings

Dressings for pressure ulcers are selected based on the stage of the ulcer identified and for the promotion of healing. Many dressings are available. The aim of the dressing may be to promote healing by debriding (removing dead tissue) the dead tissue from the pressure ulcer surface, providing a protective wall for the ulcer, or protecting the viable tissue (Table 21-3). (Tissue is viable when it is capable of developing, growing, and sustaining life.) The dressing for a pressure ulcer that drains should be designed to promote drainage and the removal of excessive exudate and loose debris without harming newly formed **granulation tissue** (soft, pink, fleshy projections that form during the healing process). This dressing is referred to as *wet-to-dry.* Dressings help debride the ulcer by removing the dead tissue when a wet dressing dries on the ulcer and is removed. Second, an environment that promotes self-digestion of the necrotic tissue may be created under the dressing (Bolander, 1994).

Once the dead tissue has been removed from the pressure ulcer wound, the focus of treatment is maintenance of the new tissue to promote healing. The best environment for healing is a clean, slightly moist ulcer surface that has little or no growth of bacteria.

Hydrophobic dressings may be ordered for an ulcer with very little drainage. **Hydrophobic dressings** are nonabsorbent and water-proof. The aim is to protect the ulcer from contamination. A second type is **hydrophilic dressings,** which are

Table 21-2 SURFACE TYPES BY PURPOSE AND ADVANTAGES

Type	Examples	Purpose	Advantages	Disadvantages	Notes
Foam overlay	Geomatt Biogard	Pressure reduction, comfort	Has low cost, is easy to use, has many sizes	Is hot, traps moisture, has limited life, loses pressure reduction with use	Usually, only one client can use it. Washing removes flame-retardant chemicals. It is easy to use at home.
Foam replacement	MaxiFloat DeCube Comfortex	Pressure reduction, comfort	Has reduced bed height, reduces nursing time, has multiple client use	Has high initial cost, is difficult to evaluate when effectiveness is lost	Some have removable sections (cubes). It may be rented or purchased.
Fluid overlay	Lotus	Pressure reduction, comfort	Is easily cleaned, has multiple client use, is readily available	Is heavy, leaks with puncture, cannot raise head of bed	It may be rented or purchased. Baffled systems control motion.
Air overlay	Sofcare Roho KoalaKare	Pressure relief	Is easy to set up, has single- or multiple-use products available	Is not comfortable, can be damaged by sharp objects, requires monitoring for inflation	It may be rented or purchased. It adapts to multiple settings.
Low air loss	KinAir Flexicair Mediscus	Pressure relief	Is easy to use, has seat that deflates for transfer, has company that offers support staff	Has noisy, portable blowers; has slippery surface	It is generally rented. Home unit is available.
Air fluidized	Clinitron Fluidair Skytron	Pressure relief	Reduces friction and shear, facilitates control of high drainage, has company that offers support staff	May cause coughing to be less effective, is heavy, may cause circulating air to dehydrate, makes transfers difficult	It is available for home, but it may be too heavy.
Kinetic	Rotokinetic treatment table	Movement, skeletal stability	Mobilizes secretions, stabilizes skeleton, supports traction, has company that offers support staff	Must be kept in rotation or no pressure reduction, causes shearing if client position is not correct	It must be in rotation 21 hours/day. It is now available as low-air-loss version.
Bariatric	Burke	Management of morbidly obese, staff safety	Facilitates client independence, converts to chair	Has standard width, so surface may not accommodate turning	It requires addition of special mattress and overlay for pressure relief.

From Potter PA, Perry AG: *Basic nursing: theory and practice,* ed 3, St Louis, 1995, Mosby.

absorbent and draw excessive drainage away from the ulcer site (Ignatavicis, Workman, Mishler, 1995).

Dressing changes

Implementing the schedule for dressing changes depends on the amount of drainage and necrotic exudate (fluid, cells, or other substances that have slowly been discharged from cells or blood vessels). Dry gauze should be changed when the outer layer of the dressing becomes saturated with drainage. This phenomenon is known as "strike through." The treatment plan for dressing change guidelines should be accessible by all staff members.

Table 21-3 TREATMENT OPTIONS BY ULCER STAGE

Ulcer Stage	Ulcer Status	Dressing	Comments	Expected Change	Adjuvant
1	Intact	None Film, adherent Hydrocolloid	Dressing allows visual assessment. Dressing protects from shear. Dressing may not allow visual assessment.	Condition resolves slowly without epidermal loss over 7 to 14 days.	Turning schedule Support hydration Nutritional support Silicone-based lotion to decrease shear Pressure-relief mattress or chair cushion
2	Clean	Composite Hydrocolloid Hydrogel sheet	It includes viasorb, film plus telfa or Exudry. It limits shear. Occlusive seal is changed every 7 days. Dressing is absorbent and requires secondary dressing of gauze or adherent film.	Condition heals through reepithelialization and epithelial budding.	See previous stage Management of incontinence
3	Clean	Hydrocolloid Hydrogel	See Stage 2. Nurse applies ¼-inch thick and covers with gauze or hydrocolloid.	Condition heals through granulation and reepithelialization. (NOTE: does not become a stage 2 ulcer as it heals.)	See previous stages Electrical stimulation Evaluation of pressure relief needs
		Exudate absorbers calcium alginate wound pastes	Nurse changes when strike through is noted on secondary dressing. Nurse covers with gauze or hydrocolloid.		
		Gauze, fluffy	Dressing is used with normal saline.		
		Growth factors	Dressing is used with gauze.		

		Adherent film	Dressing will facilitate softening of eschar.	Eschar will lift at edges as healing progresses. Cross-hatching central area of eschar with small blade will facilitate release from center.	Surgical consult for debridement
	Eschar	Hydrocolloid	Dressing will facilitate softening of eschar.		Surgical consult for closure
		Gauze plus ordered solution	Absorbs drainage.		
		None	Rarely, if eschar is dry and intact, no dressing is used, allowing eschar to act as physiologic cover.		
4	Clean	Hydrogel	See Stage 3 Clean.	Condition heals through granulation and reepithelialization. Because of contraction, surface may close more rapidly than base, leaving wound cavity.	See stages 1, 2, and 3 Clean
		Hydrocolloid plus hydrocolloid paste/beads	See Stage 3 Clean; it is critical to treat areas of undermining.		
		Calcium alginate			
		Gauze			
		Growth factors			
	Eschar	See Stage 3 Eschar	See Stage 3 Clean. Nurse packs deeply undermined ulcers. Nurse uses with gauze.	See Stage 3 Eschar.	See Stage 3 Eschar.

NOTE: As with *all* occlusive dressings, wound should *not* be clinically infected.

From Potter PA, Perry AG: *Basic nursing: theory and practice,* ed 3, St Louis, 1995, Mosby.

Whirlpool Treatment

An additional treatment in the management of pressure ulcers includes physical therapy, especially if the ulcer is associated with immobility. The physical therapist assists the patient with hydrotherapy or the whirlpool. The treatment uses warm water that continually moves and an added antiseptic solution. The movement of the water facilitates removal of necrotic tissue. Once the ulcer is rid of necotic tissue and shows granulating tissue, the whirlpool should be discontinued.

Medication Treatment

Drugs may be used in the care of pressure ulcers. With an infection an antibiotic topical medication or systemic drug may be administered to help rid the ulcer of infection. Broad-spectrum antibacterial or antibiotic drugs are usually administered until the results of the culture and sensitivity test are returned from the laboratory. A systemic antibiotic should not be administered until the culture has been obtained. Once the specific microorganisms are identified, a more specific antibiotic may be ordered (Ignatavicius, Workman, Mishler, 1995).

Nutrition

Nutrition is a fundamental part of the nursing care for patients with or patients at risk for pressure ulcers. A nutritional assessment should be performed by the nurse and dietitian to determine the nutritional needs of each patient. Laboratory data such as the level of albumin (a protein) should be used to monitor and assess the patient's response to treatment. The hemoglobin level should be at least 12 g/dl. In general, patients need 2 to 4 times more protein, extra vitamins, and minerals. Zinc is included as a valuable mineral in the repair of tissue.

Surgical Intervention

Pressure ulcers are usually a chronic problem for patients. Management and restoration of skin integrity may require longer to resolve. As a result, surgical intervention may be needed to hasten the healing process. Surgical management involves removal of the necrotic tissue by debridement, skin grafting, or both to reestablish skin integrity. A **skin graft** is a portion of skin implanted to cover areas where skin has been lost. Grafting is generally used in wounds that have not healed through the normal process of epithelialization, which is healing by the growth of epithelium.

The preoperative care for a skin graft is directed at preparing the ulcer to accept the graft. The potential donor site should be assessed for circulation and signs of infection. Pressure ulcers are not usually grafted until granulation tissue is present.

Postoperative care of the graft depends on the type of graft necessary. Regardless of the type of graft, nursing care is a challenge. The goal is to provide nursing care that promotes viability of the graft. The patient is placed on bedrest for 3 to 5 days to allow the graft to vascularize (develop vessels in a tissue). The involved area should be immobilized and elevated. The patient should not participate in any activity that could cause separation of the graft from the wound. The principles of surgical asepsis should be followed to prevent infection from developing in the graft (see Chapter 17).

EVALUATION OF TREATMENT

Monitoring the ulcer for improvement is an important step in the management of pressure ulcers. Most ulcers are inspected at least daily for signs of infection such as redness, warmth, and edema. Ulcers should be measured as often as necessary to determine improvement.

Patients are often discharged before the ulcer is completely healed. The patient and support person should demonstrate ulcer wound care for home care of the ulcer. Before discharge, the nurse should develop a checklist to evaluate home care needed by the patient. When beginning evaluation, the nurse should list the steps for the support person and family to use. Included should be the steps for removing and discarding the dressing, cleaning the wound, and applying the dressing. An assessment should also include available resources and emergency numbers for assistance. Application technique and medications should be included in discharge planning. The nurse should write the instructions for the patient.

■ NURSING CARE PLAN ■

IMPAIRED SKIN INTEGRITY

Mr. B, age 78, is admitted with a pressure ulcer requiring extensive nursing care. The ulcer is 10 cm in length, 4 cm in width, and 5.5 cm in depth.

NURSING DIAGNOSIS

Impaired skin integrity related to immobility as evidenced by destruction of skin layers, skin surface disruption, and destruction of deeper skin areas

GOAL

- Patient will develop normal skin integrity.

EXPECTED OUTCOMES

- Ulcer wound will heal.
- Skin turgor will be normal for age.
- Patient will perform preventive skin care.

NURSING INTERVENTIONS

- Assess skin once each shift to prevent further skin damage or pressure ulcer on bony prominences.
- Administer appropriate supportive measures to provide comfort and sense of well-being.
- Establish and maintain positioning schedule to reduce pressure and help prevent further skin breakdown.

EVALUATION

- Pressure ulcer has healed.
- Patient administers self-care for skin.

SKILL 21-1 CARING FOR A PRESSURE ULCER

Steps	Rationale
1. **Obtain equipment:** ▪ Cleansing agent ▪ Topical medication ▪ Sterile dressings ▪ Extra pillows ▪ Eggcrate mattress or other special devices ▪ Sterile gloves ▪ Clean gloves ▪ Drapes ▪ Ruler	Helps organize procedure.
2. **Refer to medical record, care plan, or Kardex for special interventions.**	Provides basis for care.
3. **Introduce self.**	Decreases anxiety level.
4. **Identify patient by identification band.**	Identifies correct patient for procedure.
5. **Explain procedure to patient.**	Seeks cooperation and decreases anxiety.
6. **Wash hands and don clean gloves according to agency policy and guidelines from Centers for Disease Control and Prevention and Occupational Safety and Health Administration.**	Helps prevent cross-contamination.
7. **Prepare patient for intervention:**	
a. Close door to room or pull curtain.	Provides privacy.
b. Drape for procedure if necessary.	Prevents exposure of patient.
8. **Raise bed to comfortable working level.**	Provides safety for nurse.
9. **Arrange for patient privacy.**	Shows respect for patient.

Continued.

SKILL 21-1 CARING FOR A PRESSURE ULCER—cont'd

Steps	Rationale
10. Assess pressure ulcer.	Determines success of nursing care.
11. Assess for high risk for developing pressure ulcer (see Table 21-1).	Helps prevent pressure ulcer.
12. Remove ulcer dressing and assess drainage and healing.	Provides information regarding wound status.
13. Measure pressure ulcer for length, width, and depth.	Helps indicate success of nursing care.
14. Cleanse ulcer with appropriate agent:	Assists healing process.
a. Irrigate deep ulcers.	Reaches areas of ulcer that cannot be reached by simple cleansing technique.
b. Use whirlpool as prescribed.	Cleanses and debrides ulcer.
15. Apply medication as prescribed.	Assists healing process.
16. Apply sterile dressing.	Helps prevent contamination of wound.
17. Remove gloves and wash hands.	Helps prevent cross-contamination.
18. Document.	Documents procedure and patient's response.

SUMMARY

The incidence of pressure ulcers has an immense impact on health care agencies and on the patient. The pain and discomfort, lengthy hospital stay for treatment, and possible complications from the pressure ulcer itself increase health care costs. The treatment may even increase health care costs. Immobility may cause significant problems for the patient even though it is sometimes required for treatment of the ulcer. The goals of the nurse include prevention of pressure ulcers by administration of competent nursing care, which includes care of the skin.

Key Concepts

- Pressure ulcers continue to be problematic in many types of health care agencies.
- Complications from pressure ulcers increase health care agency and patient costs.
- Pressure ulcers may be associated with many chronic health problems.
- Healthy, intact skin is a major goal of the nurse and may be brought about with preventive nursing care measures.
- A schedule for positioning the patient should be maintained and helps prevent pressure ulcers.
- Maintenance of appropriate nutritional status of the patient helps guide prevention of pressure ulcers.
- Skin assessment is vital in preventing pressure ulcers.

Critical Thinking Questions

1. The nurse has just removed an external condom catheter for routine hygiene care. What assessments are needed to determine the skin integrity of the patient's penile skin and scrotum?
2. An older woman with a new, permanent colostomy is about to be discharged from the unit to her daughter's home. The skin around her stoma has no breakdown; both she and her daughter realize the importance of maintaining this skin integrity. How should the nurse advise them?
3. The patient's mobility is severely restricted, and he is receiving a medication that causes peripheral vasoconstriction. What interventions are essential in reducing pressure ulcer formation?

REFERENCES AND SUGGESTED READINGS

Agency for Health Care Policy and Research (AHCPR): *Pressure ulcers in adults: prediction and prevention,* Publication Nos 92-0047 and 92-0050, Rockville, Md, 1992. US Department of Health and Human Services, Public Health Service.

Beare PG, Myers JL: *Principles and practice of adult health nursing,* ed 2, St Louis, 1994, Mosby.

Berger KJ, Williams MB: *Fundamentals of nursing: collaborating for optimal health,* Norwalk, Conn, 1992. Appleton & Lange.

Bolander VB: *Sorenson and Luckman's basic nursing: a psychophysiologic approach,* Philadelphia, 1994. Saunders.

Burrell LO, editor: *Adult nursing in hospital and community settings,* Norwalk, Conn, 1992. Appleton & Lange.

Ferrell BA et al: A randomized trial of low-air-loss beds for treatment of pressure ulcers, *Journal of the American Medical Association* 269(4):494, 1993.

Flory C: Perfecting the art: skin assessment, *RN* 6:22, 1992.

Hanan K, Scheele L: Albumin vs. weight as a predictor of nutritional status and pressure ulcer development, *Ostomy / Wound Management* 33:22, 1991.

Ignatavicius D, Workman ML, Mishler MA: *Medical-surgical nursing: a nursing process approach,* Philadelphia, 1995. Saunders.

Kozier B et al: *Fundamentals of nursing: concepts, process, and practice,* New York, 1995. Addison-Wesley.

Lewis SM, Collier IC, Heitkemper MM: *Medical-surgical nursing: assessment and management of clinical problems,* ed 4, St Louis, 1996. Mosby.

National Pressure Ulcer Advisory Panel: Pressure ulcers: incidence, economics, risk assessment, Consensus Development Conference, *Decubitus* 2(2):24, 1989.

Pires M, Mueller A: Detection and management of early tissue pressure indicators: a pictoral essay, *Progressions* 3(3):3, 1991.

Potter PA, Perry AG: *Basic nursing: theory and practice,* ed 3, St Louis, 1995, Mosby.

CHAPTER 22

Safety

Learning Objectives

After studying this chapter, the student should be able to . . .

- Define the key terms.
- Summarize safety precautions that may be implemented to reduce the incidence of falls.
- Discuss specific risks to safety as they pertain to the young child, the older adult, the hospitalized patient, and the health care worker.
- List four reasons for applying restraints.
- Apply restraints appropriately and safely.
- Describe nursing interventions specific to the patient requiring restraints.
- List the steps to be followed in the event of a fire.
- Discuss the role of the nurse in disaster planning.
- Describe nursing interventions in the event of accidental poisoning.

Key Terms

Carcinogen	Pathogen
Disaster	Poison
Disaster-preparedness plan	Poisoning
Parasite	Restraint

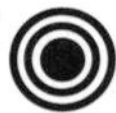

Skills

22-1 Applying restraints
22-2 Caring for victims of accidental poisoning

The need for a safe environment is constant. Environmental concerns deal with the immediate environment of a patient and the general environment in which people live and work. Issues such as water and air pollution, disposal of waste and toxic materials, safety on highways, protection of endangered species, and preservation of forests illustrate general environment concerns about safety. The hospital environment, in terms of overall safety for the patient, has traditionally been a primary concern of nursing. The focus on a safe hospital environment has now expanded to recognize and identify possible hazards and threats faced by hospital personnel.

SAFE ENVIRONMENT

A safe environment provides freedom from injury and focuses on preventing falls, electrical injuries, fires, burns, and poisoning. The nurse should be aware of possible safety problems. The nurse should also know about how to report and respond to situations that threaten safety.

The patient, visitors, and members of the health care team all share responsibility for providing and maintaining a safe environment. Protecting the health care team and patient, educating the patient, and ensuring a safe health care environment are primary nursing responsibilities. For example, the nurse should check to see that the call light or signal system being used is working and accessible to the patient.

Falls are a common problem, and nurses should be aware of patients who are prone to them (Table 22-1). Children and older adults are not the only patients at risk. Individuals who become ill or are injured are also at risk. Various safety precautions may be taken (see box).

Ensuring a safe immediate environment for the child requires protection of the child and education of the parents. Anticipating the injuries that are likely to occur can assist the nurse in individualiz-

Table 22-1 CAUSES OF FALLS IN OLDER ADULTS

Normal Aging Process	Pathologic Process
Neurologic and sensory changes	
Vision changes: presbyopia (farsightedness) or reduction in light that reaches retina	Vision changes: glaucoma or cataracts
Auditory impairment: decreased acuity	Auditory impairment: vertigo (dizziness)
Central processing: decreased proprioceptive reflexes	Central processing: senile epilepsy, cerebrovascular accident (stroke), or neurosyphilis
Musculoskeletal changes	
Fibrotic changes in joints, muscles, tendons, and ligaments	Gait abnormalities: shuffling; waddling; slow, short, deliberate steps; or muscle rigidity
Loss of muscle size, strength, and speed of contraction	Arthritis Osteoporosis
Cardiovascular changes	
Impaired regulation of cerebral blood flow	Orthostatic hypotension
Decreased baroreceptor sensitivity	Postprandial hypotension
Progressive decrease of cerebral blood flow	Carotid sinus hypersensitivity—excessive cardiac slowing or hypotension Supraventricular and ventricular dysrhythmias—sudden reduction in cardiac output or systemic blood pressure Drop attacks
Genitourinary and endocrine changes	
Low estrogen in postmenopausal women	Stress incontinence in postmenopausal women

From McFarland GK, McFarlane EA: *Nursing diagnosis and intervention: planning for patient care,* ed 2, St Louis, 1993, Mosby.

ing nursing care and providing family teaching. Growth and the acquisition of new motor skills places the child at risk for injury. For example, the inability of children to read prevents them from reading labels on house cleaners or medication containers. Young infants put almost anything into their mouths, and as infants learn to crawl, electric sockets and cords may become a danger. Providing covers for the sockets and cords protects the child while allowing exploration of the surroundings.

Changes associated with aging significantly affect the ability of older adults to protect themselves from injury. For example, irregularity in gait causes falls. Age-related eye changes may affect the individual's ability to see the height of stairs. Dizziness is often related to medications and chronic conditions. Eyeglasses, hearing aids, and other assistive devices such as canes should be used by patients with deficits. Long, loose-fitting clothing, which may cause tripping, should be avoided. Specific interventions may help ensure safe surroundings for the patient by removing possible threats to safety. If safety is threatened, agency guidelines should be available to handle the situation.

SAFETY PRECAUTIONS TO PREVENT PATIENT FALLS

- Bedside and overbed tables should be placed within patient's reach.
- Patients who have had surgery or who have been in bed for extended periods require assistance when first getting out of bed.
- Environment should be free of litter (for example, books, magazines, and shoes) that can cause patient to trip and fall.
- Nurse should follow facility policies regarding use of side rails.
- Since most facilities have adjustable beds that can be raised and lowered, bed should be kept in lowest position except when care is being given.
- Nurse should encourage ambulating patients to wear shoes with low heels. Loose-fitting, soft, or floppy shoes should be avoided.
- Nurse should ensure that spilled liquids are wiped up or mopped promptly. Nurse should pay attention to signs warning of wet or slippery floors.
- Nurse should point out and encourage use of handrails in bathrooms and halls and demonstrate how emergency call buttons and cords work.

NURSING PROCESS FOR SAFETY

Assessment

The nurse must understand that a safe environment is essential for maintaining and restoring a patient's health. Nurses in hospitals or other health care settings are the patient's first line of defense against falls, medication errors, poisoning, and other injuries. The nursing process is used to reduce the risk of injury through nursing interventions. The nurse promotes a safe environment by teaching patients and families about hazards in their homes. The nurse also assesses the environment for physical hazards such as inadequate lighting and clutter, **carcinogens** (substances that causes the development or risk of cancer), **pathogens** (organisms capable of causing illness) and **parasites** (organisms living in or on other organisms and obtaining nourishment from them), and sanitation and pollution problems.

Nursing Diagnosis

The nursing diagnosis should include specific causes of a patient's safety risks so that nursing care can be individualized. For instance, a patient's visual impairment may lead the nurse to diagnosis a risk for injury. Possible nursing diagnoses related to patient safety include the following:

Altered thought processes
Impaired physical mobility
Knowledge deficit (specify)
Risk for injury
Risk for poisoning
Risk for trauma
Sensory/perceptual alterations (specify)

Planning

The nurse should plan interventions and set goals with the patient, family, and other members of the health care team. The plan of care may identify nursing interventions that prevent threats to safety and meet safety needs (see care plan on p. 428).

Goals are prioritized based on the risk to the patient's safety and health promotion. The care plan is based on one or more of the following goals:

Goal #1: Patient learns potential threats to safety in the home.

Outcome

Patient lists hazards within the home.

Goal #2: Patient's risk of accidental poisoning is reduced.

Outcome

Syrup of Ipecac is in the home, and patient can describe its correct use.

Implementation

Nursing interventions are designed to promote the safety of the patient in the home and health care setting. These interventions include health promotion, developmental considerations, and environmental protection. In the case of children, it is important for the nurse to promote good safety habits in the home (see teaching box). The nurse can also instruct the older adult about safety measures (see gerontologic box).

Evaluation

Nursing interventions for reducing safety threats are evaluated by comparing the patient's response to the anticipated outcome. The nurse must be pre-

PATIENT TEACHING

- If there are firearms at home, instruct parents to keep them locked up, unloaded, and out of reach of children.
- Teach children how to phone for emergency help.
- Instruct children never to operate electrical appliances while alone.
- Advise parents to use back burners on stove and to turn pot handles toward wall to reduce risk of burns to children.
- Teach parents to cover electric sockets and cords to protect infants.
- Advise parents of infants to place household cleaners and medication containers out of reach of their children.

GERONTOLOGIC CONSIDERATIONS

- The nurse should teach older adult patients to keep living areas well lighted and free of clutter and to keep eyeglasses in good condition.
- Patients should be advised about drug interactions, signs and symptoms of drug toxicity, and the possibility of medication-induced dizziness.
- Patients need to be taught the proper use of assistive devices (for example, canes, rails in tub and bathroom, and elevated seats).
- Eye changes and irregularity of gait may predispose the older adult to falls.

pared to revise the plan of care if the outcomes have not been achieved. Examples of goals and evaluative measures include the following:

Goal #1: Patient learns potential threats to safety in the home.

Evaluative measure

Observe patient identifying potential hazards.

Goal #2: Patient's risk of accidental poisoning is reduced.

Evaluative measure

Observe for syrup of ipecac in the home and have patient state its proper use.

SAFETY IN THE HOSPITAL

The hospital environment itself is a source of possible safety hazards to health care workers. Various biologic, chemical, and physical hazards have been identified as safety hazards. Hazards range from smoke inhalation associated with laser use in the operating room to exposure to the human immunodeficiency virus.

The Hazard Communication Act of the Occupational Safety and Health Administration (OSHA) requires hospitals to inform employees about harmful exposures and ways to reduce the risk of exposure. The Centers for Disease Control and Prevention (CDC) also provides guidelines for working with infected patients. The nurse should request information and follow recommended guidelines and agency policy to reduce exposure to hazards in the hospital.

RESTRAINTS

Restraints are devices used to immobilize patients. Soft restraints are the most common type. These restraint devices are called *Posey restraints* in reference to the company that manufactures them.

There are various reasons for the use of restraints. Patient safety is the primary consideration. Restraints are used in the maintenance of treatment. For example, wrist restraints are used to prevent the removal of intravenous tubing and nasogastric tubes. Restraints also prevent the confused patient from wandering and prevent or reduce the risk of the patient falling out of a bed, chair, or wheelchair. Movement may also be restricted to protect other patients and the staff from harm. Guidelines for use of restraints are listed in Table 22-2.

Use of Restraints

The use of restraints is widespread in North America. From 7% to 10% of the hospital population is restrained approximately 50% of the time. Certain patient populations, such as older adults and the confused, are more likely to be restrained. Today, ethical and legal issues surround the use of restraints. The focus is on using other means of providing protection for patients.

The use of restraints may also result in increased restlessness and anxiety for the patient. Restraint use contributes to immobility and associated problems. Patients who are restrained often pull against the restraints, causing skin and circulation problems.

Documentation

Documentation about the need for restraints, the type of restraint used, and the patient's response is crucial. A comprehensive assessment that focuses on the patient's behavior, activity, and skin condition is necessary (Skill 22-1). All nursing interventions, including patient and family teaching, must be documented.

Many health care agencies have specific policies and procedures related to the use of restraints. Many agencies require a medical order. The nurse should be familiar with agency policies as well as the physician's requirements regarding the application of restraints. If questions arise, the nurse should consult the supervisor.

FIRE PREPAREDNESS

Both the home and health care agency are at risk for fires. Fires in the health care agency are often related to smoking in bed or faulty electrical equipment. Approximately 8100 hospital fires and 4300 nursing home fires are reported each year.

An established fire-safety program is mandatory for all health care agencies. Most agencies have a safety committee that is actively involved in developing fire-prevention and fire-education programs. Fire prevention includes appropriate housekeeping, maintenance, and employee discipline.

Housekeeping personnel are responsible for eliminating all unnecessary combustible material, whereas maintenance personnel address the functioning of fire-protection devices such as alarms, extinguishers, and sprinklers. All mechanical and electrical equipment should be regularly inspected and maintained to minimize fire hazards.

All employees should know the telephone number and procedure for reporting a fire as well as the lo-

Table 22-2 **GUIDELINES FOR THE USE OF RESTRAINTS**

Guidelines	Rationale
Physical restraint should be selected to reduce patient's movement only as much as necessary.	Overrestraining patient so that activities are unduly restricted can exacerbate hazards of immobility and increase patient restlessness.
If restraint is necessary, nurse should carefully explain type of restraint and reasons for its use.	Restraint can increase confusion or hostility in patient and family. Explanation of restraint can reduce or even prevent some of these negative perceptions.
Restraint should not exacerbate patient's health problem.	Restraints that are too tight can impair circulation to distal extremities.
Restraint should not interfere with treatment.	Restraints placed over intravenous sites can impede flow of fluid into circulation. Restraints attached to fractured or dislocated extremities can impair healing.
Bony prominences should be padded before application of restraint.	Padding reduces risk of injury to skin from pressure.
Restraints should be changed when they become soiled or damp.	Soiled or damp restraints increase risk of skin breakdown.
Restraints should be secured away from a patient's reach. Caregiver should be able to quickly release device.	When patient is able to undo restraints, purpose of restraint is negated. Quick-release ties ensure that patient can be released quickly to avoid injury.
Restraint applied to patient in bed should be attached to bed frame, not side rails.	Release of side rails while restraint remains attached can result in injury to patient's musculoskeletal system.
Restraints should be removed a minimum of every 2 hours (see agency policy). Patient should not be left unattended when restraints are removed.	Removal provides opportunity to assess skin integrity, circulation, respiratory function (in the case of rest restraint), and patient's behavior. Skin care is provided as needed. Previously restrained patient who is left unattended can cause self-injury or can injure others.
Frequent (up to every hour) circulation checks should be performed when extremity restraints are used (see agency policy).	Checks reduce risk of vascular extremity injury from poor distal circulation caused by tightening of restraint.

From Potter PA, Perry AG: *Basic nursing: theory and practice,* ed 3, St Louis, 1995, Mosby.

cation of the nearest alarms and firefighting equipment. In addition, health care workers should know their role in the overall hospital evacuation plan. Assessing for fire hazards should occur continuously.

An important element in a fire-safety program is knowing about types of fires and types of fire extinguishers to use for them. Paper, wood, and cloth fires require a *type A* fire extinguisher. Flammable liquid fires, such as those caused by grease and anesthetics, require a *type B* fire extinguisher. Electrical fires require a *type C* fire extinguisher. Fire extinguishers marked *ABC* may be used on any type of fire. Knowing which type of extinguisher is available before a fire occurs is vital. Most fire-safety programs allow health care workers the opportunity to handle the different types of fire extinguishers.

In the event of fire the nurse should ensure rescue of patients in immediate danger and then follow agency procedure for ringing the fire alarm and reporting the location and extent of the fire. Measures should then be taken to contain or extinguish the fire until firefighters arrive. Measures to contain or put out the fire include closing doors and windows, turning off oxygen and electrical equipment, and using the appropriate fire extinguisher.

The nurse should enforce agency smoking policy and help prevent fires from starting. For example, frayed or broken electrical cords or faulty equipment should not be used. The maintenance department should be immediately notified of defects in equipment. The safety of both the patient and the nursing staff depend on the nurse's knowledge of fire safety.

ACCIDENTAL POISONING

Poisoning is the condition or physical state produced by the ingestion, injection, or inhalation of or exposure to a poisonous substance. A **poison** is a substance that impairs health or destroys life.

Childhood poisoning is one of the major causes of death in children under 5 years of age. There are more than 500 toxic substances in the average home. Although legislation passed in the early 1970s required the use of child safety packaging for certain substances, a significant number of accidental poisonings continues to occur. Specific antidotes and treatments are not available for all types of poisons.

The older adult is also at risk. Changes associated with aging interfere with the individual's ability to absorb or excrete drugs. Because of the cost factor, older adults may share drugs with friends or save medications with plans to take them when they are needed again. Changes in eyesight may lead to an accidental ingestion, or if there is memory impairment, older patients may forget when they last took prescribed or over-the-counter drugs.

Hospitalized patients are at risk for all types of accidents. Ingestion of harmful substances should be prevented by the nurse. Drug administration procedures should be followed. Staff-development programs related to new drugs or updated information on frequently used drugs should be attended.

Prevention of Poisoning

For prevention of poisoning, toxic agents should be removed. Toxic or poisonous substances should not be removed from their original containers, since the substance may be mistaken for something else. Poisonous substances should be labeled conspicuously and put away immediately after use.

Poison control centers are valuable sources of information when poisoning is suspected or does occur. Information received from the center may aid in treatment and referral. Many health care agencies have posted instructions about how to handle cases of poisoning (Skill 22-2). The nurse should know where these instructions are located.

DISASTER PREPAREDNESS

A **disaster-preparedness plan** is a formal plan of action that enables the hospital staff and rescuers to respond effectively and efficiently when confronted with a disaster in the hospital or community. A **disaster** is an uncontrollable, unexpected, psychologically shocking event. Examples of natural threats to safety are earthquakes, hurricanes, floods, and tornadoes. Bombings, arson, riots, and hostage-taking represent acts of violence carried out by people.

Each disaster situation is unique and directly affects health agencies. Factors that affect disaster response include the time of day; the scope and duration of the triggering event; prior readiness of the health agency, personnel, equipment, and procedures; and the extent to which the various community agencies and institutions collaborate with each other. Health agencies are expected to receive victims and survivors and to assist rescuers.

Types of Disasters

Disasters can be external or internal. The external disaster originates outside the health care agency and results in an influx of casualties brought to the agency. The emergency department is the main focus of activity. There is no immediate safety threat to the staff, patients, or agency. An internal disaster is brought about by events within the health care agency. The organization's ability to function normally is threatened. The internal disaster often threatens the safety of the patients, visitors, staff, and agency.

Disaster preparedness represents the means by which health care agencies and personnel meet the responsibilities associated with managing the disaster. The conduction of disaster drills on a routine basis helps ensure that health care personnel respond effectively. Personnel should be familiar with the location and contents of the agency disaster manual. Generally, disaster manuals specify departmental responsibilities, chain of command, callback procedures, assignment procedures, patient evacuation procedures and routes, and procedures for the receipt and management of supplies and equipment.

■ NURSING CARE PLAN ■

RISK FOR POISONING

Mr. M, age 87, is admitted for intake of a caustic substance, lye. His wife told the physician that her husband has been getting confused lately and has been diagnosed with Alzheimer's disease.

NURSING DIAGNOSIS

Risk for poisoning related to internal factors (swallowed lye) as evidenced by burns in and around the mouth, pain, and dyspnea

GOAL

- Patient will respond to treatment.

EXPECTED OUTCOMES

- Patient will not be further exposed to caustic substances.
- Family will explain safekeeping of caustic substances in future.

NURSING INTERVENTIONS

- Observe patient continuously (around the clock or in a nursing home) to help prevent another incident.
- Monitor vital signs every 1 to 2 hours to assess for complications.
- Teach wife about importance of constant observation of her husband and determine wife's ability to protect husband.

EVALUATION

- Observe environment for potential threats to safety.

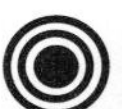

SKILL 22-1 APPLYING RESTRAINTS

Steps	Rationale
1. Obtain equipment: ▪ Clean gloves ▪ Type of restraint necessary ▪ Lotion	Helps organize procedure.
2. Refer to medical record, care plan, or Kardex for special interventions.	Provides basis for care.
3. Introduce self.	Decreases anxiety level.
4. Identify patient by identification band.	Identifies correct patient for procedure.
5. Explain procedure to patient.	Seeks cooperation and decreases anxiety.
6. Wash hands and don gloves according to agency policy and guidelines from Centers for Disease Control and Prevention and Occupational Safety and Health Administration.	Helps prevent cross-contamination.
7. Prepare patient for intervention:	
a. Close door to room or pull curtain.	Provides privacy.
b. Drape for procedure if necessary.	Prevents exposure of patient.
8. Raise bed to comfortable working level.	Provides safety for nurse.
9. Arrange for patient privacy.	Shows respect for patient.
10. Assess patient's potential for injury.	Helps protect patient injury.
11. Apply appropriate type of restraint.	
WRIST OR ANKLE (EXTREMITY RESTRAINT)	
12. Make clove hitch, if using Kerlix (Fig. 22-1), by forming a figure eight and pick up loops.	Immobilizes extremity: clove hitch does not tighten when pulled.
13. Place gauze or padding around extremity.	Decreases injury to skin.
14. Slip wrist or ankle through loops directly over padding.	Protects skin.
15. Wrap padded portion of restraint around affected extremity, thread through slit in restraint, and fasten to second tie with secure knot.	Protects skin.
16. Tie ends of restraint in bow (not to side rails).	Prevents patient injury.

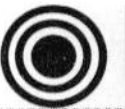

SKILL 22-1 APPLYING RESTRAINTS—cont'd

Steps	Rationale
17. Leave as much slack as possible (1 to 2 in).	Allows patient movement.
18. Palpate pulses below restraint.	Ensures that restraint is not too tight.
19. Monitor skin for irritation.	Prevents impaired skin integrity, which can be caused by excessive pressure.
20. Assess circulation to extremity distal to restraint at least every 2 hr.	Identifies problems and thus need to remove or adjust restraint.
ELBOW RESTRAINT	
21. Place restraint and piece of fabric with slots for insertion of tongue blades to keep restraint straight over elbow.	Prevents elbow flexion and keeps children from reaching equipment.
22. Wrap restraint snugly, tying restraints at top.	Prevents patient removal of restraint.
23. Monitor position of restraint, circulation, and skin condition frequently.	Helps prevent skin irritation.
VEST (JACKET OR CHEST) RESTRAINT	
24. Apply restraint over patient's gown (Fig. 22-2).	Protects patient's skin.
25. Place vest on with V-shaped opening in front or fasten with Velcro and zipper.	Prevents patient from choking.
26. Pull tie at end of vest flap across chest and slip tie through slit on opposite side of vest.	Provides appropriate and safe application of restraint.
27. Wrap other end of flap across patient and tie straps in bow to frame of bed or behind wheelchair (where patient cannot untie it) (Fig. 22-3).	Helps secure vest restraint to patient.
28. Make room for fist in space between vest and patient.	Ensures that vest is not too tight.
29. Monitor respiratory status.	Helps prevent respiratory distress.
30. Remove restraints every 2 hr according to agency policy and patient need. *(Patient should not be left unattended during removal.)*	Enables skin and circulation to be assessed and patient's position to be changed.
31. Wash, rinse, and dry skin areas and massage with lotion.	Increases circulation and prevents skin breakdown.
32. Perform range-of-motion exercises when restraints are removed.	Increases circulation and joint movement.
33. Remove gloves and wash hands.	Helps prevent cross-contamination.
34. Document.	Documents procedure and patient's response.

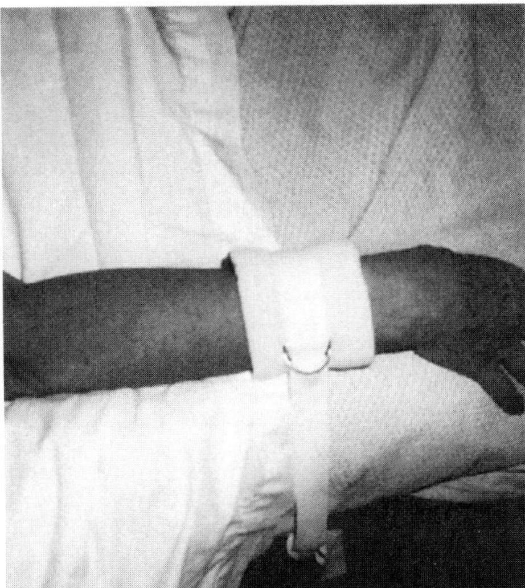

Fig. 22-1 Wrist or ankle restraint. (From Christensen BL, Kockrow EO: *Foundations of nursing,* ed 2, St Louis, 1995, Mosby.)

Continued.

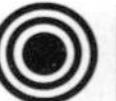

SKILL 22-1 APPLYING RESTRAINTS—cont'd

Steps	Rationale

A 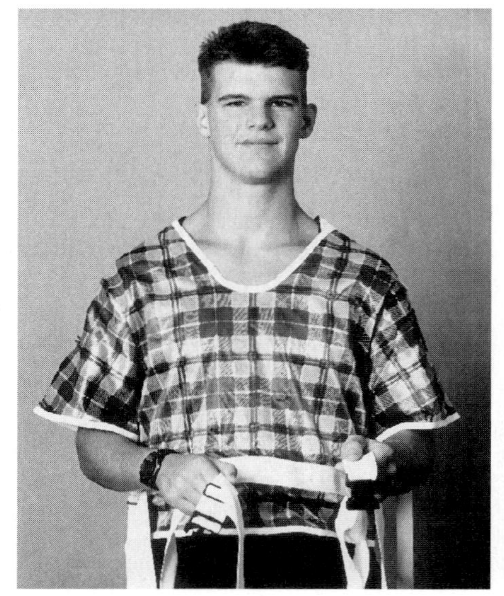 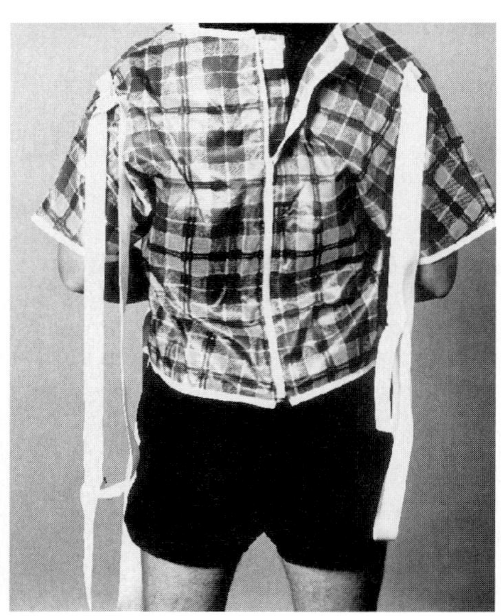 B

Fig. 22-2 Vest restraint. **A,** Front view. **B,** Rear view.

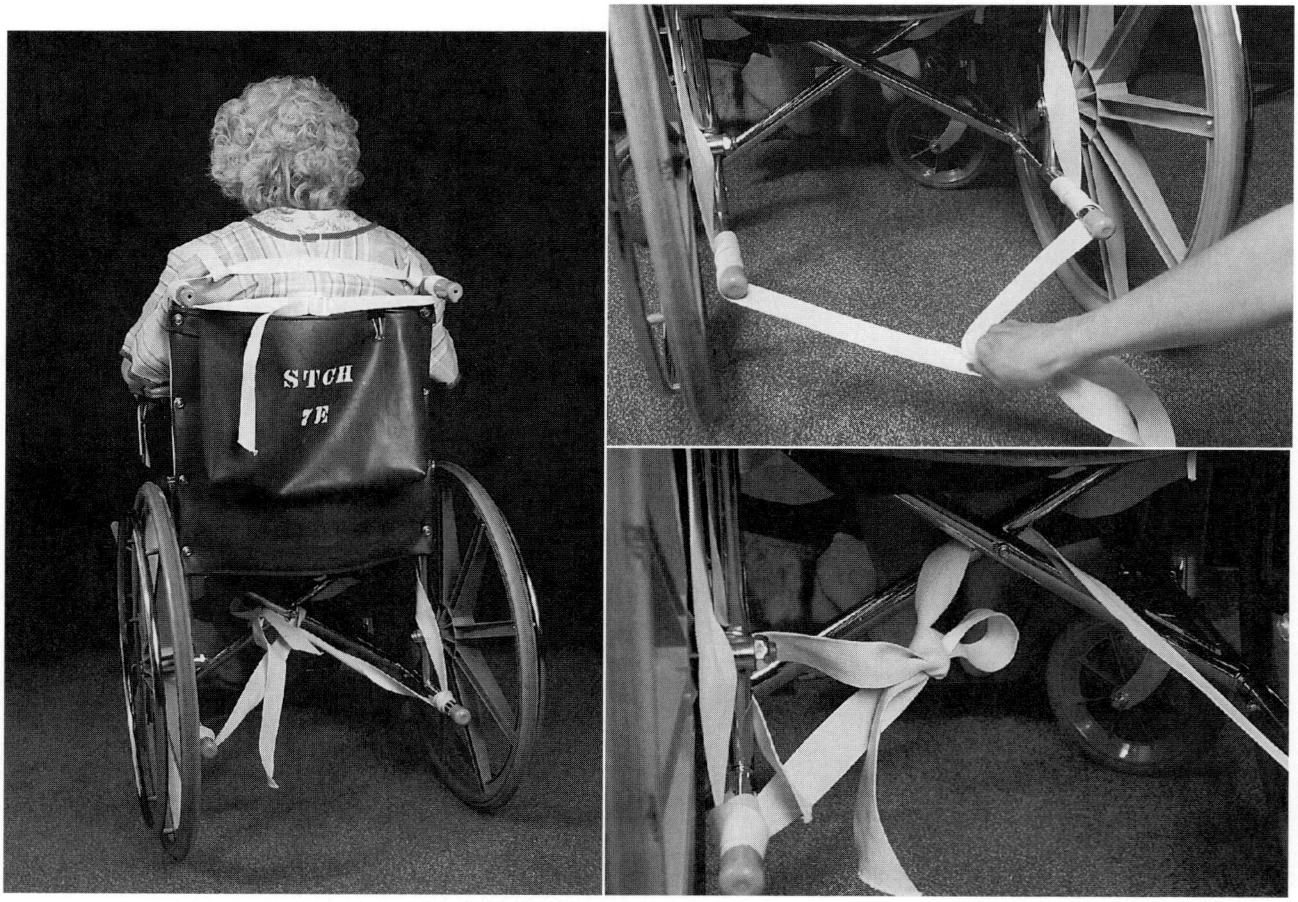

Fig. 22-3 Quick release tie for Posey vest restraint with patient in wheelchair. (From Potter PA, Perry AG: *Basic nursing: theory and practice,* ed 3, St Louis, 1995, Mosby.)

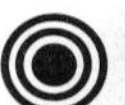

SKILL 22-2 CARING FOR VICTIMS OF ACCIDENTAL POISONING

Steps	Rationale
1. Obtain equipment: ▪ Clean gloves ▪ Ipecac ▪ Emesis basin	Helps organize procedure.
2. Refer to medical record, care plan, or Kardex for special interventions.	Provides basis for care.
3. Introduce self.	Decreases anxiety level.
4. Identify patient by identification band.	Identifies correct patient for procedure.
5. Explain procedure to patient.	Seeks cooperation and decreases anxiety.
6. Wash hands and don clean gloves according to agency policy and guidelines from Centers for Disease Control and Prevention and Occupational Safety and Health Administration.	Helps prevent cross-contamination.
7. Prepare patient for intervention:	
a. Close door to room or pull curtain.	Provides privacy.
b. Drape for procedure if necessary.	Prevents exposure of patient.
8. Raise bed to comfortable working level.	Provides safety for nurse.
9. Arrange for patient privacy.	Shows respect for patient.
10. Notify poison control center or follow agency protocols.	Furnishes treatment guidelines.
11. If instructed, use ipecac to induce vomiting, following dosage instructions, and provide adequate liquids:	Induces emesis when it is safe to do so.
a. Make certain gag reflex is intact.	Prevents aspiration.
b. If instructed, save emesis. (Note presence or absence of pill particles.)	Provides specimen for toxicologic analysis.
c. Place patient's head to one side.	Reduces risk of aspiration.
12. Do not induce vomiting if poisoning is related to household cleaners, lye, furniture polish, grease, or petroleum products.	Reduces risk of internal burns and damage.
13. Do not induce vomiting in an unconscious patient.	Reduces danger of aspiration.
14. Continue to monitor vital signs and patient's response to treatment.	Provides ongoing assessment.
15. Remove gloves and wash hands.	Helps prevent cross-contamination.
16. Document.	Documents procedure and patient's response.

SUMMARY

The need for a safe environment is constant. The hospital environment has traditionally been a primary concern of nursing, and it has expanded to recognize threats faced by hospital personnel.

Restraints are sometimes necessary for the patient's safety as well as for the safety of those around the patient. Restraints should not be used unless absolutely necessary and then for only as long as necessary.

Health care agencies and their employees should be in a state of fire preparedness. Accidental poisoning should be prevented. The child and the older adult are the most at risk for injury in this area. Disaster preparedness provides medical and nursing care for potential victims.

Key Concepts

- A safe environment in a health care agency is important to prevent injury.
- Children are at high risk, especially regarding fatal home accidents.
- Older adults are at high risk related to the aging process and the inability to function as they did at one time in their lives.
- The nurse is usually the one responsible for patient safety in the hospital.
- The patient should not be physically restrained unless there is possible risk of injury to the patient or to others.

Critical Thinking Questions

1. Mr. Jones is a disoriented older adult who likes to wander the halls in the long-term care facility. Restraining him adds to his disorientation and causes him to become agitated. Describe alternative nursing measures that could be used to ensure his safety.
2. During a clinical rotation, the nurse admits an older blind patient to the nursing unit. The patient is mobile but unaccustomed to the surroundings. What measures would the nurse take to ensure this patient's safety?
3. The fire alarm sounds, indicating that there is a fire on the unit. The nurse is giving a bath to a patient with limited mobility. Describe the sequence of actions that the nurse would take to best provide for the safety of the patients and personnel.

REFERENCES AND SUGGESTED READINGS

Christensen BL, Kockrow EO: *Foundations of nursing,* ed 2, St Louis, 1995, Mosby.

Farrell J: *Nursing care of the older person,* Philadelphia, 1994, Lippincott.

Potter PA, Perry AG: *Basic nursing: theory and practice,* ed 3, St Louis, 1995, Mosby.

Seliger JS, Simoneau JK: *Emergency preparedness,* Rockville, Md, 1994, Aspen.

CHAPTER 23

Hygiene

Learning Objectives

After studying this chapter, the student should be able to . . .

- Define the key terms.
- Explain the principles of bedmaking.
- Identify the purposes for administering oral hygiene.
- Explain the safety measures in assisting the patient on and off the bedpan.
- Make the following types of beds: open, closed, occupied, unoccupied, orthopedic, and surgical.
- Administer a bed bath, partial bath, self-bath, shower, tub bath, sitz bath, tepid sponge bath, and medicated bath.
- Perform perineal care.
- Administer care of a patient's hair, nails, feet, ears, and nose.
- Shave a male patient.

Key Terms

Alopecia
Bedpan
Bedtime care
Cerumen
Closed bed
Complete bed bath
Early AM care
Fracture pan
Hygiene
Medicated tub bath
Open bed
Oral hygiene
Partial bath
Patient unit
Pediculosis
Perineal care
Prosthesis
Sitz bath
Stimulus
Surgical bed
Tepid sponge bath
Urinal

Skills

23-1 Making a bed
23-2 Bathing a patient
23-3 Assisting with oral hygiene
23-4 Caring for the hair
23-5 Caring for the hands, feet, and nails
23-6 Shaving the male patient
23-7 Assisting with the bedpan and urinal

Hygiene is the observance of health rules and methods or means of preserving health. Appropriate physical hygiene is necessary for comfort, safety, and well-being. Whereas well people are usually capable of meeting their own hygienic needs, ill people may require assistance. Several factors influence hygiene practice (see box). The nurse determines a patient's ability to perform self-care and provides or assists with hygiene care according to the patient's needs and preferred practices.

NURSING PROCESS FOR HYGIENE

Assessment

Most assessment occurs as the nurse cares for the patient's hygienic needs. Hygiene care allows the nurse to assess for a variety of health care problems and thus helps set health care priorities. Nursing assessment is an ongoing process. However, the nurse must always first determine whether the patient can tolerate hygiene procedures, which can often be exhausting.

While bathing a patient, for example, the nurse assesses physical conditions such as skin turgor and condition, areas of potential breakdown, and tissue perfusion. Because hygiene care often requires inti-

FACTORS INFLUENCING HYGIENE PRACTICE

Body Image
- The way patients look and feel about themselves indicates the importance of hygienic practices. The nurse must not convey feelings of disapproval if the patient's hygiene is poor. When body image changes from surgery or illness, the nurse takes extra care to provide hygiene.

Economic Status
- Hygienic practices are influenced by the economic resources available to patients. The nurse determines whether patients can afford hygiene supplies.

Knowledge
- Patients' knowledge about the importance of proper hygiene influences motivation and practice. Often, learning about the illness or condition encourages patients to improve hygiene.

Sociocultural Variables
- The patient's cultural beliefs, age, personal values, and familial practices influence hygiene care. Patients from diverse cultural backgrounds follow different self-care practices.

Personal Preferences
- Each patient has individual desires and preferences concerning hygiene. The nurse incorporates the patient's schedule and care practices into the plan.

Physical Condition
- Certain illnesses, surgical procedures, and devices, such as casts or traction, may exhaust, incapacitate, or decrease the dexterity of patients. The nurse may need to assist with or perform total hygiene care.

From Potter PA, Perry AG: *Basic nursing: theory and practice,* ed 3, St Louis, 1995, Mosby.

mate contact with the patient, the nurse can use communication skills to promote the therapeutic relationship and to learn about a patient's emotional needs.

Nursing Diagnosis

Nursing assessment helps identify the patient's need for and ability to maintain personal hygiene. Care of the patient is then based on the nursing diagnoses that have been identified. Possible nursing diagnoses for hygiene include the following:

Altered health maintenance
Altered oral mucous membrane
Body-image disturbance
Bowel incontinence
Impaired physical mobility
Impaired skin integrity
Knowledge deficit (specify)
Risk for impaired skin integrity
Risk for infection
Self-care deficit: bathing/hygiene, dressing/grooming
Self-esteem disturbance

Planning

The plan for providing hygienic care should focus on types or methods of care and on the many care measures that the nurse can perform. Considering a patient's preferences before planning is important. The type of hygiene that the patient desires or requires determines the supplies and equipment that the nurse must prepare. The nurse should also schedule hygienic care around tests and procedures.

The plan of care focuses on achieving specific goals and outcomes that relate to the identified nursing diagnoses. Examples of these include the following:

Goal #1: Patient achieves relaxation and comfort.

Outcome

Patient expresses sense of comfort and cleanliness after hygienic measures.

Goal #2: Patient participates in hygiene.

Outcome

Patient begins performing hygienic measures independently 2 days before discharge.

Implementation

Hygienic measures include care of the patient's environment and personal hygiene needs. Nursing actions include bedmaking, bathing, and care of the hair, eyes, ears, nose, nails, and skin. Certain principles guide nurses in providing patient hygiene.

1. Unbroken and healthy skin and mucous membranes help the body protect itself from harm.
2. The skin and mucous membranes of different people vary in sensitivity and irritations.
3. Appropriate blood circulation is necessary for healthy cells and tissues.

While providing hygiene care, the nurse can also assess readiness to learn and teach health-promotion practices (see teaching box). The nurse must also consider patients' beliefs, values, and habits. Individual preferences do not significantly affect health and can usually be included in the plan of care. The nurse preserves as much of the patient's independence as possible, ensures privacy, and fos-

PATIENT TEACHING

- Stress the importance of daily hygienic care.
- Advise patient against putting foreign objects in ears and nose.
- Teach patient to blow nose gently.
- Stress the importance of appropriate diet to promote good oral health.
- Advise patient to brush teeth at least 4 times daily and to thoroughly rinse after brushing.
- Teach caregivers to provide personal hygiene for the patient.

GERONTOLOGIC CONSIDERATIONS

- Older adults are more likely to become chilled during bathing or when left uncovered. The room temperature should be warmer than for younger persons, and drafts should be minimized.
- Older adults should be treated with respect. Grooming, including hair care and use of cosmetics, should be age appropriate.
- Too frequent bathing and use of detergent soaps can have harmful effects on the skin of older adults. Type and frequency of baths and choice of soaps should be based on individual needs.
- Decreased production of saliva in aging necessitates more frequent oral hygiene. Appropriate cleaning of the oral cavity and teeth or dentures may help reduce the alteration in taste common with aging.

ters physical well-being (see care plan on p. 443). The special needs of the older adult must also be considered (see gerontologic box).

Evaluation

During and after hygienic care, the nurse evaluates the success of interventions. The process is dynamic because the patient's condition may change. The nurse must always be prepared to revise the care plan based on the evaluation. For example, if a patient's skin continues to be reddened over the sacrum, more frequent turning may be necessary. Systematic evaluation requires the nurse to determine whether expected outcomes have been met. The nurse refers to the goals and outcomes identified when planning care and performs measures designed to specifically evaluate the achievement of those goals. Examples of goals and their corresponding evaluative measures include the following:

Goal #1: Patient achieves relaxation and comfort.

Evaluative measure

Ask patient to describe level of comfort or fatigue after hygienic measures

Goal #2: Patient participates in hygiene.

Evaluative measure

Observe patient beginning and assisting with hygienic activities.

ENVIRONMENT

The needs of the patient include five environmental needs: space, comfort, privacy, safety, and stimuli. Each of these areas must be met to prevent discomfort and complications.

Space

Patients prize the space allotted as theirs, no matter how small. Generally, in a hospital or long-term care facility this space includes the **patient unit.** The patient unit consists of the bed, an overbed table, a bedside table, and possibly a chair. There may also be closet space or drawers. The nurse should respect the patient's space and keep it in appropriate order.

Comfort

Several areas of the patient's environment can contribute to or detract from comfort. In many facilities, rooms have been remodeled to get away from the stark white institutional colors of the past. Some facilities now have carpeting, wallpaper, house lighting, drapes, and pictures on the walls. The nurse must still be aware of the glare from lights, whether natural or artificial. The humidity (moisture) in the air is most comfortable at 30% to 60%. Some patients (for example, those with asthma or other respiratory conditions) may be more comfortable at a higher humidity. The room temperature is most comfortable at 68° to 74° F. Patients with burns or older adults may require warmer temperatures. The room air should be as free of pollen and microbes as possible.

The furniture is designed to promote comfort. Most facilities have beds with adjustable head and knee areas. The bed as a whole can be positioned higher or lower to assist the nurse in using appropriate body mechanics. The mattress is generally firm for appropriate body alignment. It is often covered with plastic to protect the mattress from moisture and microorganisms. However, this covering can cause some patients to perspire. The pillow is usually made of foam to prevent possible allergy, and it is often covered with plastic. Some institutions now issue disposable pillows for patient use.

The overbed table is provided for eating, reading, and writing. It also allows the patient to be positioned in the tripod, or forward-leaning, position. Some overbed tables have a drawer for storage of the patient's personal items for grooming.

The bedside stand holds equipment for personal care and provides space on top for placing personal items. A straight chair and a stuffed chair may also be a part of the room.

On entering the facility, the patient is usually issued some personal care items. These may include a water pitcher, glass, wash basin, soap dish, mouthwash cup, emesis basin, bedpan and urinal, mouthwash, toothpaste, toothbrush, tissues, skin lotion, and powder. Most equipment is made of plastic, making it much quieter and disposable to lessen the risk of cross-contamination.

Diversionary items may also be supplied or be made available to the patient. Television or radio; soft, melodious music on the intercom; and a telephone are items the nurse may note in the patient's room.

Privacy

Some areas of the health care facility threaten the patient's privacy. The procedures that the nurse performs may become routine for the nurse but are viewed as new and invasive by the patient. Noises may invade the patient's privacy. Overstimulation from noise may cause fatigue. The most prevalent kinds of noises in a health care facility include other patients' radios or televisions, talking in the corridors or other rooms, other patients in distress, voice paging, crying of babies and children, telephones, and noises from the unit pantry, kitchen, or utility rooms.

Odors can also invade the patient's privacy, since illness may alter the patient's sense of smell. Different odors are inherently a part of a health care facility. To help decrease the odors the nurse should empty all waste and emesis basins frequently, replace the water in old flowers frequently, change soiled linens promptly, use deodorant and offer deodorant to patients, avoid the use of heavy perfumes, and avoid the smell of cigarettes on one's own clothing.

The patient is also at risk for unnecessary body exposure. To prevent exposure, the nurse should remember to close window drapes, close the curtain between beds and in front of the room door, and provide a robe and houseslippers for the patient when out of bed.

Safety

Falls account for half the accidental deaths in the home. Scalds and other burns are second. It is reasonable to assume that accidents are even more likely in an environment with which the patient is unfamiliar and during a time of illness (see Chapter 22). Measures the nurse may take to prevent falls in the health care facility include the use of side rails. Side rails should be up at all times unless the patient is coherent or a release has been signed. The bed should be in the lowest position and with wheels locked unless the nurse is directly beside the bed. The call system is provided at the bedside, in the bathroom, in lounges, and in shower rooms. The nurse ensures that the patient understands how the system works. Nonskid stools are provided in tubs or showers so that the patient can sit if needed. Nonskid strips are placed on the floors of showers or tubs as well. The nurse should clean up spills as soon as they are noted. Waiting for someone from housekeeping to clean up a spill can lead to an accident. The patient should wear sturdy shoes or slippers whenever out of bed. Clutter is kept off the floors, and pathways are cleared before ambulation is attempted with a patient. At night, the pathways should be well lit to prevent accidents. The nurse walks with any patient who seems unsteady.

Safety measures to prevent electrical shock are also necessary. Cords are inspected for signs of fraying or breaks. Plugs are removed by holding onto the plug and not by pulling on the cord. The nurse never kinks cords or overloads a wall outlet. An appliance that feels or smells hot or gives shocks is never used. All plugs in the facility should be grounded. Water conducts electricity. Neither the nurse nor the patient should stand in water or have wet hands when handling electrical equipment. Safety risks are always reported.

Stimuli

A **stimulus** is anything in the environment that causes a response in a person. This could be a noise, odor, light, pain, or taste. *Deprivation* is the state of having too little stimuli for patient well-being. *Overload* is the state of having too much stimuli for patient well-being. The nurse should provide nursing interventions to prevent both extremes. To help relieve the monotony of a stay in a facility, the nurse uses diversionary methods, moves lights and plants, converses with patients, encourages visitors, encourages physical activity as allowed, gathers patients together when possible, and encourages the patient to use television, radio, magazines, and books.

MAKING A BED

Bath time is a good opportunity for making the patient's bed. Hospitalized patients, especially those on bedrest, spend a great deal of time in bed. Lying in bed may interfere with maintenance of skin integrity, and a vital responsibility of the nurse is to prevent skin breakdown. The patient's bed must be kept clean, dry, and free of wrinkles and food crumbs. Beds should be made well enough to remain tight even after the patient has been in the bed for a while (Skill 23-1). After meals, the bed should be assessed for food crumbs, which should be removed. The patient's clothing and the bed linens should be kept clean and dry to prevent pressure ulcers.

While handling linens, the nurse should wear clean gloves to protect against body fluids. Linens should not be shaken or come into contact with the nurse's uniform to prevent the spread of microorganisms. The side of the linens touching the patient may be rolled up inside the other linens to further decrease the spread of microorganisms.

A bed is said to be a **closed bed** if the top bed linens are pulled up over the bed with the pillow on top. This is the type of bed that is used in long-term facilities and after one patient leaves the hospital but before the next has been admitted. A bed is said to be an **open bed** when the top linens are fanfolded (folded lengthwise like a fan). This makes the bed ready for the patient. A **surgical bed** also has a fanfolded sheet, the pillow is at the foot of the bed, and a protective plastic sheet is on the bed at approximately the site of surgery (see Chapter 17).

HYGIENE

The skin is the largest of all body organs. Keeping the skin clean and dry is the responsibility of the nurse. The outer layer of skin is call the *epidermis.* This layer helps protect the inner layers from trauma. Next is the dermis, followed by the subcutaneous layer. Beneath these three layers of skin lie the fascia, muscle, and bone. Functions of the skin include protection, secretion, body temperature regulation, and sensory information (Table 23-1).

During hygienic measures, the nurse should assess all areas of the skin, especially bony promi-

Table 23-1 FUNCTION OF THE SKIN AND IMPLICATIONS FOR CARE

Function/Description	Implications for Care
Protection Epidermis is relatively impermeable layer that prevents entrance of microorganisms. Although microorganisms reside on skin surface and in hair follicles, relative dryness of surface inhibits bacterial growth. *Sebum* removes bacteria from hair follicles. Acidic pH of skin further slows bacterial growth.	Weakening of epidermis occurs by scraping or stripping its surface such as by use of dry razors, tape removal, or improper turning or positioning techniques. Excessive dryness causes cracks and breaks in skin and mucosa that allow bacteria to enter. Emollients soften and prevent moisture loss, soaking improves moisture retention, and hydration of mucosa prevents dryness. However, constant exposure to moisture causes maceration or softening, which interrupts dermal integrity and promotes ulcers and bacterial growth. Bed linen and clothing should be kept dry. Misuse of soap, detergents, cosmetics, deodorant, and depilatories can cause chemical irritation. Alkaline soaps neutralize protective acid condition of skin. Cleansing removes excess oil, sweat, dead skin cells, and dirt that can promote bacterial growth.
Sensation Skin contains sensory organs for touch, pain, heat, cold, and pressure.	Friction should be minimized to avoid loss of stratum corneum, which can result in pressure ulcers. Smoothing linen removes sources of mechanical irritation. Nurse should remove rings to prevent injuring patient's skin. Bath water should not be too hot or cold.
Temperature regulation Body temperature is controlled by radiation, evaporation, conduction, and convection.	Factors that interfere with heat loss can alter temperature control. Wet bed linen or gowns interfere with convection and conduction. Excess blankets or bed coverings can interfere with heat loss through radiation and conduction. Coverings can conserve heat.
Excretion and secretion Sweat promotes heat loss by evaporation. Sebum lubricates skin and hair.	Perspiration and oil can harbor microorganism growth. Bathing removes excess body secretions, although excessive bathing can cause dry skin.

From Potter PA, Perry AG: *Basic nursing: theory and practice,* ed 3, St Louis, 1995, Mosby.

PURPOSES OF BATHING

Cleansing of the Skin

- Cleansing removes perspiration, some bacteria, sebum, and dead skin cells, which minimizes skin irritation and reduces chance of infection.

Stimulation of Circulation

- Good circulation is promoted through use of warm water and gentle stroking of extremities.

Improved Self-Image

- Bathing promotes relaxation and feeling of being refreshed and comfortable.

Reduction of Body Odors

- Excessive secretion of sweat from apocrine glands located in axillae and pubic areas causes unpleasant body odors. Bathing and use of antiperspirants minimize odors.

Promotion of Range of Motion

- Movement of extremities during bathing maintains joint function.

From Potter PA, Perry AG: *Basic nursing: theory and practice,* ed 3, St Louis, 1995, Mosby.

nences. The skin should appear smooth, intact, and elastic. The nurse should assess for variations common in the skin of the older adult, including loss of color or skin blotches, wrinkling, and dryness. The nurse should also assess for redness and edema (abnormal accumulation of fluid in interstitial spaces of tissues).

During a stay in a health care agency, patients are much less active than at home and are at risk of developing a pressure ulcer (see Chapter 21). Some conditions also increase the patient's risk for developing pressure ulcers if the blood supply to the skin is decreased from *stasis* (condition in which the normal flow of a fluid through a vessel is slowed or halted). Pressure ulcers usually occur over a bony prominence (projecting part of a bone).

BATHS

Normal flora (microorganisms) live on the surface of the skin, but many are removed during the bath. Types of hospital baths include the complete bed bath, partial bath, tub bath, shower, sitz bath, and medicated bath. The type of bath chosen depends on the patient's diagnosis and condition, mobility, and ability to perform self-care. The patient may choose the type of bath desired if the condition permits. The nurse must provide patient safety and privacy when any type of bath is administered (Skill 23-2). The bath has three other basic benefits to the patient besides cleanliness (see box): (1) stimulation to increase circulation, (2) administration of active or passive exercise, and (3) stimulation of respirations.

The bath also has three basic benefits for the nurse:

1. It allows time for assessment and observations.
2. It promotes establishment of the nurse-patient relationship.
3. It provides a time for patient teaching.

The hospital bath is usually administered after the morning meal. The patient's preferences should be considered whenever possible. The frequency with which a person bathes depends on the type of illness, physical activities undertaken, and dryness of the skin. Some patients do not use commercial soaps because of their drying effect on the skin. If this is a problem, bath oils, creams, lotions, powder, deodorants, and antiperspirants may be used.

When a patient is seriously or critically ill, sedated, or in a weakened state, the nurse must assist by administering a **complete bed bath.** As the patient improves, a partial bath may be administered. For a **partial bath,** the nurse bathes the body parts that the patient cannot.

Patients may be allowed to take a tub bath or shower if the condition warrants and ambulation has been ordered.

The physician may order a **sitz bath** for a patient who has undergone rectal or vaginal procedures to promote healing and provide pain relief. Women who have delivered infants take sitz baths for the same reasons. A sitz bath requires a patient to sit in a tub filled to hip level with warm water (110° to 115° F or 94° to 98° F if tissues are damaged) for 15 to 20 minutes. The sitz bath may also be administered using a special pan that fits into the toilet. This pan may have a bag of warm water with a tube that is clamped and unclamped to keep the water warm. The application of warm water on the skin produces dilation of blood vessels, soothes tissue, and promotes healing. If the warm water is applied for a prolonged period, however, the blood vessels once again constrict, producing the opposite effect. The tolerance of heat varies with individuals and with different areas of the body. Therefore the nurse should assess the area often during application of heat. Moist heat feels warmer and damages tissues faster than dry heat. A debilitated, unconscious, or older patient may not easily tolerate the application

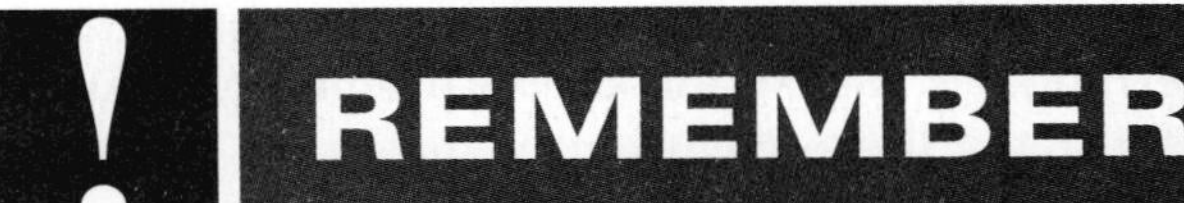

- The patient's privacy during bath time should be guarded, especially with other personnel entering and leaving the room at random.
- The nurse should use care and discretion when bathing the extremely modest patient.
- The nurse should encourage the patient to keep covered with a drape during the bath.

of heat and must be carefully assessed. The nurse also assesses all patients for faintness, pressure to the back of the legs, and chilling. These problems are reported to the charge nurse.

A **tepid sponge bath** (moderately warm, approximately 80 to 90° F) is administered to reduce an elevated temperature. When children are ill, they often have high temperatures, so sponging is often performed. The tepid sponge bath should last 25 to 30 minutes. Applying cool water to the skin immediately constricts the blood vessels. However, if the cool water is applied for a prolonged period, the vessels dilate once more and produce the opposite effect. During a tepid sponge bath, the nurse bathes each extremity for 5 minutes and the patient's back for 5 minutes. The nurse drapes the patient to prevent chilling. The nurse assesses for changes in the patient's color, chilling, or trembling. If the temperature is brought down too rapidly, the patient is at risk for shock. The tolerance for application of cold varies with individuals and with different areas of the body. Moist cold feels colder and damages tissues faster than dry cold. Debilitated, unconscious, and older patients may not easily tolerate the application of cold. Thus the nurse should assess the tissue often during the application of cold.

Medicated tub baths may be ordered from time to time. These baths include oatmeal or oatmeal extract (used to reduce tension and decrease itching), cornstarch (also used to decrease itching), Burrow's solution (used in certain skin disorders), and sodium bicarbonate (also used to decrease itching).

A whirlpool bath involves the immersion of the body or a part of the body in a tank of hot water agitated by a jet of equally hot water and air.

When assisting a patient with a tub bath or shower, the nurse may need to provide **perineal care** (cleaning of the genital and anal areas). Perineal care may also be ordered to be performed more often than a bath (that is, after the delivery of a child, after vaginal or rectal surgery, and in other conditions). Smegma is the thick, normal secretions found in the perineal area. Smegma may become foul smelling and provides an excellent medium for the growth of microorganisms if not removed quickly with bathing.

When providing perineal care for the female patient, the nurse must wash between the labia majora and the labia minora. In the male patient, the nurse must retract the uncircumsized foreskin to cleanse underneath it. The foreskin must be replaced to prevent discomfort, constriction, and edema. The scrotum must be handled gently to prevent pain. While giving perineal care, the nurse works from the inner areas to the outer areas and from the top of the perineal area to the bottom of the perineal area (from "clean to dirty").

Backrub

The backrub provides massage to areas of the skin prone to pressure and pressure ulcer formation. The massage increases circulation, keeping the skin cells healthy. The backrub is also relaxing to the patient who may be under tension related to illness and responsibilities at home.

Oral Hygiene

Oral hygiene is included in the morning bath and involves keeping the teeth and oral cavity clean and free of odor. Keeping the mouth clean encourages the patient to eat and helps food taste better. The nurse provides or assists with oral hygiene according to the patient's needs (Skill 23-3). Oral hygiene may be performed by the patient or by the nurse. The nurse may need to provide oral hygiene to the unconscious patient or to the patient with dentures. The nurse must carefully handle dentures to prevent breakage.

Many people neglect oral hygiene or inappropriately perform care of the teeth. The nurse can help the patient by teaching performance of appropriate oral hygiene and encourage its performance. Some patients may need oral hygiene every 1 to 2 hours. Older patients must be assessed often, since many may forget to perform oral hygiene. Pediatric patients should begin oral hygiene in infancy using a soft cloth to wipe the gums. As the teeth appear, the parent will need to provide oral hygiene until the child can be taught to consistently perform the procedure. Dental visits should begin no later than age 2 and should continue every 6 months to 1 year throughout life.

Hair Care

Care of the hair is a part of the patient's personal hygiene. Clean and neat hair improves the patient's self-image. Hair care is usually included with the morning bath (Skill 23-4). It is administered to pre-

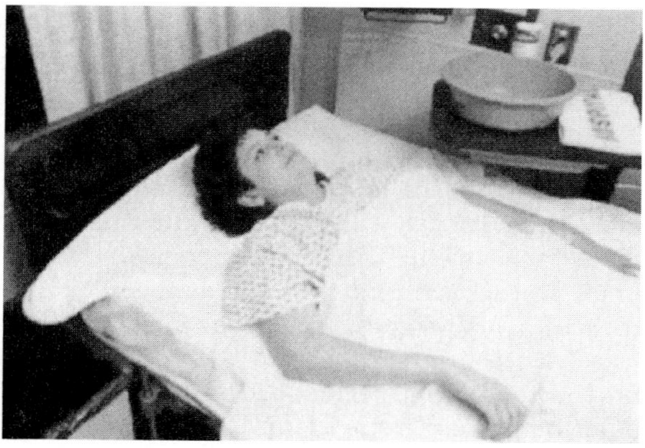

Fig. 23-1 Use of shampoo tray for patient on bedrest. (From Perry AG, Potter PA: *Clinical nursing skills and techniques,* ed 3, St Louis, 1994, Mosby.)

vent tangling and matting for the patient on bedrest. It is important that the patient's hair be combed or brushed at least every day for comfort.

During hair care, the nurse should assess for open sores, scratch marks, pressure areas, or the presence of nits. Nits are the eggs of the human louse, which attaches to the hair shaft. **Pediculosis** is an infestation of lice on the head, skin, or body or on the eyelids, eyelashes, or pubic region. Lice are treated to prevent their spread to others. Contrary to popular belief, uncleanliness is not the cause of pediculosis.

Alopecia (loss of hair) may be caused from a lack of caring for hair. It may also be related to immobility when the patient continually lies in the same position with pressure on the same area of the scalp.

A patient may be allowed to shampoo the hair with a medical order. A special type of device is used by the nurse to shampoo the hair in bed. This device allows rinse water to flow down to a receptacle on the floor (Fig. 23-1).

Care of the Hands, Feet, and Nails

Care of the hands, feet, and nails is often neglected until problems arise. Hangnails, ingrown toenails, and broken nails occur and are often ignored. (For common foot and nail problems, see Table 23-2.) Unless contraindicated, it is the responsibility of the nurse to provide this care (Skill 23-5), usually as a part of morning care after the bath and bedmaking. It is important to understand the agency policy regarding care of the nails, since inappropriate care can cause injury to tissues. During these procedures, the nurse teaches the patient how to appropriately perform this care. The patient who has diabetes mellitus must be taught hand, foot, and nail care, since these patients do not heal quickly. Patients with diabetes may suffer serious problems, including loss of limb, if great caution is not taken regarding care of the hands, feet, and nails. For this reason, the nurse should assess the facility's policy and medical orders before providing care for this patient.

During care of the hands, feet, and nails the nurse should assess carefully for any infections, hangnails, ingrown nails, breaks in the skin, corns, calluses, bunions, or pressure ulcers (see Chapter 21).

Shaving the Male Patient

The male patient is assisted to shave or is shaved by the nurse when necessary. The nurse avoids cutting or nicking the patient's skin. Before beginning shaving, the nurse searches the patient history regarding bleeding problems such as hemophilia or leukemia and possible bleeding problems from the use of anticoagulants (that is, heparin). The razor must be sharp, and appropriate strokes must be made to safely perform the skill (Skill 23-6). Shaving for the male patient benefits his self-image and can improve a sense of well-being.

Care of the Eyes

Care of the eyes is considered part of the bath. The nurse must know the procedure and ensure the patient's safety during its performance. The nurse also has the opportunity to perform an eye assessment and report findings to the physician. Care of the eyes includes washing and drying the eyes, applying medication and compresses, and protecting the eyes from injury. The nurse should know the parts of the eye to detect symptoms of eye disease.

A contact lens is a small, curved glass or plastic lens shaped to fit the eye to correct refraction or inability of the lens of the eye to focus accurately. Care should be taken by the nurse to ensure safekeeping of the patient's contact lenses. Lenses may be sent home with the family.

When the patient is unable to remove contact lenses because of serious illness or injury, the lenses are removed for the patient. Professional assistance is best, but if an ophthalmologist is not available, the procedure must be performed for the patient. In the emergency room a suction cup is available for use. Hard and soft contact lenses are removed differently. The nurse may be responsible for removing the contact lenses and must be able to perform the procedure. After removal the lenses must be stored appropriately.

If the patient wears glasses, the nurse stores the glasses in a case in a drawer during the bath. Storing the glasses on top of a table invites accidental

Table 23-2 COMMON FOOT AND NAIL PROBLEMS

Condition	Characteristics	Implications	Interventions
Callus	Thickened portion of epidermis, consisting of mass of horny, keratotic cells; usually flat, painless, and on undersurface of foot or on palm; caused by local friction or pressure	Condition may cause discomfort when wearing tight-fitting shoes.	Advise patient to wear gloves when using tools or objects that may create friction on palmar surfaces. Encourage patient to wear comfortable shoes. Soak callus in warm water and Epsom salts to soften cell layers. Use pumice stone to remove callus after it softens. Reduce reformation by applying creams or lotions.
Corns	Keratosis caused by friction and pressure from shoes; seen mainly on toes and over bony prominence; usually cone shaped, round, and raised	Conical shape compresses underlying dermis, making it thin and tender. Pain is aggravated when tight-fitting shoes are worn. Tissue can become attached to bone if allowed to grow. Patient may suffer alteration in gait because of pain.	Know that surgical removal may be necessary, depending on severity of pain and size of corn. Avoid use of oval corn pads, which increase pressure on toes and reduce circulation.
Plantar warts	Fungating lesion that appears on sole of foot; caused by papilloma virus	Warts may be contagious. They are painful and make walking difficult.	Treat per orders of physician: applications of salicylic acid, electrodesiccation (burning with an electrical spark), or freezing with solid carbon dioxide.
Athlete's foot (tinea pedis)	Fungal infection of foot; scaliness and cracking of skin between toes and on soles of feet; possible appearance of small blisters containing fluid; apparently induced by wearing constricting footwear (for example, sneakers)	Athlete's foot can spread to other body parts, especially hands. It is contagious and frequently recurs.	Keep feet well ventilated. Dry feet well after bathing and apply powder help to prevent infection. Teach patient that wearing clean socks or stockings reduces incidence. Apply griseofulvin, miconazole, or tolnaftate per physician's orders.
Ingrown nails	Toenail or fingernail growing inward into soft tissue around nail; often results from improper nail trimming	Ingrown nails can cause localized pain when pressure is applied.	Apply hot soaks in antiseptic solution. Know that other treatment may be removal of portion of nail that has grown into skin. Instruct client on proper nail-trimming techniques.
Ram's horn nails	Unusually long curved nails	Attempt by nurse to cut nails may result in damage to nail bed with risk of infection.	Refer client to podiatrist.
Paronychia	Inflammation of tissue surrounding nail after hangnail or other injury; occurs in people who frequently have their hands in water; common in diabetic patients	Area can become infected.	Apply hot compresses or soaks and locally apply antibiotic ointments. Teach careful manicuring.
Foot odors	Result of excess perspiration promoting microorganism growth	Condition may cause discomfort as result of excess perspiration.	Teach frequent washing, use of foot deodorants and powders, and wearing of clean footwear.

From Potter PA, Perry AG: *Basic nursing: theory and practice,* ed 3, St Louis, 1995, Mosby.

breakage. The glasses are washed in warm water and possibly detergent. The lenses are dried with a soft cloth. The nurse should not use tissues, which may scratch plastic lenses.

A **prosthetic** (artificial) eye also requires care. If the patient cannot care for it, the nurse must do so. The nurse extracts the prosthetic, cleanses it, and possibly irrigates the enucleated eye socket.

Care of the Ears

The ears of patients may require special care beyond simple washing during the bath. During the bed bath, the nurse should not wash beyond what is easily accessible with the washcloth. However, **cerumen** (earwax) may build up in the ear canal and cause diminished hearing and provide a medium for infection. The physician may use a syringe to remove the cerumen or order the procedure done by a registered nurse proficient with the procedure. The nurse may help the physician or another nurse perform this procedure.

The nurse teaches patients appropriate care of the ears. The use of cotton-tipped swabs are discouraged because they may lead to infection and can contribute to injury of internal tissues. The nurse teaches the patient to blow the nose gently to prevent blocking of the eustachian tube. Parents are taught that children often place small items such as beans, peas, buttons, and teddy bear eyes into their ears. Such items must be removed by the physician.

Care of the Nose

The nose may become irritated if secretions are allowed to remain on the skin. Irritation may also occur if the patient uses tissues often or blows the nose hard. Secretions may be removed gently from the nares by using a safe agent to first soften the crusts. The nose should not be irrigated because this may force matter into the sinuses, causing the spread of microorganisms. Once again, parents are taught that small children place small items in the nares.

PLACING THE BEDPAN AND URINAL

A bedpan or urinal is used when a patient is unable to use the bathroom for urination (voiding) or defecation (bowel movement). The procedure is private, and the patient should be treated with respect and allowed as much privacy as the condition allows (Skill 23-7). Pediatric patients are often very modest and need understanding regarding elimination.

A **bedpan** may be made of metal or plastic. There are two types of bedpans. One type has a high back and is larger. The second type, called a **fracture pan,** is flatter and smaller (Fig. 23-2).

A **urinal** is made of metal or plastic. There are two types. One type is used by the male for voiding (Fig. 23-3). The other has a fuller opening to fit over the vulva. It is called a *female urinal.* The urinal and the bedpan should be emptied immediately after use, cleansed, and returned to appropriate storage. The nurse must know when a patient's intake and output must be measured before emptying the receptacle.

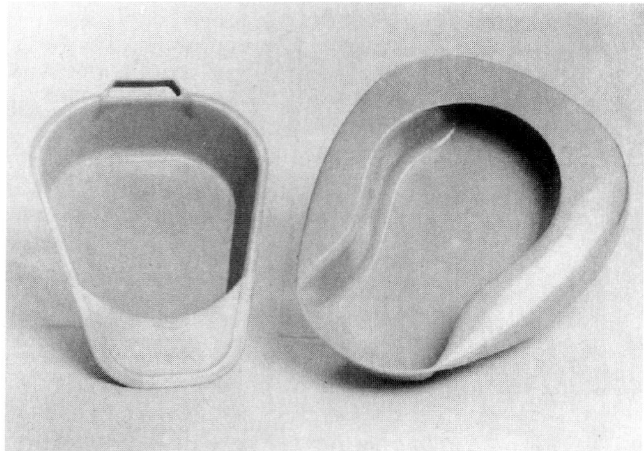

Fig. 23-2 Types of bedpans. *Left,* Fracture bedpan. *Right,* Regular bedpan. (From Perry AG, Potter PA: *Clinical nursing skills and techniques,* ed 3, St Louis, 1994, Mosby.)

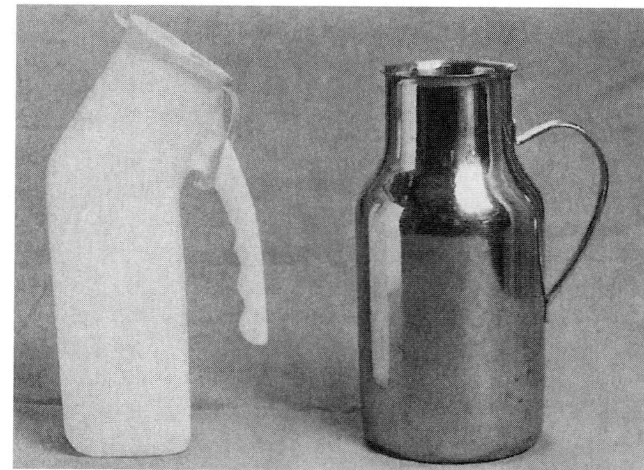

Fig. 23-3 Male urinals. (From Christensen BL, Kockrow EO: *Foundations of nursing,* ed 2, St Louis, 1995, Mosby.)

The metal bedpan is warmed, and the seat powdered. The plastic bedpan is powdered lightly around the seat. This prevents skin from pulling and possibly tearing. The patient is assured that the call light will be answered. The bedpan must not pulled carelessly from under the patient to prevent skin breakdown and spillage. Some patients may require help with cleansing after voiding or defecating. The nurse returns the patient to an appropriate body alignment after removing the bedpan.

A bedside commode may be used for patients who are too weak to walk to the bathroom but who can manage to sit at the bedside. The device is a chair with a hole in the seat area with a receptacle under the seat for receiving body wastes.

A urine or bowel movement provides an opportunity to obtain any needed specimens (see Chapter 13). The nurse should not place toilet tissue into the bedpan or urinal because this may hinder the results of the test.

Early AM Care

Before the arrival of breakfast, the nurse should visit each assigned patient to provide **early AM care.** The patient is offered the bedpan or urinal or is assisted to the bathroom. Supplies are given to the patient to wash the face and hands, or facewashing is performed for the patient. The patient may elect to brush the teeth before breakfast to improve the taste of the food. The nurse should straighten the bed linens and position the patient and the overbed table for the arrival of breakfast.

Bedtime Care

Bedtime care is usually provided between 8 and 10 PM. The nurse offers the patient the bedpan or urinal or assists the patient to the bathroom. Oral hygiene and hair care are provided. Supplies to wash the hands and face are given to the patient, or facewashing is performed for the patient. The patient may be given a backrub. The nurse should straighten the bed linens and ensure that the patient is comfortable. The nurse also offers an extra blanket and darkens the room. The bed is in the low position, the side rails are up as needed, and the call system is within easy reach of the patient.

■ NURSING CARE PLAN ■

SELF-CARE DEFICIT

Mr. J, age 71, has suffered a cerebrovascular accident (stroke). He is unable to use the left side of his body.

NURSING DIAGNOSIS

Self-care deficit: bathing/hygiene and feeding/grooming related to perceptual cognitive impairment as evidenced by lack of personal hygiene

GOAL

- Patient will provide own personal hygiene.

EXPECTED OUTCOME

- Patient will provide own daily personal hygiene by the end of the week.

NURSING INTERVENTIONS

- Assess for status of personal hygiene.
- Assess for patient's ability to help with personal hygiene.
- Provide assistance with daily bed bath; eye care; elimination; oral hygiene; hair care; care of hands, feet, and nails; and shaving.
- Assess skin areas every 2 hr for signs of pressure.
- Provide assistance to patient to turn every 2 hr.
- Assist patient to sit in chair next to bed when possible.

EVALUATION

- Patient indicates satisfaction with level of personal hygiene achieved.
- Patient does not acquire a pressure ulcer.

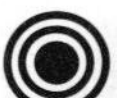

SKILL 23-1 MAKING A BED

Steps	Rationale
1. **Obtain equipment:** ▪ Pillow ▪ Pillowcase ▪ Bedspread ▪ Top sheet ▪ Drawsheet (optional some agencies) ▪ Bottom sheet ▪ Patient gown ▪ Straight chair ▪ Clean gloves	Helps organize procedure.
2. **Refer to medical record, care plan, or Kardex for special interventions.**	Provides basis for care.
3. **Introduce self.**	Decreases anxiety level.
4. **Identify patient by identification band.**	Identifies correct patient for procedure.
5. **Explain procedure to patient.**	Seeks cooperation and decreases anxiety.
6. **Wash hands and don clean gloves according to agency policy and guidelines from Centers for Disease Control and Prevention and Occupational Safety and Health Administration.**	Helps prevent cross-contamination.
7. **Prepare patient for intervention:**	
a. Close door to room or pull curtain.	Provides privacy.
b. Drape for procedure if necessary.	Prevents exposure of patient.
8. **Raise bed to comfortable working level.**	Provides safety for nurse.
9. **Arrange for patient privacy.**	Shows respect for patient.
10. **Assess for urinary or fecal incontinence.**	Causes impaired skin integrity and promotes spread of microorganisms.
11. **Assess for personal items in bed.**	Prevents loss of patient's belongings.
MAKING AN UNOCCUPIED (CLOSED) BED	
12. **Place linens in order of use on seat of a straight chair:** ▪ Pillow ▪ Pillowcase ▪ Bedspread ▪ Top sheet ▪ Drawsheet ▪ Bottom sheet ▪ Patient gown	Facilitates performance of skill because linens are placed in order of use.
13. **Place laundry bag over back of straight chair or near bed.**	Helps prevent collection of lint from loose linens.
14. **Remove pillowcase from pillow and place pillow under stack of linen.**	Places pillow out of way until ready for use.
15. **Loosen bed linens from under mattress on side of bed where nurse is standing.**	Prepares for removal of linens without tearing them on bedsprings.
16. **Remove and fold bedspread and place on pillow unless soiled (if soiled, get clean one).**	Moves bedspread out of way until ready for use.
17. **Fold soiled bed sheets inward toward middle of bed.**	Protects from spread of microorganisms.
18. **Place bundle of soiled linens into laundry bag.**	Prevents spread of microorganisms.
19. **Straighten and move mattress to head of bed.**	Aligns mattress.
20. **Lay bottom sheet on mattress and unfold from top to foot of bed (place bundle of soiled linens into laundry bag).**	Prevents dragging sheet on floor.
21. **Place bottom sheet on bed, hem-side down at edge of foot of mattress (Fig. 23-4) with excess sheet at head of bed.**	Arranges sheet for tucking and prevents skin irritation from raw hem.

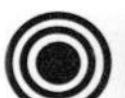

SKILL 23-1 MAKING A BED—cont'd

Steps	Rationale
22. Tuck bottom sheet in at head of bed while standing in front of work area.	Provides appropriate body mechanics for nurse while preventing back strain.
23. *Miter* (make a certain fold and tuck) corner at head of bed (Figs. 23-5 to 23-9). Then tuck sheet under one third of mattress (Fig. 23-10).	Ensures tightness of bottom sheet.
24. Place top sheet over bed with raw edge of hem facing up and with excess sheet at foot of bed.	Prevents raw edge of sheet from rubbing against patient's skin.
25. Complete one side of bed before walking to opposite side.	Saves nurse's energy level as well as time.
26. Loosen bed linen under mattress on opposite side of bed.	Prepares for removal of linens without tearing them on bedsprings.

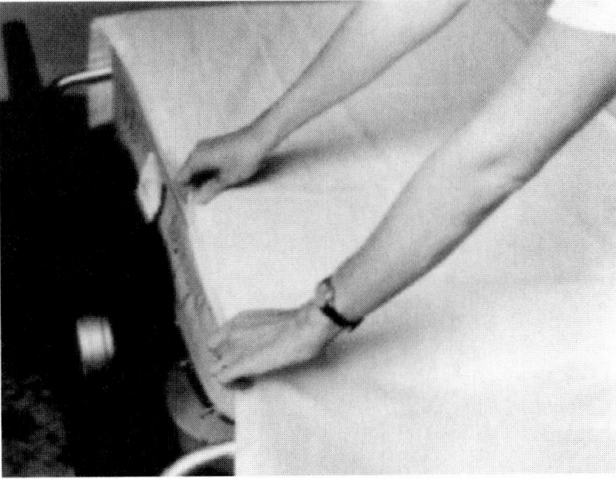

Fig. 23-4 Place bottom sheet on bed. (From Perry AG, Potter PA: *Clinical nursing skills and techniques,* ed 3, St Louis, 1994, Mosby.)

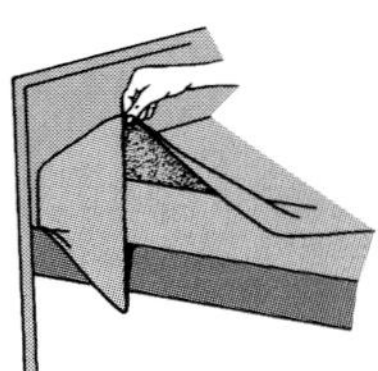

Fig. 23-5 Lift edge of top sheet approximately 45 cm (18 inches) from top of mattress. (From Perry AG, Potter PA: *Clinical nursing skills and techniques,* ed 3, St Louis, 1994, Mosby.)

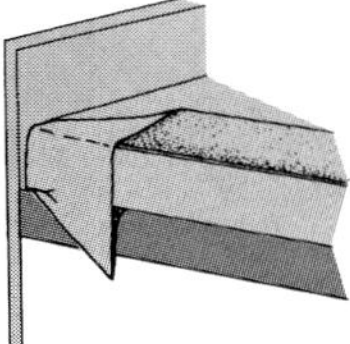

Fig. 23-6 Place sheet on top of mattress to form triangular fold, with lower base of triangle even with mattress side edge. (From Perry AG, Potter PA: *Clinical nursing skills and techniques,* ed 3, St Louis, 1994, Mosby.)

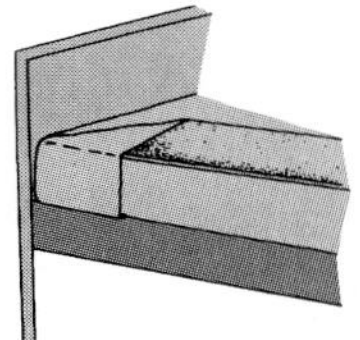

Fig. 23-7 Tuck lower edge of sheet under mattress without pulling triangular fold. (From Perry AG, Potter PA: *Clinical nursing skills and techniques,* ed 3, St Louis, 1994, Mosby.)

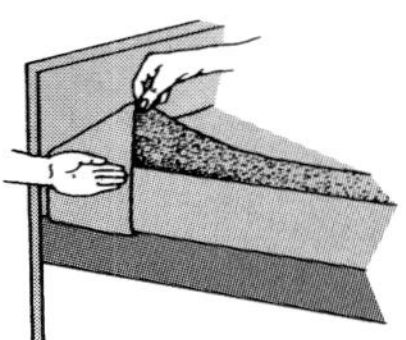

Fig. 23-8 Hold portion of sheet covering side edge of mattress in place with one hand. (From Perry AG, Potter PA: *Clinical nursing skills and techniques,* ed 3, St Louis, 1994, Mosby.)

Continued.

SKILL 23-1 MAKING A BED—cont'd

Steps	Rationale
27. Complete opposite side of bed, mitering corner at head of bed and pulling bottom sheet tight, removing all wrinkles.	Completes placement of sheets and provides patient safety and comfort.
28. Place bedspread on bed about 2 in down from hem of sheet at head of bed. Tuck in tightly at foot and miter sheet corner and bedspread together. Allow bedspread to hang below sheet on side of bed toward door (Fig. 23-11).	Completes placement of bedspread and provides a finished, neat look to bed.
29. Turn sheet hem down over bedspread about 2 in on both sides of bed.	Completes bedmaking.
30. Place clean pillow case on pillow (Fig. 23-12).	Provides finished look to bedmaking.
31. Review work to ensure neat, finished look to bed.	Completes making (unoccupied) closed bed.
OPENING A BED	
32. *Fanfold* top sheet and bedspread to foot of bed.	Prepares for patient's return to bed.
33. Replace pillow with open end away from door to room and seam edge away from where patient's head will rest.	Provides patient comfort.

Fig. 23-9 Pick up top of triangular fold, bring it over side of mattress, and tuck this portion of sheet under mattress. (From Perry AG, Potter PA: *Clinical nursing skills and techniques,* ed 3, St Louis, 1994, Mosby.)

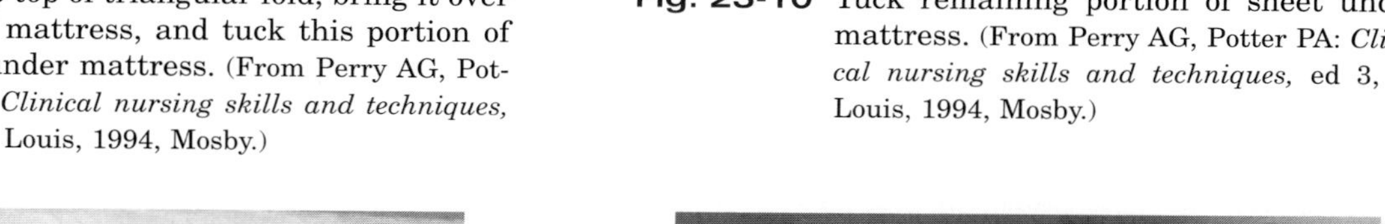

Fig. 23-10 Tuck remaining portion of sheet under mattress. (From Perry AG, Potter PA: *Clinical nursing skills and techniques,* ed 3, St Louis, 1994, Mosby.)

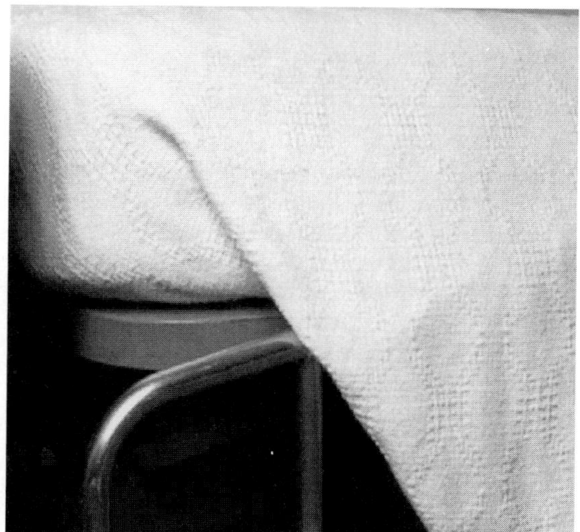

Fig. 23-11 Miter corner of sheet and bedspread together. (From Perry AG, Potter PA: *Clinical nursing skills and techniques,* ed 3, St Louis, 1994, Mosby.)

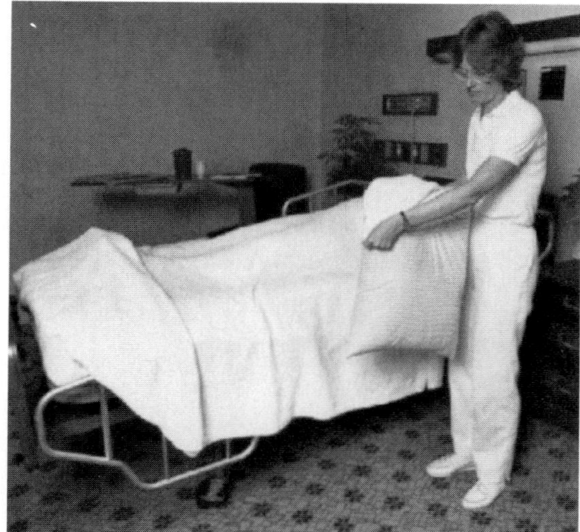

Fig. 23-12 Apply clean pillowcase without contamination from nurse's uniform. (From Perry AG, Potter PA: *Clinical nursing skills and techniques,* ed 3, St Louis, 1994, Mosby.)

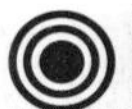

SKILL 23-1 MAKING A BED—cont'd

Steps	Rationale
MAKING AN OCCUPIED BED	
34. Remove pillow case from pillow and place it in laundry bag.	Helps prevent spread of microorganisms.
35. Place pillow under bed linen on straight chair.	Places pillow out of way until ready for use.
36. Turn patient toward opposite side of bed with side rail in up position.	Provides patient safety and comfort.
37. Straighten mattress and move to head of bed.	Aligns mattress.
38. Loosen bed linens from under mattress on side of bed where nurse is standing.	Prepares for removal of linens without tearing them on bedsprings.
39. Remove and fold bedspread and place on pillow unless soiled (if soiled get clean one).	Moves bedspread out of way until ready for use.
40. Fold soiled sheets inward toward middle of bed and gently push them under patient's back.	Prevents spread of microorganisms.
41. Lay bottom sheet on mattress and unfold from top to foot of bed.	Prevents dragging sheet on floor.
42. Place bottom sheet on bed, hem-side down at edge of foot of mattress with excess sheet at head of bed.	Arranges sheet for tucking and prevents skin irritation from raw hem.
43. Tuck bottom sheet in at head of bed while standing in front of work area. (Apply drawsheet if policy dictates.)	Provides appropriate body mechanics for nurse while preventing back strain.
44. Miter corner at head of bed. Then tuck sheet under one third of mattress. Push soiled linens toward patient and gently fanfold under patient.	Ensures tightness of bottom sheet.
45. Place top sheet over bed with raw edge of hem facing up and with excess sheet at foot of bed.	Prevents raw edge of sheet from rubbing against patient's skin.
46. Complete one side of bed before raising side rail on one side and moving to opposite side of bed.	Saves nurse's energy and time. Maintains safety.
47. Lower side rail. Assist patient to roll slowly to other side of bed.	Allows access to linens.
48. Loosen bed linen under mattress on opposite side of bed.	Prepares for removal of linens without tearing them on bedsprings.
49. Complete opposite side of bed, mitering corner at head of bed and pulling bottom sheet tight, removing all wrinkles.	Completes placement of sheets and provides patient safety and comfort.
50. Place bedspread on bed about 2 in down from hem of sheet at head of bed. Tuck in tightly at foot and miter sheet corner and bedspread together. (Bedspread should hang below sheet on side of bed toward door.)	Completes placement of bedspread and provides a finished, neat look to bed.
51. Turn sheet hem down over bedspread about 2 in on both sides of bed.	Completes bedmaking.
52. Place clean pillow case on pillow.	Provides finished look to bedmaking.
53. Replace pillow with open end away from door to room and seam edge away from where patient's head will lie.	Provides patient comfort.
54. Review work to ensure a neat and finished look to bed.	Completes making occupied bed.
55. Make toe pleat for patient.	Provides comfort, patient movement, and helps prevent footdrop.
56. Assist patient in returning to supine position.	Maintains patient comfort.

Continued.

SKILL 23-1 MAKING A BED—cont'd

Steps	Rationale
MAKING AN ORTHOPEDIC BED	
57. Place bottom sheet at head of bed, tuck, and pull sheet down under patient's shoulders, waist, and legs to foot of bed unless contraindicated.	Prevents patient pain.
58. Tuck bottom sheet and miter corners and allow top sheet to hang loose at foot if traction apparatus is attached to foot of bed, if footboard is used, or if bed cradle is in place on top of bed.	Considers need of patient and type of equipment being used.
59. Keep patient warm, especially feet, when bed sheet hangs loose from bed.	Provides warmth and comfort.
60. Dispose of dirty linens.	Provides clean environment and prevents spread of microorganisms.
61. Straighten rest of room.	Ensures that room is neat and pleasant.
62. Remove gloves and wash hands.	Helps prevent cross-contamination.
63. Document.	Documents procedure and patient's response.

SKILL 23-2 BATHING A PATIENT

Steps	Rationale
1. Obtain equipment: ▪ Bath towel ▪ Face towel ▪ Washcloth ▪ Soap ▪ Soap dish ▪ Bath basin ▪ Lotion ▪ Hospital gown or personal gown ▪ Bath blanket ▪ Warm clean water ▪ Bed linens for bedmaking ▪ Clean gloves	Helps organize procedure.
2. Refer to medical record, care plan, or Kardex for special interventions.	Provides basis for care.
3. Introduce self.	Decreases anxiety level.
4. Identify patient by identification band.	Identifies correct patient for procedure.
5. Explain procedure to patient.	Seeks cooperation and decreases anxiety.
6. Wash hands and don clean gloves according to agency policy and guidelines from Centers for Disease Control and Prevention and Occupational Safety and Health Administration.	Helps prevent cross-contamination.
7. Prepare patient for intervention:	
a. Close door to room or pull curtain.	Provides privacy.
b. Drape for procedure if necessary.	Prevents exposure of patient.
8. Raise bed to comfortable working level.	Provides safety for nurse.
9. Arrange for patient privacy.	
10. Assess patient's skin integrity.	Determines bathing and skin care needs.
11. Assess patient preferences regarding bathing depending on condition.	Helps patient to be more cooperative and more likely to allow bath.
COMPLETE BED BATH	
12. Offer bedpan or urinal and allow patient to wash hands afterward (see Skill 23-7).	Provides for elimination needs and helps patient feel refreshed and clean.

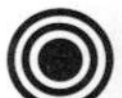

SKILL 23-2 BATHING A PATIENT—cont'd

Steps	Rationale
13. Provide oral hygiene (see Skill 23-3).	Helps prevent tooth and gum disease and refreshes patient's mouth.
14. Remove pillow unless contraindicated and place pillowcase in laundry bag.	Provides container for used linens.
15. Replace top linen with bath-blanket, placing soiled linens in laundry bag.	Provides privacy and warmth.
16. Remove patient's bed clothes and jewelry, securing their safety.	Prepares patient for bath, protects patient's privacy, and prevents jewelry from getting wet.
17. Fill bath basin one-third to one-half full with hot water (105° F). Assess patient's tolerance to temperature on skin.	Prevents spillage of water and provides safe temperature for warmth during bath.
18. Move patient to side of bed toward nurse in supine position.	Helps nurse to reach easily and use appropriate body mechanics.
19. Fold cloth to form mitt (Fig. 23-13) and wash eyes with water only from inner to outer aspect (Fig. 23-14).	Prevents wet, cold ends of cloth from dangling over patient and prevents patient from chilling.

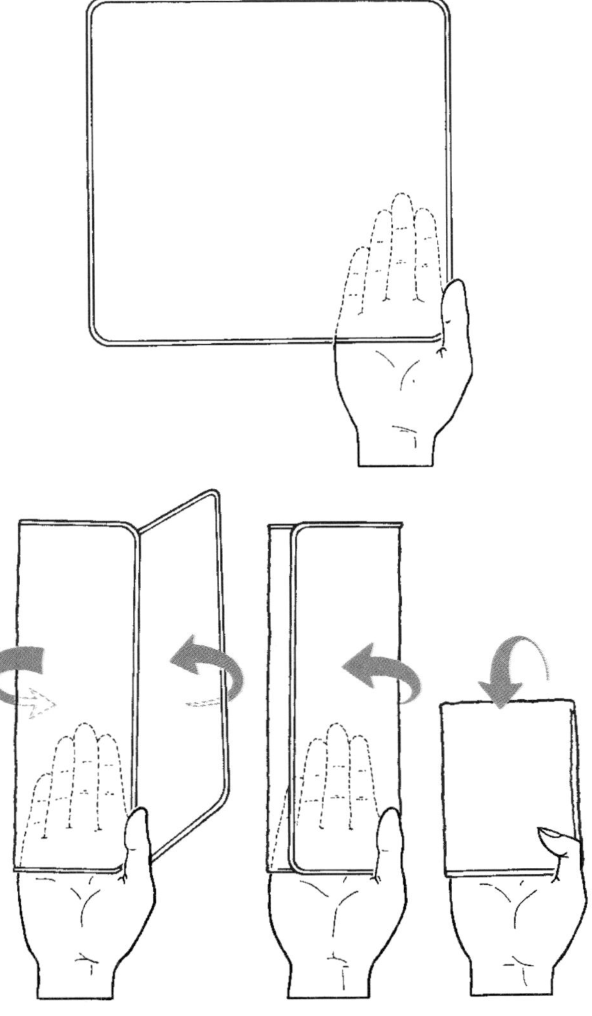

Fig. 23-13 Washcloth folded to form mitt. (From Christensen BL, Kockrow EO: *Foundations of nursing,* ed 2, St Louis, 1995, Mosby.)

Continued.

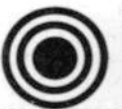

SKILL 23-2 BATHING A PATIENT—cont'd

Steps	Rationale
20. Wash, rinse, and dry face, neck, and ears. From this point on, use towel to drape area being bathed.	Begins bathing from clean to dirty parts of body.
21. Wash, rinse, and dry one arm and then the other using long, firm strokes. Then allow patient to place both hands in basin to wash and soak or have them washed with soap and water, rinsed, and dried.	Provides comfort and is soothing to patient.
22. Wash, rinse, and dry chest and breasts without exposure.	Considers patient's modesty and privacy.
23. Wash, rinse, and dry abdomen, providing attention to umbilicus, using long, firm strokes.	Provides comfort and is soothing to patient.
24. Change bath water and prepare as before.	Helps keep water clean and warm.
25. Wash, rinse, and dry one leg (Fig. 23-15). Soak and wash foot in basin by flexing knee and placing foot in bath basin, protecting heel from resting against edge of basin. Keep patient adequately draped. Assess patient for ticklishness.	Provides comfort. Prevents pressure on heel. Prevents genital area from being exposed. Prevents foot from spilling water from basin onto bed, patient, and nurse.

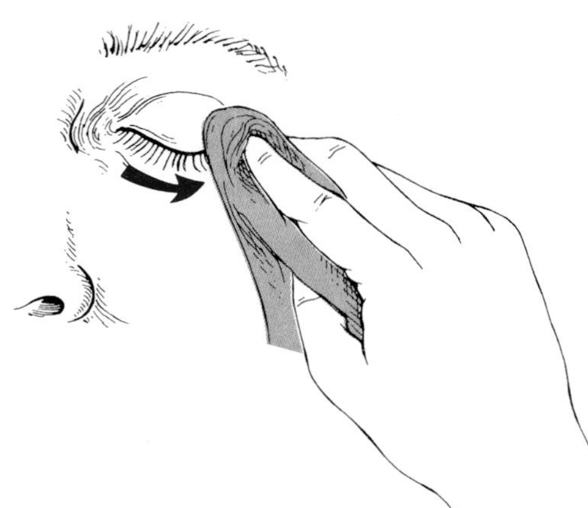

Fig. 23-14 Wash eye from inner aspect to outer aspect. (From Perry AG, Potter PA: *Clinical nursing skills and techniques,* ed 3, St Louis, 1994, Mosby.)

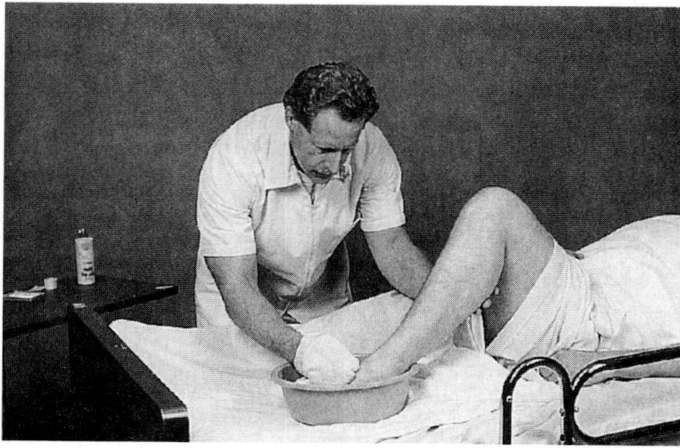

Fig. 23-15 Wash feet one at a time. (From Perry AG, Potter PA: *Clinical nursing skills and techniques,* ed 3, St Louis, 1994, Mosby.)

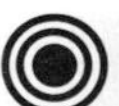

SKILL 23-2 BATHING A PATIENT—cont'd

Steps	Rationale
26. Repeat Step 25 for the opposite leg and foot.	Provides care and comfort.
27. Change bath water and prepare as before.	Helps keep water clean and warm.
28. Wash, rinse, and dry back and buttocks using long, firm strokes.	Provides comfort and increases circulation.
29. Administer 3- to 5-min backrub using lotion warmed in hands. Rub back and buttocks using circular motions (Fig. 23-16).	Provides comfort and relaxation and increases circulation.
30. Wash, rinse, and dry genitals or allow patient to finish bath if able.	Completes patient's bath.
31. Apply clean bedclothes.	Provides warmth and privacy. Provides patient comfort in case physician or family enters room.
32. Empty and clean bath basin.	Readies equipment for next use and helps prevent spread of microorganisms.
33. Provide haircare (see Skill 23-4), shave male patient (see Skill 23-4), and arrange for makeup for female. Assist as necessary with grooming.	Helps patient's body image and well-being.
34. Turn patient toward opposite side of bed with side rail in up position.	Provides patient safety.
35. Move mattress up to head of bed.	Aligns mattress.
36. Make occupied bed.	Provides patient comfort and helps prevent impaired skin integrity.
PARTIAL BATH	
37. Assist with bathing parts of body patient is unable to reach (usually back, legs, and feet). Assist with oral hygiene (see Skill 23-3).	Determines where patient needs assistance.
38. Administer a 3- to 5-min backrub using lotion warmed in hands. Rub back and buttocks using circular motions.	Provides comfort and relaxation and increases circulation.
39. Make open bed.	Prepares for easy access back to bed.
SHOWER OR TUB BATH	
40. Assist patient as necessary to tub or shower room.	Provides patient safety.
41. Arrange for oral hygiene.	Maintains oral care.
42. Make open bed (see Skill 23-1).	Prepares for easy access back to bed.

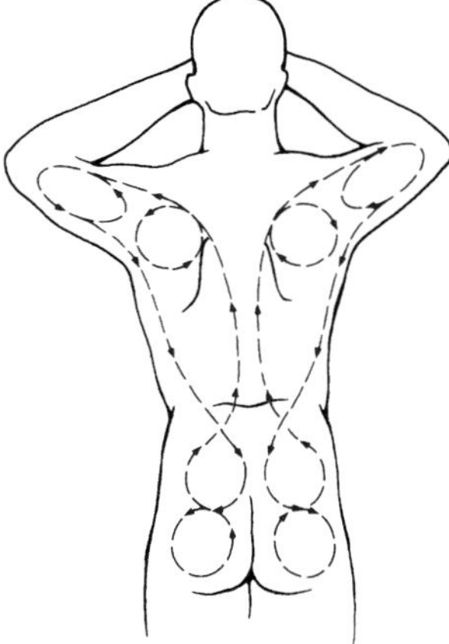

Fig. 23-16 Massage back using circular motion. (From Perry AG, Potter PA: *Clinical nursing skills and techniques,* ed 3, St Louis, 1994, Mosby.)

Continued.

SKILL 23-2 BATHING A PATIENT—cont'd

Steps	Rationale
SITZ BATH	
43. Arrange for oral hygiene (see Skill 23-3).	Maintains oral care.
44. Run appropriate amount and temperature of water in tub: ensure that water comes just to patient's hips.	Prevents burning and provides safety.
45. Assist patient into tub. Arrange more assistance if necessary.	Provides patient safety from injury.
46. Time bath for 15 to 20 min (Time depends on whether this is patient's first time for sitz bath.)	Follows procedure and prevents patient from fainting or becoming weak.
47. Assist patient from tub. Arrange more assistance if necessary. Pat skin dry.	Prevents patient injury.
48. Assist patient back to room.	Prevents patient injury or fall.
49. Assist patient to chair, if able, and make open bed.	Provides easy access back to bed.
TEPID SPONGE BATH	
50. Assess body temperature before sponging.	Provides baseline body temperature.
51. Apply bath blanket over patient.	Provides warmth and prevents chilling.
52. Place warm, wet cloth on face and warm wet towels over body for 20 to 30 min.	Helps reduce body temperature.
53. Reassess body temperature.	Determines change (lowering) of body temperature.
54. Continue sponging at 15-min intervals or until temperature returns to normal or is reduced. Assess condition of patient throughout procedure for complications.	Continues reduction of body temperature and protects patient.
55. Dry patient gently, dress, and provide warmth.	Prevents chilling.
56. Remake bed if necessary (see Skill 23-1).	Provides dry bed and causes comfort.
57. Remove gloves and wash hands.	Helps prevent cross-contamination.
58. Document.	Documents procedure and patient's response.

SKILL 23-3 ASSISTING WITH ORAL HYGIENE

Steps	Rationale
1. Obtain equipment: ▪ Dental floss ▪ Toothbrush ▪ Toothpaste or oral swabs ▪ Dentifrice for dentures ▪ Mouthwash ▪ Emesis basin ▪ Facial tissues ▪ Mouthwash cup ▪ Clean gloves ▪ Towel ▪ Water	Helps organize procedure.
2. Refer to medical record, care plan, or Kardex for special interventions.	Provides basis for care.
3. Introduce self.	Decreases anxiety level.
4. Identify patient by identification band.	Identifies correct patient for procedure.
5. Explain procedure to patient.	Seeks cooperation and decreases anxiety.

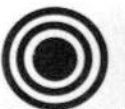

SKILL 23-3 ASSISTING WITH ORAL HYGIENE—cont'd

Steps	Rationale
6. **Wash hands and don clean gloves according to agency policy and guidelines from Centers for Disease Control and Prevention and Occupational Safety and Health Administration.**	Helps prevent cross-contamination.
7. **Prepare patient for intervention:**	
a. Close door to room or pull curtain.	Provides privacy.
b. Drape for procedure if necessary.	Prevents exposure of patient.
8. **Raise bed to comfortable working level.**	Provides safety for nurse.
9. **Arrange for patient privacy.**	Shows respect for patient.
10. **Assess patient's ability to perform oral hygiene.**	Determines amount of assistance needed.
11. **Arrange towel over patient's chest.**	Prevents soiling of bedclothes.
12. **Wet toothbrush, apply toothpaste, and allow patient to brush teeth and gums at 45-degree angle (Fig. 23-17).**	Allows brushing of all tooth surfaces.
13. **Provide patient with water for rinsing mouth.**	Rinses mouth and concludes brushing of teeth.
14. **Provide dental floss.**	Encourages removal of particles and plaque-producing materials and prevents tartar build up.
15. **Allow patient to rinse again.**	Removes particles that flossing dislodges.
16. **Clean and replace articles.**	Provides clean environment.
17. **Remove gloves and wash hands.**	Helps prevent cross-contamination.
18. **Document.**	Documents procedure and patient's response.

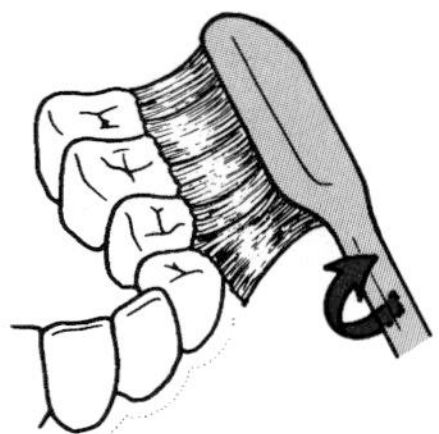

Fig. 23-17 Hold toothbrush at 45-degree angle to gum line. (From Perry AG, Potter PA: *Clinical nursing skills and techniques,* ed 3, St Louis, 1994, Mosby.)

SKILL 23-4 CARING FOR THE HAIR

Steps	Rationale
1. **Obtain equipment:** ▪ Brush ▪ Comb ▪ Face towel ▪ Hair ornaments if desired ▪ Mirror ▪ Clean gloves	Helps organize procedure.
2. **Refer to medical record, care plan, or Kardex for special interventions.**	Provides basis for care.
3. **Introduce self.**	Decreases anxiety level.
4. **Identify patient by identification band.**	Identifies correct patient for procedure.
5. **Explain procedure to patient.**	Seeks cooperation and decreases anxiety.
6. **Wash hands and don clean gloves according to agency policy and guidelines from Centers for Disease Control and Prevention and Occupational Safety and Health Administration.**	Helps prevent cross-contamination.

Continued.

SKILL 23-4 CARING FOR THE HAIR—cont'd

Steps	Rationale
7. Prepare patient for intervention:	
a. Close door to room or pull curtain.	Provides privacy.
b. Drape for procedure if necessary.	Prevents exposure of patient.
8. Raise bed to comfortable working level.	Provides safety for nurse.
9. Arrange for patient privacy.	Shows respect for patient.
10. Assess patient's hair regarding cleanliness, texture, distribution, scalp lesions, and infestation.	Determines type of hair care necessary.
11. Assess type care patient uses for hair and its appropriateness.	Helps determine importance that patient places on overall appearance and personal hygiene.
12. Place towel around shoulders if patient is able to sit or under head.	Prevents hair from falling on gown and refreshes patient to sit up.
13. Comb or assist in combing patient's hair by sections (Fig. 23-18).	Helps prevent pulling hair.
14. Remove towel by folding it away from gown.	Keeps gown clean of hair.
15. Remove gloves and wash hands.	Helps prevent cross-contamination.
16. Comb hair during bath and AM care.	Allows one documentation for several procedures.

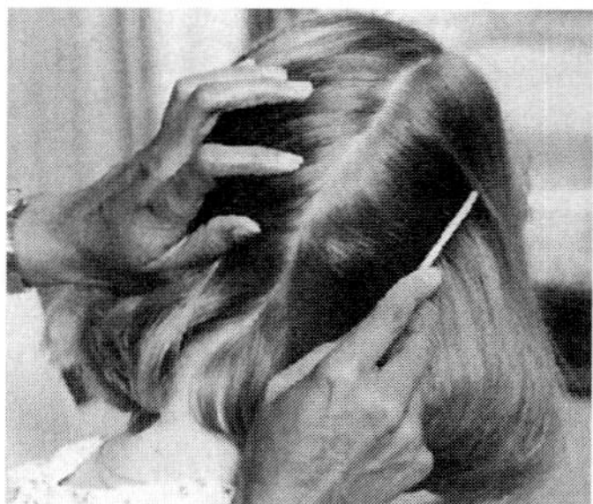
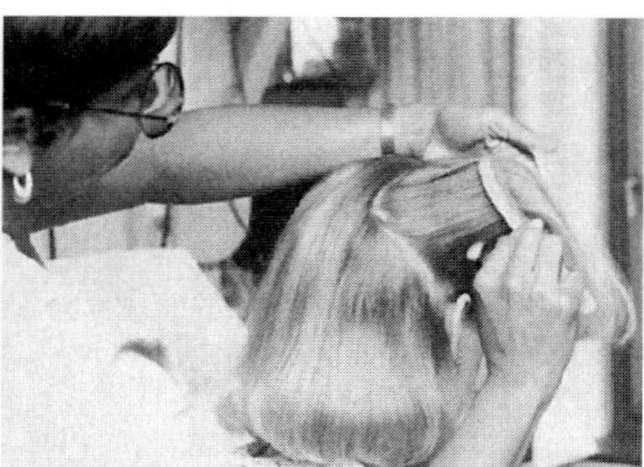

Fig. 23-18 Combing patient's hair. (From Christensen BL, Kockrow EO: *Foundations of nursing,* ed 2, St Louis, 1995, Mosby.)

SKILL 23-5 CARING FOR THE HANDS, FEET, AND NAILS

Steps	Rationale
1. Obtain equipment: ▪ Wash basin ▪ Bath thermometer ▪ Bath towel ▪ Face towel ▪ Washcloth ▪ Orange stick (2) ▪ Emesis basin ▪ Nail clippers, unless contraindicated ▪ Emery board or nail file ▪ Body lotion ▪ Paper towels ▪ Bath mat ▪ Clean gloves	Helps organize procedure.
2. Refer to medical record, care plan, or Kardex for special interventions.	Provides basis for care.
3. Introduce self.	Decreases anxiety level.

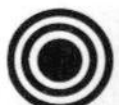

SKILL 23-5 CARING FOR THE HANDS, FEET, AND NAILS—cont'd

Steps	Rationale
4. Identify patient by identification band.	Identifies correct patient for procedure.
5. Explain procedure to patient.	Seeks cooperation and decreases anxiety.
6. Wash hands and don clean gloves according to agency policy and guidelines from Centers for Disease Control and Prevention and Occupational Safety and Health Administration.	Helps prevent cross-contamination.
7. Prepare patient for intervention:	
a. Close door to room or pull curtain.	Provides privacy.
b. Drape for procedure if necessary.	Prevents exposure of patient.
8. Raise bed to comfortable working level.	Provides safety for nurse.
9. Arrange for patient privacy.	Shows respect for patient.
10. Assess color and sensation of fingers, nails, and feet.	Determines circulation to parts.
11. Assess for breaks in skin or cracking of fingers, nails, feet, and toes.	Determines type of care necessary.
12. Assess patient's knowledge of care of fingers, nails, feet, and toes.	Determines need for patient teaching.
13. Fill basin half full of warm water.	Facilitates procedure.
FEET AND TOENAILS	
14. Assist patient in placing feet in warm water to soak.	Softens areas needing care.
15. After soaking nails and feet for 10 to 15 min, dry feet by patting and carefully clean nails with orange stick. Clip nails straight across (Fig. 23-19) or file with nail file unless contraindicated.	Protects patient's skin.
HANDS AND FINGERNAILS	
16. Soak hands for 10 to 15 min in warm water (may soak while caring for feet) (Fig. 23-20).	Softens areas needing care.
17. Dry hands by patting and carefully clean nails with orange stick. Clip nails straight across or file with nail file unless contraindicated.	Protects patient's skin.
18. Remove gloves and wash hands.	Helps prevent cross-contamination.
19. Document special care of hands, feet, and nails but not routine care. Follow agency policy.	Documents care.

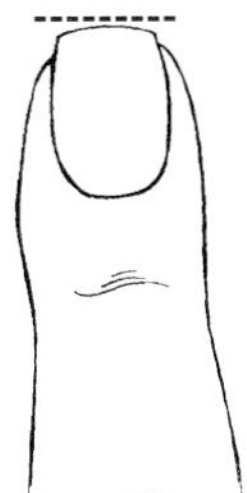

Fig. 23-19 Clip nails straight across. (From Perry AG, Potter PA: *Clinical nursing skills and techniques,* ed 3, St Louis, 1994, Mosby.)

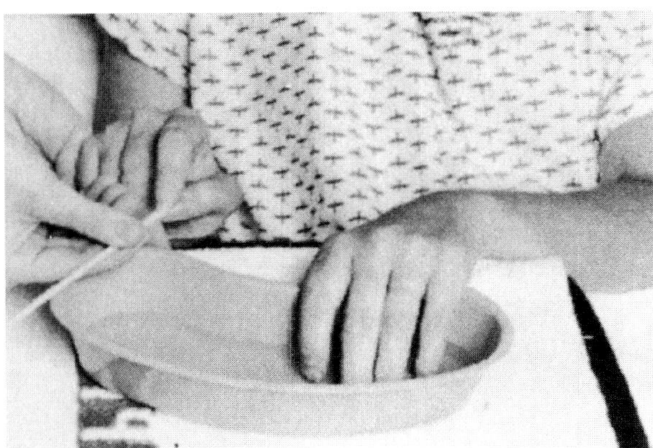

Fig. 23-20 Soak hands in warm water. (From Perry AG, Potter PA: *Clinical nursing skills and techniques,* ed 3, St Louis, 1994, Mosby.)

SKILL 23-6 SHAVING THE MALE PATIENT

Steps	Rationale
1. **Obtain equipment:** ▪ Razor (regular or electric) ▪ Bath towel ▪ Washcloths (2) ▪ Bath basin ▪ Shaving agent (patient preference if possible) ▪ After-shave lotion if desired ▪ Clean gloves	Helps organize procedure.
2. **Refer to medical record, care plan, or Kardex for special interventions.**	Provides basis for care.
3. **Introduce self.**	Decreases anxiety level.
4. **Identify patient by identification band.**	Identifies correct patient for procedure.
5. **Explain procedure to patient.**	Seeks cooperation and decreases anxiety.
6. **Wash hands and don clean gloves according to agency policy and guidelines from Centers for Disease Control and Prevention and Occupational Safety and Health Administration.**	Helps prevent cross-contamination.
7. **Prepare patient for intervention:**	
a. Close door to room or pull curtain.	Provides privacy.
b. Drape for procedure if necessary.	Prevents exposure of patient.
8. **Raise bed to comfortable working level.**	Provides safety for the nurse.
9. **Arrange for patient privacy.**	Shows respect for patient.
10. **Assess for bleeding problems.**	Determines which shaving device to use.
11. **Assess patient's emotional status in case patient needs assurance.**	Provides emotional comfort and safety.
12. **Place patient in semi-Fowler's position unless contraindicated.**	Provides safe, convenient work area.
13. **Place very warm wet washcloth over patient's face, avoiding burning. Remove washcloth.**	Helps soften whiskers and skin.
14. **Apply shaving cream to face.**	Further softens whiskers and skin.
15. **Begin shaving from ear downward to near mouth (Fig. 23-21). Rinse razor.**	Sets pattern to follow to ensure that entire face is shaved.
16. **Continue step 15 until face is completely shaved, rinsing razor often.**	Ensures that entire face is shaved.
17. **Shave upper lip from under nose downward. Rinse razor.**	Helps prevent cuts.
18. **Rinse face and dry by patting.**	Provides comfort.
19. **Apply after-shave if patient desires.**	Helps prevent chapping of skin.
20. **Reposition patient as required.**	Promotes comfort.
21. **Remove gloves and wash hands.**	Helps prevent cross-contamination.
22. **Document according to policy (considered part of bath in some agencies).**	Documents procedure and patient's response.

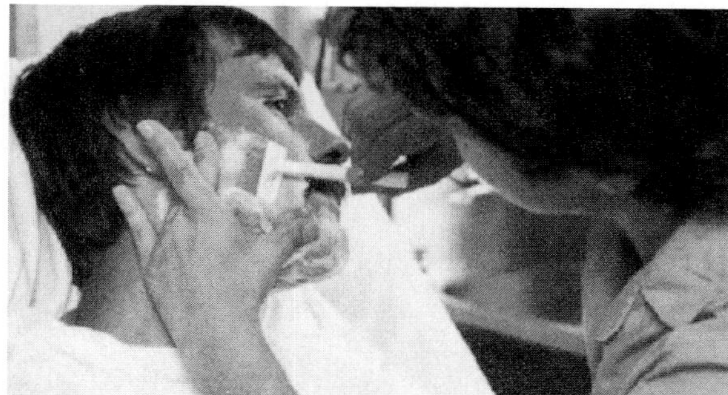

Fig. 23-21 Shaving the male patient. (From Perry AG, Potter PA: *Clinical nursing skills and techniques,* ed 3, St Louis, 1994, Mosby.)

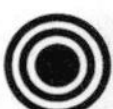

SKILL 23-7 ASSISTING WITH THE BEDPAN AND URINAL

Steps	Rationale

1. Obtain equipment:
▪ Bedpan or urinal
▪ Toilet tissue
▪ Bed protector
▪ Clean gloves
▪ Supplies for washing patient if necessary:
  ▪ Towel
  ▪ Washcloth
  ▪ Bath basin
  ▪ Soap
  ▪ Warm water
	Organize procedure.

2. Refer to medical record, care plan, or Kardex for special interventions.	Provides basis for care.
3. Introduce self.	Decreases anxiety level.
4. Identify patient by identification band.	Identifies correct patient for procedure.
5. Explain procedure to patient.	Seeks cooperation and decreases anxiety.
6. Wash hands and don clean gloves according to agency policy and guidelines from Centers for Disease Control and Prevention and Occupational Safety and Health Administration.	Helps prevent cross-contamination.
7. Prepare patient for intervention:	
a. Close door to room or pull curtain.	Provides privacy.
b. Drape for procedure if necessary.	Prevents exposure of patient.
8. Raise bed to comfortable working level.	Provides safety for nurse.
9. Arrange for patient privacy.	Shows respect for patient.
10. Assess patient's need for assistance.	Assesses need for nursing care.
11. Place protector under patient.	Prevents patient's bed from getting wet.
12. Warm metal bedpan or metal urinal under running warm water.	Provides patient comfort.
HELPING PATIENT UNABLE TO ASSIST SELF ON BEDPAN	
13. Turn patient away from nurse toward opposite side rail, moving linens out of way.	Provides patient safety.
14. Fit bedpan to patient buttocks (Fig. 23-22).	Helps put patient on bedpan without damaging skin.
15. Assist patient to turn over with bedpan while nurse holds bedpan securely. Raise head of bed to 30 degrees.	Keeps bedpan in place for patient comfort and prevents injury to nurse.
16. Place toilet tissue and call light within easy reach.	Provides convenience for patient to clean area or seek assistance.

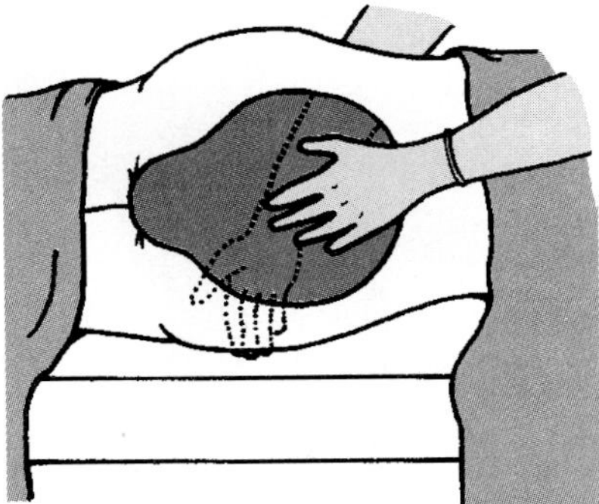

Fig. 23-22 Fit bedpan to patient's buttocks. (From Perry AG, Potter PA: *Clinical nursing skills and techniques,* ed 3, St Louis, 1994, Mosby.)

Continued.

SKILL 23-7 ASSISTING WITH THE BEDPAN AND URINAL—cont'd

Steps	Rationale
17. Allow patient time for elimination or remain in room (if condition warrants), allowing as much privacy as possible.	Provides privacy and safety.
18. Assist in cleaning perineal area if needed.	Helps prevent impaired skin integrity.
19. Remove bedpan as it was applied.	Prevents skin shearing and spillage of urine.
HELPING PATIENT ABLE TO ASSIST SELF ON BEDPAN	
20. Move bed linens out of way.	Prevents linen from getting wet.
21. Ask patient to raise buttocks off bed while nurse supports back (Fig. 23-23, *A*).	Positions patient for placement on bedpan.
22. Slide warmed bedpan under patient's buttocks (Fig. 23-23, *B*).	Provides comfort and prevents shock of cold bedpan.
23. Ask patient to sit on bedpan while nurse adjusts comfort level.	Prevents pressure on bony prominences and impaired skin integrity.
24. Raise head of bed up to tolerance, arrange toilet tissue, and place light within reach of patient.	Positions patient for more natural position for elimination.
PLACING URINAL	
25. Move linens away from genital area without patient exposure.	Prevents exposing patient and from getting bed linens wet.
26. Lift male penis gently and place in urinal if patient unable to do so. If patient is able, allow to handle urinal for voiding.	Prevents injury to male genitals.
27. Replace bed linens over patient.	Provides warmth and prevents exposure.
28. Allow patient to void unless assistance is needed.	Provides freedom to void in privacy.
29. Remove urinal and assist patient as needed.	Determines need for assistance.
30. Measure urine as indicated. Empty bedpan or urinal into graduated container or toilet. Cleanse and replace bedpan or urinal.	Provides part of intake and output if needed.
31. Remove gloves and wash hands.	Helps prevent cross-contamination.
32. Document.	Documents procedure and patient's response.

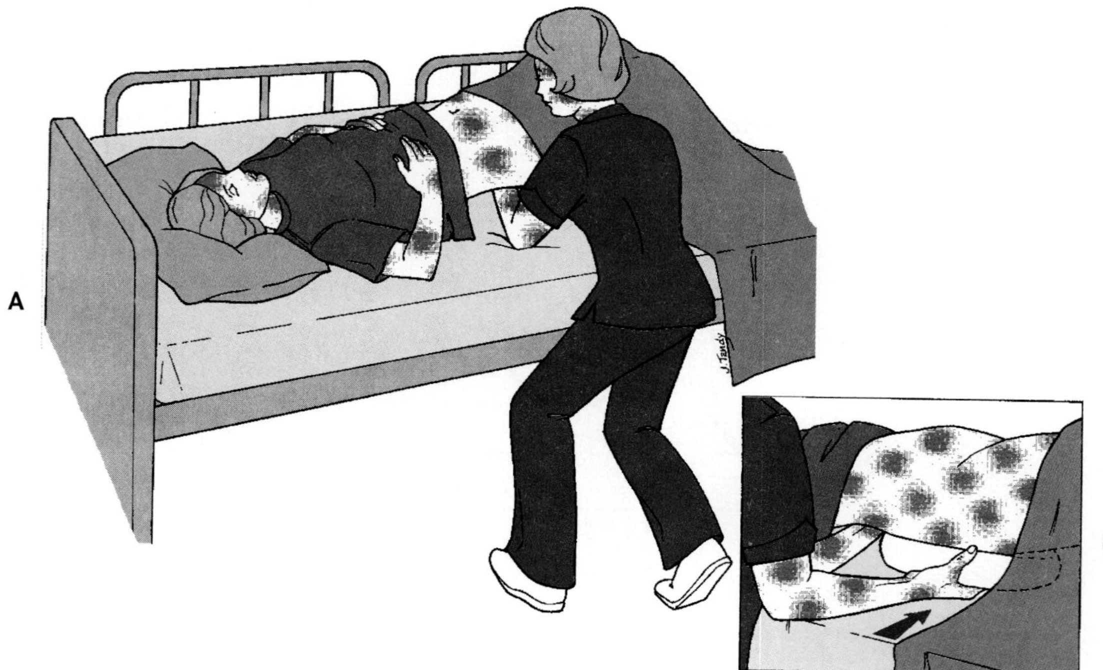

Fig. 23-23 Place bedpan under patient's buttocks.

SUMMARY

The skin is the largest organ of the body and should be kept clean to prevent skin problems. Personal hygiene should be regularly maintained by the patient with assistance from the nurse. The nurse assesses the skin as part of the physical assessment. The patient's immediate environment should also be kept clean to prevent problems while the patient returns to wellness. The nurse is responsible for the patient's comfort, privacy, and safety. Bathing the patient promotes comfort and increases the patient's well-being.

Key Concepts

- The nurse administers a patient's bath when necessary.
- The patient is encouraged to provide personal care as soon as the condition warrants.
- Bath time provides the opportunity to completely assess the patient's problems and needs.
- The patient is allowed to control hygiene situations whenever possible.
- Providing personal hygiene allows the nurse to care for the physical and emotional needs of the patient.
- Patient teaching may be provided during hygienic care once the patient is comfortable and the nurse has had time to develop an appropriate nurse-patient relationship.
- Patient privacy is a must during administration of personal care because it reduces embarrassment and shows respect.
- A backrub should be administered during bath time.
- The patient who has diabetes mellitus should have nail and foot care administered, and the patient should be taught prevention of complications.

Critical Thinking Questions

1. Mrs. Jones, a 70-year-old widow who lives alone, has been admitted to the unit. She is frail and unkempt. Her skin is extremely dry and cracked, with some reddened areas on the sacrum. Describe appropriate nursing interventions that the nurse would take in the situation. What other assessments are required in this situation?
2. Mr. Johns is unconscious after a fall. The plan of care requires good oral hygiene. What measures will ensure safe oral hygiene?
3. Mrs. Lee, a 50-year-old newly diagnosed diabetic patient, has long toenails and asks the nurse to cut them. Describe the sequence of actions the nurse would take and give a rationale for each.

REFERENCES AND SUGGESTED READINGS

Anderson KN, Anderson LE, Glanze WD, editors: *Mosby's medical, nursing, and allied health dictionary,* ed 4, St Louis, 1994, Mosby.

Brunner LS, Suddarth DS: *The Lippincott manual of nursing practice,* ed 6, Philadelphia, 1994, Lippincott.

Lewis SM, Collier IC, Heitkemper MM: *Medical-surgical nursing: assessment and management of clinical problems,* ed 4, St Louis, 1996, Mosby.

McFarland GK, McFarlane EA: *Nursing diagnosis and intervention: planning for patient care,* ed 2, St Louis, 1993, Mosby.

Phipps WJ et al, editors: *Medical-surgical nursing: concepts and clinical practice,* ed 5, St Louis, 1995, Mosby.

Scanlon VC, Sanders T: *Essentials of anatomy and physiology,* Philadelphia, 1995, Davis.

CHAPTER 24

Fluids and Electrolytes

Learning Objectives

After studying this chapter, the student should be able to . . .

- Define the key terms.
- State the difference between intracellular and extracellular fluid.
- Describe the process of electrolyte distribution in the body.
- Identify major electrolytes and their functions.
- Discuss the process of edema formation.
- List signs and symptoms of selected fluid and electrolyte imbalances.
- State nursing interventions related to fluid and electrolyte imbalances.
- State the significance of maintaining a normal acid-base balance in the body.
- Demonstrate the recording of intake and output.

Key Terms

Acid
Acid-base balance
Active transport
Anion
Base
Buffer
Cation
Diffusion
Electrolyte
Extracellular fluid
Hydrostatic pressure
Insensible loss
Interstitial fluid
Intracellular fluid
Intravascular fluid
Oncotic pressure gradient
Osmosis
Plasma

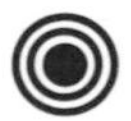

Skill

24-1 Measuring and recording fluid intake and output

Monitoring and maintaining fluid and electrolyte balance is a major responsibility of the nurse when rendering nursing care to patients, particularly the very young and the very old, both of whom are at high risk (see box). Fluid and electrolyte balance is essential for maintaining optimal health. The imbalance of fluids and electrolytes may contribute to altered physiologic function. For example, an increase in the *sodium* level causes fluid retention, and a decrease in the *potassium* level causes a decrease in muscle contractility, eventually leading to paralysis or cardiac dysrhythmias.

BODY FLUIDS

Body fluids are distributed between two major parts (Fig. 24-1). **Intracellular fluid** is found in all cells of the body and is crucial to fluid and electrolyte balance and metabolism. **Extracellular fluid** is all fluid outside a cell and divides into two smaller components. One is **interstitial fluid,** which is found in the spaces between cells of the body and outside of the blood vessels. This fluid accounts for a major percentage of total body fluid. The second component is **intravascular fluid,** or blood plasma. **Plasma** is the fluid portion of the lymph and blood. Other components of plasma are erythrocytes, leukocytes, water, electrolytes, and proteins.

There are three methods by which body fluids and electrolytes move throughout the body. One method is **osmosis,** the movement of a solvent, such as water, through a membrane from a solution that has a lower solute concentration (Fig. 24-2). A second method is **diffusion,** the process in which solid particles of matter in a fluid move from an area of higher concentration to an area of lower concentration, resulting in an even distribution of the particles in the fluid. The third method, **active transport,** is the movement of materials across the membrane of a cell by means of chemical activity that allows the cell to admit larger molecules than would

RISK FACTORS FOR FLUID, ELECTROLYTE, AND ACID-BASE IMBALANCES

- Age
  - Very young
  - Very old
- Chronic diseases
  - Cancer
  - Cardiovascular disease such as congestive heart failure
  - Endocrine disease such as Cushing's disease and diabetes mellitus
  - Malnutrition
  - Chronic obstructive pulmonary disease
  - Renal disease such as progressive renal failure
  - Decreased level of consciousness
- Trauma
  - Crush injuries
  - Head injuries
  - Burns
- Therapies
  - Diuretics
  - Steroids
  - Intravenous therapy
  - Total parenteral nutrition
- Gastrointestinal losses
  - Gastroenteritis
  - Nasogastric suctioning
  - Fistulas

From Potter PA, Perry AG: *Basic nursing: theory and practice,* ed 3, St Louis, 1995, Mosby.

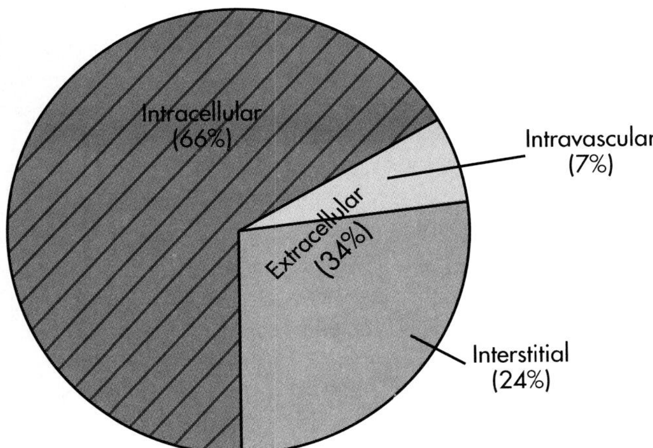

Fig. 24-1 Volumes of body fluids in each fluid compartment. (From Christensen BL, Kockrow EO: *Foundations of nursing,* ed 2, St Louis, 1995, Mosby.)

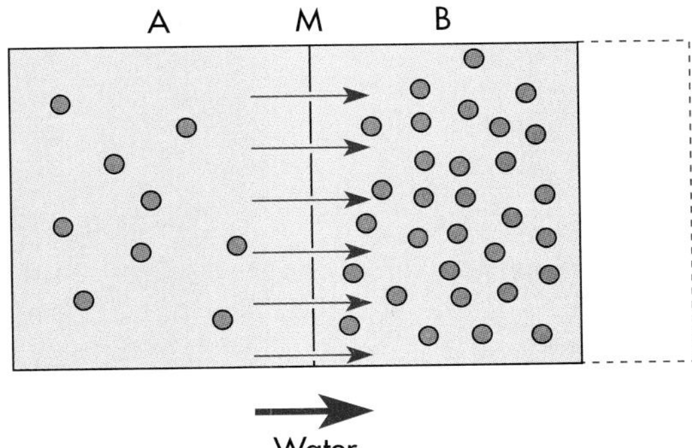

Fig. 24-2 Osmosis: Water moves from an area of lesser solute concentration *(A)* through a membrane *(M)* to an area of greater solute concentration *(B)* until the concentration of solute on both sides of the membrane is equal. Compartment *B* will have to expand *(dotted lines)* to accept the additional water. (From Christensen BL, Kockrow EO: *Foundations of nursing,* ed 2, St Louis, 1995, Mosby.)

otherwise be able to enter. This method also absorbs glucose and other substances needed to sustain life and health.

ELECTROLYTES

Electrolytes are elements or compounds that, when dissolved in water or another solvent, dissociate [separates] into ions and are able to conduct an electric current. They are found in plasma, interstitial fluid, and cell fluid. They are also found in body secretions and excretions. Excessive loss of electrolytes (that is, vomiting, diarrhea, or gastric suction) may cause a fluid or electrolyte imbalance. An **insensible loss,** a continuous, nonvisible form of water loss, may also affect fluid and electrolyte balance. For example, continuous water loss occurs through the skin by evaporation (500 to 600 ml each day). Insensible losses also occur in the lungs through the elimination of water vapor through breathing (300 to 400 ml each day). The water loss through the lungs is much greater with increased respiratory rate and depth. Many illnesses have the potential for accelerating insensible water loss. Some examples are febrile states, major burns, and recurrences of chronic obstructive pulmonary disease.

Fluid and electrolyte imbalances may occur through excessive intake of electrolytes. That is, increased sodium levels cause edema, and increased potassium concentrations adversely affect muscle contractility. Primary serum electrolytes, related bodily functions, normal serum values, definitions of electrolyte imbalances, and signs and symptoms of excesses and deficits can be found in Table 24-2.

ACID-BASE BALANCE

Acid-base balance occurs when the rate at which the body produces acids or bases is balanced with the rate at which acids or bases are excreted. **Acids** are compounds that yield (give up) hydrogen ions in solution, and that turn blue, have a sour taste, and react with bases to form salts. **Bases** are chemical compounds that combine with acid to form salts and that relate to or contain alkaline compounds. The result of acid-base balance is a stable concentration of hydrogen ions in body fluids. The body uses chemical, biologic, and physiologic regulatory mechanisms to maintain acid-base balance. These regulators act as buffers to maintain acid-base balance. A **buffer** is a substance or group of substances that can absorb or release hydrogen ions to correct an acid-base imbalance.

NURSING PROCESS

Assessment

During assessment of fluid, electrolyte, and acid-base balances, the nurse identifies patients at risk for imbalances and the extent to which body systems are involved. Nursing care measures provided for the patient depend on information obtained during assessment. Assessment includes nursing history, measurement and recording of intake and output, laboratory tests, and consideration of factors that influence fluid and electrolyte balance.

Nursing Diagnosis

Nursing diagnoses are established after the nurse reviews data gathered during assessment. Data to determine potential problem areas include oral fluid intake, urine output, inappropriate skin turgor resulting from dry skin, and results of laboratory tests. The presence of a nursing diagnosis in the areas of fluid, electrolyte, and acid-base balance may be subtle. The nurse must be aware that many body systems are involved.

Possible nursing diagnoses related to fluid and electrolyte imbalance include the following:

Decreased cardiac output
Diarrhea
Fluid volume deficit
Fluid volume excess
Impaired gas exchange
Impaired oral mucous membrane
Impaired skin integrity
Ineffective breathing pattern
Risk for fluid volume deficit

PATIENT TEACHING 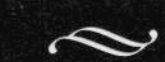

- Instruct patient and caregivers about fluid and dietary measures for fluid, electrolyte, and acid-base imbalances.
- Explain fluid volume deficit and the importance of seeking medical attention to prevent severe illness.
- Explain fluid intake and output and how to measure it accurately.

Planning

The plan of care should focus on the priority problems identified through assessment and diagnosis to prevent life-threatening conditions. It is important for the nurse to collaborate with the patient and family when establishing the plan of care. Often the family can identify subtle behavioral changes associated with fluid, electrolyte, and acid-base imbalances, such as anxiety, irritability, or confusion. The patient and family must know preventive measures, signs and symptoms to report, and measures to implement if an imbalance occurs (see teaching box).

The plan of care may include the following goal:

Goal: Patient's fluid and electrolyte balances are restored and maintained.

Outcomes

Vital signs return to baseline normals.
Urine output equals intake.

Implementation

When implementing the plan of care, the nurse removes or treats the cause of the imbalance if possible. For the patient with an imbalance, the nurse provides appropriate dietary measures and administers supplements if ordered (see care plan on p. 471). The nurse should use special considerations for the older adult (see gerontologic box).

Evaluation

The nurse evaluates the interventions by comparing the patient's responses to the expected outcomes of the established goals. The nurse should be prepared to revise the plan of care based on the evaluation. Evaluative measures may include the following:

Goal: Patient's fluid and electrolyte balances are restored and maintained.

Evaluative measures

Obtain patient's vital signs.
Measure all routes of intake and output.

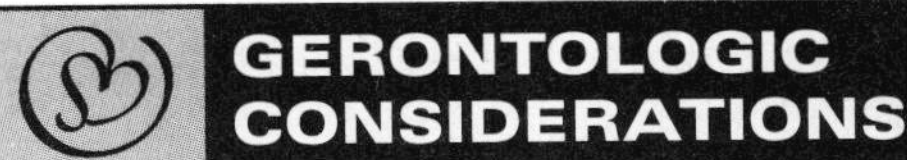

- To compensate for taste changes, older adults may use too much salt on foods, resulting in fluid and electrolyte imbalance.
- Decreased fluid intake increases the risk of constipation.
- The older adult's kidneys are less able to concentrate urine, leading to fluid loss.
- Decreased mobility may result in decreased fluid intake.

REGULATING BODY FLUIDS

Body fluids must be regulated by fluid intake, fluid output, and hormones to maintain balance of the body systems. However, there are variables that influence electrolytes and acid-base (see box).

Thirst controls fluid intake. The hypothalamus controls thirst. The amount of fluid intake needed by a man in 24 hours totals 2600 ml: 1300 ml from fluid intake, 1000 ml from foods, and 300 ml from metabolism.

Fluid output occurs through four organs of water loss, which are the kidneys, skin, lungs, and gastrointestinal tract. Water lost from the kidneys through the excretion of urine provides the greatest amount of output. Water loss from the skin is regulated by the sympathetic nervous system by activation of the sweat glands. The amount that a person sweats in a given time depends on several factors such as muscular exercise, high environmental temperature, and increased metabolic activity. The lungs lose approximately 400 ml of water during a day. The average loss of water is 100 ml in 24 hours. Fluid is lost through the gastrointestinal tract through vomiting and diarrhea.

Two major hormones affecting fluid and electrolyte balance are antidiuretic hormone (ADH) (hormone that decreases the production of urine) and aldosterone (steroid hormone produced by the adrenal cortex to regulate sodium and potassium balance in the blood). Fluid deficits stimulate the secretion of aldosterone into the blood.

Fluid Needs

The nurse plays a major role in assessing the patient's fluid needs. Of particular importance is assessing for the presence of edema. Edema is the excessive accumulation of fluid in the interstitial spaces. Edema occurs when there is an imbalance between the **hydrostatic pressure** (pressure exerted by a fluid) within the capillary network and the **oncotic pressure gradient** (the pressure difference between osmotic pressure and that of tissue fluid or lymph) within the interstitial spaces. This problem may occur when there are protein shifts or electrolyte imbalances, which can occur in conditions such as renal failure, venous obstruction, congestive heart failure, or any insult to body tissues. Edema is measured in millimeters (mm) with a numerical value of 1+ to 4+. A 1+ (2-mm) finding indicates slight pitting edema, whereas a 4+ (8-mm) finding indicates a severe excess of fluid. The nurse may use several techniques to evaluate the status of fluid and electrolyte balance. An assessment guide, with rationales and nursing interventions, is found in Table 24-1.

REGULATING ELECTROLYTES

Electrolyte regulation involves sodium, potassium, calcium, and magnesium. For regulation of these **cations** (positively charged ions) and **anions** (negatively charged ions), these elements must be in balance.

Sodium is one of the most important elements in the body. Sodium ions are involved in acid-base balance, water balance, transmission of nerve impulses, and contraction of muscles. *Potassium* salts are necessary for the life of all plants and animals. In the body, potassium helps regulate neuromuscular excitability and muscle contraction. Sources of potassium are whole grains, meat, legumes, fruit such as bananas and apricots, and vegetables.

Potassium is important in glycogen formation, protein synthesis, and the correction of imbalances of acid-base metabolism. Most of the dietary potassium in the body is absorbed form the gastrointestinal tract, and the amount of potassium excreted in the urine is essentially equal to the amount of potassium in the diet.

Calcium is the fifth most abundant element in the human body and occurs mainly in the bones. The body requires calcium ions for the transmission of nerve impulses, muscle contraction, blood coagulation, cardiac functions, and other processes. More than 90% of the calcium in the body is stored in the skeleton, which constantly changes its supplies with the calcium of the interstitial fluids.

Magnesium occurs abundantly in nature, always in combination with other elements; in sea, water, bones, and seeds; in chlorophyll in plants, and in minerals such as magnesite. It is obtained chiefly by

VARIABLES INFLUENCING FLUID, ELECTROLYTE, AND ACID-BASE BALANCES

Fluid and Electrolyte Balances

Age

- Infants' proportion of total body water is greater than that of children or adults, but they are not protected from fluid loss (for example, as a result of diarrhea) because they ingest and excrete relatively greater daily water volume than adults (Mollohan, Riddle, 1992). They are at greater risk for fluid volume deficit and hyperosmolar imbalance because body water loss is proportionately greater than per kilogram of weight.
- Low-birth-weight infants are at risk for fluid volume deficit and hypertonic fluid imbalances because of increased insensible water losses and immature renal function. These infants are also at risk for hypernatremia and hyperkalemia (Davis, 1992).
- In children, regulatory responses to imbalances are less stable and there is narrow range of tolerance for severe balance changes. Children also respond to illness with high fevers.
- Adolescents have increased metabolic processes and increased water production. Girls have greater fluid changes because of hormonal changes.
- Pregnant women have increased aldosterone secretion and excretion, which increases circulating blood volume. This increased blood volume decreases rapidly after delivery.
- In older adults, fluid, electrolyte, and acid-base alterations can occur because of age-related changes such as decreased ability to produce maximally concentrated urine. Older adults are at risk for decreased excretion of medications, which can affect fluid, electrolyte, or acid-base balances, resulting in metabolic or respiratory acidosis, fluid volume deficit and hyperosmolar imbalance, and hyponatremia and hypernatremia (Kee, 1992).

Body size

- Obese patients have proportionately less body water because fat contains no water.
- Because women have more fat deposits than men, they have less total body water.

Environmental temperature

- Overall body response to environmental temperatures exceeding 28° to 30° C (82.4° to 86° F) is increased water loss by sweating. The healthy adult can tolerate sweating 1 L/hr for 2 hours, losing 5% of body weight. Body weight loss over 7% decreases ability of cooling mechanism to conserve water.
- Exposure to excessive environmental temperatures causes increase in peripheral vasodilation (blood comes to the surface for cooling), increase in body fluid loss through sweating accompanied by loss of sodium and chloride ions, increase in cardiac output and pulse rate, and increase in aldosterone secretion (causing sodium retention and potassium excretion by kidneys).

Life-style

- When nutritional intake is inadequate, body tries to preserve protein stores by breaking down glycogen and fat stores. Eventually, however, body destroys protein stores, which results in hypoalbuminemia, decreased serum colloid oncotic pressure, and edema.
- Stress causes increase in aldosterone, resulting in sodium and water retention. Increased ADH secretion decreases urine output. Stress response increases fluid volume, cardiac output (within limits), blood pressure, and perfusion to major organs.
- Exercise increases water loss through sweat.

Level of health

- Stress response causes fluid balance changes in second to fifth postoperative day. Aldosterone, glucocorticoids, and ADH are increasingly secreted, causing sodium and chloride retention, potassium excretion, and decreased urinary output.
- Severe second- or third-degree burns cause fluid loss by one of five routes: (1) plasma leaves intravascular spaces and becomes trapped as edema, (2) plasma and interstitial fluids are lost as burn exudate, (3) water vapor and heat are lost because burned skin is no longer a barrier, (4) blood leaks from damaged capillaries, or (5) sodium and water shift into cells.
- In patients with heart disease, reduced cardiac output decreases perfusion to kidneys, glomerular filtration rate, and urinary output. Patients retain sodium and water, causing fluid volume excess and peripheral and pulmonary edema.
- Failing kidneys cause abnormal buildup of sodium, chloride, potassium, phosphorus, and extracellular fluid. Serum calcium will be decreased. Acute renal failure is reversible; chronic renal failure can be treated.
- All types of fluid and electrolyte imbalances can be caused by cancers. Patients with cancer may also develop third-space fluid accumulations that increase total body water, with decrease in extracellular fluid volume.

Acid-Base Balance

Age

- Very young and very old are most susceptible to imbalances because of limited adaptive reserve in these age-groups.
- Aging process changes lung function and can lead to respiratory acidosis and the inability to compensate for metabolic acidosis.

Life-style

- Dieting can lead to acidosis because rapid water loss can lead to hyperosmolar fluid imbalance. Near-starvation diets alter normal metabolic processes and cause metabolic acidosis.
- Anxiety can lead to hyperventilation and respiratory alkalosis.

From Potter PA, Perry AG: *Basic nursing: theory and practice,* ed 3, St Louis, 1995, Mosby.

VARIABLES INFLUENCING FLUID, ELECTROLYTE, AND ACID-BASE BALANCES—cont'd

- Alcoholism leads to acidosis because of its association with malnutrition.

Medications

- Diuretics and steroids can cause metabolic alkalosis. Respiratory center depressants such as narcotics can cause decreased rate and depth of respirations, and stimulants can cause hyperventilation, which may result in respiratory acidosis or alkalosis, respectively.

Level of health

- Patients with pulmonary disease or diabetes mellitus are at risk for acidosis.
- Normal metabolism requires a 20:1 ratio between bicarbonate and carbonic acid. Any alteration of either element can lead to imbalances.
- During illness, metabolic activities are altered, and imbalances can rapidly occur.

Table 24-1 MAINTAINING FLUID BALANCE AND RECORDING FLUID INTAKE AND OUTPUT

Nursing Intervention	Rationale
Assess for overhydration.	Assessment detects presence of peripheral or sacral edema. Adventitious lung sounds (crackles, rhonchi, and wheezes) are detected. Hemoglobin level and hematocrit for decreased values are monitored. Vital signs are monitored for elevated blood pressure and increased pulse and respiratory rates.
Assess for dehydration.	Assessment reveals excessive thirst. Assessment detects dry lips and oral mucosa. Skin turgor is evaluated. Hemoglobin level and hematocrit are monitored for increased values. Vital signs are monitored for variations in baseline.
Obtain baseline body weight.	Same scale is used for additional weights.
Know totals of I&O record.	Patient's 24-hour fluid I&O is monitored.
Monitor intravenous fluids for correct solution, flow rates, and timely absorption. (Intravenous solutions are isotonic, hypotonic, or hypertonic.)	Isotonic solution is prescribed when there is fluid volume deficit: Ringer's lactate and 0.9% normal saline. Hypotonic solution is prescribed when there is need for basic fluid maintenance: 0.45% sodium chloride, D5W. Hypertonic solution is prescribed for severe sodium losses: 3% sodium chloride. NOTE: This solution has a great potential for causing fluid volume excess and must be closely monitored.
Know agency laboratory reference values for primary electrolyte readings.	Each agency may differ in number of readings.
Monitor laboratory values such as electrolytes, arterial blood gases, and hematocrit as appropriate.	Abnormal levels indicate a problem involving fluid balance.
Follow medical orders and agency policy for recording I&O.	Physicians may differ on what is wanted.
Know amount of fluid in oral intake containers as well as all output measuring devices.	Water, milk, juice, jello are included in intake.
Assess for all sources for I&O recording.	Intake includes intravenous solutions, oral fluid, and tube feedings. Output includes emesis, urine, nasogastric tube drainage, diarrhea stools, and surgical wound-collecting receptacles.
Assess patient's cooperation and ability to assist in record keeping.	Cooperation helps ensure accurate I&O recordings.
Follow agency policy for placement and documentation of all recordings.	Agencies may differ on policy.

I&O, Intake and output.

the electrolytes. Magnesium is the second most abundant cation of the intracellular fluids in the body and is essential for many enzyme activities. It is also important for muscular excitability.

Chloride is a compound in which the negative element is chlorine. Chlorides are salts of hydrochloric acid, the most common being sodium chloride (table salt). It has been recommended that the salt content in food be lowered to prevent heart problems.

Bicarbonate or *sodium bicarbonate* is an antacid, electrolyte, and urinary alkalinizing agent. It is used to treat acidosis, gastric acidity, peptic ulcer, and indigestion. The patient should use discretion in the use of bicarbonate because of its potential side effects such as gastric distention, acid rebound, hypernatremia, and hyperkalemia.

Phosphate is a salt of phosphoric acid. Phosphates are extremely important in living cells, particularly in the storage and use of energy and the transmission of genetic information within a cell and from one cell to another.

Electrolyte Imbalance

Sodium imbalance occurs with the seriously ill patient when there is an excess or deficit of extracellular fluid. With a loss of sodium, it becomes diluted in extracellular fluids and may cause shock or vascular collapse. Electrolyte imbalances may be seen in Table 24-2.

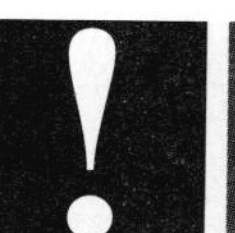

REMEMBER

- It is the responsibility of the nurse to make certain that the fluid intake and output is assessed for all patients, regardless of whether there is a medical order.
- When emptying any body excretion, the nurse uses a graduate or calibrated measuring device for accuracy.

Table 24-2 ELECTROLYTE IMBALANCES

Causes	Signs and Symptoms
Hyponatremia Kidney disease resulting in salt-wasting Adrenal insufficiency Gastrointestinal losses Increased sweating Use of diuretics, especially when combined with low-sodium diet Psychogenic polydipsia Secretion of inappropriate ADH (SIADH)	*Physical examination:* apprehension, personality change, postural hypotension, postural dizziness, abdominal cramping, nausea and vomiting, diarrhea, tachycardia, convulsions and coma, and fingerprints remaining on sternum after palpation *Laboratory findings:* serum sodium level <135 mEq/L, serum osmolality <280 mOsm/kg, and urine specific gravity <1.010 (if not caused by SIADH)
Hypernatremia Ingestion of large amounts of concentrated salt solutions Iatrogenic administration of hypertonic saline solution parenterally Excess aldosterone secretion Diabetes insipidus Increased sensible and insensible water loss Water deprivation	*Physical examination:* thirst, dry and flushed skin, dry and sticky tongue and mucous membranes, fever, agitation, convulsions, restlessness, and irritability *Laboratory findings:* serum sodium levels >145 mEq/L, serum osmolality >295 mOsm/kg, and urine specific gravity >1.030 (if not caused by diabetes insipidus)
Hypokalemia Use of potassium-wasting diuretics Diarrhea, vomiting, or other gastrointestinal losses Alkalosis Excess aldosterone secretion Polyuria Extreme sweating Excessive use of potassium-free intravenous solutions Treatment of diabetic ketoacidosis with insulin	*Physical examination:* weakness and fatigue, decreased muscle tone, intestinal distention, decreased bowel sounds, ventricular dysrhythmias, paresthesias and weak, irregular pulse *Laboratory findings:* serum potassium level <3.5 mEq/L and electrocardiogram (ECG) abnormalities (for example, ventricular dysrhythmias [likely when potassium level is <2.6 mEq/L*])

Table 24-2 ELECTROLYTE IMBALANCES—cont'd

Causes	Signs and Symptoms
Hyperkalemia Renal failure Fluid volume deficit Massive cellular damage such as from burns and trauma Iatrogenic administration of large amounts of potassium intravenously Adrenal insufficiency Acidosis, especially diabetic ketoacidosis Rapid infusion of stored blood Use of potassium-sparing diuretics	*Physical examination:* anxiety, dysrhythmias, paresthesia, weakness, abdominal cramps, and diarrhea *Laboratory findings:* serum potassium level >5.3 mEq/L and ECG abnormalities (bradycardia, heart block, dysrhythmias† usually appear with serum potassium level >7 mEq/L‡)
Hypocalcemia Rapid administration of blood transfusions containing citrate Hypoalbuminemia Hypoparathyroidism Vitamin D deficiency Pancreatitis Alkalosis	*Physical examination:* numbness and tingling of fingers and circumoral region, hyperactive reflexes, positive Trousseau's sign (carpopedal spasm with hypoxia), positive Chvostek's sign (contraction of facial muscles when facial nerve is tapped), tetany, muscle cramps, and pathologic fractures (chronic hypocalcemia) *Laboratory findings:* serum calcium level <4.0 mEq/L or 8.5 mg/dl and ECG abnormalities
Hypercalcemia Hyperparathyroidism Malignant neoplastic disease Paget's disease Osteoporosis Prolonged immobilization Acidosis	*Physical examination:* anorexia, nausea and vomiting, weakness, lethargy, low back pain (from kidney stones), decreased level of consciousness, personality changes, and cardiac arrest *Laboratory findings:* serum calcium level >5 mEq/L or 10.5 mg/dl; x-ray examination showing generalized osteoporosis, widespread bone cavitation, radiopaque urinary stones; and elevated blood urea nitrogen level >25 mg/dl and elevated creatinine level >1.5 mg/dl caused by fluid volume deficit or renal damage caused by urolithiasis; ECG abnormalities
Hypomagnesemia Inadequate intake: malnutrition and alcoholism Inadequate absorption: diarrhea, vomiting, nasogastric drainage, fistulas; diseases of small intestine Excessive loss resulting from thiazide diuretics Aldosterone excess Polyuria	*Physical examination:* muscular tremors, hyperactive deep tendon reflexes, confusion and disorientation, dysrhythmias, and positive Chvostek's and Trousseau's sign *Laboratory findings:* serum magnesium level <1.5 mEq/L
Hypermagnesemia Renal failure Excess oral or parenteral intake of magnesium	*Physical examination:* physical findings that are more frequent in acute elevations in magnesium levels: hypoactive deep tendon reflexes, decreased depth and rate of respirations, hypotension, and flushing *Laboratory findings:* serum magnesium level >2.5 mEq/L

*Data from DeAngelis R, Lessig L: Hypokalemia, *Critical Care Nurse* 11(7):71, 1991.
†Levels >8.5 mEq/L are frequently fatal as a result of cardiac standstill (Horne MM, Heitz UE, Swearingen PL: *Fluid, electrolyte and acid-base balance: a case study approach,* St Louis, 1991, Mosby).
‡Data from Metheny NM, *Fluid and electrolyte balance: nursing considerations,* ed 2, Philadelphia, 1992, Lippincott.
From Potter PA, Perry AG: *Basic nursing: theory and practice,* ed 3, St Louis, 1995, Mosby.

A problem caused by sodium loss is hyponatremia (loss of sodium in the blood). It occurs frequently in seriously ill clients. Hypernatremia is a greater-than-normal concentration of sodium in the blood.

In hypokalemia an inadequate amount of potassium in the circulating bloodstream occurs. Diuretics such as thiazides and loop diuretics remove potassium from the blood. Hyperkalemia (too much potassium in the blood) and cardiac conditions may also occur.

A calcium imbalance results from severe illness and causes hypocalcemia, or reduced calcium in the blood. Hypercalcemia is an increase of calcium in the blood and most often results from excessive bone resorption and release of calcium.

An imbalance of magnesium tends to depress the action of skeletal muscle, and excessive amounts (hypermagnesemia) interferes with the action of motor nerve impulses. Insufficient magnesium in extracellular fluid (hypomagnesemia) increases muscular excitability and may cause tetany (condition characterized by cramps, convulsions, muscle twitching, and sharp flexion of the wrist and ankle joints).

A decrease of chloride in the blood may be caused from prolonged vomiting resulting from loss of hydrochloric acid. The same may occur from prolonged diarrhea illness in the newborn.

REGULATING ACID-BASE BALANCE

Respiratory acidosis is an abnormal increase in the hydrogen ion concentration in the body resulting from an accumulation of an acid or the loss of a base. This type of acidosis results from respiratory retention of carbon dioxide. Conditions causing this problem are pneumonia, drug overdose, and hypoxemia.

Respiratory alkalosis is indicated by a pH level greater than 7.44 (Fig. 24-3). This problem may be caused by hyperventilation and dehydration.

Other acid-base imbalances may be seen in Table 24-3.

INTAKE AND OUTPUT

Measuring and recording fluid intake and output helps determine fluid, electrolyte, and acid-base status of the patient. The nurse is responsible for assessing and recording fluid intake and output (Fig. 24-4). Fluid intake includes liquids taken orally, by tube feedings, or by the parenteral route (intravenously). Liquid output includes urine, diarrheal

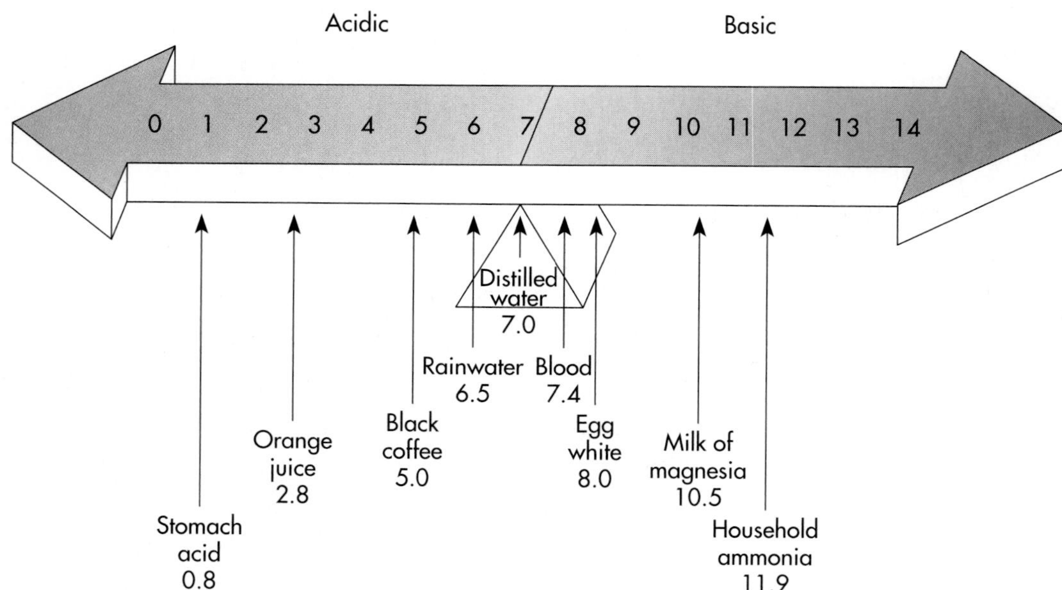

Fig. 24-3 pH scale. A pH of 7 is considered neutral, so the scale is depicted as balancing at that point. Values to the left (below 7) are acidic (the lower the number, the more acidic). Values to the right (above 7) are basic (the higher the number, the more basic). Representative fluids and their approximate pHs are listed below the figure. (From Christensen BL, Kockrow EO: *Foundations of nursing,* ed 2, St Louis, 1995, Mosby.)

Table 24-3 ACID-BASE IMBALANCES

Causes	Signs and Symptoms
Respiratory acidosis	
Hypoventilation resulting from primary respiratory problems	
Atelectasis (obstruction of small airways often caused by retained mucus) Pneumonia Cystic fibrosis Respiratory failure Airway obstruction Chest wall injury	*Physical examination:* confusion, dizziness, lethargy, headache, ventricular dysrhythmias, warm and flushed skin, muscular twitching, convulsions, and coma *Laboratory findings:* arterial blood gas alterations: pH <7.35, partial pressure of carbon dioxide in arterial blood ($Paco_2$) >45 mm Hg, arterial partial pressure of oxygen (Pao_2) <80 mm Hg, and bicarbonate level normal (if uncompensated) or >26 mEq/L (if compensated)
Hypoventilation resulting from factors outside of respiratory system	
Drug overdose with respiratory depressant Paralysis of respiratory muscles caused by various neurologic alterations Head injury Obesity	
Respiratory alkalosis	
Hyperventilation resulting from primary respiratory problems	
Asthma Pneumonia Inappropriate mechanical ventilator settings *Hyperventilation resulting from factors outside of respiratory system* Anxiety Hypermetabolic states Disorders of central nervous system (head injuries, infections) Salicylate overdose	*Physical examination:* dizziness, confusion, dysrhythmias, tachypnea, numbness and tingling of extremities, convulsions, and coma *Laboratory findings:* arterial blood gas alterations: pH >7.45, $Paco_2$ <35 mm Hg, Pao_2 normal, and bicarbonate level normal (if short lived or uncompensated) or <22 mEq/L (if compensated)
Metabolic acidosis	
High anion gap Starvation Diabetic ketoacidosis Renal failure Lactic acidosis Use of drugs (methanol, ethanol, formic acid, paraldehyde, aspirin) *Normal anion gap* Renal tubular acidosis Diarrhea	*Physical examination:* headache, lethargy, confusion, dysrhythmias, tachypnea with deep respirations, abdominal cramps, and flushed skin *Laboratory findings:* arterial blood gas alterations: pH <7.35, $Paco_2$ normal (if uncompensated) or <35 mm Hg (if compensated), Pao_2 normal or increased (with rapid, deep respirations), and bicarbonate level <22 mEq/L
Metabolic alkalosis	
Excessive vomiting Prolonged gastric suctioning Hypokalemia or hypercalcemia Excess aldosterone Use of drugs (steroids, sodium bicarbonate, diuretics)	*Physical examination:* dizziness, dysrhythmias, numbness and tingling of fingers, toes, and circumoral region, muscle cramps; tetany *Laboratory findings:* arterial blood gas alterations: pH >7.45, $Paco_2$ normal (if uncompensated) or >45 mm Hg (if compensated), Pao_2 normal, and bicarbonate level >26 mEq/L

From Potter PA, Perry AG: *Basic nursing: theory and practice,* ed 3, St Louis, 1995, Mosby.

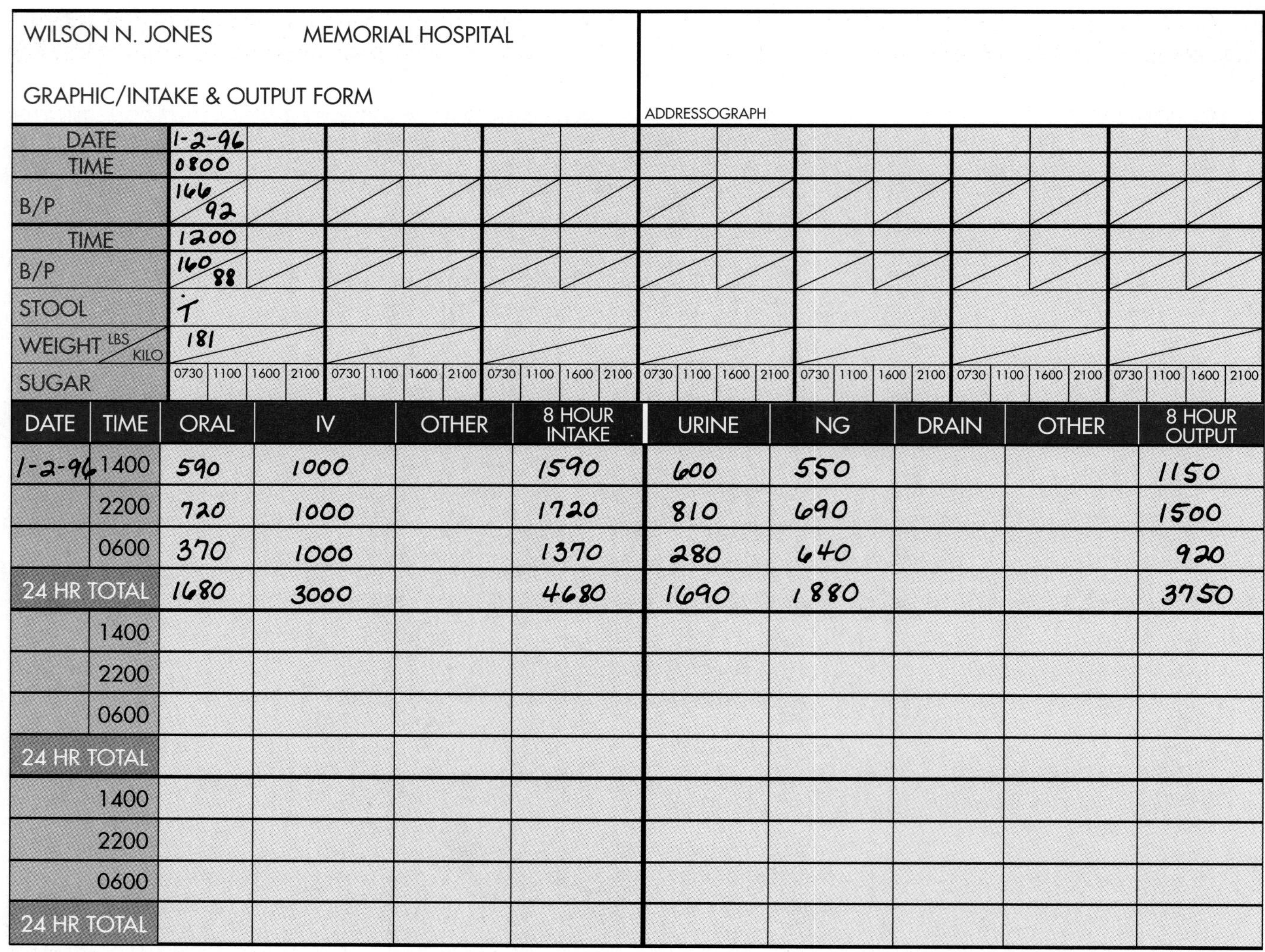

WILSON N. JONES MEMORIAL HOSPITAL

GRAPHIC/INTAKE & OUTPUT FORM

ADDRESSOGRAPH

DATE	1-2-96						
TIME	0800						
B/P	166/92						
TIME	1200						
B/P	160/88						
STOOL	T̈						
WEIGHT LBS/KILO	181						
SUGAR	0730 1100 1600 2100	0730 1100 1600 2100	0730 1100 1600 2100	0730 1100 1600 2100	0730 1100 1600 2100	0730 1100 1600 2100	0730 1100 1600 2100

DATE	TIME	ORAL	IV	OTHER	8 HOUR INTAKE	URINE	NG	DRAIN	OTHER	8 HOUR OUTPUT
1-2-96	1400	590	1000		1590	600	550			1150
	2200	720	1000		1720	810	690			1500
	0600	370	1000		1370	280	640			920
24 HR TOTAL		1680	3000		4680	1690	1880			3750
	1400									
	2200									
	0600									
24 HR TOTAL										
	1400									
	2200									
	0600									
24 HR TOTAL										

Fig. 24-4 Intake and output form. (Courtesy Wilson N. Jones Memorial Hospital, Sherman, Texas.)

stool, vomitus (emesis), gastric suction, and drainage from surgical wound receptacles (that is, Hemovac or Jackson-Pratt devices).

The physician may order intake and output to be monitored, or the nurse may request the staff to monitor and record all fluid intake and liquid output on a special form. The nurse should ensure accuracy of intake and output by teaching the staff its importance, and ensure accurate documentation of the intake and output record in the medical record. Intake and output is usually ordered every 8 hours but may be ordered hourly if urine output is decreased to a dangerous state (less than 30 ml). Intake and output totals should be totaled every 24 hours to accurately evaluate the patient (Skill 24-1). The intake and output process is crucial for the safety of the patient.

Measurement of intake and output is automatically performed for the hospitalized child because body metabolism may change rapidly when ill. The child does not have the physical reserve of the adult and, for example, may become seriously ill from dehydration. Such a problem may be life threatening to a child.

■ NURSING CARE PLAN ■

FLUID VOLUME DEFICIT

Mrs. C, age 69, has had diarrhea for 36 hours and is admitted for treatment. The patient is confused and not certain where she is. A neighbor brought Mrs. C. to the hospital emergency unit.

NURSING DIAGNOSIS

Fluid volume deficit related to active loss (diarrhea) as evidenced by altered electrolyte levels, dry mucous membranes, tympanic fever measurement of 102.6° F, nonelastic skin turgor, and rapid and shallow respirations

GOAL

- Fluid volume will be adequate.

EXPECTED OUTCOMES

- Patient will have normal skin turgor.
- Body temperature will remain normal.
- Patient will revert to elastic skin turgor.

NURSING INTERVENTIONS

- Assess and monitor vital signs every 2 hr or as necessary.
- Administer oral and intravenous fluids.
- Assess skin turgor continuoually.

EVALUATION

- Patient's vital signs are within normal limits.
- Body temperature remains normal.
- Body fluid status remains normal.
- Electrolytes remain in normal range.

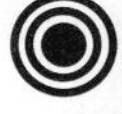

SKILL 24-1 MEASURING AND RECORDING FLUID INTAKE AND OUTPUT

Steps	Rationale
1. Obtain equipment: ▪ Ink pen (usually black) ▪ Intake and output record form ▪ Calibrated container for accurate measurement of urine ▪ Clean gloves	Helps organize procedure.
2. Refer to medical record, care plan, or Kardex for special interventions.	Provides basis for care.
3. Introduce self.	Decreases anxiety level.
4. Identify patient by identification band.	Identifies correct patient for procedure.
5. Explain procedure to patient.	Seeks cooperation and decreases anxiety.
6. Wash hands and don clean gloves according to agency policy and guidelines from Centers for Disease Control and Prevention and Occupational Safety and Health Administration.	Helps prevent cross-contamination.
7. Prepare patient for intervention:	
a. Close door to room or pull curtain.	Provides privacy.
b. Drape for procedure if necessary.	Prevents exposure of patient.
8. Raise or lower bed to comfortable working level for nurse.	Provides safety for nurse.
9. Arrange for patient privacy.	Shows respect for patient.

Continued.

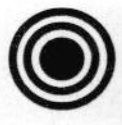

SKILL 24-1 MEASURING AND RECORDING FLUID INTAKE AND OUTPUT—cont'd

Steps	Rationale
10. Measure and record all fluids taken orally, including tube feedings, parenteral fluids, blood components, total parenteral nutrition, and foods that melt at room temperature.	Ensures accurate record of fluid intake.
11. Inform patient not to empty any body excreta but to contact nurse as needed.	Ensures accurate record of intake and output.
12. Instruct patient to inform nurse of all oral intake or record amounts on form.	Provides for more accurate measuring of intake and output.
13. Measure and record drainage from Foley catheter drainage system, nasogastric suction, surgical wound receptacles, emesis, and diarrheal stools every 8 hr.	Maintains accurate output for each shift.
14. Remove gloves and wash hands.	Helps prevent cross-contamination.
15. Document.	Documents procedure and patient's response.

SUMMARY

Monitoring and maintaining fluid, electrolyte, and acid-base balance for the patient is a major responsibility of the nurse. Imbalances are serious and may be fatal if not treated. The patient should receive appropriate nursing care to help prevent imbalances. When these problems arise, the nurse should restore balance.

Key Concepts

- Body fluid is distributed between extracellular and intracellular fluid.
- The nurse plays a major role in assessing and meeting the fluid needs of the patient.
- Body fluids should be regulated to maintain a balance of body systems.
- Body fluids are regulated by fluid intake, liquid output, and hormonal controls.
- Fluid output occurs through the kidneys, skin, lungs, and gastrointestinal tract.
- Fluid intake and liquid output helps determine fluid and electrolyte balance.
- The nurse may provide a nursing order to place a patient on intake and output.
- Children and the older adult should be closely assessed for fluid, electrolyte, and acid-base imbalance because they are at risk.

Critical Thinking Questions

1. Mr. Jackson is 72 years old. He now has an infection and has had a fever of 102° F for 36 hours. He has been vomiting, and he reports that he has been profusely diaphoretic. For what fluid imbalance is he at risk at this time? What further assessment data is needed to confirm the type of fluid imbalance that he is experiencing?
2. Mr. Norman is 65 years old. He has had diabetes mellitus since he was 10 years old and requires insulin injections twice each day to control the diabetes. He has had an infection for 2 days with a fever of 104° F, and he is admitted to the hospital to determine the cause of the infection. On admission, he is lethargic and arouses to answer questions only with difficulty. It is found that his blood glucose level is 680 mg/dl. His respirations are 32/breaths/min and deep. His arterial blood gas levels reveal pH of 7.30, Pa_{CO_2} of 28 mm Hg, and bicarbonate of 15 mEq/L. Which acid-base imbalance does Mr. Norman have? Are his respiratory characteristics a cause of or compensatory mechanisms for this imbalance?

REFERENCES AND SUGGESTED READINGS

Bolander V: *Sorensen and Luckmann's basic nursing: a psychophysiologic approach,* ed 3, Philadelphia 1994, Saunders.

Carpenito LJ: *Nursing diagnosis,* ed 5, Philadelphia, 1993, Lippincott.

Davis M: Fluids, electrolytes, and nutrition in the low-birth-weight infant, *NAACOG's Clin Iss Perinatal Women's Health Nursing* 3(1):45-61, 1992.

Ellis J, Nowlis E, Bentz P: *Basic nursing skills,* ed 3, Philadelphia, 1992, Lippincott.

Kee CC: Age-related changes in the renal system: causes, consequences, and nursing implications, *Geriatric Nurs* 13(2):80-93, 1992.

Metheney N: *Fluid and electrolyte balance: nursing considerations,* ed 2, Philadelphia, 1992, Lippincott.

Mollohan J, Riddle II: Fluid balance in infants and children. In Metheny N, editor: *Fluid and electrolyte balance: nursing considerations,* ed 3, Philadelphia, 1992, JB Lippincott.

Mosby's medical, nursing, and allied health dictionary, ed 4, St Louis, 1994, Mosby.

Perry AG, Potter PA: *Clinical nursing skills and techniques,* ed 3, St Louis, 1994, Mosby.

Phillips L: *Manual of IV therapeutics,* Philadelphia, 1993, Davis.

Potter PA, Perry AG: *Fundamentals of nursing: concepts, process, and practice,* ed 3, St Louis, 1993, Mosby.

Smith S, Duel D: *Clinical nursing skills,* ed 3, Norwalk, Conn, 1992, Appleton & Lang.

Taylor C, Little C, LeMone P: *Fundamentals of nursing,* ed 2, Philadelphia, 1993, Lippincott.

CHAPTER 25

Nutrition

Learning Objectives

After studying this chapter, the student should be able to . . .

- Define the key terms.
- List essential nutrients in a diet.
- Describe the components and purposes of specific therapeutic diets.
- Serve nutritious meals to a patient in a safe, pleasant environment.
- Assist in feeding or feed patients nutritious meals.
- Explain the purpose of enteral nutrition.
- Administer gastric gavage (nasogastric tube) feedings.
- Administer a gastrostomy feeding.
- Identify the principles and purposes of total parenteral nutrition.
- Administer total parenteral nutrition.
- Encourage the drinking of fluids, especially water.

Key Terms

Amino acid
Carbohydrate
Chyme
Enteral nutrition
Fat
Gastrostomy
Mineral
Nasogastric tube feeding
Nasointestinal tube feeding
NPO
Protein
Total parenteral nutrition (TPN)
Villi
Vitamin

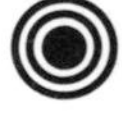

Skills

25-1 Serving food and assisting with feeding a patient
25-2 Administering nasogastric tube and gastrostomy feedings
25-3 Administering total parenteral nutrition

The nutritional status of a patient must be considered in all aspects of health care. Nutrition is an indicator of the patient's potential for optimal health and the ability to cope with illness or disease. Therefore sound nursing care considers nutrition in assessing, planning, implementing, and evaluating a patient's total health and nursing care.

Physiologically, food provides energy, builds and maintains body tissues, and regulates body processes. Good nutrition also helps people feel emotionally alert, energetic, and capable of handling stress and decisions. On the other hand, inadequate nutrition makes people feel tired, run-down, listless, or depressed. Food is also used to express feelings. It can help people feel loved and secure, or it can be unpleasant. Eating can be pleasurable when an attractive meal is served at a happy social occasion with family or friends. Eating can be unpleasant when the food is improperly prepared, unattractive, or served in a stressful social context.

NURSING PROCESS

Assessment

The nurse obtains a diet history to assess the patient's actual or potential nutritional needs. The diet history includes intake of foods and liquids and information about preferences, allergies, and digestive problems (see care plan on p. 485). The nurse also gathers information about activity levels to determine the patient's energy needs. The energy needed is then compared to food intake.

PATIENT TEACHING

- Help patient learn to plan menus and ensure nutrition within a budget.
- Give patient a list of community resources that provide help in adhering to prescribed diets.
- Provide information about Meals on Wheels program for the patient unable to prepare meals at home.

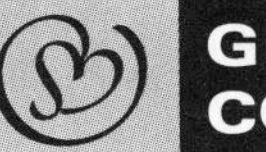

GERONTOLOGIC CONSIDERATIONS

- Water and dietary fiber play an important role in preventing constipation in older adults.
- Age-related changes in taste, medication use, loss of teeth, loneliness, and forgetfulness can affect the eating habits of older adults.
- Because of a decrease in muscle, the basal metabolic rate decreases with aging.

Nursing Diagnosis

The nurse reviews all data gathered during assessment to determine whether nutritional problems exist. Specific nursing diagnoses are then identified. The nursing diagnosis may also involve a general nutritional deficiency or problems that place the patient at risk for nutritional deficiencies. Nursing diagnoses related to nutritional problems include:

Altered nutrition: less than body requirements
Altered nutrition: more than body requirements
Altered nutrition: risk for more than body requirements
Constipation
Fluid volume deficit
Fluid volume excess
Impaired swallowing
Noncompliance: preparing balanced diet
Risk for aspiration
Risk for fluid volume deficit
Self-care deficit: feeding

Planning

After identifying patients at risk for nutritional problems, the nurse develops a plan of care designed to prevent or minimize nutritional problems. It is important for the patient and family to participate in planning care. The nurse can collaborate with the dietician to provide correct nutritional education and counseling (see box).

The plan of care may include the following goal:

Goal: The patient states which foods to select for a properly balanced diet.

Outcome

The patient states appropriate foods for balanced nutritional intake.

Implementation

The nurse must understand the influences that reduce appetite and be willing to do everything possible to improve a patient's intake. It is important for the nurse to conduct ongoing monitoring of a patient's overall nutritional status. Special considerations should be given to the older patient (see box).

Evaluation

The nurse evaluates the success of interventions and must be prepared to revise the care plan based on the evaluation. The nurse uses the established expected outcomes to evaluate the interventions.

Goal: The patient states which foods to select for a properly balanced diet.

Evaluative measure

Review the patient's 24-hour diet history.

NUTRIENTS

The nutrients from food are divided into six classifications: carbohydrates, fats, proteins, vitamins, minerals, and water. An appropriate balance of these nutrients is essential for the prevention and treatment of illness or disease.

Carbohydrates

Carbohydrates are a relatively inexpensive source of many nutrients and are the major source of the body's energy. A **carbohydrate** is any of a group of organic compounds, the most important being the saccharides, starches, cellulose, and gum. The main sources of carbohydrates include cereals, vegetables, fruits, rice, potatoes, legumes (peas), and flour products.

Carbohydrates also function as a constituent of many body compounds and nonessential amino acids. Carbohydrates also play a supportive role in normal fat metabolism; protein sparing; maintenance of gastric motility; and increase in the dietary intake of protein, minerals, and B vitamins. Carbohydrates consist of simple sugars (monosaccharides) in the form of glucose, fructose, and galactose; double sugars (disaccharides) in the form of sucrose, lactose, and maltose; and complex carbohydrates (polysaccharides), such as starch, glycogen, and cellulose.

Symptoms of deficiency of carbohydrates are fatigue, depression, breakdown of essential body protein, and electrolyte imbalance. Excessive consumption of carbohydrates is associated with tooth decay, obesity, diabetes mellitus, and cardiovascular disease.

Fats

Fats (lipids) are important in maintaining the health and structure of all body cells. **Fat** provides a continuous fuel supply that helps keep the body's lean tissue from being depleted. Body fat also protects the organs from temperature extremes and mechanical shock. When it is used for fuel in the absence of glucose, it forms ketones that can meet about half of the energy needs of the brain and nervous system. In the presence of starvation, the body uses fat to maintain life. Fat is also important in the transport of the fat-soluble vitamins A, D, E, and K.

The major classifications of lipids are listed below:

1. *Triglycerides* make up most animal, vegetable, and body fats (adipose tissue).
2. *Phospholipids* are important for the transportation of water-soluble lipids in the blood.
3. *Fatty acids* are composed of saturated fatty acids, which come from animal sources, and essential fatty acids, such as linoleic and arachidonic acids, which are obtained in food and are necessary for growth and metabolism.
4. *Cholesterol* is a structural component of cell membranes, a precursor in the formation of body steroids, and a prognostic characteristic of a patient's health.
5. *Lipoproteins* are the circulating form of body lipids.
6. *Glycolipids* are a constituent of nerve tissue.

Proteins

Proteins are complex organic compounds composed of 22 amino acids essential for the growth, maintenance, and regulatory functions of the body. **Amino acids** contain the elements carbon, hydrogen, nitrogen, oxygen; usually sulfur, and occasionally phosphorus, iron, iodine, or other essential constituents of living cells.

The amino acids that can be synthesized by the body are called *nonessential amino acids,* and the nine amino acids that must be supplied by food are called *essential amino acids.* Most protein foods, such as meat and milk, contain all the essential amino acids and are therefore able to support life and normal growth. These foods are called *complete proteins.* Other protein foods, such as legumes, peanuts, and grains, have limited or insufficient amino acids and are called *incomplete proteins.* An insufficient protein intake depletes the body of reserves and decreases resistance to infection.

Specific functions of protein include the following:

1. Building new body tissue (Proteins are particularly needed during periods of increased growth [for example, childhood, adolescence, pregnancy] and during periods of wound healing or illness.)
2. Repairing body tissue
3. Producing essential compounds (Amino acids are components of enzymes, hormones, and other body secretions.)
4. Regulating water balance (Protein attracts water and helps maintain fluid and electrolyte balance.)
5. Regulating acid-base balance (Plasma proteins act as buffers to maintain a correct pH.)
6. Providing resistance to disease (Antibodies are proteins.)
7. Providing transport mechanisms (Proteins help transport insoluble lipid substances.)
8. Providing energy

Vitamins

Vitamins are organic chemicals that are required by the body so that it can use proteins, fats, and carbohydrates for energy, growth, and cell maintenance. Vitamins are classified according to their solubility in water or fat. Vitamins A, D, E, and K, which are stored in the body, are fat soluble and are much more stable with ordinary cooking methods than water-soluble vitamins. The water-soluble vitamins, C and B complex, are destroyed by high cooking temperatures and are not readily stored in the body. Although vitamins have no caloric value, they are essential for normal body development and function.

Minerals

Minerals are inorganic substances of essential food nutrients. Minerals are divided into groups depending on the amounts found in the body. Those found in large amounts are called *macronutrients.* Essential macronutrients are calcium, phosphorus, sodium, potassium, magnesium, chloride, and sulfur. Minerals found in minute amounts are called *micronutrients* or *trace elements.* Essential micronutrients include iron, copper, cobalt, zinc, manganese, iodine, molybdenum, fluorine, selenium, and chromium. Minerals have many functions and are part of the skeleton and teeth (calcium, phosphorus, and magnesium), vitamin B_{12} (cobalt), hemoglobin (iron), thyroid hormone (iodine), and enzyme systems (trace elements). Minerals also function in transmitting nerve impulses and maintaining acid-base balance, osmotic pressure (pressure exerted on a semipermeable membrane, separating a solution from a solvent), and cell permeability (ability of a substance to pass through the cell wall).

Water

Water is second only to oxygen in its importance for the survival of life. Water must be supplied regularly for metabolic use and compensation for body losses. Body fluids consist almost entirely of water and dissolved substances, including the electrolytes sodium, potassium, calcium, magnesium, bicarbonate, chloride, sulfate, protein, and organic acids. The healthy man is composed of 60% water, and the healthy woman is composed of 50% water. Daily water loss occurs continuously through urination, perspiration, respiration, and defecation. Almost all food contains water, particularly fruits, vegetables, dairy products, and meat. During illness, body fluids are lost faster, which may lead to a life-threatening fluid and electrolyte imbalance.

DIGESTIVE PROCESS

Nourishment of the body requires six physiologic processes. These processes are ingestion, digestion, absorption, transportation, cell metabolism, and excretion. These processes occur in the digestive system, which includes the alimentary canal (tube lined with mucous membranes that extend from the mouth to the anus) and accessory organs (Fig. 25-1).

In the mouth the mechanical actions of the teeth and tongue crush and tear food. The food is mixed

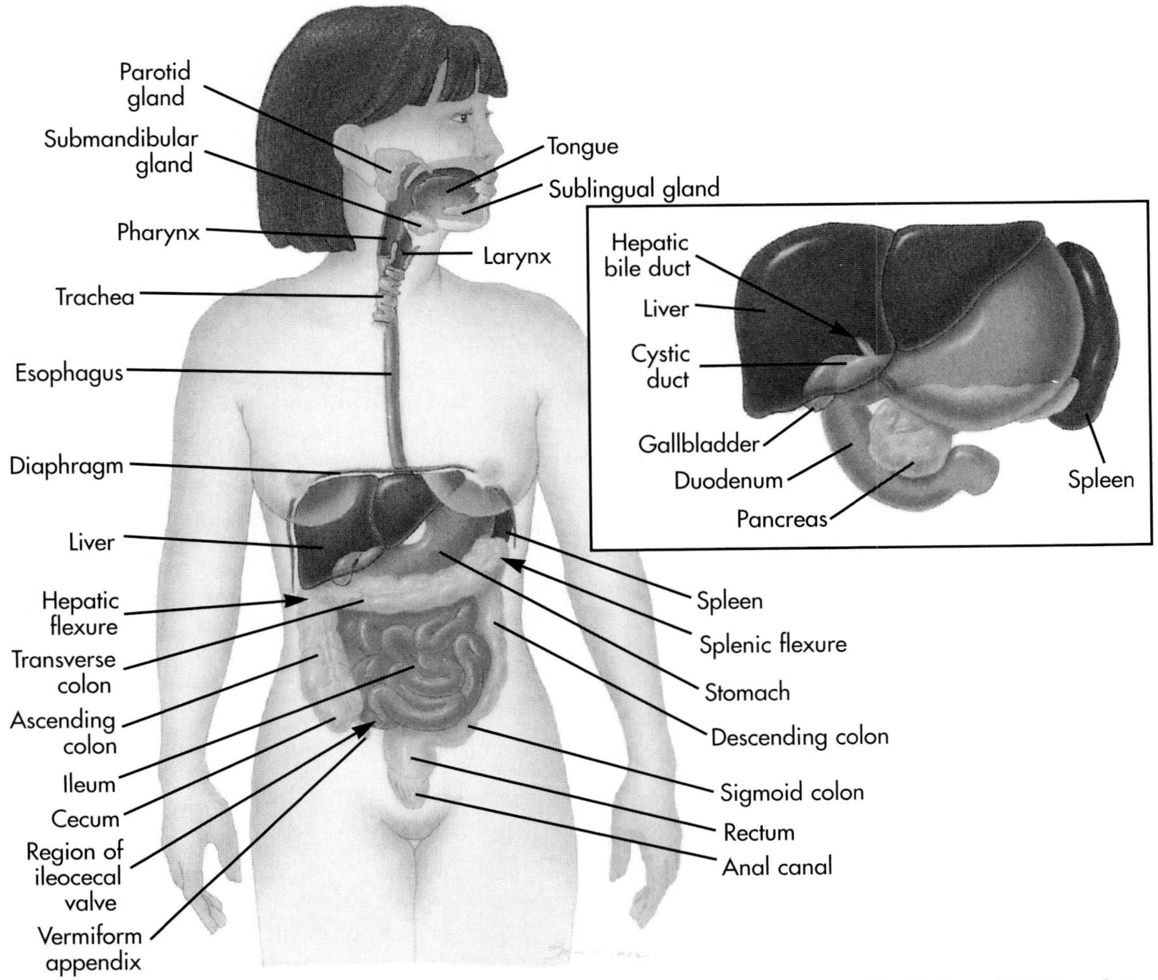

Fig. 25-1 Organs of the digestive system and assorted structures. (From Christensen BL, Kockrow EO: *Foundations of nursing,* ed 2, St Louis, 1995, Mosby.)

with saliva, and the salivary enzyme, amylase, begins breaking down starches. The taste buds detect sweet, salty, sour, and bitter sensations and work with aromas, which stimulate the olfactory nerves (pair of nerves associated with the sense of smell) to determine the acceptability of the food.

Swallowing moves the food into the esophagus, a 10-inch tube, which in turn moves food to the stomach by gravity and peristalsis (rhythmic contractions of the intestine that propel gastric contents through the gastrointestinal tract). Food entering the stomach is mixed with mucus, hydrochloric acid, the enzymes pepsin and lipase, and the intrinsic factor, which is essential for the absorption of vitamin B_{12}. The mixture in the stomach is called ***chyme,*** a viscous (sticky) paste.

Through peristalsis, the chyme is passed to the small intestine, where most absorption takes place through the **villi** (fingerlike projections that arise out of the mucosa). Chyme is then mixed with mucus, pancreatic juices (carbohydrases), and bile from the liver. Within the villi are specific enzymes that are responsible for completing the digestion of carbohydrates, fats, and protein. Cellulose, a carbohydrate, is not digestible. The duodenum and jejunum are principally responsible for the absorption of simple sugars, amino acids, glycerol, vitamins, minerals, and electrolytes. The small intestine absorbs 80% to 90% of the water content by osmosis.

The remaining chyme in the ileum is passed through the ileocecal valve and into the cecum. Peristalsis continues to propel the chyme into the ascending, transverse, and descending large intestine, where water and electrolytes are reabsorbed.

The remaining material, feces, consists of food that cannot be digested or absorbed, bile pigments, and water. Bacteria in the colon, called *flora,* help synthesize vitamins K, B_{12}, B (thiamine), and B_2 (riboflavin and biotin). Bacterial action also produces flatus (gas) and the odor of feces. Peristalsis propels the excrement into the rectum, where it is discharged from the body.

1990 DIETARY GUIDELINES

- *Eat a variety of foods.*
  - Choose fruits and vegetables.
  - Choose whole grain and enriched breads, cereals, and other grain products.
  - Choose milk, cheese, yogurt, and other milk products.
  - Choose meat, poultry, fish, eggs, and dry peas and beans.
- *Maintain healthy weight.*
- *Choose a diet low in fat, saturated fat, and cholesterol.*
  - Choose lean meat, fish, and poultry.
  - Use dry peas and beans as protein sources.
  - Use low-fat milk and milk products.
  - Use egg yolk and organ meats moderately.
  - Limit consumption of butter, cream, heavily hydrogenated fats and oils, and foods high in palm and coconut oil.
  - Trim off excess fat on meats.
  - Broil, bake, or boil rather than fry.
- *Choose a diet with plenty of vegetables, fruits, and grain products.*
  - Eat three or more servings of vegetables each day.
  - Consume two or more servings of fruits daily.
  - Eat six or more servings of grain products each day.
- *Use sugar in moderation.*
  - Use less sugar and eat fewer high-sugar foods.
  - Avoid between-meal sweets.
  - Avoid foods whose labels contain sucrose, glucose, and lactose.
  - Select foods canned without syrup or with light syrup.
- *Use salt in moderation.*
  - Learn to enjoy unsalted food.
  - Cook with only a small amount of added salt.
  - Add little or no salt at the table.
  - Limit intake of salty foods.
  - Read food labels.
  - Use new, lower-sodium products.
- *If you drink alcohol, do so in moderation.*

From Potter PA, Perry AG: *Basic nursing: theory and practice,* ed 3, St Louis, 1995, Mosby. Data from USDA and USDHHS: *Nutrition and your health: dietary guidelines for Americans.* USDA/DHHS Home and Garden Bulletin No. 232, Washington, DC, 1990, US Government Printing Office.

FOOD GROUPS AND NUTRITION EDUCATION

The 1990 dietary guidelines of the U.S. Department of Agriculture (USDA) (see box) were devised to assist people in selecting food items that meet essential nutritional requirements. Food categories with similar nutrients are grouped together. Recommended servings vary according to age and stages of life.

The most recent nutritional guideline established by the USDA is the Food Guide Pyramid (Fig. 25-2). It replaces the basic four food groups in use since the 1950s. The pyramid is designed as a guide for buying food and meal preparation.

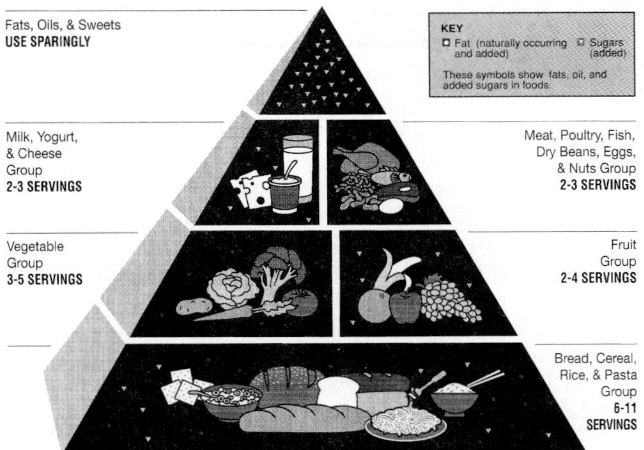

Fig. 25-2 Food Guide Pyramid. (From US Department of Agriculture: *USDA's food guide pyramid,* USDA Human Nutrition Information Pub No 249, Washington, DC, 1992, US Government Printing Office.)

INFLUENCES ON NUTRITION

Culture

Nutritional habits are often influenced by cultural beliefs and traditions. The diversity of ethnic groups in the United States necessitates special consideration to adequately meet individual nutritional needs. A hospitalized patient may refuse to eat a particular food or adhere to a therapeutic diet because of cultural or religious beliefs. Socioeconomic factors and geographical location may also influence food choices. An adequate diet can be planned if preferred foods can be determined.

African-American Generally the dietary habits of African-Americans are influenced by their geographic location (for example, North or South). Some African-Americans are in a low socioeconomic group, which necessitates choosing inexpensive sources of food that may lead to iron, calcium, and vitamin deficiencies. Soul food is often cooked for a long time and is highly seasoned. Some food preferences may include black-eyed peas, collard greens with fatback; sweet potatoes, pork products such as chitterlings; fried chicken, and fish.

Mexican-American Mexican food reflects a blend of Spanish and Indian preferences. Because of the limited availability and high cost of animal-protein foods, the traditional diet is based on plant foods: beans, corn, tomatoes, avocados, and chile peppers. Typical dishes, such as tortillas and tamales, are made with corn meal. Also enjoyed are tacos, tostitos, enchiladas, and frijoles (refried beans). Beef and chicken are enjoyed in combination dishes, whereas fish is infrequently eaten.

Asian-American Although the food patterns of the Chinese, Japanese, Korean, and Filipino are different, they do share some commonalities. A wide variety of meat, eggs, legumes, fruits, and vegetables are preferred. Plant foods, such as seaweed, bamboo shoots, and bean sprouts, are enjoyed. Polished white rice is considered a staple food. Quick-cooking techniques, such as stir-frying and steaming, leave the vegetables crisp. Soy sauce is a frequent ingredient. Few desserts and little cheese are eaten.

Religion

Jewish Judaism observes dietary laws based on biblical and rabbinical regulations. Jewish families differ in food practices according to their group affiliation. Orthodox members observe strict adherence, conservative members have a nominal adherence, and reformed members place less ceremonial emphasis on general dietary laws and practice minimal observance. Food restrictions may include eating meat only from cattle, sheep, goats, or deer; not serving meat and dairy products at the same meal; and eating only fish with fins and scales—no shellfish. Other regulations restrict cooking of food on the Sabbath, prohibit consumption of unleavened bread during Passover, and encourage fasting on Yom Kippur.

Catholic Catholics commonly abstain from eating meat on Ash Wednesday and Fridays during Lent.

Mormon Mormons do not drink alcoholic beverages or take stimulants such as coffee, tea, and most carbonated beverages that contain caffeine.

Moslem Moslems eat no pork or gelatin-based foods. No alcoholic products, including flavoring extracts, are consumed. Preferred foods are honey, dates, milk, meat, seafood, and olive oil.

THERAPEUTIC NUTRITION

Illnesses and disease processes create many physiologic and psychologic changes that may predispose a person to malnutrition. Hospitalized patients who are critically ill or are confined to bed for a long period may have special nutritional problems for which a nursing care plan must be developed. Patients who are nutritionally compromised or refuse

GUIDELINES FOR ADEQUATE NUTRITION

- Appropriate balance of carbohydrates, fats, proteins, vitamins, minerals, and trace elements is essential for health and treatment of illness or disease. Nutritious meals should be planned based on Food Guide Pyramid.
- Cultural and religious influences must be considered when planning patient's diet.
- All forms of nutrition (oral, enteral, or total parenteral nutrition) should be given in clean, nonstressful environment. Courteous, concerned attitude helps ensure dietary compliance.
- Patients must understand type of diet prescribed and importance of nutritional regimen. Some diets may include foods such as chicken broth or pureed foods that patient may not particularly like. Other forms of nutrition, such as tube feedings, may be frightening to patient. Nurse is responsible for teaching patient and concerned family members about prescribed diet or form of nutrition. When necessary, consultation with nutritionist should be obtained.
- Enteral and total parenteral nutrition may be life-maintaining forms of nutrition but may also be hazardous to patient's health. Nurse must carefully follow established protocol when administering these forms of nutrition.

to eat must be assessed to determine the source of the problem. Common problems may include the absence or poor condition of teeth, poorly fitted dentures, the presence of abdominal gas pains and cramping, nausea and vomiting, unpleasant treatments before meals, adverse effects of certain medications, and depression. In addition, the food itself may be unattractive. Guidelines for providing adequate nutrition can be seen in the box.

Therapeutic nutrition should correct nutritional deficiencies and promote optimal nutritional status, even in the presence of illness or disease. Generally, the physician prescribes the type of diet. The patient may have a regular diet or a modified diet specific to the disease or medical-surgical treatment, or the patient may have nothing by mouth **(NPO).** Frequently, as the patient's condition improves, the diet is changed to a more normal meal. Common hospital therapeutic diets are described in Table 25-1.

Assessing Nutritional Status

Nursing assessment of a patient's nutritional status begins with a dietary history and examination of the patient's physical status. The purpose of a nutritional assessment is to determine the patient's current nutritional status and the cause of any problems. Because a variety of physical and psychosocial factors may influence nutritional status, the assessment must be comprehensive and must consider individual aspects such as financial, cultural, physical, educational, and psychologic factors. The process begins with a health history (see box) and a physical assessment (Table 25-2). The physical assessment may identify signs and symptoms of a nutritional problem.

HEALTH HISTORY

- Patient recall of items eaten in last 24 hours (This information will provide overview of patient's dietary habits and allows evaluation of nutritional adequacy.)
- Recent changes in patient's diet
- Recent weight gain or weight loss
- Changes in appetite or bowel habits
- Patient intake of alcoholic beverages or tobacco use
- Patient use of prescription, over-the-counter, or street drugs and use of vitamins and health-food supplements
- Significant stress or changes in financial status that may affect dietary intake
- Use of financial assistance, such as food stamps, WIC program, discount lunches at school, or Meals-on-Wheels
- Environmental problems, such as transportation problems for shopping, adequacy of cooking facilities, or ability to prepare foods
- History of food allergies
- History of illness, dental work, or chronic medical conditions that may influence dietary intake
- Cultural or religious factors that may specify dietary intake

Serving Food to a Patient

Nutrition is essential for normal body functioning and recovery from illness. Eating also serves as a psychosocial function that requires a clean, pleasant environment. Food is served to a patient to promote growth and healing, maintain adequate intake of essential nutrients and fluids, improve the patient's sense of well-being, and maintain the patient's energy level.

The person serving food should be neat, clean, and pleasant, thereby encouraging the patient to eat. When serving food to a patient, the nurse ensures that the correct food tray is delivered to the patient and that the correct food is on the tray (Skill 25-1). The nurse follows up by assessing the type and amount of food eaten. Food eaten is documented in percentages, such as 0% to 100%.

Table 25-1 HOSPITAL THERAPEUTIC DIETS

Diet	Description
Regular	Is ordered for patients requiring no specific modifications. Generally, allows patients to select their food choices based on normal nutritional requirements for patient's age, sex, and activity level.
Clear-liquid	Allows clear, bland liquids, such as chicken broth, gelatin, and apple juice, that leave little residue and are easily absorbed. Is commonly ordered for short-term use (24 to 48 hours) after episodes of vomiting, diarrhea, or surgery.
Full-liquid	Consists of foods that liquefy at room or body temperature and are easily digested and absorbed. Includes foods allowed on clear-liquid diet plus milk and some milk-containing foods, such as creamed, strained soups. Is commonly ordered before or after surgery for patients who are acutely ill from infection or for patients who cannot chew or tolerate solid foods.
Pureed	Includes easily swallowed foods that do not require chewing. May be ordered for patients with head and neck abnormalities or who have had surgery.
Mechanical or dental-soft	Consists of foods that do not need chewing, such as chopped or ground foods. Avoids tough meats, nuts, bacon, and fruits with tough skins or membranes. May be ordered for patients who have chewing problems caused by lack of teeth or sore gums.
Soft	Includes foods that are low in fiber, easily digested, easy to chew, and simply cooked. Does not permit fatty, rich, and fried foods. Is sometimes referred to as *low-fiber diet.*
High-fiber	Includes sufficient amounts of indigestible carbohydrate to relieve constipation, increase gastrointestinal motility, and increase stool weight. May be ordered for patients with diverticulosis or irritable bowel syndrome.
Sodium-restricted	Allows low levels of sodium and may include a 4-g (no added salt), 2-g (moderate), 1-g (strict), or 500-mg (very strict) diet. May be ordered for patients with congestive heart failure, renal failure, cirrhosis, or hypertension.
Prudent (low-cholesterol)	Is ordered to reduce high serum lipid levels. Reduces cholesterol intake to 300 mg daily and fat intake to 30% to 35% by eliminating or reducing fatty foods.
Diabetic	Is ordered as essential treatment for patients with diabetes mellitus. Provides patients with exchange list of foods recommended by American Diabetes Association, which allows patient to select set amount of food from basic food groups.

Table 25-2 PHYSICAL ASSESSMENT

Physical Characteristic	Normal	Abnormal
Weight	Weight appropriate for age, gender, height, body build	Underweight, overweight
Hair	Shininess, firmness	Dullness, patchiness
Eyes	Clearness, shininess	Dullness, red sclera, pale conjunctiva
Lips	Smoothness, moisture	Swelling, cracking
Tongue	Red color, moisture	Dark red color, swelling, coating, or very smooth surface
Gums	Pink color, firmness	Red color, sponginess
Skin	Clear with good turgor	Rash, bruises, flakiness, swelling, poor turgor
Nails	Firmness, pink color	Cracking, brittleness, spoon shape
Musculoskeletal system	Normal gait, good muscle tone, appropriate posture for age	Wasted appearance, abnormal gait, abnormal prominences on bones, poor muscle tone

! REMEMBER

- Patients should be assessed for religious, cultural, or any other food preferences before the nurse orders the tray from the dietary department. If the patient is unable to respond appropriately, the family or caregiver should be asked about to the patient's preferences.
- A large syringe may be used instead of a feeding bag for enteral nutrition. The syringe is filled with the formula and allowed to infuse by gravity for 20 to 30 minutes.

Assisting with Feeding a Patient

To support a patient's self-esteem and promote independence, the nurse should encourage the patient to eat without assistance as much as possible. The nurse must be observant and knowledgeable about the patient's physical condition to determine the extent of assistance needed. If a patient is not eating the nurse should assist the patient and even provide different foods agreeable to the patient's likes and dislikes. The nurse may need to arrange a nutritional consultation.

Handicapped patients or patients who have had strokes may need adaptive devices, such as silverware with enlarged handles or plates on suction cups, to feed themselves. Patients with poor eyesight may be able to feed themselves if they know where the food is located on the tray. Food for the blind is placed in order of the clock. For example, the nurse may tell the patient that the peas are at 1:00 on the plate. When feeding a blind patient, the nurse should describe and identify each food before placing it in the patient's mouth.

When feeding a patient, the nurse should remember to offer small bites of food and allow the patient enough time for appropriate chewing of the food. Pleasant surroundings are important to encourage the patient to eat. As soon as the condition warrants, the patient should be encouraged to self-feed.

Administering Nasogastric Tube Feedings

Nasogastric tube feeding is a type of enteral nutrition (that is, tube feeding) and refers to the delivery of nutrients directly into the gastrointestinal tract. **Enteral nutrition** is used for patients who have normal gastrointestinal motility and absorp-

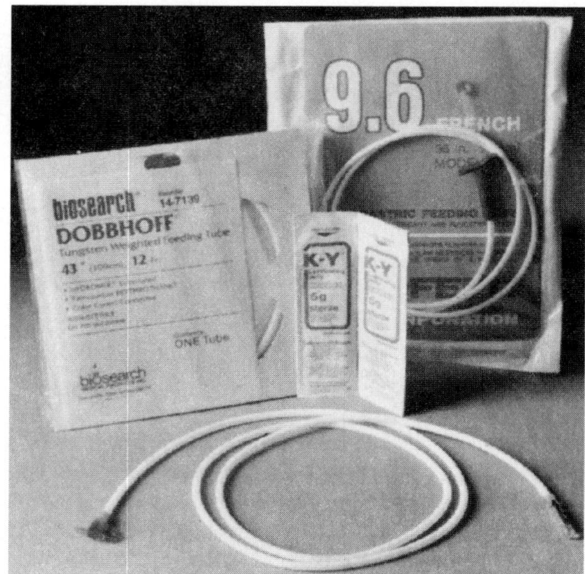

Fig. 25-3 Supplies for nasogastric tube feeding. (From Perry AG, Potter PA: *Clinical nursing skills and techniques,* ed 3, St Louis, 1994, Mosby.)

tion but cannot meet nutritional needs orally because of an underlying illness or disease. Patients with physiologic conditions that may lead to malnutrition (that is, cerebral vascular accident [stroke], head trauma, cancer of the head or neck, multiple sclerosis, or severe cardiopulmonary problems necessitating the assistance of a ventilator) are candidates for enteral feeding. These patients may have inhibited swallowing mechanisms related to mandibular fractures, may have had head or neck surgery or head or neck irradiation, or may be unconscious or comatose.

Enteral nutrition should not be administered to patients who do not have sufficient bowel function to absorb nutrients or to patients who have had abdominal trauma or surgery resulting in intestinal obstruction, ileus (obstruction of the bowel), or intractable (unrelieved) vomiting.

All liquid formulas used for nasogastric tube feeding consist of proteins, carbohydrates, fats, electrolytes, vitamins, and trace elements. A variety of commercial formulas are available (Skill 25-2). All differ in nutritional composition and are designed to meet the needs of different patient conditions. Commonly used formulas include Ensure, Compleat, Vivonex, and Isocal.

Nasogastric tube feeding is accomplished via a *nasogastric tube,* which is a French size 12 to 18 plastic or rubber tube placed through the nose and esophagus into the stomach (Fig. 25-3). The tubes are made of pliable polyurethane, silicone, or polyvinyl chloride. Commonly used tubes include the

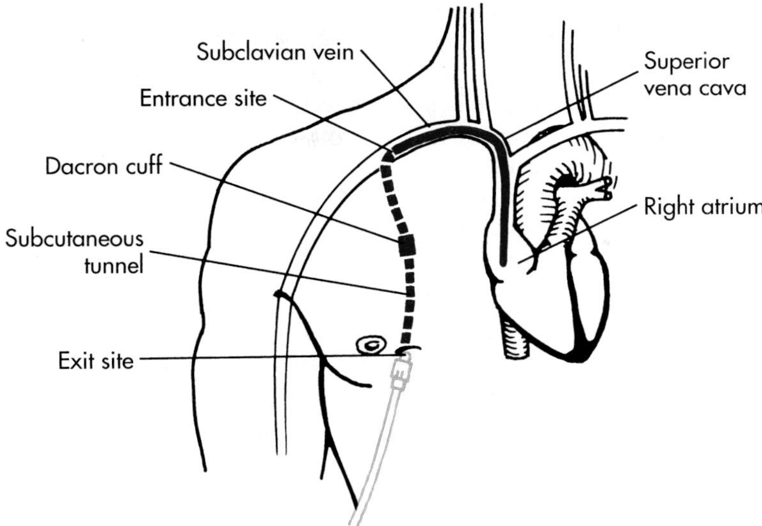

Fig. 25-4 Placement of Hickman catheter for administration of TPN solutions.

Levin tube, a single-lumen tube; the Salem sump tube, a double-lumen tube with airway; or the Dobbhoff tube, a thin, single-lumen tube with a small amount of tungsten (a metallic element) weighted in the end (distal tip).

Feeding schedules may be continuous or intermittent. An intermittent schedule is usually preferred because the stomach normally receives food intermittently. The average individual can tolerate between 240 and 400 ml of formula per feeding. Generally, feedings should be delivered by a gravity drip and regulated with a roller clamp to infuse over 30 to 60 minutes. Some systems are set up to infuse constantly and are slowly administered. This system helps prevent quick infusion and, in turn, prevents diarrhea as well as other complications.

Patients may also be given a **nasointestinal tube feeding,** which supplies nutrients directly into the small intestine. This method may be used for patients who are at risk for aspiration or have a dysfunctional gastric outlet. A French size 6 to 12 flexible tube with a weighted distal tip is placed by the physician with x-ray assistance. Formula delivered by this route should be administered by constant infusion with an enteral feeding pump to maintain a constant, consistent flow.

Administering Gastrostomy Feedings

Patients requiring long-term enteral nutrition may be fed by a **gastrostomy.** Gastrostomy tubes are directly inserted into the stomach through the abdominal wall by surgery or endoscopy. This access to the stomach may be needed by patients who have head and neck cancer, esophageal cancer, or neurologic impairments. Patients who are at risk for aspiration or aspiration pneumonia are not candidates for a gastrostomy.

A permanent gastrostomy may be surgically performed by suturing the stomach to the abdominal wall, creating a stoma through which a Foley or gastrostomy tube is inserted. Unlike the Foley or mushroom catheter, the MIC tube has an external anchoring device that inhibits downward migration of the catheter. Another type of gastrostomy is percutaneous catheter placement, whereby an endoscope pulls a mushroom catheter down to the stomach with the long end of the tube exiting through a small hole in the abdominal wall.

Enteral formulas used for gastrostomy feeding are the same as those used for nasogastric tube feedings. In addition, the nurse assesses the catheter insertion site for signs of infection, wound separation, or hernia and changes the dressing as necessary.

A responsibility of the nurse administering gastrostomy feeding is to ensure that the skin around the tubing is kept dry and intact to prevent skin breakdown (see Chapter 21).

Administering Total Parenteral Nutrition

Total parenteral nutrition (TPN) is the administration of nutritionally complete solutions intravenously. Central total parenteral nutrition (CTPN) is the administration of the solution through a central vein, commonly the subclavian or cephalic vein (Fig. 25-4). Peripheral total parenteral nutrition (PTPN) is the administration of the solution through a peripheral vein, usually reserved for patients needing TPN for 7 to 10 days to prevent malnutrition.

TPN is indicated when the gastrointestinal tract cannot absorb nutrients, the bowel needs a complete rest, or the patient has persistent vomiting and diarrhea. These symptoms occur in patients who have been severely burned or traumatized, postoperative cardiac patients, patients who are septic, patients who require mechanical ventilation, patients with acute renal disease or cancer, and patients with inflammatory bowel disease or pancreatitis (inflammation of the pancreas). If these conditions are present, the patient will not be able to tolerate oral or enteral feedings.

TPN formulas contain all the essential nutrients for weight gain, wound healing, growth, and anabolism (metabolism characterized by the conversion of simple substances into more complex substances). The essential nutrients in TPN formulas include water, protein, carbohydrates, fats, electrolytes, vitamins, and trace elements. The calories and proportion of these nutrients vary according to the solution used and the patient's physical condition. Usually intravenous fats are administered in a separate container. However, a new method of TPN, named total nutrient admixture (TNA), combines a 24-hour supply of all nutrients, including fats, in one solution. TNA is also referred to as *all-in-one TPN*.

The TPN solution is initiated slowly, and as the patient's fluid and glucose tolerance permits, the solutions are advanced. Infusion pumps must be used to maintain a constant infusion rate and reduce the possibility of fluctuations in blood glucose levels. TPN solutions that have fallen behind schedule are *never* increased to catch up. TPN solutions are also never terminated abruptly because of the possibility of rebound hypoglycemia (less-than-normal amount of glucose in the blood). Instead, a solution of 5% dextrose may be used temporarily.

TPN solutions containing 15% to 50% dextrose (high osmolarity) are infused in a central vein, such as the subclavian vein, using a silicone rubber tube called a Broviac or Hickman catheter. These catheters must be flushed with heparin solution several times a day to prevent clogging. The Groshong CV catheter has valves that are located at the tip and that are closed when the catheter is not in use to eliminate the need for heparin flushes. Currently, the central-line catheters have single, double, triple, or quadruple lumens for patients requiring multiple infusions or blood samples. The multilumen catheters should be color coded to indicate their use or should be capped with a heparin infusion lock cap and clearly marked with tape.

Implantable ports are used for long-term access. These ports are implanted in the subcutaneous tissue and require the percutaneous use of a Huber needle to access the catheter. The implantable ports reduce the risk of infection and may be helpful for TPN administered at home.

Patients receiving CTPN require careful monitoring for complications. Problems arising from the insertion of the catheter include pneumothorax, hemothorax, hydrothorax, arterial puncture, air embolism, injury to brachial plexus, catheter embolism, cardiac perforation, and dysrhythmia. Complications that may arise after catheter insertion and during infusion appear in the box.

TPN must be performed under rigid, sterile technique (Skill 25-3). Some facilities allow only registered nurses to perform this procedure. The licensed practical/vocational nurse may be allowed to care for TPN or to assist with the skill, depending on agency policy. The licensed practical/vocational nurse can also be trained to perform TPN.

POTENTIAL COMPLICATIONS AFTER CATHETER INSERTION IN TPN

- *Air embolism:* abnormal presence of air in cardiovascular system, resulting in obstruction of flow of blood through vessel
- *Arterial puncture:* puncture of artery
- *Cardiac perforation:* puncture in heart
- *Catheter embolism:* blood clot that forms at insertion site of intravenous feeding, breaks loose, and invades circulation
- *Catheter occlusion:* blockage in catheter, rendering it unusable
- *Deep vein thrombosis:* blood clot in deep vein
- *Dysrhythmia:* disturbance or abnormality in normal rhythmic pattern
- *Hemothorax:* blood and fluid in pleural cavity
- *Hydrothorax:* noninflammatory accumulation of serous fluid in one or both pleural cavities
- *Infection:* invasion of body by pathogenic microorganisms that reproduce and multiply
- *Injury to brachial plexus:* injury to network of nerves in neck that pass under clavicle and into axilla; originate in the fifth, sixth, seventh, and eighth cervical nerves and first two thoracic spinal nerves; and innervate muscles and skin of chest, shoulders, and arms
- *Pneumothorax:* collapsed lung

■ NURSING CARE PLAN ■

ALTERED NUTRITION: LESS THAN BODY REQUIREMENTS

Mrs. J, age 65, is admitted for the loss of 25 pounds in 3 months. She is to receive a nutritional workup and tests beginning in the morning.

NURSING DIAGNOSIS

Altered nutrition: less than body requirements related to inability to digest or absorb nutrients because of biologic factors as evidenced by weight loss, abdominal pain, diarrhea, nonelastic skin turgor, and poor muscle tone

GOAL

- Patient will gain weight lost.

EXPECTED OUTCOMES

- Patient will show no further evidence of weight loss.
- Patient will gain 3 pounds weekly.

NURSING INTERVENTIONS

- Record patient's weight daily.
- Provide and encourage diet prescribed.
- Determine food preferences and make sure that patient receives those foods.
- Arrange a diet consultation.

EVALUATION

- Patient shows no further evidence of weight loss.
- Patient does not exhibit signs of diarrhea.
- Patient gains weight appropriately.

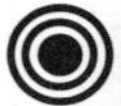

SKILL 25-1 SERVING FOOD AND ASSISTING WITH FEEDING A PATIENT

Steps	Rationale
1. **Obtain equipment:** ▪ Water ▪ Soap ▪ Towel ▪ Washcloth ▪ Oral hygiene supplies ▪ Food tray ▪ Clean gloves	Helps organize procedure.
2. **Refer to medical record, care plan, or Kardex for special interventions.**	Provides basis for care.
3. **Introduce self.**	Decreases anxiety level.
4. **Identify patient by identification band.**	Identifies correct patient for procedure.
5. **Offer pain medication or other medication, if indicated.**	Provides for patient comfort.
6. **Offer bedpan or urinal, if needed.**	Provides for patient comfort.
7. **Wash hands and don clean gloves according to agency policy and guidelines from Centers for Disease Control and Prevention and Occupational Safety and Health Administration.**	Helps prevent cross-contamination.

Continued.

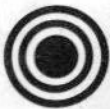

SKILL 25-1 SERVING FOOD AND ASSISTING WITH FEEDING A PATIENT—cont'd

Steps	Rationale
8. Prepare patient for intervention:	
a. Close door to room or pull curtain.	Provides privacy.
b. Drape for procedure if necessary.	Prevents exposure of patient.
9. Raise bed to comfortable level for eating.	Provides comfort for patient.
10. Arrange for patient privacy.	Shows respect for patient.
11. Assist with oral hygiene or dentures, if needed.	Allows patient to feel clean and ready to eat.
12. Provide water, soap, and towel for patient's hands and face, if needed. Wash patient's hands and face if patient is unable.	Freshens patient for mealtime and promotes eating.
13. Clear off over-bed table.	Provides neat environment.
14. Obtain tray and assess for correct diet (Fig. 25-5).	Ensures that correct patient receives diet as ordered.
SERVING FOOD	
15. Assist with food preparation as needed. Open milk carton, spread butter or jelly on bread, cut meat, open any prepackaged items, and place items within convenient reach of patient. Encourage patient to do as much as possible for self.	Aids patient, who may have physical impairment that necessitates assistance.
ASSISTING WITH FEEDING A PATIENT	
16. Assess patient's ability to self-feed and assist as necessary.	Determines amount and type assistance needed by nurse.
17. Lower side rail, if necessary.	Allows access to patient.
18. Place napkin under patient's chin.	Prevents soiling of patient's clothing.
19. Butter bread and cut meat, if needed. Open liquid cartons. Pour hot liquids, and prepare tea or coffee as patient desires. Provide drinking straw for liquids.	Prepares food.
20. Encourage patient to eat without assistance.	Encourages independence.

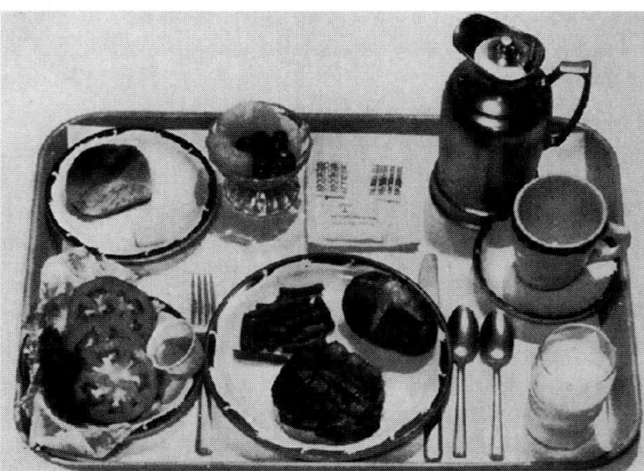

Fig. 25-5 Regular diet.

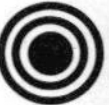

SKILL 25-1 SERVING FOOD AND ASSISTING WITH FEEDING A PATIENT—cont'd

Steps	Rationale
21. Give solid foods from point of spoon or fork (Fig. 25-6). Alternate solids and liquids. Alternate types of food given to patient. Never blow on food to cool it or taste patient's food. Allow patient to hold bread or assist if possible. Allow for rest periods as needed. Use napkin to wipe patient's mouth as needed.	Allows eating process to be as normal as possible. Keeps food neat and uncontaminated by nurse.
22. Remove tray when finished.	Provides clean environment.
23. Offer oral care, bedpan, or handwashing as needed.	Allows patient to feel clean and neat.
24. Raise side rail, if needed.	Keeps environment safe.
25. Remove gloves and wash hands.	Helps prevent cross-contamination.
26. Document.	Documents procedure, patient's response, and intake and output.

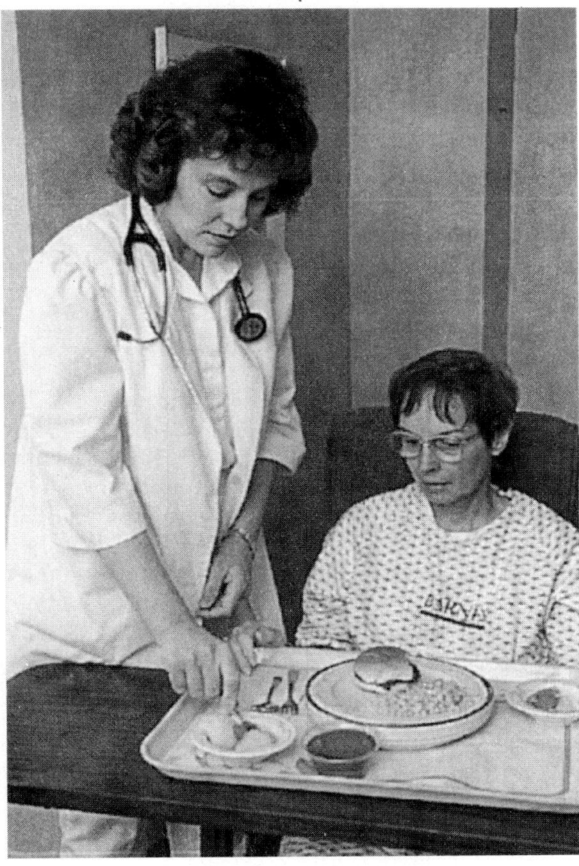

Fig. 25-6 Feeding a patient. (From Perry AG, Potter PA: *Clinical nursing skills and techniques,* ed 3, St Louis, 1994, Mosby.)

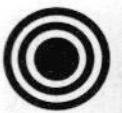

SKILL 25-2 ADMINISTERING NASOGASTRIC TUBE AND GASTROSTOMY FEEDINGS

Steps	Rationale
1. Obtain equipment: *NG tube feeding:* ▪ Towel ▪ Feeding syringe (Asepto or Toomey) or feeding bag ▪ 30 ml of tap water ▪ Required amount of formula ▪ Clean gloves ▪ Stethoscope ▪ Warm, soapy water *Gastrostomy tube feeding:* ▪ Oral hygiene supplies (see Chapter 23) ▪ 50-ml syringe ▪ Feeding bag and tubing for gravity drip or enteral infusion pump ▪ Formula ▪ Water in glass or cup ▪ Dressing change tray ▪ Clean gloves ▪ 30 ml of tap water	Helps organize procedure.
2. Refer to medical record, care plan, or Kardex for special interventions.	Provides basis for care.
3. Introduce self.	Decreases anxiety level.
4. Identify patient by identification band.	Identifies correct patient for procedure.
5. Explain procedure to patient.	Seeks cooperation and decreases anxiety.
6. Wash hands and don clean gloves according to agency policy and guidelines from Centers for Disease Control and Prevention and Occupational Safety and Health Administration.	Helps prevent cross-contamination.
7. Prepare patient for intervention:	
a. Close door to room or pull curtain.	Provides privacy.
b. Drape for procedure if necessary.	Prevents exposure of patient.
8. Raise bed to comfortable working level.	Provides safety for nurse.
9. Arrange for patient privacy.	Shows respect for patient.
10. Place patient in high semi-Fowler's position.	Allows gravity to aid in digestion and reduces risk of aspiration.
11. Assess bowel sounds.	Evaluates functioning of gastrointestinal tract.
NASOGASTRIC TUBE FEEDING	
12. Verify tube placement:	
a. Unclamp tube and aspirate stomach contents. Determine amount of residual fluid. According to hospital or physician policy, return the residual fluid to stomach.	Verifies tube placement and determines amount of residual fluid in stomach. Prevents fluid and electrolyte imbalance. (If residual fluid is over 50 to 100 ml, physician may not want patient to be fed at this time.)
b. Connect syringe with tube and push in approximately 20 ml of air while listening over the epigastric area with stethoscope for gurgling. Remove syringe.	Verifies tube placement.
13. For intermittent feeding, fill feeding bag and tubing with formula.	Provides correct feeding for patient.
14. Attach feeding bag to nasogastric tube, regulating drip rate with roller clamp.	Provides appropriate drip rate for tube feeding.
15. Hang feeding bag on intravenous pole 18 in above patient.	Allows feeding to infuse by correct drip method.
16. Allow feeding to infuse slowly for 20 to 30 min.	Keeps tube patent.

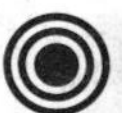

SKILL 25-2 ADMINISTERING NASOGASTRIC TUBE AND GASTROSTOMY FEEDINGS—cont'd

Steps	Rationale
17. When feeding is completed, flush nasogastric tube with 30 to 50 ml of water as ordered.	Clears tubing, prevents clogging, and provides extra water for intake.
18. Clamp nasogastric tube. Keep patient comfortable in Fowler's position.	Aids digestion and prevents aspiration.
19. Wash feeding bag and tubing with warm, soapy water, rinse well, and dry. Change bag and tubing every 24 to 48 hr, depending on hospital policy.	Prevents transmission of bacteria.
20. Give water between feedings as ordered.	Provides adequate intake.
21. If the patient is receiving continuous tube feeding, after filling bag and pump tubing, attach tubing to nasogastric tube. Set enteral infusion pump to deliver ordered volume and rate, unclamp tubing, and start pump. Check volume every 1 to 2 hr.	Provides appropriate volume and fluid rates.
22. Irrigate tube every 3 to 4 hr with 20 to 30 ml of water as ordered.	Keeps tube patent (open) for use.
GASTROSTOMY TUBE FEEDING	
23. Verify tube placement by unclamping tube and aspirating stomach contents.	Verifies tube placement and determines amount of residual fluid in stomach.
24. Determine amount of residual fluid. According to hospital or physician policy, return residual fluid.	Prevents fluid and electrolyte imbalance. (If residual is 50 ml to 100 ml, physician may not want patient to be fed at this time.)
25. Return residual fluid to stomach.	
26. For intermittent feeding, fill feeding bag and tubing with formula.	Prepares formula for feeding.
27. Attach feeding bag to gastrostomy tube, regulating drip rate with roller clamp.	Sets appropriate amount of feeding.
28. Hang feeding bag on pole 18 in above patient's abdomen.	Allows infusion to drip.
29. Allow feeding to infuse slowly for 20 to 30 min.	Allows appropriate time to ensure absorption.
30. Assess patient for signs of discomfort, such as abdominal cramping. If necessary, slow or stop infusion.	Provides patient assistance.
31. When feeding is completed, flush gastrostomy tube with 30 ml of tap water as ordered.	Keeps tube patent.
32. Clamp gastrostomy tube.	Prevents leakage.
33. Wash, rinse, and dry skin around tube insertion site as needed.	Keeps wound site clean and dry to prevent infection.
34. Apply clean gauze dressing as needed.	Prevents contamination.
35. Maintain patient in high semi-Fowler's position.	Aids digestion.
36. Wash feeding bag and tubing, rinse, and dry. Bag and tubing are changed every 24 to 48 hr, depending on hospital policy.	Prevents transmission of bacteria.
37. Give water between feedings as ordered.	Allows patient enough fluids.
38. If patient is receiving a continuous tube feeding, attach tubing to gastrostomy tube after filling bag and pump tubing. Set enteral infusion pump to deliver ordered volume and rate and start pump. Check volume every 1 to 2 hr. Irrigate tube with water as ordered.	Provides appropriate volume and fluid rates.
39. Remove gloves and wash hands.	Helps prevent cross-contamination.
40. Document.	Documents procedure and patient's response.

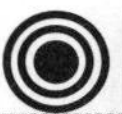

SKILL 25-3 ADMINISTERING TOTAL PARENTERAL NUTRITION

Steps	Rationale
1. Obtain equipment: ▪ TPN solution ▪ Intravenous tubing with filter for TPN solution ▪ Intravenous tubing without filter for lipids ▪ Infusion pump ▪ Extension tubing, if needed ▪ Intake and output record ▪ TPN record sheet ▪ Sterile gloves ▪ Clean gloves	Helps organize procedure.
2. Refer to medical record, care plan, or Kardex for special interventions.	Provides basis for care.
3. Introduce self.	Decreases anxiety level.
4. Identify patient by identification band.	Identifies correct patient for procedure.
5. Explain procedure to patient.	Seeks cooperation and decreases anxiety.
6. Wash hands and don clean gloves according to agency policy and guidelines from Centers for Disease Control and Prevention and Occupational Safety and Health Administration.	Helps prevent cross-contamination.
7. Prepare patient for intervention:	
a. Close door to room or pull curtain.	Provides privacy.
b. Drape for procedure if necessary.	Prevents exposure of patient.
8. Raise bed to comfortable working level.	Provides safety for nurse.
9. Arrange for patient privacy.	Shows respect for patient.
10. Compare TPN label with patient's identification band.	Verifies correct patient.
11. Identify catheter port for TPN and, if necessary, close it with infusion plug.	Prevents contamination.
12. Remove cap from filtered tubing to expose spike.	Prepares tubing.
13. Remove cover or cap from TPN bottle or bag.	Prepares solution.
14. Insert tubing spike.	Prepares solution.
15. Open drip controller, prime drip chamber, and run solution through tubing.	Eliminates air from tubing.
16. Close drip controller.	Prevents leakage.
17. Hang feeding bag on pole attached to infusion pump.	Allows solution to flow according to ordered amount.
18. Slide tubing into infusion pump.	Prepares solution for infusing.
19. If ordered, prepare lipid solution by inserting vented, nonfiltered tubing spike into lipid bottle. Open drip chamber and run solution through tubing. Place 21-gauge needle on end of tubing and plug into distal port of TPN tubing.	Allows TPN solution and lipids to be administered simultaneously.
20. Attach TPN tubing to central catheter port.	Allows flow into correct site.
21. Set infusion pump for appropriate volume per hour.	Sets correct infusion rate.
22. Calculate and assess drip rate for TPN solution (and lipids, if ordered).	Verifies infusion rate.
23. Assist patient to comfortable position.	Promotes comfort and well-being.
24. Remove used disposable supplies.	Cleans environment.
25. Remove gloves and wash hands.	Helps prevent cross-contamination.
26. Document.	Documents procedure and patient's response.

SUMMARY

Appropriate nutrition helps ensure wellness. The nurse should teach the patient about appropriate nutrition when necessary. Cultural influences of patients should be considered: Many people will not eat foods that interfere with cultural and religious beliefs and practices. Illness and disease affect nutrition, sometimes to the point of malnutrition. When patients have special nutritional problems, the nurse is responsible for assessing and treating those problems. The nurse is also responsible for teaching patients about hospital diets and making certain that the patient receives the correct diet at mealtime.

Key Concepts

- Therapeutic nutrition prevents malnutrition.
- A nursing care plan should be developed to assist the patient with nutrition problems.
- Encouraging the drinking of adequate fluids, especially water, is a responsibility of the nurse.
- Mealtime should be a pleasant as well as a social event.
- It is important to consider and provide likes and dislikes when encouraging the patient to eat.
- Special nutrition problems may be corrected by nasogastric tube feedings, gastrostomy feedings, and total parenteral nutrition therapy before or after surgery or illness.

Critical Thinking Questions

1. With a partner, role play the following situation: The nurse assists the patient in developing a weekly diet plan based on the food guide pyramid. The patient is a vegetarian or must follow specific ethnic-cultural dietary guidelines. The nurse must help the patient incorporate personal preferences and restrictions into a healthy diet plan.
2. Student nurses have many stressors specific to their academic situations. Keep a log of your own nutrition and rest patterns for 7 days. Compare your lifestyle to the recommendations for a healthy lifestyle given in the text. Can you recognize modifications necessary to reduce stress?
3. Dietary fiber is increasingly being recognized for its therapeutic effects. Identify and explain two of these.

REFERENCES AND SUGGESTED READINGS

Burtis G et al: *Applied nutrition and diet therapy,* Philadelphia, 1992, Saunders.

Caldwell E, Hegner B: *Nursing assistant,* New York, 1993, Delmar.

Flynn J, Hackel R: *Technological foundations in nursing,* Norwalk, Conn, 1994, Appleton & Lange.

Lederer J: *Care planning pocket guide,* ed 3, Redwood City, Calif, 1994, Addison-Wesley.

Morton P: *Health assessment in nursing,* Springhouse, Penn, 1993, Springhouse.

Perry AG, Potter PA: *Clinical nursing skills and techniques,* ed 3, St Louis, 1994, Mosby.

Potter PA, Perry AG: *Fundamentals of nursing: concepts, process, and practice,* ed 3, St Louis, 1993, Mosby.

Smith A, Johnson J: *Nurse's guide to clinical procedures,* Philadelphia, 1994, Lippincott.

Smith S, Duell D: *Clinical nursing skills,* ed 3, Norwalk, Conn, 1993, Appleton & Lange.

CHAPTER 26

Sleep

Learning Objectives

After studying this chapter, the student should be able to:

- Define the key terms.
- Compare the characteristics of sleep and rest.
- Promote rest and sleep in all phases of illness and recovery.
- Identify four age-specific interventions for promoting rest and sleep.
- Document the patient's rest and sleep activities.
- Describe common sleep disorders.
- List nursing measures to promote comfort and relaxation.
- Describe the effects of sleep loss.
- Differentiate the stages of sleep.

Key Terms

Dream
Electroencephalogram (EEG)
Enuresis
Insomnia
Narcolepsy
Nonrapid eye movement (NREM)
Rapid eye movement (REM)
Sleep
Sleep apnea
Sleep deprivation
Sleep terrors
Somnambulism
Sudden infant death syndrome (SIDS)

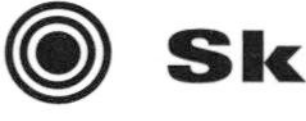

Skill

26-1 Promoting sleep

Sleep is a state marked by reduced consciousness, diminished activity of the skeletal muscles, and depressed metabolism.

Obtaining adequate rest and sleep are important in promoting general health and ensuring recovery from illness. Throughout the life cycle, rest and sleep aid in healing and are necessary for maintaining optimal health. Sleep also increases the ability to learn and to recall knowledge.

People have different needs regarding the amount and quality of sleep required. When people have difficulty sleeping, the ability to concentrate, make usual judgments, and work optimally is reduced, and the lack of sleep may cause irritability. Sleep is also essential in preserving emotional stability and helps a person to be socially adaptable. Inadequate rest and short- and long-term sleep deprivation may have serious consequences, depending on a person's existing health status. Sleep disturbance may cause a patient to seek assistance from a physician. The nurse provides nursing care to patients who have sleep disturbances before being hospitalized and whose problems are compounded by illness.

The need for rest and sleep varies from person to person and throughout an individual's life cycle. These needs also change in response to different types of stressors. Illness, hospitalization, and surgery may all adversely affect a person's ability to obtain adequate amounts of sleep. The responsibility of the nurse in assessing the patient's sleep needs include diagnosing sleep problems, implementing nursing measures to promote rest and sleep, and evaluating the patient's response to the effectiveness of intervention.

Specific brain wave patterns occur in each stage of sleep. An **electroencephalogram (EEG)** is an examination that records electrical impulses in the brain. The test itself does not diagnose illness, but it does give information that shows the need for further testing. However, sleep patterns may be determined by this examination.

NURSING PROCESS

Assessment

The first step in assessing the patient's sleep status is to determine how much sleep is needed for optimal functioning and how the illness or hospitalization will affect sleep requirements (see box). Nursing history forms usually require information about the patient's sleep patterns. This may include the number of hours of sleep needed, usual bedtime, usual wake time, number of times that the patient urinates during the night, measures practiced to promote sleep, and medications taken. This information assists the nurse in identifying sleep disturbances and developing a plan of care.

Careful physical assessment may lead to practical solutions for decreasing discomfort related to sleep disturbance. For example, loosening a tight binder or assisting the patient to urinate may promote sleep. The nurse also assesses the patient's environment for factors that may interfere with sleep, such as noise, light, odors, and temperature.

Nursing Diagnosis

The nurse reviews the data gathered during assessment. Clustering defining characteristics reveals a diagnosis. Possible nursing diagnoses for sleep disturbance include the following:

Altered thought processes
Fatigue
Ineffective breathing pattern
Sleep pattern disturbance

Planning

An individualized plan of care can be developed only after the nurse understands the patient's normal and current sleep patterns and the factors disrupting the patient's sleep. It is also important for the nurse to understand the effect of the sleep disturbance on other health problems. The nurse should work with the patient to develop interventions to promote rest and sleep (see teaching box).

The plan of care may include the following goal:

Goal: Patient establishes a regular healthy sleep pattern within 2 weeks.

Outcome

Patient reports no episodes of awakening during the night.

PATIENT TEACHING 

- Instruct patient to exercise daily.
- Advise patient to follow a regular schedule of sleep and wake times.
- Suggest that the patient's bedroom be darkened and soundproofed to provide a restful environment.

GERONTOLOGIC CONSIDERATIONS

- The sleep of the older adult is less deep. This increases the risk of early awakening and complaints of sleep disturbance.
- Insufficient sleep may lead to memory and personality changes in the older adult.
- The older adult may take medications that interfere with sleep. Times of administration should be assessed and modified when possible.
- If the patient cannot go to sleep, the nurse may sit with the patient for a few minutes to help relaxation and remove any fears.

Implementation

When implementing the plan of care, the nurse must consider the patient's routines and preferences. The selection of appropriate sleep therapies lessens interruptions of the sleep cycle and promotes a more normal, restful environment for the patient. Special consideration should be given to the older adult (see gerontologic box).

Evaluation

The nurse determines whether the established plan of care is effective. The patient is the best source for evaluating whether the quality of sleep has improved or whether other health care problems have been eliminated through the improvement of sleep (see care plan on p. 500). The nurse uses evaluative measures for each expected outcome. The information gathered determines the status of each goal.

Goal: Patient establishes a regular healthy sleep pattern within 2 weeks.

Evaluative measure

Nurse asks patient each morning about any occurrences of awakening.

STAGES OF SLEEP

Sleep normally follows a pattern of four to six cycles, each of which is composed of five stages (see

FACTORS AFFECTING SLEEP

Physical Illness

- Pain or physical discomfort results in difficulty falling or staying asleep.
- Chronic pain may have circadian rhythm* of increasing intensity at night, thus disrupting sleep (Glyn et al, 1976).
- Illness may force patients to sleep in positions to which they are unaccustomed.
- Respiratory diseases interfere with rhythm of breathing or influence position person must assume to breathe easily. Both factors can disturb sleep.
- Patients with heart disease are often afraid to go to sleep at night.
- Hypertension causes early morning awakening and fatigue.
- Nocturia and "restless leg syndrome" disrupt sleep, causing patients to awaken during night and often result in difficulty resuming sleep.
- Conditions that increase intracranial pressure or alter central nervous system physiology alter sleep patterns and can cause excessive daytime sleeping.

Anxiety and Depression

- As anxiety and depression increase, so does lack of sleep, and as sleep decreases, anxiety and depression increase (Hodgson, 1991).
- Bereaved people often experience sleep problems related to fear of intruders, loneliness, and dreams or nightmares that occur involving lost loved one.

Drugs and Substances

- Various drugs and substances affect pattern and quality of sleep (see box on p. 498).
- Older adults often take several drugs, combined effects of which disrupt sleep.
- L-Tryptophan, protein found in foods such as milk, cheese, and meats, may help induce sleep.

Life-style

- Daily routines such as working rotating shifts influence sleep patterns. Only after several weeks of working a night shift does person's biologic clock adjust.
- Performing unaccustomed heavy work, late-night social activities, and changing evening mealtimes are activities that can disrupt sleep.

Sleep Patterns

- Sleep patterns include starting time and duration of sleep.
- Most significant cause of daytime sleepiness is inadequate or abnormal sleep at night (Berman et al, 1990).
- Everyone has increased sleep tendency from 2 to 7 AM and to lesser degree from 2 to 5 PM (Mitler et al, 1988). When sleep patterns are disrupted, natural tendency to be sleeping at select times increases.
- Sleep patterns influence succeeding attempts to fall asleep because of changes in circadian rhythm. Sleeping 1 hour later results in falling asleep 1 hour later next night.
- Chronic lack of sleep can alter ability to perform daily functions such as driving.

Stress

- Stress resulting from personal problems or situational crises causes tension and may cause person to try too hard to fall asleep, to awaken frequently, or to oversleep.
- Stress causes release of corticosteroids and adrenalin, which leads to catabolism and sleeplessness.
- Patients with advanced cancer or chronic illness often are afraid to sleep in case they might die.
- Older patients experience losses such as retirement or death of loved one. Thus older adults can suffer delays in falling asleep, earlier REM sleep, frequent awakening, increased total bed time, and feelings of sleeping poorly (Colling, 1983).

Environment

- Environmental factors influence ability to fall and remain asleep. Significant factors include ventilation, lighting, type of bed, sound level, and presence or absence of bed partner.
- In hospitals, unfamiliar noises and higher noise levels such as those created by wall suction, opening packages, ringing alarms, and flushing toilets can cause sleep deprivation.
- Intensive care units are sources for high noise levels.

Exercise and Fatigue

- Exercise and fatigue in moderation usually facilitate restful sleep, but excess fatigue from exhausting or stressful work can make falling asleep difficult.
- Exercise 2 hours before bedtime allows body to cool down and promotes relaxation.

Nutrition

- Weight gain causes longer sleep periods with fewer interruptions and later awakening.
- Weight loss can cause reduction in total sleep along with broken sleep and earlier awakening.

From Potter PA, Perry AG: *Basic nursing: theory and practice,* ed 3, St Louis, 1995, Mosby.
*Circadian rhythm is pattern based on 24-hour cycle, especially repetition of certain physiologic phenomena such as eating and sleeping.

STAGES OF SLEEP

Stage 1: NREM
- This is lightest level of sleep.
- Stage lasts a few minutes.
- Decreased physiologic activity begins with gradual fall in vital signs and metabolism.
- Person is easily aroused by sensory stimuli such as noise.
- If awakened, person feels as though daydreaming has occurred.
- Autonomic activities (for example, heart rate) are reduced.

Stage 2: NREM
- This is period of sound sleep.
- Relaxation progresses.
- Arousal is still easy.
- Stage lasts 10 to 20 minutes.
- Body functions are still slowing.

Stage 3: NREM
- This is initial stages of deep sleep.
- Sleeper is difficult to arouse and rarely moves.
- Muscles are completely relaxed.
- Vital signs decline but remain regular.
- Stage lasts 15 to 30 minutes.
- Hormonal response includes secretion of growth hormone.

Stage 4: NREM
- This is deepest stage of sleep.
- It is very difficult to arouse sleeper.
- If sleep loss has occurred, sleeper will spend most of night in this stage.
- Stage restores and rests body.
- Vital signs are significantly lower than during waking hours.
- Stage lasts approximately 15 to 30 minutes.
- Sleepwalking and enuresis may occur.
- Hormonal response continues.

REM Sleep
- This is stage of vivid, full-color dreaming. (Less vivid dreaming may occur in other stages.)
- Stage first occurs approximately 90 minutes after sleep has begun and thereafter occurs at end of each NREM cycle
- Stage is typified by autonomic response of rapidly moving eyes, fluctuating heart and respiratory rates, and increased or fluctuating blood pressure.
- Loss of skeletal muscle tone occurs.
- Stage is responsible for mental restoration.
- This is stage in which sleeper is most difficult to arouse.
- Duration increases with each cycle and averages 20 minutes.

From Potter PA, Perry AG: *Basic nursing: theory and practice,* ed 3, St Louis, 1995, Mosby.

box). The entire five-stage process occurs approximately every 90 to 120 minutes throughout the period of sleep. Stages 1 through 4 are referred to as **nonrapid eye movement (NREM)** sleep. NREM is characterized by the progression of relaxation. **Rapid eye movement (REM)** is considered to be stage 5. This stage is essential in the sleep cycle, involves increased activity, and is characterized by a rapid, horizontal movement of both eyes, profound muscular relaxation, and vivid dreaming. After REM sleep, the person returns to stage 2 sleep and begins the cycle again. Stage 1 is not repeated unless the person is awakened. The normal adult sleep cycle and the stages of sleep are summarized in Fig. 26-1.

Presleep Before stage 1 sleep, the person becomes drowsy. This stage lasts about 10 to 30 minutes before falling asleep and is a normal stage in the routine sleep pattern.

Stage 1 sleep During stage 1, the person is still alert and is able to respond to events taking place within the body (i.e., thirst) and in the surrounding environment (i.e., a ringing telephone). This stage acts as a brief adjustment period from being awake to the later stages of sleep.

Stage 2 sleep During stage 2, general relaxation and reduction of activity in the brain and body take place. The person has decreased responses to both internal (bodily) and external (environmental) events. Sensory responses are greatly reduced. Hearing is the last fully functional sense to diminish before the person enters stages of deep sleep.

Stage 3 sleep Stage 3 is the initial stage of deep sleep and is characterized by a general lowering of body functions. All vital signs—temperature, pulse, respiration, and blood pressure—are decreased but remain regular. As the muscles completely relax, the person is difficult to arouse and rarely moves.

Stage 4 sleep Stage 4 is very deep sleep. The person may be awakened only by strong or painful stimuli. This stage is necessary for the restoration of body tissue. Any period of extreme physical tiredness or exertion increases the amount of time spent in stage 4 sleep. The hormone responsible for growth is released during this stage, and sleepwalking and enuresis may also occur. About 20 to 30 minutes into sleep, the process is reversed. The sleeper moves from stage 4 to stage 3 to stage 2 and then enters the most profound stage of sleep, or REM sleep.

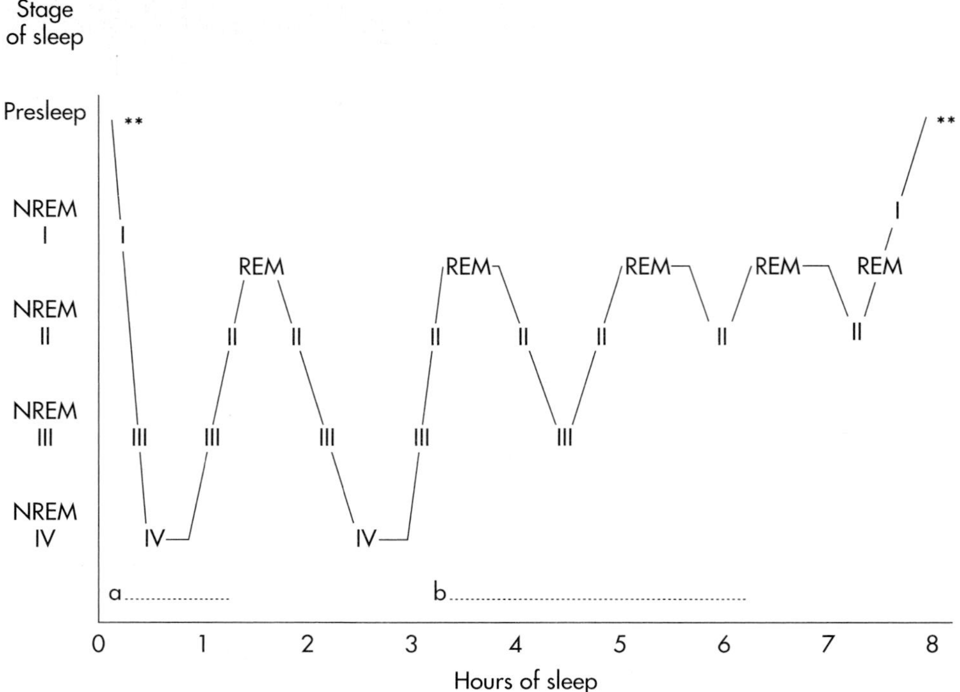

Fig. 26-1 Normal adult sleep cycle and the stages of sleep. (From Potter PA, Perry AG: *Basic nursing: theory and practice,* ed 3, St Louis, 1995, Mosby; modified from Biddle C, Oaster TRF: The nature of sleep, *Journal of the American Association of Nurse Anesthetists* 58(1):36, 1990.)

REM sleep During this part of the sleep cycle, the muscles remain relaxed, but there is increased activity in several other body systems, especially the sympathetic nervous system. This extra activity causes vital signs, the need for oxygen, and the breathing rate to increase. Irregular heart rhythms, chest pain, convulsion, myocardial infarction (heart attack), and abdominal pain are more likely to occur because of the increased activity of the sympathetic nervous system. Dreams in this stage are colorful and intense. REM sleep is necessary for the maintenance of psychologic health and adaptation, for sorting information attained while awake, and for the processes of learning and memory.

DREAMS

A **dream** is a sequence of ideas, thoughts, emotions, or images that pass through the mind during NREM and REM sleep. Dreams are more vivid and elaborate during REM sleep. People dream about many things but often dream about current issues such as a fight with a loved one. A person may also dream about things that are frightening. A psychotherapist may gain access to the unconscious mind by examining the content of dreams. People who have certain mental illnesses and are under a great deal of stress may not dream and are treated so that they can dream.

DEVELOPMENTAL CONSIDERATIONS

The length of sleep necessary to maintain physical and psychologic health gradually diminishes with age from as much as 20 hours a day in infants to as little as 6 hours a day in older adults.

The *newborn* sleeps 15 to 20 hours a day. Short waking periods occur approximately every 2 hours. During sleep, there are spontaneous movements of the face and body. Some 50% of sleep is REM sleep. Awakening is usually related to hunger, a wet diaper, or the need for attention. The rapid rate of growth and development that occurs at this age increases the need for rest and sleep.

The *infant* (1 month to 1 year of age) sleeps approximately three fourths of the time, an average of 15 to 18 hours a day. The infant usually takes one or two naps during the day. The infant may resist going to sleep because of wanting the parents.

A *toddler* (1 through 3 years of age) sleeps less than the infant. The sleep pattern is broken into several periods and is adapted to the family routine.

This child resists going to sleep after being put to bed by requesting a drink of water or some other form of attention. The toddler enjoys taking a favorite toy or blanket to bed for comfort and relaxation. The child sleeps approximately 12 to 14 hours a day, which includes a nap of 1 to 2 hours. The amount of REM sleep decreases as additional opportunities to interact with the environment occur.

The *preschool-age* child (3 to 5 years of age) spends about half of the time napping and sleeping at night. Children in this age group often have difficulty sleeping after long, intensely active days. They also have frightening, intense dreams because of an increased imagination. It is common for the child to awaken from nightmares. A child who is frequently disturbed at night by frightening dreams should have a daytime nap. Otherwise, the preschooler no longer requires a nap.

The *school-age* child (6 to 11 years of age) still sleeps about half of the time but does not need naps. It is common for children in this age group to have difficulty falling asleep. The older child may resist going to bed because of increased needs for independence and autonomy. The youngster may demand a later bedtime. The child requires 10 to 12 hours sleep a day and may experience night terrors or nightmares.

The *adolescent* (12 to 18 years of age) averages 8 to 9 hours sleep a day. The young person usually does not resist going to sleep because of increased mental and physical activity. Social activities may interfere with sleep patterns because the adolescent desires to spend more time with peers.

The *adult* (18 to 60 years of age) spend only about 25% of total sleep time in REM. Approximately one third of adults report some type of sleep disturbance, and most of these involve complaints of difficulty sleeping or not feeling adequately rested on arising in the morning. The adult also reports increased irritability, restlessness, inability to concentrate, and general feelings of tiredness. The adult is easily awakened and has more difficulty returning to sleep in an unfamiliar environment.

The *older adult* (60 years of age and older) sleeps approximately one fourth of the time or less. The people in this age group often have decreased amounts of REM sleep and stage 4 sleep. The older adult awakens more often, an average of 6 times a night. The person takes longer to go to sleep and usually awakens earlier. This patient requires frequent monitoring during the night because of disorientation from an unfamiliar environment. Restraints may be necessary to prevent the patient from wandering or receiving an injury at night. Older adults may experience sleep disturbance at home and especially while in the hospital.

CONTROLLING NOISE IN THE HOSPITAL

- Close doors to patient's room.
- Reduce volume of nearby telephone and paging equipment.
- Wear rubber-soled shoes and avoid wearing clogs.
- Turn off bedside equipment not in use, such as oxygen or suction equipment.
- Avoid abrupt loud noise, such as flushing toilet or moving beds.
- Keep necessary conversations at low levels, particularly at night.
- Conduct discussions or nursing report in private, separate area away from patient rooms.
- Turn off television or radio unless patient prefers soft music.

From Potter PA, Perry AG: *Fundamentals of nursing: concepts, process, and practice,* ed 3, St Louis, 1993, Mosby.

NURSING INTERVENTIONS

To promote adequate rest and sleep during hospitalization, the nurse should assist the patient in following familiar routines and make necessary changes in the hospital environment that do not interfere with nursing care (Skill 26-1). Meeting the basic needs of the patient and controlling unnecessary environmental stimuli help the patient obtain as much sleep as possible.

The inability to sleep during hospitalization is often related to the lack of a familiar environment, anxiety, pain, changes in routine, separation from family, and repeated awakenings for procedures, medications, and assessments of vital signs. A common complaint of the hospitalized patient is the noise, especially at night. It is the responsibility of the nurse to help control noise (see box). Sleeping medication causes a lack of REM sleep. Medications such as sedatives, tranquilizers, and antidepressants may shorten or prevent REM sleep (see box). When administered for an extended time, these drugs should be slowly withdrawn, since they may cause increased restlessness, anxiety, and difficulty sleeping.

To meet the basic needs of the patient, the nurse should ensure that the patient is not hungry, has an empty bladder, is comfortably positioned, and has been given medication for pain, if necessary. The nurse should administer comfort measures for promoting sleep (see box). The older adult may have difficulty sleeping despite comfort measures, so the

DRUGS AND THEIR EFFECTS ON SLEEP

- Hypnotics
  - Interfere with reaching deeper sleep stages
  - Provide only temporary (1-week) increase in quantity of sleep
  - Eventually cause "hangover" during day: excess drowsiness, confusion, decreased energy
  - May worsen sleep apnea in older adults
- Diuretics
  - Cause nocturia (excessive urination at night)
- Antidepressants and stimulants
  - Suppress REM sleep
- Alcohol
  - Speeds onset of sleep
  - Disrupts REM sleep
  - Awakens person during night and causes difficulty returning to sleep
- Caffeine
  - Prevents person from falling asleep
  - May cause person to awaken during night
- Digoxin
  - Causes nightmares
- Beta blockers
  - Cause nightmares
  - Cause insomnia
  - Cause awakening from sleep
- Valium
  - Decreases stages 2, 4, and REM sleep
  - Decreases awakenings
- Narcotics (Morphine/Demerol)
  - Suppress REM sleep
  - If discontinued quickly, can increase risk of cardiac dysrythmias because of "rebound REM" periods
  - Cause increased awakenings and drowsiness

From Potter PA, Perry AG: *Basic nursing: theory and practice,* ed 3, St Louis, 1995, Mosby.

COMFORT MEASURES FOR PROMOTING SLEEP

- Administer analgesics, sedatives, or both about 30 minutes before bedtime.
- Encourage patients to wear loose-fitting nightwear.
- Remove any irritants against patient's skin, such as moist or wrinkled sheets or drainage tubing.
- Position and support body parts to protect pressure points and aid muscle relaxation.
- Offer massage just before bedtime.
- Administer necessary hygiene measures.
- Keep bed linen clean and dry.
- Provide comfortable mattress.
- Encourage patient to void hour before sleep.

From Potter PA, Perry AG: *Fundamentals of nursing: concepts, process, and practice,* ed 3, St Louis, 1993, Mosby.

SAFETY MEASURES FOR PROMOTING SLEEP

- Use night lights.
- Place bed in low position.
- Use side rails as appropriate.
- Place call bell within reach.
- Teach patient how to obtain assistance.
- Teach patient how to move around in bed with intravenous or drainage tubing.
- Ascertain that tubing is long enough to allow patient to move.

nurse should provide time during the day for rest and perhaps a nap. However, this patient should not be allowed to sleep too long during the day because it often prevents sleeping at night. Safety measures (see box) should be provided for the older adult during sleeping hours.

SLEEP DISORDERS

Sleep deprivation **Sleep deprivation** occurs when a patient fails to acquire an adequate amount of sleep and when the person is unable to complete all five stages of sleep. Patients who have psychiatric illness, who are recovering from surgery, or who are in critical care units are most likely to develop sleep deprivation. Sleep deprivation symptoms are listed in the box. Children, older adults, and patients with multisystem or severe, debilitating illnesses (that is, patients with acquired immune deficiency syndrome) also experience severe stress during hospitalization and are susceptible to sleep deprivation.

Narcolepsy and sleep apnea Narcolepsy and sleep apnea are two types of sleep disorders found in only a small percentage of the population. If present, these problems require medical intervention, and it is important that the nurse report complaints or assessments regarding these disorders.

Narcolepsy is a syndrome that causes a sudden, uncontrollable desire to sleep. Attacks may occur at any time and last from a few minutes to a few hours. The patient is not in control of the urge to sleep, and narcolepsy cannot be successfully treated with adjustments to the sleep schedule or additional sleep time. The patient requires medication, usually stimulants, and must be treated throughout the life span.

Sleep apnea is the absence of respiration and may occur one to several times during sleep, most often during NREM sleep. These periods of apnea may last a few seconds to a few minutes and are often accompanied by snoring and restlessness. Many patients are unaware that they are experiencing sleep apnea unless it is brought to their attention by spouses or caregivers. Sleep apnea may develop at any time and may be associated with sinus conditions or other nose and throat problems. Adults with sleep apnea may sometimes be treated with surgery if the cause if a correctable nose or throat problem.

This type of apnea occurs more often in overweight middle-aged or older men. It is important for the nurse to remember that patients are deprived of oxygen during periods of sleep apnea. Administration of analgesics or anesthetics may make it more difficult for the body to respond when respiration has temporarily ceased. Therefore patients recovering from anesthesia or from taking pain medication should be monitored carefully if they also have sleep apnea.

Sleep apnea in infants has been implicated as the cause of death in some cases of **sudden infant death syndrome (SIDS),** the unexpected and sudden death of an apparently normal and healthy infant that occurs during sleep and with no physical or autopsic evidence of disease. There is a newer finding that SIDS may be directly related to malfunction of the brainstem of the infant. Research is being conducted regarding this finding. Infants who are diagnosed with sleep apnea are usually sent home with special monitors to alert the parents. Infants usually outgrow the problem by approximately 1 year of age.

Other sleep disorders **Sleep terrors** is a condition characterized by repeated episodes of abrupt awakening, usually with panicky screams. It is accompanied by intense anxiety, confusion, agitation, disorientation, unresponsiveness, marked motor movements, and total amnesia concerning the event. This disorder is seen usually in children and is more common in boys than girls. It is more likely to occur if the individual is fatigued or under stress.

Somnambulism, or sleepwalking, is a condition characterized by complex motor activity, usually culminating in leaving the bed and walking, with no recall of the episode on awakening. The condition is seen primarily in children and is more common in boys than in girls. The problem is more likely to occur if the individual is fatigued or under stress.

Enuresis is the abnormal inability to control urination, especially in bed at night. It occurs most often in children who are very sound sleepers or who have small bladder capacities. In some cases, enuresis is related to emotional or physical causes.

Insomnia is the chronic inability to sleep or to remain asleep throughout the night. The causes of sleeplessness may be physical, psychologic, or most often, both. Some causes include noises, lights, sharing of a bed, consumption of beverages containing caffeine (coffee, tea, and cola) or a heavy meal before bedtime, distended bladder, uncomfortable bedding, personal problems, and worries.

SLEEP DEPRIVATION SYMPTOMS

Physiologic Symptoms
- Hand tremors
- Decreased reflexes
- Slowed response time
- Reduction in word memory
- Decreased reasoning and judgment
- Cardiac dysrhythmias

Psychologic Symptoms
- Moodiness
- Disorientation
- Irritability
- Decreased motivation
- Fatigue
- Sleepiness
- Hyperactivity

From Potter PA, Perry AG, *Fundamentals of nursing: concepts, process, and practice,* ed 3, St Louis, 1993, Mosby.

■ SAMPLE NURSING CARE PLAN ■

SLEEP PATTERN DISTURBANCE

Mr. R, age 79, is hospitalized for chronic obstructive pulmonary disease. He has been unable to sleep since admission and is complaining about nursing care, nurses, laboratory technicians, and respiratory therapy staff.

NURSING DIAGNOSIS

Sleep pattern disturbance related to change in behavior, including irritability, as evidenced by complaints about the hospital staff, interrupted sleep, wandering in the unit hall during the night, and verbal comments about not feeling rested on arising

GOAL

- Patient will sleep 7 hours at night.

EXPECTED OUTCOMES

- Patient will state that he feels rested after sleeping.
- Patient will be relaxed and will talk freely to hospital staff.

NURSING INTERVENTIONS

- Ask about what helps to induce sleep at home.
- Teach patient relaxation techniques.
- Make changes, if possible, in immediate environment to help patient sleep.

EVALUATION

- Patient continues to be relaxed.
- Patient verbalizes feeling rested.
- Patient sleeps through the night, without interruption.

SKILL 26-1 PROMOTING SLEEP

Steps	Rationale
1. **Obtain equipment:** ▪ Notepaper or appropriate form ▪ Ink pen ▪ Clean gloves	Helps organize procedure.
2. **Refer to medical record, care plan, or Kardex for special interventions.**	Provides basis for care.
3. **Introduce self.**	Decreases anxiety level.
4. **Identify patient by identification band.**	Identifies correct patient for procedure.
5. **Explain procedure to patient.**	Seeks cooperation and decreases anxiety.
6. **Wash hands according to agency policy and guidelines from Centers for Disease Control and Prevention and Occupational Safety and Health Administration.**	Helps prevent cross-contamination.
7. **Prepare patient for intervention:**	
a. Close door to room or pull curtain.	Provides privacy.
8. **Raise bed to comfortable working level.**	Provides safety for nurse.
9. **Arrange for patient privacy.**	Shows respect for patient.
10. **Assess the following:**	
a. Question patient about sleep habits.	Elicits problems with sleep patterns.
b. Determine patient's general level of health.	Determines patient's health status, which affects sleep patterns.
c. Identify medications that patient may be taking.	Reduces chance that certain medications will affect sleep patterns.
d. Identify rituals or routines used at home to aid sleep.	Allows nurse to duplicate home routines to help patient sleep better in hospital.
e. Assess for signs and symptoms of sleep deprivation or disturbance.	Helps nurse use appropriate nursing interventions to help patient sleep.

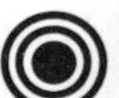

SKILL 26-1 PROMOTING SLEEP—cont'd

Steps	Rationale
11. Explain importance of adequate rest and sleep to patient, especially in relation to healing and restorative functions.	Encourages patient to work with nurse to ensure adequate rest and sleep.
12. Interview patient for revelation of sleep disturbances.	Identifies need for intervention.
13. Decide which patient routines that aid in producing sleep at home that may be used while in hospital.	Allows patient to maintain familiar routine, such as drinking glass of milk before bed, and thus may assist patient in attaining normal sleep pattern.
14. Ensure that patient's bedtime is quiet and unhurried and that basic physical and safety needs are met before sleep (see boxes on p. 498).	Helps patient become calm and helps ensure decreased interruptions once sleep is attempted.
15. Wash hands.	Helps prevent cross-contamination.
16. Document.	Documents procedure and patient's response.

SUMMARY

Basic physiologic and psychologic processes depend on the amount and type of sleep obtained for continued, healthy function. Sleep is essential in preserving emotional stability and the ability of a person to be socially adaptable. The responsibility of the nurse includes assessing the patient's need for sleep, diagnosing sleep problems, implementing nursing measures to promote rest and sleep, and evaluating the patient's response to the effectiveness of nursing interventions.

Key Concepts

- Rest is a period of inactivity and relaxation, whereas sleep is a state of reduced consciousness.
- The need for sleep varies from person to person and usually diminishes with age.
- Sleep usually follows a pattern of four stages referred to as nonrapid eye movement sleep and then rapid eye movement sleep.
- The nurse should promote adequate rest and sleep during hospitalization by helping the patient follow familiar routines, meeting the patient's basic needs, and controlling unnecessary environmental stimuli.
- Sleep deprivation occurs when the patient fails to get an adequate amount of sleep or when the patient is unable to complete the five stages of sleep. Sleep deprivation may have serious consequences for the patient's physical and mental health.
- The nurse should assess for and report manifestations of sleep disorders such as narcolepsy, sleep apnea, and somnambulism because they often require medical intervention.

Critical Thinking Questions

1. The nurse is working in the outpatient medical clinic for a small community hospital. A patient who has recently been diagnosed with cancer is in for testing and is accompanied by his wife. The patient has had a great deal of pain lately. The wife's appearance is listless. She has difficulty following the conversation with her husband. What areas of assessment would the nurse include for this family? What is the potential sleep problem that they may be experiencing?
2. Take a tour of a general nursing division. After doing so, answer the following question: Consider a patient newly admitted to this nursing

division. What factors on the division have you identified that may serve as barriers to this patient's ability to receive adequate sleep?

3. Ms. Sims is a 32-year-old account executive with a major corporation. She has been moving up the corporate ladder for a number of years. She travels frequently, sometimes to Europe. She freely admits that her sleep schedule is erratic because of frequent meetings in the late evening. She has trouble falling asleep at night because she is so "wound up." She knows that she needs to be getting more sleep. "I just don't feel that well in the morning. It takes me a while to get energized." Ms. Sims drinks at least 10 cups of coffee daily. What factors in Ms. Sim's history suggest that a sleep disturbance problem may exist? What additional factors would the nurse assess about her? Develop a plan of care based on these findings.

REFERENCES AND SUGGESTED READINGS

Berman TM et al: Sleep disorders: take them seriously, *Patient Care* 24:85, 1990.

Christensen BL, Kockrow EO: *Foundations of nursing,* ed 2, St Louis 1995, Mosby.

Colling J: Sleep disturbances in aging: a theoretical and empiric analysis, *Advances in Nursing Science* 6:36, 1983.

DeWit SC: *Keane's essentials of medical-surgical nursing,* ed 3, Philadelphia, 1992, Saunders.

Doenges ME: *Nurses' pocket guide: nursing diagnoses with interventions,* ed 4, Philadelphia, 1993, Davis.

Glyn CJ et al: The diurnal variation in perception of pain, *Proceedings of the Royal Society for Medicine* 69:369, 1976.

Harkness G, Dincher JR: *Medical-surgical nursing: total patient care,* ed 9, St Louis, 1996, Mosby.

Hodgson LA: Why do we need sleep? Relating theory to nursing practice, *Journal of Advanced Nursing* 16:1503-1510, 1991.

Jaffe MS: *Medical-surgical nursing care plans,* Norwalk, Conn, 1992, Appleton & Lange.

Mitler MM et al: Catastrophies, sleep and public policy: consensus report, *Sleep* 11:100, 1988.

Perry AG, Potter PA: *Clinical nursing skills and techniques,* ed 3, St Louis, 1994, Mosby.

Thompson JM et al: *Mosby's clinical nursing,* ed 3, St Louis, 1993, Mosby.

CHAPTER 27

Managing Pain

Learning Objectives

After studying this chapter, the student should be able to . . .

- Define the key terms.
- Identify sources of pain.
- Explain pain reception, perception, and reaction.
- Differentiate between acute and chronic pain.
- Identify and explain the types of pain.
- List information obtained during pain assessment.
- Identify signs and symptoms of pain.
- Give an example of a nursing diagnosis for the patient in pain.
- Explain comfort measures used to help relieve pain.
- Explain the use of distraction to alleviate pain.

Key Terms

Acute pain
Analgesic
Chronic pain
Distraction
Endorphins
Epidural analgesia
Intractable pain
Pain
Patient-controlled analgesia (PCA)
Perception
Phantom pain
Radiating pain
Reception
Referred pain
Superficial pain
Threshold
Tolerance
Transcutaneous electrical nerve stimulation (TENS)
Visceral pain

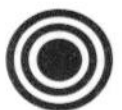

Skill

27-1 Relieving pain with equipment and comfort measures

PAIN EXPERIENCE

According to the International Association for the Study of Pain, **pain** is "an unpleasant, subjective sensory and emotional experience associated with actual or potential tissue damage, or described in terms of such damage."

Sources of Pain

The sources of pain include mechanical, chemical, thermal, and electrical. *Mechanical pain* refers to pain caused by an alteration in body fluids (for example, edema) duct distention, a tumor, or pressure. Chemical pain is derived from a perforated visceral organ, such as a ruptured appendix. Thermal pain occurs because of a burn from heat or extreme cold. Electrical pain results from burns severe enough to destroy layers of tissue.

Reception, Perception, and Reaction

Pain receptors are free nerve endings that warn a person of potentially harmful changes in the environment, such as excessive pressure or temperature. These free nerve endings, constituting most of the pain receptors, occur chiefly in the epidermis and in the epithelial covering of certain mucous membranes. This process is called ***reception.*** **Threshold** is the amount of noxious stimuli needed for a person to sense pain. It is an individual, subjective response. **Tolerance** is the ability of the person to endure pain. The amount of pain tolerated differs from person to person, depending on attitudes, values, and previous experience with pain.

Perception is the point at which a person feels pain. Painful stimuli are first received by special receptors in the endings of sensory nerve fibers. These fibers are found in the skin and subcutaneous tissue, bone, muscle, and internal organs. Stimuli then pass through the spinal cord to the brainstem. From

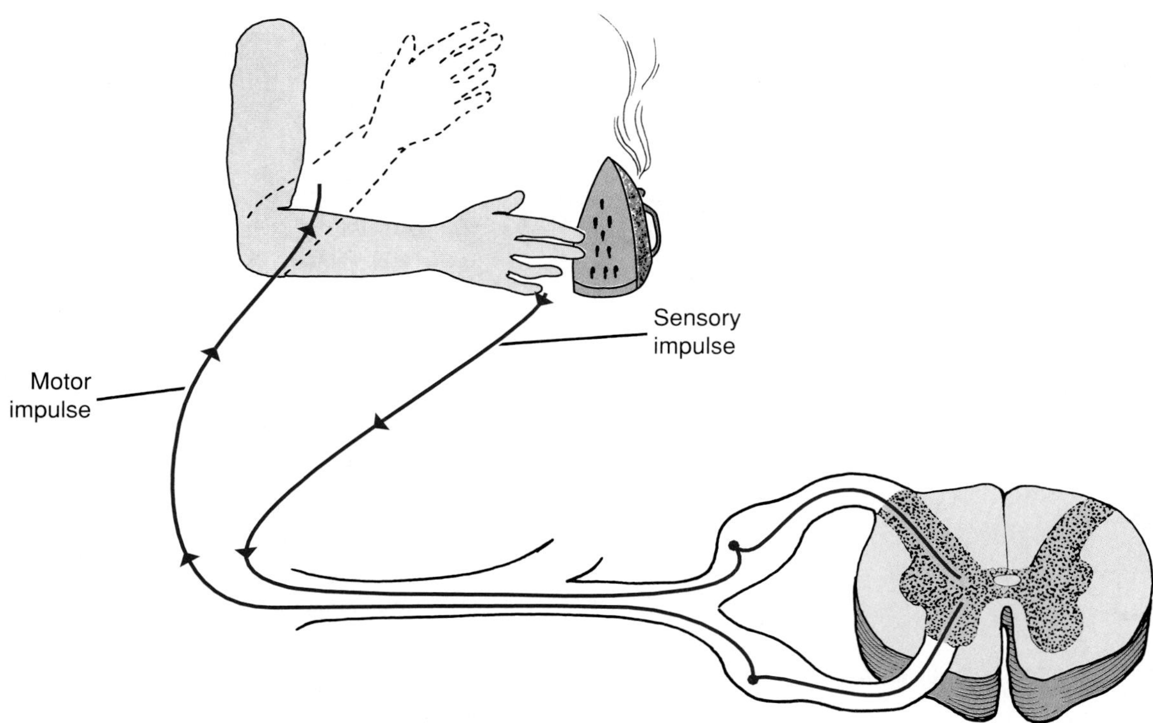

Fig. 27-1 Protective reflex to pain stimulus. (From Potter PA, Perry AG: *Fundamentals of nursing: concepts, process, and practice,* ed 3, St Louis, 1993, Mosby.)

the brainstem the stimuli move to the cortex, where the impulses are perceived. At this point, the impulses travel through motor nerve fibers to the muscle near the site of pain stimulation, resulting in a protective withdrawal response (Fig. 27-1). A theory that receives much attention and most realistically explains pain transmission is the gate-control theory.

Gate-control theory

According to the gate-control theory, the transmission of pain impulses is controlled at the spinal cord (the "gate"). Pain impulses flow freely when the gate is open and become blocked when the gate is closed. Interventions for pain relief, such as massage or heat to the involved area, may close the gate to painful stimuli because of the stimulation of naturally occurring chemicals called ***endorphins.*** The spinal cord has receptor sites for these chemicals that inhibit pain impulses. The gate-control theory is shown in Fig. 27-2.

Reaction

Reaction is a response to a stimulus such as pain. Physiologic response to pain includes increased pulse and heart rates, a rise in blood pressure, perspiration, pupil dilation, flushing, and tense muscles. A patient's behavior changes: The patient may cry, become anxious, verbalize the pain, and grimace.

Acute and Chronic Pain

Acute pain is characterized by rapid onset and varying intensity. It may last no more than 6 months. The pain serves as a warning of tissue damage or a high risk thereof. The pain resolves when healing occurs. Patients in acute pain often respond by crying or moaning or by rubbing or guarding the painful area.

Chronic pain lasts longer than 6 months. The pain may be continuous or intermittent (coming and going at intervals). It may be as intense as acute pain. Chronic pain is not an indicator of tissue damage. The patient may exhibit few, if any, symptoms. Patients do not adapt to chronic pain, but seem to suffer from physical and mental exhaustion. Symptoms of chronic pain include fatigue, insomnia, anorexia, weight loss, depression, helplessness, and anger. The patient in chronic pain often has periods of remission (partial or complete disappearance of symptoms) and exacerbation (increase in severity of symptoms) (Table 27-1).

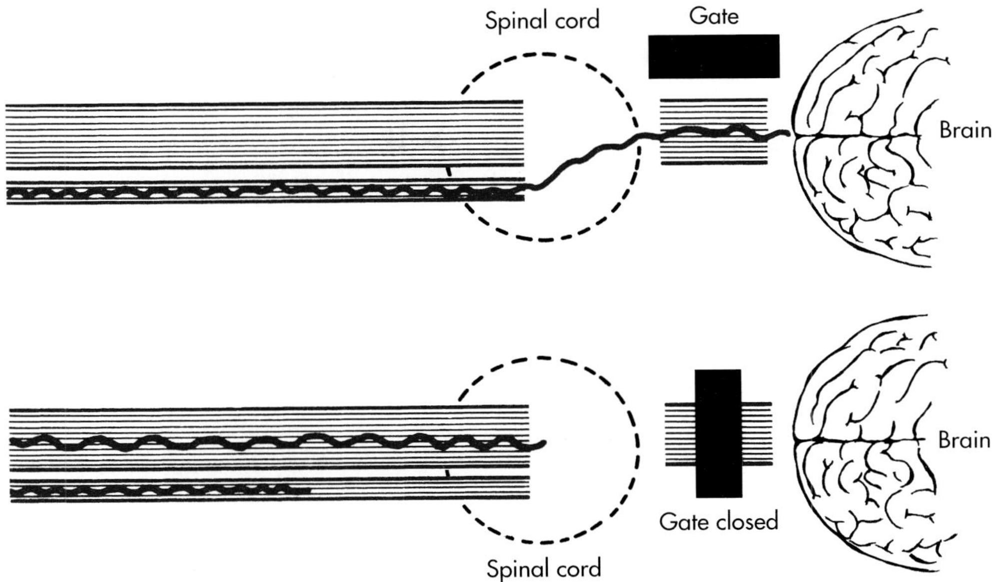

Fig. 27-2 Gate-control theory of pain. (From Christensen BL, Kockrow EO: *Foundations of nursing,* ed 2, St Louis, 1995, Mosby.)

Table 27-1 COMPARISON OF ACUTE AND CHRONIC PAIN

Characteristic	Acute Pain	Chronic Pain
Onset	Usually sudden	May be sudden or develop insidiously
Duration	Transient (up to 3 months)	Prolonged (months to years)
Pain localization	Pain vs. nonpain areas generally well identified	Pain vs. nonpain areas less well identified; intensity becomes more difficult to evaluate (change in sensations)
Clinical signs	Signs of sympathetic overactivity (such as increased blood pressure)	Usually no change in vital signs (adaptation)
Purpose	Warning that something is wrong	Meaningless; no purpose
Pattern	Self-limiting or readily corrected	Continuous or intermittent; intensity may vary or remain constant
Prognosis	Likelihood of eventual complete relief	Complete relief usually not possible

From Phipps WJ et al: *Medical-surgical nursing: concepts and clinical practice,* ed 5, St Louis, 1995, Mosby.

Other Types of Pain

Superficial pain, or cutaneous pain, originates in surface areas such as the skin or subcutaneous tissues. It is usually sharp and confined to a specific area. For example, superficial pain occurs when a person is given an injection. **Visceral pain,** or deep pain, originates in deeper body structures such as the bones and muscles. It is usually dull and diffuse or spread to a wider area of the body. It occurs with an ulcer or with angina.

Referred pain is pain felt in an area other than the site of the injury or damage (Fig. 27-3). This type of pain occurs often with injury to visceral organs and is felt on the skin surfaces. For example, a patient suffering from a myocardial infarction (heart attack) may complain of pain in the arm or jaw but not in the area of the heart.

Radiating pain is perceived at a source and extends to surrounding or nearby tissues. For example, the pain of a inflammed appendix is felt throughout the abdomen.

Phantom pain is pain felt in a body part that is no longer present, such as an amputated limb.

Pain may also be classified by intensity or severity. **Intractable pain** cannot be relieved. This pain may result from severe arthritis or uncontrolled cancer.

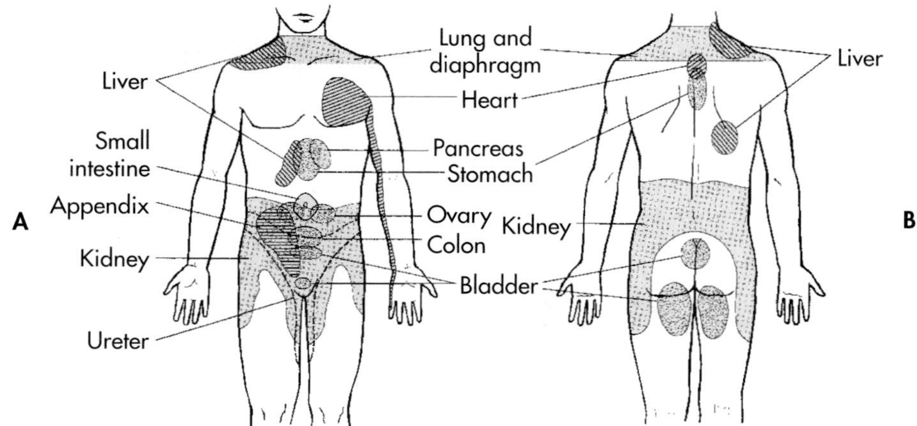

Fig. 27-3 Referred pain. **A,** Front. **B,** Back. (From Phipps WJ et al: *Medical-surgical nursing: concepts and clinical practice,* ed 5, St Louis, 1995, Mosby.)

NURSING PROCESS AND PAIN

Assessment

Pain assessment is one of the most common and most difficult activities a nurse performs. The nurse assesses the pain experience from the patient's perspective. Patients must understand that informed reporting of pain is valuable and necessary if the health care team is to manage pain effectively.

Specific terms are used when assessing pain. *Onset* indicates when the problem begins. *Duration* is how long the pain lasts from the onset until it is resolved. Pain is also classified by *location* (Table 27-2). *Severity* indicates whether the pain is mild, moderate, or intense in nature. Sample pain scales can assist the nurse in assessing pain (Fig. 27-4). The patient may also describe the pain as sharp, stabbing, dull, achy, or throbbing.

The patient experiencing pain may exhibit symptoms such as a rise in the pulse rate and blood pressure, perspiration, and dilated pupils. Pain can make a patient fatigued or exhausted, which should be avoided when possible. The patient may be fearful and restless when in pain.

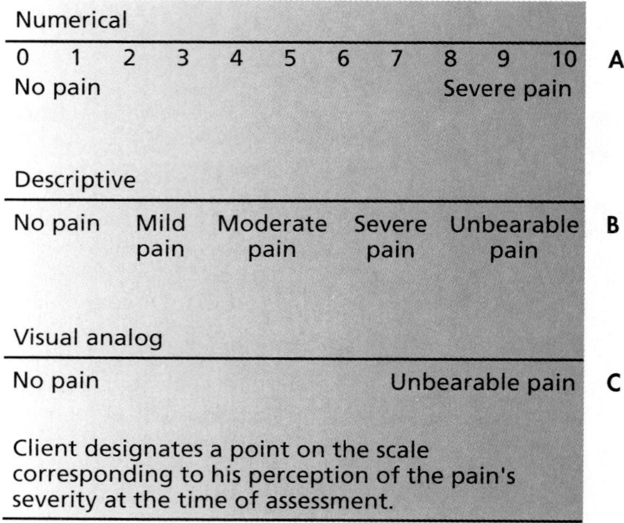

Fig. 27-4 Sample pain scales. **A,** Numerical. **B,** Verbal descriptive. **C,** Visual analog. (From Potter PA, Perry AG: *Fundamentals of nursing: concepts, process, and practice,* ed 3, St Louis, 1993, Mosby.)

Nursing Diagnosis

An accurate diagnosis of the patient with pain will enable the nurse to effectively plan and implement relief measures. Possible nursing diagnoses for pain include the following:

Anxiety
Chronic pain
Fatigue
Fear
Pain
Self-care deficit: bathing/hygiene
Self-care deficit: dressing/grooming
Sleep pattern disturbance

Planning

When developing the plan of care, the nurse establishes priorities based on the patient's level of

Table 27-2 CLASSIFICATION OF PAIN BY LOCATION

Definition	Characteristics	Examples
Superficial or cutaneous Pain resulting from stimulation of skin	Pain is of short duration and is localized. It is usually sharp sensation.	Needlestick; small cut or laceration
Visceral or deep Pain resulting from stimulation of internal organs	Pain is diffuse and may radiate in several directions. Duration varies, but pain usually lasts longer than superficial pain. Pain may be sharp, dull, or unique to organ involved.	Crushing sensation (for example, angina pectoris); burning sensation (for example, gastric ulcer)
Referred Perception of pain in unaffected areas: common phenomenon in visceral pain because many organs have no pain receptors; entrance of sensory neurons from affected organ into same spinal cord segment as neurons from areas where pain is felt	Pain is felt in part of body separate from source of pain and may assume any characteristic.	Myocardial infarction, which may cause referred pain to jaw, left arm, and left shoulder; kidney stones, which may refer pain to groin
Radiating Sensation of pain extending from initial site of injury to another body part	Pain feels as though it travels down or along body part. It may be intermittent or constant.	Low-back pain from ruptured intravertebral disk accompanied by pain radiating down leg from sciatic nerve irritation

From Potter PA, Perry AG: *Fundamentals of nursing: concepts, process, and practice,* ed 3, St Louis, 1993, Mosby.

pain and its effect on the patient's condition (see care plan on p. 509). The nurse and patient set realistic expectations for pain relief and discuss the degree of pain relief to expect. Patient-centered goals and outcomes may include the following:

Goal #1: Patient obtains a sense of well-being and comfort within 3 days.

Outcome

Patient demonstrates nonverbally (that is, via facial expression, tone of voice) relief from pain within 48 hours.

Goal #2: Patient regains ability to perform self-care independently within 48 hours.

Outcome

Patient bathes and grooms self without hesitancy or restriction of movement within 48 hours.

PATIENT TEACHING 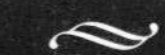

- Explain the characteristics of pain and pain behaviors.
- Elicit the patient's participation in pain-relief measures.
- Instruct the patient and family about the types of pain therapies.
- Explain techniques often used as adjuncts to medications.
- Explain the pain-management program that may be used in the patient's home.
- Discuss and have the patient practice pain-management techniques to use after discharge.

Implementation

It is important that a trusting nurse-patient relationship be established for the patient to believe that relief measures will work. The nurse can best help by seeing the patient as a total person, listening carefully to concerns, attending promptly to patient needs, and respecting any response to pain. In a successful nurse-patient relationship, the nurse understands that the patient knows more about personal pain and its relief.

The nurse may teach various measures to help

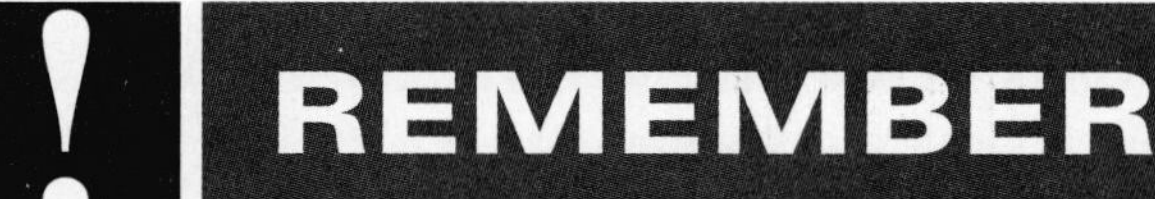

- Assess pain for type, onset, location, duration, severity, and intensity, since intervention may depend on this information. For example, the nurse must know if the patient needs pain relief for surgical pain or for a headache. The amount of medication administered for surgical pain is greater than that administered for a mild headache.
- Keep in mind that pain not only is physical, but also is related to psychogenic (psychologic), sociocultural, and environmental factors.

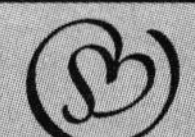

GERONTOLOGIC CONSIDERATIONS

- With some narcotic-analgesics, the older patient may have a reverse action (reaction opposite to that intended). The older adult thus may become confused and combative. The nurse must be aware of and assess for this problem.
- Many older patients can withstand a good deal of pain, but they still need to be assessed and offered pain-relief measures.

the patient and family prevent and deal with pain (see teaching box). These comfort measures can sometimes prevent the need for pain medication. Some measures are appropriate positioning and alignment in bed, washing and massaging the back, ambulation unless contraindicated, and prevention of constipation (Skill 27-1).

Distraction

Distraction may prevent the need for pain medication and other more invasive techniques. Distraction is used to help the patient think about things other than the pain. The nurse and patient may need to explore which methods work best. Techniques that may be used are music, special breathing, meditation, reading, and talking about family.

Relaxation

Some people find it difficult to relax, which in itself may cause pain. Relaxation techniques can help the patient avoid pain. The nurse should elicit information about the patient's usual relaxation techniques and use them to help control pain.

The patient may also be taught relaxation techniques. Meditation or yoga may be used, if there are no contraindications. The patient can continue to use this technique after discharge.

Medications

Sometimes, distraction and relaxation do not help the patient's pain, so analgesic drugs must be used. An **analgesic** provides pain relief. It alters the perception and interpretation of pain by depressing the central nervous system. There are three major classifications of analgesics:

1. Narcotic (for example, morphine, codeine, and meperidine [Demerol]). Before administration of a narcotic, the patient's respiratory rate and level of consciousness must be assessed for baseline data, since respiratory depression and decreased awareness are major adverse effects. Naloxene (Narcan) is a narcotic antagonist that reverses untoward effects.
2. Nonnarcotic (for example, nonsteroidal antiinflammatories [NSAIDs], aspirin, and acetaminophen [Tylenol]). The nurse must assess the patient for baseline data for gastrointestinal symptoms such as nausea and vomiting before administration.
3. Combination (for example, Tylenol No. 3, which combines Tylenol and Codeine). These drugs are a combination of narcotic and nonnarcotic analgesics.

Surgical pain usually requires the strongest intravenous (within the vein) dosages, but these are usually used for only a few days. Then the patient is placed on an oral medication. Management of pain consists of dependent and collaborative action, and a medical order is necessary.

Pain relief is also administered through **patient-controlled analgesia (PCA).** This is a portable, programmable intravenous (within the vein) infusion pump that allows the patient to self-administer intermittent doses of pain medication as they are needed. The patient pushes a button on a cord attached to the pump, and a small, preset dose of analgesia is administered.

Transcutaneous electric nerve stimulation (TENS) provides a portable unit with electrodes that attach to the skin near the area of pain. The mild electric current interrupts the pain-conduction impulse and relieves pain.

Epidural analgesia involves an anesthetic injected around major nerves at the base of the spinal cord outside the dura mater. It produces prolonged, intense segmental analgesia without the side effect of respiratory depression.

A child often needs less analgesia than an adult because of a more rapid metabolism. However, older children may need an adult dose, depending on their size and weight. Young children may have difficulty expressing pain other than by acting fussy or crying, so the nurse must carefully assess for objective data that may indicate pain.

Older patients may require less analgesia because of their slower metabolism and a slower functioning of the liver and kidneys, which metabolize medications. Pain is an additional risk for the older adult. Stress, fatigue, and impaired respiration compromise the cardiopulmonary system. The older person may have chronic pain that goes unreported. Therefore the nurse may be required to take extra steps to help this patient in pain (see gerontologic box).

Evaluation

Close communication between the nurse and patient is essential in achieving pain control. Continuous evaluation allows the nurse to determine whether new or revised therapies are required. The nurse refers to the goals and outcomes identified when planning care and performs evaluative measures to determine whether the goals have been reached. Examples of goals and evaluative measures may include the following:

Goal #1: Patient obtains a sense of well-being and comfort within 3 days.

Evaluative measure

Observe patient's facial expression and body movements, noting whether there is spontaneous freedom of movement.

Goal #2: Patient regains ability to perform self-care independently within 48 hours.

Evaluative measure

Observe patient perform grooming activities.

■ NURSING CARE PLAN ■

PAIN

Ms. W, age 41, underwent a cholecystectomy (removal of the gallbladder) because of gallstones. On the first postoperative day, the patient is having moderate to severe incisional pain.

NURSING DIAGNOSIS

Pain related to physical agents (midline surgical incision) as evidenced by facial mask of pain, pulse and blood pressure changes, verbal communication of pain, moaning, and guarding of incision

GOAL

- Patient will be free of surgical pain within 72 hours.

EXPECTED OUTCOME

- Patient will express feeling of comfort and relief of pain by discharge.

NURSING INTERVENTIONS

- Assess pain for correct intervention.
- Administer pain medication every 3 to 4 hours as necessary (prn).
- Evaluate patient for relief of pain within 30 to 45 minutes after administration of medication.

EVALUATION

- Patient indicates total pain relief within 35 minutes after administration of pain medication.

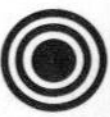

SKILL 27-1 RELIEVING PAIN WITH EQUIPMENT AND COMFORT MEASURES

Steps	Rationale
1. Obtain equipment: ▪ TENS unit ▪ PCA pump and supplies ▪ Lotion for back massage	Helps organize procedure.
2. Refer to medical record, care plan, or Kardex for special interventions.	Provides basis for care.
3. Introduce self.	Decreases anxiety level.
4. Identify patient by identification band.	Identifies correct patient for procedure.
5. Explain procedure to patient.	Seeks cooperation and decreases anxiety.
6. Wash hands and don clean gloves according to agency policy and guidelines from Centers for Disease Control and Prevention and Occupational Safety and Health Administration.	Helps prevent cross-contamination.
7. Prepare patient for intervention:	
a. Closed door to room or pull curtain.	Provides privacy.
b. Drape for procedure if necessary.	Prevents exposure of patient.
8. Raise bed to comfortable working level.	Provides safety for nurse.
9. Arrange for patient privacy.	Shows respect for patient.
10. Assess pain for onset, location, duration, and severity.	Determines which intervention is necessary.
TENS	
11. Position electrodes.	Prepares procedure.
12. Lower settings before turning unit on.	Avoids initial unpleasant sensations.
13. Increase settings on unit until patient experiences mild to moderate tingling, buzzing, or vibrating sensations.	Avoids unpleasant sensations, which may discourage patient from continuing therapy.
PCA	
14. Attach PCA tubing to syringe and fill tubing to Y-connector.	Avoids injecting air into bloodstream.
15. Attach intravenous solution tubing to PCA tubing and fill to Y-connector.	Connects intravenous solution to PCA infuser.
16. Insert syringe into PCA infuser.	Stabilizes syringe in pumping mechanism.
17. Program infuser with beginning dose (bolus), maintenance dose, and lockout interval. Program intravenous pump as to volume and rate.	Prevents medication overdose and fluid overload.
18. Close security cover and lock with key.	Safeguards medication from theft and infuser from setting changes.
19. Perform venipuncture if intravenous access does not already exist.	Allows flow of solution to keep vein open between medication administrations.
20. Connect PCA to intravenous device and begin intravenous infusion. Unclamp PCA tubing.	Prevents blood from clotting.
BACK MASSAGE	
21. Help patient to assume prone position.	Enhances relaxation. (Side-lying position may be used if patient is unable to lie prone.)
22. Drape patient to expose only area to be massaged.	Provides patient privacy.
23. Apply liberal amount lotion to hands and rub palms to warm lotion. (Reapply lotion as needed throughout procedure.)	Prevents musle tensing from coldness.
24. Begin massage in lower back, moving up spine and over shoulders in circular motion, using long, firm strokes for 3 to 5 min (Fig. 27-5).	Promotes relaxation and stimulates circulation. Avoids loss of skin integrity.
25. Massage buttocks using palm of hand, rubbing with circular motion.	Promotes relaxation and stimulates circulation.
26. Remove excess lotion from skin.	Helps prevent skin breakdown.
27. Reposition and realign patient.	Promotes comfort and relaxation.
28. Remove gloves and wash hands.	Helps prevent cross-contamination.
29. Dispose of waste materials.	Helps prevent spread of microorganisms.
30. Document.	Documents procedure and patient's response.

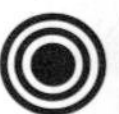

SKILL 27-1 RELIEVING PAIN WITH EQUIPMENT AND COMFORT MEASURES—cont'd

Steps	Rationale

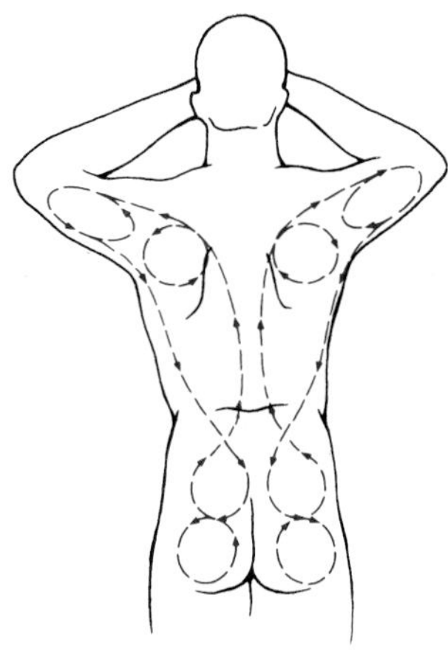

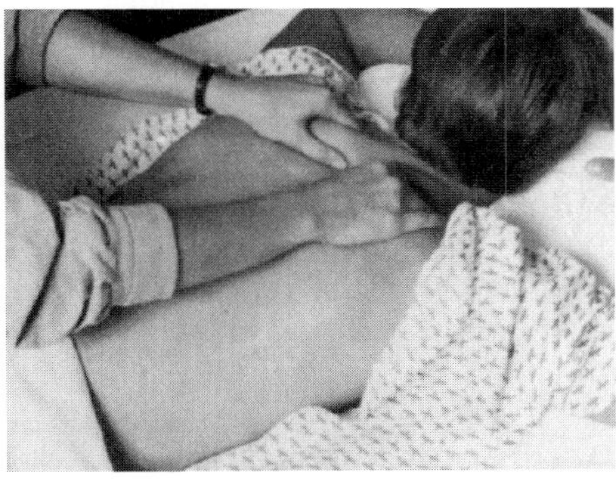

Fig. 27-5 Motions used for back massage. (From Perry AG, Potter PA: *Clinical nursing skills and techniques,* ed 3, St Louis, 1994, Mosby.)

SUMMARY

Pain is experienced in an individual manner by patients. It is a problem faced by patients in all health care settings. The nurse can provide comfort by understanding the nature of pain and the patient's perceptions, eliminating personal prejudices about pain, and working closely with the patient to find the best relief measures.

Key Concepts

- The patient has a right to experience pain as real and to expect relief of the pain.
- Pain threshold is an individual, subjective response.
- Acute pain indicates possible tissue damage.
- Endorphins inhibit pain impulses.
- The nurse must avoid doubting the degree of the patient's pain and must not refuse to administer pain-relief measures.
- Patients do not adapt to chronic pain but suffer from physical and mental exhaustion.
- Characteristics of pain include its onset, location, duration, and severity.
- The nurse must carefully assess the child who is unable to express pain.
- Older patients often do not report pain and must be carefully assessed for it.
- The use of comfort measures can sometimes prevent the need for pain medication.
- The nurse must assess the patient's pain relief within 30 to 45 minutes after the administration of pain medication.

Critical Thinking Questions

1. Mrs. Wells is a 40-year-old woman whose presenting symptoms included acute low back pain that radiated down the left leg, with numbness in the left lateral calf. On a scale of 1 to 10, the patient verbalized pain to be at a severity of 9. The patient was unable to walk without limping. Pain was aggravated when the patient sat. Lying in a supine position minimized the discomfort. A nursing diagnosis of *decreased physical mobility related to pain* was made with the goal of "patient will gain freedom of back movement without pain within 4 weeks." Identify expected outcomes to be incorporated into the plan of care. What evaluative measures would you use to judge the patient's success in meeting outcomes?
2. Mr. Jasper and Mr. Stern are patients experiencing back pain. Mr. Jasper's pain resulted after a fall from a ladder 48 hours ago. Mr. Stern's pain has been bothering him for more than 8 months with no known cause. As the nurse caring for both patients, how might you anticipate differences in assessment and treatment?
3. Ms. Rogers is receiving morphine by way of a PCA device after abdominal surgery for a hysterectomy. During your assessment, you note Ms. Rogers to be more drowsy and her respirations have decreased from 16 a minute to 10. What actions should you take?
4. Mr. Lake is a 45-year-old man who experienced a traumatic injury to his left arm after an industrial accident 24 hours ago. His arm is in a very bulky dressing, and pain is aggravated when he lies on his left side. He has an intravenous line witha continuous infusion of fluids in his right arm. What nonpharmacologic pain relief measures might be helpful for Mr. Lake?

REFERENCES AND SUGGESTED READINGS

International Association for the Study of Pain, Subcommittee on Taxonomy: Pain terms: a list with definitions and notes on usage, *Pain* 6:249, 1979.

Lewis SM, Collier IC, Heitkemper MM: *Medical-surgical nursing: assessment and management of clinical problems,* ed 4, St Louis, 1996, Mosby.

Perry AG, Potter PA: *Clinical nursing skills and techniques,* ed 3, St Louis, 1994, Mosby.

Potter PA, Perry AG: *Fundamentals of nursing: concepts, process, and practice,* ed 3, St Louis, 1993, Mosby.

Thibodeau GA, Patton KT: *The human body in health and disease,* St Louis, 1992, Mosby.

CHAPTER 28

Mobility

Learning Objectives

After studying this chapter, the student should be able to . . .

- Define the key terms.
- Identify the implications for using each assistive device.
- Maintain skeletal traction.
- Maintain skin traction.
- Describe guidelines for performing cast care.
- Outline steps of the four major crutch gaits.
- Apply a brace for a patient.
- Apply an abduction pillow.
- Assist with mobility by assisting a patient using a cane, walker, and wheelchair.
- Turn a patient on a Stryker wedge frame, CircOlectric bed, and a Roto Rest Bed.
- Provide nursing care to a patient on a Clinitron bed.
- Identify teaching needs of a patient with altered mobility.
- Perform patient teaching for use of three assistive mobility devices.
- Maintain a Continuous Passive Motion machine for a patient.

Key Terms

Abduction
Abduction pillow
Activities of daily living (ADLs)
Adduction
Bivalved cast
Brace
Cast
Continuous passive motion (CPM) machine
Crutches
External rotation
Hemiplegia
Internal rotation
Mobility
Neutral alignment
Paraplegia
Sling
Traction
Weight bearing

Skills

28-1 Assisting with applying skeletal traction
28-2 Assisting with applying skin traction
28-3 Caring for a cast
28-4 Applying braces
28-5 Applying an abduction pillow
28-6 Teaching crutch gaits
28-7 Teaching use of a cane
28-8 Teaching use of a walker
28-9 Using a wheelchair
28-10 Using a therapeutic frame or bed

Mobility is a person's ability to move about freely. It affects a patient's physiologic and psychologic well-being. The ability to move freely has a strong influence on family relationships, occupation, and leisure time activities. Also, children interrelate with their world through activity. When disease or accidents alter mobility, a patient experiences helplessness, dependence, and some degree of social isolation. The nurse assumes responsibility to assist patients in achieving an optimal (most desirable or satisfactory) level of mobility. This type of assistance may require that the patient learn to use assistive devices. Encouragement and patience from the nurse and family should help the patient overcome some of the frustration of learning new ambulation techniques. For the immobilized patient, the nurse supports patient involvement in meeting daily living needs as well as strives to minimize the risk of immobility complications.

There are useful devices that enable the nurse to assist the patient in achieving optimal mobility. The nurse should consider the patient's prior level of independence in accomplishing **activities of daily living (ADLs),** which are activities usually performed in the course of a normal day in the patient's life, such as eating, dressing, brushing the teeth, or grooming. Then the nurse helps the patient be realistic yet strive for as normal activity as possible according to the disability. The nurse should be certain to incorporate the patient's personal goals into the plan of care.

The patient's medical history of cardiovascular and respiratory problems as well as existing conditions, such as arthritis and diabetes, should be noted to determine appropriate nursing diagnoses and the resulting plan of care. Also, knowing the patient's preexisting medical conditions should assist the nurse in determining the potential for complications of immobility. The nurse should understand the patient's limitations and potential energy level before ambulation is undertaken. The nurse should consider the patient's dietary preferences. Wound healing and fractures require a well-balanced diet for children and adults. The patient may need assistance in choosing nutritious foods. The dietician should be consulted when necessary.

NURSING PROCESS

Assessment

Assessment of the patient's mobility focuses on range of motion, muscle strength, activity tolerance, gait, and posture. Observing the patient perform ADLs helps the nurse estimate the patient's fatigability, muscle strength, and range of motion. Observing posture and gait helps the nurse determine the type of assistance that the patient may require when changing positions or transferring from a bed to a chair. This information enables the nurse to assess the patient's overall level of mobility and coordination.

When assessing a young child who is immobilized, the nurse determines whether the child is able to meet developmental tasks and is progressing normally. Developmental assessment is also important with the older adult. The nurse assesses this adult patient's ability to meet needs independently and to adapt to developmental changes.

Nursing Diagnosis

Assessment reveals data that indicate whether a problem or potential problem exists. These data identify characteristics that reveal a diagnosis. Possible nursing diagnoses for immobility include the following:

Activity intolerance
Altered body image
Altered patterns of urinary elimination
Fear
Impaired physical mobility
Impaired skin integrity
Ineffective individual coping
Risk for impaired gas exchange
Risk for impaired skin integrity
Risk for infection
Self-care deficit: bathing/hygiene, dressing/grooming, feeding, toileting
Sleep pattern disturbance
Social isolation
Total incontinence

PATIENT TEACHING 

- Explain the importance of maintaining independence in movement and ADLs.
- Describe the risk factors for and signs and symptoms of pressure ulcers (see Chapter 21).
- Encourage the patient's participation in care and decision making.
- Demonstrate range-of-motion exercises.

Planning

The nurse should develop goals and expected outcomes to increase the patient's mobility as soon as possible. This is important in preventing problems from becoming chronic. The immediacy of any problem is determined by the effect that it has on the patient's mental and physical health. For example, breathing problems generally take precedence over recreational activity deficits when the nurse is setting priorities.

It is important for the patient and family to participate in planning care. The nurse can teach health-promotion practices and care (see teaching box). The plan of care may include one or more of the following goals:

Goal #1: Patient regains appropriate or optimal body alignment.

Outcome

Patient maintains range of motion in all joints.

Goal #2: Patient performs self-care activities.

Outcomes

Patient uses assistive devices for self-feeding and self-toileting.

Patient participates in self-care by washing upper body.

Implementation

Nursing interventions for the immobilized patient focus on preventing the hazards of immobility. The nurse should observe the patient for failure to cope with restricted mobility. If interventions from the care plan are not improving the patient's coping

GERONTOLOGIC CONSIDERATIONS

- Older patients may require arm-strengthening exercises to facilitate the use of an assistive device.
- Older patients may be hesitant to use a healed extremity after the cast is removed.
- An external catheter may be ordered if the patient is incontinent and soiling of the cast is likely.

patterns, outside assistance may be required. Recommendations of consultants should be incorporated into the plan of care. The nurse should remember that the older adult is extremely susceptible to all hazards of immobility (see gerontologic box).

Evaluation

The plan of care is evaluated by comparing the patient's response to the expected outcomes for each goal. The nurse revises the care plan if the outcomes are not achieved. Examples of goals and corresponding evaluative measures include the following:

Goal #1: Patient regains proper or optimal body alignment.

Evaluative measure

Inspect musculoskeletal system for joint contractures.

Goal #2: Patient performs self-care activities.

Evaluative measures

Observe patient for increased activity tolerance.

Observe patient for increased ability and willingness to feed, bathe, dress, and complete ADLs.

TRACTION

Traction is the application of equipment that permits pull on the long axis of the fractured or congenitally impaired bone, overcoming muscle tension and shortening and resulting in alignment, union, or both. Traction is generally applied by using slings, ropes, pulleys, and weights. The counterpull is usually provided by the patient's own body weight. The purpose of traction is to immobilize fractures in adults and children, reduce muscle spasm and pain, and prevent deformity. There are three basic types of traction: manual traction, skin traction, and skeletal traction. The nurse should be aware of the basic principles governing each type of traction to ensure establishment of appropriate nursing diagnoses and a plan of care.

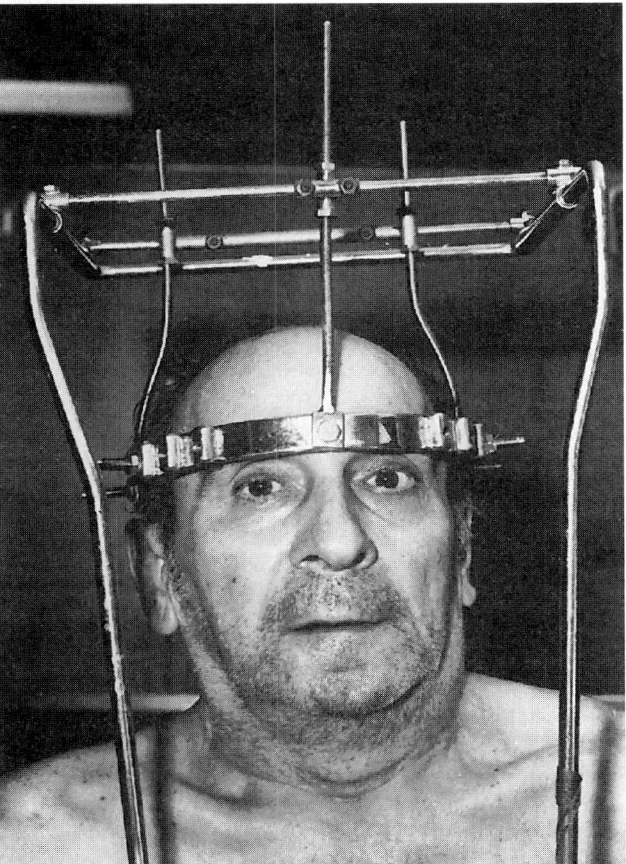

Fig. 28-1 Halo traction. (From Christensen BL, Kockrow EO: *Foundations of nursing,* ed 2, St Louis, 1995, Mosby.)

Manual Traction

Manual traction is generally performed immediately after the injury to reduce a fracture or replace a dislocated bone into its proper position in the joint. Manual traction is the direct pull on a body part by the physician's hands while manipulating the bone ends into correct alignment. Often a cast is applied to maintain alignment until healing occurs.

Skeletal Traction

Skeletal traction applies direct pull on bones of up to 30 pounds of force through the use of tongs, pins, or wires connected to a system of ropes, pulleys, and weights. Skeletal traction permits the use of a greater amount of weight for pull than can be applied to skin tissues using skin traction. This type of traction is used primarily for immobilization of the spine after cervical fractures or for femoral fractures. Cervical traction is maintained by inserting Crutchfield or Gardner-Wells traction tongs into the skull. The halo apparatus (Fig 28-1) also promotes

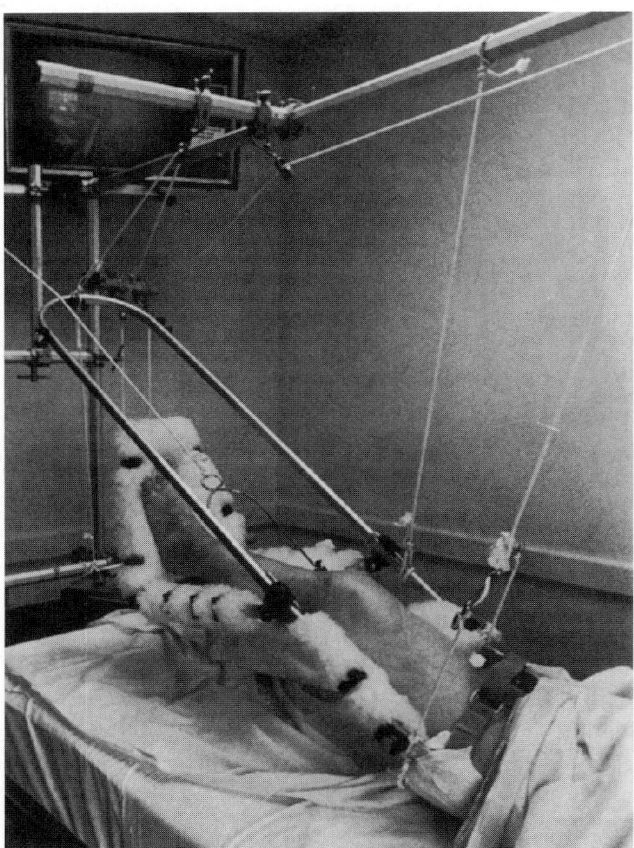

Fig. 28-2 Pearson attachment and Thomas splint.

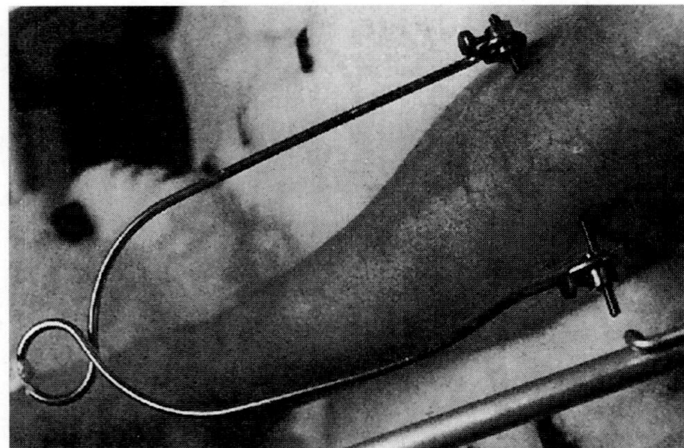

Fig. 28-3 Site of pin or tong insertion. (From Christensen BL, Kockrow EO: *Foundations of nursing,* ed 2, St Louis, 1995, Mosby.)

PREVENTING COMPLICATIONS FROM IMMOBILITY

Assessing the Five Ps

- *Pulselessness:* Lack of peripheral perfusion for some of heart contractions
- *Paralysis:* Loss of muscle function, loss of sensation, or both
- *Pallor:* Unnatural paleness or absence of skin color
- *Pain*
- *Paresthesia:* Numbness, tingling, or "pins-and-needles" sensation

spine immobilization while allowing the patient independent ambulation. Femoral fractures are stabilized with balanced suspension traction, which consists of a Thomas splint and a Pearson attachment (Fig. 28-2). The use of countertraction, or a force that counteracts the pull of traction, such as the force of body weight resulting from the pull of gravity, is sometimes used and allows more movement for the patient. A Steinmann pin or a Kirschner wire is inserted into the distal end of the femur or calf and then attached to traction (Fig. 28-3). The Thomas splint is a padded ring that encircles and supports the thigh. The Pearson attachment contains a canvas sling for supporting the calf. Balance suspension fosters mobility in bed without disrupting alignment.

Skeletal traction must be applied by a physician. The traction is constant and should not be discontinued without a specific medical order. Skeletal traction is most frequently used for adults because more weight must be applied to align and reduce fractures. This type of treatment may be necessary for up to 4 months.

The primary role of the nurse in caring for patients with skeletal traction is to maintain traction alignment and prevent complications from immobility, which include the five Ps (see box). Frequent assessment of the traction equipment and the patient's respiratory, neurovascular, skin, and elimination status is performed. Because skeletal traction provides an entry site for infection, meticulous pin care should be performed (Skill 28-1).

Skin Traction

Skin traction applies a pulling force on the skin and soft tissues that immobilizes a body part. The pulling force is maintained through a system of ropes, pulleys, and weights attached by nonadhesive tapes, belts, halters, or boots. The primary types of skin traction are cervical, humerus, pelvic, Buck's, Russell, and Bryant's. In *cervical traction,* a sling or halter is applied under the patient's chin to relieve muscle spasms. *Humerus* traction is used for a fracture of the humerus or for shoulder dislocations. *Pelvic* traction is established by use of a Velcro pelvic binder (Fig. 28-4). It may be used continuously or intermittently to relieve muscle spasms in the patient experiencing low back pain. *Buck's* extension traction (Fig. 28-5) is ordered for a patient with a

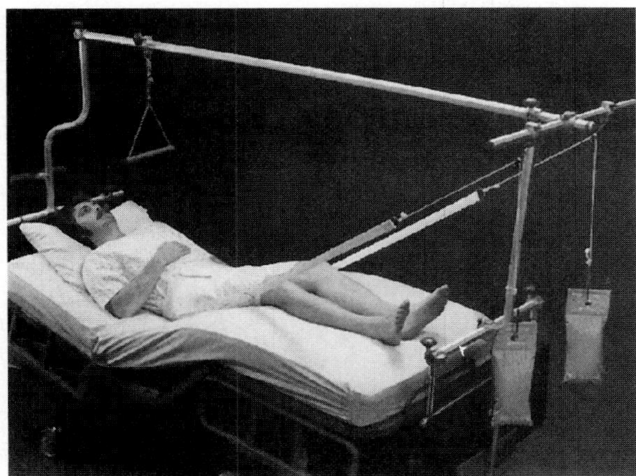

Fig. 28-4 Pelvic belt.

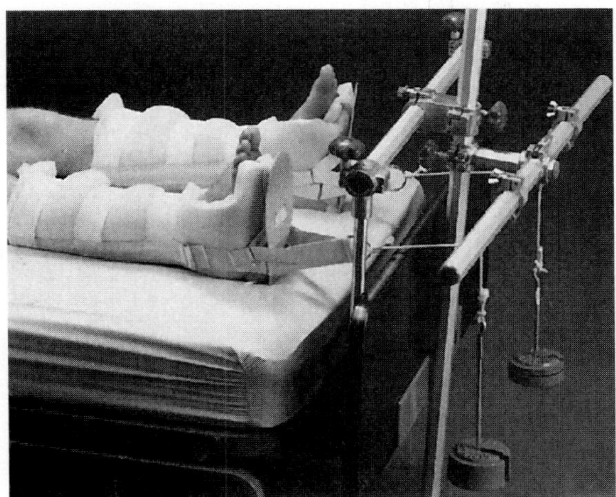

Fig. 28-5 Buck's extension traction. (From Christensen BL, Kockrow EO: *Foundations of nursing,* ed 2, St Louis, 1995, Mosby.)

fractured hip until surgery may be performed. Often, this patient needs a medical workup to be prepared to physically withstand the surgery. *Russell's* traction (Fig. 28-6) resembles Buck's traction but is used for a patient with a fractured femur who is awaiting surgery. The use of *Bryant's* traction (Fig. 28-7) is limited to young children who have congenital hip dislocations or fractured femurs.

The state nurse practice act and agency policy determine whether the application of skin traction is performed by the physician or nurse. Generally, the nurse assists with and maintains the application of traction (Skill 28-2).

CASTS

Casts are used to immobilize an extremity or joint for patients with sprains, fractures, or structural defects (that is, hip deformities). A **cast** is a stiff, solid dressing formed with plaster of paris or another material around a limb or another body part to immobilize it during healing. Serial casting is a method used in rehabilitation health care to progressively decrease the amount of contracture in an extremity. The cast is applied for 24 hours and then bivalved. The **bivalved cast** is cut in half to monitor and detect pressure under the cast. It is applied according to a strict schedule developed by the occupational or physical therapist. A split or bivalved cast may also be applied to allow for edema (swelling) associated with a fracture. When the swelling subsides, a permanent cast is then applied. The cast is usually molded to the contour of the body part being covered. (Figs. 28-8 and 28-9). Casting materials include plaster of paris or the newer synthetics, such as fi-

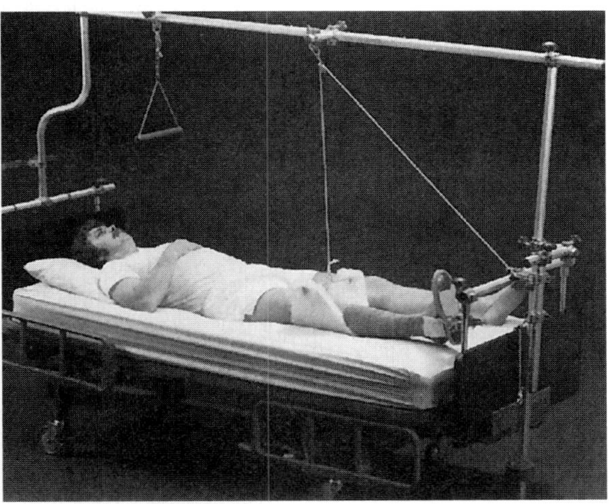

Fig. 28-6 Russell's traction. (From Christensen BL, Kockrow EO: *Foundations of nursing,* ed 2, St Louis, 1995, Mosby.)

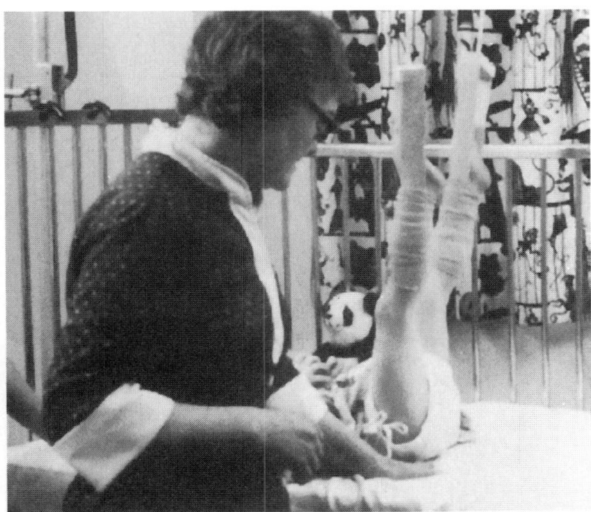

Fig. 28-7 Bryant traction.

berglass and polyester. Plaster of paris casts have a smooth exterior and are less expensive but have prolonged drying times, are difficult to keep clean, and become soft and heavy when wet. In contrast, synthetic casts have quicker drying times, are lighter weight, and do not soften with activities such as showering and swimming. However, these casts are more expensive, have a rough exterior, and may cause skin softening with frequent exposure to moisture.

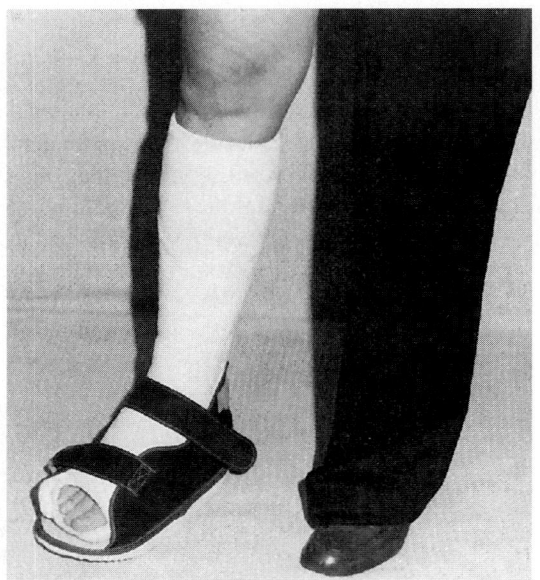

Fig. 28-8 Short leg walking cast with cast shoe. (From Christensen BL, Kockrow EO: *Foundations of nursing,* ed 2, St Louis, 1995, Mosby.)

There are basically three types of casts: cylinder cast, body cast, and hip spica cast. A cylinder cast is a rigid mold generally applied to one of the extremities. The location of the fracture dictates the length of the cast. The joints above and below the fracture site are usually immobilized by the cast. Toes or fingers are exposed to enable assessment of circulation, motion, and sensation (CMS). The body cast is similar to a cylinder cast, but it encircles the trunk of the body, extending from the nipple line to the hips. This cast may be bivalved and worn as a clam shell. A hip spica cast extends from the lower trunk to one or both of the lower extremities. A bar frequently extends from one leg to the other, resulting in increased cast strength. This bar should not be used as a position turning bar.

One of the nurse's roles in providing cast care is to prevent neuromuscular damage in the casted part of the body (Skill 28-3). CMS to the distal portion of the extremity should be continually assessed. As described earlier, the five Ps should be assessed. The nurse also performs cast care to maintain immobilization of the injured extremity or joint, prevent skin breakdown and infection, and decrease pain associ-

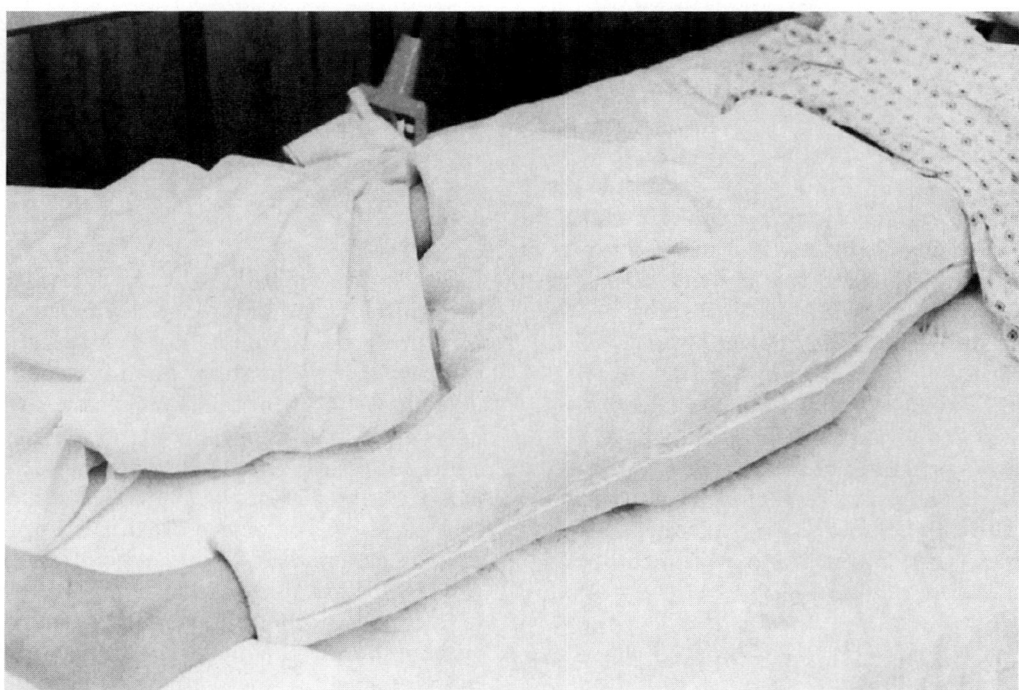

Fig. 28-9 Hip spica cast, applied to provide immobilization of left femoral fracture, was bivalved when patient developed severe pain and swelling of left leg several hours after cast was applied. Ace bandages wrapped over cast to provide support have been removed for picture.

ated with the injury. The amount of bleeding should also be evaluated. When blood is observed on the cast, the nurse should circle the drainage and include the date, time, and initials of the nurse. The nurse should know whether there is a drain in the skin but should still mark the cast. The nurse should notify a physician if bleeding continues or if neurovascular impairment occurs. A cast may need to be removed if the situation warrants. Cast cutters should be available at all times on the nursing unit. Occasionally a small, square piece of the cast is removed. This is called a *cast window.* A window enables direct visualization of the skin without complete removal of the cast. A window also permits treatments such as application of medication to be completed. The piece of the cast (the window) is replaced as soon as possible to prevent tissue bulging through the window and skin breakdown.

After removal of the cast, the skin appears scaly and pale. Patches of dead skin may be noted. Because of the prolonged period of immobility, the muscle usually appears smaller and is weak. Assistive devices such as a cane, braces, or crutches may be necessary until the patient regains strength assisted by physical and occupational therapy.

ASSISTIVE DEVICES

Braces **Braces** primarily consist of metal bars and leather straps and are designed for a particular body part. Short and long leg braces may be used for patients with **hemiplegia** (paralysis of one side of the body) or **paraplegia** (paralysis of the lower limbs), respectively. Short leg braces are attached to an orthopedic shoe and provide ankle support. A similar spring-loaded brace (Fig. 28-10) aids plantar flexion and dorsiflexion (see Chapter 20). Long leg braces extend to the top of the thigh and have ankle and knee joints. The Milwaukee brace assists in correcting the spinal deformity of scoliosis. This brace extends from the chin to the pelvis and is worn 23 hours a day for 1 to 2 years. The brace is removed for 1 hour a day for hygiene and skin care. The fiberglass brace may be used for adults and children to provide support to weakened muscles after back surgery. Patients with cervical disk injury or whiplash may be fitted with neck braces for support. Knee immobilizers are frequently used after hip surgery.

The nurse teaches the patient to apply and maintain the brace. The patient's family or parents should learn the application and care of the brace to oversee the child's care and application and to assist the patient when needed. The nurse's role in brace application is outlined in Skill 28-4.

Slings **Slings** are bandages or devices used to elevate and support an injured area. Many types and sizes of slings are available. A sling is used primarily to position an arm across the chest, leaving the hand higher than the elbow or to suspend the lower extremity when the patient is in bed. Appropriate application needs to be reviewed with the patient.

Abduction pillow An abduction pillow (Fig. 28-11) is used for patients who have undergone total hip replacement surgery. (**Abduction** is movement away from the body.) The **abduction pillow** keeps the repaired hip and leg in **neutral alignment** (that is, in appropriate anatomic position), thus preventing **external rotation** (turning away from the midline of the body) or **internal rotation** (turning

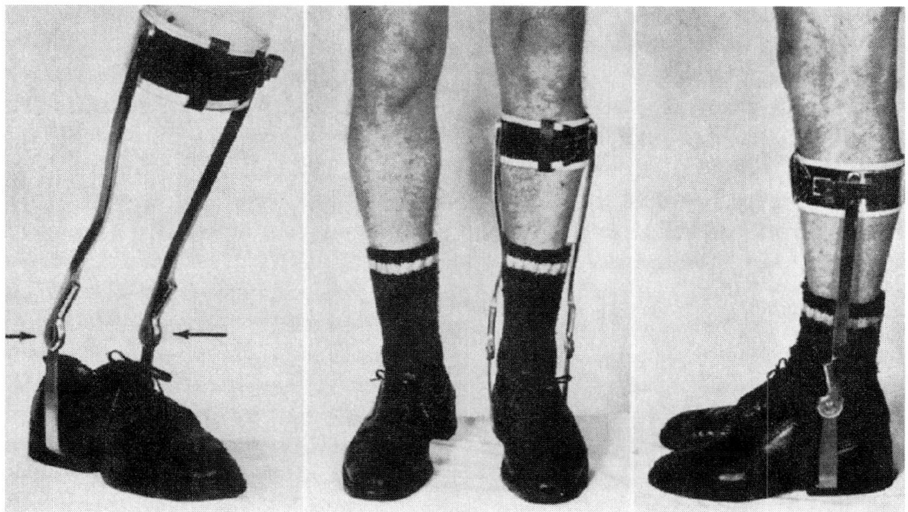

Fig. 28-10 Spring-loaded brace.

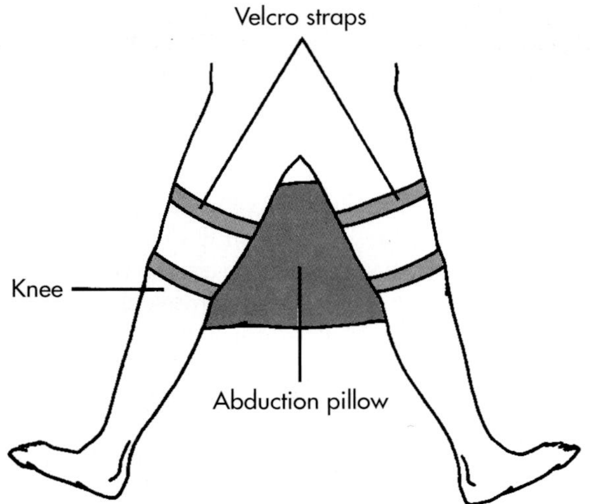

Fig. 28-11 Abduction pillow.

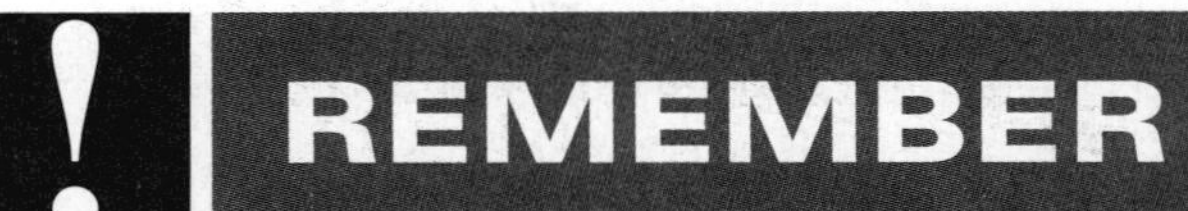

- Continually pay careful attention to skin breakdown.
- When a patient is in traction, change the linen from top to bottom rather than from side to side.
- If Ace bandages are used alone to secure traction, rewrap them every 8 hours.

toward the midline of the body) of the hip and **adduction** (movement toward the body) of the leg.

The pillow does not resemble the foam or feather pillow used under a patient's head. It is a fairly rigid, triangular box encased in a plastic covering that permits easy care and maintenance. The abduction pillow is sometimes referred to as an *abduction box* because of its sturdiness. A variation of this pillow is the abduction splint. Physician preference determines which device is ordered for the patient.

The role of the nurse in caring for patients with abduction pillows is to prevent external rotation and adduction of the affected hip and leg (Skill 28-5). The patient needs assistance and encouragement in maintaining this position. Another nursing responsibility is monitoring neurovascular damage in the affected extremity.

Knee immobilizers and trochanter rolls Other assistive devices may be used to maintain alignment. A *knee immobilizer* may be used with the abduction pillow. However, the pillow does not prevent adduction from occurring. A *trochanter roll* may also be used to prevent external rotation. The commercial trochanter roll is made out of sponge rubber and is often improvised with a rolled bath blanket or towel. The device is placed along the upper thigh and hip area to prevent external rotation of the hips when the patient is in the supine position.

Continuous passive motion machine

A **continuous passive motion (CPM) machine** is an electrical device that provides passive range of motion to an impaired extremity. It is frequently used after orthopedic joint replacement surgery. The machine can be programmed to exercise the involved joint to a specific degree of flexion and extension. The degree is increased as the patient's condition warrants. The CPM machine helps restore range of motion, prevents pooling of blood and resulting formation of blood clots, and accelerates wound healing by increasing synovial fluid circulation around the joint.

Walking belts

Walking belts or gait belts are used in many agencies to enhance the supportive feeling of the patient and to promote safe transfers. Handles on the side and back of the belt enable the caregiver to have a firm grip when assisting with a transfer or ambulation.

Crutches

Crutches are wooden or metal staffs that aid a person in walking and are used by patients who are allowed no or only partial weight bearing but who need support for coordination and balance. **Weight bearing** is the force exerted on the body. A physical therapist measures the patient for appropriate crutch fit and, with the physician, determines the appropriate crutch gait according to the patient's ability and limitation. The nurse reinforces the physical therapy assessment and instructions.

Correct crutch height is attained when the crutch pad is at least a three fingerwidths from the axilla (Fig. 28-12) and the handgrips allow 30-degree flexion. The basic crutch stance is the tripod position. The recommended placement of the crutches is 6 inches in front of and to the side of the toes to provide a broad base of support and balance. Patients are taught to support weight on their hands instead of resting the arm pads in the axillary area of the body. Weight bearing on the axillae may damage the brachial nerve, causing numbness, tingling, and possibly paralysis. Before assisting ambulation with crutches, the nurse determines the patient's fears and willingness to learn crutchwalking. By knowing the patient's goals, the nurse may ease fears as well as encourage goal accomplishment.

A variety of crutches are available. However, all crutches require significant physical strength and

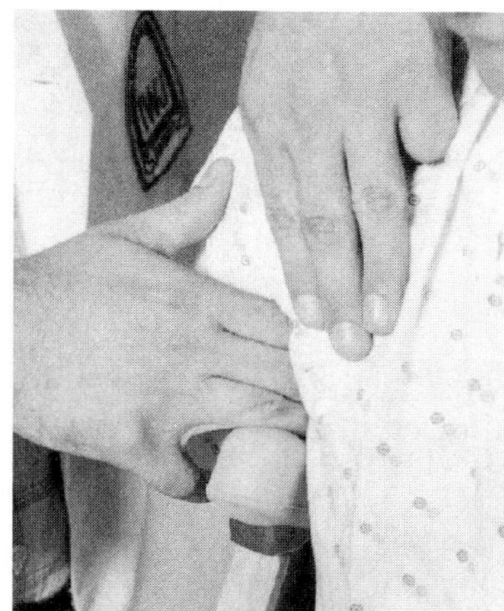

Fig. 28-12 Verifying correct distance between crutch pads and axilla. (From Perry AG, Potter PA: *Clinical nursing skills and techniques,* ed 3, St Louis, 1994, Mosby.)

stamina. Thus many of older adults are not candidates for crutches and use a walker. Axillary crutches are fitted under the axillae, require upper extremity strength and mobility, and are used on a temporary basis. Examples of crutches with no axillary support are Lofstrand or Canadian crutches. This type of crutch has a metal band around the forearm and a handgrip. This crutch is used on a long-term basis. A platform crutch supports the forearms and is usually used for patients with limited hand and wrist mobility and strength. The patient's weight is distributed over the entire forearm. Many arthritic patients successfully use this type of crutch.

There are several gaits for crutch walking (Skill 28-6). The two-point gait is used by patients who can bear partial weight on both legs. The three-point gait is used by patients whose weight bearing is limited to one leg. The four-point gait is used by patients who can bear partial weight on both legs and yet can move each leg separately. The swing-through gait is used by paraplegic patients who use supporting braces.

Canes

Patients who have one-sided weakness or who need help with balance may use canes for walking and additional support. The patient's mobility needs determine whether a single-tipped or a four-point (quad) cane is used (Fig. 28-13). Canes are made of wood or aluminum with rubber-tipped ends. Wood or aluminum canes are made in a variety of sizes, but wooden ones are not adjustable.

The grip may vary in shape and texture to make the grasp easier for the patient. The cane should be held on the patient's unaffected or strong side and placed 6 inches in front of the foot. The patient's elbow should be slightly flexed during weight bearing, and the hand grip should be at the height of the hip joint. The patient is encouraged to incorporate the cane as part of the normal gait. The nurse or physical therapist should recommend a quad cane for the patient who uses a cane on uneven surfaces or is unsteady on the feet. The nurse should assist the patient in ambulating (Skill 28-7) and, when necessary, in modifying ADLs.

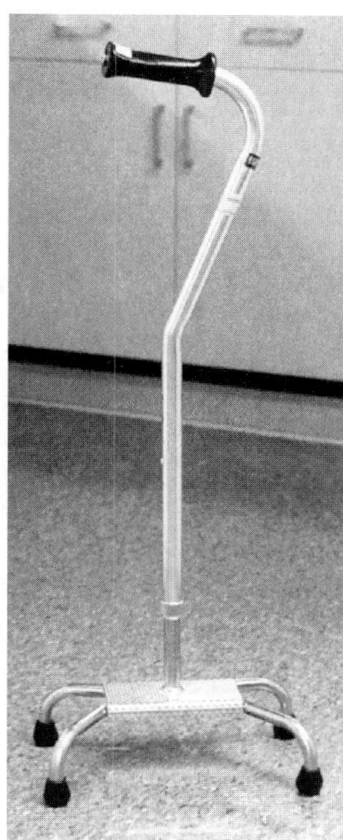

Fig. 28-13 Four-point (quad) cane. (From Christensen BL, Kockrow EO: *Foundations of nursing,* ed 2, St Louis, 1995, Mosby.)

Walkers

The walker is a four-legged assistive device designed for use by the patient who is unable to bear complete weight on one or both legs or who has balance problems. The patient's arms must be strong enough to bear partial weight. Two primary types of walkers are the stationary walker (Fig. 28-14) and the rolling walker. The stationary walker provides greater stability than the rolling walker. This type of walker is picked up or slid forward for movement and is available in a collapsible form for ease of travel and storage. The rolling walker has four wheels and may be dangerous for the patient with coordination and balance problems.

A physical therapist adjusts the walker for the patient's height. The recommended height is slightly

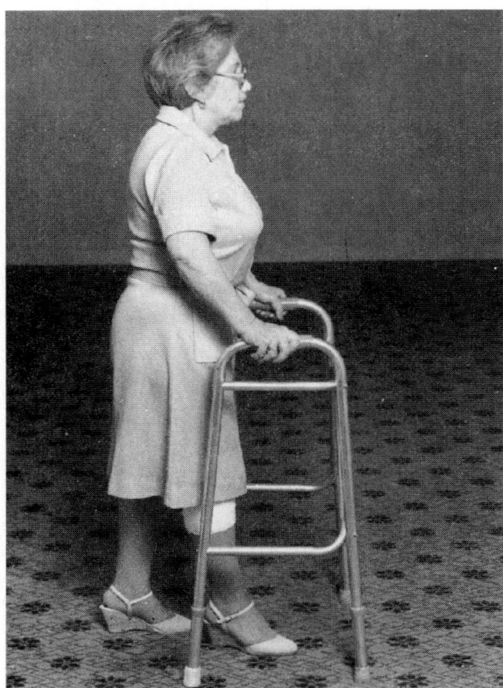

Fig. 28-14 Patient using stationary walker. (From Perry AG, Potter PA: *Clinical nursing skills and techniques,* ed 3, St Louis, 1994, Mosby.)

below the patient's waist level so that the elbows are flexed as a 30-degree angle while the patient grasps the handgrips. The physical therapist also determines whether a stationary or rolling walker is appropriate. The nurse should assist the patient to walk and adapt patient activities for use of the walker (Skill 28-8).

Wheelchairs

The wheelchair provides independent mobility for the patient who would otherwise be bedridden temporarily or permanently. The wheelchair may be operated by hand or battery. The chair comes in various sizes and is made of aluminum or wood. Most aluminum wheelchairs are collapsible for easier transportation and storage. Numerous accessories, such as gel-foam cushions, removable armrests, adjustable backs, intravenous pole holders, oxygen carriers, or lap trays, may be purchased. The needs of each patient should be assessed by the nurse before the most suitable type of wheelchair and accessories are determined.

The standard wheelchair has large wheels in the back and smaller wheels in the front, a design that facilitates indoor and outdoor use. The amputee wheelchair, a variation of the standard model, is specially designed for bilateral amputee victims who require altered centers of balance to prevent tipping backward.

The nurse should assist the patient in a dependent (lifting) or partially dependent (pivoting) transfer to the wheelchair (Skill 28-9). The patient's physical ability and personal goals determine whether the patient is able to accomplish independent wheelchair maneuverability.

THERAPEUTIC FRAMES OR BEDS

Stryker Wedge Frame

Stryker wedge frames (Fig. 28-15) are used for patients with unstable spinal cord injuries that require cervical traction and for patients who have had back surgery. The primary purpose of the Stryker frame is to provide immobilization while allowing the patient to be turned laterally from the prone to supine positions and vice versa. The frame consists of two metal frames, anterior and posterior, that are covered with stretched canvas and a thin mattress. Numerous accessories, such as armboards, footboards, bedpan holders, traction pulleys, and adjustable facepieces, have been designed to assist the totally immobilized patient. The Stryker frame is contraindicated for patients who weigh more than 200 pounds, are taller than 6 feet, and are wider than the width of the frame.

Nursing care is administered to the patient in either the prone or supine position (Skill 28-10). Position changes are achieved by briefly "sandwiching" the patient between the anterior and posterior frame. The newer version of the frame, known as the *Stryker wedge turning frame,* has a circular turning mechanism that allows the frame to be turned by one nurse. However, two nurses are recommended for the procedure to ensure safety and to decrease patient fear.

The nurse is responsible for safely and competently turning patients on the Stryker frame as well as preventing complications from immobility. If possible, the nurse should demonstrate use of the equipment. When the condition of the patient does not allow a demonstration, the purpose of operation of the frame should be explained to the patient. The nurse should also explain that the sensation of falling is not uncommon and that everything possible is done to prevent this from occurring.

CircOlectric Bed

The CircOlectric bed (Fig. 28-16) is used for the patient with stable spinal cord injury and burns. The bed, like the Stryker frame, enables the patient

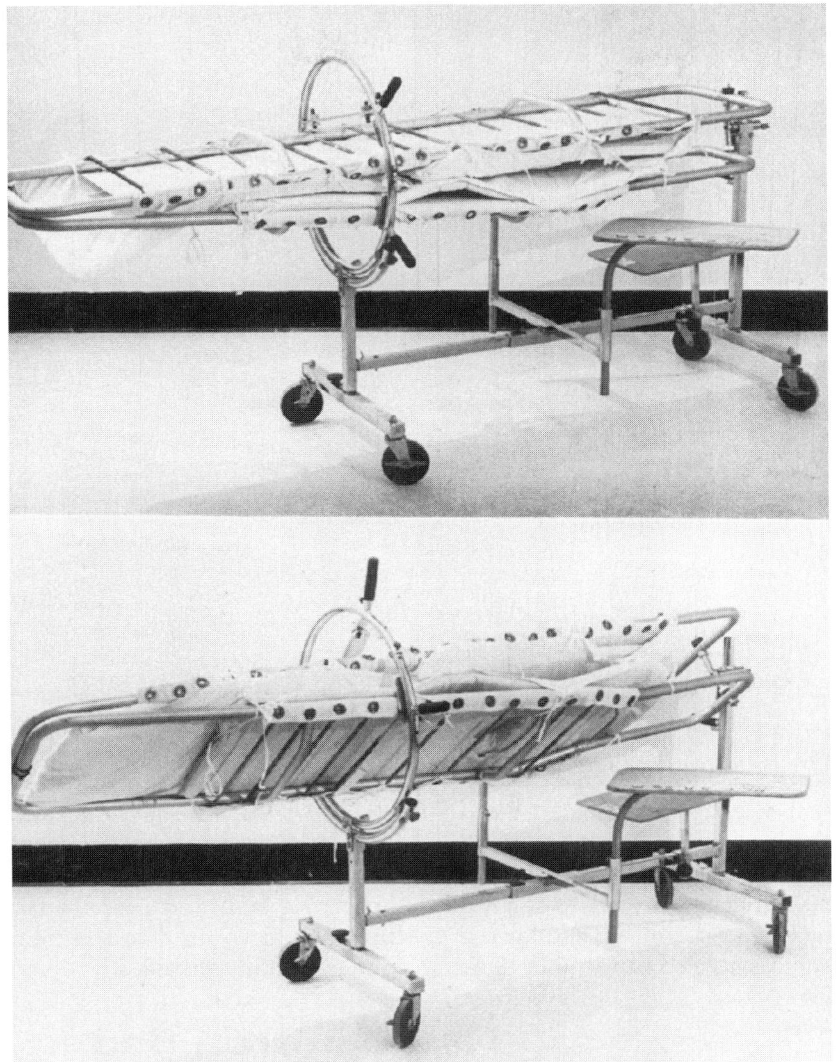

Fig. 28-15 Stryker frame.

to be turned while maintaining immobilization. The bed rotates vertically from the supine to prone positions. The bed improves vascular tone. In addition, the bed may be placed in Trendelenburg's position. The standing position is used to facilitate weight bearing as well as increase the patient's tolerance for being in an upright position when possible. Standard accessories include armrests, footboards, traction bars, headrests, and bedpan attachments. The patient is positioned between two mattresses much like the Stryker frame, but the bed is rotated with an electric control. Patients may find turning in this type bed quite frightening and need encouragement from the nurse.

When first assigned to care for a patient in a CircOlectric bed, the nurse may feel overwhelmed. However, once the nurse understands and has practiced the mechanics of the bed, administering nurs-

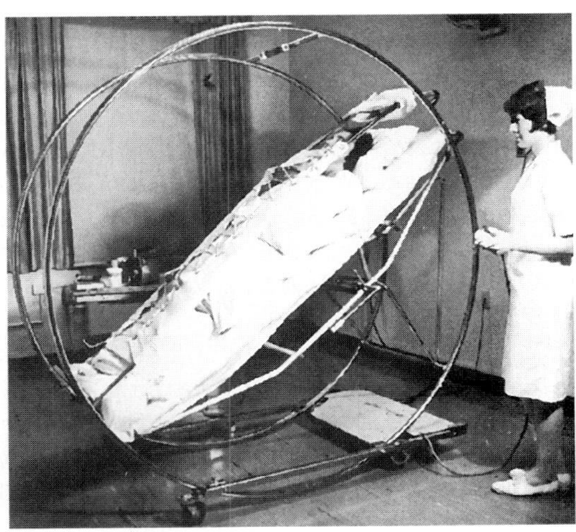

Fig. 28-16 CircOlectric bed.

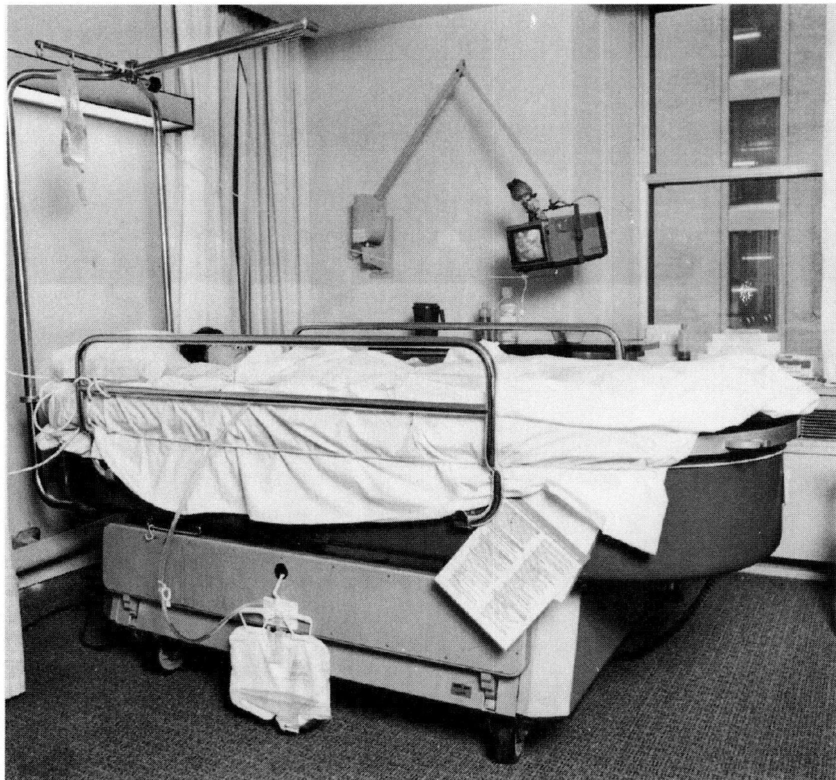

Fig. 28-17 Clinitron bed. (From Perry AG, Potter PA: *Clinical nursing skills and techniques,* ed 3, St Louis, 1994, Mosby.)

ing care to the immobilized patient is easier than anticipated. When turning a patient on this bed for the first few times, another experienced nurse should be present to assist.

Rotation Bed

The rotation bed (that is, Roto Rest) is used to promote postural drainage of the severely injured patient and to prevent complications of immobility. The bed rotates from side to side in a cradlelike motion, achieving a maximum elevation of 62 degrees and full side-to-side turning approximately every 4½ minutes. The bed holds the patient motionless. Thus it is useful for the patient with spinal cord injury, multiple trauma, severe burns, hypostatic pneumonia, and other pulmonary and neurologic conditions. Rotation beds are contraindicated for the patient who has severe fracture without the complications of immobility.

This type of bed is driven by a silent motor. Several hatches provide access for nursing care of the cervical, thoracic, perineal, and rectal areas. The bed is radiolucent, allowing x-rays studies to be done without moving the patient. The nurse should review the manufacturer's instructions, carefully inspect the bed, and prepare the bed for the patient precisely according to the instructions. Special linens may be required.

Clinitron Bed

The Clinitron bed (Fig. 28-17) is a rectangular bed filled with thousands of lime soda glass beads. By blowing air through the beads, a process known as *fluidization,* the beads are set in motion. The patient lies on a filter sheet that allows drainage of secretions and exudates and keeps the skin clean and dry. Patients who have large pressure ulcers or burns, as well as those who are immobilized or experiencing severe pain, receive the greatest benefit from this type of bed. For repositioning, coughing, and deep breathing, the bed must be turned off. Cardiopulmonary resuscitation must be performed with the bed defluidized. Although the bed maintains the patient's body at a constant temperature, the continuous flow of air promotes fluid and electrolyte loss with subsequent dehydration.

The patient placed on a Clinitron bed needs continual nursing care to prevent further impairment of skin integrity as well as other complications of immobility. Attention must also be given to the significant problem of fluid loss. In addition, because patients may be confined to a Clinitron bed for long periods, the nurse should address the patient's psychosocial needs.

NURSING INTERVENTIONS

Nursing interventions are specific according to the mobility or assistive device being used. For the patient in traction, interventions are directed toward maintaining appropriate traction and counter traction, preventing complications of immobility, and maintaining the use of the mechanical equipment. A cast should remain intact, dry, and rigid during its use. It may be cleansed with a damp cloth and a small amount of cleanser. The cast may not be immersed in water and must be covered with plastic when the patient showers. If cast edges become sharp, the nurse may petal (smooth) its edges to prevent skin breakdown. The nurse repairs the cast edges by applying petals made from tape. If CMS is impaired, the nurse or authorized person should remove the cast. Each agency has a policy regarding this problem, and it should be followed.

The patient requires individual instruction for ambulation assistive devices. Appropriate fit is essential for use of the devices. Ongoing periodic assessment ensures continued correct use of the assistive device. A patient placed on a therapeutic frame often requires extensive nursing care. The patient usually depends on the nurse for position changes and all daily activities. Emotional and psychologic support is a primary intervention. The patient is often frightened of the bed and terrified of the diagnosis and potential prognosis. Relaxation techniques should be taught to the patient.

Mobility and Assistive Devices for Children

A child in traction must be frequently assessed to ensure appropriate positioning related to frequent movement and smaller body weight. Explanations at the child's age of development help increase compliance. Visual stimuli and age-related play activities should be provided for the young patient. The child must be carefully fed if supine to prevent aspiration.

Assistive devices are available in pediatric sizes. The nurse should obtain the correct size to ensure appropriate body alignment. Walkers should be chosen based on strength of the child and the level of mobility. Milwaukee braces require periodic adjustment to accommodate growth. The nurse should discuss with the parents and child the importance of continuously wearing the brace. The parents and child should be taught the care of the brace, since it has several parts and is an expensive device.

The nurse should carefully assess a small child or infant who has a plaster cast. The heat produced by the drying cast may affect the child's body temperature. Parents should be instructed to prevent the child from placing small objects in the cast. The parents should prevent the child from putting anything in the cast such as a coat hangar to scratch itchy skin. Urine and stool must not irritate the skin around the cast in a child who has not been toilet trained.

Assistive Devices for Older Adults

Older adults should be assessed carefully for the risks of immobility. Preventive measures should be implemented early to maintain skin integrity during the period of mechanical immobilization. Constipation and circulatory and respiratory complications should also be carefully monitored. Older adults should be carefully assessed for their ability to use assistive devices. Walkers frequently replace the use of crutches.

Assistive Devices in Home Care

Home care follow-up is frequently required for immobile patients. Patients who have had hip surgery may need a toilet extender and a high, firm chair to prevent hip flexion greater than 90 degrees. Assistance with ADLs may also be necessary. Shower and toilet bars may need to be installed. The patient should be instructed to clean a brace daily and inspect all equipment daily for safety. Throw rugs or waxed floors may need to be altered to promote safety. Detailed written instructions regarding traction and assistive devices should be provided to the patient and caregiver. The name and number for a contact should be provided for problems that cannot be handled at home.

■ NURSING CARE PLAN ■

IMPAIRED PHYSICAL IMMOBILITY

Mr. W, age 52, fell and sustained a fracture of the right distal femur. The swelling was reduced and a cast applied to the limb.

NURSING DIAGNOSIS

Impaired physical mobility related to neuromuscular impairment as evidenced by impaired coordination and reluctance to move

GOALS

- Patient will develop no impaired neuromuscular dysfunction.
- Patient will move freely.

EXPECTED OUTCOMES

- Patient has no complications from casted right femur.
- Patient moves freely from bed to wheelchair.

NURSING INTERVENTIONS

- Assess presence and quality of distal peripheral pulse and compare with unimpaired limb.
- Assess capillary return, skin color, and warmth distal to fracture.
- Maintain affected extremity in elevated position.
- Encourage active range of joint motion distal to injury.

EVALUATION

- Neurovascular movement is intact.
- Pedal pulses are palpable.
- Toes of the right foot are warm to the touch.
- Patient is mobile and has sensation in right toes.

SKILL 28-1 ASSISTING WITH APPLYING SKELETAL TRACTION

Steps	Rationale
1. **Obtain equipment:** ▪ Sterile/clean gloves ▪ Hydrogen peroxide ▪ Sterile saline ▪ Povidine-iodine swabs or ointment ▪ Cotton-tip applicators ▪ Antiseptic ointment (if ordered)	Helps organize procedure.
2. **Refer to medical record, care plan or Kardex for special interventions.**	Provides basis for care.
3. **Introduce self.**	Decreases anxiety level.
4. **Identify patient by identification band.**	Identifies correct patient for procedure.
5. **Explain procedure to patient.**	Seeks cooperation and decreases anxiety.
6. **Wash hands and don clean gloves according to agency policy and guidelines from Centers for Disease Control and Prevention and Occupational Safety and Health Administration.**	Helps prevent cross-contamination.
7. **Prepare patient for intervention:**	
a. Close door to room or pull curtain.	Provides privacy.
b. Drape for procedure if necessary.	Prevents exposure of patient.
8. **Raise bed to comfortable working level.**	Provides safety for nurse.
9. **Arrange for patient privacy.**	Shows respect for patient.
10. **Assess patient for pain; immobility problems; CMS of the distal extremity; skin condition around pin or tong insertion sites; cleanliness and dryness of dressing; and traction alignment**	Determines baseline data. Determines which intervention is necessary.

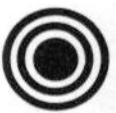

SKILL 28-1 ASSISTING WITH APPLYING SKELETAL TRACTION—cont'd

Steps	Rationale
11. **Inspect traction apparatus for direction of pull, unobstructed ropes, appropriate alignment of ropes and pulleys, free-moving weights, appropriate weight poundage, and secure knots.**	Ensures that patient is receiving appropriate traction therapy. (Weights that touch floor or bed reduce amount of traction.)
12. **Perform CMS assessment bilaterally every 2 hr for initial 24 hr, then every 2-4 hr.**	Alerts nurse to high-risk neurovascular problems.
13. **Maintain extremity in neutral alignment.**	Promotes appropriate traction force.
14. **Assess position of Pearson attachment.**	Assesses for pressure on heel and Achilles tendon.
15. **Assess skin around Thomas splint.**	Prevents skin breakdown.
16. **Inspect skin or tong sites for localized warmth, redness, odor, and drainage every 4-8 hr.**	Alerts nurse to risk for infection.
17. **Assess vital signs every 4-8 hr.**	Allows nurse to note elevated vital signs, which may indicate infection.
18. **Use sterile technique to clean pin sites every shift according to agency policy with hydrogen peroxide or saline.**	Prevents infection at pin sites and thus osteomyelitis.
19. **Cleanse around pin entrance and exit sites with sterile cotton applicators (avoid digging at pin sites):**	Helps prevent infection and skin breakdown.
a. Use a separate applicator at each site.	Cleanses once at site, which is sterile technique.
b. Leave sites uncovered unless significant drainage is present.	
20. **Apply antibacterial ointment if prescribed.**	Helps prevent infection.
21. **Instruct patient or perform range-of-motion exercises to unaffected muscles and joints every 4 hr.**	Maintains muscle strength and prevents atrophy (wasting or dimuation of size) or degeneration.
22. **Teach patient strengthening exercises for quadriceps, gluteus triceps, and biceps and have patient perform 10 repetitions every 2-4 hr.**	Maintains muscle strength, joint function, and peripheral circulation.
23. **Dispose of equipment or waste materials.**	Helps prevent spread of microorganisms.
24. **Remove gloves and wash hands.**	Helps prevent cross-contamination.
25. **Document.**	Documents procedure and patient's response.

SKILL 28-2 ASSISTING WITH APPLYING SKIN TRACTION

Steps	Rationale
1. **Obtain equipment:** ▪ Standard bed with traction frame ▪ Trapeze ▪ Weights ▪ Pulleys ▪ Ropes ▪ Padding ▪ Spreader bar ▪ Nonadhesive tape traction ▪ Ace bandages ▪ Solutions ▪ Boot, harness, or halter, depending on type of traction ▪ Tincture of benzoin ▪ Clean gloves	Helps organize procedure.

Continued.

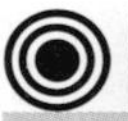

SKILL 28-2 ASSISTING WITH APPLYING SKIN TRACTION—cont'd

Steps	Rationale
2. **Refer to medical record, care plan, or Kardex for special interventions.**	Provides basis for care.
3. **Introduce self.**	Decreases anxiety level.
4. **Identify patient by identification band.**	Identifies correct patient for procedure.
5. **Explain procedure to patient.**	Seeks cooperation and decreases anxiety.
6. **Wash hands and don clean gloves according to agency policy and guidelines from Centers for Disease Control and Prevention and Occupational Safety and Health Administration.**	Helps prevent cross-contamination.
7. **Prepare patient for intervention:**	
a. Close door to room or pull curtain.	Provides privacy.
b. Drape for procedure if necessary.	Prevents exposure of patient.
8. **Raise bed to comfortable working level.**	Provides safety for nurse.
9. **Arrange for patient privacy.**	Shows respect for patient.
10. **Assess patient for CMS distal to extremity; redness of the skin and bony prominences; appropriate body alignment; and risk of immobility problems.**	Determines baseline data. Determines which interventions are necessary.
11. **Place bed in appropriate position: flat.**	Promotes appropriate line of traction pull.
12. **Cleanse skin with warm, soapy water, rinse; and dry skin thoroughly. (If ordered, apply tincture of benzoin to affected extremity).**	Protects skin from nonadhesive tapes.
13. **Assist physician in applying nonadhesive traction tapes lengthwise on opposite sides of affected extremity leaving 4-6 in beyond foot.**	Applies tapes, which are used to attach spreader bar and traction weights.
14. **Place padding over bony prominences.**	Protects skin from irritation.
15. **Have second nurse elevate extremity and wrap it in ace bandages.**	Secures nonadhesive tape to extremity.
16. **Assist with attachment of spreader bar to distal end of nonadhesive traction tapes.**	Prevents pressure on side of foot.
17. **Thread rope through pulleys and tie correct traction knots.**	Ensures that ropes have secure knots to prevent traction discontinuance.
18. **Tie rope to spreader bar, slowly and gently attach 4 to 7 lbs of weight to distal end of rope.**	Traction begins when weights are added. Gradual weight release prevents causing pain.
19. **Palpate area over adhesive tapes daily.**	Detects pressure areas that could irritate skin.
20. **While second nurse applies manual traction, remove Ace bandages every shift (if prescribed).**	Maintains traction during skin and neurovascular assessments.
21. **Perform checks of circulation, motion, and sensation bilaterally every 2-4 hr.**	Alerts nurse to potential neurovascular problems.
22. **Assess for pressure over peroneal nerve and Achilles tendon every shift.**	Prevents pressure on nerve and tendon, which can cause footdrop and other musculoskeletal problems.
23. **Maintain extremity in neutral alignment.**	Promotes correct traction force.
24. **Assess for complaints of burning sensation. Notify charge nurse and physician immediately.**	Alerts health care team to potential problems.
25. **Assess traction apparatus for direction of pull, unobstructed ropes, free-moving weights, and secure knots.**	Promotes effective traction therapy.
26. **Assess patient's comfort and position.**	Alerts nurse to potential problems.
27. **Place call light and personal articles within reach.**	Allows patient to call nurse in case turning from side to side disrupts traction and moves bone fragments.
28. **Dispose of or return equipment to be cleaned.**	Helps prevent spread of microorganisms.
29. **Remove gloves and wash hands.**	Helps prevent cross-contamination.
30. **Document.**	Documents procedure and patient's response.

SKILL 28-3 CARING FOR A CAST

Steps	Rationale
1. Obtain equipment: ▪ Pillows ▪ Ice packs ▪ Clean gloves	Helps organize procedure.
2. Refer to medical record, care plan or Kardex for special interventions.	Provides basis for care.
3. Introduce self.	Decreases anxiety level.
4. Identify patient by identification band.	Identifies correct patient for procedure.
5. Explain procedure to patient.	Seeks cooperation and decreases anxiety.
6. Wash hands and don clean gloves according to agency policy and guidelines from Centers for Disease Control and Prevention and Occupational Safety and Health Administration.	Helps prevent cross-contamination.
7. Prepare patient for intervention	
a. Close door to room or pull curtain.	Provides privacy.
b. Drape for procedure if necessary.	Prevents exposure of patient.
8. Raise bed to comfortable working level.	Provides safety for nurse.
9. Arrange for patient privacy.	Shows respect for patient.
10. Assess patient for newly applied cast, CMS distal to extremity; and pain in area where cast is applied.	Determines baseline data. Determines which interventions are necessary. Determines need for intervention. Determines need for pain medication.
11. Use palm of hands to move extremity or body with newly applied cast.	Prevents creating indentations in cast and causing subsequent pressure areas on skin.
12. Remove bed covers from cast until dried.	Exposes cast to air, causing it to dry faster.
13. Elevate casted extremity above level of heart on firm pillows, placing them from furrow of buttocks to foot.	Helps promote drying of cast and decreases edema, which could cause excess cast tightness.
14. Perform CMS assessment bilaterally every 1-2 hr for initial 24 hr and then perform checks every 2-4 hr.	Alerts nurse to high-risk neurovascular problems.
15. Assess for signs and symptoms of infection (that is, drainage or foul odor at distal end of cast and fever).	Promotes prompt intervention.
16. Assess for blood stains over fracture site and chart date, time, and size of area.	Determines amount of drainage.
17. Inspect for skin irritation around cast edges and petal edges if necessary.	Prevents rough edges of cast from irritating skin.
18. Assess for increased pain on passive movement of digits.	Indicates compartment syndrome.
19. Assist patient to change positions and perform range-of-motion exercises on unaffected extremities.	Prevents immobility complications and facilitates drying of all cast surfaces.
20. Dispose of equipment.	Helps prevent spread of microorganisms.
21. Remove gloves and wash hands.	Helps prevent cross-contamination.
22. Document.	Documents procedure and patient's response.

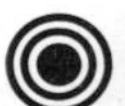

SKILL 28-4 APPLYING BRACES

Steps	Rationale
1. Obtain equipment: ▪ Brace ▪ Flat, nonskid shoes ▪ Thin undershirt if required for brace ▪ Robe ▪ Clean gloves	Helps organize procedure.
2. Refer to medical record, care plan, or Kardex for special interventions.	Provides basis for care.
3. Introduce self.	Decreases anxiety level.
4. Identify patient by identification band.	Identifies correct patient for procedure.
5. Explain procedure to patient.	Seeks cooperation and decreases anxiety.
6. Wash hands and don clean gloves according to agency policy and guidelines from Centers for Disease Control and Prevention and Occupational Safety and Health Administration.	Helps prevent cross-contamination.
7. Prepare patient for intervention:	
a. Close door to room or pull curtain.	Provides privacy.
b. Drape for procedure if necessary.	Prevents exposure of patient.
8. Raise bed to comfortable working level.	Provides safety for nurse.
9. Arrange for patient privacy.	Shows respect for patient.
10. Assess patient for skin breakdown, safety of brace device (that, rough edges, twisting, loose screws, worn straps, and cracked plastic), and need for other assistive devices.	Determines which interventions are necessary.
11. Have patient wear flat, nonskid shoes.	Promotes balance and helps prevent falls and footdrop.
12. With back brace, have patient wear thin, knitted undershirt.	Protects patient's skin and keeps brace clean.
13. Have patient lie on bed, fit brace over appropriate body part, and fasten in place.	Gives full back support before patient gets out of bed. Allows brace to be applied in supine position, which is easier.
14. Assist patient to sitting position on side of bed.	Allows nurse to adjust brace before patient stands.
15. Assist patient to ambulate with brace in place.	Determines patient's balance and difficulty in ambulating.
16. Assess CMS to distal extremity every 4-8 hr.	Prevents pressure of brace from altering distal circulation.
17. After removing brace, inspect skin areas.	Determines whether brace is causing skin irritation.
18. Place brace against wall or on a table.	Prevents distortion of brace.
19. Teach patient to apply and remove brace.	Fosters patient independence.
20. Dispose of or clean and store equipment.	Helps prevent spread of microorganisms.
21. Remove gloves and wash hands.	Helps prevent cross-contamination.
22. Document.	Documents procedure and patient's response.

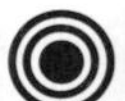

SKILL 28-5 APPLYING AN ABDUCTION PILLOW

Steps	Rationale
1. Obtain equipment: ▪ Abduction pillow ▪ One or two extra pillows ▪ Clean gloves	Helps organize procedure.
2. Refer to medical record, care plan, or Kardex for special interventions.	Provides basis for care.
3. Introduce self.	Decreases anxiety level.
4. Identify patient by identification band.	Identifies correct patient for procedure.
5. Explain procedure to patient.	Seeks cooperation and decreases anxiety.
6. Wash hands and don clean gloves according to agency policy and guidelines from Centers for Disease Control and Prevention and Occupational Safety and Health Administration.	Helps prevent cross-contamination.

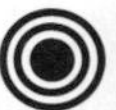

SKILL 28-5 APPLYING AN ABDUCTION PILLOW—cont'd

Steps	Rationale
7. Prepare patient for intervention:	
a. Close door to room or pull curtain.	Provides privacy.
b. Drape for procedure if necessary.	Prevents exposure of patient.
8. Raise bed to comfortable working level.	Provides safety for nurse.
9. Arrange for patient privacy.	Shows respect for patient.
10. Assess patient for appropriate body posture and neutral alignment of affected leg and hip; redness or open areas of lower extremities; and CMS bilaterally of lower extremities.	Determines which intervention is necessary.
11. Place patient in appropriate posture with hip and leg in neutral alignment.	Appropriate position necessary before pillow is placed.
12. Move patient's nonoperative leg away from legs.	Allows room for pillow to be placed between operative site.
13. With Velcro straps unfastened, place narrow (top) end of abduction pillow near top of patient's thigh but below perineum.	Appropriate positioning of abduction pillow.
14. Place Velcro straps around legs and fasten to top of abduction pillow (see Fig. 28-11).	Secures positioning of abduction pillow.
15. Assess patient's level of comfort.	Determines whether straps are too tight or pillow is pinching skin. Also could indicate whether hip is in wrong position.
16. Dispose of any waste materials.	Helps prevent spread of microorganisms.
17. Remove gloves and wash hands.	Helps prevent cross-contamination.
18. Document.	Documents procedure and patient's response.

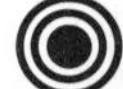

SKILL 28-6 TEACHING CRUTCH GAITS

Steps	Rationale
1. Obtain equipment: ▪ Crutches with rubber tips ▪ Hand grips ▪ Axillary pads ▪ Flat nonskid shoes ▪ Straight chair. ▪ Clean gloves	Helps organize procedure.
2. Refer to medical record, care plan, or Kardex for special interventions.	Provides basis for care.
3. Introduce self.	Decreases anxiety level.
4. Identify patient by identification band.	Identifies correct patient for procedure.
5. Explain procedure to patient.	Seeks cooperation and decreases anxiety.
6. Wash hands and don clean gloves according to agency policy and guidelines from Centers for Disease Control and Prevention and Occupational Safety and Health Administration.	Helps prevent cross-contamination.
7. Prepare patient for intervention:	
a. Close door to room or pull curtain.	Provides privacy.
b. Drape for procedure if necessary.	Prevents exposure of patient.
8. Raise bed to comfortable working level.	Provides safety for nurse.
9. Arrange for patient privacy.	Shows respect for patient.
10. Assess patient for arm and upper-body strength and visual acuity.	Determines ability of patient and directs interventions.
11. Assess crutches for secure attachment of rubber tips, cracks in wooden crutches, and abnormal bends in aluminum crutches.	Ensures safety of equipment.
12. Have patient wear flat, nonskid shoes.	Fosters balance and prevents helps prevent injury.

Continued.

SKILL 28-6 TEACHING CRUTCH GAITS—cont'd

Steps	Rationale
STANDING	
13. Instruct patient to place crutches in hand on side, slide forward in straight chair, grasp chair arm with opposite hand, and push up to standing position.	Facilitates safe movement from sitting to standing position.
14. Have patient assume tripod stance (Fig. 28-18). (Crutches are placed 6 in in front and 6 in to side of each foot).	Promotes balance and support.
TWO-POINT GAIT	
15. Have patient move right foot and left crutch forward.	Movements simulate normal walking pattern.
16. Instruct patient to move left foot and right crutch forward (Fig. 28-19).	Movements simulate normal walking pattern.
THREE-POINT GAIT	
17. Instruct patient to stand on stronger leg while moving crutches as well as weaker leg forward 6 in.	Allows stronger leg to support movement.
18. Have patient shift weight to crutches and move stronger leg forward (Fig. 28-20).	Ensures weight is shifted to arms and handgrips—not to axillae.
SWING-THROUGH GAIT	
19. Teach patient to move crutches forward and then swing legs forward in front of crutches.	Provides support while moving forward.
20. Ask patient to rapidly move crutches forward,	Maintains patient's balance.
FOUR-POINT GAIT	
21. Instruct patient to move right crutch forward, advance left foot, move left crutch forward, and advance right foot (Fig. 28-21).	Prevents full weight-bearing to each leg during ambulation.

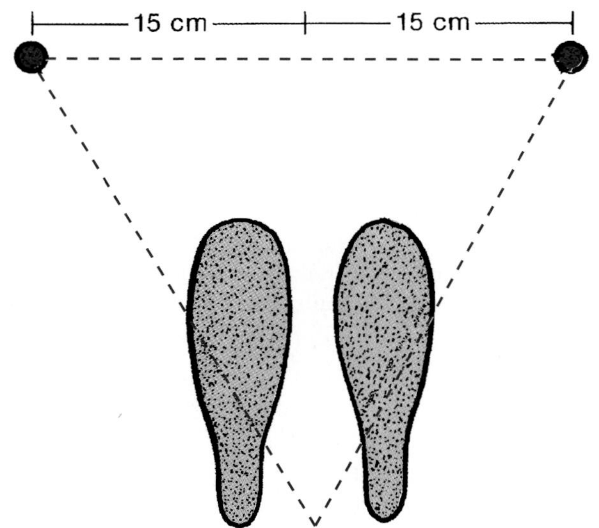

Fig. 28-18 Tripod stance. (From Perry AG, Potter PA: *Clinical nursing skills and techniques,* ed 3, St Louis, 1994, Mosby.)

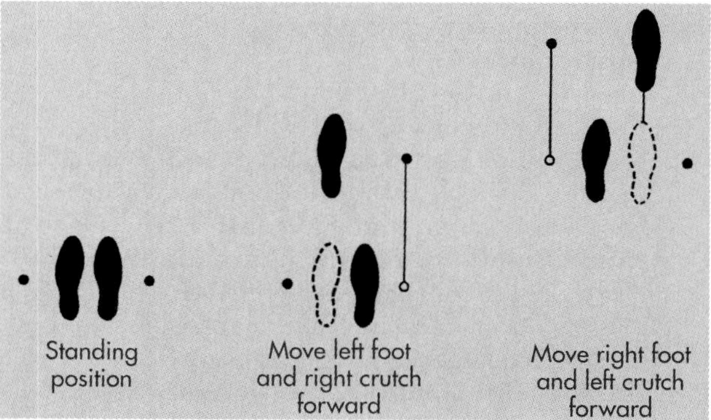

Fig. 28-19 Two-point gait. (From Christensen BL, Kockrow EO: *Foundations of nursing,* ed 2, St Louis, 1995, Mosby.)

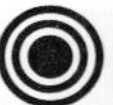

SKILL 28-6 TEACHING CRUTCH GAITS—cont'd

Steps	Rationale
CLIMBING STAIRS	
22. Have patient place body weight on hand rests of crutches (Fig. 28-22, *A*) and then move strong leg up to next step (Fig. 28-22, *B*).	Crutches can support weaker side while ascending stair.
23. With patient's weight placed on strong leg, have patient move crutches and weaker leg to next step (Fig. 28-22, *C*).	Stronger leg and crutches provide support to move weaker side.
24. Repeat sequence until stairs are ascended.	
DESCENDING STAIRS	
25. Have patient move crutches to lower step (Fig. 28-23, *A*) and then place weaker leg first, followed by stronger leg (Fig. 28-23, *B*).	Stronger leg is used to provide support when descending stairs.
26. Repeat sequence until stairs are descended.	
SITTING	
27. Have patient turn around and back toward chair until legs touch chair seat (Fig. 28-24, *A*).	Allows patient to feel chair seat.
28. Ask patient to place crutches in hand on strong side and use other hand grasp chair arm to lower body into chair (Fig. 28-24, *B*).	Arms used for support, weight bearing, and balance.
29. Remove gloves and wash hands.	Helps prevent cross-contamination.
30. Document.	Documents procedure and patient's response.

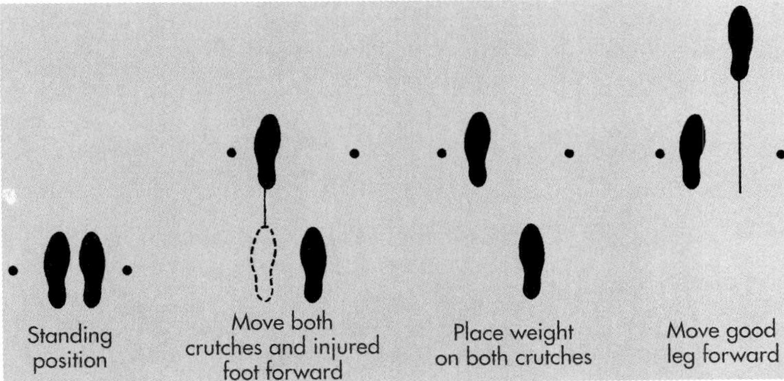

Fig. 28-20 Three-point gait. (From Christensen BL, Kockrow EO: *Foundations of nursing,* ed 2, St Louis, 1995, Mosby.)

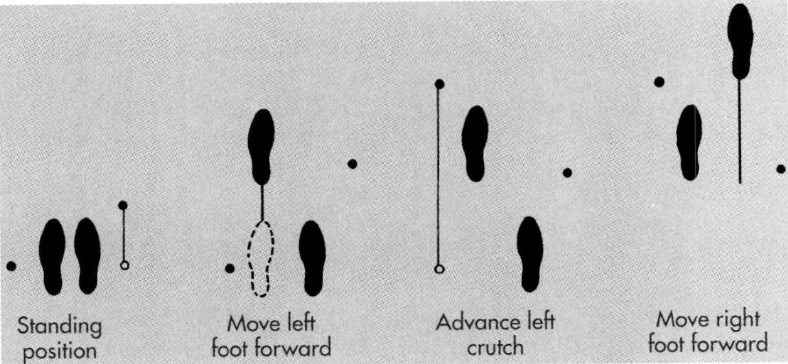

Fig. 28-21 Four-point gait. (From Christensen BL, Kockrow EO: *Foundations of nursing,* ed 2, St Louis, 1995, Mosby.)

Continued.

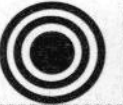

SKILL 28-6 TEACHING CRUTCH GAITS—cont'd

Steps **Rationale**

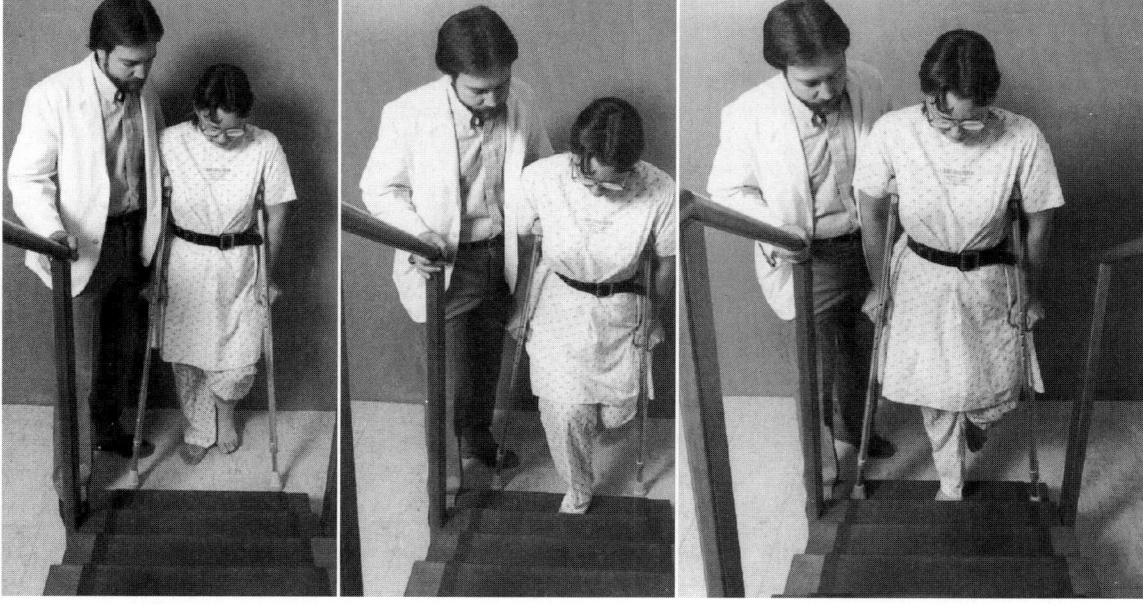

Fig. 28-22 **A,** Patient's body weight placed on hand rests of crutches. **B,** Moving strong leg up to next step. **C,** With weight placed on strong leg, crutches and weaker leg are moved up to next step. (From Perry AG, Potter PA: *Clinical nursing skills and techniques,* ed 3, St Louis, 1994, Mosby.)

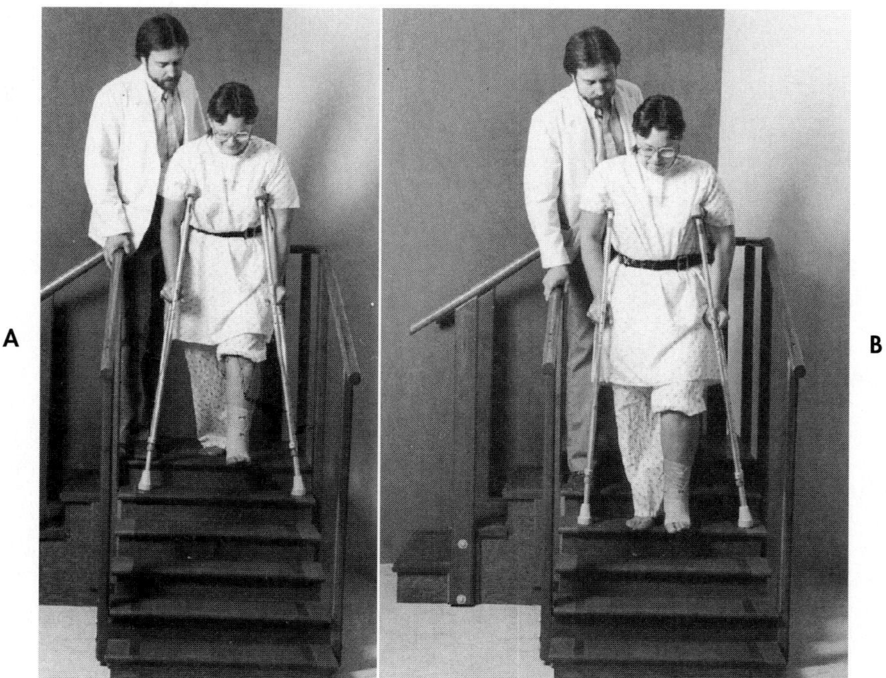

Fig. 28-23 **A,** Moving crutches to lower step. **B,** Weaker leg is placed first, followed by stronger leg. (From Perry AG, Potter PA: *Clinical nursing skills and techniques,* ed 3, St Louis, 1994, Mosby.)

SKILL 28-6 TEACHING CRUTCH GAITS—cont'd

Steps	Rationale

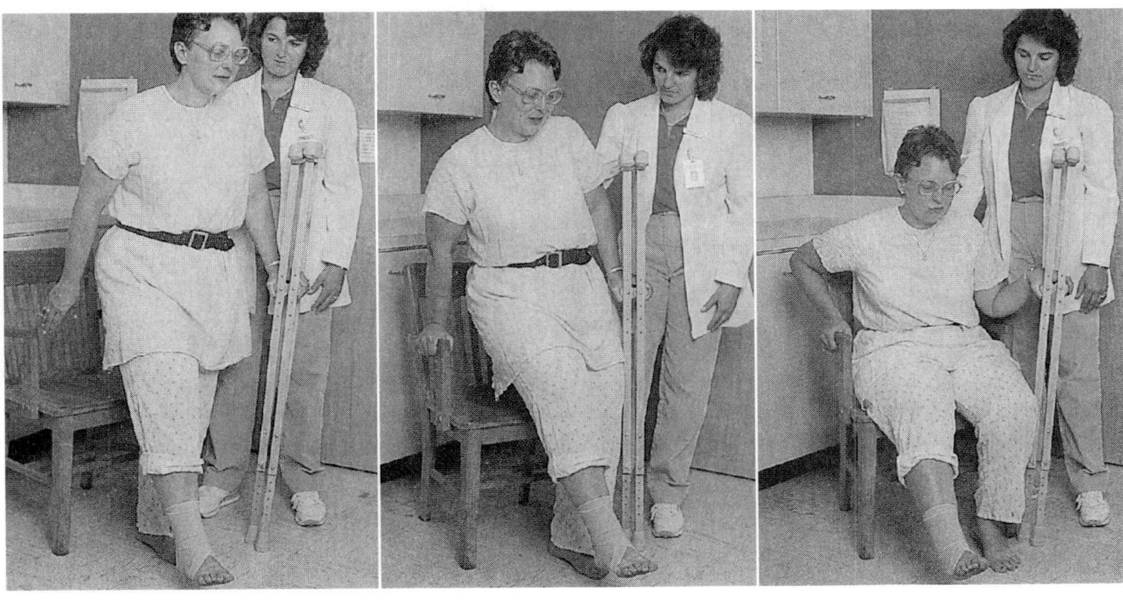

Fig. 28-24 Sitting in a chair. **A,** Both crutches are held by one hand. Patient transfers weight to crutches and unaffected leg. **B,** Patient grasps arm of chair with free hand and begins to lower herself into chair. **C,** Patient completely lowers herself into chair. (From Potter PA, Perry AG: *Basic nursing: theory and practice,* ed 3, St Louis, 1995, Mosby.)

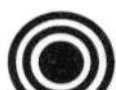

SKILL 28-7 TEACHING USE OF A CANE

Steps	Rationale
1. Obtain equipment: ▪ Cane ▪ Flat, nonskid shoes ▪ Robe ▪ Clean gloves	Helps organize procedure.
2. Refer to medical record, care plan, or Kardex for special interventions.	Provides basis for care.
3. Introduce self.	Decreases anxiety level.
4. Identify patient by identification band.	Identifies correct patient for procedure.
5. Explain procedure to patient.	Seeks cooperation and decreases anxiety.
6. Wash hands and don clean gloves according to agency policy and guidelines from Centers for Disease Control and Prevention and Occupational Safety and Health Administration.	Helps prevent cross-contamination.
7. Prepare patient for intervention:	
a. Close door to room or pull curtain.	Provides privacy.
b. Drape for procedure if necessary.	Prevents exposure of patient.
8. Raise bed to comfortable working level.	Provides safety for nurse.
9. Arrange for patient privacy.	Shows respect for patient.

Continued.

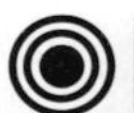

SKILL 28-7 TEACHING USE OF A CANE—cont'd

Steps	Rationale
10. Assess patient for strength and tightness of patient's handgrip, balance and coordination, strength of unaffected side, visual acuity, and integrity of cane being used.	Determines baseline ability of patient and which interventions are necessary.
11. Measure and adjust height of cane. (Adjustment is limited to aluminum canes.)	Allows cane to extend from floor to patient's hip joint.
12. Have patient wear flat, nonskid shoes.	Helps prevent falls.
STANDING AND WALKING	
13. Instruct patient to place cane in hand opposite affected leg and slide forward in chair.	Provides support and makes standing easier.
14. Have patient grasp one arm of chair with free hand and, if possible, grasp cane and chair arm with opposite hand. If not possible, tell patient to grasp cane only.	Increases balance and reduces possibility of falling.
15. Have patient use chair arms and cane to push directly downward to a standing position.	Develops muscle strength and balance. (Pushing at angle would throw patient off balance.)
16. Once standing, have patient pause to attain balance before positioning cane.	Assesses for dizziness and keeps patient from tripping on cane.
17. Have patient stand straight and look ahead.	Ensures appropriate posture, which provides more stability for walking.
18. Have patient move cane forward 4-6 in and bear weight on unaffected foot, while moving cane and affected foot forward simultaneously.	Allows strength of unaffected side to be used for support of weakened side.
19. Have patient transfer weight to affected foot and cane while moving unaffected foot forward.	Provides support for weight bearing on affected extremity.
20. Walk to side and slightly behind patient.	Provides support when patient is unsteady.
21. Advise patient to take small steps.	Increases sense of balance.
SITTING	
22. Have patient use cane to turn around and back into chair until legs touch chair seat.	Enables patient to sense edge of chair.
23. Have patient grasp both chair arms while holding cane in one hand and lower body into chair.	Supports body weight into sitting position.
24. Teach patient to place cane on chair arm.	Prevents cane from being misplaced.
CLIMBING STAIRS	
25. Have patient place cane on affected side.	Allows stronger hand to assist in climbing stairs.
26. Have patient place stronger foot on step while grasping handrail with stronger hand.	Promotes patient safety because stronger leg is used.
27. Have patient shift weight to stronger leg and then move weaker leg onto same step.	Promotes safe stair negotiation.
28. Repeat sequence until stairs have been ascended.	
DESCENDING STAIRS	
29. Have patient place cane on weaker side and grasp handrail with stronger hand.	Promotes using stronger hand to assist in descending stairs.
30. Have patient move weaker leg and cane to next step.	Stronger side supports weaker side during descent.
31. Have patient move strong leg to same step using cane and handrail.	Promotes safe stair descent.
32. Repeat sequence until stairs have been descended.	
33. Dispose of any waste materials.	Helps prevent spread of microorganisms.
34. Remove gloves and wash hands.	Helps prevent cross-contamination.
35. Document.	Documents procedure and patient's response.

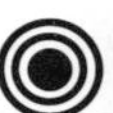

SKILL 28-8 TEACHING USE OF A WALKER

Steps	Rationale
1. Obtain equipment: ▪ Walker ▪ Flat, nonskid shoes ▪ Robe ▪ Clean gloves	Helps organize procedure.
2. Refer to medical record, care plan, or Kardex for special interventions.	Provides basis for care.
3. Introduce self.	Decreases anxiety level.
4. Identify patient by identification band.	Identifies correct patient for procedure.
5. Explain procedure to patient.	Seeks cooperation and decreases anxiety.
6. Wash hands and don clean gloves according to agency policy and guidelines from Centers for Disease Control and Prevention and Occupational Safety and Health Administration.	Helps prevent cross-contamination.
7. Prepare patient for intervention:	
a. Close door to room or pull curtain.	Provides privacy.
b. Drape for procedure if necessary.	Prevents exposure of patient.
8. Raise bed to comfortable working level.	Provides safety for nurse.
9. Arrange for patient privacy.	Shows respect for patient.
10. Select appropriate walker.	Ensures patient safety.
▪ Adjust walker height, if necessary.	Provides correct walker height to approximate patient's hip joint when elbows are flexed 30 degrees while holding handgrips.
11. Have patient wear flat, nonskid shoes.	Helps prevent falls.
12. Place walker in front of patient.	Prepares patient for walker ambulation.
13. Have patient place both hands on chair arms, slide forward, and push up to standing position.	Because chair is lower, allows patient to push with more force. Prevents walker from falling onto patient because it is less stable.
14. Have patient place one hand at time on walker handgrips.	Prevents patient from losing balance during transfer.
15. Have patient shift weight to unaffected leg while simultaneously moving walker and affected leg forward 4-6 in (see Fig. 28-14).	Promotes patient's stability while moving walker forward.
16. Have patient shift weight to walker and affected leg and move stronger leg forward.	Allows arms and walker to support patient's weight while moving stronger leg forward.
17. Repeat sequence for anticipated distance.	
18. Walk closely behind and slightly to side of patient.	Provides support in case patient becomes unsteady.
SITTING	
19. Have patient turn around in front of chair and back up until legs touch chair.	Places patient in correct position to sit directly into chair.
20. Have patient shift weight to stronger leg and reach behind with one hand and then other hand to grasp chair arms.	Allows patient to safely transfer weight from walker to chair.
21. Have patient bear weight on chair arms and lower into chair.	Promotes balance and shifts patient's weight to chair arms.
22. Place walker beside chair.	Makes walker convenient for patient and prevents others from tripping over it.
23. Remove gloves and wash hands.	Helps prevent cross-contamination.
24. Document.	Documents procedure and patient's response.

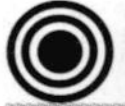

SKILL 28-9 USING A WHEELCHAIR

Steps	Rationale
1. Obtain equipment: ▪ Wheelchair ▪ Slippers ▪ Robe ▪ Pillow if needed ▪ Clean gloves	Helps organize procedure.
2. Refer to medical record, care plan, or Kardex for special interventions.	Provides basis for care.
3. Introduce self.	Decreases anxiety level.
4. Identify patient by identification band.	Identifies correct patient for procedure.
5. Explain procedure to patient.	Seeks cooperation and decreases anxiety.
6. Wash hands and don clean gloves according to agency policy and guidelines from Centers for Disease Control and Prevention and Occupational Safety and Health Administration.	Helps prevent cross-contamination.
7. Prepare patient for intervention:	
a. Close door to room or pull curtain.	Provides privacy.
b. Drape for procedure if necessary.	Prevents exposure of patient.
8. Raise bed to comfortable working level.	Provides safety for nurse.
9. Arrange for patient privacy.	Shows respect for patient.
10. Assess patient for arm and shoulder strength, leg strength, redness of skin and bony prominences, and motivation to regain independence.	Determines which interventions are necessary.
TRANSFER BY LIFTING	
11. Position wheelchair beside bed, lock brakes, and lift up footrests.	Provides for patient safety: Keeps wheelchair from moving because brakes are not locked prior to moving a patient in or out of a wheelchair. Keeps patient from accidentally stepping on footrests and flipping chair forward.
12. Remove armrests, raise patient's head, and raise bed above level of chair.	Decreases energy required to transfer patient.
13. Cross patient's hands over chest. Have one nurse stand behind patient, slide hands under axillae, and grasp patient's wrists.	Provides full support of upper body.
14. Have other nurse move beside patient in front of wheelchair, lifting patient's knees and thighs.	Provides full support of lower body.
15. Count to three. Have both nurses simultaneously lift patient into wheelchair.	Allows nurses to move simultaneously to maintain equal weight distribution and patient's feeling of security.
16. Place patient in correct body alignment: upper body straight, feet on footrests, and arms on chair arms or supported by pillows.	Prevents muscle strain and contractures and promotes comfort.
17. Apply restraining device or lap belt on patients with altered levels of consciousness or patients who are quadriplegics.	Prevents patient from falling out of wheelchair.
TRANSFER BY PIVOTING	
18. Position wheelchair beside bed on patient's stronger side, lock brakes, and lift up footrests.	Enables patient to pivot with stronger side. Prevents injury to patient.
19. Assist patient to a sitting position on side of bed.	Facilitates easier transfer.

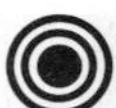

SKILL 28-9 USING A WHEELCHAIR—cont'd

Steps	Rationale
20. Moving in front of patient, place arms under axillae and grasp hands behind patient's back.	Provides stronger support in case patient becomes weak or dizzy.
21. Have patient use strong leg to assist in standing.	Increases independence and prevents muscle strain to nurse.
22. Allow patient few seconds to gain balance.	Gives patient time to gain balance especially after prolonged recumbency.
23. Pivot with patient. Back patient up to chair. Have patient grasp chair arms and lower into wheelchair.	Promotes patient safety in transfer from bed to wheelchair.
24. Unlock brakes and push wheelchair in direction patient is facing.	Enables nurse and patient to see potential hazards.
25. If descending gently sloped ramp, push wheelchair in normal manner.	Allows nurse to safely maintain control of patient and wheelchair.
26. If descending steep ramp, turn wheelchair around and descend backward.	Prevents patient from falling out of wheelchair. Promotes patient feeling of security.
27. Remove gloves and wash hands.	Helps prevent cross-contamination.
28. Document.	Documents procedure and patient's response.

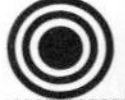

SKILL 28-10 USING A THERAPEUTIC FRAME OR BED

Steps	Rationale
1. Obtain equipment: *For Stryker Frame:* ▪ Anterior and posterior frame with sheets ▪ Armboards ▪ Footboard ▪ Bedpan holder ▪ Facepiece ▪ Two safety straps ▪ Pillows *For CircOlectric Bed:* ▪ Anterior and posterior frame with sheets ▪ Armrests ▪ Footboard ▪ Two safety straps ▪ Pillows ▪ Clean gloves *For Roto Rest Bed:* ▪ Rotation bed with appropriate accessories ▪ Pillow cases or linen-saver pads ▪ Flat sheet *For Clinitron Bed:* ▪ Clinitron bed	Helps organize procedure.
2. Refer to medical record, care plan, or Kardex for special interventions.	Provides basis for care.
3. Introduce self.	Decreases anxiety level.
4. Identify patient by identification band.	Identifies correct patient for procedure.
5. Explain procedure to patient.	Seeks cooperation and decreases anxiety.
6. Wash hands and don clean gloves according to agency policy and guidelines from Centers for Disease Control and Prevention and Occupational Safety and Health Administration.	Helps prevent cross-contamination.

Continued.

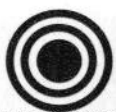

SKILL 28-10 USING A THERAPEUTIC FRAME OR BED—cont'd

Steps	Rationale
7. Prepare patient for intervention:	
a. Close door to room or pull curtain.	Provides privacy.
b. Drape for procedure if necessary.	Prevents exposure of patient.
8. Raise bed to comfortable working level.	Provides safety for nurse.
9. Arrange for patient privacy.	Shows respect for patient.
10. Assess patient for level of anxiety and apprehension, level of pain, need for elimination, vital signs and respiratory status, intake within last 15 to 20 min, and safety of bed being used (that is, worn joints, screws, bolts, canvas, and electrical defects).	Helps provide nursing care for patient needs.
STRYKER WEDGE FRAME	
11. Remove all accessories, including bedpan, and secure intravenous bags and lines, urinary catheter bags, or other drainage bags.	Prevents equipment from being dislodged and patient from being injured during turn. Prevents accessories from prohibiting turning.
12. Place pillows across patient's chest and any areas where side sliding is possible.	Assists in relieving chest discomfort and prevents patient from sliding.
13. With two people, place anterior or posterior frame over patient and fasten ends of frame together with screws.	Follows policy of most facilities, which require two people to perform safe turning procedure.
14. Place two safety straps around anterior and posterior frames and patient: one over chest and other over thighs.	Provides additional safety and makes patient feel more secure.
15. Double-check all screws, bolts, and straps.	Ensures safe turn.
16. Inform patient of direction of turn.	Promotes greater feeling of safety.
17. Arrange signal so patient will know when frame will be turned.	Decreases patient's anxiety.
18. On count of 3, turn patient in smooth uninterrupted motion at moderate speed.	Decreases potential for vertigo and nausea.
19. Remove safety straps and uppermost frame.	Allows patient to breathe easier.
20. Check patient's position and alignment. (If prone, adjust facepiece and place straps over patient. Remove wrinkles from sheets.) (see Fig. 28-15).	Prevents deformities and skin breakdown and increases patient's comfort. (Prevents patient from falling off frame. Promotes comfort.)
21. Reposition accessories (that is, armboards and footboard). Place personal articles and call light within easy reach.	Promotes patient comfort. Reduces frustration and involves patient in ADLs.
22. Store frame securely in upright position in clean area.	Prevents frame from becoming dirty or accidentally falling on someone.
23. Repeat turning at least every 2 hr unless physician orders different schedule.	Assists in preventing complications of immobility.
CIRCOLECTRIC BED	
24. Remove footboard and armrests, secure traction, intravenous bags and lines, urinary catheter bags, other drainage bags, and electric cord.	Prevents footboard and armrests from interfering with turning. Prevents dislodgment of lines, bags, and cord. Allows traction to hang freely to side.
25. Remove nuts and bolts from both ends of frame.	Allows two people to place frame appropriately. Prevents patient falls.
26. With another nurse lift frame over patient, replace bolts, and tightly secure frame with nuts (see Fig. 28-16).	
27. If patient is supine, adjust headrest and pad footboard on uppermost frame.	Increases patient's comfort to assume prone position.

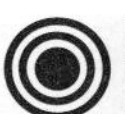

SKILL 28-10 USING A THERAPEUTIC FRAME OR BED—cont'd

Steps	Rationale
28. Instruct patient to grasp sides of frame or cross arms over chest.	Prevents patient's arms from being injured.
29. Double-check nuts and bolts.	Ensures safety.
30. Inform patient of turning direction.	Promotes patient understanding and lessens anxiety.
31. Using control switch, turn bed without stopping until it reaches desired position.	Helps decrease nausea, vertigo, spatial disorientation, and fear of falling.
32. Have second nurse observe closely for signs of cardiac and respiratory arrest, as well as intravenous line and tube entanglement.	Helps nurse detect cardiac and respiratory instability, which occur frequently during first few days after spinal cord injury. Prevents intravenous line and tube dislodgement.
33. If patient is prone, release uppermost frame and apply two safety straps. Otherwise remove uppermost frame.	Allows nurse to provide care. Prevents patient from falling.
34. Assess patient's position, alignment, and face support and remove wrinkles from sheets.	Prevents skin breakdown and deformities and promotes patient comfort.
35. Assess patient's vital signs.	Determines whether patient's vital signs have decreased because of postural hypotension.
36. Reposition accessories and place personal articles and call light within reach.	Promotes patient performance of ADLs.
37. Store frame securely in upright position in clean area.	Keeps frame clean and prevents injury to other staff.
38. Repeat procedure every 2 hr unless contraindicated.	Assists in preventing immobility complications.
ROTO REST BED	
39. Before positioning in bed, be sure bed is turned off. Lock bed in horizontal position, lock wheels, and latch all hatches.	Ensures safety of patient and staff to prevent falls and back injury.
40. Move patient to center of bed. Smooth pillowcase under hips. Place tubes through designated areas in hatches and ensure that traction is free hanging.	Prevents contact with pillar posts and ensures proper balance during bed operation. Prevents restricted flow resulting from kinking or compression. Allows weights to be free hanging to apply desired force.
41. Insert thoracic side supports and allow 1-in space between axillae and supports.	Avoids pressure on brachial plexus and blood vessels.
42. Push supports against chest and lock cam arms securely.	Provides support and ensures safety.
43. Place disposable supports under patient's legs.	Removes pressure from heels and prevents pressure ulcers from developing.
44. Install and adjust foot supports to maintain correct position. Keep in place only 2 hr every shift.	Prevents footdrop and pressure ulcers.
45. Place abductor packs in appropriate supports, allowing 6-in space between packs and patients groin.	Prevents pressure on groin.
46. Tighten associated knobs.	Provides support and prevents pressure ulcers.
47. Apply leg supports against hips. Position knee assemblies slightly above knees. Tighten cam arms for leg and knee assemblies. Position knee packs until they rest slightly on top of hand covering patient's knees.	Maintains correct lateral position of shoulder clamp assembly and head-support pack.
48. Loosen retaining rings on cross bar and carefully slide head-and-shoulder assembly in place, just touching patient's head. Move shoulder packs till it touches hand on patient's shoulders. Tighten in place. Do not allow head pack to touch patient's ears.	Prevents development of pressure ulcers.

Continued.

SKILL 28-10 USING A THERAPEUTIC FRAME OR BED—cont'd

Steps	Rationale
49. Tighten head-and-shoulder assembly tightly so that it will not move off bed. Tighten restraining rings next to shoulder-assembly bracket.	Provides safety for patient.
50. Place patient's arms on disposable supports. Apply side arm supports and secure safety straps across shoulder assembly and thoracic supports.	Ensures patient is safe when being turned.
51. Balance bed as directed in manufacturers instructions.	Balancing bed is necessary for appropriate bed use.
52. Check that all packs are securely in place.	Ensures safety of patient.
53. Hold footboard firmly and remove locking pin to start motor.	Allows bed to continue to rotate until pin is reinserted.
54. Raise connecting arm cam handle until connecting assembly locks in place.	Locks bed in automatic rotation.
55. Remain with patient for three complete turns side to side.	Provides emotional support and safety and ensures comfort.
56. Refer to manufacturer's instructions for placement of drainage tubes through hatches.	Promotes gravity drainage of tubes.
57. Perform scheduled range-of-motion exercises as ordered.	Allows full access to extremities without disturbing spinal alignment.
58. Lock bed in extreme lateral position for access to back of head, thorax, and buttocks through appropriate hatches.	Allows easy access for personal hygiene and treatments.
CLINITRON BED	
59. Transfer patient to bed using appropriate transfer techniques (see Fig. 28-17).	Prevents injury to personnel and patient.
60. Assess patient's position and alignment.	Prevents development of contractures.
61. Turn on control for activating fluidization.	Decreases shearing force on skin.
62. Adjust temperature control.	Makes adjustment based on patient's condition.
63. Replace covers and place personal items and call light within reach.	Promotes comfort and access to personal belongings.
64. Assess for nausea.	Assesses for complications of treatment.
65. Remove gloves and wash hands.	Helps prevent cross-contamination.
66. Document.	Documents procedure and patient's response.

SUMMARY

An alteration in mobility status may result from a variety of conditions. The nurse prevents complications and assists the patient in achieving an optimal level of independence. The amount of independence achieved is often dictated by preexisting illnesses. The patient must be an active participant in the plan of care. Immobility may lead to complications affecting almost every body system. The nurse should provide nursing care while maintaining the mechanical equipment and assessing for potential complications.

Key Concepts

- The nurse assesses for skin breakdown.
- The nurse assesses for circulation, motion, and sensation of distal extremities.
- The nurse evaluates equipment for appropriate, safe functioning.
- Weights must not rest on the floor or bed, and patient must be prevented from slipping to the base of the bed.
- Patients in cervical traction may not be placed in a Stryker wedge frame or CircOlectric bed.
- Transfer board may be used for patients with limited lower extremity strength. Adequate upper extremity strength is necessary.
- The nurse removes as many portions of the wheelchair as possible to enhance transfer technique (that is, footrests, headrest).
- Wheelchair push-ups should be performed every 20 minutes to prevent skin breakdown.
- Transfer belt may be worn to prevent injury to the nurse.
- Patients should use their own assistive devices to ensure correct fit and height.
- Chairs with firm, hard seats facilitate rising from sitting positions.
- The nurse logrolls a patient when turning with an abduction pillow in place.
- The nurse avoids adduction of the legs or flexion of more than 90 degrees at the hip joint after hip surgery.
- It may take up to 3 days for a cast to dry. The patient must be turned every 2 hours to facilitate this process.
- If the arm has a cast above the elbow, the nurse pads the axilla area to prevent irritation.

Critical Thinking Questions

1. Identify the appropriate placement of equipment, positioning of the patient, and movement of the nurse in the following situations.
   a. While the nurse helps a patient walk to the bathroom, the client states that she feels faint and starts to fall to the floor.
   b. The nurse is moving a heavy patient from a stretcher to the bed.
   c. The nurse is giving an intramuscular injection into the left dorsogluteal muscle of a patient in bed.
2. The nurse is caring for an 80-year-old woman with a fractured hip who has been healthy and independent until this hospitalization. What are the priorities for reducing the risk of complications from immobility?

REFERENCES AND SUGGESTED READINGS

Brunner LS, Suddarth DS: *Textbook of medical-surgical nursing,* ed 7, Philadelphia, 1992, Lippincott.

Doenges M, Moorhouse MF, Geissler A: *Nursing care plans: guidelines for planning and documenting patient care,* ed 3, Philadelphia, 1993, Davis.

Earnest V: *Clinical skills in nursing practice,* ed 2, Philadelphia, 1993, Lippincott.

Ellis J, Nowlis E, Bentz P: *Modules for basic nursing skills,* ed 5, Philadelphia, 1992, Lippincott.

Loeb S: *Nursing procedures,* Springhouse, Penn, 1992, Springhouse.

Long BC, Phipps WJ: *Medical-surgical nursing: a nursing process approach,* ed 3, St Louis, 1993, Mosby.

Nichol D: Preventing infection: patients with skeletal pins, *Nursing Times* 89(13):78, 1993.

Perry AG, Potter PA: *Clinical nursing skills and techniques,* ed 3, St Louis, 1994, Mosby.

Potter PA, Perry AG: *Fundamentals of nursing: concepts process, and practice,* ed 3, St Louis, 1994, Mosby.

Strength D: *Clinical manual of gerontological nursing,* St Louis, 1992, Mosby.

Thompson JM et al: *Mosby's clinical nursing,* ed 3, St Louis, 1993, Mosby.

Wong DL: *Whaley and Wong's essentials of pediatric nursing,* ed 4, St Louis, 1993, Mosby.

CHAPTER 29

Oxygenation

Learning Objectives

After studying this chapter, the student should be able to . . .

- Define the key terms.
- Recognize and report the signs and symptoms of respiratory distress.
- Describe diagnostic tests of the respiratory system.
- Relate the rationales for positioning the patient, providing mouth care, and encouraging deep breathing and fluids for a patient with decreased respiratory function.
- Teach deep breathing exercises to a patient with or without a cough.
- Explain postural drainage.
- Explain percussion and vibration techniques.
- Describe the positions used when performing postural drainage.
- Explain the use of a vaporizer.
- Recognize and report the signs and symptoms of oxygen deficiency.
- Perform appropriate nursing care for a patient receiving oxygen.
- Describe safety precautions associated with the use of oxygen therapy.
- Perform oropharyngeal, nasopharyngeal, and endotracheal suctioning.
- Provide care of a tracheostomy, including suction and cleansing of the outer tube and cannula.
- Perform nursing care of a patient with water-seal drainage.

Key Terms

Atelectasis
Bronchoscopy
Dyspnea
Hypoxia
Incentive spirometry
Laryngoscopy
Negative pressure
Nonproductive cough
Oxygen toxicity
Oxygenation
Pleural space
Pneumothorax
Postural drainage
Productive cough
Sputum
Subcutaneous emphysema
Tachycardia
Tidal volume
Tracheostomy
Vaporizer
Vital capacity

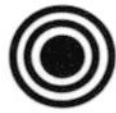 Skills

29-1 Using incentive spirometry
29-2 Performing postural drainage and percussion
29-3 Using the vaporizer
29-4 Administering oxygen
29-5 Performing oropharyngeal suctioning
29-6 Performing nasopharyngeal suctioning
29-7 Performing endotracheal suctioning
29-8 Performing tracheostomy care and suctioning
29-9 Caring for closed chest drainage systems

When the patient is having difficulty breathing the nurse must use the principles of respiration in the assessment, planning, intervention, and evaluation of nursing care to help the patient. Some of the procedures are performed by nursing personnel. However, in many hospitals, a respiratory therapy department often directs and performs some of the tests and procedures. Nevertheless, the nurse should know how the procedures are performed and must document the results of the procedures and response of the patient.

RESPIRATION

For the patient to receive adequate **oxygenation** (process of combining or treating with oxygen), the air passages must remain clear of mucus, drainage, and objects. The muscles of respiration, the diaphragm and the intercostals, must be capable of contracting and relaxing. Pressure changes must take place inside the lungs for air to pass into and out of the lungs. The patient's fluid intake must be adequate to keep respiratory secretions liquid. Perfusion of the body tissues by the circulatory system must be maintained to ensure adequate oxygenation of organs and tissues. If any of these principles are violated, the patient's respiratory status is said to be *compromised* (less effective).

Diagnostic Tests

Pulmonary function test Many tests are used in diagnosing respiratory conditions. One of the most common is the pulmonary function test. This test requires the patient to breathe into a machine via a special adaptive mouthpiece and tubing. The machine measures the adequacy of respiration.

Tidal volume is one type of pulmonary function test. **Tidal volume** is the total amount of air the patient breathes in or out with normal respiration. **Vital capacity** is the greatest amount of air that the patient can breathe out after a maximal inspiration.

During the testing, the patient may need to breathe very rapidly or very deeply. Each measurement may need to be performed several times before an appropriate result can be accomplished. The patient may feel dizzy during some parts of the testing and often complains of fatigue afterward.

Arterial blood gases Testing for arterial blood gas (ABG) levels is also called *blood gas analysis*. For this test, a sample of arterial blood is extracted and tested for the content of oxygen, carbon dioxide, and pH. The nurse needs to be aware that a blood sample has been obtained. The site of injection needs to be assessed closely for bleeding. The site may be more tender than the sites of venous blood samples.

Laryngoscopy Laryngoscopy is the insertion of a lighted instrument (laryngoscope) into the larynx to view its structures. An anesthetic is used to temporarily paralyze the gag reflex (see Chapter 19). After the test, the nurse should not give the patient food or water until the gag reflex has returned. The nurse also documents accurate assessments of the patient's respiratory status after the test.

Bronchoscopy A **bronchoscopy** is the insertion of a lighted instrument (bronchoscope) into the bronchi to view their structures. Follow-up precautions are the same as for a laryngoscopy. This patient may be sent to the surgical unit or to a special examination room. Emergency equipment should be on hand at all times during and after the test in case of respiratory distress.

Other diagnostic tests Other respiratory diagnostic tests include chest, sinus, and lateral (side) neck x-ray studies; magnetic resonance imaging (MRI) (see Chapter 13); and computerized tomography (CAT or now CT scan) (see Chapter 13). Another test is a radiologic uptake scan. These tests usually need no patient preparation.

Breath Sounds

The nurse also assesses the patient's respirations, color, and breath sounds. The nurse should listen to all lobes of the lungs using an S-shaped pattern. The order of the pattern is less important than its completion. Neglecting one area of the lungs could result in missing a vital assessment. The nurse should listen to each site through one entire respiratory cycle, carefully assessing where and when abnormal sounds occur. A great deal of practice is required to become proficient at assessing breath sounds. Abnormal breath sounds should be documented and reported to the physician. The terminology used to describe breath sounds depends on the policies of the facility (see the box).

SYSTEMS USED TO DESCRIBE ABNORMAL LUNG Sounds

Rales
Bubbling or crackling sound
- *Fine*
Sound like fizzing of soda in bottle
- *Coarse*
Sound like blowing bubbles in milk

Rhonchi
- Musical sounds
- *Sibilant*
High-pitched sound, usually on expiration
- *Sonorous*
Low-pitched sound

Crackles
Crackling sound
- *Fine*
Sound like fizzing of soda in bottle
- *Coarse*
Sound like blowing bubbles in milk

Wheeze
- High-pitched musical sound, usually on expiration

Snoring
- Low-pitched musical sounds

Coughs

The nurse should assess for coughing, with special emphasis on the type of cough. **Productive coughs** remove **sputum** (mucus, cellular debris, and microorganisms coughed up from the lungs). The nurse determines whether the specimen is from deep in the respiratory tree (lung) or merely from the back of the throat. Saliva alone is not an acceptable specimen for testing. A **nonproductive cough** is a dry, hacking cough. It is irritating to the patient and does not accomplish any clearing of the lungs or air passages.

NURSING PROCESS AND OXYGENATION

Assessment

The nursing assessment of a patient's cardiopulmonary functioning should include a nursing history, a physical examination, and diagnostic tests. The nursing history includes the patient's cough, shortness of breath, wheezing, pain, past respiratory problems, smoking history, and medication use. Inspection, palpation, auscultation, and percussion are used during a physical examination when the level of tissue oxygenation is assessed. Diagnostic tests may be performed to determine the adequacy of the patient's cardiac conduction system, myocardial (heart muscle) contraction and blood flow, adequacy of ventilation and oxygenation, and respiratory tract infections.

Nursing Diagnosis

The nurse reviews data gathered during assessment and identifies characteristics that determine nursing diagnoses. These may include the following:

Activity intolerance
Decreased cardiac output
Impaired gas exchange
Ineffective airway clearance
Ineffective breathing pattern
Risk for infection

Planning

The plan of care should include measures to promote optimal oxygenation and to help allay fear the patient experiences when unable to breathe (see care plan on p. 558). The patient should be assured that the nurse will do everything possible to correct breathing problems. The patient and family members may participate in developing the plan of care. The nurse should include the patient's family when teaching health promotion (see teaching box).

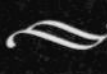

PATIENT TEACHING

- Instruct patient to report changes in sputum color, amount, and thickness to physician.
- Teach patient deep breathing and coughing exercises (see Chapter 17).
- Encourage patient to drink plenty of fluids, since they help keep secretions liquified and loose.

GERONTOLOGIC CONSIDERATIONS

- When assessing for respiratory status, the nurse should remember that the older adult may have altered skin coloration resulting from other physical conditions.
- The nurse should not assume that confusion is due to age. Instead, it may be related to inadequate oxygenation.
- The older patient who requires postural drainage and percussion may need more time to rest between steps.
- Many older adults have difficulty expectorating and may require suctioning to remove respiratory secretions.

The care plan may include the following goals:

Goal #1: Patient achieves improved activity tolerance.

Outcome

Patient reports less discomfort with exercise.

Goal #2: Patient maintains a patent airway.

Outcome

Patient clears airway by coughing.

Implementation

Maintaining the patient's optimal level of health is important in reducing respiratory symptoms. Nursing interventions may include improving the patient's activity tolerance. This results in the patient's increased ability to perform activities of daily living while not increasing cardiac workload or the work of breathing. The nurse should remember that ventilation and gas exchange decline with age, lowering oxygenation levels in the older adult. Special consideration should be given to this patient (see gerontologic box).

Evaluation

The nurse evaluates the expected outcomes and determines their effectiveness. A revision of the plan and interventions may be necessary. The nurse should not hesitate to notify the physician if the patient's breathing does not immediately improve. The patient may suddenly worsen and require emergency interventions. Goals and evaluative measures for oxygenation may include the following:

Goal #1: Patient achieves improved activity tolerance.

Evaluative measure

Observe patient exercise.

Goal #2: Patient maintains a patent airway.

Evaluative measure

Auscultate airways after patient coughs.

NURSING CARE

Comfort Measures

Repositioning

Sometimes, simply repositioning the patient improves oxygenation. It is easier for the patient to breathe sitting up than lying down. The tripod position also eases breathing. This position is referred to as the *orthopneic position.* In this position, the patient sits up or leans over a table or stand, with the weight of the upper body supported on the elbows. This provides space for the respiratory muscles to expand and contract.

Oral hygiene

Mouth and oral care may improve respiratory status. If the patient has a productive cough, suctioning has been performed, or a specimen has been obtained, mouth care may help remove any bad taste from the mouth. Appropriate mouth and oral hygiene decreases the number of bacteria in the mouth and may help prevent nosocomial infection (see Chapter 14).

Increased fluids

The nurse should encourage fluids for the patient with a respiratory condition. Fluids help keep the respiratory secretions more liquid and ease removal by coughing or suctioning. The nurse may offer a variety of fluids, including fruit juices, carbonated beverages, flavored waters, ice chips, and water, to encourage the patient to drink. Involving the patient in keeping track of the amount taken and setting goals may also encourage a larger intake of fluid.

Deep Breathing and Coughing

Deep breathing and coughing exercises often help clear air passages and lungs of excess mucus or drainage. Appropriately positioning the patient for ease of breathing aids respiration. The nurse should instruct the patient to take three or four deep breaths through the mouth. The patient should hold each breath for a count of 3 before exhaling through the mouth. If coughing is to be performed, the patient should cough forcefully after the last inhalation. The nurse must make certain to have the patient cough into a tissue and, wearing gloves, assesses any sputum for amount, color, and consistency. Mouth care should be offered afterward. Coughing may be contraindicated for some patients (for example, patients with hernias and head injuries or those who have had some back surgeries). Medical orders should be assessed for contraindications.

Incentive Spirometry

Some patients are predisposed to having **atelectasis,** which is a collapsed lung caused by mucous plugs or excessive secretions. A more measurable method of providing deep breathing and coughing exercises for the patient is **incentive spirometry.** A device called a *spirometer* measures the air capacity of the lungs. The mouthpiece of the spirometer is placed in the mouth. The patient inhales deeply from a tubing connected to a gauge that measures the deep breaths. Different methods are used to "inspire" the patient to breathe more deeply each breath. Some spirometers have a ball that can be floated higher and longer. Others use lights or signals. In still others, the patient's breath raises the bottom of a collapsed cylinder along a calibrated volume meter (see p. 559). The results are assessed and documented.

Incentive spirometry is ordered by the physician, but the nurse is responsible for encouraging the patient to use the device (Skill 29-1). Some patients do not have the motivation to perform the procedure thoroughly and must be monitored to make certain that they appropriately perform the procedure. Patients should be supervised periodically even though they are compliant. The nurse should also monitor patients to ensure they do not become too fatigued from the procedure.

Postural Drainage and Percussion

Postural drainage is usually performed by respiratory therapy personnel, but the nurse assesses the patient's response and provides the follow-up care needed for recovery. In **postural drainage** the patient is placed in various positions so that gravity moves secretions from the bronchial tree for removal through coughing and expectoration. During this procedure (Skill 29-2), vibration and percussion of the back and chest wall may be used to assist in loosening secretions (Table 29-1).

Table 29-1 POSITIONS AND PROCEDURES FOR DRAINAGE, PERCUSSION, AND VIBRATION

Area and Procedure	Percussion	Vibration	Bronchial Lobe
Left and right upper lobe anterior apical bronchi Have patient sit in chair, leaning back. Percuss and vibrate with heel of hands at shoulders and fingers over collarbones (clavicles) in front (can do both sides at same time). Note body posture and arm position of nurse. Keep back straight and elbows and knees slightly flexed.	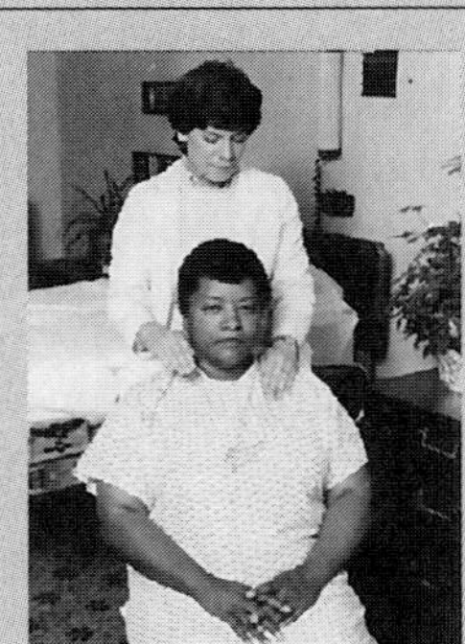	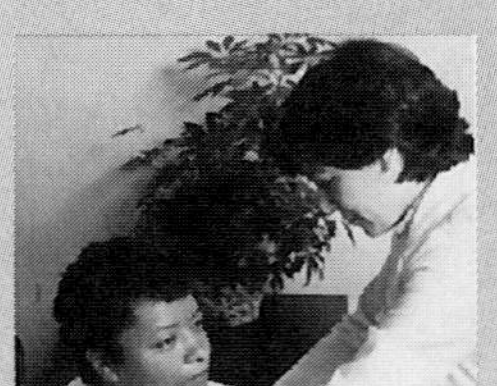	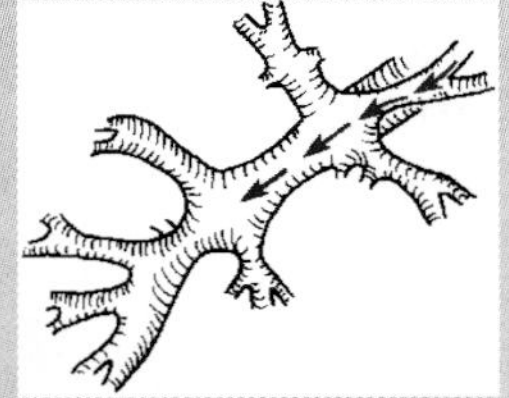
Left and right upper lobe posterior apical bronchi Have patient sit in chair, leaning forward on pillow or table. Percuss and vibrate with hands on either side of upper spine (can do both sides at same time).	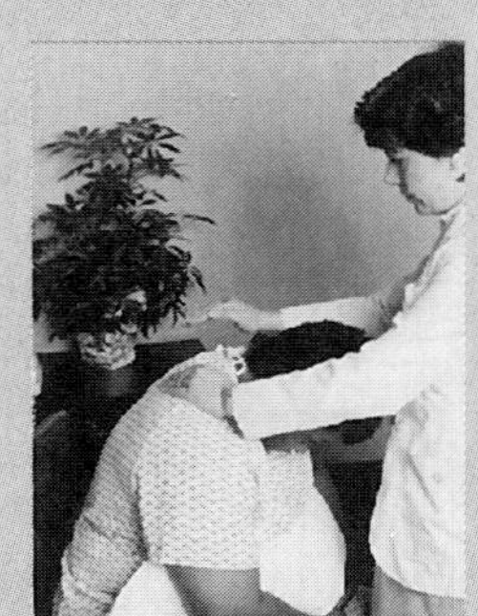	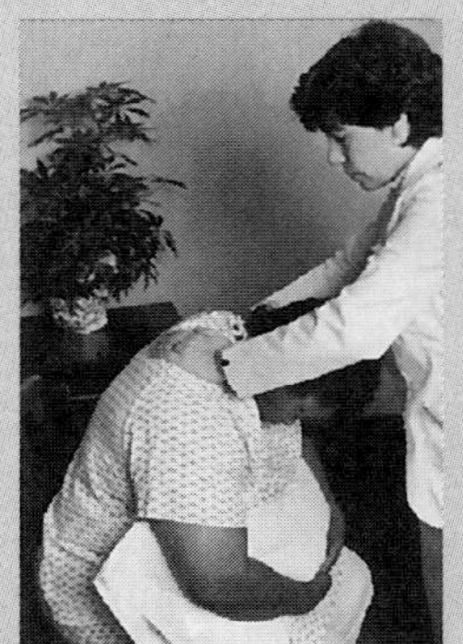	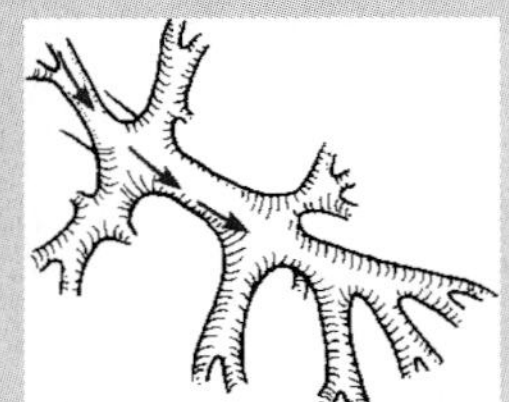
Right and left anterior upper lobe bronchi Have patient lie flat on back with small pillow under knees. Percuss and vibrate just below clavicle on either side of sternum.	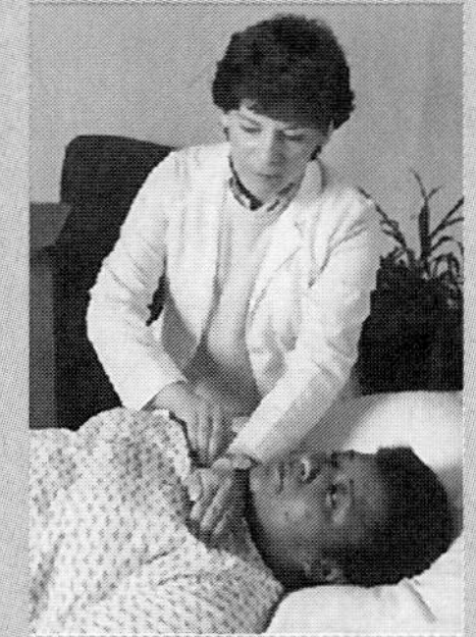	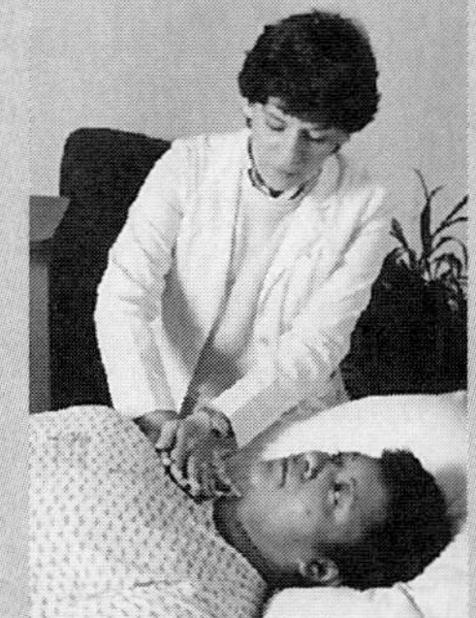	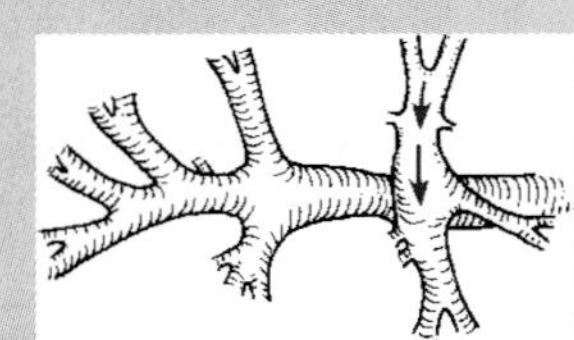
Left upper lobe lingular bronchus Have patient lie on right side with arm over head in Trendelenburg's position, with foot of bed raised 30 cm (12 in). Place pillow behind back, and roll patient one-fourth turn onto pillow. Percuss and vibrate lateral to left nipple below axilla.	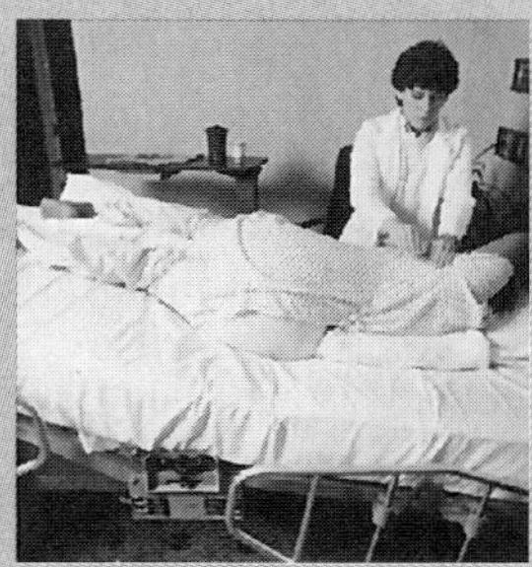	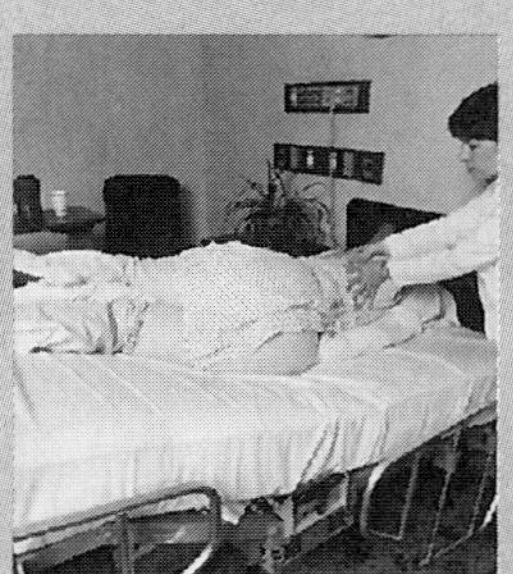	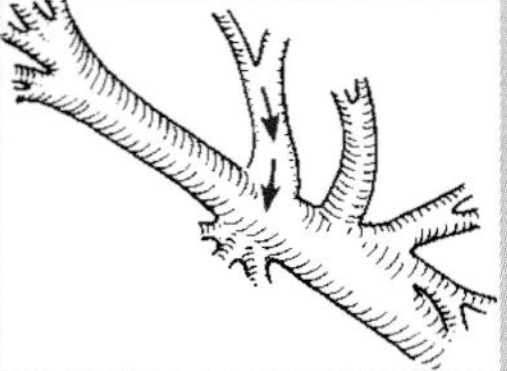

Table 29-1 POSITIONS AND PROCEDURES FOR DRAINAGE, PERCUSSION, AND VIBRATION—cont'd

Area and Procedure	Percussion	Vibration	Bronchial Lobe
Right middle lobe bronchus Have patient lie on left side and raise foot of bed 30 cm (12 in). Place pillow behind back and roll patient one-fourth turn onto pillow. Percuss and vibrate lateral to right nipple below axilla.	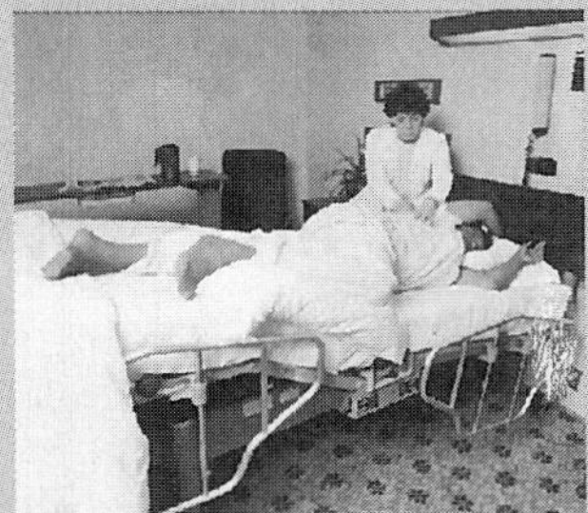	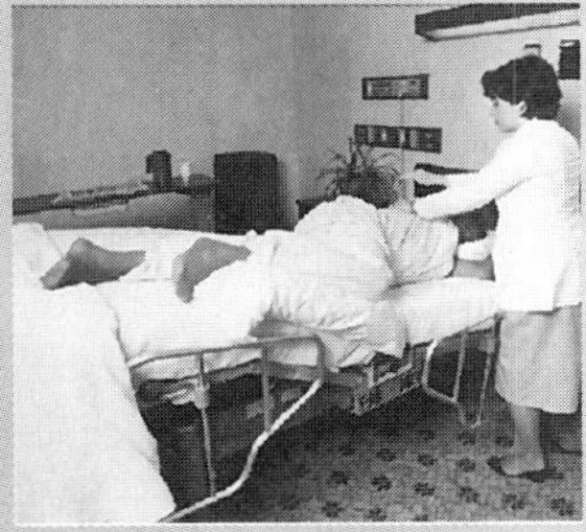	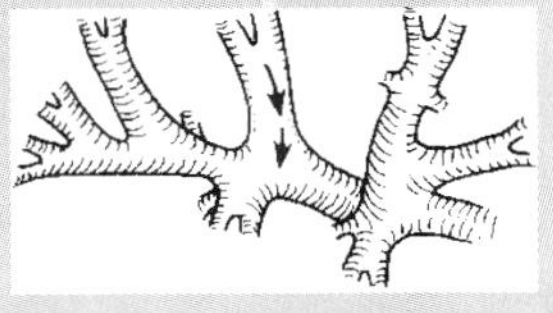
Left and right anterior lower lobe bronchi Have patient lie on back in Trendelenburg's position with foot of bed elevated 45-50 cm (18-20 in). Have knees bent on pillow. Percuss and vibrate over lower anterior ribs on both sides.	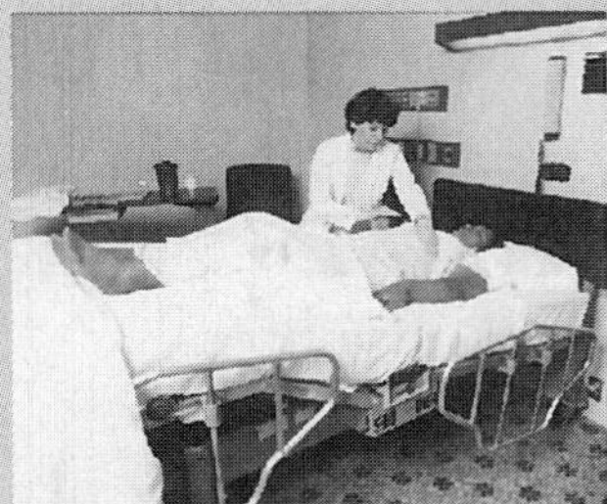	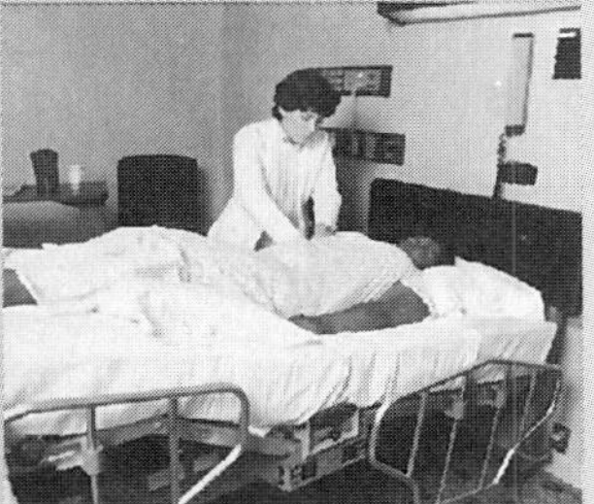	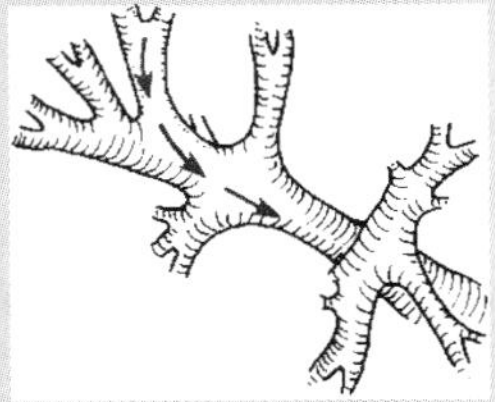
Right lower lobe lateral bronchus Have patient lie on left side in Trendelenburg's position with foot of bed raised 45-50 cm (18-20 in). Percuss and vibrate on right side of chest below shoulder blades (scapulas) posterior to midaxillary line.	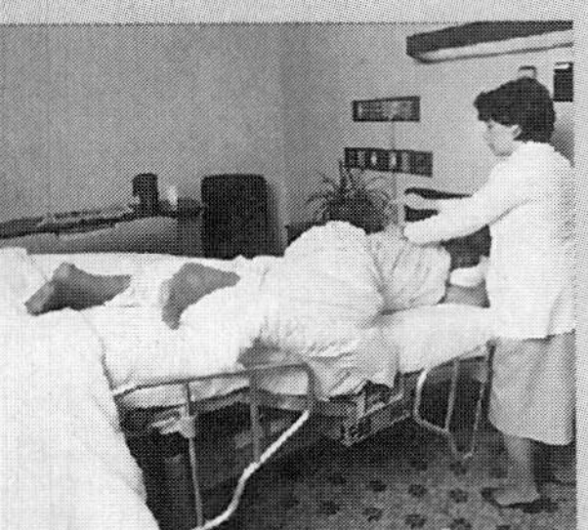	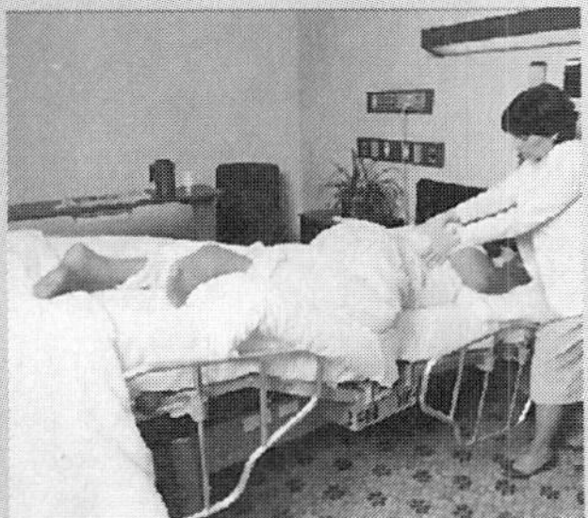	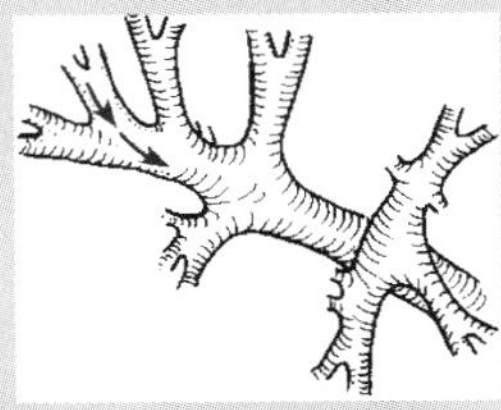
Left lower lobe lateral bronchus Have patient lie on right side in Trendelenburg's position with foot of bed raised 45-50 cm (18-20 in). Percuss and vibrate on left side of chest below scapulas posterior to midaxillary line.	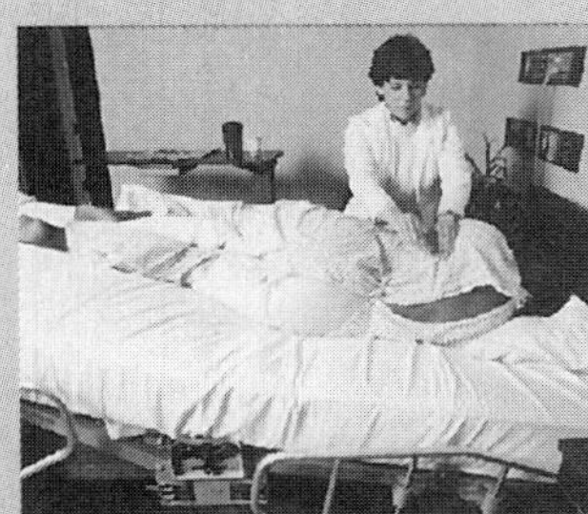	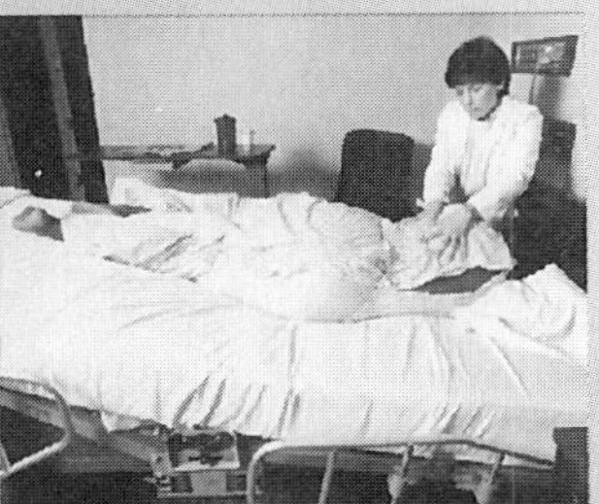	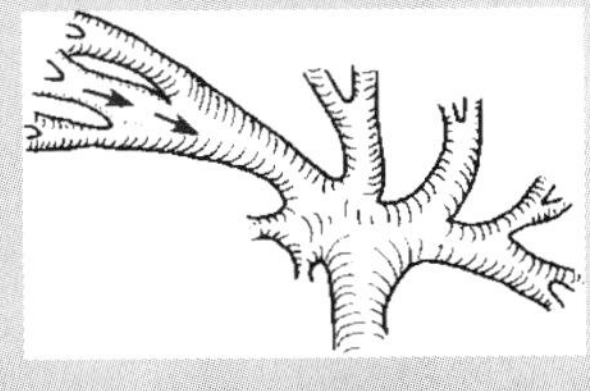

Continued.

The exercises are usually performed 2 to 4 times a day, including before meals and at bedtime. If complications such as chest pain, **dyspnea** (difficulty breathing), or **tachycardia** (rapid heartbeat) occur, the procedure should be stopped immediately and reported to the assigned nurse and physician. Auscultation should be used to locate the involved areas. The therapist avoids percussion over soft tissue areas, such as the kidneys, spine, spleen, and breasts, since this may cause injury to these areas.

Table 29-1 POSITIONS AND PROCEDURES FOR DRAINAGE, PERCUSSION, AND VIBRATION—cont'd

Area and Procedure	Percussion	Vibration	Bronchial Lobe
Right and left lower lobe superior bronchi Have patient lie flat on stomach with pillow under stomach. Percuss and vibrate below scapulas on either side of spine.	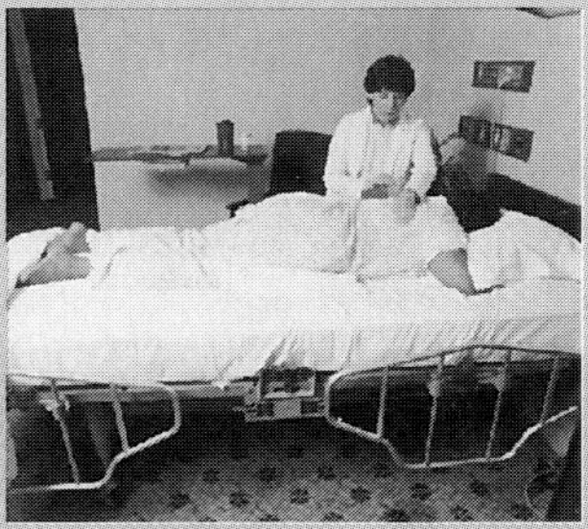	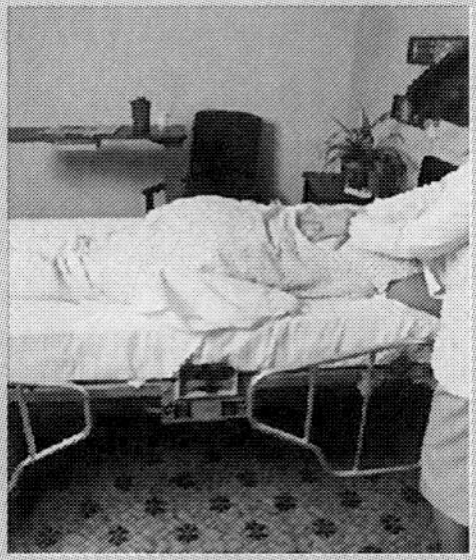	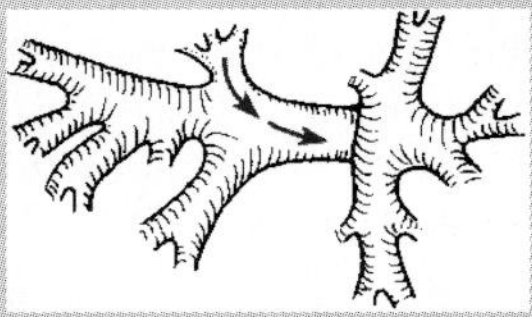
Left and right posterior basal bronchi Have patient lie on stomach in Trendelenburg's position with foot of bed elevated 45-50 cm (18-20 in). Percuss and vibrate over lower posterior ribs on either side of spine.	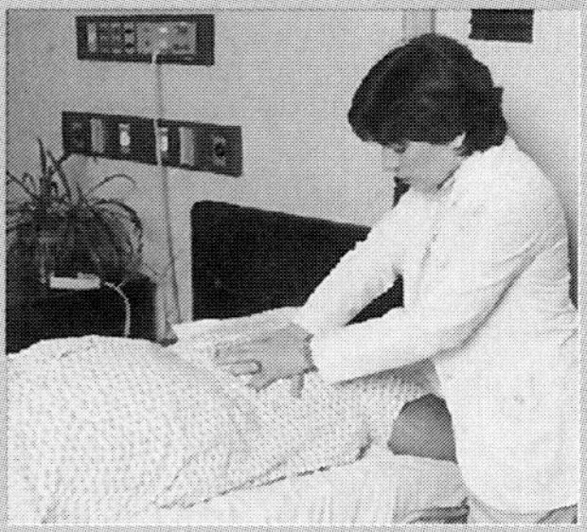	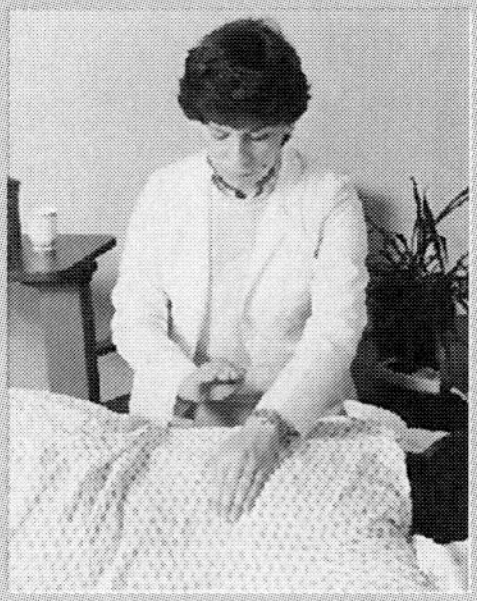	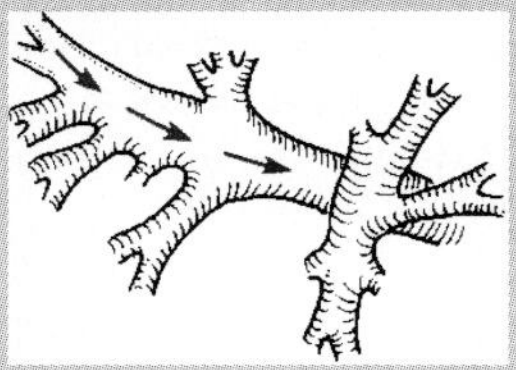

The patient should be monitored throughout the procedure for signs or symptoms of airway obstruction. Patients with chest pain or copious (extremely huge amount) production of mucus need closer assessment to indicate further complications or the need for emergency procedures.

Vaporizer

A **vaporizer** is a device that adds moisture to room air to aid in loosening and thus removing secretions. Distilled or tap water is used to fill the unit, which should be placed near the bedside. Infants and small children with minor upper respiratory conditions may be helped with this treatment. A vaporizer is also helpful for adults and older children. It is used to maintain high humidity to keep the upper respiratory passages moist and to liquefy and loosen secretions for removal by expectoration. The vaporizer is not used as much now as in the past.

A vaporizer requires a medical order, but the nurse may be responsible for the set up and maintenance of the equipment (Skill 29-3). The nurse must also monitor the patient throughout use to ensure that clothing and hair do not become saturated with moisture, which can cause chilling, and to assess the respiratory status of the patient. Patients with excessive secretions should be monitored closely to determine the need for emergency procedures. The nurse should assess the vaporizer often for the level of fluid to ensure the appropriate functioning of the unit.

Oxygen Therapy

Oxygen is an odorless, tasteless, colorless gas that supports combustion. Safety factors regarding the use of oxygen include avoiding the use of electrical equipment, grease or oil (such as petroleum jelly on the lips), and alcohol or ether around oxygen. "No smoking" signs should be posted on the patient's door and the policy enforced for both patient and visitors. A fire extinguisher should be available for use in case of emergency. Do's and don'ts for oxygen use are listed in the box.

Most oxygen is piped into the hospital, but it may also be dispensed from a cylinder or collected from room air by an oxygen concentrator (Fig. 29-1). A

OXYGEN SAFETY PRECAUTIONS

Do's

Place "no smoking" sign on door.
Enforce smoking regulation with visitors and patients.
Keep fire extinguisher nearby.

Don'ts

Use no grease or oil.
Use no alcohol or ether.
Avoid use of ungrounded electrical equipment

flowmeter regulates the amount of oxygen delivered to the patient. Oxygen is usually ordered in liters per minute (L/m). Generally, lower flow rates (1 or 2 L/m) are ordered for a patient with a chronic respiratory problem to avoid overriding the body's internal mechanism that prompts the next respiration. Another patient may have a flow rate much higher. It is not unusual to see an order for 3 to 5 L/m. Oxygen is administered to relieve **hypoxia,** which is inadequate cellular oxygenation that may result from a deficiency in the delivery or use of oxygen at the cellular level. There are several methods of administering oxygen (Skill 29-4). One is by use of the nasal cannula, a two-pronged, plastic tubing device that may be fitted around the patient's head or over the ears (Fig. 29-2).

Oxygen has a drying effect on the mucosa of the nares and air passages. Often, the oxygen is run through a bottle of saline or water before being delivered to the patient. The nurse should ensure that the bottle of liquid is at least two-thirds full.

Care must be taken to prevent the cannula from resting directly on the nasal mucosa. The nurse maintains oxygen, prevents breakdown of the skin on the nares, and ensures a patent airway. The concentration of oxygen administered through a cannula varies from 24% to 40%.

Another method for administering oxygen is the face mask, which covers the nose and mouth and has an elastic piece that fits around the head or over the ears (Fig. 29-3). The use of a mask provides control of oxygen concentration. A patient may feel closed in when wearing the mask, so the nurse must help the patient become adjusted to its use. There are several types of face masks such as a simple face mask without aerosol and a nonrebreathing mask (Fig. 29-4). The concentration of oxygen administered by mask varies from 60% to 100%.

A third method of administering oxygen is the oxygen tent. Its use has greatly decreased in the past years and is seen usually now with the use of a Croupette for small children. A higher oxygen concentration may be administered with this method, and the Croupette provides a constant temperature, usually about 70° F. A child may move about and see out of the tent for diversion (Fig. 29-5). Clothing and bed linens must be frequently changed to keep the patient dry and comfortable.

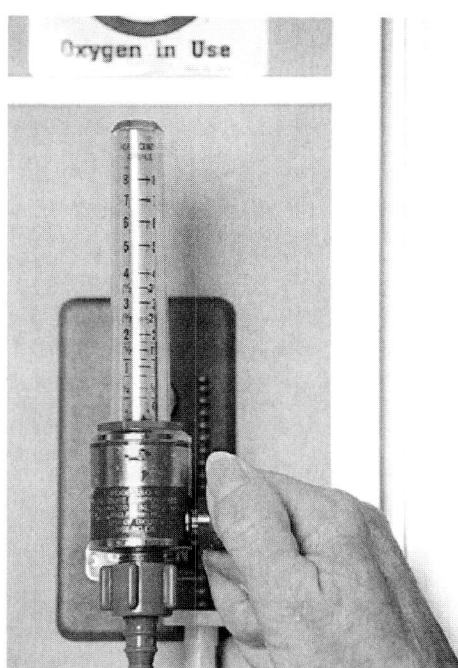

Fig. 29-1 Oxygen flowmeter. (From Potter PA, Perry AG: *Basic nursing: theory and practice,* ed 3, St Louis, Mosby.)

Oxygen may also be administered for a tracheostomy tube through a tracheostomy collar (Fig. 29-6). The flow rate is adjusted to meet the patient's needs. The device fits over the tracheostomy and administers oxygen and humidity. Most patients find this device more comfortable than other devices.

The nurse should also be alert to the signs or symptoms of **oxygen toxicity** (oxygen overdosage that can result in pathologic tissue changes) in the patient receiving oxygen. These changes may include reduced vital capacity or respiratory distress, irritation of the mucous membranes of the respiratory tract, and with increasing toxicity, neurologic symptoms such as confusion and hallucinations. The nurse should notify the physician of these symptoms.

The nurse should frequently assess the function of equipment used to provide oxygen to a patient. The nurse should also ensure that the administration of oxygen is restarted when a patient returns from other areas of a facility or receives other therapies in the room. Measures should be provided to keep the patient's nares clean for comfort and to allow more oxygen to be administered.

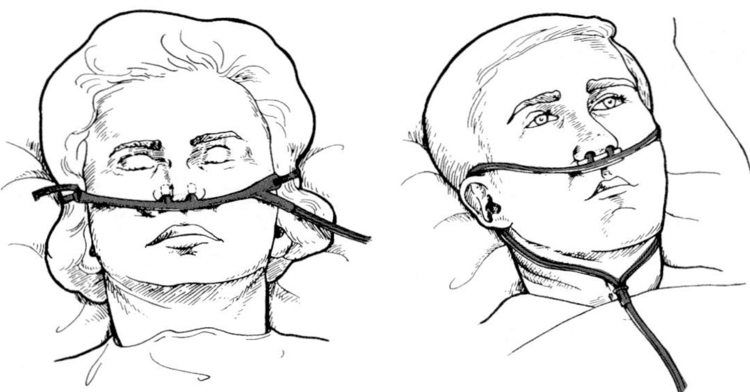

Fig. 29-2 Nasal cannula fits around patient's head or over the ears. (From Perry AG, Potter PA: *Clinical nursing skills and techniques,* ed 3, St Louis, 1994, Mosby.)

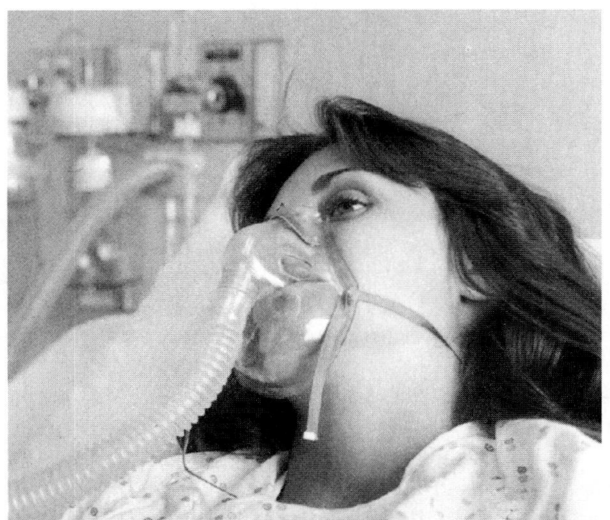

Fig. 29-3 Simple face mask. (From Perry AG, Potter PA: *Clinical nursing skills and techniques,* ed 3, St Louis, 1994, Mosby.)

Suctioning

Oropharyngeal suctioning

Oropharyngeal suctioning is required when a patient is unable to expectorate secretions that accumulate in the back of the throat and mouth. The frequency of suctioning depends on the amount of secretion accumulated. At this point, the nurse should ensure a patent (open) airway for the patient. The area suctioned is from the center of the pharynx to the oral cavity (Skill 29-5). The nurse should suction gently, since these delicate tissues may be easily injured. It is also important to note that suctioning may often break down these tissues.

Patients with copious amounts of secretions should be closely assessed for the need of a tracheostomy. The physician makes the decision to perform a tracheostomy.

An unconscious patient who needs suctioning is placed in a side-lying position toward the nurse. This helps prevent aspiration of secretions. Being unable to breathe is a frightening experience for the patient, and the nurse must reassure the patient that the staff will help. If suctioning becomes necessary, the nurse talks to the patient in a low, calm voice. The nurse may take this opportunity to explain what is being done. If the patient is aware of the procedure, the nurse may simply continue to reassure the patient.

The nurse must recognize the signs and symptoms of respiratory or cardiac arrest, such as the absence of a palpable carotid or femoral pulse, immediate loss of consciousness, absence of breath sounds, limpness, ashen color, excessive use of sternal and intercostal muscles in an effort to breath, and nasal flaring. Cardiopulmonary resuscitation (CPR) may be necessary at any time with a patient who has excessive secretions or is in a serious condition.

Nasopharyngeal suctioning

The physician may also order nasopharyngeal suctioning to remove secretions. If a patient is not alert enough to cooperate, this method of suctioning is used to prevent the patient from biting the suction catheter. In nasopharyngeal suctioning the nurse inserts the catheter through the nose and into the nasopharynx (Skill 29-6). The nurse should monitor for signs or symptoms of airway obstruction throughout the procedure.

Endotracheal suctioning

Performing *endotracheal suctioning* removes deep secretions in the tracheobronchial tree and stimulates deep coughing to help the patient remove secretions. Some patients are unable to readily cough up secretions and must be assisted. Endotracheal suctioning is not performed on patients with bleeding disorders, laryngeal edema or spasm, or esophageal varices (varicose veins of the esophagus) to prevent bleeding. The nurse should take care to

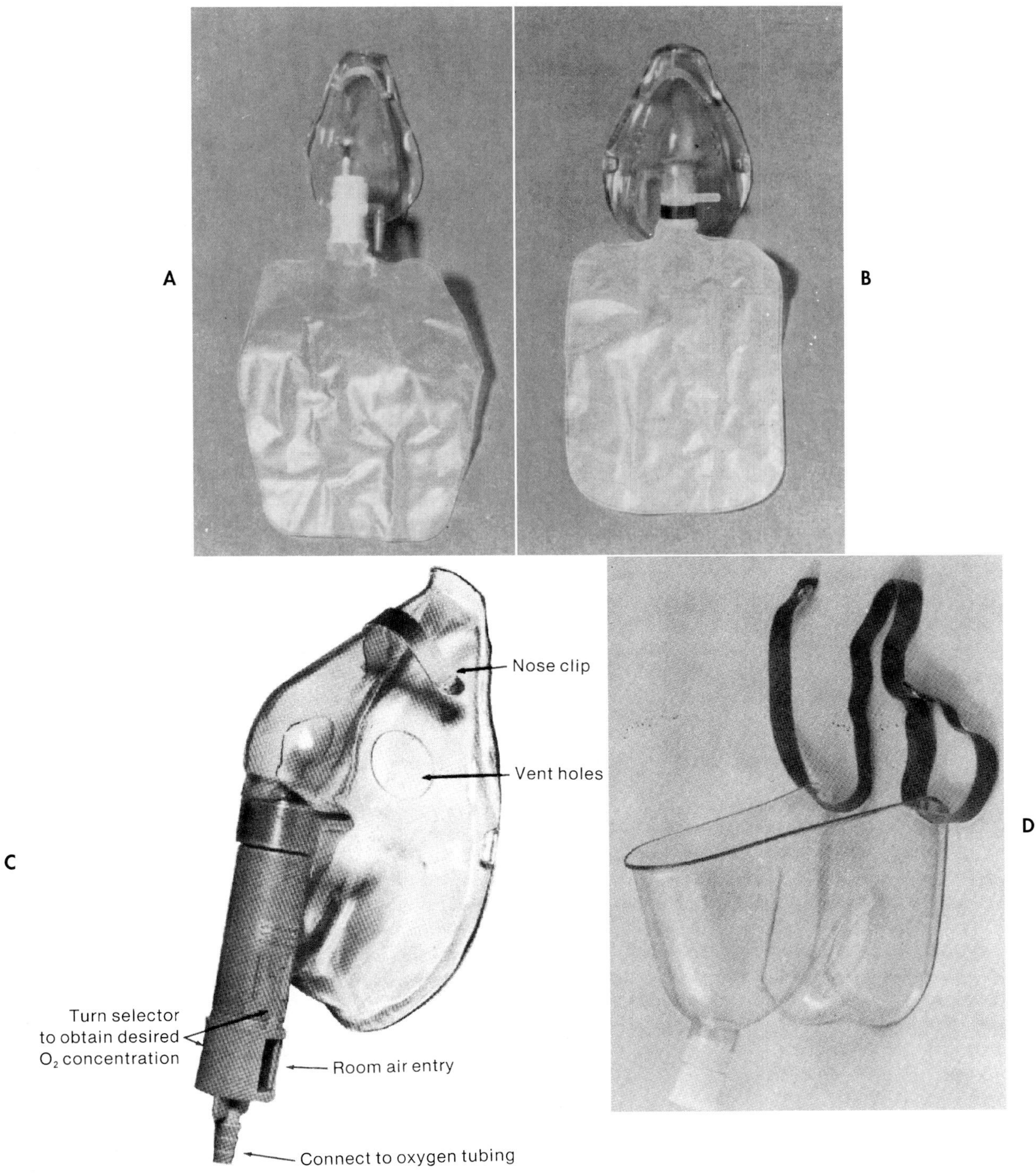

Fig. 29-4 Types of face masks. **A,** Nonrebreathing mask. **B,** Partial rebreathing mask. **C,** Venturi mask. **D,** Face tent. (From Perry AG, Potter PA: *Clinical nursing skills and techniques,* ed 3, St Louis, 1994, Mosby.)

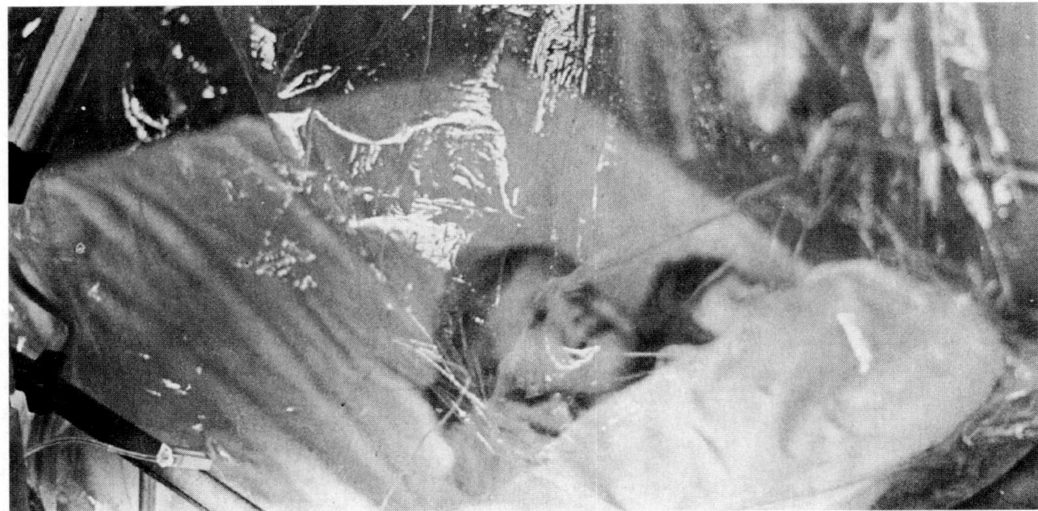

Fig. 29-5 Oxygen tent or Croupette. (From Perry AG, Potter PA: *Clinical nursing skills and techniques,* ed 3, St Louis, 1994, Mosby.)

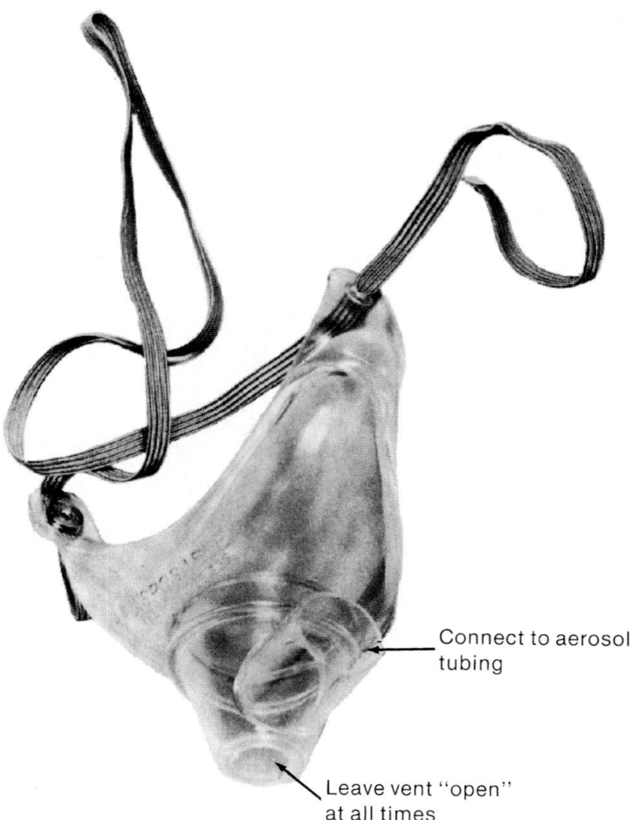

Fig. 29-6 Tracheostomy collar. (From Perry AG, Potter PA: *Clinical nursing skills and techniques,* ed 3, St Louis, 1994, Mosby.)

prevent trauma or injury to the nasal passages (Skill 29-7). For example, the catheter should never be forced if resistance is met when suctioning because hemorrhage could occur through the nasal area. Suctioning too often may cause edema or swelling of the larynx, or voice box, as well as cause tissue damage.

As with the other types of suctioning, the nurse should closely assess the patient who has copious amounts of secretions. The physician may have to perform a tracheostomy. The nurse must remain alert for signs and symptoms of respiratory or cardiac arrest, anxiety, or unconsciousness. The nurse provides reassurance before and during the procedure and is prepared to provide CPR if necessary.

Laryngeal spasms may occur during this type of suctioning. This is an emergency situation in which the larynx closes tightly and does not allow respirations. Immediate medical attention is required, or the patient will die.

Tracheostomy care and suctioning

A **tracheostomy** is a surgical incision made into the trachea for opening the airway. The procedure is performed to relieve an obstruction of the trachea. A tracheostomy tube is inserted into the trachea so that the patient can breathe. This procedure is nearly always performed in an emergency situation to save a patient's life. Occasionally, it is an elective procedure in which the patient must have time to heal or in which an airway must be maintained during healing.

The nurse performs tracheostomy care and suctioning to maintain a patent airway (Skill 29-8). Care includes keeping the skin around the tube clean and dry, preventing skin breakdown (see Chapter 21), and preventing infection (see Chapter 14) (Fig. 29-7). Tracheostomy stoma care is generally administered every 8 hours or when necessary. It includes cleansing the area around the stoma, cleansing the tube, and replacing the gauze dressing

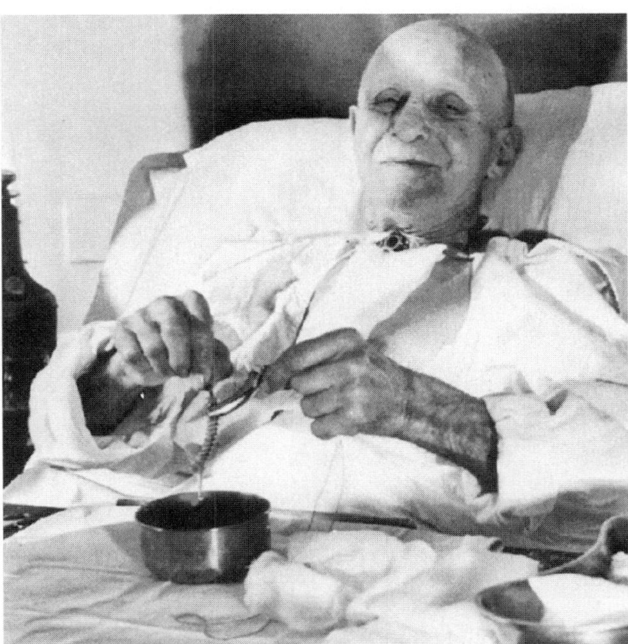

Fig. 29-7 This 82-year-old man cares for his own tracheostomy tube. He is about to clean the inner tube with a small tube brush.

around the stoma and tube. The items used in tracheostomy care are seen in Fig. 29-8. Tracheostomy suctioning is provided as necessary and involves suctioning secretions from the tube and portions of the bronchial tree. However, suctioning should be administered infrequently to prevent tissue damage.

There are two main types of tracheostomy tubes: cuffed and noncuffed (Fig. 29-9). Tracheostomy tubes may be made of metal, such as silver, but today they are more likely to be made of plastic. Unless contraindicated, a cuffed tracheostomy tube is inflated if the patient receives positive-pressure ventilation, which is any technique in which compressed air is delivered to the respiratory passages at greater than ambient pressure. If the patient has a problem with aspiration, the cuff remains inflated. The cuff is maintained inflated at 18 mm Hg to prevent obstruction of capillary circulation, which results in tissue necrosis (death). Parts of the noncuffed tracheostomy tube consist of the outer tube and the cannula (semiflexible tube that fits inside the outer tube). The obturator is another part of the tube. It is the device that fits inside the tracheostomy tube during insertion to ease passage and to prevent displaced tissues from blocking the opening. The cuffed tube includes the outer tube with the cuff and tube for inflation, cannula, and obturator (Fig. 29-10).

The reasons for performing a tracheostomy include obstruction of the mouth or throat, edema, trauma from injuries causing severe respiratory difficulty, and radical surgery in the area of the trachea. Tracheostomy patients can use paper and pencil to communicate until they can hold their fingers over the tracheostomy tubes. Special devices are also available to produce artificial speech if the vocal chords have been removed (Fig. 29-11).

Closed Chest Drainage

Normal breathing depends on what is referred to as ***negative pressure*** (pressure inside the chest cavity lower than pressure outside the body.) The outside pressure is called *atmospheric pressure.* If the chest is opened, such as in surgical intervention or in an open chest wound, the negative pressure becomes lower and causes the lung to collapse. ***Pneumothorax*** is the medical term for a collapsed lung in which a collection of air or gas occurs in the pleural cavity.

The procedure used to reexpand the lung is referred to as *closed chest drainage.* The physician inserts a chest tube into the **pleural space** (space between the lungs and thorax), sutures the tube to the skin, and then connects it to some type of drainage system. Often, this is an underwater-seal drainage method. The underwater-seal drainage system works by attaching the chest tubing or catheter to one bottle using a one-way valve. The tip of the tube is placed at least 1 inch below water level (Fig. 29-12, *A*). The water in the bottle acts as a seal and allows air and fluid to drain from the chest, preventing air from reentering the tip of the tube.

There are three types of systems used for chest drainage. In one system the water fluctuates as the patient breathes; it rises when the patient inhales and lowers when the patient exhales. If constant bubbling occurs, there may be leakage of air from the lung or a leak in the drainage system.

Another type of chest drainage system is called the *two-bottle system.* This system uses the same water-seal chamber as the system previously described as well as a fluid-collection bottle. When the pleural fluid drains, the water-seal system is not affected, and suction can be provided by a wall unit (Fig. 29-12, *B*).

The third type of chest drainage system is the three-bottle system, which is similar to the two-bottle system but adds a third bottle to control the amount of suction applied. Suction is controlled by varying the depth to which the tip of the glass stem is placed under water. The wall suction unit makes and maintains negative pressure throughout the system (Fig. 29-12, *C*).

Many commercial and disposable chest drainage devices that use the water-seal principle are available (Fig. 29-13). The closed chest drainage is provided by a single enclosed unit. Generally, these units use the three-bottle system. The chamber for chest drainage is calibrated for easy measurement.

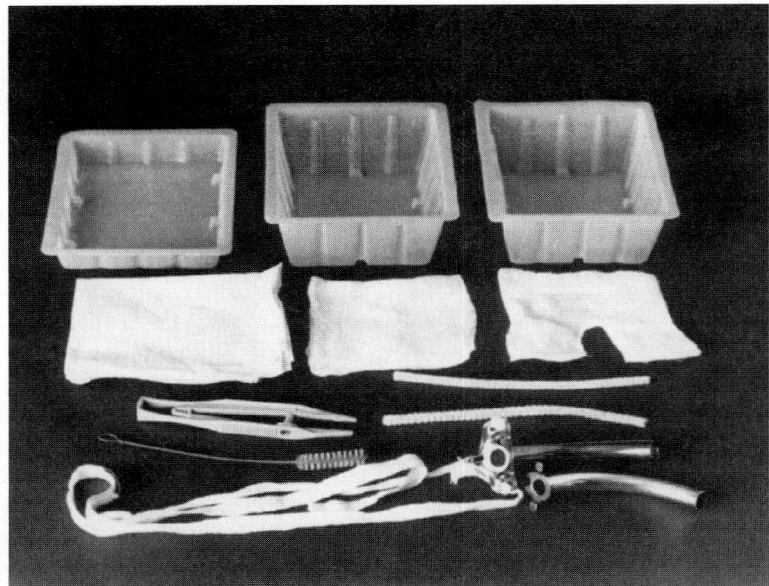

Fig. 29-8 Disposable tracheostomy care kit.

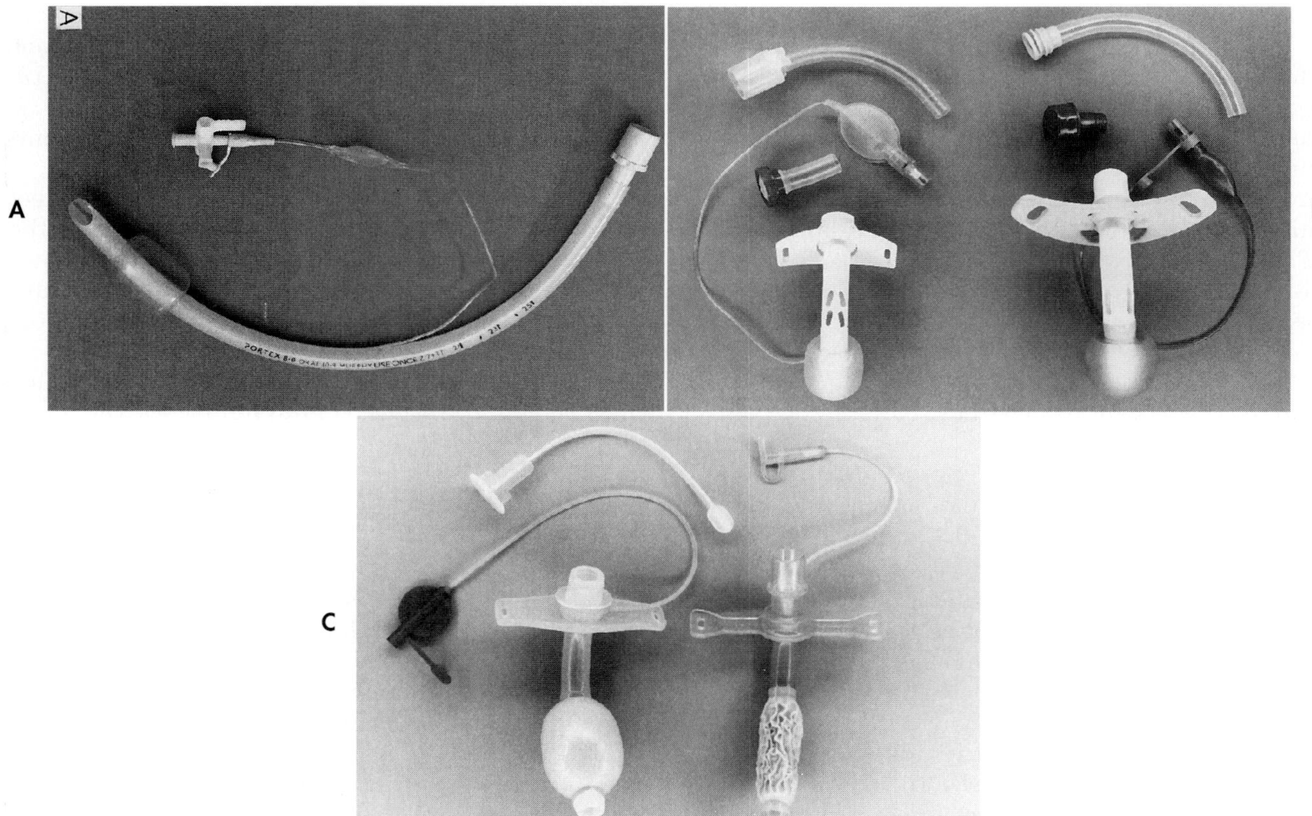

Fig. 29-9 Types of endotracheal and tracheostomy tubes. **A,** Disposable oral/nasal tube with cuff, stopcock, and pilot balloon. **B,** Shiley and Portex fenestrated tracheostomy tube with cuff, inner cannula, decannulation plug, and pilot balloon. **C,** Bivona (Fome-Cuf) tracheostomy tube with foam cuff and obturator (one cuff is deflated on tracheostomy tube). (From Lewis SM, Collier IC: *Medical-surgical nursing: assessment and management of clinical problems,* ed 3, St Louis, 1992, Mosby.)

The nurse maintains the chest drainage system (Skill 29-9). The patient is encouraged to move and learn to compensate with the chest tube in place while relieving the patient's fear that normal, controlled movement should not dislodge the tube. The nurse maintains the patient's comfort. The chest tube may be painful with movement. There is controversy regarding stripping the chest tubes, which means to force secretions out by pushing down the tubing, holding the tube pressed closed (pinched off) by the thumb and index finger and then reversing the hands and repeating the process. Some research indicates this may cause excessive negative pressure and that the chest tube may damage the pleura. The nurse follows the medical order and agency policy regarding this portion of the procedure.

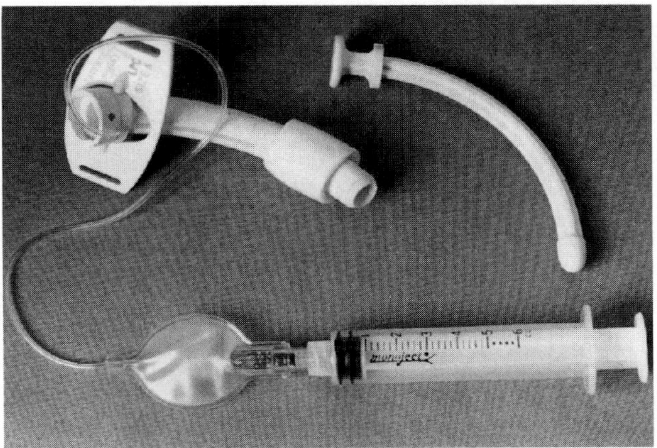

Fig. 29-10 Parts of tracheostomy tube. (From Perry AG, Potter PA: *Clinical nursing skills and techniques,* ed 3, St Louis, 1994, Mosby.)

The nurse should also assess the insertion site of the chest tube for signs of subcutaneous emphysema. **Subcutaneous emphysema** occurs when air or another gas is present under the skin, specifically in the subcutaneous layer. The tissue may be painful to the touch, and the nurse may hear crackling or snapping as the air moves under touch. The face, neck, and chest may become edematous. In severe cases the patient becomes dyspneic and cyanotic (bluish). The nurse should report any signs of subcutaneous emphysema immediately. The physician may need to change the positioning of the chest tube, and incision of the affected skin may be necessary.

Although chest tubes rarely become dislodged or disconnected, the nurse should be prepared to provide emergency assistance if it occurs. The nurse should immediately place the end of a disconnected tube into water, thus completing a seal once again. The registered nurse can then reconnect the tube using a sterile connector. If the chest tube becomes dislodged, the nurse can provide emergency treatment by placing petrolatum gauze over the opening to create a seal. Petrolatum gauze should be kept at the bedside of the patient with a chest tube at all times for this emergency.

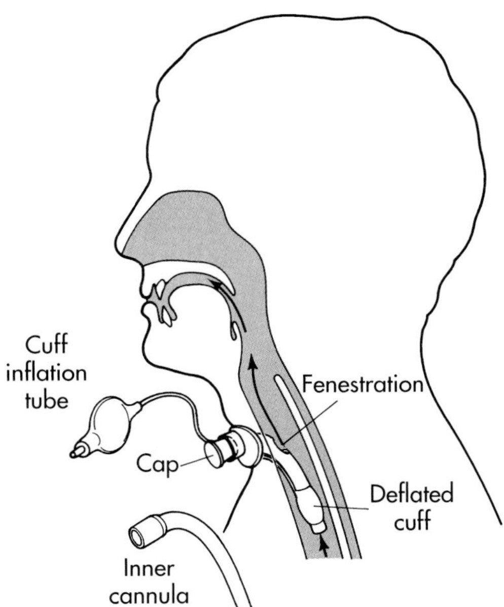

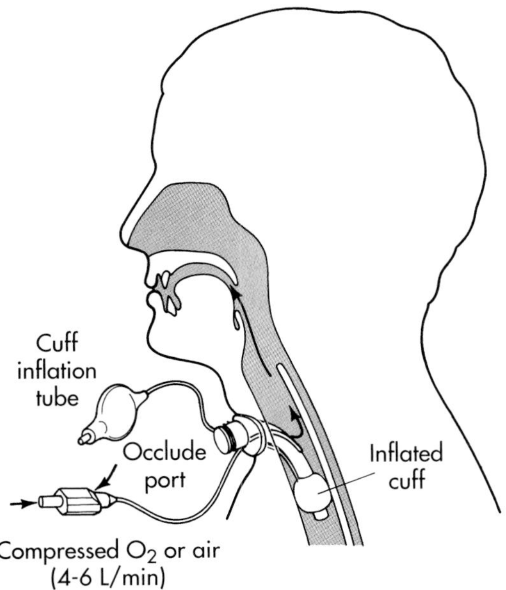

Fig. 29-11 Speaking tracheostomy tube. One tubing is used for cuff inflation. The second tubing is connected to a source of compressed air or oxygen. When the port on the second tubing is occluded, air flows up over the vocal cords, allowing speech with an inflated cuff. (From Lewis SM, Collier IC: *Medical-surgical nursing: assessment and management of clinical problems,* ed 3, St Louis, 1992, Mosby.)

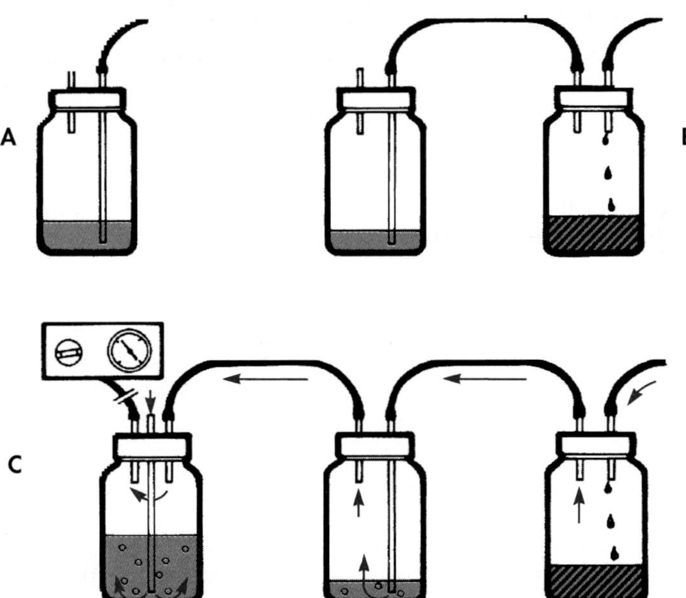

Fig. 29-12 Three types of chest tube bottle systems. **A,** One-bottle system. **B,** Two-bottle system. **C,** Three-bottle system with suction. (From Christensen BL, Kockrow EO: *Foundations of nursing,* ed 2, St Louis, 1995, Mosby.)

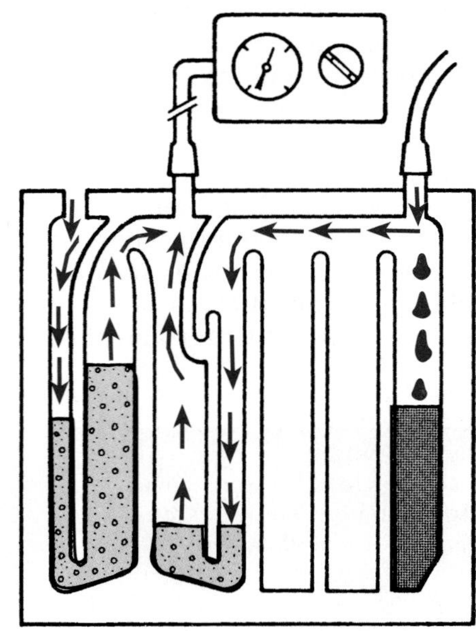

Fig. 29-13 Disposable, commercial chest drainage system. (From Perry AG, Potter PA: *Clinical nursing skills and techniques,* ed 3, St Louis, 1994, Mosby.)

■ NURSING CARE PLAN ■

IMPAIRED GAS EXCHANGE

Mr. L, age 78, was brought to the emergency room with air hunger, cyanosis, and confusion, and he is anxious. He has been admitted for further treatment. Mr. L has a history of emphysema.

NURSING DIAGNOSIS

Impaired gas exchange related to altered oxygen supply as evidenced by severe dyspnea, decreased mental acuity, restlessness, and tachycardia

GOALS

- Patient will have normal arterial blood gas levels.
- Patient will have as near-normal activity as possible.

EXPECTED OUTCOMES

- Patient maintains respiratory rate with +5 of baseline.
- Patient has normal breath sounds.

NURSING INTERVENTIONS

- Assess and record pulmonary status every 2 to 4 hr or more often as necessary.
- Monitor vital signs and cardiac rhythm at least every 4 hr.
- Position patient for best gas exchange.
- Administer medications to improve oxygenation.

EVALUATION

- Patient's respiratory status remains within established limits.
- Patient performs activities of daily living without dyspnea.
- Patient has normal breath sounds.

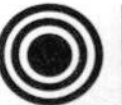

SKILL 29-1 USING INCENTIVE SPIROMETRY

Steps	Rationale
1. Obtain equipment: ▪ Spirometer ▪ Tissues ▪ Emesis basin ▪ Mouth care supplies ▪ Clean gloves.	Helps organize procedure.
2. Refer to medical record, care plan, or Kardex for special interventions.	Provides basis for care.
3. Wash hands and don clean gloves according to agency policy and guidelines from Centers for Disease Control and Prevention and Occupational Safety and Health Administration.	Helps prevent cross-contamination.
4. Introduce self.	Decreases anxiety level.
5. Identify patient by identification band.	Identifies correct patient for procedure.
6. Explain procedure to patient.	Seeks cooperation and decreases anxiety.
7. Raise bed to comfortable working level.	Provides safety for nurse.
8. Arrange for patient privacy.	Shows respect for patient.
9. Assess respiratory status.	Determines patency of airway and need for spirometry.
10. Place patient in semi-Fowler's position unless contraindicated.	Assists respirations.
11. Teach steps for using spirometer, especially before surgery.	Helps patient follow instructions when groggy from anesthesia or pain medication.
12. Request that patient insert mouthpiece and inhale slowly and deeply (Fig. 29-14).	Teaches best method for loosening secretions. Encourages patient to obtain maximal inspiration.
13. Have patient repeat steps required number of times according to medical orders or agency policy.	Increases loosening of secretions.
14. Offer mouth care.	Removes foul taste and reduces transmission of microorganisms.
15. Clean and store spirometer.	Prevents growth of microorganisms and contamination of other personnel.
16. Dispose of waste materials.	Helps prevent spread of microorganisms.
17. Remove gloves and wash hands.	Prevents cross-contamination.
18. Document.	Documents procedure and patient's response.

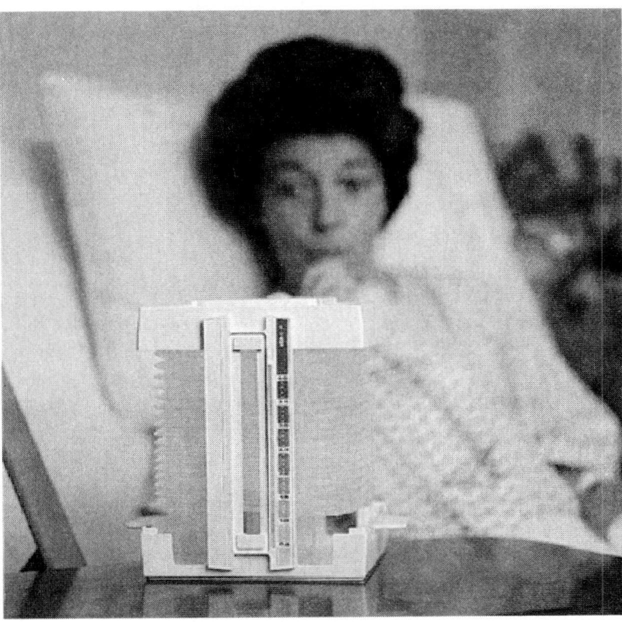

Fig. 29-14 Volume-oriented spirometer. (From Potter PA, Perry AG: *Basic nursing: theory and practice,* ed 3, St Louis, 1995, Mosby.)

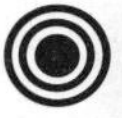

SKILL 29-2 PERFORMING POSTURAL DRAINAGE AND PERCUSSION

Steps	Rationale
1. Obtain equipment: ▪ Adjustable hospital bed ▪ Emesis basin ▪ Tissues ▪ Stethoscope ▪ Straight chair ▪ Watch with sweep second hand ▪ Clean gloves	Helps organize procedure.
2. Refer to medical record, care plan, or Kardex for special interventions.	Provides basis for care.
3. Introduce self.	Decreases anxiety level.
4. Identify patient by identification band.	Identifies correct patient for procedure.
5. Explain procedure to patient.	Seeks cooperation and decreases anxiety.
6. Wash hands and don clean gloves according to agency policy and guidelines from Centers for Disease Control and Prevention and Occupational Safety and Health Administration.	Helps prevent cross-contamination.
7. Prepare patient for intervention.	
a. Close door to room or pull curtain.	Provides privacy.
b. Drape for procedure if necessary.	Prevents exposure of patient.
8. Raise bed to appropriate level for performance of procedure.	Provides safety for patient and nurse.
9. Arrange for patient privacy.	Shows respect for patient.
10. Assess respiratory status, including breath sounds.	Determines areas where drainage is needed.
11. Position patient in ordered positions.	Assists drainage of secretions.
12. Percuss chest wall and back with cupped hand or percussion device (see Table 29-1).	Helps dislodge secretions.
13. Vibrate chest wall by placing one hand over the other while patient slowly exhales (see Table 29-1).	Helps dislodge secretions.
14. Provide rest period.	Prevents fatigue and allows completion of therapy.
15. Repeat procedure as prescribed.	Increases production of secretions.
16. Dispose of waste materials.	Helps prevent spread of microorganisms.
17. Remove gloves and wash hands.	Prevents cross-contamination.
18. Document.	Documents procedure and patient's response.

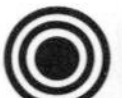

SKILL 29-3 USING THE VAPORIZER

Steps	Rationale
1. Obtain equipment: ▪ Vaporizer ▪ Distilled water ▪ Clean gloves	Helps organize procedure.
2. Refer to medical record, care plan, or Kardex for special interventions.	Provides basis for care.
3. Wash hands and don clean gloves according to agency policy and guidelines from Centers for Disease Control and Prevention and Occupational Safety and Health Administration.	Helps prevent cross-contamination.

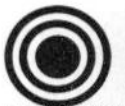

SKILL 29-3 USING THE VAPORIZER—cont'd

Steps	Rationale
4. **Introduce self.**	Decreases anxiety level.
5. **Identify patient by identification band.**	Identifies correct patient for procedure.
6. **Explain procedure to patient.**	Seeks cooperation and decreases anxiety.
7. **Arrange for patient privacy.**	Shows respect for patient.
8. **Assess respiratory status.**	Determines patency of airway and need for spirometry.
9. **Fill vaporizer with distilled water up to indicated line.**	Prepares vaporizer for use.
10. **Direct flow of mist toward patient but not directly on patient.**	Gives maximal therapy without making clothing wet.
11. **Adjust flow and temperature.**	Provides appropriate therapy and patient comfort.
12. **Monitor patient and change moist clothing as necessary.**	Provides comfort and prevents chilling.
13. **Remove gloves and wash hands.**	Prevents cross-contamination.
14. **Document.**	Documents procedure and patient's response.

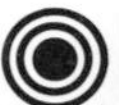

SKILL 29-4 ADMINISTERING OXYGEN

Steps	Rationale
1. **Obtain equipment:** ▪ Device to be used to administer oxygen ▪ Source of oxygen ▪ Flowmeter ▪ Humidifier bottle if applicable ▪ "No smoking" signs ▪ Nebulizer and distilled water ▪ Tracheostomy device if needed ▪ Clean gloves	Helps organize procedure.
2. **Refer to medical record, care plan, or Kardex for special interventions.**	Provides basis for care.
3. **Wash hands and don clean gloves according to agency policy and guidelines from Centers for Disease Control and Prevention and Occupational Safety and Health Administration.**	Helps prevent cross-contamination.
4. **Introduce self.**	Decreases anxiety level.
5. **Identify patient by identification band.**	Identifies correct patient for procedure.
6. **Explain procedure to patient.**	Seeks cooperation and decreases anxiety.
7. **Raise bed to comfortable working level unless emergency exists.**	Provides safety for nurse.
8. **Arrange for patient privacy.**	Shows respect for patient.
9. **Assess respiratory status.**	Determines patency of airway and need for oxygen.
10. **Assess laboratory reports of arterial blood gas levels.**	Determines need for oxygen.
11. **Apply appropriate type of oxygen (Fig. 29-15).**	Physician determines type.
12. **Provide oral care frequently as needed.**	Provides patient comfort and moistens mucous membranes.
13. **Remove gloves and wash hands.**	Prevents cross-contamination.
14. **Document.**	Documents procedure and patient's response.

Continued.

SKILL 29-4 ADMINISTERING OXYGEN—cont'd

Steps	Rationale

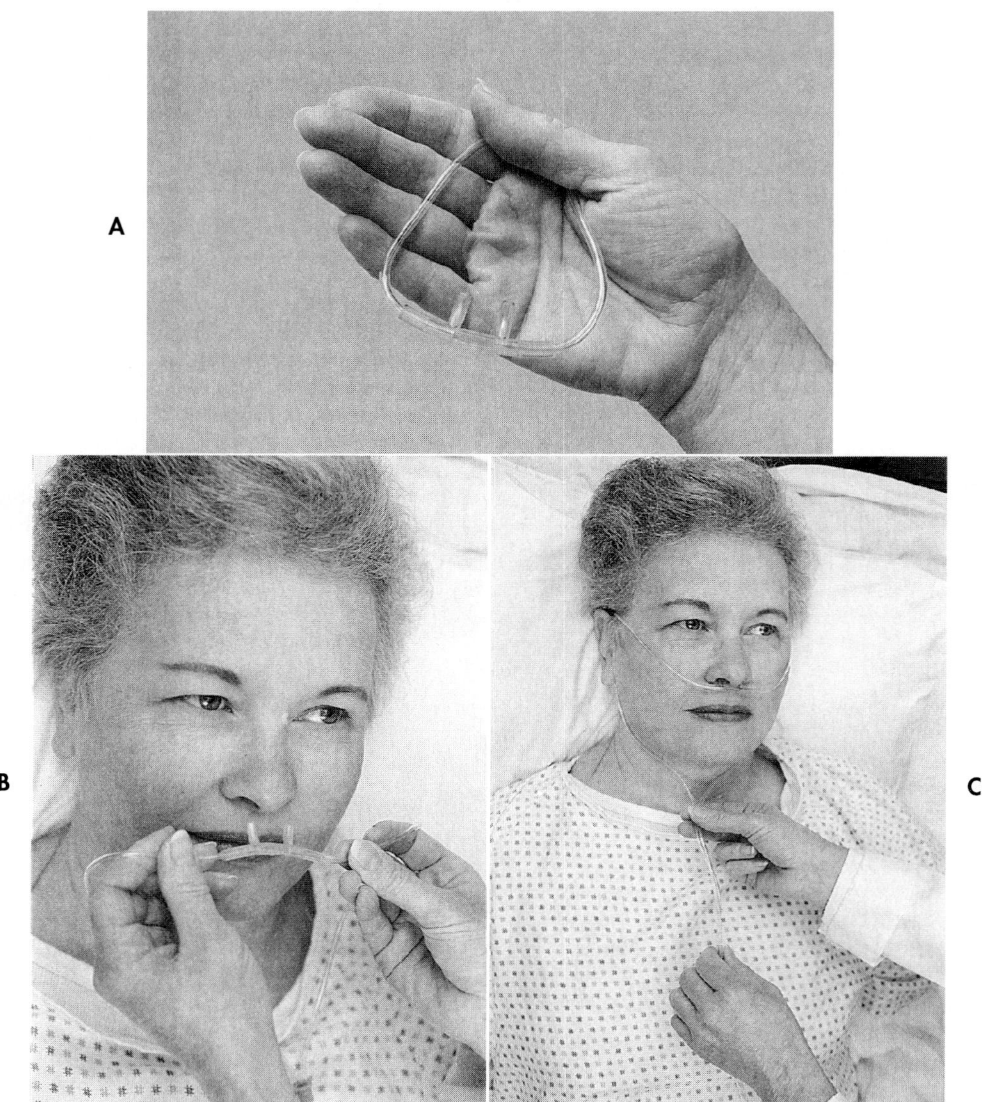

Fig. 29-15 Applying oxygen. **A,** Nasal cannula. **B,** Placing tips of cannula into patient's nares. **C,** Adjusting elastic headband or plastic slide until cannula fits snugly and comfortably. (From Potter PA, Perry AG: *Basic nursing: theory and practice,* ed 3, St Louis, 1995, Mosby.)

SKILL 29-5 PERFORMING OROPHARYNGEAL SUCTIONING

Steps	Rationale
1. **Obtain equipment:** ▪ Suction apparatus, either wall or portable type ▪ Sterile suction catheter with thumb-control tip ▪ Sterile water and normal saline ▪ Sterile gloves ▪ Clean gloves ▪ Clean, water-repellant gown, goggles, and mask	Helps organize procedure.

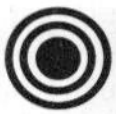

SKILL 29-5 PERFORMING OROPHARYNGEAL SUCTIONING—cont'd

Steps	Rationale
2. Refer to medical record, care plan, or Kardex for special interventions.	Provides basis for care.
3. Wash hands and don clean gloves according to agency policy and guidelines from Centers for Disease Control and Prevention and Occupational Safety and Health Administration.	Helps prevent cross-contamination.
4. Introduce self.	Decreases anxiety level.
5. Identify patient by identification band.	Identifies correct patient for procedure.
6. Explain procedure to patient.	Seeks cooperation and decreases anxiety.
7. Raise bed to comfortable working level.	Provides safety for nurse.
8. Arrange for patient privacy.	Shows respect for patient.
9. Assess respiratory status.	Determines patency of airway and need for suctioning.
10. Assess for indications of airway obstruction.	Indicates need for suctioning (Secretions in oropharynx produce gurgling sound.)
11. Select appropriate suction pressure: ▪ Adults: 110-115 mm Hg ▪ Children: 95-110 mm Hg ▪ Infants: 50-95 mm Hg	Prevents trauma to tissues from too much pressure.
12. Pour sterile solutions into sterile containers.	Maintains sterile technique.
13. Attach suction catheter to suction apparatus (Fig. 29-16), touching only thumb-control end and leaving suction tip in package. Turn suction machine on.	Prepares equipment for suctioning and maintains sterile technique.
14. Measure approximate length of catheter to insert by noting distance from patient's mouth to ear lobe and from ear lobe to Adam's apple.	Ensures appropriate placement of catheter tip.
15. Remove one clean glove and replace with sterile glove.	Allows nurse to use sterile glove to touch sterile tip of suction tube.
16. Hold suction tip in sterile hand, and thumb-control end in clean hand.	Maintains sterile technique.
17. Lubricate suction end by inserting into sterile solution or water-soluble lubricant.	Prevents tissue trauma and pain.
18. Insert suction catheter gently into one side of mouth.	Avoids stimulating cough reflex.
19. Glide catheter toward oropharynx. Stop procedure if resistance is met.	Ensures appropriate placement of catheter. (Resistance may indicate stricture of oropharynx.)

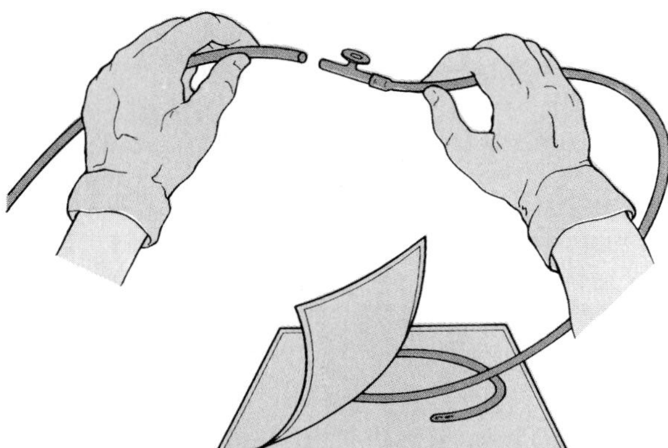

Fig. 29-16 Attaching suction catheter to suction apparatus. (From Perry AG, Potter PA: *Clinical nursing skills and techniques,* ed 3, St Louis, 1994, Mosby.)

Continued.

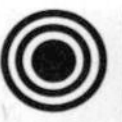

SKILL 29-5 PERFORMING OROPHARYNGEAL SUCTIONING—cont'd

Steps	Rationale
20. Place thumb of clean hand over thumb-control tip, rotating slightly and twisting catheter gently back and forth, as it is withdrawn.	Allows suction to occur and secretions to be removed. Also prevents tissue trauma and hemorrhage.
21. Limit suction time to 10-15 sec by releasing thumb-control.	Allows patient to breathe and prevents tissue trauma. Allows approximately same amount of time patient would normally breathe.
22. Allow patient to rest and repeat suctioning if necessary.	Allows further oxygenation.
23. Rinse suction catheter between suctionings by running sterile saline or water through tubing.	Cleanses suction tubing.
24. Allow patient to cough deeply.	Brings up more secretions to suction.
25. Suction between gum line and under tongue.	Removes final secretions from oral cavity.
26. Rinse catheter with sterile water.	Cleans suction tubing.
27. Discard contaminated suction catheter.	Prevents contamination of other health care workers.
28. Remove gloves and wash hands.	Prevents cross-contamination.
29. Replace sterile suction catheter for next use.	Keeps catheter ready for emergency use.
30. Document.	Documents procedure and patient's response.

SKILL 29-6 PERFORMING NASOPHARYNGEAL SUCTIONING

Steps	Rationale
1. Obtain equipment: ▪ Suction apparatus, either wall or portable type ▪ Sterile suction catheter with thumb-control tip ▪ Sterile water and sterile saline ▪ Sterile gloves ▪ Clean gloves ▪ Clean, water-repellant gown, goggles, and mask	Helps organize procedure.
2. Refer to medical record, care plan, or Kardex for special interventions.	Provides basis for care.
3. Wash hands and don clean gloves according to agency policy and guidelines from Centers for Disease Control and Prevention and Occupational Safety and Health Administration.	Helps prevent cross-contamination.
4. Introduce self.	Decreases anxiety level.
5. Identify patient by identification band.	Identifies correct patient for procedure.
6. Explain procedure to patient.	Seeks cooperation and decreases anxiety.
7. Raise bed to comfortable working level.	Provides safety for nurse.
8. Arrange for patient privacy.	Shows respect for patient.
9. Assess respiratory status.	Determines patency of airway and need for suctioning.
10. Assess for indications of obstruction.	Indicates need for suctioning. (Secretions in nasopharynx produce gurgling sound.)
11. Select appropriate suction pressure: ▪ Adults: 110-115 mm Hg ▪ Children: 95-110 mm Hg ▪ Infants: 50-95 mm Hg	Prevents trauma to tissues from too much pressure.
12. Pour sterile solutions into sterile containers.	Maintains sterile technique.
13. Attach suction apparatus to thumb-control end of suction catheter without touching suction end of catheter.	Prepares equipment and maintains sterile technique.

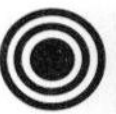

SKILL 29-6 PERFORMING NASOPHARYNGEAL SUCTIONING—cont'd

Steps	Rationale
14. Measure approximate length of catheter by noting distance from patient's nares to earlobe and from earlobe to Adam's apple.	Ensures appropriate placement of catheter tip.
15. Leave suction end of catheter in sterile package. Turn on suction machine.	Maintains sterile technique.
16. Remove clean gloves and don sterile glove on dominant hand.	Maintains sterile technique.
17. Handle suction end of catheter with sterile hand. Handle thumb-control end with clean hand.	Maintains sterile technique.
18. Lubricate suction catheter by inserting end into sterile solution.	Prevents tissue trauma.
19. Insert suction catheter gently through nose into nasopharynx (Fig. 29-17). Stop procedure if resistance is met at lower point.	Permits suctioning of this area. Indicate stricture or another obstruction.
20. Place thumb over thumb-control, rotating slightly and twisting catheter back and forth as it is withdrawn.	Allows suction to occur and removes secretions and prevents tissue trauma or hemorrhage.
21. Limit suction time to 10-15 sec. Remove thumb from thumb-control every 2-3 sec. Never suction during insertion of catheter.	Allows patient to breathe normally and prevents tissue trauma or hemorrhage.
22. Allow patient to rest and repeat suctioning as necessary. Administer oxygen between suctionings, if ordered.	Allows further oxygenation.
23. Allow patient to cough deeply.	Often brings up more secretions.
24. Suction between gum line and under tongue.	Removes final secretions from oral cavity.
25. Rinse catheter by suctioning sterile solution through tubing after each suctioning.	Maintains patency of tubing.
26. Discard contaminated suction catheter.	Prevents contamination of other health care workers.
27. Arrange sterile suction catheter for next use.	Keeps catheter ready for use immediately, if necessary.
28. Provide oral care as needed.	Provides patient comfort and removes foul tastes.
29. Remove gloves and wash hands.	Prevents cross-contamination.
30. Document.	Documents procedure and patient's response.

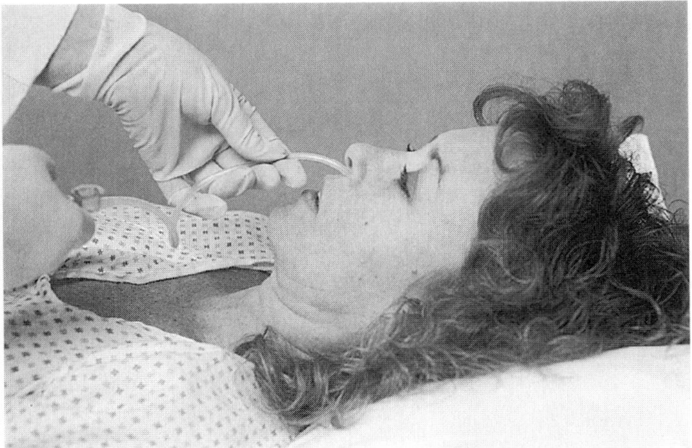

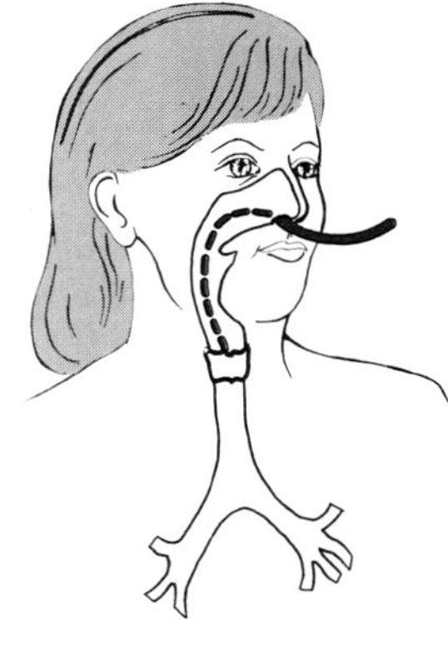

Fig. 29-17 Nasopharyngeal suctioning. (From Potter PA, Perry AG: *Basic nursing: theory and practice,* ed 3, St Louis, 1995, Mosby.)

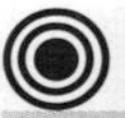

SKILL 29-7 PERFORMING ENDOTRACHEAL SUCTIONING

Steps	Rationale
1. Obtain equipment: ▪ Suction apparatus, either wall or portable type ▪ Sterile suction catheter with thumb-control tip ▪ Sterile water and sterile saline ▪ Sterile gloves ▪ Clean gloves ▪ Clean, water-repellant gown, goggles, and mask	Helps organize procedure.
2. Refer to medical record, care plan, or Kardex for special interventions.	Provides basis for care.
3. Wash hands and don clean gloves according to agency policy and guidelines from Centers for Disease Control and Prevention and Occupational Safety and Health Administration.	Helps prevent cross-contamination.
4. Introduce self.	Decreases anxiety level.
5. Identify patient by identification band.	Identifies correct patient for procedure.
6. Explain procedure to patient.	Seeks cooperation and decreases anxiety.
7. Raise bed to comfortable working level.	Provides safety for nurse.
8. Arrange for patient privacy.	Shows respect for patient.
9. Assess respiratory status.	Determines patency of airway and need for suctioning.
10. Assess for indications of airway obstruction.	Indicates need for suctioning. (Secretions in nasopharynx produce gurgling sound.)
11. Select appropriate suction pressure: ▪ Adults: 110-115 mm Hg ▪ Children: 95-110 mm Hg ▪ Infants: 50-95 mm Hg	Prevents trauma to tissues from too much pressure.
12. Pour sterile solutions into sterile containers.	Maintains sterile technique.
13. Attach suction apparatus to thumb-control end of suction catheter without touching suction end and leave suction end of catheter in sterile package. Turn on suction machine.	Maintains sterile technique and prepares equipment.
14. Measure approximate length of catheter needed by noting distance from patient's nares to earlobe and from earlobe to midsternum.	Ensures appropriate placement of catheter tip.
15. Remove one clean glove and replace with sterile glove.	Maintains sterile technique.
16. Hold thumb-control end with clean hand and suction end of catheter with dominant sterile hand.	Maintains sterile technique.
17. Lubricate catheter by inserting suction end into sterile solution.	Prevents tissue trauma or hemorrhage.
18. Insert suction catheter gently through nose into trachea. Stop procedure if resistance is met.	Permits suctioning of correct area. Prevents tissue trauma and hemorrhage.
19. Place thumb over thumb-control end, rotating slightly and twisting catheter gently back and forth as it is withdrawn.	Allows suction to occur and removes secretions. Prevents tissue trauma and hemorrhage.
20. Limit suction time to 10-15 sec and lift thumb from control every 2-3 sec. Do not suction during insertion.	Allows patient to breathe and prevents tissue trauma and hemorrhage.
21. Allow patient to rest and repeat suctioning if necessary.	Allows further oxygenation.
22. Allow patient to cough deeply.	Often brings up more secretions.
23. Suction between gum line and under tongue.	Removes final secretions from oral cavity.

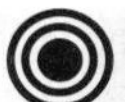

SKILL 29-7 PERFORMING ENDOTRACHEAL SUCTIONING—cont'd

Steps	Rationale
24. Rinse catheter by suctioning sterile solution after each suctioning.	Maintains tubing patency.
25. Discard contaminated suction catheter.	Prevents contamination of other health care workers.
26. Dispose of other waste materials.	Helps prevent spread of microorganisms.
27. Arrange sterile suction catheter for next use.	Keeps catheter ready for immediate use if needed.
28. Provide oral care.	Provides patient comfort and removes foul tastes.
29. Remove gloves and wash hands.	Prevents cross-contamination.
30. Document.	Documents procedure and patient's response.

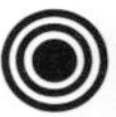

SKILL 29-8 PERFORMING TRACHEOSTOMY CARE AND SUCTIONING

Steps	Rationale

1. Obtain equipment:
▪ Sterile, disposable tracheostomy care kit containing: (see Fig. 29-8)
  ▪ Two basins
  ▪ Pipe cleaners
  ▪ Forceps
  ▪ Gauze pads
  ▪ Cotton tape
  ▪ Sterile towel
▪ Hydrogen peroxide
▪ Sterile water or saline
▪ Sterile gloves if not in kit
▪ Clean gloves
▪ Wall or portable suction apparatus
▪ Sterile suction catheter
▪ Clean, water-repellant gown, goggles, and mask
	Helps organize procedure.

2. Refer to medical record, care plan, or Kardex for special interventions.	Provides basis for care.
3. Wash hands and don clean gloves. according to agency policy and guidelines from Centers for Disease Control and Prevention and Occupational Safety and Health Administration.	Helps prevent cross-contamination.
4. Introduce self.	Decreases anxiety level.
5. Identify patient by identification band.	Identifies correct patient for procedure.
6. Explain procedure to patient.	Seeks cooperation and decreases anxiety.
7. Raise bed to comfortable working level.	Provides safety for nurse.
8. Arrange for patient privacy.	Shows respect for patient.
9. Assess respiratory status.	Determines patency of airway and need for spirometry.
10. Assess stoma for redness, edema, character of secretions, and bleeding.	Determines need for suctioning and cleaning of area.
11. Place sterile hemostat, sterile obturator, and sterile tracheostomy set at bedside.	Ensures that emergency equipment is close at hand.
12. Attach suction apparatus to thumb-control end of catheter without touching suction end. Leave suction end in sterile package.	Readies equipment.
13. Pour sterile solutions into sterile containers, including hydrogen peroxide into one basin of tracheostomy cleaning kit and sterile water or saline into other.	Readies equipment.

Continued.

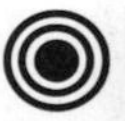

SKILL 29-8 PERFORMING TRACHEOSTOMY CARE AND SUCTIONING—cont'd

Steps	Rationale
14. Place sterile drape on patient's chest under tracheostomy without touching upper surface of drape.	Prevents contamination of stoma, patient's bed clothing, and bed linens.
15. Turn on suction machine and adjust to appropriate level for age: ▪ Adults: 110-115 mm Hg ▪ Children: 95-110 mm Hg ▪ Infants: 50-95 mm Hg	Prevents tissue injury.
16. Unlock and remove cannula and place in basin with hydrogen peroxide.	Begins cleaning of tracheostomy tube by soaking.
17. Remove one clean glove and replace with sterile glove.	Maintains sterile technique.
18. Hold thumb-control end with clean hand and suction end with sterile hand.	Maintains sterile technique.
19. Lubricate catheter by placing suction end in sterile solution. Instill small amount of sterile solution into tracheostomy per medical order.	Prevents tissue trauma and hemorrhage. May help loosen secretions.
20. Insert suction catheter into tracheostomy slowly and gently with no suction applied. Stop if resistance is felt.	Avoids tissue trauma and hemorrhage. (Resistance may indicate stricture.)
21. Hold thumb over thumb-control end and pull catheter out of tracheostomy tube, turning slightly and twisting catheter back and forth gently.	Applies suction, removes secretions, and prevents tissue trauma and hemorrhage.
22. Limit suctioning to 10-15 sec and remove thumb from control every 2-3 sec.	Avoids tissue trauma and allows patient to breathe.
23. Allow patient to rest and repeat suctioning if needed. Administer oxygen between suctionings if needed.	Allows further oxygenation.
24. Allow patient to cough deeply.	Often brings up more secretions.
25. Suction around outside edge of tracheostomy tube.	Removes secretions from all areas of tube and prevents skin breakdown around stoma edges.
26. Rinse catheter by suctioning sterile solution after each suctioning.	Maintains patency of catheter.
27. Discard contaminated catheter.	Prevents contamination of other health care workers.
28. Remove clean gloves and replace with sterile gloves.	Maintains sterile technique.
29. Arrange pipe cleaners, brush, gauze pads, forceps, and cotton tapes on sterile field.	Readies materials for use.
30. Pick up inner cannula from peroxide with forceps. Use brush and pipe cleaners to thoroughly cleanse inside and outside of cannula. Twist pipe cleaners together or bend double to provide appropriate thickness to fit inside cannula.	Maintains sterile technique and rids cannula of secretions. Ensures removal of all secretions from cannula.
31. Rinse cannula in sterile water.	Completes cleansing of cannula.
32. Dry cannula with gauze pads.	Prevents water droplets from entering trachea.
33. Inspect to ensure cannula is clean and dry inside.	Prevents contamination of trachea and prevents choking and aspiration.
34. Replace and lock cannula.	Secures cannula to prevent dislodging.
35. Cleanse skin and surrounding area of stoma with gauze pads moistened with peroxide.	Protects skin from breakdown and prevents growth of microorganisms.

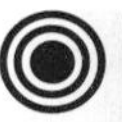

SKILL 29-8 PERFORMING TRACHEOSTOMY CARE AND SUCTIONING—cont'd

Steps	Rationale
36. Change tracheostomy tie tapes if soiled. Insert new tapes before removing old tapes. If this is not possible, have helper hold tracheostomy tube in place with clean, gloved hand while ties are replaced.	Provides comfort, prevents growth of microorganisms, and prevents dislodgement of tube.
37. Replace soiled gauze pad under tracheostomy tube without dislodging.	Protects skin and stoma from breakdown.
38. Provide oral hygiene.	Provides comfort, provides moisture, and removes foul tastes.
39. Dispose of all waste materials and solutions.	Helps prevent spread of microorganisms.
40. Remove gloves and wash hands.	Prevents cross-contamination.
41. Document.	Documents procedure and patient's response.

SKILL 29-9 CARING FOR CLOSED CHEST DRAINAGE SYSTEMS

Steps	Rationale
1. Obtain equipment: ▪ Closed drainage system ▪ Clean gloves ▪ Suction apparatus if necessary ▪ Sterile connector for emergency use ▪ Rubber-shod clamps (kept at bedside)	Helps organize procedure.
2. Refer to medical record, care plan, or Kardex for special interventions.	Provides basis for care.
3. Wash hands and don clean gloves according to agency policy and guidelines from Centers for Disease Control and Prevention and Occupational Safety and Health Administration.	Helps prevent cross-contamination.
4. Introduce self.	Decreases anxiety level.
5. Identify patient by identification band.	Identifies correct patient for procedure.
6. Explain procedure to patient.	Seeks cooperation and decreases anxiety.
7. Raise bed to comfortable working level.	Provides safety for nurse.
8. Arrange for patient privacy.	Shows respect for patient.
9. Assess respiratory status.	Determines patency of airway.
10. Assess insertion site of chest catheter for leakage, subcutaneous emphysema, and signs of infection.	Ensures lack of complications.
11. Assess all equipment for appropriate working order.	Ensures correct suction, seal, and drainage from system.
12. Assess water level in bottles.	Ensures appropriate levels for adequate suction and seal.
13. Mark level of drainage, giving date and time.	Ensures accurate measurement of amount of drainage and provides baseline for further assessment.
14. Make certain tubing does not loop, is not kinked, and does not prevent patient movement.	Prevents problems that can impede or stop chest drainage system.
15. Encourage patient movement as allowed and deep breathing and coughing exercises as ordered. Splint chest to decrease pain.	Promotes mobility of secretions.
16. Keep drainage bottle below chest.	Prevents backflow of fluid into pleural space, thus collapsing lung.

Continued.

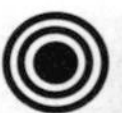

SKILL 29-9 CARING FOR CLOSED CHEST DRAINAGE SYSTEMS—cont'd

Steps	Rationale
17. Strip chest catheter according to agency policy or medical orders.	Prevents plugging with clots and other materials, possibly obstructing system.
18. Make certain there is fluctuation of fluid level in water chamber.	Ensures that there is no leakage in system.
19. Make certain there is *not* continuous stream of air bubbles in water chamber.	Ensures that there is no leakage in system.
20. Report shallow breathing, cyanosis, pressure in chest, and hemorrhage immediately.	Denotes need for emergency treatment.
21. If chest tube becomes disconnected, notify registered nurse to use sterile connector to reconnect drainage system.	Prevents backflow of fluid into pleural space.
22. If chest tube becomes dislodged from chest wall, apply pressure with gloved hand and sterile gauze and call for help.	Prevents further collapse of lung and denotes need for emergency treatment.
23. Dispose of waste materials.	Helps prevent spread of microorganisms.
24. Remove gloves and wash hands.	Prevents cross-contamination.
25. Document.	Documents procedure and patient's response.

SUMMARY

The nurse must recognize the signs and symptoms of respiratory distress because without intervention the patient will die. It is fearful not to be able to take a breath, and the fear often causes additional respiratory problems.

The nurse assesses for a patent airway or establishes one. The patient often completely depends on the nurse for breathing assistance. The nurse must accurately assess lung sounds and respiration. Many tests assist in discovering the cause of alterations in oxygenation, but it is often the nurse who discovers that the patient is in distress.

Key Concepts

- The nurse should understand the procedures that the respiratory therapy department performs on patients to assess their effectiveness and the patient's progress.
- For adequate oxygenation the muscles of respiration, the diaphragm and the intercostals, must be capable of contracting and relaxing.
- Pressure changes must take place inside the lungs for air to pass into and out of the lungs.
- If the principles of respiration are violated, the patient's respiratory status is compromised.
- Drinking plenty of fluids is necessary to liquify secretions for removal.
- Postural drainage and percussion techniques and exercises help loosen secretions from the bronchial tree for easier removal.
- Patient teaching is important to help the patient learn to take personal responsibility for respiratory care.

Critical Thinking Questions

1. The nurse is caring for a patient who had abdominal surgery 24 hours ago. This patient has a 10-year history of chronic obstructive pulmonary disease. What assessments and interventions are necessary to maintain a patent airway?
2. The patient is back from the recovery room after abdominal surgery. She is awake and alert and asking for something for pain. Her respirations are diminished in the lower bases. What other evaluations of her respiratory system must be made?

REFERENCES AND SUGGESTED READINGS

Anderson K, Anderson L, Glanze W, editors: *Mosby's medical, nursing, and allied health dictionary,* ed 4, St Louis, 1994, Mosby.

Brunner LS, Suddarth DS: *The Lippincott manual of nursing practice,* ed 5, Philadelphia, 1994, Lippincott.

Harkness G, Dincher JR: *Medical-surgical nursing: total patient care,* ed 9, St Louis, 1996, Mosby.

McFarland GK, McFarlane EA: *Nursing diagnosis and intervention: planning for patient care,* ed 2, St Louis, 1993, Mosby.

Phipps WJ et al, editors: *Medical-surgical nursing: concepts and clinical practice,* ed 5, St Louis, 1995, Mosby.

Potter PA, Perry AG: *Basic nursing: theory and practice,* St Louis, 1995, Mosby.

Potter PA, Perry AG: *Fundamentals of nursing: concepts, process, and practice,* ed 3, St Louis, 1993, Mosby.

■ CHAPTER 30 ■

Urinary Elimination

Learning Objectives

After studying this chapter, the student should be able to . . .

- Define the key terms.
- Trace the pathway of a drop of urine from formation to elimination.
- Identify nursing techniques used in assessing urinary alterations.
- Compare the characteristics of normal and abnormal urine.
- Describe various nursing measures for assisting the patient with urinary elimination, including using the bathroom, a commode, a urinal, and a bedpan.
- Identify factors that influence urinary elimination.
- Explain measures to protect the patient from urinary infections.
- Strain the urine of a patient.
- Identify various types of catheters used for urinary elimination.
- Perform catheterization.
- Discuss the management of an indwelling catheter.
- Explain the steps of bladder training.
- Explain the procedures for collecting urine specimens.

Key Terms

Anuria
Bacteriuria
Credé's maneuver
Dysuria
Glycosuria
Hematuria
Kegel exercises
Micturition
Oliguria
Polyuria
Proteinuria
Pyuria
Renal calculi
Residual urine
Retention
Specific gravity
Stoma
Ureterostomy
Urinalysis
Urinary incontinence
Urinary tract infection (UTI)

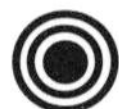

Skills

30-1 Performing male and female catheterization
30-2 Performing bladder irrigation and instillation
30-3 Collecting a sterile urine specimen from a Foley catheter

Urinary elimination is a basic function of the body whereby waste products and materials not needed for normal body function are excreted. Elimination depends on the normal structure and functioning of the kidneys, ureters, bladder, urethra, and other related structures (Fig. 30-1). *Urination, micturition,* and *voiding* are all terms used to describe the process by which urine is eliminated from the urinary bladder. This process is very personal and private to the patient. Interference or interruption of the patient's urinary process requires physiologic and psychologic assistance by the nurse to maintain homeostasis (balance) of the body's functioning as well as the comfort and well-being of the patient.

URINARY STRUCTURE AND FUNCTION

Kidneys The kidneys are two bean-shaped organs that lie on either side of the vertebral column, just above the waistline and under the back muscles, at approximately the twelfth thoracic and third lumbar vertebrae. Every minute the kidneys filter 25% of the blood volume pumped by the heart. The kid-

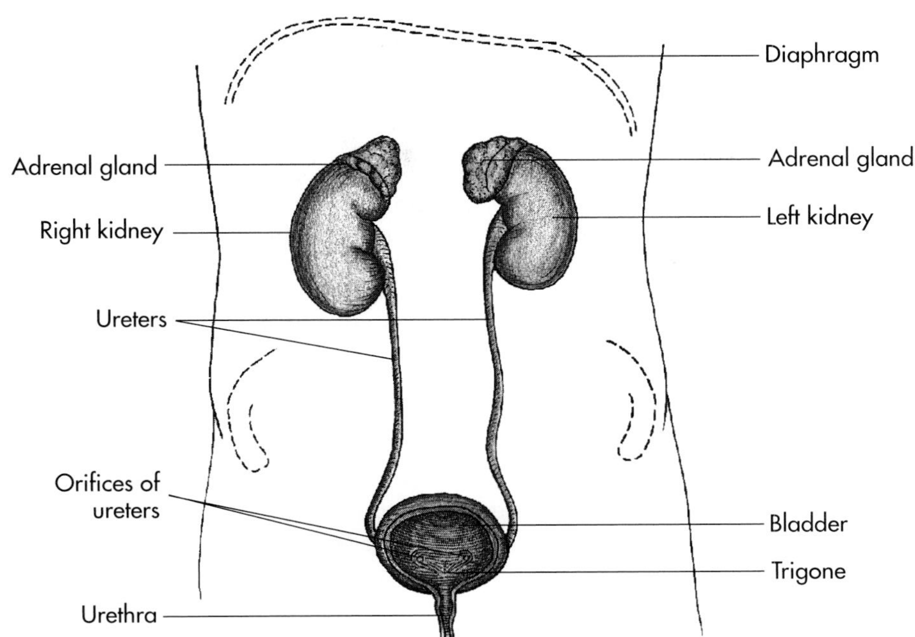

Fig. 30-1 Organs of the urinary system. (From Potter PA, Perry AG: *Fundamentals of nursing: concepts, process, and practice*, ed 3, St Louis, 1993, Mosby.)

neys normally produce 1 to 2 L of urine a day. Within the renal cortex (outer layer of kidney containing glomeruli, which remove body wastes via the urine), microscopic nephrons selectively filter wastes and resorb fluid and other needed substances. The kidneys determine the composition and amount of urine to be excreted. Urine drains through the collecting tubules into the renal pelvis at the lower portion of the kidney. From there it enters the ureters.

Ureters The ureters are tubes, 10 to 12 inches long, that look like uncooked spaghetti and connect the renal pelvis portion of the kidney to the bladder. These tubes are lined with mucous membranes and have a muscular layer that produces peristaltic movements to move the urine into the bladder. The mucous lining contains sensory nerve endings.

Urinary bladder The bladder is the storage chamber for urine. Composed of elastic, muscular fibers, it has the ability to expand and contract to hold and empty variable amounts of urine. When empty, the urinary bladder lies behind the symphysis pubis, but when full, it expands into the lower abdomen. The ureters enter the bladder from above, and the urethra exits below. Nerve impulses signal the need to empty the bladder at approximately 350 to 400 ml of capacity.

Urethra Leaving the bladder, urine drains down the urethra through the external opening, the urinary meatus. In women, this narrow tube is about 1½ inches long. However, in men the urethra is approximately 8 inches long and serves a dual role. The male urethra serves as a passageway for both urine and reproductive fluid (semen). Two rings of muscular tissue surround the urethra. They are called *sphincters.* The internal sphincter is at the exit of the bladder and is involuntary. The external sphincter lies around the bladder neck and is under voluntary control.

Micturition When the bladder signals increased pressure, an emptying reflex is initiated, and relaxation of the internal sphincter occurs involuntarily, allowing urine to enter the urethra. Voluntary contraction of the external sphincter suppresses urination, whereas voluntary relaxation of the external sphincter permits emptying of the bladder **(micturition).** Voluntary control of the external sphincter allows suppression of the emptying reflex until the bladder capacity is filled. However, attempting to suppress bladder emptying beyond its capacity may result in loss of voluntary control.

FACTORS INFLUENCING MICTURITION

Multiple factors influence urinary elimination. Urine amounts, content, and characteristics and elimination patterns are variable. External as well as internal influences effect urinary elimination. By understanding factors that influence urination, the nurse can anticipate problems and assist patients to maintain homeostasis. When taking a patient's health history, the nurse assesses elimination patterns and symptoms of urinary alterations. Important areas of assessment include normal urination pattern, symptoms of alterations, and factors that may affect urinary elimination.

Fluid intake Increased fluid intake or ingestion of foods or fluids containing alcohol or caffeine usually increase urination. Diminished fluid intake or excess excretion of fluid through the lungs, skin, or intestine decreases urination.

Medications Drugs may increase or decrease urine production. Some medications may change the color of urine.

Growth and development Infants, young children, and older adults may not have voluntary control over urinary elimination. They may not have large bladders and thus have diminished ability to concentrate urine. Weak muscle tone, problems of mobility, and chronic diseases make toileting problematic.

Psychologic factors Anxiety; stress; and social, cultural, and gender factors influence urinary elimination. Sufficient privacy and time to relax may be necessary to void. Standing for men and sitting with the knees flexed for women are preferred positions that may enable successful bladder emptying. Normal patterns may be altered by social constraints such as long meetings, travel, and school or work schedules. In some cultures, elimination is a very private matter, whereas in others communal toileting facilities are acceptable.

Surgical and diagnostic procedures Trauma to the urinary system may cause interruptions in normal urinary patterns. Cystoscopy (examination of cells), intravenous pyelography (radiographic technique for examining the structures of the urinary tract), abdominal or pelvic trauma, anesthetics, pain-killing drugs, and decreased circulatory volume to the kidneys may reduce urine production or elimination.

Pathologic conditions Voluntary bladder control may be lost because of spinal cord injuries, stroke, multiple sclerosis, or any paralyzing illness. Altered bladder functioning results from diabetes mellitus, renal disease, febrile conditions, and chronic conditions that slow mobility and reaction time.

NURSING PROCESS

Assessment

When assessing a patient's urinary elimination problem and gathering data for a plan of care, the nurse obtains a nursing history. This includes the patient's urinary elimination patterns and any symptoms of urinary alterations. The nurse may assess urinary function by examining the renal laboratory work. Assessment of the external urinary meatus and palpation of the suprapubic (above the pubis) area for bladder distention may be done. The patient's fluid intake and urine output may also be measured (see care plan on p. 588). The nurse inspects the patient's urine for consistency, color, amount, and odor. A urine specimen may be collected for diagnostic testing when ordered.

Nursing Diagnosis

The nurse assesses the patient's urinary function and identifies characteristics that reveal a diagnosis. Nursing diagnoses for urinary elimination may include the following:

Altered patterns of urinary elimination
Body-image disturbance
Functional incontinence
Knowledge deficit (specify)
Pain
Reflex incontinence
Risk for impaired skin integrity
Risk for infection
Self-care deficit: toileting
Stress incontinence
Total incontinence
Urge incontinence
Urinary retention

Planning

The nurse plans interventions for patients with urinary elimination problems. Preventive interventions may be required for patients with potential problems. Planning should include consideration of the patient's home and normal elimination routines. Teaching throughout the hospital stay and when preparing for discharge is important (see teaching box). Reinforcement of good health habits improves the likelihood for compliance with the plan of care.

Patient-centered goals may include the following:

Goal: Patient understands how to help prevent urinary tract infection.

PATIENT TEACHING

- Explain signs and symptoms of urinary infections.
- Teach correct perineal hygiene care to reduce the risk of urinary tract infection.
- Encourage fluid intake to flush the urinary system.

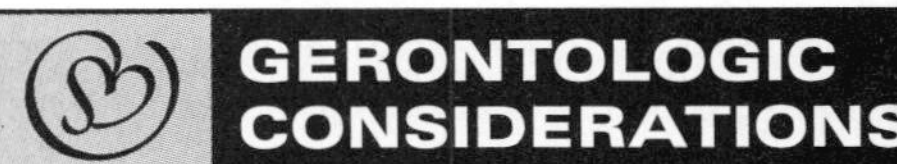

GERONTOLOGIC CONSIDERATIONS

- Inadequate fluid intake and immobility may increase the risk of urinary infection in the older adult.
- Older women are particularly at risk for stress incontinence because of hormonal changes and weakened pelvic muscles.
- Urinary incontinence can lead to a loss of self-esteem and result in decreased participation in social activities.

Outcome

Patient demonstrates appropriate hygiene measures to prevent infection.

Implementation

When implementing the plan of care, the nurse should provide patient teaching related to normal voiding, complete emptying of the bladder to help prevent infection and other related problems, and maintenance of skin integrity. The nurse should give special attention to the older adult (see gerontologic box).

Evaluation

The nurse evaluates the success of the goals established for the plan of care. The process is dynamic because the patient's condition may change. The nurse must always be prepared to revise the care plan based on the evaluation.

Goal: Patient understands how to prevent urinary tract infection.

Evaluative measure

Observe patient's techniques for cleansing perineum.

ASSESSMENT OF URINARY ELIMINATION

Observing the characteristics of urine—its amount, color, consistency, and odor—and measuring the patient's intake and output give the nurse important information about the patient's urinary functioning. The nurse's assessment provides important information that guides health care treatment and early nursing interventions and helps prevent complications.

The color of normal urine ranges from amber to bright yellow to a pale straw yellow, depending on the time of day and the patient's hydration status. Usually, urine is more concentrated in the morning, after having collected in the bladder all night. During the day, when the patient is moving and taking in fluids, the urine becomes more diluted. At certain times, urine may look clear, like water.

Beets, blackberries, rhubarb, and some medications may turn the urine red or orange. Dyes from diagnostic procedures or certain medications may color the urine blue or green. Patients with liver disease may experience dark amber urine. In **hematuria** (blood in the urine), the color of the blood may indicate the organ from where the bleeding is occurring. Dark red blood usually indicates bleeding in the kidneys or ureters, whereas bleeding from the bladder or urethra is usually bright red. Small amounts of blood in the urine may make it appear smoky or brownish. Urine may be contaminated with blood from the vagina of a menstruating woman or may occur from the rectum.

Normal, freshly voided urine appears transparent. A urine specimen that has been kept at room temperature may become cloudy. Fresh urine that has a cloudy appearance may contain bacteria **(bacteriuria),** pus **(pyuria),** or protein **(proteinuria).**

Normal urine has a faintly aromatic odor that can be affected by foods, medications, and fluid intake. The ammonia breakdown of standing urine in specimen containers, urine collection bags, bedpans, or urinals causes the odor to become stronger. Nursing measures to ensure emptying and cleansing of these receptacles maintains patient dignity while helping decrease contamination and infection.

Intake and Output

The nurse keeps a record of the patient's fluid volume intake and urinary output to ensure fluid balance. In a health care agency and at home the nurse and patient work together to keep accurate intake and output records. Oral fluids are measured by calculating the volume of the glass or cup used by the patient, in milliliters which is then multiplied by the number of glasses of fluid taken. Any intravenous fluids must also be calculated and documented in the total fluid intake.

Output may be measured using bedpans, urinals,

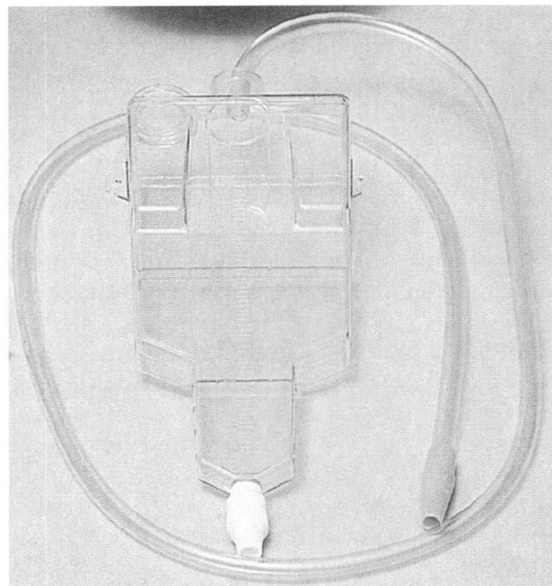

Fig. 30-2 Urimeter. (From Potter PA, Perry AG: *Basic nursing: theory and practice,* ed 3, St Louis, 1995, Mosby.)

or other plastic receptacles. When the patient has a catheter, the urinary output can be calculated from the collection bag or special urimeter attachments on the catheter tubing for more precise measurements (Fig. 30-2). Urinary output should not fall below 30 ml per hour. When urine production falls below this rate, **oliguria** (scanty urine) or **anuria** (cessation of urine production) occurs, and the nurse should immediately notify the physician and assess for other signs of shock. **Polyuria** (excretion of large amounts of urine) indicates diabetes mellitus or the use of diuretics. After measuring urinary output, the nurse appropriately disposes of the urine and cleanses or replaces the receptacle for continued use by the patient.

ASSISTING WITH TOILETING

Patient safety is always a priority while assisting the patient with toileting. The nurse's responsibility depends on the patient's condition and any medical orders restricting activities. If the patient is allowed bathroom access, the nursing assessment of the patient's ability to reach the bathroom safely dictates the amount of nursing assistance required. The nurse should orient the patient to the bathroom, indicating the location of supplies and ensuring that the call light is within reach. The nurse instructs the patient concerning any measuring device to collect excreta. The bathroom door should remain unlocked, and the nurse remains nearby to promptly assist if the need arises. In some instances, it is necessary to remain in the bathroom with the patient. For some patients, elimination sounds cause embarrassment and inhibit the ability to void. Running water may mask embarrassing noises and stimulate the voiding reflex.

A nurse may be required on each side to assist the weakened male patient to a standing position for voiding. The patient usually requires time to void. Integrating the patient's normal habits, including normal voiding times, reading material, music, or certain liquids (for example, juice, tea, or coffee) helps maintain a normal elimination pattern. Nursing measures to stimulate the voiding reflex include putting the patient's hand in warm water, pouring warm water over the perineum (this water is measured and subtracted from the output total), offering oral fluids, running water in the sink, and having the patient stroke the inner thigh.

After toileting, the nurse provides an opportunity for cleansing of the perineum and handwashing. The patient is assisted back to bed as necessary, leaving a clean, comfortable, and safe environment. The nurse documents any necessary information immediately.

Assistive Devices

Bedside commode

Some patients may not be able to navigate the distance to the bathroom. A bedside commode, a chairlike structure with a toilet seat and a removable collection receptacle, may enable the patient to maintain normal elimination habits. The commode can be placed at the bedside and the patient safely assisted to it. Some commodes have wheels that allow the patient to be wheeled into the bathroom and the commode seat, with the receptacle removed, placed over the toilet. A graduated measurement receptacle must be used when the patient needs accurate output measurement.

Urinal

Although a urinal is usually used by men, there are female adapters that make urinals useful for women. For patients confined to bed, urinals provide a means for collecting urine. Many patients find using the urinal a necessary but embarrassing experience. The nurse is responsible for reducing the unpleasantness by providing easy access to the urinal and safe, clean disposal of the urine (Fig. 30-3). Some patients may require assistance with repositioning to facilitate use of the urinal. Guidelines for assisting the patient to use a urinal follow:

1. Hand the clean, dry urinal to the alert patient.

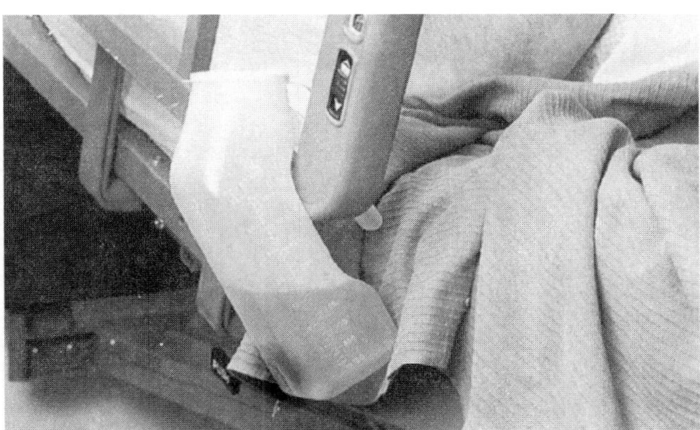

Fig. 30-3 Male urinal.

2. If the patient is not alert, don gloves and place the urinal between the patient's legs, placing the penis in the opening.
3. Place the call light, tissue, and wet washcloth within the patient's reach. If patient is not alert, return frequently to assess for urination.
4. After the patient has voided, remove the urinal carefully to avoid spilling.
5. Assess the amount, color, consistency, odor, and abnormalities. Test, measure, or save urine specimen as needed.
6. Empty and clean urinal according to agency policy and place it within patient's reach or store it appropriately.
7. Document promptly.

Bedpan

A bedpan may be used for urine or stool elimination. The use of a bedpan is usually reserved for patients unable to leave the bed. One type, called a *fracture pan,* is shaped like a wedge. The flat end slides up under the buttocks to assist patients who cannot sit or elevate their hips (Fig. 30-4).

Incontinence

Urinary incontinence is the inability to control micturition. Depending on its cause, incontinence may be temporary or permanent. Various types of incontinence exist, and nursing approaches vary with causes and symptoms. Incontinence causes embarrassment and change in body image. The patient experiencing incontinence is at risk for impaired skin integrity and pressure ulcers. Recognizing the type of incontinence the patient is experiencing enables the nurse to plan nursing care that diminishes embarrassment, enhances self-esteem, and prevents skin breakdown. Table 30-1 describes symptoms and causes of and nursing approaches for the different types of incontinence.

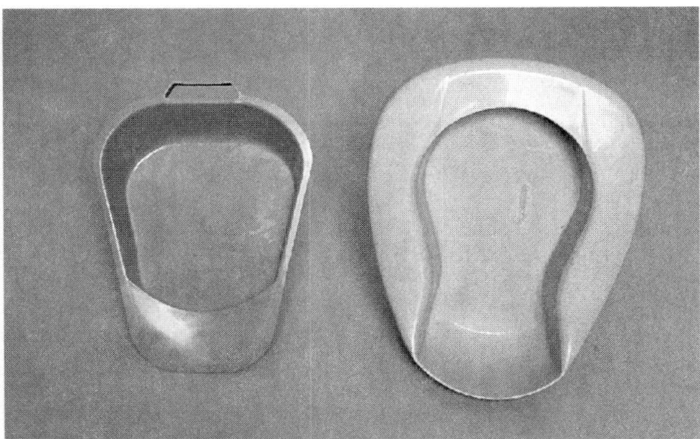

Fig. 30-4 Types of bedpans. *Left,* Fracture bedpan. *Right,* Regular bedpan. (From Christensen BL, Kockrow EO: *Foundations of nursing,* ed 2, St Louis, 1995, Mosby.)

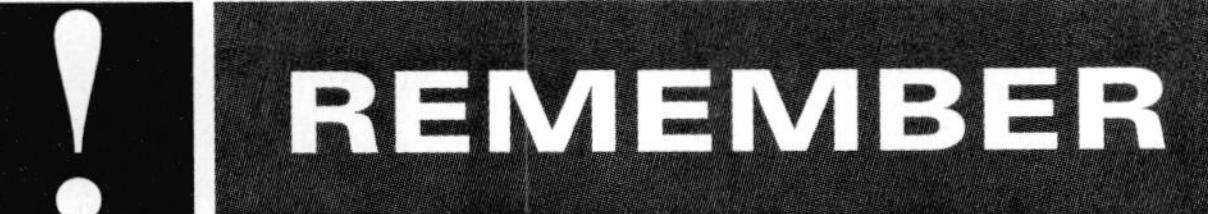

- Kinked or twisted drainage tubes obstruct urine flow.
- Traction on the catheter may cause irritation and injury internally.
- The collection bag should remain lower than the bladder to prevent backflow.

The nurse should be familiar with techniques used to strengthen pelvic floor muscles, triggering mechanisms to elicit the voiding reflex, and methods of facilitating bladder emptying. Instructing patients and their families in methods that facilitate effective bladder emptying encourages self-care and maintains the patient's dignity and self-esteem.

Kegel exercises

For patients experiencing stress incontinence (urination precipitated by coughing, sneezing, and other straining), exercises that strengthen the pelvic muscle may provide a greater level of control. Also called ***Kegel exercises,*** these isometric exercises increase the tone of the pelvic floor muscles that voluntarily control the passage of urine, flatus, and stool. Consistent, repetitive Kegel exercises help the patient regain and maintain increased control. The patient should be instructed to follow the following steps:

1. Tighten the rectal and urinary muscles as though trying to stop urinating.
2. Hold these muscles tight for 10 to 15 seconds.
3. Relax the muscles for 10 to 15 seconds.
4. Repeat relaxing and contracting the muscles for 10 to 25 repetitions.
5. During the day, perform three to five sets of 10 to 25 repetitions (one repetition on awakening,

Table 30-1 TYPES OF URINARY INCONTINENCE

Symptoms	Causes	Nursing Approaches
Overflow		
Full bladder, urine leaking around catheter, dribbling	Kinked catheter, overdistended bladder, lack of sensation indicating bladder fullness	Maintenance of catheter patency; frequent bladder palpation and assessment; use of trigger mechanisms, including Credé's maneuver, to stimulate voiding.
Stress		
Involuntary leakage of urine during increased abdominal pressure, frequency and urgency	Coughing, sneezing, lifting, laughing, vomiting, pregnancy, weak pelvic muscles, obesity	Weight loss; delivery; pelvic muscle strengthening exercises
Reflex		
Involuntary escape of urine without sensation of bladder pressure, lack of urge to void	Spinal cord injury, trauma, tumor, neurologic impairment	Straight intermittent catheterization; use of triggering mechanisms
Total		
Complete and continuous loss of urine, lack of ability to control	Trauma, disease or neuropathy of sensory nerves, urethral or vaginal fistula, loss of sphincter control	Patient education about absorbent undergarments; indwelling or external catheter
Functional		
Urgency with loss of urine before reaching toilet or urine receptacle	Deficits of mobility, cognition, communication, and sensation; unfamiliar environment	Clothing modifications, improved accessibility to toileting receptacle, frequently scheduled assistance to toilet
Urge		
Urgency, frequency, bladder spasm, nocturia, frequent and small amounts	Increased fluid intake, ingestion of alcohol or caffeine, bladder irritation, decreased bladder capacity	Decreased amounts of caffeine or alcohol; treatment for bladder infections; maintenance of balanced fluid intake; diuretics in early morning; frequent toileting

one before or after each meal, and one at bedtime).

As the perineal musculature tone improves, the patient may assess the progress by attempting to stop the urine flow several times during voiding. Consistent Kegel exercise, even after stress incontinence is eliminated, maintains muscle tone to counter the relaxing effects of aging.

Cutaneous triggering

Triggering mechanisms may be used effectively in patients who experience reflex incontinence. It is important for the nurse to assess whether a voiding reflex is present before using techniques to manually stimulate voiding. If the anal sphincter contracts with genital stimulation or insertion of a thermometer, the voiding reflex is present. Spinal cord–injured and other paralyzed patients may learn to trigger the voiding reflex, although they cannot neurologically initiate or control it. The bladder should be palpated for distention every 2 to 3 hours. When the bladder is full, the patient should be seated on a bedpan, toilet, or commode. Continuous tapping over the suprapubic area for 45 to 60 seconds may be successful. If initially unsuccessful, tapping over an adjacent area may prove more effective. When voiding begins, tapping is ceased.

For some patients, stroking the inner thigh, gently pulling the pubic hairs, or massaging the inguinal area may be successful. The stimulus may take several minutes to be successful. Once a successful method has been found, the patient continues its use to initiate subsequent urination. If an attempted method is not successful, a pause of 1 to 2 minutes should be allowed before attempting a new stimulus.

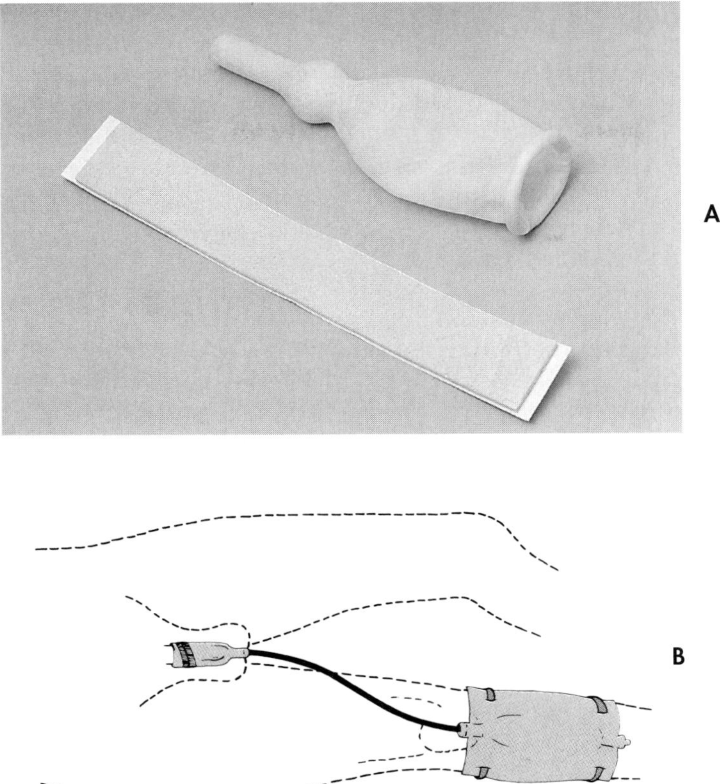

Fig. 30-5 **A,** Condom catheter and elastic tape. **B,** Condom catheter with leg drainage bag. (From Potter PA, Perry AG: *Basic nursing: theory and practice,* ed 3, St Louis, 1995, Mosby.)

Finding a successful method of triggering the voiding reflex enables the paralyzed or spinal cord injured patient to avoid the embarrassment of reflex incontinence and the complications of odor, impaired skin integrity, irritation, and infection. Triggering mechanisms may eliminate the need for intermittent straight catheterization, indwelling catheters, external catheter appliances, and their complications. Patients may be taught to perform their own triggering mechanism, allowing them a measure of independence in caring for their toileting needs.

Credé's maneuver

Credé's maneuver may be helpful for patients who experience retention and overflow incontinence. This maneuver is a technique for promoting the expulsion of urine by manual compression of the bladder through pressure on the lower abdominal wall. It is manually performed by placing the hands or fists below the naval and slowly pressing inward and downward over the bladder in wavelike motions. Having the patient hold the breath and lean forward while performing this maneuver assists in increasing intraabdominal pressure and expelling the bladder's contents.

Condom catheters

When other methods have proved unsuccessful for the male patient with incontinence, a condom catheter may be used. This is an external appliance that diverts the urine away from clothing and skin into a collection receptacle.

Medical supply companies manufacture and sell different types of condom catheters with various features (Fig. 30-5). For its effective and safe use, it is best to follow the manufacturer's instructions that accompany the device. A simple condom catheter may be assembled, however, with a condom, flexible tubing (¼-inch diameter), and a collection receptacle. This homemade appliance is less costly and as effective as commercial products.

Assembling a condom catheter

1. Unwrap the condom and inspect it for tears.
2. Place the end of the tubing into the reservoir end of the condom.
3. Secure tubing into reservoir with a small rubber band or dental floss.
4. Pierce a small hole for urine drainage in the condom where it attaches to the tubing.
5. Invert the condom so that the connection is inside.

6. Resecure the outside of the connection with a rubber band or dental floss.

Applying a condom catheter

1. Assemble equipment, provide privacy, wash hands, and don gloves.
2. Explain the procedure to the patient and assist him to a supine position.
3. Wash and dry the penis appropriately.
4. Spiral wrap a strip of double-sided tape along the penis shaft.
5. Gently pinch 1 inch of the condom balloon end to prevent the drainage connection from irritating the meatus.
6. Unroll the remainder of the condom over the shaft of the penis toward the body.
7. Gently but firmly press the condom against the spiral tape along the penis.
8. Gently secure the upper end of the condom with another tape strip. (Be careful not to constrict the blood supply.)
9. Connect the drainage tube to the collection receptacle.
10. Assess frequently for twists or kinks impeding urine flow.
11. Readjust or change the appliance if it is too tight or too loose.
12. Change the condom catheter daily for cleansing and appropriate personal hygiene.

Soap and water cleansing and a mild vinegar solution for rinsing to eliminate odors keep the equipment fresh for further use. The equipment may be cleaned and reused as long as it remains intact.

URINARY DIVERSIONS

Suprapubic Catheterization

Because of trauma or disease it may be necessary to divert the flow of urine from the normal pathway. The surgeon may place a catheter through the skin, through the abdominal wall, over the suprapubic region, and directly into the bladder. This catheter is inserted surgically through a small incision just above the pubic bone and into the urinary bladder. The catheter is anchored in place with sutures or a commercially prepared body seal to prevent drainage around the catheter. This temporary catheter allows the urine to drain from the bladder into a collection receptacle attached to the catheter. Because it becomes a surgical site, care should be taken to perform catheter care under sterile conditions to prevent introducing microorganisms into the urinary tract. The nurse and patient are careful to care for the skin around the catheter and report urine leakage to the surgeon.

The surgeon may also place a catheter directly into the kidney and through the abdominal wall and skin. The nurse assesses the characteristics and measures the amounts of urine from these diversions separately.

Surgical Diversions

For some patients with spinal cord injuries, birth defects, or removal of the bladder because of severe trauma or malignancy, a permanent surgical diversion, called a ***ureterostomy,*** is performed (see Chapter 32). The ureters are brought out to the abdomen through an artificial opening called a ***stoma.*** The urine drains out the stoma into a stomal pouch, an appliance that fits over the stoma, protecting the surrounding skin and keeping the patient's clothing dry (Fig. 30-6, *A*). The patient empties the pouch as necessary through a drainage valve at the bottom of the appliance.

Various types of ureterostomies are possible (Fig. 30-6, *B*). To avoid the need for two appliances the ureters may be joined and brought out through one stoma. This is called a *transureterostomy.* In patients with only one functional kidney, a single ureterostomy may be performed. An ileal conduit involves a loop of intestinal ileum to which the surgeon attaches the ureters. This loop of intestine is brought out to the skin to form one stoma. The conduit is only a channel for urine, not a collection chamber. The nurse may also care for patients with double ureterostomies. These patients present a challenge in fitting the appliances comfortably.

Nurses with specialized training may become enterostomal therapists. These therapists are valuable resources to both the nurse and patient in all aspects of stomal care and life with an ostomy. The patient with a ureterostomy may engage in sports and physical activities, work, travel, date, marry, and have sexual intercourse. Ostomy support groups are beneficial in providing assistance in coping with body-image and lifestyle adaptations.

Catheterization

Urinary elimination is a normal process whereby urine is expelled from the urinary bladder. Bacteria entering the urinary tract is normally prevented from doing so by the forceful flow of urine through the urinary ureters, the mucous membrane lining of the urethra, and the mucous secretion of the urethral glands. Failure or interference of this process requires manual intervention to drain urine from

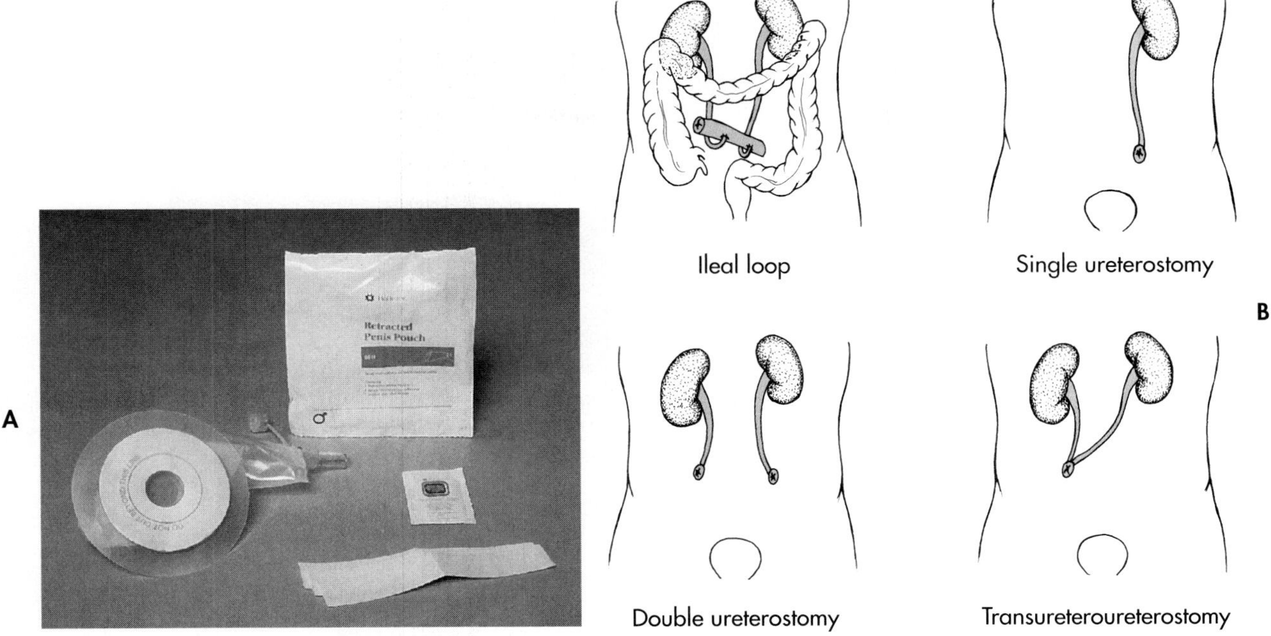

Fig. 30-6 **A,** External urinary device. **B,** Types of ureterostomies. (From Potter PA, Perry AG: *Fundamentals of nursing: concepts, process, and practice,* ed 3, St Louis, 1993, Mosby.)

Table 30-2 INTERMITTENT AND INDWELLING CATHETERS

Indications	Nursing Considerations
Intermittent	
Patients unable to void 6-8 hr after surgery	Obtain a sterile urine specimen.
Patients unable to void because of sedation or analgesics	Assess for residual urine.
Patients with urethral trauma with urinary retention	
Patients with progressive neuromuscular degeneration	
Patients with spinal cord injuries	
Indwelling	
Patients with obstruction from prostate enlargement or urethral stricture	Obtain output measurement in critically ill or comatose patients.
Patients who have had surgical repair of urethra or transurethral surgery or who have bladder tumors	Prevent impaired skin integrity in comatose patients.
	Provide continuous bladder irrigation.
	Watch for medical order to leave catheter in place.

the bladder by inserting a catheter into the bladder using sterile technique. This procedure should be performed only after every effort has been made to assist the patient to void, since catheterization poses a risk for **urinary tract infection (UTI)** (infection of one or more structures of the urinary tract). The two types of catheterization are intermittent and indwelling. Indications for each use are described in Table 30-2. A urinary catheter is a rubber or plastic tube that is inserted through the urinary meatus and urethra and into the bladder. Catheters can be used to provide a continuous flow of urine in patients who have obstructions, **retention** (abnormal accumulation of urine in the bladder), or incontinence. Catheters are available in many sizes and types. A straight catheter is a single-lumen tube inserted for bladder emptying and immediate withdrawal (Fig. 30-7). An indwelling, retention, or Foley catheter is a double-lumen tube. One lumen connects to an inflatable balloon that secures or anchors the catheter in the bladder. The other lumen provides a passageway for the urine to drain from the

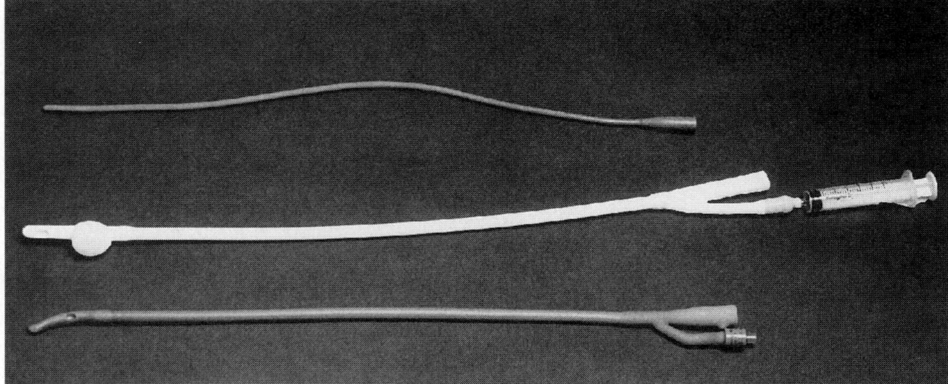

Fig. 30-7 Types of catheters. *Top:* straight catheter; *middle,* indwelling, double-lumen catheter with inflated balloon; *bottom,* Coudé catheter. (From Potter PA, Perry AG: *Fundamentals of nursing: concepts, process, and practice,* ed 3, St Louis, 1993, Mosby.)

bladder. Catheters used for bladder irrigation have a third lumen, which is used to instill irrigating solution into the bladder.

A medical order is required for catheterization (Skill 30-1). Strict aseptic technique must be used to prevent infection (see Chapter 14). The steps are the same for inserting a straight catheter intermittently or placing an indwelling catheter. The difference involves testing of the balloon and inflating it to secure the indwelling catheter in the bladder, which is unnecessary when performing a straight catheterization.

Many agencies stock prepackaged kits containing the necessary supplies for performing catheterization. If the package looks like it has been opened or is damaged, it should not be used. The nurse must assess the list of contents to ensure that all the necessary equipment is included. Gathering other essential equipment before opening the kit helps maintain aseptic technique. Once opened, the kit should be used immediately and discarded appropriately after use.

The patient should be taught that insertion of the catheter should cause only a sensation of pressure on insertion. Infection or swollen, injured tissue may cause discomfort, and the patient's report of pain should be carefully assessed and reported.

Catheter care provides comfort and cleanliness for a patient with an indwelling catheter. In addition, preventing infection and maintaining a continual flow of urine is achieved. Catheter care should be performed under clean conditions to prevent introduction of microorganisms into the urinary tract system. Clean technique is carried out for catheter care to provide cleanliness and prevent infection. The nurse is responsible for catheter care, which may be performed during the morning bath

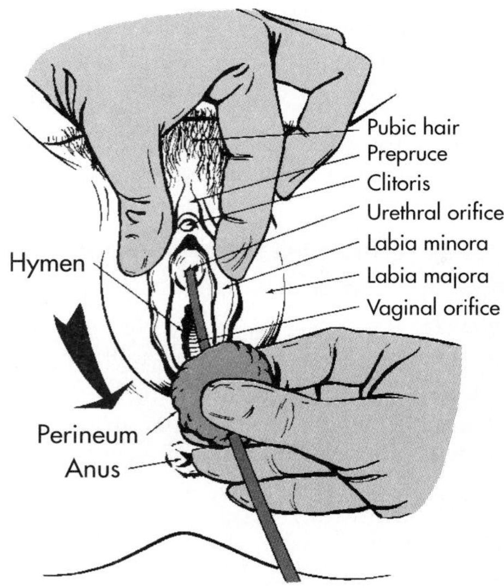

Fig. 30-8 Catheter care.

(see Chapter 23). Integrating catheter care into daily bath time enables the nurse to assess the function of the catheter and inspect the urinary meatus for odor, irritation, crust formation, or swelling.

Agencies have written policy and procedure manuals listing steps for cleansing. The nurse is responsible for knowing agency policy. Although some facilities use antiseptic solutions for catheter care, others use mild soap and water. It is important to perform perineal hygiene around the catheter insertion site and several inches down the catheter (Fig. 30-8). Any abnormalities should be documented and reported to prevent complications.

Teaching of self-catheterization

Self-catheterization is an option for some patients with irreversible disease or spinal cord injuries. Intermittent self-catheterization gives the patient some control over bladder function and promotes dignity and self-esteem. When instructing the patient in self-catheterization, the nurse also teaches medical asepsis. Although surgical asepsis is required in health care agencies, research has shown that the patient using medical asepsis at home is usually safe. The procedure for inserting the catheter is listed in Skill 30-1. The following factors are important for the patient to know:

1. Handwashing is the most important step of infection control.
2. The catheter may be washed in soap and water, rinsed, dried, and stored in a covered container.
3. The patient should be instructed to attempt to empty the bladder before beginning the procedure.
4. Adequate lighting and a comfortable position encourage success.
5. A woman may need a mirror to locate the meatus.
6. Cleansing the perineum and urinary meatus is performed with clean hands, soap and water, and cotton balls.
7. The lubricated catheter is inserted until urine begins to flow into the container.
8. The catheter is held in place until the flow stops and then is slowly and gently withdrawn to drain urine in the lower bladder area.
9. The patient may perform Credé's maneuver to assist in emptying the bladder.
10. Pinching the catheter before removing it prevents leaking of the urine from the catheter.
11. Perineal hygiene, cleansing the catheter for future use, and thorough handwashing complete the procedure.

Irrigation and instillation

A well-draining catheter does not need to be irrigated. However, some catheters become clogged or obstructed by blood clots, mucus, or sediment and require irrigation to maintain patency. Occasionally, the nurse needs to introduce medication into the bladder (bladder instillation), and the procedure for catheter irrigation is performed before the instillation.

There are three methods of irrigation: open, intermittent, and continuous. The open method is performed when occasional irrigation is required. It is the least desirable method, since the potential for transmitting microorganisms into the urinary tract is greatest. As the catheter is separated from the drainage system, the exposure of both open ends of the system doubles the opportunity for contamination (Fig. 30-9). Strict adherence to aseptic principles helps avoid complications. Within closed systems, there is less potential for contamination if strict aseptic technique is followed. Intermittent irrigation is performed when specified periods of irrigation are required, and the continuous method is performed when a constant flow of irrigating solution is necessary.

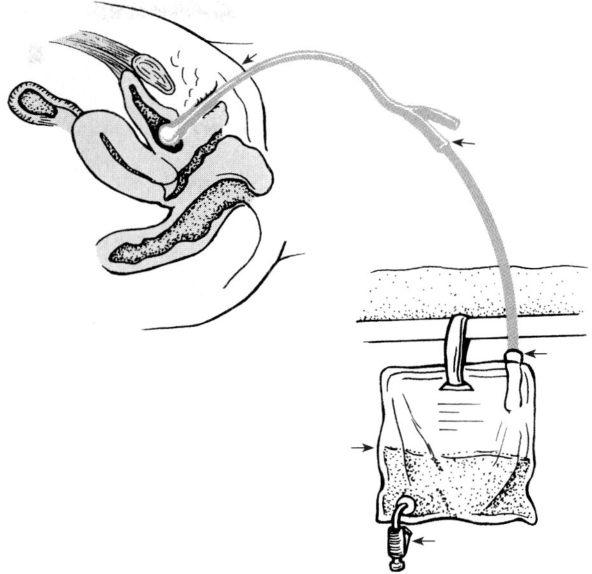

Fig. 30-9 Opportunity for contamination from disconnection of catheter. (From Potter PA, Perry AG: *Fundamentals of nursing: concepts, process, and practice,* ed 3, St Louis, 1993, Mosby.)

Performing catheter irrigation is the responsibility of the nurse. In most instances, however, a medical order is required before the procedure is performed. The solution should be at least at room temperature but preferably at body temperature to prevent bladder spasms. Irrigating solutions should be measured and calculated accurately to determine the patient's actual output total. Supplies needed include sterile irrigating solution, sterile Asepto syringe, antiseptic wipes, sterile connecting tubing covers, a collecting basin, gloves, and a waterproof pad (Fig. 30-10).

When irrigating a closed-system indwelling catheter the nurse performs the following steps:

1. Perform appropriate handwashing.
   a. Don clean gloves.
2. Assemble supplies: 50-ml syringe with needle connection hub; antiseptic wipes; large-bore, 18- to 19-gauge, 1½- to 2-inch needle; and sterile irrigation solution.
3. Attach needle and fill syringe with 30 to 50 ml of irrigation solution.
4. Cleanse catheter access port with antiseptic wipe.

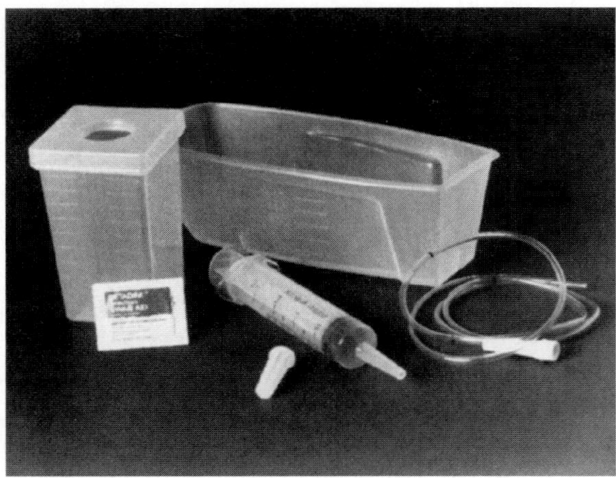

Fig. 30-10 Supplies for catheter irrigation.

5. Enter port with needle at 45-degree angle, assessing needle lumen of tubing.
6. Clamp the drainage tube, promoting movement of the irrigant toward the bladder, not the drainage receptacle.
7. Inject the irrigation solution slowly into the catheter toward the bladder.
8. Remove the needle from the port when all solution is instilled.
9. Discard the contaminated needle in an approved puncture-resistant container.
10. Unclamp the drainage tube and assess the draining fluid.
11. Remove gloves and wash hands.
12. Document the amount of irrigation fluid on the intake record.
13. Document the procedure and results.

Continuous bladder irrigation Frequent intermittent or continuous bladder irrigation is usually managed through a triple-lumen catheter. While the first and second lumen maintain the balloon and drainage systems, the third lumen is attached to the bag of irrigation solution suspended from an intravenous pole. The solution flow rate is controlled manually or by an infusion flow-control pump. The solution enters the bladder at a controlled rate and drains by gravity into the drainage receptacle. The bladder irrigation prevents blood clots from forming; flushes out purulent, stagnant urine; prevents other sediment from building up; and prevents blood retention in the bladder.

The physician usually orders bladder irrigation for patients who have had bladder or prostate surgery. Keeping the system functioning without obstructions is the nurse's responsibility (Skill 30-2). Other important nursing responsibilities include documenting the amount of irrigant infused and the amount and characteristics of the drainage, ensuring that the drainage receptacles are emptied frequently, and replacing the irrigation solution is as necessary.

Bladder instillation Occasionally the physician orders a bladder instillation. The instillation of an antiseptic solution or antibiotic directly into the urinary bladder should be performed using sterile technique (Skill 30-2). Caution should be taken to instill the solution slowly, by gravity, to avoid bladder spasms and injury. The temperature of the solution should be warmed to body temperature before instillation to prevent bladder spasms. The steps to performing a bladder instillation are similar to those for bladder irrigation. However, the solution is introduced into the bladder by gravity rather than injection, and the catheter is clamped to retain the medication in the bladder for a prescribed time. At the end of the prescribed time, the catheter is unclamped, and the solution is allowed to drain out by gravity. The volume of the solution instilled is deducted from the the output for accuracy.

Discontinuing a Foley catheter

Eventually an indwelling catheter must be removed. Whether it is to be removed and replaced by a new catheter or removed and the patient allowed to excrete urine through the normal route, the nurse follows the following steps:

1. Assess the label on the catheter to determine the volume of the balloon.
2. Assemble gloves, waterproof pad, tissues, alcohol swab, and a sterile syringe for the volume of the balloon.
3. Ensure privacy and protect the patient's modesty.
4. Position the patient the same as for catheterization, keeping the patient appropriately draped.
5. Obtain sterile urine specimen, if required.
6. Wash hands, don gloves, and place pad between the patient's legs.
7. Remove the tape or commercial device for anchoring the catheter to thigh.
8. Insert the syringe into the balloon valve and deflate the balloon.
9. Explain that patient should feel nothing except perhaps slight pressure on withdrawal of the catheter.
10. Slowly and smoothly pull the catheter out, wrapping it in the waterproof pad.
11. Offer the tissue to the patient to wipe the perineal area or cleanse the genital area.
12. Dispose of the catheter, tubing, and drainage bag according to agency policy.
13. Remove gloves, wash hands, and assist patient to a position of comfort
14. Provide and encourage fluids.
15. Instruct the patient that frequency, urgency,

and dribbling may occur and will subside as the bladder regains muscle tone.

16. Document the time of catheter removal and characteristics of urine.
17. Instruct the patient to measure the first voiding and to inform the nurse.
18. Notify the physician if the patient has not voided within 8 hours.

Bladder training

Because muscle tone is lost when the muscle is not used, the bladder that experiences continual draining from an indwelling catheter losses its ability to expand and contract with different volumes of urine. When the catheter is removed, the patient may experience **dysuria** (painful urination), hesitancy, and frequency because of decreased capacity. This loss of muscle tone is a common problem after prolonged catheter use. Bladder training or reconditioning may assist the patient to regain some muscle tone before removal of the catheter, thus restoring normal voiding habits sooner.

Requiring a medical order, and beginning 8 to 10 hours or more before the catheter is removed, this technique stimulates the bladder to accommodate volumes of urine in readiness for natural urinary elimination. The nurse clamps the catheter, allowing urine to accumulate in the bladder for several hours, stretching the bladder walls. At the end of this time the nurse unclamps the catheter and allows the bladder to drain 5 to 15 minutes. The procedure is repeated several more times, allowing the filling and emptying of the bladder to simulate natural voiding patterns while reconditioning the muscle tone. When the nurse removes the catheter, the patient usually returns to normal voiding patterns sooner than one who has had no bladder training. Another term for this procedure is *tidal drainage*.

COLLECTING URINE SPECIMENS

Laboratory testing of urine **(urinalysis)** gives the health care team important information that influences nursing care and treatment decisions. The nurse is usually responsible for specimen collection. Specimens should be collected, labeled, and handled appropriately to provide accurate information and avoid false measurement and interpretation of results. The type of test ordered dictates the method of collection. All specimens should be clearly labeled according to agency policy. This policy usually includes the patient's name, date, and collection time. It may also include the type of test ordered, type of collection used, and any medications that the patient may be taking. If there is a possibility that the specimen may have been contaminated by menstrual or rectal bleeding, this should be noted.

Urine specimens should be stored in a refrigerator, kept on ice, or immediately taken to the laboratory to prevent bacterial growth and ammonia breakdown, which occurs when urine is left at room temperature. Analysis of urine that has been left standing at room temperature gives altered results that may lead to inappropriate and unnecessary treatments.

When handling body fluids the nurse should follow universal precautions provided by the Centers for Disease Control and Prevention, and guidelines from the Occupational Safety and Health Administration, and agency policy.

Routine Urine Tests

As blood is filtered through the kidneys, urine is formed. The examination of urine provides important information concerning many body processes. Laboratory tests not only determine **glycosuria** (glucose in the urine), pyuria, hematuria, proteinuria, and bacteriuria but may also determine kidney functioning and the presence of renal disease. Various urine tests are used to assess for substances such as electrolytes, enzymes, hormones, protein, vitamins and minerals, and drugs.

Urinalysis Routine urinalysis screens for urinary tract alterations, fluid imbalance, and metabolic and renal disease. The nurse may perform simple tests for glucose, ketones, albumin, bile, pH, and blood by using commercially prepared test strips that are dipped into the urine and read according to the manufacturer's instructions on the package.

Specific gravity **Specific gravity** is the weight of the concentration of waste products in the urine. A higher specific gravity indicates a greater concentration of urine, and conversely a lower specific gravity indicates a lesser concentration. Normal specific gravity may range from 1.005 to 1.035. A urinometer is a calibrated, enclosed glass cylinder with a weighted bulb at the bottom. The nurse places urine into a clean, dry cylinder and suspends the urinometer in the urine. The urinometer floats in the urine, and the reading is taken at eye level. The place where the level of the urine meniscus crosses the urinometer calibrations indicates the specific gravity reading. A newer instrument, the refractometer, requires only that the nurse place a drop of urine on the inside flat surface of the instrument. The nurse then closes the refractometer and looks through it like a telescope. The reading is recorded where the line crosses the numbered scale. Each method requires that the nurse understand how to use and clean the instrument appropriately according to agency policy.

Urine culture A sterile urine specimen is required for performing an accurate urine culture. Because it takes time to grow and identify bacteria, the results of urine cultures are not immediately available. When culture and sensitivity are ordered, the laboratory determines not only the infecting microorganisms, but also the most effective antibiotic or antibacterial medications to destroy them. This part of the test is called *sensitivity.* It may take 3 to 4 days before the final results are determined.

Renal calculus When the patient has **renal calculi** (kidney stones), it may be necessary to strain all urine excreted. The patient should void in a bedpan or urinal. All urine is strained through a fine mesh sieve. The patient and the family should be told how to strain the urine or to notify the nurse after each voiding. Any small particle or suspicious residue should be saved and sent to the laboratory for diagnostic testing. Calculi are formed of various minerals, and the laboratory determines the type of stone, enabling appropriate interventions and treatment. To ensure that all urine is strained, the nurse places a reminder sign at the patient's bedside or at the bathroom door.

Specimen Collection

Timed collection

Urine may need to be collected over a period of time. Timed urine collection may last 2, 8, 12, or 24 hours. A specimen collected over a period of time will contain measurable, diagnostic amounts of substances that are normally excreted in such minute amounts that their detection in small volumes is impossible.

The nurse explains each test to the patient and ensures understanding to reduce anxiety. The patient is cautioned to avoid contamination of the urine with stool or toilet tissue. Loss of one small urine specimen during the collection time invalidates the test and requires that it be repeated. This may result in longer hospitalization as well as personal and financial difficulties for the patient and family. The nurse contacts the laboratory for any specific directions, preservatives, or dark containers that may be required for the test. The container is labeled with the patient's name, room number, and date. When the test begins, the exact time is documented in the patient's medical record and on the container. The test must begin and end with an empty bladder.

The patient voids and discards the urine specimen. The time of this voiding is recorded as the beginning time of the test. The nurse offers the patient sufficient fluids for hydration and stimulation of urine production during the test, unless contraindicated. The nurse shares any instructions concerning dietary, drug, or activity restrictions to encourage cooperation. All urine is placed in the designated container, which may be refrigerated or kept on ice to prevent decomposition and odor. The nurse may need to frequently replenish the ice supply to keep the specimen chilled. If the patient has an indwelling catheter, the collection bag should be placed on ice and emptied frequently.

At the end of the designated test time, the patient voids. This final voiding is added to the container, and the testing ends. This ensures that the patient began and ended the test with an empty bladder and that all urine produced within the test time was included in the specimen. The ending time is documented on the container, the patient's medical record, and any other paperwork required by the agency.

Double-voided specimens

Double- or second-voided specimens require that the patient void and drink a glass of water. About 15 to 20 minutes later, the patient voids a second time. This ensures that the second specimen is freshly formed by the kidneys and is a valid indication of current urine production for accuracy of the test.

Freshly voided urine from a urinal or bedpan may be transferred into a collection container. The alert patient may be able to void directly into the container. If a bedpan specimen is used, the nurse ensures that no tissue or fecal contamination accompanies the specimen. The nurse collects the specimen and then labels it and takes it to the laboratory. This method of collection is subject to contamination by microorganisms and cells from surfaces of the perineum and containers.

Midstream specimens

The advantage of midstream (clean-catch) collection is that, if performed appropriately, it provides a specimen relatively free of microorganisms from the lower urinary tract and surrounding skin. The nurse instructs the patient that thorough handwashing is the first step. After receiving further instruction, the patient takes the sterile container and antiseptic wipes into the bathroom.

Before voiding, the patient cleanses the meatus. For women, this involves spreading the labia with one hand and wiping from the meatus toward the rectum with a soap- or disinfectant-saturated wipe.

The area must then be rinsed. This decreases the surface microorganisms surrounding the meatus that could be picked up by the urine as it passes into the container. Male patients are instructed to use the soap or disinfectant-saturated wipe to cleanse using a circular motion, starting at the meatus and moving in circular motions down around the glans. The patient is to use each provided wipe only once and then discard it to prevent carrying and depositing microrganisms back to the meatus.

After cleansing the site, the patient is instructed to begin to urinate and allow the first part of the stream to be discarded into the toilet. This helps to flush the resident bacteria from the urethra and meatus. The patient should try to "catch" urine from the "midstream" in the sterile container provided without stopping the urine flow, taking care not to place the fingers inside the container or lid and not to contaminate the container by placing it against the perineum or meatus.

Depending on the patient's mobility, agility, or alertness, the nurse may need to assist the patient with this collection method. The nurse secures the top of the container, labels it appropriately, and sends it to the laboratory for testing. On receiving abnormal results, the nurse promptly communicates with the nursing care provider to ensure prompt intervention and treatment.

Collection of urine from a stoma

The nurse may be required to collect a urine specimen from a patient with a urinary stoma. Two methods are frequently used. After cleansing the stoma and the skin around it, the nurse or patient holds the collection container under the stoma until a sufficient amount of urine has been obtained. Another method, when the patient has an appliance in place, is to first empty the appliance container. The container is held under the appliance drainage port until the needed volume of urine has been obtained.

Sterile specimen collection

A sterile urine specimen may be obtained by inserting a sterile straight catheter into the patient's bladder or collecting a specimen from an indwelling catheter. Urine that has been lying in the drainage tubing or collection receptacle should not be used for testing. This urine has been standing at room temperature, is old, and may thus provide false laboratory results.

A medical order is required to catheterize a patient for a urine specimen. The nurse follows the steps in Skill 30-3 for inserting the straight catheter. When setting up the sterile field, the nurse places the exit end of the catheter into a sterile container to ensure specimen collection even if the patient has very little urine in the bladder. The nurse withdraws the catheter after the specimen has been collected and the bladder has been completely emptied.

If an indwelling catheter is to be inserted and a sterile specimen collected on insertion, the nurse may, when using an open system, collect the specimen before connecting the catheter to the drainage system. When using a closed system, the nurse may immediately collect the first urine that flows through the sterile system. This is the only time that a sterile urine specimen may be collected from an indwelling catheter drainage bag.

Collection of residual urine

Some patients may require sterile straight catheterization for **residual urine** (urine remaining in the bladder after urination). This may be performed to measure the urine remaining in the bladder directly after voiding. The patient may be voiding in small, frequent amounts or feel as though the bladder is not completely empty after urinating. After securing a medical order, the nurse assembles the necessary equipment to perform a straight catheterization. The patient is instructed to empty the bladder as completely as possible. Catheterization for residual urine must be performed immediately after voiding. Waiting 10 to 20 minutes allows the bladder to begin to refill with newly produced urine, giving an erroneous perception of the amount left immediately after voiding.

■ NURSING CARE PLAN ■

URINARY RETENTION

Mr. M, age 46, has difficulty voiding and is scheduled for intravenous pyelography in the morning.

NURSING DIAGNOSIS
Urinary retention related to obstruction as evidenced by dysuria, urgency, severe flank pain, frequency, hematuria, and hesitancy

GOAL
- Patient will be free of infection.

EXPECTED OUTCOMES
- Patient will maintain fluid balance. Intake will equal output.
- Patient will voice increased comfort.
- Patient will voice understanding of treatment.

NURSING INTERVENTIONS
- Assess patient's voiding habits.
- Document characteristics of urine: amount, color, and consistency.
- Provide supportive measures such as pain medication.

EVALUATION
- Patient's intake and output are appropriate.
- Patient verbalizes feelings of comfort.
- Patient maintains normal urinary practice.

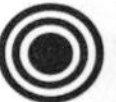

SKILL 30-1 PERFORMING MALE AND FEMALE CATHETERIZATION

Steps	Rationale
1. **Obtain equipment:** ▪ Sterile Foley catheterization tray (Fig. 30-11) ▪ Sterile gloves if not in tray ▪ Bed protector ▪ Drape ▪ Light ▪ Bedpan ▪ Device for anchoring catheter ▪ Graduated container ▪ Clean gloves	Helps organize procedure.
2. **Refer to medical record, care plan, or Kardex for special interventions.**	Provides basis for care.
3. **Introduce self.**	Decreases anxiety level.
4. **Identify patient by identification band.**	Identifies correct patient for procedure.
5. **Explain procedure to patient.**	Seeks cooperation and decreases anxiety.
6. **Wash hands and don clean gloves according to agency policy and guidelines from Centers for Disease Control and Prevention and Occupational Safety and Health Administration.**	Helps prevent cross-contamination.
7. **Prepare patient for intervention:**	
a. Close door to room or pull curtain.	Provides privacy.
b. Drape for procedure if necessary.	Prevents exposure of patient.
8. **Raise bed to comfortable working level.**	Provides safety for nurse.

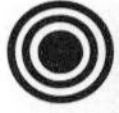

SKILL 30-1 PERFORMING MALE AND FEMALE CATHETERIZATION—cont'd

Steps	Rationale
9. Arrange for patient privacy.	Shows respect for patient.
10. Assist patient to position: ▪ Female: dorsal-recumbent or side-lying ▪ Male: supine	Prepares patient for procedure and for easy access to site.
11. Arrange light.	Assists nurse to locate urinary meatus.
12. Wash, rinse, and dry perineum of female, if necessary.	Decreases microorganisms at site.
13. Remove gloves and wash hands.	Helps prevent cross-contamination.
14. Place supplies at foot of bed.	Allows easy access to supplies.
15. Open sterile supplies.	Arranges for sterile field for working.
16. Don sterile gloves.	Provides for sterile work area.
17. Place sterile drape under patient's buttocks and cleansing tray near perineum.	Establishes sterile work area.
18. Open cleansing agent and pour on all but one or two cotton balls.	Prepares for cleansing site.
19. Remove cap from syringe containing sterile water.	Readies use of syringe.
20. Squirt water-soluble lubricant on side near perineum.	Prepares use of lubricant for catheter insertion.
21. Place tray with Foley catheter touching cleansing tray.	Provides easy access to supplies.
22. Place sterile fenestrated drape over perineum and over upper thighs.	Drapes work area.
MALE	
23. Grasp penis in nondominant hand at shaft below glans with one hand holding it up. Continue to hold throughout procedure (Fig. 30-12, *A*).	Positions for cleansing.
24. With dominant hand, use forceps to clean penis with cotton balls.	Reduces microorganisms.
25. Cleanse meatus in circular motions without touching meatus with same cotton ball.	Decreases introduction of organisms into bladder.
26. Repeat cleansing twice more, using sterile cotton balls each time.	Decreases introduction of organisms into bladder.

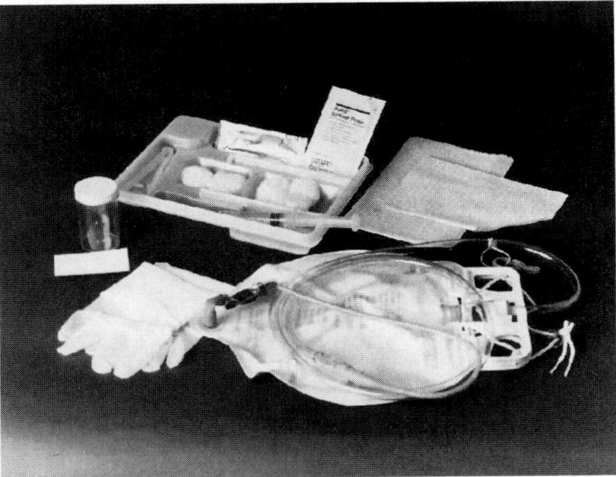

Fig. 30-11 Sterile Foley catheterization tray.

Continued.

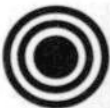

SKILL 30-1 PERFORMING MALE AND FEMALE CATHETERIZATION—cont'd

Steps	Rationale
FEMALE	
27. Spread labia minora with thumb and index finger of nondominant hand to expose urinary meatus. (Once hand is placed inside labia, it may not be moved until the catheter is inserted into the bladder to prevent contamination.)	Provides full view of area.
28. With dominant hand, use forceps to hold soaked cotton ball.	Prepares cleansing of genitals.
29. Cleanse area from clitoris down past anus. Next, cleanse down right side of labia and down left side of labia. Cleanse down center once more if necessary. (If meatus is not readily seen or is difficult to find, take dry cotton ball and place where meatus should be and brush upward.)	Cleanses least contaminated area to most contaminated area. (Opens tissue that may cover the meatal opening.)
30. Pick up catheter near tip with dominant hand. Keep distal end of catheter in container with closed drainage system (Fig. 30-12, *B*).	Allows easy manipulation and insertion of catheter.
31. Lubricate tip of catheter and gently insert it 2-4 in (female) and 7-9 in (male) until urine begins to flow. Then insert catheter another inch.	Provides easy insertion and flow of urine.
32. Collect urine specimen if needed by placing open end of catheter into specimen container.	Obtains sterile urine specimen.
FOLEY CATHETER	
33. Inflate balloon with required amount sterile water (Fig. 30-13).	Anchors catheter in bladder to to prevent slipping.
34. Pull catheter gently to ensure feeling of resistance.	Ensures anchorage.
35. Attach closed drainage system to appropriate place on bed below level of bladder.	Ensures that system is not contaminated.
36. Secure catheter to patient's thigh (female) or abdomen (male) or according to agency policy.	Prevents pulling against catheter.
37. Clip drainage tubing to bed linen. Allow slack for body movement (Fig. 30-14).	Minimizes tension and trauma of urethral and meatal openings.

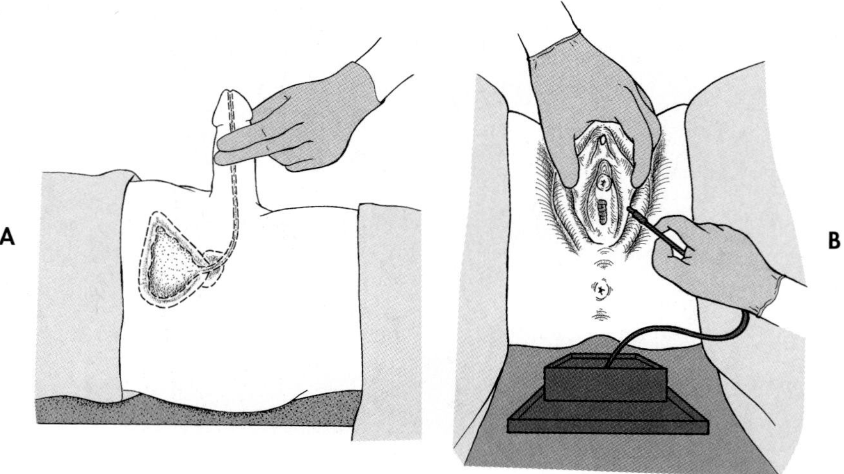

Fig. 30-12 **A,** Grasping male penis and holding for position for cleaning and insertion of catheter. **B,** Holding tip of catheter toward urinary meatus. (From Christensen BL, Kockrow EO: *Foundations of nursing,* ed 2, St Louis, 1995, Mosby.)

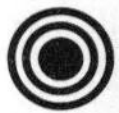

SKILL 30-1 PERFORMING MALE AND FEMALE CATHETERIZATION—cont'd

Steps	Rationale
STRAIGHT CATHETER	
38. Hold coiled catheter in hand with opening over basin.	Prevents spillage of urine.
39. Empty bladder completely and remove catheter.	Prevents complications such as urinary tract infection.
40. Dry perineal area.	Prevents impaired skin integrity.
41. Dispose of supplies.	Helps prevent spread of microorganisms.
42. Label urine specimen and take it to laboratory.	Provides correct specimen to laboratory.
43. Reposition patient.	Promotes patient comfort.
44. Assess urine flow in drainage bag. Note characteristics of urine.	Ensures appropriate functioning.
45. Remove gloves and wash hands.	Helps prevent cross-contamination.
46. Document.	Documents procedure and patient's response.

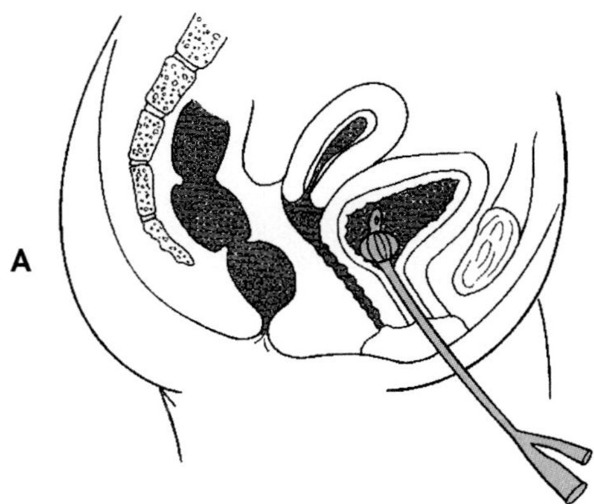

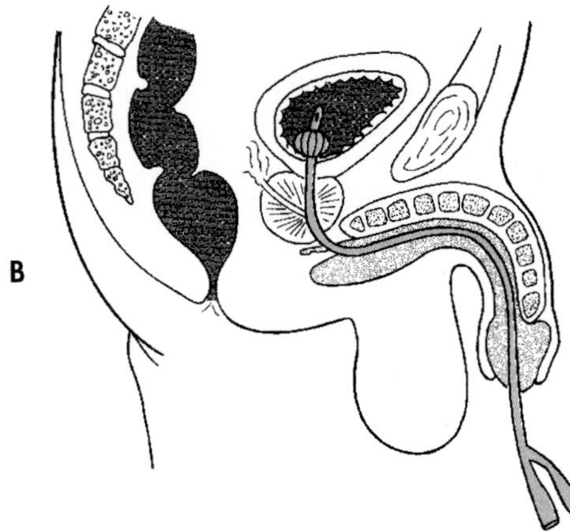

Fig. 30-13 **A,** Foley catheter in the female bladder. The inflated balloon at the top prevents the catheter from slipping through the urethra. **B,** Foley catheter with balloon inflated in the male bladder.

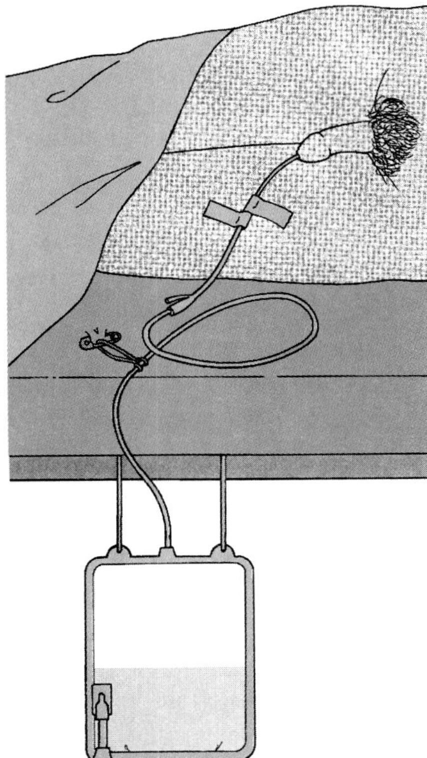

Fig. 30-14 The collecting tube is coiled on the bed and pinned to the bottom linens. A rubber band is placed around the tubing with a clove hitch. The safety pin is passed through the loops and pinned to the linens. The catheter is taped as shown. Enough slack is left on the catheter to prevent friction at the urethra.

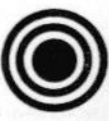

SKILL 30-2 PERFORMING BLADDER IRRIGATION AND INSTILLATION

Steps	Rationale
1. Obtain equipment: ▪ Irrigation set-up or: ▪ Clean gloves ▪ Sterile gloves ▪ Sterile irrigating solution ▪ Sterile graduated container ▪ Sterile Asepto syringe or plastic irrigating syringe ▪ Sterile basin ▪ Antiseptic preparations ▪ Sterile plug ▪ Waterproof pad	Helps organize procedure.
2. Refer to medical record, care plan, or Kardex for special interventions.	Provides basis for care.
3. Introduce self.	Decreases anxiety level.
4. Identify patient by identification band.	Identifies correct patient for procedure.
5. Explain procedure to patient.	Seeks cooperation and decreases anxiety.
6. Wash hands and don clean gloves according to agency policy and guidelines from Centers for Disease Control and Prevention and Occupational Safety and Health Administration.	Helps prevent cross-contamination.
7. Prepare patient for intervention:	
a. Close door to room or pull curtain.	Provides privacy.
b. Drape for procedure if necessary.	Prevents exposure of patient.
8. Raise bed to comfortable working level.	Provides safety for nurse.
9. Arrange for patient privacy.	Shows respect for patient.
10. Place waterproof pad under patient.	Protects bed linen and provides patient comfort.
11. Position patient to supine.	Provides easy access to site.
12. Open sterile supplies and arrange on bedside table.	Arranges supplies near at hand.
13. Pour sterile solution into sterile graduated container and recap solution bottle.	Maintains sterility.
14. Don sterile gloves.	Protects patient from microorganisms.
15. Place sterile basin between patient's legs, near perineal area.	Provides for drainage from catheter.
16. Disconnect catheter from drainage system and plug end of catheter or use port of closed drainage system.	Prepares for procedure.
17. Cleanse end of catheter with antiseptic swab.	Reduces chance of contamination.
IRRIGATION	
18. Draw 30 ml of sterile solution into syringe.	Prepares for use of irrigant.
19. Place tip of syringe into end of catheter and inject solution slowly.	Injects solution into bladder.
20. Withdraw syringe, allowing solution to drain by gravity into basin.	Cleanses and withdraws refuse from bladder.
21. Repeat until either all solution has been used or solution is clear.	Determines success of procedure.
22. Reattach drainage system, if needed.	Reestablishes drainage system.
23. Assess and measure drainage.	Allows documentation.
24. Dispose of waste materials.	Helps prevent contamination.
INSTILLATION	
25. Draw medication or solution into syringe.	Prepares for instillation.
26. Place tip of syringe into end of catheter and slowly inject solution.	Injects solution into bladder.
27. Clamp off end of catheter for period of time necessary.	Allows solution or medication to be absorbed by bladder.
28. Remove gloves and wash hands.	Helps prevent cross-contamination.
29. Document.	Documents procedure and patient's response.

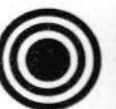

SKILL 30-3 COLLECTING A STERILE URINE SPECIMEN FROM A FOLEY CATHETER

Steps	Rationale
1. **Obtain equipment:** ▪ 10-ml syringe ▪ 1-inch needle ▪ Antiseptic swabs ▪ Sterile collection container ▪ Clean gloves	Helps organize procedure.
2. **Refer to medical record, care plan, or Kardex for special interventions.**	Provides basis for care.
3. **Introduce self.**	Decreases anxiety level.
4. **Identify patient by identification band.**	Identifies correct patient for procedure.
5. **Explain procedure to patient.**	Seeks cooperation and decreases anxiety.
6. **Wash hands and don clean gloves according to agency policy and guidelines from Centers for Disease Control and Prevention and Occupational Safety and Health Administration.**	Helps prevent cross-contamination.
7. **Prepare patient for intervention:**	
a. Close door to room or pull curtain.	Provides privacy.
b. Drape for procedure if necessary.	Prevents exposure of patient.
8. **Raise bed to comfortable working level.**	Provides safety for nurse.
9. **Arrange for patient privacy.**	Shows respect for patient.
10. **Clamp tubing to allow urine to collect.**	Ensures fresh urine for specimen.
11. **Cleanse catheter port with antiseptic swabs.**	Removes microorganisms from port.
12. **Insert needle into port at 30- to 45-degree angle, watching for needle tip to enter tubing lumen (Fig. 30-15).**	Ensures placement of needle tip into urine.
13. **Aspirate 5 to 10 ml of urine into syringe (more if needed) and remove needle.**	Collects specimen for testing.
14. **Place urine in sterile container.**	Ensures sterility of specimen.
15. **Dispose used syringe into required container.**	Prevents injury.
16. **Rewipe port with swab.**	Removes contaminant.
17. **Unclamp catheter tubing.**	Allows urine to flow appropriately.
18. **Label specimen appropriately.**	Ensures appropriate identification of specimen.
19. **Remove gloves and wash hands.**	Helps prevent cross-contamination.
20. **Document.**	Documents procedure and patient's response.

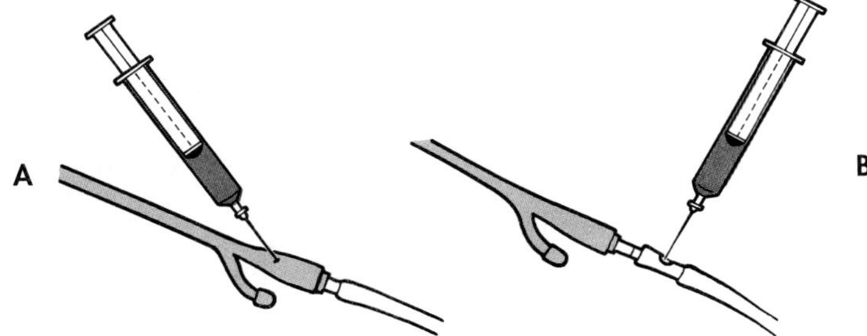

Fig. 30-15 Urine specimen collection from an indwelling catheter. **A,** Aspiration of a urine specimen from a catheter. **B,** Aspiration of a urine specimen from a collection port in the drainage tubing of an indwelling catheter. (From Potter PA, Perry AG: *Fundamentals of nursing: concepts, process, and practice,* ed 3, St Louis, 1993, Mosby. Redrawn from McConnell EA: *Care of patients with urologic problems,* Philadelphia, 1983, Lippincott.)

SUMMARY

The nurse assists the patient to maintain normal urinary function whenever possible. When urinary problems occur, the nurse uses a variety of nursing interventions to promote return to normal functioning. The nurse applies external devices and appliances and instructs the patient in self-care procedures to maintain patient safety and promote self-esteem. Helping the patient maintain normal elimination patterns includes an understanding of and sensitivity to the patient's need for privacy and dignity.

Key Concepts

- Urinary catheters carry a risk for urinary infections.
- The risk for impaired skin integrity is greater with incontinence and urinary diversion.
- The nurse instructs the patient in the importance of fluid balance and handwashing.
- Normal urinary elimination helps flush microorganisms out of the urinary system.
- A clamped, kinked, or obstructed catheter causes urine back flow into the bladder.
- Retention catheters must be secured to the patient's thigh or abdomen to prevent tugging on the urethra and meatus.
- Young children and infants require smaller catheters, but the technique is the same as catheterizing an adult.
- First specimens of timed urinary collections are always discarded.
- Urine specimens must be handled promptly and appropriately to provide accurate information.
- Nursing interventions for incontinence depend on the type of incontinence.
- A clean-catch or midstream urine specimen, when collected appropriately, does not contain bacteria from the lower urinary tract.
- The urinary system is a sterile system.
- Factors influencing urination include fluid intake, medications, growth and development, psychologic factors, surgical and diagnostic procedures, and pathologic conditions.
- The nurse assesses urine characteristics—amount, color, consistency, odor—and intake and output.
- Nursing interventions support the patient's privacy and dignity.

Critical Thinking Questions

1. Mrs. J is 8 hours postpartum and has not voided. The physician has written an order for catheterization. What criteria does the nurse use to determine whether to use a straight or indwelling catheter?
2. When inserting a retention catheter into a female patient, the nurse follows the appropriate steps. Urine does not begin to flow even though the catheter has been inserted approximately 3 to 4 inches. What should the nurse do?
3. The second-shift nurse finds a labeled urine specimen container filled with clear yellow urine on the utility room counter. The label includes the patient's name, room number, and today's date. What is the nurse's responsibility in this situation?

REFERENCES AND SUGGESTED READINGS

Blaylock B et al: A catheter anchoring device, *Ostomy and Wound Management* 39(6):36, 1993.

Dalton J: Urologic management of the patient with spinal cord injury, *Trauma Quarterly* 9(2):72, 1993.

Dille C, Kirchhoff K: Decontamination of vinyl urinary drainage bags with bleach, *Rehabilitation Nursing* 18(5):292, 1993.

Flack S: Finding the best solution: encrustation of indwelling urethral catheters: how effective are bladder washout solutions, *Nursing Times* 89(11):68, 1993.

Garibaldi RA: Catheter associated urinary tract infection, *Current Opinion in Infectious Diseases* 5(4):517, 1992.

Getliffe K: Care of urinary catheters, *Nursing Standard* 7(44):31, 1993.

Moore C, Raiwet C: A home care teaching tool: care of an indwelling catheter at home, *AARN Newsletter* 50(2):29, 1994.

Nursing procedures: student version, Springhouse Penn, 1993, Springhouse.

Potter PA, Perry AG: *Basic nursing: theory and practice,* ed 3, St Louis, 1995, Mosby.

Roe B: Catheter associated urinary tract infection: a review, *Journal of Clinical Nursing* 2:197, 1993.

Sims L, Ballard N: A comparison of two methods of catheter cleansing and storage used with clean intermittent catheterization, *Rehabilitation Nursing Research* 2(2):87, 1993.

CHAPTER 31

Bowel Elimination

Learning Objectives

After studying this chapter, the student should be able to . . .

- Define the key terms.
- Promote appropriate bowel elimination.
- Remove a fecal impaction.
- Implement bowel training.
- Insert a rectal tube.
- Administer a cleansing, carminative, and retention enema.
- Teach a patient to use natural measures for bowel elimination.
- Measure abdominal girth.
- Explain peristalsis.
- Perform an assessment of bowel elimination patterns.

Key Terms

Bowel training
Carminative enema
Cathartic
Cleansing enema
Constipation
Defecation
Diarrhea
Enema
Fecal impaction
Fecal incontinence
Feces
Flatulence
Laxative
Peristalsis
Rectal tube
Retention enema

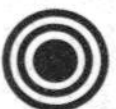

Skills

31-1 Removing a fecal impaction
31-2 Performing bowel training
31-3 Inserting a rectal tube
31-4 Administering an enema

Elimination of bowel waste **(defecation)** is a basic human need and is essential for normal body function. Normal bowel elimination depends on several factors: a balanced diet, including high-fiber foods; a daily fluid intake of 2000 to 3000 ml; and activity to promote muscle tone and **peristalsis** (rhythmic contractions of the intestines that propel gastric contents through the gastrointestinal tract). Normal stool **(feces)** is described for documentation as moderate in amount, brown, and soft in consistency and is expelled every 1 to 3 days. However, each patient has an individual pattern of defecation.

Promotion of normal patterns of elimination includes establishing a routine time for defecation, heeding the urge to defecate, sitting on a commode, and having privacy during elimination. Many people have their own established rituals to promote elimination, such as drinking warm water with lemon juice or drinking black coffee with breakfast.

Bowel elimination is a private activity, and affording the patient privacy is the responsibility of the nurse. The nurse should respect the patient's embarrassment, provide supportive nursing measures, and allow as much privacy as possible.

During the physical assessment for admission, the nurse should assess the patient's abdomen to determine nursing diagnoses related to alterations in bowel elimination, including patterns and habits. The nurse should be alert to patient habits that are detrimental to normal bowel function. The long-term, routine use of **laxatives** and **cathartics** (substances that produce bowel movements) eventually causes the intestines to lose the ability to respond to the presence of stool, often resulting in chronic constipation. The routine use of mineral oil may cause reduced absorption of fat-soluble vitamins. Overcoming cathartic dependency is often difficult to accomplish and requires patient teaching by the nurse.

NURSING PROCESS

Assessment

The nurse begins assessment of bowel elimination patterns by obtaining a nursing history. Identification of normal and abnormal patterns and habits allows the nurse to determine the patient's problems and anticipate potential problems. Much of the nursing history can be organized around the factors that affect elimination. The nurse then assesses the abdomen and notes the character and frequency of bowel sounds. The patient's feces should be inspected for color, odor, consistency, amount, and shape. Laboratory and diagnostic tests may also be performed to obtain information concerning a patient's elimination problems.

Nursing Diagnosis

Assessment of the patient's bowel function reveals data that may indicate an actual or potential problem. The nurse reviews the data and clusters defining characteristics to reveal a diagnosis. Possible nursing diagnoses for bowel elimination problems include the following:

Bowel incontinence
Colonic constipation
Constipation
Diarrhea
Impaired skin integrity
Pain
Perceived constipation
Risk for impaired skin integrity
Self-care deficit: toileting

Planning

The plan of care should include the patient's elimination habits or routines as much as possible and reinforce those that promote health. The nurse and patient should work together to plan effective interventions, since defecation patterns vary among individuals. Education is important so that the patient understands normal patterns and the relatively easy ways to promote elimination (see care plan on p. 600). If the patient is physically unable to follow hygiene elimination practices, the family should be included in the plan of care. The nurse should be sensitive and understanding in discussing bowel elimination, a topic that may cause embarrassment.

Goals and expected outcomes for patients with elimination problems may include the following:

Goal #1: Patient achieves regular defecation habits within 2 weeks.

Outcome

Patient defecates on a predictable schedule by 1 week.

Goal #2: Patient understands normal elimination.

Outcome

Patient verbalizes understanding of expected defecation pattern.

Implementation

The success of the interventions depends on improving the patient's and family's understanding of bowel elimination. The patient should be taught effective bowel habits (see teaching box). The nurse should give special consideration to the older adult (see gerontologic box). It is important for the nurse to preserve as much of the patient's independence as possible, ensure privacy, and promote physical well-being.

Evaluation

The nurse evaluates the success of the interventions by determining whether the established goals and expected outcomes have been met. The nurse

PATIENT TEACHING 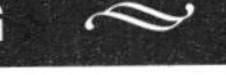

- Explain the importance of heeding the urge to defecate to promote normal bowel elimination.
- Instruct the patient about cleansing the anal area with mild soap and water after elimination to maintain skin integrity.
- Assure the patient that privacy will be given when a bedpan or bedside commode is used.
- Teach the patient that dependence on laxatives and cathartics can result in chronic constipation and that the overuse of mineral oil can reduce the body's absorption of vitamins A, D, E, and K.

GERONTOLOGIC CONSIDERATIONS

- The older adult may make a self-diagnosis of constipation (perceived constipation) and believe that a laxative must be taken to have a daily bowel movement.
- It is important for the older adult to maintain a proper diet to reduce the risk of constipation.
- Decreased muscle tone can cause difficulty in controlling defecation. Age-appropriate exercises should be encouraged to maintain healthy bowel elimination patterns.

must be prepared to revise the care plan based on the evaluation. Examples of goals and evaluative measures follow:

Goal #1: Patient achieves regular defecation habits within 2 weeks.

Evaluative measure

Observe a recorded defecation pattern over several days.

Goal #2: Patient understands normal elimination.

Evaluative measure

Ask patient to describe factors affecting elimination.

COMMON ALTERATIONS

Alterations in bowel elimination often occur, causing the patient distress and discomfort. Such alterations include constipation, fecal impaction, loss of muscle tone of the bowel, flatulence, incontinence, and diarrhea.

Constipation and Fecal Impaction

Constipation (difficulty passing stool or infrequent passage of hard stool) may occur when there is reduced peristalsis or when stool is retained in the lower colon or rectum. Constipation usually results from irregular bowel habits such as ignoring the defecation reflex. It can also result from inadequate fluid intake, a low-fiber diet, lack of exercise, and immobility. Pregnancy can also cause constipation.

Since water is reabsorbed from stool in the colon, feces that remains in the colon or rectum because of constipation may become dry and hard, forming an obstructive mass called a ***fecal impaction.*** Factors that predispose a patient to this problem include dehydration, nutritional deficit, prolonged immobility, x-ray studies using barium, and certain constipating medications such as narcotics, iron preparations, or antidepressants.

A fecal impaction may cause a small amount of liquid, oozing diarrheal stool. The nurse should assess the patient's rectum, palpating for the impaction, unless it is higher in the tract. If an impaction is confirmed, an oil retention or a cleansing enema is administered in an attempt to break up the stool for removal. Often, at least part of the impacted stool may be removed at the time of assessment (Skill 31-1). This activity aids the removal of more stool when the enema is administered. Removal of a fecal impaction requires a medical order, and in some agencies, only the physician or registered nurse may remove one.

Loss of Muscle Tone

Loss of muscle tone of the bowel causes sluggishness and makes it more difficult to evacuate stool. Once this problem occurs, the nurse should begin bowel training to increase the muscle tone so that the patient can evacuate stools normally and thus prevent fecal incontinence.

Flatulence

Flatulence (presence of air or gas in the intestinal tract) may be caused when a person consumes gas-producing liquids and foods such as carbonated beverages, cabbage, or beans; swallows excessive amounts of air; or is constipated. In hospitalized patients, flatulence is often caused by decreased peristalsis, abdominal surgery, some narcotic medications, and decreased physical activity. Flatulence may cause distention (swelling) of the stomach and abdomen and in some cases mild to moderate abdominal cramping and pain. One of the most effective measures to promote peristalsis and passage of flatus is walking. When the discomforts of flatulence are not relieved by eliminating the cause or by walking, a rectal tube may be used. The presence of the tube in the rectum stimulates peristalsis and the movement of flatus.

Fecal Incontinence

Fecal incontinence is the inability to control the passage of feces and gas from the anus. Causes may include multiple sclerosis, cerebrovascular accidents (strokes), spinal cord trauma, loss of muscle tone, and tumors or growths of the anal sphincter. The patient may be unaware of the need to defecate because of mental conditions such as dementia, severe depression, and schizophrenia or because of the use of sedatives. There is a risk of skin breakdown (see Chapter 21) in the patient with fecal incontinence.

Diarrhea

Diarrhea is the passage of liquid feces as well as an increase in the number of stools. It is a symptom of gastrointestinal disorders such as enteritis, colitis, Crohn's disease, and irritable bowel syndrome. It can also be caused by stress, allergies, food intolerance, medications, and surgery.

Diarrheal feces is liquid because it passes too quickly through the small and large intestines, thus preventing the body from absorbing fluid. The loss of fluid can cause fluid and electrolyte imbalances, especially in infants and older adults (see Chapter 24). There is also a risk of impaired skin integrity (see Chapter 21).

NURSING CARE

Bowel Training

Bowel training is a method of establishing regular evacuation by reflex conditioning and is used in the treatment of fecal incontinence, impaction, and chronic diarrhea. In this method the patient's previous bowel habits are assessed, and a program is begun to induce an evacuation at the same time each day or every other day (Skill 31-2), a time that is also called *habit time*. Exercises to strengthen abdominal muscles, such as pushing up, bearing down, and contracting the musculature, are demonstrated. A bedside commode is provided, and privacy is ensured. The nurse instructs the patient to recognize and respond promptly to signals indicating a full bowel, such as goose pimples and perspiration, and to develop cues to stimulate the urge to defecate, such as drinking coffee, massaging the abdomen, pressing the inner thigh, or stroking the anus. A daily fluid intake of 3000 ml is encouraged. Prune juice, orange juice, and coffee are included in the daily diet, and the importance of having well-balanced meals that include bulk and roughage and of avoiding constipating foods such as bananas, beans, and cabbage is discussed. A total of 4 to 10 ounces of prune juice may be required each night or 12 hours before the time set for evacuation. A glycerin suppository may be required before the set time. Reflex conditioning is often an effective method of developing regular bowel habits, especially if the patient is highly motivated.

Insertion of a Rectal Tube

A **rectal tube** is a flexible, small tube inserted into the rectum to assist in the relief of flatus. The nurse has the patient assume a side-lying position during the insertion of a rectal tube (Skill 31-3). The tube is inserted 15 cm (6 inches) for an adult and 5 to 10 cm (2 to 4 inches) in a child. It is taped to the buttocks, and the patient is instructed to lie quietly in bed. A gauze dressing or waterproof pad is placed around the open end of the tube to catch liquid feces. A rectal tube should not be left in place longer than 30 minutes.

Administration of Enemas

An **enema** is a procedure in which a warm solution or a solution at body temperature is introduced into the rectum for cleansing, therapeutic, or diagnostic purposes. An enema is often used to promote bowel elimination. When an enema solution enters the rectum and descending colon, it causes irritation of the mucosa and distends the intestines, thereby stimulating peristalsis and bowel evacuation.

! REMEMBER

- If flatulence is not relieved by a rectal tube, more aggressive therapy may be necessary.
- Liquid enema soap should be added to the water for an enema to prevent soap bubbles.
- If the enema solution is not expelled, the nurse should try repositioning the patient in bed or should have the ambulatory patient walk. The enema tubing may also be reinserted in an attempt to stimulate peristalsis.

Table 31-1 TYPES OF ENEMAS AND THEIR PURPOSES

Type	Purpose
Cleansing	
Tap water	Removes stool from intestines before surgery
Normal saline	Removes stool from intestines before diagnostic testing
Soapsuds	
Hypertonic (commercially prepared)	Relieves flatulence, constipation and fecal impaction
Carminative	Relieves flatulence
MGW (magnesium, 30 ml; glycerin, 60 ml, water, 90 ml)	
Milk and molasses (equal parts)	
Retention	
Oil (mineral oil)	Lubricates intestines and stool to make feces softer and easier to move

There are several types of enemas, but those included in this chapter are categorized as cleansing, carminative, and retention (Table 31-1). A **cleansing enema** is usually composed of soapsuds and tap water or tap water alone administered to remove all formed fecal material from the colon. A **carminative enema** consists of a combination of milk and molasses that relieves flatulence and abdominal distention. The **retention enema** is a medicinal or nutrient enema specially formed so that it remains in the bowel without stimulating the nerve endings that would ordinarily result in evacuation immediately after administration or within a few minutes of administration.

Enemas may be commercially prepared, disposable units or reusable equipment prepared just before use (Skill 31-4). Commercially prepared enemas contain approximately 4 ounces (120 ml) of solution.

Side effects

Each enema solution has its own adverse effects. Tap water enemas may cause electrolyte imbalances. Soap solution enemas may irritate and damage the intestinal mucosa. Hypertonic solutions in commercially prepared enemas may produce sodium retention. Because of these potential problems, the patient should be taught the adverse effects of taking frequent enemas and should be encouraged to learn to have bowel movements by normal measures.

Enema solution

The amount of fluid used in administering an enema depends on the medical order and the individual. Most adults may hold between 500 and 1000 ml successfully. The least amount of solution that receives the best results should be used.

When a medical order reads "cleansing enemas until clear," enemas are continued until the fluid returned is clear of feces. If the "return" is not clear after three enemas, the physician or immediate supervisor should be consulted. This type of procedure requires a larger amount of fluid.

An enema solution is warmed to a safe temperature, usually 105° to 110° F for an adult and 100° F for a child. The temperature for younger children should be directed by the physician.

The warmer the fluid, the better results from the enema. However, not all patients can stand the same amount of heat. Therefore the nurse should take care not to burn a patient. A discussion about the temperature of the solution should occur before the patient's first enema is administered. The nurse follows agency policy for the correct, safe temperature and listens to the patient who says that the solution is too hot.

Administration

Many patients have had enemas administered by a nurse or family member or have administered one themselves. Others have never had an enema and need teaching and support from the nurse because they are probably anxious about the procedure. The nurse should explain how the procedure is done and what is expected from the patient. The patient often fears not being able to hold the solution as instructed. To help, the nurse suggests deep breathing with the mouth open and keeps a bedpan nearby for patient use.

A left side-lying position (Sims') is used because it is usually more conducive to relaxation and longer retention of fluid. However, the patient may be placed on the right side-lying position if necessary. If the patient cannot hold the solution, the nurse may position the patient on a bedpan during administration.

■ NURSING CARE PLAN ■

PERCEIVED CONSTIPATION

Mrs. Y, age 78, has developed constipation 4 days after surgery. The nurse discovers that Mrs. Y has been using strong over-the-counter laxatives for the past several months to have daily bowel movements.

NURSING DIAGNOSIS

Perceived constipation related to use of laxatives as evidenced by daily use of laxatives and the belief of necessity to have daily bowel movement

GOAL

- Elimination pattern will return to normal.

EXPECTED OUTCOMES

- Patient will have bowel movement every 2 days.
- Patient will drink recommend oral fluids daily.
- Patient will eat well-balanced meals.

NURSING INTERVENTION

- Assess frequency and character of stool.
- Monitor fluid intake and output.
- Instruct patient regarding diet and exercise.

EVALUATION

- Patient resumes normal bowel elimination.
- Patient stops laxative use after learning new information.
- Patient exercises and drinks recommended fluids.

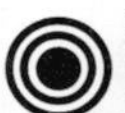

SKILL 31-1 REMOVING A FECAL IMPACTION

Steps	Rationale
1. Obtain equipment: ▪ Bedpan ▪ Water-soluble lubricant ▪ Waterproof pad ▪ Toilet tissue ▪ Washcloth ▪ Towel ▪ Soap ▪ Bath basin ▪ Clean gloves	Helps organize procedure.
2. Refer to medical record, care plan, or Kardex for special interventions.	Provides basis for care.
3. Introduce self.	Decreases anxiety level.
4. Identify patient by identification band.	Identifies correct patient for procedure.
5. Explain procedure to patient.	Seeks cooperation and decreases anxiety.
6. Wash hands and don clean gloves according to agency policy and guidelines from Centers for Disease Control and Prevention and Occupational Safety and Health Administration.	Helps prevent cross-contamination.
7. Prepare patient for intervention:	
a. Close door to room or pull curtain.	Provides privacy.
b. Drape for procedure if necessary.	Prevents exposure of patient.
8. Raise bed to comfortable working level.	Provides safety for nurse.
9. Arrange for patient privacy.	Shows respect for patient.
10. Place patient in left Sims' position.	Places patient in position of choice for rectal procedures.
11. Place waterproof pad under patient's buttocks.	Protects bed from getting wet and soiled.
12. Place bedpan on bed near foot of bed.	Allows easy access to bedpan, which is used for holding feces as it is removed.
13. Arrange patient's gown and top linen so that they are out of way but provide privacy.	Avoids exposure and soiling of gown and linen.
14. Count radial pulse.	Provides baseline cardiovascular status.
15. Lubricate dominant forefinger liberally.	Reduces pain and irritation of mucosa.
16. Insert forefinger gently. Slowly move finger into and around fecal mass.	Helps reduce patient discomfort.
17. As pieces of stool are broken off, remove them to bedpan.	Removes small amounts of stool to aid patient discomfort.
18. Continue procedure until as much as possible of impaction is removed.	Allows for almost complete removal of fecal impaction.
19. During procedure, stop for few minutes if patient complains of discomfort.	Provides rest for patient.
20. After procedure, wash and dry perineal area thoroughly.	Prevents tissue irritation and skin breakdown.
21. Remove waterproof pad and place patient in position of comfort.	Provides patient comfort and safety.
22. Dispose of equipment.	Reduces transmission of microorganisms.
23. Remove gloves and wash hands.	Helps prevent cross-contamination.
24. Count radial pulse.	Detects deviation from baseline pulse rate.
25. Document.	Documents procedure and patient's response.

SKILL 31-2 PERFORMING BOWEL TRAINING

Steps	Rationale
1. **Obtain equipment:** ▪ Suppository, if prescribed ▪ Waterproof pad ▪ Bedpan or bedside commode ▪ Clean gloves	Helps organize procedure.
2. **Refer to medical record, care plan, or Kardex for special interventions.**	Provides basis for care.
3. **Introduce self.**	Decreases anxiety level.
4. **Identify patient by identification band.**	Identifies correct patient for procedure.
5. **Explain procedure to patient.**	Seeks cooperation and decreases anxiety.
6. **Wash hands and don clean gloves according to agency policy and guidelines from Centers for Disease Control and Prevention and Occupational Safety and Health Administration.**	Helps prevent cross-contamination.
7. **Prepare patient for intervention:**	
a. Close door to room or pull curtain.	Provides privacy.
b. Drape for procedure if necessary.	Prevents exposure of patient.
8. **Raise bed to comfortable working level.**	Provides safety for nurse.
9. **Arrange for patient privacy.**	Shows respect for patient.
10. **Ask patient what measures have promoted bowel elimination in past.**	Provides baseline to begin training.
11. **Assess patient's ability to understand and cooperate with program.**	Allows patient participation, which increases likelihood of success.
12. **Administer cathartic rectal suppository, if prescribed, 30 min before normal time of defecation.**	Stimulates peristalsis.
13. **Provide for factors that normally precede patient's bowel elimination.**	Stimulates peristalsis.
14. **Within 30 min of suppository administration or earlier if patient expresses urge to defecate, assist patient to bedpan, bedside commode, or preferably, commode.**	Stimulates peristalsis, usually within 30 min, and enhances bowel elimination.
15. **Ensure patient privacy and safety by leaving alone no longer than 15 to 30 min, if condition warrants.**	Aids patient relaxation, thus promoting elimination.
16. **Provide encouragement and positive reinforcement for patient success.**	Encourages patient to remain on program.
17. **Assist in cleaning rectal area and helping patient back to bed.**	Enhances patient comfort and safety.
18. **Dispose of equipment.**	Reduces transmission of microorganisms.
19. **Remove gloves and wash hands.**	Helps prevent cross-contamination.
20. **Document.**	Documents procedure and patient's response.

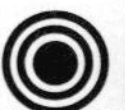

SKILL 31-3 INSERTING A RECTAL TUBE

Steps	Rationale
1. **Obtain equipment:** ▪ Rectal tube (22 to 34 Fr) ▪ Specimen container or urinal ▪ Water-soluble lubricant ▪ Waterproof pad ▪ Nonallergenic tape ▪ Tape measure ▪ Toilet tissue	Helps organize procedure.

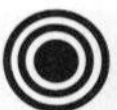

SKILL 31-3 INSERTING A RECTAL TUBE—cont'd

Steps	Rationale
▪ Washcloth ▪ Towel ▪ Bedpan or bedside commode ▪ Clean gloves	
2. Refer to medical record, care plan, or Kardex for special interventions.	Provides basis for care.
3. Introduce self.	Decreases anxiety level.
4. Identify patient by identification band.	Identifies correct patient for procedure.
5. Explain procedure to patient.	Seeks cooperation and decreases anxiety.
6. Wash hands and don clean gloves according to agency policy and guidelines from Centers for Disease Control and Prevention and Occupational Safety and Health Administration.	Helps prevent cross-contamination.
7. Prepare patient for intervention:	
a. Close door to room or pull curtain.	Provides privacy.
b. Drape for procedure if necessary.	Prevents exposure of patient.
8. Raise bed to comfortable working level.	Provides safety for nurse.
9. Arrange for patient privacy.	Shows respect for patient.
10. Have patient assume left side-lying position.	Provides access to rectum.
11. Arrange gown and top linens so that they are out of way but drape patient.	Prevents soiling and provides privacy.
12. Place waterproof pad under patient's buttocks.	Protects bottom linen from soiling.
13. Lubricate rectal tube thoroughly.	Reduces irritation of mucosa.
14. Expose anus to view and insert rectal tube 4 to 6 in (10 to 15 cm), avoiding injury.	Allows anus to be clearly identified so that hemorrhoids may be protected and so that discomfort of unsuccessful attempts to insert rectal tube is minimized.
15. Tape tube to buttocks and insert end into receptacle or use commercially prepared setup.	Helps prevent dislodgment of rectal tube and prevents soiling from drainage of stool that may accompany flatus.
16. Instruct patient to lie still.	Helps prevent dislodgment of rectal tube.
17. Leave rectal tube in place no longer than 30 min at one time.	Prevents reduced stimulation of peristalsis caused by continued insertion beyond 30 min.
18. Remove rectal tube and assist patient to bedpan, bedside commode, or commode.	Allows stimulation of peristalsis, which may result in bowel movement.
19. Provide for hygiene and assist patient to bed or chair.	Provides for patient comfort.
20. Reinsert rectal tube later or as prescribed.	Ensures effectiveness of treatment, since single insertion may not relieve all flatus and discomfort.
21. Dispose of equipment.	Reduces transmission of microorganisms.
22. Remove gloves and wash hands.	Helps prevent cross-contamination.
23. Document.	Documents procedure and patient's response.

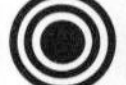

SKILL 31-4 ADMINISTERING AN ENEMA

Steps	Rationale
1. Obtain equipment: ▪ Commercially prepared kit or enema set (Fig. 31-1) ▪ Solution ▪ Additive (that is, soap packet) ▪ Bath thermometer ▪ Bedpan ▪ Toilet tissue ▪ Waterproof pad ▪ Intravenous pole ▪ Washcloth	Helps organize procedure.

Continued.

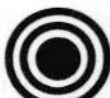

SKILL 31-4 ADMINISTERING AN ENEMA—cont'd

Steps	Rationale
▪ Towel ▪ Soap ▪ Bath blanket ▪ Bedside commode, if prescribed ▪ Clean gloves	
2. Refer to medical record, care plan, or Kardex for special interventions.	Provides basis for care.
3. Introduce self.	Decreases anxiety level.

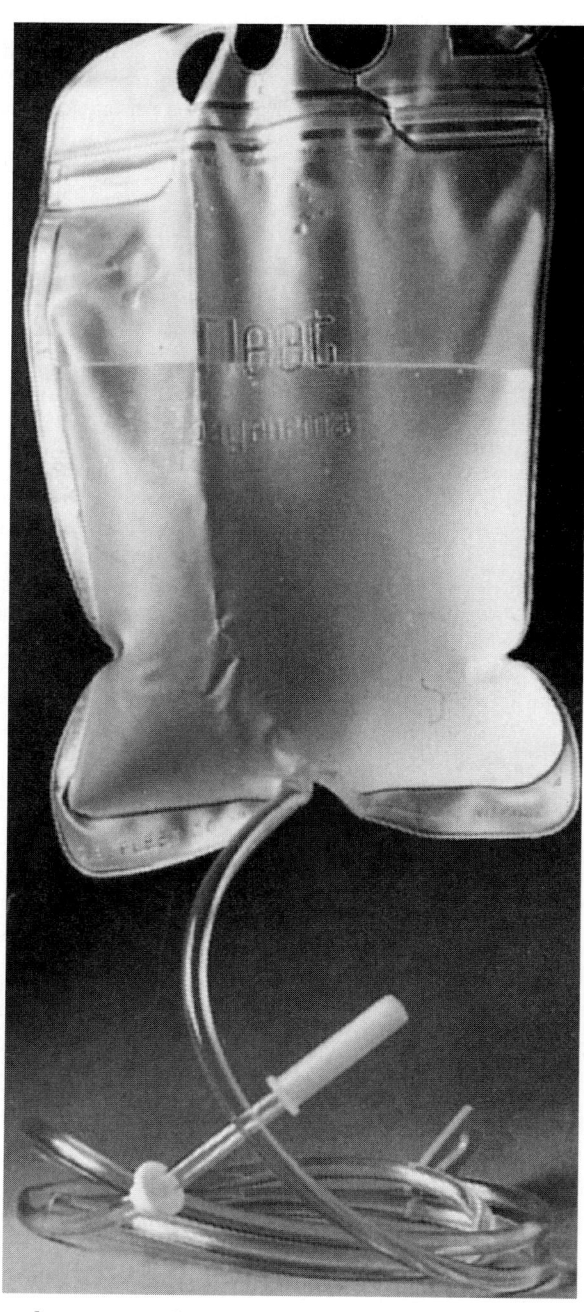

Fig. 31-1 High-volume enema bag with tubing. (From Perry AG, Potter PA: *Clinical nursing skills and techniques,* ed 3, St Louis, 1994, Mosby.)

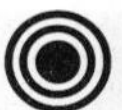

SKILL 31-4 ADMINISTERING AN ENEMA—cont'd

Steps	Rationale
4. Identify patient by identification band.	Identifies correct patient for procedure.
5. Explain procedure to patient.	Seeks cooperation and decreases anxiety.
6. Wash hands and don clean gloves according to agency policy and guidelines from Centers for Disease Control and Prevention and Occupational Safety and Health Administration.	Helps prevent cross-contamination.
7. Prepare patient for intervention:	
a. Close door to room or pull curtain.	Provides privacy.
b. Drape for procedure if necessary.	Prevents exposure of patient.
8. Raise bed to comfortable working level.	Provides safety for nurse.
9. Arrange for patient privacy.	Shows respect for patient.
10. Place waterproof pad under patient's buttocks.	Protects bottom linen.
11. Place patient in Sim's (side-lying) position.	Facilitates relaxation and enhances effectiveness of enema.
12. Arrange top linen and patient gown so that they are out of way but provide privacy.	Protects top linen and gown from soiling.
CLEANSING ENEMA	
13. Clamp enema tubing 7 in (28 cm) from end of tubing.	Keeps clamp out of way.
14. Fill enema container with appropriately warmed solution and required additive.	Provides for patient comfort.
15. Read disposable package instructions.	Ensures correct procedure.
16. Release tubing clamp, allowing solution to flow through tubing to clear tubing of air. Reclamp tubing.	Removes air from tubing.
17. Hang enema container on intravenous pole so that bottom of container is 12 to 18 in (30 to 45 cm) above level of patient's anus.	Allows solution to flow at appropriate rate.
18. Lubricate 4 in (10 cm) of end of tubing.	Provides for easy insertion of tubing.
19. Spread patient's buttocks with nondominant hand.	Provides view of anus before insertion of enema tubing is attempted.
20. While rotating enema tubing, gently insert it 3 to 4 in (7 to 10 cm) (Fig. 31-2).	Reduces trauma to tissues.

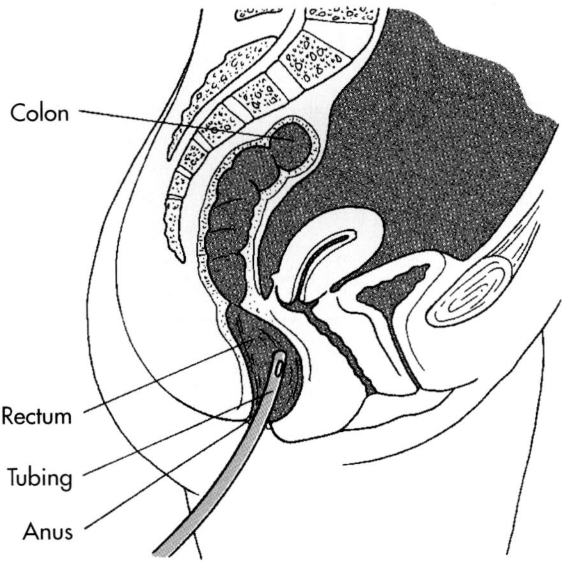

Fig. 31-2 Insertion of enema tubing.

Continued.

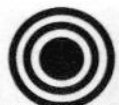

SKILL 31-4 ADMINISTERING AN ENEMA—cont'd

Steps	Rationale
21. Release tubing clamp and allow solution to flow slowly while holding tube. Allow solution to flow 5 to 10 min.	Keeps tubing in place. Allows intestines to distend without producing immediate urge to defecate.
22. Lower enema container or clamp tubing if patient complains of cramping and encourage slow, deep breathing with mouth open.	Allows sufficient solution to be administered and retained.
23. Clamp and remove enema tubing when all or enough solution has been administered. Encourage patient to retain solution at least 5 min.	Promotes peristalsis and enhances defecation.
COMMERCIALLY PREPARED ENEMA	
24. Remove cover from prelubricated enema tip (Fig. 31-3) and insert entire tip into rectum.	Provides for patient comfort, safety of patient, and convenience of nurse.
25. Squeeze container until it can no longer introduce solution.	Prevents introduction of air into rectum because container cannot be completely emptied of solution.
26. Encourage patient to retain solution.	Provides better results from enema.
27. When patient can no longer retain solution or all solution has been introduced, assist patient to bedpan, bedside commode, or commode. Remind patient not to flush commode.	Enhances defecation and allows nurse to assess enema results.
28. Provide patient hygiene.	Prevents skin breakdown and provides patient comfort.
29. Assist patient back to bed.	Allows patient to rest after procedure.
30. Dispose of equipment.	Reduces transmission of microorganisms.
31. Remove gloves and wash hands.	Helps prevent cross-contamination.
32. Document.	Documents procedure and patient's response.

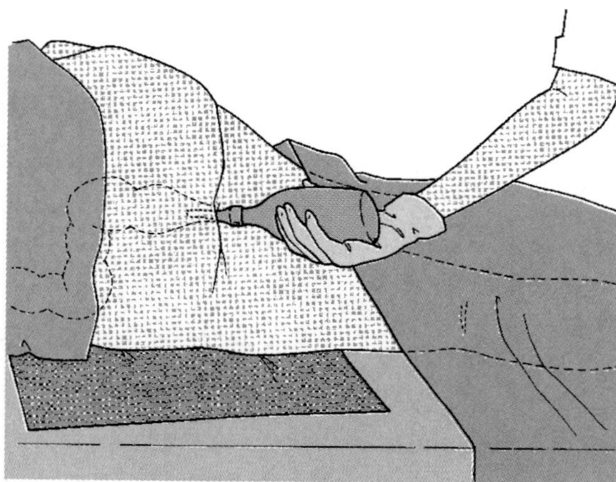

Fig. 31-3 Insertion of commercial enema.

SUMMARY

Elimination of feces is a basic human need, and the patient needs to be respected and accepted and made comfortable when the nurse must be in attendance. A well-balanced diet, adequate fluid intake, and exercise are essential to the promotion of regular bowel function.

Key Concepts

- Normal stool is moderate in amount, brown, and soft in consistency and is expelled every 1 to 3 days.
- The routine use of laxatives or cathartics may cause the intestines to lose the ability to respond to the presence of stool, often resulting in chronic constipation.
- Regular bowel elimination depends on factors such as a high-fiber diet, a daily fluid intake of 2000 to 3000 ml, and physical activity to promote peristalsis.
- The promotion of regular patterns of elimination include establishing a routine time for defecation, heeding the urge to defecate, sitting on a commode, and having privacy during elimination.
- Fecal impaction is evident by the lack of bowel movement for several days or by frequent, small, watery, unformed, and perhaps diarrheal stool.

Critical Thinking Questions

1. A 25-year-old man with a history of good health is admitted to the unit after a motor vehicle accident. His injuries and treatments are such that he has been prescribed bedrest for the next 2 weeks. What type of plan would the nurse design to prevent him from becoming constipated during this period of immobility?
2. The nurse is asked to provide an outpatient with material and instructions for three stool guaiac tests. Identify and explain four important points of information that the nurse would want to include in the instructions.
3. This is the nurse's first day of caring for a bedridden, comatose, 87-year-old man. In reviewing his chart, the nurse can find no entry of a bowel movement for the past 10 days. How would the nurse proceed with the bowel assessment?

REFERENCES AND SUGGESTED READINGS

Kim MJ, McFarland GK, McLane AM: *Pocket guide to nursing diagnoses,* ed 6, St Louis, 1995, Mosby.

Long BC, Phipps WJ, Cassmeyer VL: *Medical-surgical nursing: a nursing process approach,* ed 3, St Louis, 1993, Mosby.

Mosby's medical, nursing, and allied health dictionary, ed 4, St Louis, 1994, Mosby.

Perry AG, Potter PA: *Clinical nursing skills and techniques,* ed 3, St Louis, 1994, Mosby.

Potter PA, Perry AG: *Basic nursing: theory and practice,* ed 3, St Louis, 1995, Mosby.

CHAPTER 32

Ostomy Care

Learning Objectives

After studying this chapter, the student should be able to . . .

- Define the key terms.
- Identify the guidelines used in performing ostomy care.
- Compare similarities in caring for a colostomy, an ileostomy, and a ureterostomy.
- Assist a patient in accepting and adjusting to an ostomy.
- Implement care for a colostomy, an ileostomy, and a ureterostomy.
- Perform colostomy irrigation.
- Teach a patient ostomy self-care.

Key Terms

Anastomosis
Colostomy
Conduit
Enterostomal therapist (ET)
Excoriation
Herniation
Ileostomy
Ostomate
Ostomy
Peristomal
Prolapse
Stoma
Ureterostomy

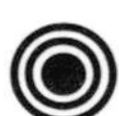

Skills

32-1 Caring for a colostomy or an ileostomy
32-2 Performing colostomy irrigation
32-3 Caring for a ureterostomy

ANATOMY REVIEW

Intestines

The adult human body contains approximately 23 feet of small intestine and 6 feet of large intestine.The small intestine begins at the base of the stomach, where the pyloric sphincter opens and admits waste into the small intestine. The beginning section of the small intestine, called the *duodenum,* is C-shaped and is approximately 10 inches in length. The next section, called the *jejunum,* is approximately 9½ feet in length. The remaining section, the ileum, follows the jejunum and is approximately 12½ feet in length. The small intestine is the major site of digestion and absorption of essential nutrients in the body.

The large intestine begins at the end of the small intestine in an area called the *ileocecal valve.* Sections of this portion of the large intestine are called the *ascending, transverse, descending,* and *sigmoid* colon. The rectum and anus complete the large bowel. The large intestine completes the digestive process begun in the small intestine. It plays a critical role in water resorption. The contents of the colon are gradually dehydrated until the consistency of a normal stool is achieved.

Urinary System

The ureters are two tubes that carry urine from the kidney to the bladder. The organs are 28 to 34 cm long and consist of three layers. The ureters originate at the pelvis of the kidney and empty into the bladder. When the bladder fills, urine is evacuated through the urethra and out from the urinary meatus (external opening of the urethra).

OSTOMIES

An **ostomy** is a surgical procedure that creates an abdominal opening originating in the bowel or urinary tract through which feces or urine is eliminated. The abdominal opening is called a ***stoma.*** It should protrude approximately 2.5 cm (1 inch) above the abdominal wall. The word ***ostomate*** refers to a person on whom an ostomy has been performed. The **enterostomal therapist (ET)** is a nurse specialist in ostomy and wound care management. The ET nurse directs the care of the ostomy after surgery.

NURSING PROCESS

Assessment

The stoma and surrounding area must be assessed at least every shift during the patient's hospital stay. The nurse should be alert for the following complications: excessive bleeding, darkening or extreme lightening of the color of the stoma (indicating lack of blood supply); drying, edema, or **prolapse** (pulling back into abdomen) of the stoma; skin irritations around the stoma; signs of infection; or **herniation** (protrusion of an organ through an abdominal opening). These conditions require physician notification. Other routine assessments include intake and output; daily weight; electrolyte monitoring; amount, color, consistency, odor, and frequency of stool or urine; vital signs; and diet.

The type and adherent ability of the appliance should be assessed on a regular basis. The appliance must be large enough that it does not cut off circulation but small enough to prevent leakage and resultant skin irritation (see care plan on p. 615). Because of stoma edema, the size of the pouch decreases during the first 4 to 6 weeks after surgery.

Nursing Diagnosis

The nurse reviews all data collected during assessment and clusters defining characteristics to reveal a diagnosis. Examples of nursing diagnoses related to ostomy care include the following:

Altered nutrition: less than body requirements
Altered patterns of urinary elimination
Body-image disturbance
Constipation
Diarrhea
Fluid volume deficit
Impaired skin integrity
Pain
Risk for impaired skin integrity
Risk for infection

PATIENT TEACHING

- Have the patient demonstrate ostomy self-care at least twice before discharge.
- Teach the patient to inspect the appearance of the stoma and surrounding area on a routine basis.
- Instruct the patient to report excessive bleeding, abnormal color, or edema to the nurse or physician.
- Teach the patient to avoid the use of peroxide on or around the stoma because it irritates tissue.
- Instruct the patient to avoid the use of alcohol to cleanse around a stoma because it dilates capillaries and causes bleeding of the stomal margin.

GERONTOLOGIC CONSIDERATIONS

- Manual dexterity should be assessed in the older patient. Simple measures, such as precutting the ostomy bag, can assist the patient who has limited dexterity.
- Family members may need to assist the older adult with ostomy care.
- The older patient should be closely monitored for signs of fluid and electrolyte imbalance.

Planning

The nurse and the patient should collaborate in planning goals and expected outcomes for ostomy care. The initial interaction of the nurse is critical in determining the patient's eventual acceptance of the stoma. The nurse should approach the patient with an accepting, professional attitude. Forming a trusting nurse-patient relationship assists the patient in believing that the skills necessary for self-care of the ostomy can be learned. It is important for the nurse to provide patient teaching (see teaching box). Teaching needs should be continually reevaluated. The patient's psychologic and emotional adjustment should not be overlooked.

The plan of care may include the following goal:

Goal: Patient's skin integrity is maintained.

Outcome

Patient expresses understanding of proper periostomal hygiene to prevent skin breakdown.

Implementation

While implementing the plan of care, the nurse does not hurry the patient's acceptance of the ostomy. Supportive nursing care respects the patient's privacy and emotional needs. The nurse should be especially sensitive to the special needs of the older patient (see gerontologic box).

Evaluation

The effectiveness of nursing interventions is measured by the success of meeting the established goals of care. If the goals have not been achieved, the nurse may need to revise the plan of care. An evaluative measure may include the following:

Goal: Patient's skin integrity is maintained.

Evaluative measure

Ask patient to explain skin care measures.

COLOSTOMY AND ILEOSTOMY

A **colostomy** is the surgical creation of an artificial anus on the abdominal wall by incising (cutting) the colon and bringing it out to a stoma on the abdominal surface. The procedure is performed for patients with cancer of the colon, intestinal obstructions, intestinal trauma, or inflammatory diseases of the colon. The colostomy may be permanent or temporary until intestinal healing occurs.

The colostomy diverts stool through the stoma. The stool may be liquid, semiformed, or formed, depending on the area of the colon incised.

When the ostomy is placed in the ascending colon, the consistency of the stool is always liquid. The patient cannot be certain when the stool will evacuate and must constantly wear a collection device for safety from eruption. An ostomy along the ascending colon is called an *ascending colostomy* (Fig. 32-1). If the stoma is along the transverse colon, the ostomy is referred to as a *transverse colostomy.* The stool in this portion of the colon is semisoft. When the colostomy is performed at the lower part of the descending colon, it is called a *sigmoid colostomy.* The stool in this part of the colon is formed. The patient with a sigmoid colostomy can usually gain control of routine fecal evacuation through a regimen of irrigation, diet, and exercise. In some cases, routine evacuation eliminates the need to wear a pouch continuously.

A fecal stoma is usually constructed in one of three ways. A loop colostomy is created when the bowel is brought to the exterior with a plastic rod supporting it. The bowel has only one layer incised. The distal and proximal ends remain intact. The

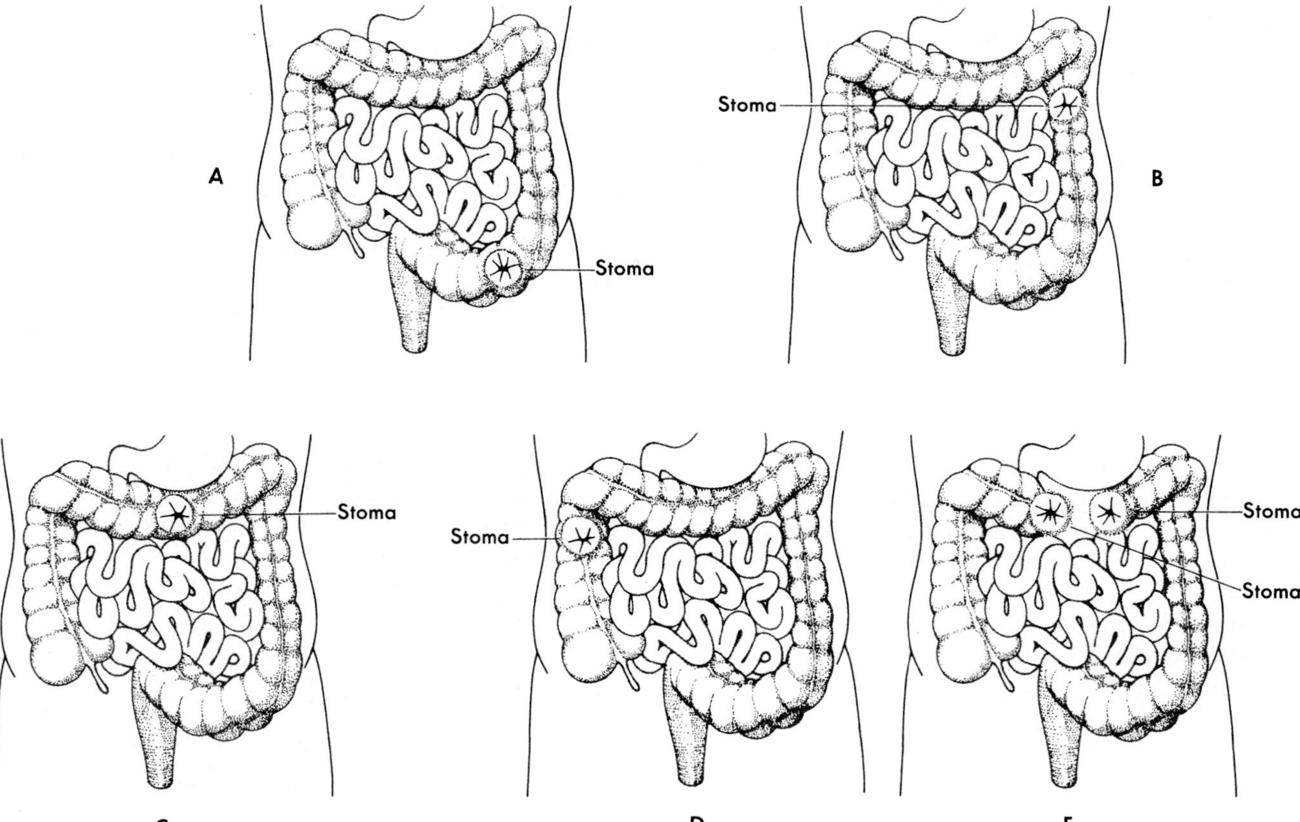

Fig. 32-1 **A,** Sigmoid colostomy. **B,** Descending colostomy. **C,** Transverse colostomy. **D,** Ascending colostomy. **E,** Double-barrel colostomy.

proximal end of this temporary colostomy drains stool. The distal end drains mucus.

An end stoma is a procedure in which the proximal bowel is brought out to the abdominal wall. The distal end is removed. The anus is closed. The end stoma is a permanent colostomy.

A double-barrel colostomy is created when the bowel is severed, and both ends are brought to the exterior, resulting in two abdominal stomas. The proximal end, which is pouched, drains feces. The distal end, covered with a petrolatem gauze that is changed daily, drains mucus. The double-barrel colostomy can be permanent or temporary. A temporary colostomy can be reversed when the bowel heals and normal bowel function is resumed.

An **ileostomy** (Fig. 32-2) is the surgical formation of an opening of the ileum onto the surface of the abdomen, through which fecal matter is emptied. It is performed for patients with inflammatory bowel conditions and cancer of the large intestine. Although the stoma looks like that of a colostomy, it is somewhat smaller and is located lower on the abdomen. After surgery, the patient wears a temporary disposal bag to collect the semiliquid fecal matter. An ileostomy may be temporary or permanent, depending on the reason for performing the surgery.

In normal bowel elimination, water is absorbed from stool in the large intestines, resulting in the passage of formed stool. An ileostomy places the stoma in the small intestine, causing an almost constant elimination of liquid stool.

The steps for caring for a colostomy and an ileostomy are listed in Skill 32-1.

Irrigation

A colostomy irrigation is essentially the same as administration of an enema with the exception of the site. The patient is unable to control the expulsion of fluid contents. Colostomy irrigation assists the patient in achieving specific, timed elimination of stool; cleanses the colon of gas, stool, and intestinal bacteria; and promotes ostomy self-care by the patient. Colostomies may also be irrigated to cleanse the bowel in preparation for diagnostic tests or surgery. The colostomy of a child or infant is rarely irrigated. These irrigations are generally performed by the ET.

The decision regarding whether to irrigate a colostomy depends on the location of the stoma and the patient's preference. Patients with sigmoid colostomies are often able to regulate elimination of stool to the time and place of their choosing. Thus the patient controls defecation, which reduces the fear of eruption of fecal contents at an inconvenient time. Ileostomies are not irrigated. The passage of stool is generally liquid and constant. Therefore blockage is not a problem, and control of evacuation is not usually possible.

An irrigation sleeve is used to direct the flow of contents into the toilet or bedpan (Fig. 32-3). Cone-shaped irrigation tips are used for irrigation to prevent bowel perforation (Fig. 32-4). Colostomy irrigation may be performed in bed. However, an upright position in the bathroom is usually preferred by the patient. When a catheter is inserted (no more than 3 to 4 inches), the procedure takes 10 to 15 minutes to complete. When completed with the irrigation, the cone and sleeve are removed, the peristomal skin is cleansed, and a clean pouch or gauze dressing is reapplied (Skill 32-2).

Some patients choose not to irrigate because they do not have the time, find it unpleasant, or are physically unable to perform the task. Since colostomy irrigation should be performed every day or every other day at the same time of day, a support person should be taught how to perform the procedure.

When performing or teaching colostomy irrigation, it is important for the nurse to consider the patient's feelings and emotions in trying to deal realistically with the alteration in body image. Assisting the patient in caring for and accepting the co-

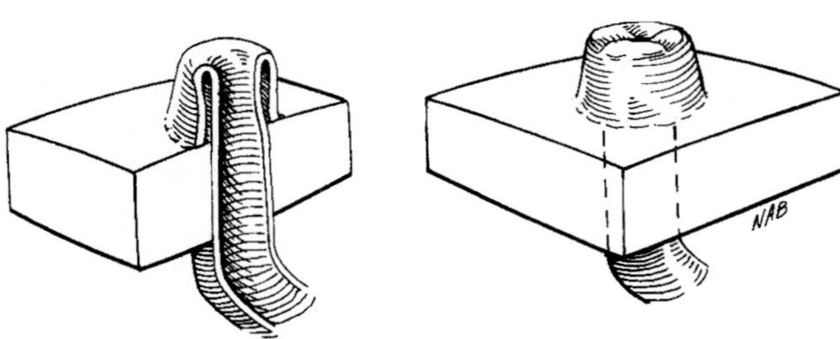

Fig. 32-2 Ileostomy stoma (Brooke's procedure) with 1-inch stoma.

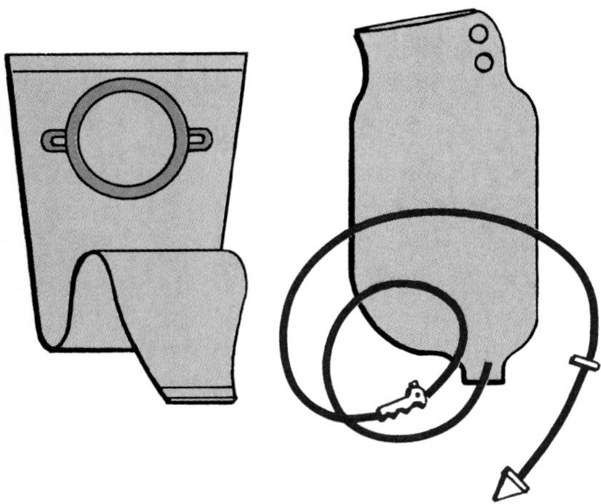

Fig. 32-3 Colostomy irrigating sleeve and irrigating bag with cone attachment.

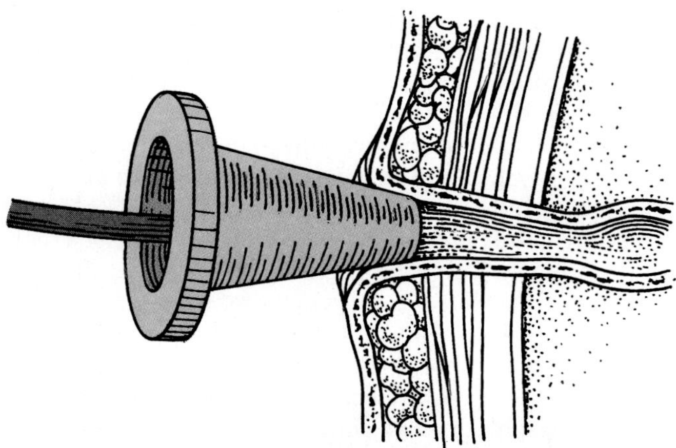

Fig. 32-4 Cone attachment. (From Perry AG, Potter PA: *Clinical nursing skills and techniques,* ed 3, St Louis, 1994, Mosby.)

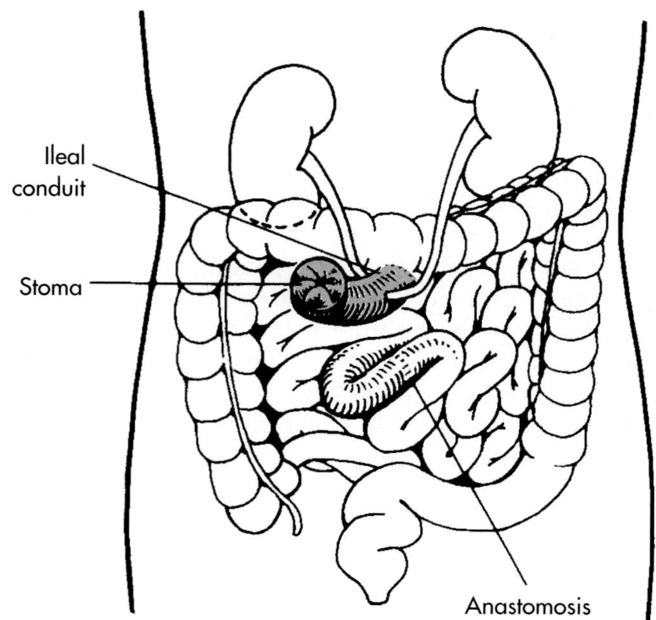

Fig. 32-5 Ileal conduit or ileal loop.

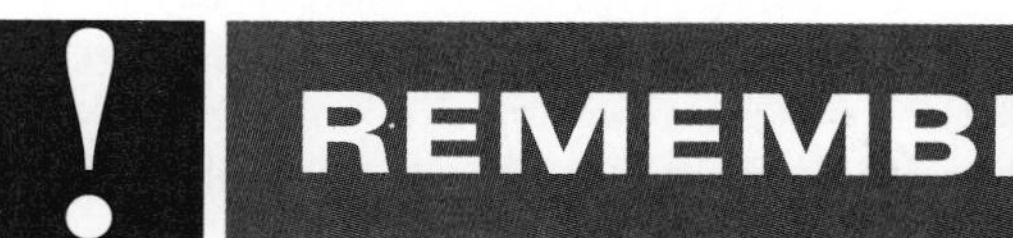

REMEMBER

- Colostomy irrigation is simply an enema through the stoma.
- The type of output produced by a colostomy varies according to the site at which the colostomy is located.
- The stoma should always appear wet and dark and pink to beefy red in color.
- Complaints of burning or discomfort at the peristomal area should be investigated immediately.
- Changes in the characteristics of the stool such as constipation or diarrhea and color may result from illness, medications, or chemotherapy.

lostomy is an important function of the nurse. The manner in which the patient is first approached helps facilitate acceptance of the new responsibilities and some of the changes in lifestyle.

URETEROSTOMY

Because of congenital abnormalities, malignancy, or other diseases of the urinary tract, urine may have to be diverted from its normal path of excretion, creating a **ureterostomy.** The most common urinary diversion created is the ileal conduit (Bricker Loop) (Fig. 32-5). A **conduit** is an artificial channel or passage that connects two organs or different parts of the same organ. An ileal conduit is created by severing the ureters from the bladder and **anastomosing** (rejoining) them to a 15- to 20-cm section of terminal ileum separated from the intestinal tract. The distal end of the ileal segment is brought through the lower right quadrant of the abdominal wall to create a stoma. The proximal end is closed. This technique creates a conduit through which urine passes as it exits the body. The urinary bladder is bypassed because of surgical removal, disease, or malfunction, making the conduit an exit route, not a reservoir like the bladder. Infection is always a threat after this procedure, since bacteria can enter through the skin opening and ascend to the kidneys. The newly created conduit has no sphincter to control urine flow. A urinary pouching appliance must be worn at all times because the patient is incontinent of urine.

Because the urinary pouch constantly fills with urine, it has a valve at the end through which it is emptied. At night the valve can be attached to a gravity drainage bag so that sleep is not interrupted to empty the pouch.

A variety of pouches are available. Many come with the skin barrier already attached. A starter hole or presized stomal measurement may also be available in the pouch chosen for each patient.

The nurse should make every effort to keep the stoma clean, dry, and free of urine leakage (Skill 32-3). This intervention prevents skin irritation and unnecessary embarrassment.

Recent advances in science and reconstructive bowel surgery have led to the development of the continent urinary diversion. In these procedures, the small or large bowel is used to form a reservoir that holds urine until evacuation.

Kock's pouch is the most prominent continent urinary diversions (Fig. 32-6). It is the creation of a reservoir from a portion of small bowel. The reservoir may be attached to the urethra or to an abdominal

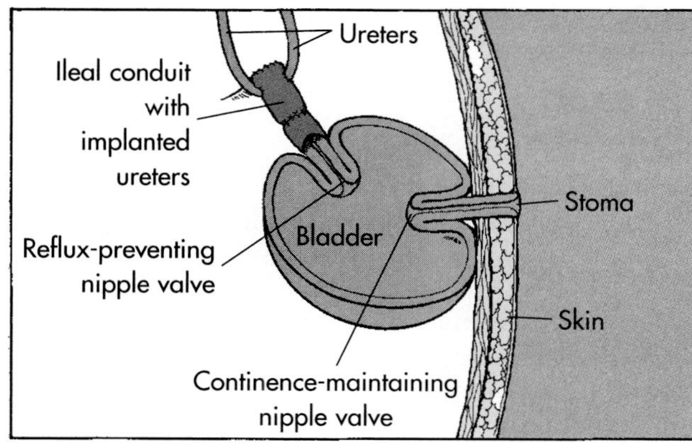

Fig. 32-6 Kock's pouch. (From Belcher AE: Cancer nursing: *Mosby's clinical nursing series,* St Louis, 1992, Mosby.)

stoma. In either case, the reservoir is emptied by catheterization. Approximately 56 cm of terminal ileum is used to construct Kock's pouch. The nipple valves make the pouch continent. They are created by inverting the ileum into the pouch.

Other forms of continent urinary diversions have been developed since Kock's pouch was introduced. With this type of ureterostomy, the stoma is smaller, is less obvious beneath the clothing, and can frequently be covered by a small bandage. This convenience facilitates psychosocial adjustment.

NURSING CARE

Care of the Stoma and Pouch

Depending on the type of pouch used, the pouch should be changed 1 or 2 times per week. Stoma edema occurs after surgery, so the pouch should be cut to fit for approximately 4 weeks. After shrinkage of the stoma, the patient can be measured for a precut pouch. A support adhesive holds the pouch in place on the skin. The use of a skin barrier is often recommended to protect the skin and form a seal with the pouch. The stoma and the **periostomal** (around the stoma) area are cleansed with water and soap that is free of creams and oils, are rinsed, and are patted dry. The stoma should be shiny, wet, and dark pink.

Some bleeding may occur because of the rich blood supply. If bleeding is prolonged or the discharge is bloody, the physician should be contacted. The bottom of the pouch is closed with a type of clamp called a *tail closure.* A pouch a third to half full with stool or flatus requires emptying. Intake and output is monitored during the hospital stay.

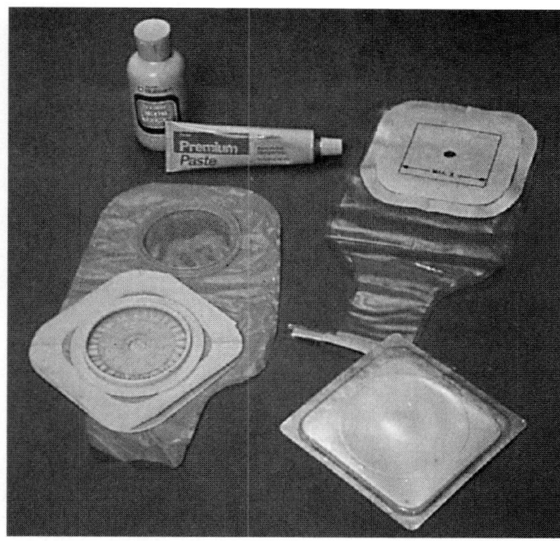

Fig. 32-7 Drainable pouches. (From Perry AG, Potter PA: *Clinical nursing skills and techniques,* ed 3, St Louis, 1994, Mosby.)

Most insurance companies cover at least part of the cost of ostomy appliances.

Skin Care

Excoriation is the injury of skin caused by scratching or abrasion. The digestive enzymes present in liquid stool are very irritating to the skin. Therefore pouch adherence care is important in preventing leakage onto abdominal skin. Preventive skin care should be performed to prevent skin breakdown. Skin barrier substances can be used.

Various types and styles of pouches are available (Fig. 32-7) to cover the stoma and serve as a reservoir for stool or urine. Many products are available (Fig. 32-8) to protect skin, promote pouch adherence, promote healing of irritated periostomal skin, and reduce odor.

Activities of Daily Living

Normal clothing may be worn with an ostomy. If the ostomy is at waistline, suspenders may be worn instead of a leather belt to prevent irritation. Pouching systems are constructed to be waterproof. The patient may take a shower or go swimming with the pouch in place. Heavy lifting is prohibited the first 6 to 8 weeks after surgery. No activity limitations persist beyond this time unless complications occur.

Nutrition

A low-fiber diet is recommended immediately after bowel surgery. Beyond this time, the colostomy patient may usually return to a regular diet. However, gas-forming foods such as cabbage, onions,

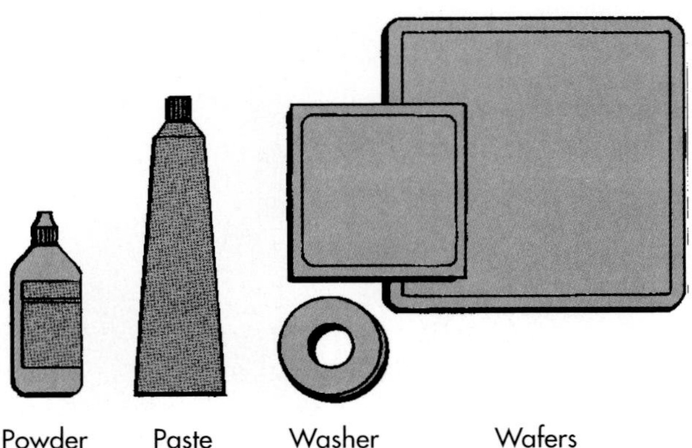

Fig. 32-8 Skin barriers.

beans, cucumbers, radishes, and beer should be avoided to assist odor control. Odor-forming foods such as cheese, eggs, fish, beans, onions, and cabbage as well as some vitamins and medications may be a nuisance. Odor may be reduced by the consumption of cranberry juice, buttermilk, or yogurt. The patient with an ileostomy needs to avoid foods that could cause blockage. These foods include dried fruits, popcorn, nuts, hotdogs, raw vegetables, and meats in casings. The patient with an ileostomy must slowly and completely chew food and increase liquid intake because of the lack of resorption in the large intestine. Fluids containing electrolytes (for example Gatorade and broth) are encouraged. This patient must also check for undissolved pills and capsules in stool.

The pH of the urine is an important factor in the patient with a ureterostomy. The degree of acidity or alkalinity is expressed in pH values. Acidity is expressed in numbers less than 7, and alkalinity is expressed in numbers greater than 7. Acidification of the urine, which is the conversion of the urine to an acid state, is desirable. A patients who has a ureterostomy should adhere to an acid ash diet, which includes cranberries, prunes, plums, cereals, rice, peanuts, noodles, cheese, poultry, and fish. If sulfa drugs are prescribed, this diet is discontinued, since alkaline urine is necessary for optimal drug absorption. This diet is useful in acidifying urine to decrease the risk of stone or crystal formation. The patient should avoid salt substitutes, antacids, and products containing calcium. These products may increases the risk of stone formation.

Psychologic Concerns

People with stomas may lead active lives. The degree of difficulty experienced in adjusting to this alteration in body image varies from person to person. Caring for this patient presents physical, emotional, psychologic, social, and spiritual challenges. Expressions of feelings and emotions should be encouraged. The patient has usually experienced the diagnosis of a life-threatening disease, major surgery, and a resultant alteration in body image. The patient may question the meaning of life. Grief is common when a body part is altered or lost (see Chapter 10). The patient may express denial, anger, disgust, depression, withdrawal, or acceptance. The changes in body image may affect others with whom a close relationship is shared. Feelings of loss of sexuality are common. The nurse should encourage questions and dispel any myths or misconceptions. The nurse should be attentive to the patient as well as the newly created stoma. To lead a normal, productive, independent life, the patient should be able to assume complete care of the ostomy. In the first week after surgery, complete ostomy care may seem impossible to the patient. Sutures and surgical edema (swelling) make initial pouch adherence difficult, resulting in leakage. Acceptance of the stoma may take several days to weeks. However, the patient may be able to physically care for it in 4 to 5 days. The nurse should be prepared to listen, offer support, give encouragement, teach where needed, and understand the patient's feelings. Local ostomate self-help groups provide a base of support and encouragement after discharge. These groups also discuss common problems and solutions.

Some patients are never able to completely care for the ostomy. In this case, family members must assume partial or complete responsibility for ostomy care. If the patient is allowed to remain in denial, acceptance of the stoma takes longer. The patient should not be allowed to go too long without accepting the ostomy and its care. If too much time passes, the patient may never accept the reality of having a stoma. Patience and kind firmness is often required by the nurse to help the patient reach acceptance of the stoma.

The nurse must examine personal feelings about ostomies. The nurse's initial approach can have a critical impact on the patient's feelings. The patient observes the nurse's facial expression during ostomy care. The nurse's words of encouragement are meaningless if the patient observes an expression of distaste or disgust.

Nursing Care for Special Patients

Children

The child ostomate requires care similar to the adult. However, there are some differences. Pediatric pouches are smaller than adult pouches. Frequent nighttime leakage may result because of collection of flatus and feces in the small pouches. To prevent leakage, a small pinhole can be placed in the pouch to allow flatus to escape. Pediatric stomas frequently prolapse. This problem is not an emergency as long as the stoma remains pink. Frequently the prolapse may be reduced by having the child lie down and suck a pacifier while a cold, moist cloth is placed over the stoma. Stomas of infants and children rarely require irrigation. Such irrigations should be performed by the ET. The parents and child require continuous teaching and encouragement to accept the situation.

Older adults

Manual dexterity may be a problem for older adults. Postoperative stomal swelling usually subsides in approximately 6 to 8 weeks. Thereafter, the patient can be fitted for a pouch with a presized opening precut into the skin barrier. Colostomy irrigation is less apt to be successful in regulating elimination. Activity, adequate diet, and adequate fluid consumption should be monitored for successful bowel elimination in the older adult.

Referral to Home Health Care

The patient should have a referral to a home health agency or a visiting nurse before hospital discharge. Pouches that wear well in the hospital may not wear well when the patient assumes a normal routine. A visiting nurse can ensure optimal wear and comfort after discharge, ensure compliance with irrigation routine, and assist in problem solving when necessary. For example, the nurse may suggest that the irrigation solution container hang from a hook on the wall or from a shower curtain rod instead of an intravenous pole. Ureterostomy, colostomy, and ileostomy products may usually be purchased at local pharmacies. The patient should be encouraged to become involved with local ostomy organizations.

■ NURSING CARE PLAN ■

RISK FOR IMPAIRED SKIN INTEGRITY

Ms. D, age 62, underwent ileostomy surgery for colon cancer 3 days ago. Slight redness was assessed around the stoma during pouch change. No open skin areas were assessed.

NURSING DIAGNOSIS

Risk for impaired skin integrity related to frequent flow of loose stools as evidenced by slight redness of the skin surrounding the stoma site

GOAL

- Skin integrity will be maintained.

EXPECTED OUTCOMES

- Patient will demonstrate behaviors that prevent skin breakdown.
- Skin around stoma will be clean, dry, and intact.

NURSING INTERVENTIONS

- Inspect stoma and surrounding skin with each pouch change.
- Cleanse skin with soap and water. Assess for redness, rash, or excoriation.
- Measure stoma with each pouch and dressing change.
- Apply an effective skin barrier.
- Apply pouch with opening approximately ⅛-inch larger than stoma size.
- Empty and irrigate pouch every 8 hours and when needed.
- When change is scheduled, remove old pouch carefully while supporting surrounding skin.
- Change appliance immediately if patient complains of burning or itching. Investigate problem.
- Assess appliance fit as ongoing procedure.

EVALUATION

- Skin surrounding stoma remains clean, dry, and intact.
- No excoriation is assessed.
- Patient verbalizes comfort regarding stoma area.

SKILL 32-1 CARING FOR A COLOSTOMY OR AN ILEOSTOMY

Steps	Rationale

1. Obtain equipment:
▪ Pouch with preattached skin barrier
▪ Pouch clamp
▪ Pouch belt
▪ Skin protectant
▪ Warm water
▪ Cleansing agent according to agency policy or medical order
▪ Towel and wash cloth or soft paper towel
▪ Plastic bag
▪ Toilet tissue
▪ Clean gloves
▪ Any additional ostomy products such as:
  ▪ Paste
  ▪ Pouch deodorant
  ▪ Measuring card
  ▪ Scissors
  ▪ Bedpan or collection device
	Helps organize procedure.

2. Refer to medical record, care plan, or Kardex for special interventions.	Provides basis for care.
3. Introduce self.	Decreases anxiety level.
4. Identify patient by identification band.	Identifies correct patient for procedure.
5. Explain procedure to patient.	Seeks cooperation and decreases anxiety.
6. Wash hands and don clean gloves according to agency policy and guidelines from Centers for Disease Control and Prevention and Occupational Safety and Health Administration.	Helps prevent cross-contamination.
7. Prepare patient for intervention:	
a. Close door to room or pull curtain.	Provides privacy.
b. Drape for procedure if necessary.	Prevents exposure of patient.
8. Raise bed to comfortable working level.	Provides safety for nurse.
9. Arrange for patient privacy.	Shows respect for patient.
10. Inspect adherence and type of pouch.	Denotes appropriate pouching technique or need for change.
11. Assess stoma for color, size, and shape.	Assesses for adequate circulation and general condition.
12. Examine peristomal skin for signs of irritation.	Assesses skin integrity.
13. Assess stool for color, odor, amount, consistency, and frequency.	Assesses bowel elimination and function.
14. Inspect, auscultate, percuss, and palpate abdomen.	Assesses bowel motility and function.
15. Ask patient if there are any concerns or discomfort.	Indicates acceptance, need for teaching, or intervention.
16. Assess ability of patient or significant other to perform ostomy care.	Denotes acceptance or identifies need for further teaching.
17. Position patient for access to stoma and for patient comfort.	Maintains appropriate body alignment and accessibility to work area.
18. Unfasten and remove belt (if in use).	Eases pouch removal.
19. Carefully push skin away from pouch. (Wet cotton balls may be used to decrease shearing if necessary.)	Prevents alteration in peristomal skin integrity.
20. Place reusable pouch on clean area and disposable pouch in plastic bag.	Prevents cross-contamination.
21. Gently cleanse stoma and peristomal skin with warm water and gently pat dry.	Prevents odor and infection from feces, enhances pouch adherence, and promotes skin integrity.

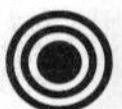

SKILL 32-1 CARING FOR A COLOSTOMY OR AN ILEOSTOMY—cont'd

Steps	Rationale
22. Apply skin prep to peristomal skin and allow to dry.	Provides protection against shearing during pouch changes and for pouch adherence.
23. Measure stoma using measuring card or custom-made pattern.	Ensures that skin barrier will be cut to protect peristomal skin without rubbing stoma.
24. Place toilet tissue over stoma.	Absorbs excrement expelled before pouch is applied.
25. Using pattern or measuring guide, cut opening in pouch skin barrier ⅛ in larger than measurement.	Prevents stomal lesions caused by rubbing of skin barrier against stomal mucosa.
26. Remove tissue from stoma.	Ensures exposure of area to pouch.
27. Remove paper cover from pouch skin barrier, center pouch with skin barrier or flange with skin barrier over stoma, and press gently but firmly to skin. (Most one-piece pouches have preattached skin barrier. All of two-piece pouch systems have skin barrier made into flange.)	Establishes contact between barrier adhesive and skin and ensures that pouch will adhere.
28. Snap pouch to flange if using two-piece system. Attach pouch clamp to bottom of pouch for both one- and two-piece pouches.	Ensures appropriate collection of feces into pouch reservoir.
29. Attach belt if used.	Supports pouch and enhances feelings of security.
30. Assist patient to comfortable position in bed or chair.	Promotes comfort.
31. Remove equipment from bedside.	Reduces transmission of microorganisms.
32. Empty, wash, rinse, and dry reusable pouch.	Reduces odor and extends usefulness.
33. Dispose of soiled supplies.	Reduces transmission of microorganisms.
34. Remove gloves and wash hands.	Helps prevent cross-contamination.
35. Document.	Documents procedure and patient's response.

SKILL 32-2 PERFORMING COLOSTOMY IRRIGATION

Steps	Rationale
1. Obtain equipment: *Irrigation set:* ▪ Container ▪ Tubing with clamp ▪ Catheter with cone ▪ Irrigation sleeve with or without belt ▪ Clamps ▪ Water-soluble lubricant ▪ New pouch or patch and related supplies ▪ Clean gloves ▪ Bedpan ▪ Bed protector ▪ Washcloth and towel ▪ Water and basin ▪ Gentle soap	Helps organize procedure.
2. Refer to medical record, care plan, or Kardex for special interventions.	Provides basis for care.
3. Introduce self.	Decreases anxiety level.
4. Identify patient by identification band.	Identifies correct patient for procedure.

Continued.

SKILL 32-2 PERFORMING COLOSTOMY IRRIGATION—cont'd

Steps	Rationale
5. Explain procedure to patient.	Seeks cooperation and decreases anxiety.
6. Wash hands and don clean gloves according to agency policy and guidelines from Centers for Disease Control and Prevention and Occupational Safety and Health Administration.	Helps prevent cross-contamination.
7. Prepare patient for intervention:	
a. Close door to room or pull curtain.	Provides privacy.
b. Drape for procedure if necessary.	Prevents exposure of patient.
8. Raise bed to comfortable working level.	Provides safety for nurse.
9. Arrange for patient privacy.	Shows respect for patient.
10. Assess ability of patient or significant other to perform irrigation.	Reveals areas in which teaching is needed.
11. Position patient:	
a. In bathroom, have patient sit on toilet or on chair in front of toilet.	Allows irrigating sleeve to drain into commode.
b. In bed, have patient lie comfortably with head elevated slightly.	Assists with drainage.
12. Remove pouch or patch. Cleanse skin.	Provides access to stoma.
13. Place irrigation sleeve over stoma and attach belt, if appropriate.	Allows return to flow into commode and secures sleeve to abdomen.
14. Place end of sleeve in commode.	Allows contents to escape into commode.
15. Close clamp on irrigating tubing and fill irrigation container with 500 to 1000 ml of tepid water (or as prescribed).	Prevents irrigating fluid from flowing as container is filled.
16. Hang tubing on intravenous pole so that bottom of container is at level of patient's shoulder.	Permits slow infusion.
17. Holding end of tubing over commode and allow small amount of water to flow through tubing to remove air.	Flushes air from tubing.
18. Attach cone to tubing and lubricate cone.	Reduces trauma to stoma.
19. Insert cone into stoma through top of sleeve.	Prevents backflow of fluid during irrigation and keeps return in sleeve.
20. While holding cone in place, allow solution to flow slowly into colon. If patient complains of cramping, slow or stop flow without removing cone until cramps subside.	Allows better distention of colon and thus more effective irrigation.
21. After all solution has been introduced, remove cone and close top of sleeve.	Prevents spillage of contents.
22. Have patient sit about 15 min while return flows into commode. Clean and clamp bottom of sleeve so that patient can move around freely until drainage stops.	Allows most of return to occur. (Complete emptying generally takes 30 min to 1 hr.)
23. Drain, rinse, and remove sleeve.	Allows sleeve to be reused.
24. Assess patient and fecal return and flush commode.	Reveals effectiveness of irrigation and patient's response to procedure.
25. Apply new pouch or patch.	Provides sealing and prevents leakage of fecal material.
26. Dispose of equipment.	Reduces transmission of microorganisms.
27. Removes gloves and wash hands.	Helps prevent cross-contamination.
28. Document.	Documents procedure and patient's response.

SKILL 32-3 CARING FOR A URETEROSTOMY

Steps	Rationale

1. **Obtain equipment:**
▪ Pouch with valve closed
▪ Belt
▪ Skin protector
▪ Nonallergic tape
▪ Gauze pads
▪ Water and gentle soap
▪ Towel
▪ Washcloth
▪ Plastic bag
▪ Clean gloves
▪ Graduated pitcher
▪ Measuring card
▪ Scissors
▪ Ostomy products:
  ▪ Solvent
  ▪ Commercial skin cleanser
  ▪ Paste
  ▪ Powder
  ▪ Cream
	Helps organize procedure.

2. **Refer to medical record, care plan, or Kardex for special interventions.**	Provides basis for care.
3. **Introduce self.**	Decreases anxiety level.
4. **Identify patient by identification band.**	Identifies correct patient for procedure.
5. **Explain procedure to patient.**	Seeks cooperation and decreases anxiety.
6. **Wash hands and don clean gloves according to agency policy and guidelines from Centers for Disease Control and Prevention and Occupational Safety and Health Administration.**	Helps prevent cross-contamination.
7. **Prepare patient for intervention:**	
a. Close door to room or pull curtain.	Provides privacy.
b. Drape for procedure if necessary.	Prevents exposure of patient.
8. **Raise bed to comfortable working level.**	Provides safety for nurse.
9. **Arrange for patient privacy.**	Shows respect for patient.
10. **Position patient so that stoma is easily accessible and patient is comfortable.**	Promotes use of proper body mechanics and provides patient comfort, which aids in patient readiness for teaching.
11. **Empty urine into graduated pitcher and unfasten and remove belt (if in use).**	Reduces possibility of spilling urine.
12. **Carefully peel pouch from skin. (Moist cotton balls may be needed.)**	Prevents damage to skin.
13. **Cover stoma with rolled gauze.**	Absorbs urine flow during cleaning.
14. **Place pouch in plastic bag.**	Prevents soiling of linens and gown.
15. **Cleanse patient's skin with warm water. Pat skin dry.**	Ensures that soap is not left on skin, which can cause irritation and interfere with pouch adherence. Avoids rubbing and irritating skin.
16. **Measure stoma using measuring card.**	Determines size of pouch and skin barrier openings.
17. **If using wafer-type skin barrier, cut opening hole ⅛ in larger than stoma.**	Prevents pressure on stoma.
18. **Assess that skin is free from urine. Remove backing from barrier protectant and gauze from stoma. Center opening hole over stoma and press against skin for 1 to 2 min, smoothing outward with fingers to remove air bubbles.**	Detects presence of urine on skin, which prevents formation of a seal and irritates skin. Allows protectant to form seal.

Continued.

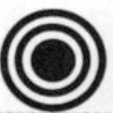

SKILL 32-3 CARING FOR A URETEROSTOMY—cont'd

Steps	Rationale
19. Attach belt to one end of pouch, adjust around waist, and attach to opposite end.	Helps support pouch and promotes adherence.
20. Assist patient to comfortable position in chair.	Promotes comfort.
21. Dispose of equipment.	Reduces transmission of microorganisms.
22. Wash and dry reusable pouch.	Reduces odors and extends usefulness of reusable pouch.
23. Measure and assess urine.	Allows for analysis of fluid balance.
24. Remove gloves and wash hands.	Helps prevent cross-contamination.
25. Document.	Document's procedure and patient's response.

SUMMARY

The patient with an ostomy has special needs based on the location of the ostomy, the prognosis, complications, and the response to nursing care. The nurse should assess the patient, plan and implement interventions, and continually evaluate the effectiveness of the nursing care plan. The nurse should also examine personal feelings about ostomies and ostomy care. The initial nurse-patient interaction is critical in determining the patient's acceptance of the ostomy and resultant change in body image.

Key Concepts

- Until all postoperative edema is relieved, the stoma should be measured at each pouch change to determine the size of the opening needed in the barrier and pouch.
- The barrier opening should be approximately ⅛ inch larger than the stoma size.
- A reusable pouch may be used only after all postoperative edema is relieved.
- Even when a pouch is adhering well, it should be changed at least every 5 to 7 days or according to pouch recommendations so that the skin and stoma can be examined.
- Intact pouches are emptied when they are one-third to one-half full.
- Scheduled colostomy irrigations may help some patients achieve control of bowel movements.
- Stoma should be dark pink to beefy red in color and moist.
- Some dietary restrictions apply primarily to patients who have an ileostomy.
- Patients who have ureterostomies should be taught to drink 2000 to 3000 ml of liquids every day and to maintain a diet that helps acidify the urine.
- Emotional support of the patient is vital for eventual acceptance of the change in body image.

Critical Thinking Questions

1. Mr. G had an ileostomy performed. He is being discharged and is questioning why he can not perform ostomy irrigations daily and achieve controlled bowel emptying. Prepare a teaching plan and present it to Mr. G. Explain why this usually will not be possible in his situation.
2. Assessing the stoma after ostomy surgery is a vital nursing function. Explain why the stoma is assessed by color and what the different colors assessed may indicate.
3. Mr. T, a patient who has an ileostomy, is being assessed on a home care visit. He states he has been following the prescribed dietary restrictions and feels fine now and would like to eat popcorn and hotdogs again. Include in the response the reasons that these restrictions are particularly important for an ileostomy patient and help plan menus that will be satisfying as well as appealing.
4. Mrs. K has a new colostomy. On the third postoperative day, she complains of burning and itching surrounding the stoma site. Describe the nursing assessments and interventions that should be implemented.

REFERENCES AND SUGGESTED READINGS

Beare PG, Myers JL: *Principles and practice of adult health nursing,* ed 2, St Louis, 1994, Mosby.

Bolander VB: *Sorensen and Luckmann's basic nursing: a psychophysiologic approach,* ed 3, Philadelphia, 1994, Saunders.

Doenges ME, Moorhouse MF, Geissler AC: *Nursing care plans: guidelines for planning and documenting patient care,* ed 3, Philadelphia, 1993, Davis.

Doughty DB: *Gastrointestinal disorders: Mosby's clinical series,* St Louis, 1993, Mosby.

Long BC, Phipps WJ, Cassmeyer VL: *Medical-surgical nursing: a nursing process approach,* St Louis, 1993, Mosby.

Potter PA, Perry AG: *Basic nursing: theory and practice,* ed 3, St Louis, 1995, Mosby.

Rosdahl CB: *Textbook of basic nursing,* ed 6, Philadelphia, 1995, Lippincott.

APPENDIX A

Resource Data

RESOURCE INFORMATION

Resources for reference and referral are an essential part of the nurse's repertoire. Assisting patients in seeking needed information is central to community health nursing practice. The following is a selected group of resources to help the nurse in working with patients and families.

COMMUNITY RESOURCES

The following is a list of resources on many different health-related topics, from alcoholism to water safety. The list includes names, addresses, and telephone numbers that can be used to obtain further information. It is not by any means a complete list but is meant to serve as a starting point.

Acquired Immunodeficiency Syndrome (AIDS)

National Gay Task Force Crisisline
(800)221-7044
(212)807-6016 in
NY, AK, and HI

Public Health Service AIDS Information Hotline
(800)342-AIDS
(202)245-6867 in AK, HI only
(call collect)

From Stanhope M, Knollmueller RN: *Handbook for community and health nursing: tools for assessment, intervention, and education,* St Louis, 1992, Mosby.

Advocacy

American Civil Liberties Union
132 W. 43rd St.
New York, NY 10036
(212)944-9800

Occupational Safety and Health Administration (OSHA)
Office of Public and Consumer Affairs
US Department of Labor,
Room N3637
200 Constitution Ave. NW
Washington, DC 20210
(202)523-8148

Alcohol and Drug Abuse

AL-ANON Family Group Headquarters, Inc.
P.O. Box 182,
Madison Square Station
New York, NY 10010

Alcohol and Drug Problems Association of North America, Inc.
1101 15th St. NW, Suite 204
Washington, DC 20005

Alcoholics Anonymous
Call local chapters (see White
Pages of phone directory).

Drug Information Association, Inc.
1050 George St., Suite 5-L
New Brunswick, NJ 08901

Friday Nite Live
c/o Sacramento County Office of Education
9738 Lincoln Village Dr.
Sacramento, CA 95827
(916)366-2180

International Commission for Prevention of Alcoholism
6830 Laurel St. NW
Washington, DC 20012

MADD—Mothers Against Drunk Driving
National Headquarters
669 Airport Freeway, Suite 310
Hurst, TX 76053
(817)268-6233 or
311 Main St., Suite C
Roseville, CA 95678
(800)443-6233

National Association on Drug Abuse Problems, Inc.
355 Lexington Ave.
New York, NY 10017

National Clearinghouse for Alcohol Information
P.O. Box 2345
Rockville, MD 20852
(301)468-2600

National Clearinghouse for Drug Abuse Information
P.O. Box 416
Kensington, MD 20795
(301)443-6500

National Cocaine Hotline
(800)COCAINE

National Committee for the Prevention of Alcoholism and Drug Dependency
6830 Laurel St. NW
Washington, DC 20012

National Council on Alcoholism, Inc.
733 Third Ave.
New York, NY 10017

National Council on Drug Abuse
571 West Jackson Blvd.
Chicago, IL 60606

National Institute on Drug Abuse Prevention Branch
(301)443-2450

SADD—Students Against Driving Drunk
P.O. Box 800
Marlboro, MA 01752
(617)481-3568 or
(state office in CA; Gaye Soroka, Director)
505 N. Tustin Ave.
Santa Ana, CA 92705
(714)542-8155
(Also Chapters in high schools)

Synanon Foundation, Inc.
P.O. Box 786
Marshall, CA 94940

Volunteers and Victim Assistance (VIVA)
5716 J St.
Sacramento, CA 95819
(916)457-VIVA

Alzheimer's Disease

Alzheimer's Disease and Related Disorders Association, Inc.
700 East Lake St.
Chicago, IL 60601
(312)853-3060;
(800)621-0379;
(800)572-6037 in IL only

Arthritis

Arthritis Foundation
1314 Spring St. NW
Atlanta, GA 30309
(404)873-3389

Arthritis Information Clearinghouse
P.O. Box 9782
Arlington, VA 22209
(703)558-8250

Arthritis Information Clearinghouse
P.O. Box 34427
Bethesda, MD 20034
(301)881-9411

Arthritis Society
920 Yonge St., Suite 420
Toronto, Canada M4W 3J7

Asthma and Allergies

Association for the Care of Asthma, Inc.
Spring Valley Rd.
Ossining, NY 10562

Asthma and Allergy Foundation of America
19 West 44th St.
New York, NY 10036

Asthma-Allergy Hotline
(800)624-0044
(414)272-1004 in WI only
(call collect)

Bereavement*

Bereavement Outreach Network
127 Arundel Rd.
Pasadena, MD 21122

The Candlelighters Foundation
2025 I St. NW
Washington, DC 20006

The Compassionate Friends
P.O. Box 3696
Oak Brook, IL 60522-3696

Growing Through Grief
P.O. Box 1664
Annapolis, MD 21404

Pregnancy and Infant Loss Center
1415 E. Wayzata Blvd.
Suite 22
Wayzata, MN 55391

SHARE
St. Johns Hospital
800 E. Carpenter
Springfield, IL 62702

Survivors of Suicide (SOS): Directory of Survivor Groups, American Association of Suicidology
2459 S. Ash St.
Denver, CO 80222

Widowed Persons Service, AARP
1909 K St. NW
Washington, DC 20049

Widow to Widow Program
58 Fernwood Rd.
Boston, MA 02115

Blindness

American Council of the Blind
1010 Vermont Ave. NW,
Suite 1100
Washington, DC 20005
(202)393-3666

Association for Education of the Visually Handicapped
919 Walnut St., 4th Floor
Philadelphia, PA 19107

American Foundation for the Blind, Inc.
15 W. 16th St.
New York, NY 10011
(212)620-2000

Braille Institute
741 N. Vermont Ave.
Los Angeles, CA 90029

Guide Dogs for the Blind
P.O. Box 1200
San Rafael, CA 94915
(415)479-4000

Guide Dog Users, Inc.
12 Riverside St., Apt. 1-2
Watertown, MA 02172
(617)926-9198

Guiding Eyes for the Blind
Yorktown Heights, NY 10598
(914)245-4024

National Association for Visually Handicapped
22 W. 21st St.
New York, NY 10010
(212)889-3141

National Eye Institute
Information Officer
Building 31, Room 6A32
Bethesda, MD 20205

National Retinitis Pigmentosa Foundation
(800)638-2300
(301)655-1011 in MD only

National Society to Prevent Blindness
500 E. Remington Rd.
Schaumburg, IL 60173
(312)843-2020

Recording for the Blind, Inc.
20 Roszel Rd.
Princeton, NJ 08540
(609)452-0606

*From Gifford B, Cleary B: Supporting the bereaved. *American Journal of Nursing,* 90(2):53, 1990.

The Library of Congress
Division of the Blind and
Physically Handicapped
1291 Taylor St. NW
Washington, DC 20542
(202)287-5100

Burns

American Burn Association
c/o William Curreri, MD
New York Hospital
Cornell Medical Center
New York, NY 10021

National Burn Federation
3737 Fifth Ave., Suite 206
San Diego, CA 92103

Cancer

AMC Cancer Information
(800)525-3777

American Cancer Society
90 Park Ave.
New York, NY 10016
(212)599-3600

Cancer Information Service (CIS)
(800)4-CANCER:
(800)638-6070 in AK only
(202)636-5700 in DC area only
(808)524-1234 in Oahu, HI
(neighbor islands call collect)

International Association Cancer Victims and Friends, Inc.
7740 W. Manchester Ave.
Suite 110
Playa del Rey, CA 90291

Leukemia Society of America, Inc.
733 3rd Ave.
New York, NY 10017
(212)573-8484

National Cancer Information Clearinghouse
Office of Communications
National Cancer Institute
Room 10A18
9000 Rockville Pike
Bethesda, MD 20205
(301)496-4070

Child Abuse

Child Abuse Listening Mediation, Inc.
P.O. Box 718
Santa Barbara, CA 93102

Child Help USA
(800)422-4453

Children's Defense Fund
(202)628-8789

Clearinghouse on Child Abuse and Neglect Information
P.O. Box 1182
Washington, DC 20013
(301)251-5157

Parents Anonymous Hotline
(800)421-0353
(800)352-0386 in CA only

Children

American Association for Maternal and Child Health, Inc.
P.O. Box 965
Los Altos, CA 94022

American Pediatric Society
David Goldring, MD
P.O. Box 14871
St. Louis, MO 63178

Child Health Associate Program
4200 E. Ninth Ave.
Box C219
Denver, CO 80262

National Sudden Infant Death Syndrome Foundation
310 S. Michigan Ave.
Chicago, IL 60604

National Tay-Sachs and Allied Disease Association
122 E. 42nd St.
New York, NY 10017

Pediatric Pulmonary Association of America
150 N. Pond Way
Roswell, GA 30076

Shriners Hospital Referral Line
(800)237-5055
(800)282-9161 in FL only

The Children's Foundation
1420 New York Ave. NW
8th Floor
Washington, DC 20005

Diabetes

American Association of Diabetes Educators
500 N. Michigan Ave.
Suite 1400
Chicago, IL 60611
(312)661-1700

American Diabetes Association
505 8th Ave.
New York, NY 10018
(212)947-9707

Juvenile Diabetes Foundation International Hotline
(800)223-1138;
(212)889-7575 in NY only

National Diabetes Information Clearinghouse
Box NDIC
Bethesda, MD 20205
(301)468-2162

The Juvenile Diabetes Foundation
23 E. 26th St.
New York, NY 10010

Down Syndrome

National Association for Down's Syndrome
P.O. Box 63
Oak Park, IL 60303

National Down Syndrome Society Hotline
(800)221-4602
(212)764-3070 in NY only

Elder Abuse Agencies and Resource Groups*

Natalie Dunlap
Bureau of Maine's Elderly
Station 11
State House
Augusta, ME 04333
(207)289-2561
(Maine has a mandatory reporting law for elder abuse)

Dr. Rosalie Wolfe
Center on Aging
University of Massachusetts
Medical Center
55 Lake Ave. N
Worcester, MA 01605

Lisa Neyenberg
Consortium for Elder
Abuse Prevention
Mt. Zion Hospital and
Medical Center
P.O. Box 7921
San Francisco, CA 94102
(415)885-7850

Mary Joy Quinn, Director
Court Investigation Unit,
Room 416
City Hall
San Francisco, CA 94102

Vernon Proctor
Institute of Gerontology
Wayne State University
205 Library Ct.
Detroit, MI 48202
(313)577-2297

Susan K. Tomita, MSW
Assistant Director of Social Work
Harborview Medical Center
325-9th Ave.
Seattle, WA 98104
(206)223-3331

Elderly. See Older Adulthood

Epilepsy

American Epilepsy Society
38238 Glenn Ave.
Willoughby, OH 44094

Epilepsy Foundation of America
4351 Garden City Dr., Suite 406
Landover, MD 20785
(301)459-3700

Epilepsy Information Line
(206)323-8174

*From Ebersole P, Hess P: *Toward healthy aging: human needs and nursing response,* ed 4, St. Louis, 1994, Mosby.

Family Planning/ Pregnancy

Abortion Information Service
(800)321-0575
(800)362-1205 in OH only

American Fertility Society
1608 13th Ave., Suite 101
Birmingham, AL 35205

American Genetic Association
818 18th St. NW
Washington, DC 20006

Bethany Lifeline
(800)238-4269

International Childbirth Education Association, Inc.
8635 Fremont Ave. S
Minneapolis, MN 55420

La Leche League International, Inc.
9616 Minneapolis Ave.
Franklin Park, IL 60131

Maternity Center Association
48 E. 92nd St.
New York, NY 10028

National Abortion Federation
(800)772-9100
(202)546-9060 in DC area only

National Clearinghouse for Family Planning Information
P.O. Box 2225
Rockville, MD 20852
(301)251-5153

National Maternal and Child Health Clearinghouse
3520 Prospect St. NW
Suite 1
Washington, DC 20057
(202)625-8410

National Pregnancy Hotline
(800)344-7211
(800)831-5881

Planned Parenthood Federation of America, Inc.
810 Seventh Ave.
New York, NY 10019

Pregnancy Crisis Center
(800)368-3336
(800)847-6828 in VA only

Southwest Maternity Center
(800)255-9612
(800)292-7021 in TX only
(512)696-7021 in TX for adoption information

The Edna Gladney Home
(800)433-2922
(817)772-2740 in TX only

Food. See also Nutrition

Food and Drug Administration
Office of Consumer Affairs
5600 Fishers Ln.
Rockville, MD 20857
(301)443-3170

Food and Nutrition Information Center
National Agricultural
Library Building,
Room 304
Beltsville, MD 20705
(301)344-3719

Gastrointestinal Disorders

Help for Incontinent People
P.O. Box 544
Union, SC 29379
(803)585-8789

International Association for Enterostomal Therapy, Inc.
2081 Business Circle Dr.
Suite 290
Irvine, CA 92715

National Digestive Diseases Education and Information Clearinghouse
1555 Wilson Blvd, Suite 600
Rosslyn, VA 22209
(301)496-9707

National Foundation for Ileitis and Colitis
444 Park Ave. S
New York, NY 10016
(212)685-3440

United Ostomy Association, Inc.
2001 W. Beverly Blvd.
Los Angeles, CA 90057
(213)413-5510

Handicaps

Architectural and Transportation Barriers Compliance Board
330 C St. SW, Room 1010
Washington, DC 20202
(202)245-1591

Association for Children with Learning Disabilities
4156 Library Rd.
Pittsburgh, PA 15234

Association for Children with Retarded Mental Development, Inc.
902 Broadway, 5th Floor
New York, NY 10010

Boy Scouts of America
Scouting for the
Handicapped Division
New Brunswick, NJ 08902

Clearinghouse on Disability Information
Department of Education,
Room 3132
330 C St. SW
Washington, DC 20202-2524
(202)732-1723

Council of World Organizations Interested in the Handicapped
432 Park Ave. S
New York, NY 10016

Directory of National Information Sources on Handicapping Conditions and Related Services
c/o Office of Handicapped
Individuals
Hubert H. Humphrey Building
Washington, DC 20201

Directory of Organizations Interested in the Handicapped
c/o People-to-People Programs
LaSalle Building, Suite 610
Connecticut Ave. and L St.
Washington, DC 20036

Disability Rights Center
1616 P St. NW, Suite 435
Washington, DC 20036
(202)328-5198

Farmers (services and devices for handicapped farmers)

FARM (Easter Seal Society of Iowa, Inc.)
P.O. Box 4002
Des Moines, IA 50333

Income tax services for people with disability Federal Internal Revenue Service
(for TDD Users)
(800)428-4732
(800)382-4059 in IN only

Independent Living for the Handicapped
Department of Housing and
Urban Development
HUD Building
Washington, DC 20410
(202)755-5720

Information Center for Individuals with Disabilities
20 Park Plaza, Room 330
Boston, MA 02116
(617)727-5540

Library of Congress National Library Services for the Blind and Physically Handicapped
(800)424-8567
(202)287-5100 in DC area only

National Amputation Foundation
12-45 150th St.
Whitestone, NY 11357
(718)767-0596

National Association of Councils of Stutterers
Speech and Hearing Center
O'Boyle Hall, Room 100
Catholic University
Washington, DC 20064

National Association of Retarded Citizens
2709 Avenue E East
Arlington, TX 76011

National Association of the Physically Handicapped, Inc.
76 Elm St.
London, OH 43140

National Congress of Organizations of the Physically Handicapped
16630 Beverly
Tinley Park, IL 60477

National Easter Seal Society
2023 W. Ogden Ave.
Chicago, IL 60612
(312)243-8400 (voice)
(312)243-8880 (TTY)

National Foundation March of Dimes
1275 Mamaroneck Ave.
White Plains, NY 10605
(914)428-7100

National Head Injury Foundation
333 Turnpike Rd.
Southborough, MA 01772
(617)431-7032

National Information Center for Handicapped Children and Youth
P.O. Box 1492
Washington, DC 20013

National Society for Autistic Children
1234 Massachusetts Ave. NW
Suite 1017
Washington, DC 20005

President's Committee on Employment of the Handicapped
111 20th St. NW, Room 636
Washington, DC 20036
(202)653-5044

Stroke Club International
805 12th St.
Galveston, TX 77550
(409)762-1022

United Cerebral Palsy Association, Inc.
66 E. 34th St.
New York, NY 10016
(212)481-6300

Health

American Association for Vital Records and Public Health Statistics
c/o Utah Dept of Health
P.O. Box 2500
Salt Lake City, UT 84110

American Health Care Association
1200 Fifteenth St. NW
Washington, DC 20005
(202)833-2050

American Health Foundation
320 E. 43rd St.
New York, NY 10018

American Holistic Nurses' Association
205 St. Luis St #506
Springfield, MO 65806-1317

American Hospital Association Center for Health Promotion
840 N. Lake Shore Dr.
Chicago, IL 60611
(312)280-6050

American Medical Radio News
(800)621-8094

American Nurse's Association
600 Maryland Ave. SW
Washington, DC 20024-2571
(202)554-4444

American Physical Fitness Research Institute
824 Moraga Dr.
Los Angeles, CA 90049

American Public Health Association
1015 15th St. NW
Washington, DC 20005
(202)789-5600

Center for Health Promotion and Education Centers for Disease Control
Building 1 South,
Room SSB249
1600 Clifton Rd. NE
Atlanta, GA 30333
(404)329-3492
(404)329-3698

Clearinghouse on Health Indexes
National Center for
Health Statistics
Division of Epidemiology and
Health Promotion
3700 East-West Highway,
Room 2-27
Hyattsville, MD 20782
(301)436-7035

Health and Education Resources
4733 Bethesda Ave., Suite 735
Bethesda, MD 20014

Health Sciences Communications Association
2343 N. 115th St.
Wauwatosa, WI 53226

Healthright, Inc.
41 Union Square, Room 206-8
New York, NY 10003

Healthy America, National Coalition for Health Promotion and Disease Prevention
1015 15th St. NW
Suite 424
Washington, DC 20005

International Council on Health, Physical Education and Recreation
1201 16th St. NW
Room 417
Washington, DC 20036

National Council on Health Care Services
1200 15th St. NW,
Suite 601
Washington, DC 20005

National Health Council, Inc.
1740 Broadway
New York, NY 10019

National Health Federation
P.O. Box 688
Monrovia, CA 91016

National Health Information Clearinghouse
P.O. Box 1133
Washington, DC 20013-1133
(800)336-4797
(703)522-2590 in VA only
(call collect)

National Indian Health Board, Inc.
1602 S. Parker Rd
Suite 200
Denver, CO 80231

National Institutes of Health
9000 Rockville Pike
Bethesda, MD 20814
(301)496-4000

National League of Nursing
350 Hudson St.
New York, NY 10014
(212)989-9393
(800)669-1656

National Wellness Association/National Wellness Institute
University of Wisconsin-
Stevens Point Foundation
South Hall
Stevens Point, WI 54481
(715)346-2172

The Aerobics and Fitness Foundation
(800)233-4886

U.S. Department of Health and Human Services
Office of Disease Prevention
and Health Promotion
Washington, DC 20201
(202)245-7611

Health—Dental

American Dental Association
211 E. Chicago Ave.
Chicago, IL 60611

Health—Eyes

American Optometric Association
243 Lindbergh Blvd.
St. Louis, MO 63141

Health—Mental

American Art Therapy Association
P.O. Box 11604
Pittsburgh, PA 15228

American Mental Health Foundation, Inc.
2 E. 86th St.
New York, NY 10028

American Psychiatric Association
1400 K St. NW
Washington, DC 20005
(202)682-6000

American Psychological Association
1200 17th St. NW
Washington, DC 20036
(202)955-7600

Mental Health Association, National Headquarters
1800 N. Kent St.
Arlington, VA 22209

National Clearinghouse for Mental Health Information
National Institute of
Mental Health
5600 Fishers Ln.,
Room 11A33
Rockville, MD 20857
(301)443-4517

Hearing and Speech

Alexander Graham Bell Association for the Deaf
3417 Volta Pl. NW
Washington, DC 20007
(202)337-5220

American Deafness and Rehabilitation Association
Box 55369
Little Rock, AR 55369
(501)663-4617

American Speech, Language, and Hearing Association
10801 Rockville Pike
Rockville, MD 20852
(301)897-5700

AT&T Communications
Reston, VA
(800)222-4474
(800)833-3232 (TDD)
(800)233-1222 (voice only)

Better Hearing Institute
Box 1840
Washington, DC 20013
(703)642-0580
(800)424-8576

National Association for Hearing and Speech Action Line
(800)638-8255
(301)897-8682 in HI, AK, and
MD only (call collect)

National Center for Stuttering
(800)221-2483
(212)532-1460; NY only

National Hearing Aid Helpline
(800)521-5247
(313)478-2610 in MI only

National Hearing Aid Society
20361 Middlebelt Rd.
Livonia, MI 48152

Self-Help for Hard of Hearing People
7800 Wisconsin Ave.
Bethesda, MD 20814
(301)657-2248
(301)657-2249 (TTY)

Telecommunications for the Deaf
814 Thayer Ave.
Silver Spring, MD 20785
(301)589-3006

Heart

American Heart Association
7320 Greenville Ave.
Dallas, TX 75231
(214)373-6300

Amyotrophic Lateral Sclerosis Association
15300 Ventura Blvd., Suite 315
Sherman Oaks, CA 91403
(818)990-2151

Association of Heart Patients
(800)241-6993
(800)282-3119 in GA only

Council on Arteriosclerosis of the American Heart Association
7320 Greenville Ave.
Dallas, TX 75231

Mended Hearts, Inc.
7320 Greenville Ave.
Dallas, TX 75231
(214)706-1442

Hospital Care

Association for the Care of Children in Hospitals
3615 Wisconsin Ave. NW,
Washington, DC 20016

Hill-Burton Hospital Free Care
(800)638-0742
(800)492-0359 in MD only

Huntington's Disease

Huntington's Disease Society of America, Inc.
140 W. Twenty-second St.
New York, NY 10011-2420
(212)242-1968

Hypertension

High Blood Pressure Information Center
120 '80 National Institutes
of Health
Bethesda, MD 20205
(301)496-1809

Kidney Disease

American Kidney Fund
(800)638-8299
(800)492-8361 in DC only

National Kidney Foundation
2 Park Ave., Room 908
New York, NY 10016

Lung

American Lung Association
1740 Broadway
New York, NY 10019
(212)315-8700

National Asthma Center
National Jewish Hospital and
Research Center
(800)222-5864
(303)398-1477 in CO only

National Jewish Center for Immunology and Respiratory Medicine
1400 Jackson St.
Denver, CO 80206
(303)388-4461

Medicare/Medicaid

DHHS Inspector General's Hotline
(800)368-5779
(301)597-0724 in MD only

Multiple Sclerosis

National Multiple Sclerosis Society
205 E. 42nd St.
New York, NY 10017
(212)986-3240

Muscular Dystrophy

Muscular Dystrophy Association, Inc.
810 7th Ave.
New York, NY 10019
(212)586-0808

Myasthenia Gravis

Myasthenia Gravis Foundation, Inc.
53 W. Jackson Blvd., Suite 909
Chicago, IL 60604
(312)427-6252

Nutrition. See also Food

American Dietetic Association (ADA)
Journal of the American
Dietetic Association
430 N. Michigan Ave.
Chicago, IL 60611
312-899-0046

Center for Adolescent Obesity
Balboa Publishing Corporation
101 Larkspur Landing
Larkspur, CA 94939
(415)461-8884

Consumer Information Center
Pueblo, CO 81009
(303)544-5277, ext. 370

Human Nutrition Center SEA
Room 421A
U.S. Department of Agriculture
Washington, DC 20250
(202)447-7854

National Dairy Council
Rosemont, IL 60018-4233

Office of Consumer Communications (HFG-10)
Food and Drug Administration
Room 15B32 Parklawn Building
5600 Fishers Ln.
Rockville, MD 20857

Older Adulthood—Care Organizations

American College of Nursing Home Administrators
4650 East-West Highway
Washington, DC 20014

Council of Nursing Home Nurses
American Nurses' Association
2420 Pershing Rd.
Kansas City, MO 64108

National Association for Home Care
519 C St. NE
Washington, DC 20002
(202)547-7424

National Association of Adult Day Care
180 East 4050 S
Murray, UT 84107
(801)262-9167 or
(801)359-3077

National Association of Home Health Agencies
426 C St. NE, Suite 200
Washington, DC 20002
(202)547-1717

National Citizen's Coalition for Nursing Home Reform
1424 16th St. NW, Suite 204
Washington, DC 20036
(202)797-8227

National HomeCaring Council
235 Park Ave. S
New York, NY 10003

National Hospice Organization
301 Maple Ave. W, Suite 506
Vienna, VA 22180
(703)938-4449

National Institute on Adult Day Care
National Council on the Aging
600 Maryland Ave. SW
Washington, DC 20024
(202)479-1200

Older Adulthood—General

Administration on Aging
330 Independence Ave. SW
Washington, DC 20201
(202)245-0724

American Association for Geriatric Psychiatry
P.O. Box 376A
Greenbelt, MD 20770
(301)220-0952

American Association of Retired Persons
1909 K St. NW
Washington, DC 20049
(202)872-4700

American Geriatrics Society
770 Lexington Ave. Suite 400
New York, NY 10021
(212)308-1414

American Psychological Association
(Division of Adult Development and Aging)
1200 Seventeenth St. NW
Washington, DC 20036
(202)955-7600

American Public Health Association
(Section of Gerontological Health)
1015 15th St. NW
Washington, DC 20005
(202)789-5600

American Society for Geriatric Dentistry
211 E. Chicago Ave
Chicago, IL 60611
(312)353-6547
(312)664-8270

American Society on Aging
833 Market St. Suite 512
San Francisco, CA 94103
(415)543-2617

Association for Gerontology in Higher Education
600 Maryland Ave. SW
West Wing 204
Washington, DC 20024
(202)484-7505

Children of Aging Parents
2761 Trenton Rd.
Levittown, PA 19056
(215)547-1070

Gerontological Society of America
1411 K St. NW, Suite 300
Washington, DC 20005
(202)393-1411

International Senior Citizens Association, Inc.
11753 Wilshire Blvd.
Los Angeles, CA 90025

National Association for Spanish Speaking Elderly
2025 I St. NW, Suite 219
Washington, DC 20006
(202)293-9329

National Caucus of the Black Aged
1424 K St. NW, Suite 500
Washington, DC 20005

National Council of Senior Citizens
925 15th St. NW
Washington, DC 20005

National Council on Aging
600 Maryland Ave. SW
West Wing 100
Washington, DC 20024
(202)479-1200

National Geriatrics Society
212 W. Wisconsin Ave.
Third Floor
Milwaukee, WI 53203
(414)272-4130

National Gerontological Nursing Association
1818 Newton St. NW
Washington, DC 20010

National Indian Council on Aging
P.O. Box 2088
Albuquerque, NM 87103

National Institute of Mental Health
Mental Disorders of the
Aging Research Branch, DCR
Room 11C-03
5600 Fishers Ln.
Rockville, MD 20857
(301)443-1185

National Institute on Aging
National Institutes of Health
Building 31, Room 5C35
9000 Rockville Pike
Bethesda, MD 20105
(301)496-1752

National Senior Citizens Law Center
1302 18th St. NW, Suite 701
Washington, DC 20036

Older Womens' League (OWL)
National Office
1325 G St. NW, Lower Level-B
Washington, DC 20005

The Association for Humanistic Gerontology
1711 Solano Ave.
Berkeley, CA 94707

The Institute of Retired Professionals
The New School of
Social Research
60 W. 12th St.
New York, NY 10011

The International Federation on Aging
1909 K St. NW
Washington, DC 20006

Older Adulthood—Services

American Association of Homes for the Aging
1129 Twentieth St. NW
Suite 400
Washington, DC 20036
(202)296-5960

Design for Aging
American Institute of Architects
1735 New York Ave. NW
Washington, DC 20006

Gray Panthers
311 South Juniper St. Suite 601
Philadelphia, PA 19107
(215)545-6555

National Association of Meal Programs
204 E St. NE
Washington, DC 20002
(202)547-6157

Organ Donors

Organ Donor Hotline
(800)24-DONOR

The Living Bank International
P.O. Box 6725
Houston, TX 77265
(800)528-2971
(713)528-2971 in TX only

Pain

National Committee on Treatment of Intractable Pain
P.O. Box 9553
Friendship Station
Washington, DC 20016-1553
(202)944-8140

Parkinson's Disease

American Parkinson Disease Association
116 John St., Suite 417
New York, NY 10038
(212)732-9550

National Parkinson Foundation
(800)327-4545
(800)433-7022 in FL only
(305)547-6666 in Miami area only

Parkinson's Disease Foundation
William Black Medical Research Building
Columbia University Medical Center
640-650 W. 168th St.
New York, NY 10032
(212)923-4700

Poison/Toxic Substances

National Pesticide Information Clearinghouse
(800)858-7378

Poison Control Branch
Food and Drug Administration
Parklawn Building, Room 15B-23
5600 Fishers Ln.
Rockville, MD 20857
(301)443-6260

Toxic Substances Control Act Hotline
(800)424-9065
(202)554-1404 in DC area only

Pregnancy. See Family Planning/Pregnancy

Product Safety

Consumer Product Safety Commission
Washington, DC 20207
(800)638-CPSC
(800)638-8270 TDD
(800)492-8104 TDD in MD only

Rape

National Center for the Prevention and Control of Rape
Parklawn Building, Room 6C-12
5600 Fishers Ln.
Rockville, MD 20857
(301)443-1910

Rehabilitation

National Rehabilitation Information Center
4407 8th St. NE
Catholic University of America
Washington, DC 20017-2299
(202)635-5826
(202)635-5884 (TDD)

Rehabilitation International
22 E. 21st St.
New York, NY 10010
(212)420-1500

Rehabilitation Services Administration
Office of Special Education and Rehabilitative Services
Department of Education
330 C St. SW, Room 3431
Washington, DC 20202
(202)723-1282

Society for the Rehabilitation of the Facially Disfigured
550 First Ave.
New York, NY 10016
(212)340-5400

Safety

Clearinghouse for Occupational Safety and Health Information
Technical Information Branch
4676 Columbia Parkway
Cincinnati, OH 45226
(513)684-8326

HUD User (Housing)
P.O. Box 280
Germantown, MD 20874
(301)251-5154

Medic Alert Foundation International
P.O. Box 1009
Turlock, CA 95380

National Highway Traffic Safety Administration
NTS-11, U.S. Department of Transportation
400 7th St. SW
Washington, DC 20590
(202)426-9294
(800)424-9393 (auto hotline)
(202)426-0123 in DC area only

National Injury Information Clearinghouse
5401 Westbard Ave.,
Room 625
Washington, DC 20207
(301)492-6424

United States Coast Guard 2nd District
(800)325-7376
(800)392-7780 in MO only

Sexually Transmitted Diseases

American Venereal Disease Association
Box 385
University of Virginia Hospital
Charlottesville, VA 22908

Sex Information and Education Council of the U.S.
32 Washington Pl.
New York, NY 10003
(212)673-3850

Sexually Transmitted Diseases
(800)227-8922

Smoking

Office on Smoking and Health
Technical Information Center
Park Building, Room 1-16
5600 Fishers Ln.
Rockville, MD 20857
(301)443-1690

Spinal Cord

National Spinal Cord Injury Association
600 W. Cummings Pk.
Suite 2000
Woburn, MA 01801
(617)935-2722

National Spinal Cord Injury Foundation
369 Elliot St.
Newton Upper Falls, MA 02169

National Spinal Cord Injury Hotline
(800)526-3456
(800)688-1733 (in Md.)

Paralyzed Veterans of America
7315 Wisconsin Ave.
Suite 301-W
Washington, DC 20014

Paraplegia News
5201 No. 19th Ave.
Suite 108
Phoenix, AZ 85015

Spina Bifida

Spina Bifida Information and Referral
(800)621-3141
(312)663-1562 in IL only

Surgery

National Second Surgical Opinion Program Hotline
(800)638-6833
(800)492-6603 in MD only

GLOSSARY

abduction Movement of a limb away from the midline or body.

abduction pillow A rigid, triangular box encased in a plastic covering used by patients who have undergone total hip replacement surgery. Designed to keep the repaired hip and leg in neutral alignment.

accountability Assuming or taking responsibility for one's behavior or performance, as in a profession or vocation.

acid A substance that liberates hydrogen ions in a solution; for example, carbonic acid.

acid-base balance A state of balance between the acidity and alkalinity (base) of body fluids.

active euthanasia Deliberately bringing about the death of a person who is suffering from an incurable disease or condition, actively such as by administering a lethal drug.

active transport A process that helps maintain the electrolyte composition between intracellular and extracellular fluids. This process requires the use of metabolic energy, in contrast to osmosis or diffusion.

activities of daily living (ADLs) Activities usually performed in the course of a normal day in the patient's life, such as eating, dressing, bathing, brushing the teeth, or grooming.

acute pain Severe pain, as may follow surgery or trauma or accompany myocardial infarction or other conditions and diseases.

adduction Movement of a limb toward the axis (center) of the body.

admission The entry of a patient into a health care facility.

advance directive An advance declaration by a patient adjudged to be terminally ill and one who does not want to be connected to life support equipment.

affective learning The acquisition of behaviors involved with expressing feelings in attitudes, appreciations, and values.

against medical advice (AMA) A patient's leaving a health care facility without a physician's order for discharge.

agar A dried hydrophilic, colloidal product obtained from certain species of red algae used as the basic ingredient in solid culture media in bacteriology.

air embolus A rare but life-threatening complication that occurs when a large amount of air enters a vein.

alopecia Baldness; a partial or complete loss of hair.

ambulatory surgery Type of surgery generally reserved for patients who need minor surgical procedures, who are in excellent health, and whose surgical outcome is expected to be uneventful. Also called *outpatient surgery, one-day surgery,* and *same-day surgery.*

amino acid Organic chemical compounds composed of one or more basic amino groups and one or more acidic carboxyl groups.

amniocentesis An obstetric procedure in which a small amount of amniotic fluid is removed for laboratory analysis.

ampule A small, sterile glass container of medication; usually a single dose given parenterally.

analgesic A drug that relieves pain.

anastomosis A surgical joining of two ducts, blood vessels, or bowel segments to allow flow from one to the other.

angiocatheter A needle covered with a plastic catheter used to perform venipuncture.

angiogram A radiographic image of a blood vessel after the injection of a contrast medium.

anion A negatively charged ion that is attracted to the positive electrode (anode) in electrolysis.

anorexia Lack or loss of appetite, resulting in the inability to eat.

antibody A protein molecule, essential to the immune system, produced in response to bacteria, viruses, or other foreign substances.

anticipatory grieving Feelings of grief that develop before rather than after a loss.

antiembolism stockings Elasticized stockings worn to prevent the formation of emboli and thrombi, especially in patients after surgery or those restricted to bed.

antigen A substance produced within the body that causes the formation of an antibody and reacts specifically with that antibody; helps form immunity.

antineoplastic Agent used to treat neoplastic (cancerous) diseases.

antipyretics Of or pertaining to a substance or procedure that reduces fever.

antiseptic Substance that inhibits growth and reproduction of microorganisms.

anuria The cessation of urine production, or a urinary output of less than 100 ml per day.
apnea Absence of breathing; a sign of approaching death.
asepsis The absence of microorganisms.
aspiration The act of withdrawing a fluid, such as mucus or serum, from the body by a suction device.
assault Unlawful threat or harm of another person.
assessment An evaluation of appraisal of a patient's condition; the process of making such an evaluation; in nursing, an identification by a nurse of the needs, preferences, and abilities of a patient.
atelectasis The collapse of lung tissue from plugs of mucus or excessive secretions, preventing the respiratory exchange of carbon dioxide and oxygen.
auscultation Method of physical examination; listening to the sounds produced by the body, usually with a stethoscope.
autocratic leadership A situation in which the leader controls all the information and makes all the decisions.
autologous transfusion The collection of the patient's blood for reinfusion after a surgical procedure.
autonomy The ability or tendency to function independently.
autopsy A postmortem (after death) examination of body organs to confirm or determine the cause of death.
autotransfusion A transfusion of the patient's own body substances.
bacteriuria Presence of bacteria in the urine.
balance A normal state of physiologic equilibrium.
bandaging Applying a strip or roll of cloth or other material to secure a dressing, maintain pressure over a compress, or immobilize a part of the body.
barium enema A rectal infusion of barium sulfate, a radiopaque contrast medium, which is retained in the lower intestinal tract during diagnostic studies for obstruction, tumors, or other abnormalities.
base A chemical compound that combines with an acid to form a salt.
base of support A manner of placing the feet securely on the floor to provide protection and support to muscle groups, enabling one to lift heavier objects.
battery Legal term for touching of another's body without consent.
bedpan A shallow vessel used by a person in bed for urination and defecation.
bedtime care Nursing care of a patient just before bedtime that includes providing oral hygiene, removing crumbs from the bed linens, and retightening the bed sheets.
binder Bandages make of large pieces of material to fit specific body parts.
bioethics committee Groups of health care workers who routinely meet to address ethical issues.
bivalve cast An orthopedic cast used for immobilizing a section of the body for the healing of one or more broken bones or for correcting or maintaining correction of an orthopedic deformity.
blanching To whiten or pale.
blood pressure The pressure exerted by the circulating volume of blood on the walls of the arteries, veins, and chambers of the heart.
blood transfusion Infusion of whole blood through a vein.
body alignment Maintaining of body structures in their appropriate anatomic positions.
body mechanics The field of physiology that studies muscular actions and the function of muscles in maintaining the posture of the body.
body temperature The level of heat produced and sustained by body processes.
bolus Round mass of chewed food ready to be swallowed.
bone marrow aspiration The removal of bone marrow from the sternum or iliac crest for testing or to infuse it intravenously into a patient.
bone marrow depression Reduction in blood cells produced within the bone marrow; results in altered immunity.
bony prominence Areas of the body where bones can be easily palpated; bony areas have skin break down more easily than other areas over the body.
brace An orthotic device, sometimes jointed, to support and hold any part of the body in the correct position to allow function, such as a leg brace that permits walking and standing.
bradycardia A slowed heartbeat, usually below 60 beats per minute.
bradypnea An abnormally slow rate of breathing.
breast self-examination A procedure in which a woman examines her breasts and their accessory structures for evidence of change that could indicate a malignant process.
bronchography An x-ray examination of the bronchi after they have been coated with a radiopaque substance.
bronchoscopy The visual examination of the tracheobronchial tree.
bruit Abnormal sound or murmur created by turbulent blood flow heard during auscultation of an organ, a gland, or an artery.

buccal Placed between the gums and inner cheek.

buffer A substance or group of substances that tends to control the hydrogen ion concentration in a solution by absorbing hydrogen ions when an acid is added to the system and releasing hydrogen ions upon the addition of a base.

capillary refill The amount of time required for color to return to the nailbed of the toes or fingers after the nail is briefly and gently compressed.

carbohydrate Any of a group of organic compounds, the most important being sugar, starch, cellulose, and gum. Carbohydrates constitute the main source of energy for all body functions and are necessary for metabolism of other nutrients.

carcinogen Substance or agent that causes the development or increases the incidence of cancer.

cardiac arrest A sudden cessation of cardiac output and effective circulation, usually precipitated by ventricular fibrillation or ventricular asystole.

cardiopulmonary resuscitation (CPR) A basic emergency procedure for life support consisting of artificial respiration and manual external cardiac (heart) massage.

carminative enema Enema consisting of a combination of milk and molasses that relieves flatulence and abdominal distention.

cast A stiff, solid dressing formed with plaster of Paris or other material placed around a limb or other body part to immobilize it during healing.

cathartic A substance that causes evacuation of the bowel.

cation A positively charged ion that in solution is attracted to a negative electrode.

cellular debris Remains of cell breakdown.

Celsius (C) A temperature scale in which 0 is the freezing point of water and 100° is the boiling point of water at sea level. Also called *centigrade scale.*

cephalocaudal From the head toward the feet.

cerumen Earwax; a yellowish or brownish waxy secretion in the external ear canal.

charting by exception A type of documentation that documents for exceptions to the norm (normal).

chemotherapy Pertaining to a chemical form of treatment, such as drug therapy.

Cheyne-Stokes respirations An abnormal pattern of respiration, characterized by alternating periods of apnea and deep, rapid breathing.

cholecystogram An x-ray film of the gallbladder, made after the ingestion or injection of a radiopaque substance, usually a contrast material containing iodine.

chronic pain Pain that continues or recurs over a prolonged period, caused by various diseases or abnormal conditions, such as rheumatoid arthritis.

chyme Viscous, semifluid contents of the stomach present during digestion of a meal that eventually pass into the intestines.

cleansing enema An enema, usually composed of soapsuds, administered to remove all formed fecal material from the colon.

clinical nurse specialist A registered nurse who holds a master's degree in nursing and who has acquired advanced knowledge and clinical skills in a specific area of nursing practice.

closed bed A hospital bed made with all linens pulled toward the head of the bed.

closed drainage system A method of collecting drainage from a wound by use of a drain or tube connected to a vacuum (e.g., Hemovac, Jackson-Pratt).

code of ethics Formal statement that delineates a profession's guidelines for ethical behavior; a code of ethics sets standards or expectations for the professional to achieve.

codependency A term applied to the individual in the family whose spouse is addicted to alcohol or other drugs or behavior. The family member enables the addicted spouse to continue the addictive behavior through caretaking activities instead of allowing the spouse to take responsibility.

cognitive Pertaining to the mental processes of comprehension, judgment, memory, and reasoning, as contrasted with emotional and volitional processes.

cognitive learning Learning that is concerned with acquisition of problem-solving abilities and with intelligence and conscious thought.

colostomy The surgical creation of an artificial anus by incising the colon and bringing it out to the abdominal surface.

communicable disease Any disease transmitted from one person or animal to another directly or indirectly.

communication Any process in which a message is transferred, especially from one person to another, via various media (speech, writing, symbol, or picture).

community A group of species who reside in a designated geographic area and who share common interests or bonds.

community health nursing A field of nursing that is a blend of primary health care and nursing practice with public health nursing. The philosophy of care is based on the belief that care directed to the individual, family, and group contributes to the health care of the population as a whole.

complete bed bath A bath administered entirely by the nurse while the patient remains in bed, usually given to the seriously ill, sedated, or weakened patient.

compress A soft pad, usually made of cloth, used to apply heat, cold, or medications to a body surface area.

compression The act of pressing, squeezing, or otherwise applying pressure to an organ, a tissue, or a body area.

computerized axial tomography An x-ray technique that produces a film representing a detailed cross section of tissue structure; may detect tumor masses, infraction, bone displacement, and accumulations of fluid.

conduit An artificial channel or passage that connects two organs or different parts of the same organ.

confidentiality Privacy; a nurse must not disclose information related to a patient's care.

constipation Difficulty in passing stools or an incomplete or infrequent passage of hard stools.

consumer One who uses goods or services.

continuing education Formal or informal educational programs designed to further knowledge, skills, and professional attitudes of practicing nurses.

continuity of care The continuing of care in another setting.

continuous passive motion (CPM) machine An electrical device that passively exercises a joint. Frequently used after joint replacement surgery.

contracture An abnormal flexion and fixation of a joint caused by muscle disuse or loss of normal skin elasticity.

contrast medium A radiopaque substance injected into the body to facilitate radiopaque imaging of internal structures that otherwise are difficult to visualize on x-ray films.

controlled substances Psychoactive drugs and narcotics that are stored in locked devices because of high risk for abuse of these medications. Federal law governs their dispensing.

coping A process by which a person deals with stress, solves problems, and makes decisions.

core temperature Temperature of deep body tissues and organs.

Credé's maneuver A technique for promoting the expulsion of urine by manual compression of the bladder through pressure on the lower abdomen wall.

crime An act that violates a law and that may include criminal intent.

crossmatching A laboratory test that determines whether the donor's and recipient's bloods are compatible.

crutches Wooden or metal staffs, the most common kinds of which reach from the ground almost to the axilla, to aid a person in walking.

cultural assessment Nursing assessment of patient behaviors based on cultural beliefs, values, and practices.

culture (1) Sample taken from a wound or other drainage, obtained by sterile technique, and sent to the laboratory for identification of microorganisms; (2) similar learned patterns of behavior, values, and attitudes shared by a group of people and passed from one generation to the next.

cyanosis Bluish discoloration of the skin and mucous membranes caused by a decreased level of oxygen in the blood.

cystoscopy The direct visualization of the urinary tract by means of a cystoscope inserted in the urethra. Also used for obtaining biopsies of tumors or other growths and for the removal of polyps.

data base A large store or bank of information, especially in a form that can be processed by computer.

data clustering Categorizing of related data into groups.

death Cessation of life as indicated by the absence of heartbeat or respiration. Legally, death is total absence of activity in the brain and central nervous, cardiovascular, and respiratory systems.

debridement To remove dirt, foreign objects, damaged tissue, or cellular debris from a wound or a burn to prevent infection and promote healing.

decompression The removal of pressure caused by gas or fluid in a body cavity, as in the stomach or intestinal tract.

defamation of character Any communication, written or spoken, that is untrue and that injures the good name or reputation of another or that in any way brings that person into disrepute.

defecation The elimination of feces from the digestive tract through the rectum.

dehiscence The separation of a surgical incision or the rupture of a wound closure.

democratic leadership A people-centered leadership style in which the group participates openly in decision making for group goals.

dependent edema A fluid accumulation in the tissues influenced by gravity. It is usually greater in the lower part of the body than in tissues above the level of the heart.

dependent nursing action Actions based on the instruction or written orders of another professional.

development The gradual process of change that allows adaptation to the environment and function within society through growth, maturation, and learning.

developmental tasks A physical or cognitive skill that a person must accomplish during a particular age period to continue developing, such as walking, which precedes the development of a sense of autonomy in the toddler period.

diarrhea The frequent passage of loose, watery stools.

diastolic pressure The minimum level of blood pressure measured between contractions of the heart. Diastolic pressures for an individual may vary with age, gender, body weight, emotional state, and other factors.

diffusion The process in which substances move through a cell membrane from an area of higher concentration to an area of lower concentration; exchanges nutrients and end products of cellular metabolism between intracellular and extracellular fluid.

diluent A substance, usually fluid, that makes a solution mixture thinner, less viscous, or more liquid.

dimpling Small, abnormal indentations or depressions on the surface of a body or an organ.

disaster An uncontrollable, unexpected, psychologically shocking event.

disaster-preparedness plan A formal plan of action, usually in written form, for coordinating the response of hospital staff in the event of a disaster within the hospital or in the surrounding community.

discharge The release of a patient from a health care facility.

discharge planning The activities that facilitate a patient's movement from one health care setting to another or to home.

disengagement stage A time in family life when children move out, leaving the couple or single parent to live alone.

disinfection The destruction of disease-causing microorganisms.

distention The state of being bloated or swollen.

distraction (1) Procedures that prevent or lessen perception of pain by focusing attention on sensations unrelated to pain; (2) a method of straightening a spinal column by the forces of axial tension pulling on the joint surfaces, such as applied by a Milwaukee brace.

do not resuscitate (DNR) An order written by a physician after discussion with the patient or family.

documentation Written material associated with a computer or documentation on a patient's medical record (chart).

dorsal (supine) Pertaining to the back or posterior.

dorsal-recumbent The supine position with the patient lying on the back, head, and shoulders with the knees flexed. Used in administering catheterization or genital care or for a vaginal examination.

drainage The removal of fluids from a body cavity, wound, or other source. Open drainage occurs when discharge passes through an open-ended tube into a receptacle (or dressing). Suction drainage uses a pump or other mechanical device to assist in extracting fluid.

dream A sequence of ideas, thoughts, emotions, or images that pass through the mind during the rapid eye movement stage of sleep; a visionary creation.

dressing A clean or sterile covering applied directly to wounded or diseased tissue for absorption of secretions, protection from trauma, or administration of medications or to stop bleeding.

drop factor Number of drops that equal 1 ml delivered by an IV tubing.

durable power of attorney for health care A document that designates an agent or a proxy to make health care decisions for a patient who is unable to do so.

duty (in law) An obligation owed by one party to another. Duty may be established by statute or other legal process, as by contract or oath supported by statute, or it may be voluntarily undertaken.

dying The process of nearing death followed by the cessation of life.

dysfunctional grieving The ineffective resolution of a loss. May be the loss of a loved one.

dysphagia Difficulty in swallowing, commonly associated with obstructive or motor disorders of the esophagus.

dyspnea Shortness of breath or difficulty in breathing that may be caused by certain heart conditions, strenuous exercise, or activity.

dysrhythmia Any disturbance or abnormality in the normal rhythmic pattern of the heartbeat. May also be called *arrhythmia.*

dysuria Painful urination resulting from bacterial infection of the bladder and obstructive conditions of the urethra.

early AM care Assisting the patient with oral hygiene, washing of the face and hands, toileting, and combing of the hair, if desired, just before eating breakfast.

edema The abnormal accumulation of fluid in the interstitial spaces of tissues.

ego A part of the mind that learns to deal with reality. It mediates the drives of the id with the demands of society according to Freud. The decision-making part of the personality.

elective surgery A surgical procedure that is not

an emergency and may not be essential but is performed by choice.

electrocardiography A method of recording electrical activity generated by the heart muscle.

electroencephalogram (EEG) A test that records brain-wave activity that is used to diagnose seizure disorders, brainstem disorders, focal lesions, and impaired consciousness.

electroencephalography The process of recording brain-wave activity, used to diagnose seizure disorders, brainstem disorders, focal lesions, and impaired consciousness.

electrolyte A chemical substance that, when dissolved in water or other fluids, dissociates into ions and is capable of conducting an electrical current.

electromyography A record of the intrinsic electric activity in a skeletal muscle to assist in diagnosing neuromuscular problems.

empathy The ability to recognize and partly share the emotions and states of mind of another person and to understand the meaning and significance of that person's behavior.

enculturation The process of learning the concepts, values, and behavioral standards of a particular culture.

endorphins Any one of the neuropeptides composed of many amino acids, elaborated by the pituitary gland and acting on the central and peripheral nervous systems to reduce pain.

endorsement A statement of recognition of the license of a health practitioner in one state by another state. The nurse may receive a license in another state without retaking the licensing examination.

endoscope An illuminated optic instrument for the visualization of the interior of a body cavity or an organ.

enema Procedure in which a solution is introduced into the rectum for cleansing or evacuation of the bowel.

engagement stage A stage of family development that usually precedes establishment of the family unit. The couple prepares for marriage and becomes free of parental domination.

enteral feedings Providing food or nutritive material through the gastrointestinal tract when the patient cannot ingest, chew, or swallow food.

enteral nutrition Nutrition for patients who have normal gastrointestinal motility and absorption but cannot eat naturally; tube feeding.

enteric coated A coating added to oral medications that are designed to be absorbed from the intestinal tract.

enterostomal therapist (ET) A nurse trained to provide wound-drainage services.

enuresis Involuntary passage of urine; incontinence.

epidural analgesia The process of achieving regional anesthesia of the pelvic, abdominal, genital, or other area by the injection of a local anesthetic into the epidural space of the spinal cord.

epistaxis Bleeding from the nose; nosebleed.

erythroblastosis fetalis A type of hemolytic anemia that occurs in newborns as a result of maternal-fetal blood group incompatibility.

eschar A scab or dry crust resulting from excoriation of the skin as in burns and infections.

esophagogastroduodenoscopy Visual examination of the esophagus, stomach, and duodenum by means of an endoscope.

establishment stage A stage that begins when the couple lives together and works on deepening the relationship.

ethical dilemma A situation involving a choice between equally unsatisfactory alternatives.

ethics Principles or standards that govern appropriate conduct.

etiology The cause of a disease.

euthanasia Deliberately bringing about the death of a person who has an incurable disease or condition either actively, by administering a lethal drug, or passively, by withholding treatment and allowing the person to die.

evaluation The fifth step in the nursing process. A category of nursing behavior in which a determination is made and recorded regarding the extent to which the established goals of care have been met.

evisceration The protrusion of an internal organ through a wound or surgical incision, especially in the abdominal wall.

excoriation An injury to the surface of the skin or other part of the body caused by trauma, such as scratching, abrasion, or chemical or thermal burns.

expectant stage A time in family life when the woman is pregnant, necessitating some changes in lifestyle.

extended family Nuclear family plus other relatives who live together.

external rotation Turning of a limb laterally or to the side.

extracellular fluid A fluid located outside the cell comprising interstitial fluid and blood plasma. Two of the most important ionized components of this fluid are sodium and chloride.

exudate Fluid that escapes from a cavity, usually during inflammation.

Fahrenheit (F) A temperature scale in which the boiling point of water is 212° and the freezing point of water is 32° at sea level.

false imprisonment Unlawful restraint of a person from exercising the right of freedom of movement.

family Two or more persons who are related by blood, marriage, or adoption and who live together over a period of time.

family interaction Sum total of all roles and behaviors shown in a family at a given time.

fanfold Folded like a fan lengthwise, such as the top linen on a hospital bed.

fat A substance composed of lipids or fatty acids and occurring in various consistencies from oil to tallow.

febrile Characterized by an elevated body temperature.

fecal impaction An accumulation of hardened feces in the rectum or sigmoid colon that the individual is unable to move.

fecal incontinence Involuntary defecation.

feces Waste or excrement from the gastrointestinal tract.

felony A serious crime that usually carries a penalty of imprisonment or death.

fidelity Loyalty to something to which one is bound by a pledge or duty.

fixation An arrest (stoppage) at a particular stage of psychosexual development, such as anal fixation.

flatulence The presence of an excessive amount of air or gas in the stomach and intestinal tract, causing distention of the organs and in some cases mild to moderate pain.

focus charting A documentation format focusing on patient needs that deviate from the norm (normal).

fomites Nonliving material, such as bed linens, that may convey pathogenic microorganisms.

fracture pan A small bedpan often used for patients with fractures to help prevent pain on movement.

fraud The act of intentionally misleading or deceiving another person by any means so as to cause legal injury, usually the loss of something valuable or the surrender of a legal right.

French (Fr) Term used to denote the size of the lumen of a feeding tube.

friction The act of rubbing one object against another.

gastrostomy Surgical creation of an artificial opening into the stomach through the abdominal wall for feeding purposes.

gastrostomy feeding tube The insertion of a feeding tube through a stoma into the stomach for the purpose of providing enteral nutrition.

gauge The diameter of a needle.

gavage The process of feeding a patient through a nasogastric tube.

general survey Clinical observation or assessment of the patient's general appearance. It includes general information such as gender, ethnic origin, and age.

glycosuria Abnormal presence of a sugar, especially glucose, in the urine. Glycosuria can result from the ingestion of large amounts of carbohydrate, or it may be the result of endocrine or renal disorders.

goal The purpose toward which an endeavor is directed, such as the outcome of diagnostic, therapeutic, and educational management of a patient's health problem. A goal reflects what the patient should be able to do.

Good Samaritan law Legislation enacted in some states to protect health care professionals from liability in rendering emergency aid, unless there is proven willful wrong or gross negligence.

gram staining The method of staining microorganisms using a violet stain followed by an iodine solution, decolorizing with an alcohol or acetone solution, and counterstaining with safranin. Used as a means of identifying and classifying bacteria.

granulation tissue Small, fleshy, beadlike projections found on the surface of a wound while healing.

grief A nearly universal pattern of physical and emotional responses to bereavement, separation, or loss.

grieving process Sequence of affective, cognitive, and physiologic states through which the person responds to and finally accepts an irretrievable loss.

growth An increase in physical size and capabilities until maturity.

health care proxy A person designated to make health care decisions for a patient who has become incapacitated.

health care team All the people, departments, and ancillary services that collectively render care and services to the client.

health history (in nursing and medicine) A collection of information obtained from the patient and from other sources concerning the patient's physical status and psychologic, social, and sexual functions. The nurse conducts a patient interview.

hematoma A localized collection of blood, usually clotted, in an organ, a space, or a tissue.

hematuria Abnormal presence of blood in the urine.

hemiplegia Paralysis of one side of the body.

hemoccult test A test used to detect occult blood in feces.

hemolysis Destruction of red blood cells.

hemorrhage A loss of a large amount of blood in a short period of time, either externally or internally. Hemorrhage may be arterial, venous, or capillary.

heredity The process by which particular traits or conditions are genetically transmitted from parents to offspring, resulting in resemblance of individuals related by descent.

herniation A protrusion of a body organ or portion of an organ through an abnormal opening in a membrane, muscle, or other tissue.

hierarchy of needs Maslow's order of physiologic needs of a person.

high Fowler's Placement of a patient in a semisitting position by raising the head of the bed more than 20 inches.

high-risk problem A patient problem in which conditions are right for its occurrence. The patient is at risk for developing a problem.

holistic care Care of the whole person, including physiologic, psychologic, and sociologic needs.

hospice System of family-centered care designed to help terminally ill persons be comfortable and maintain a satisfactory lifestyle throughout the terminal phase of their illness.

host The organism on which a parasite lives and receives nourishment.

hydrophilic dressing Absorbent dressing designed to draw excessive drainage away from the site of a pressure ulcer.

hydrophobic dressing Nonabsorbent, waterproof dressing designed to protect a pressure ulcer from contamination.

hydrostatic pressure The pressure exerted by a liquid.

hygiene Conditions or practices conducive to cleanliness and health.

hyperemia Increased blood in part of the body caused by increased blood flow, as in the inflammatory response, local relaxation of arterioles, or obstruction of the outflow of blood from an area. Skin overlying a hyperemic area usually becomes reddened and warm.

hyperpyrexia An extremely elevated temperature sometimes occurring in acute infectious diseases, especially in young children.

hypertension A common, often asymptomatic disorder characterized by elevated blood pressure persistently exceeding 140/90; high blood pressure.

hypotension An abnormal condition in which blood pressure is not adequate for normal blood supply needs and oxygenation of the tissues; low blood pressure.

hypovolemia An abnormal decrease in extracellular fluid, specifically plasma.

hypoxia Lack of oxygen to the tissues.

id Unconscious part of the mind involving basic biologic drives and reflexes according to Freud. The pleasure-seeking part of the personality.

ileostomy The surgical formation of an opening in the ileum onto the surface of the abdomen through which fecal matter is emptied.

immobility Inability to move about freely.

immunization A process by which resistance to an infectious disease is induced or augmented.

immunoglobulin Proteins capable of acting as antibodies present in serum or watery body fluid and in body secretions.

implementation A deliberate action performed to achieve a goal, such as carrying out a plan in caring for a patient.

incentive spirometry A type of therapy that encourages increased inspiration through a means of visible reward.

incident report A confidential document that describes any patient accident occurring on the premises of a health care agency.

independent nursing action Actions pertaining to certain aspects of professional nursing practice that are encompassed by applicable licensure and law and require no supervision or direction from others.

infiltration Dislodging an intravenous catheter or a needle from a vein into the subcutaneous space.

inflammation The protective response of body tissues to irritation or injury, such as pain, swelling, redness, heat, and lack of function.

informed consent Permission from a patient to perform a specific test or procedure after hearing about all risks, side effects, and benefits.

infusion pump An apparatus designed to deliver measured amounts of a drug or intravenous solution through injection over a period of time. Some kinds of infusion pumps can be implanted surgically.

inhalation The act of breathing in or drawing in with the breath.

injection An act of forcing a liquid into the body by means of a syringe.

insensible loss A nonvisible form of water loss.

inservice education Informal instruction provided by an agency or institution to employed nurses.

insomnia Chronic inability to sleep or remain asleep.

inspection Visual examination of the external surface of the body as well as of its movements and posture.

instillation A procedure in which a fluid is slowly introduced into a cavity or passage of the body and allowed to remain for a specific length of time before being drained or withdrawn.

interagency transfer A transfer to another health care facility.

interdependent nursing action Actions carried out by the nurse in collaboration with another health care professional.

internal rotation Turning of a limb medially or to the middle.

interstitial fluid Part of the extracellular fluid that bathes the cells. Primary function is to transport nutrients and waste products.

intraagency transfer A transfer within a health care facility.

intracellular fluid A fluid within the cells of the body containing ions and electrolytes, such as magnesium and potassium.

intractable pain Pain not easily relieved, such as that occuring with some types of cancer.

intradermal Injection given between layers of the skin into the dermis. Injections are given at a 5- to 15-degree angle.

intramuscular Injections given into muscle tissue. The intramuscular route provides a fast rate of absorption that is related to the muscle's greater vascularity. Injections are given at a 90-degree angle.

intravascular fluid Fluid inside a blood vessel.

intravenous Injection directly into the bloodstream. Action of the drug begins immediately when given intravenously.

intravenous pyelogram A technique in radiology for examining the structures and evaluating the function of the urinary system.

invasion of privacy The violation of another person's right to be left alone and free from unwarranted publicity and intrusion.

irrigation The process of washing out a body cavity or wounded area with a stream of water or other fluid.

ischemia Lack of blood flow to an area resulting in hypoxia.

isolation techniques Techniques used to prevent the spread of an infection or protect the patient from irritating environmental factors.

jaundice A yellow discoloration of the skin, mucous membranes, and sclerae of the eyes caused by greater than normal amounts of bilirubin in the blood.

jejunostomy feeding tube The insertion of a feeding tube usually by the nasal route and allowing the tube to pass into the patient's jejunum for the purpose of providing enteral nutrition.

justice Fairness or equity.

Kardex A card filing system usually kept at the nursing station that allows quick reference to the particular needs of each patient for nursing care.

Kegel exercises A regimen of isometric exercises in which a woman executes a series of voluntary contractions of the muscles of her pelvic diaphragm and perineum in an effort to increase the contractility of her vaginal introitus or to improve her retention of urine.

kinesics The study of body position and movement in relation to communication.

knee-chest (genupectoral) Knee-chest position. To assume this position, the person kneels so that the weight of the body is supported by the knees and chest with the abdomen raised. The head is turned to one side and the arms are flexed so that the upper part of the body can be supported in part by the elbows.

Korotkoff sounds Sounds heard during the taking of blood pressure using a sphygmomanometer and stethoscope.

Kussmaul's respirations Abnormally deep and rapid sighing respirations characteristic of accumulated ketones and associated with poorly controlled diabetes.

laissez-faire leadership Passive, permissive, nondirect style of leadership in which decisions are made by the group and the leader provides no suggestions or direction.

laryngoscopy The use of a laryngoscope to view the larynx.

lavage The therapeutic washing out of an organ.

laxative A substance that causes evacuation of the bowel.

learning Acquiring knowledge, attitudes, or skills through experience or practice.

legal death A total absence of activity in the brain as assessed and pronounced by a physician.

libel Written false statement about a person that may injure the reputation.

libido A person's general sexual energy. An underlying force in development according to Freud.

licensure The granting of permission by a competent authority (usually a government agency) to an organization or individual to engage in a practice or an activity that would otherwise be illegal.

lithotomy The surgical excision of a calculus, especially one from the urinary tract.

living will Instrument by which a dying person makes wishes known.

loss Absence of a significant other, an object, or a state of health to which the person must adapt through the grieving process.

lumbar puncture The introduction of a hollow needle and stylet into the subarachnoid space of the lumbar portion of the spinal cord.

magnetic resonance imaging Medical imaging

that uses radiofrequency radiation as its source of energy.

maleficence The act of committing harm or evil.

malpractice Professional negligence that is the most likely cause of injury or harm to a patient, resulting from a lack of professional knowledge, experience, skill, or caution.

matrilocal/matriarchal family Family in which a woman has the main authority and power.

maturation Process or condition of attaining complete development.

medical asepsis The removal or destruction of disease microorganisms or infected material.

medical diagnosis The determination of the cause of a patient's illness or suffering by the combined use of physical examination, patient interview, laboratory tests, review of the patient's medical records, knowledge of the cause of observed signs and symptoms, and differential elimination of similar possible causes.

medical record The portion of a patient's health record that is made by physicians and is a written or transcribed history of various illnesses or injuries requiring medical care. It provides an accurate description of nursing care from the time of admission to the time of discharge.

medicated tub bath A therapeutic bath in which medication is dispersed in water, usually when treating dermatologic disorders.

menopause Cessation of menses.

menses Normal flow of blood and decidua that occurs during menstruation.

microorganism A microscopic animal or plant capable of carrying on life functions.

micturition The act of passing urine.

mineral An inorganic substance occurring naturally in the Earth's crust that has a characteristic chemical composition and (usually) crystalline structure.

misdemeanor A crime less serious than a felony; the penalty is usually a fine or imprisonment for less than a year.

mobility Person's ability to move about freely.

moral A principle on which definitions of right and wrong in behavior are based.

multicultural nursing Caring for people from all ethnic and cultural backgrounds with respect and caring.

myelogram (1) An x-ray film taken after the injection of a radiopaque medium into the subarachnoid space to demonstrate any distortion of the spinal cord, spinal nerve roots, and subarachnoid space; (2) a graphic representation of a count of the different kinds of cells in a stained preparation of bone marrow.

narcolepsy Syndrome involving sudden sleep attacks that a person cannot inhibit; an uncontrollable desire to sleep may occur several times during a day.

narcotic A drug substance derived from opium or produced synthetically that alters perception of pain and with repeated use may result in physical and psychologic dependence.

nasogastric (NG) intubation The insertion of a tube passed into the stomach through the nose for the purpose of emptying the stomach of its contents or for delivering medication and/or nourishment.

nasogastric tube Any tube passed into the stomach through the nose. Used to relieve gastric distention by removing gas, gastric secretions, or food; used to instill medication, food, or fluids or to obtain a specimen for laboratory analysis.

nasogastric tube feedings The process of introducing nutrients in a liquid form directly into the stomach via a nasogastric tube.

nasointestinal tube feeding Method of supplying nutrients directly into the small intestine; may be used for patients who are at risk for aspiration or have a dysfunctional gastric outlet.

necrosis Changes in tissue related to death of cells.

negative nitrogen balance The state in which the amount of nitrogen ingested that is related to protein intake is less than that excreted every day. The result is an elevation of serum albumin, which increases the oncotic pressure and pulls fluid to the interstitial spaces resulting in edema.

negative pressure Suction.

negligence Careless act of omission or commission that results in injury to another.

neutral alignment The positioning of an extremity in a straight line without internal or external rotation.

nonproductive cough A sudden, noisy expulsion of air from the lungs that may be caused by irritation or inflammation and does not remove sputum from the respiratory tract.

nonrapid eye movement (NREM) The four stages in which there is relatively no rapid eye movement.

nonverbal communication The transmission of a message without the use of words. It may involve any or all of the five senses.

normovolemic hemodilution Removal of the patient's blood immediately before or after administration of the anesthesia. A colloid solution is given intravenously to the patient to help replace the volume of blood and maintain normal volume. The blood can be reinfused.

nosocomial infection An infection acquired during hospitalization.

NPO Nothing by mouth over a period of hours of a patient who is about to undergo surgery or special diagnostic procedures requiring that the digestive tract be empty.

nuclear family Mother, father, and child(ren) in the family unit.

nurse administrator A nurse who performs in an administrative position instead of performing nursing care (e.g., a director of nursing).

nurse anesthetist A registered nurse qualified by advanced training in an accredited program in the specialty of nurse anesthesia to manage the care of the patient during the administration of anesthesia in selected surgical situations.

nurse educator A registered nurse whose primary area of interest, competence, and professional practice is the education of nurses.

nurse midwife A registered nurse qualified by advanced training in obstetric and neonatal care and certified by the American College of Nurse Midwives. The nurse midwife manages the perinatal care of women having a normal pregnancy, labor, and childbirth.

Nurse Practice Act Statute enacted by the legislature of any of the states or by appropriate officers of the districts or possessions.

nurse practitioner A nurse who by advanced education and clinical experience in a specialized area of nursing practice, such as in a master's degree program in nursing, has acquired expert knowledge in the special branch of practice.

nurse researcher A registered nurse who specializes in nursing research to help improve nursing care through problem solving and working with others.

nursing Profession concerned with the diagnosis and care of human responses to actual and potential health problems.

nursing care plan A written plan based on a nursing assessment and nursing diagnosis, devised by a nurse. Should be part of every patient's chart; an abbreviated form should be available for quick reference, as in a Rand or Kardex file.

nursing diagnosis The second step in the nursing process. A statement of a health problem or potential problem in the patient's health status that a nurse is licensed and competent to treat. Diagnosis has three parts: the term that closely describes the problem, the probable cause, and the defining characteristics.

nursing intervention Any act by a nurse that implements any part of the nursing care plan.

nursing process The process that serves as an organizational framework for the practice of nursing. It encompasses all the steps taken by the nurse in caring for a patient: data collection, diagnosis, planning, implementation, and evaluation.

objective data Information or findings that can be measured by the observations of the nurse. Includes physical assessment and results of laboratory, radiologic, or other studies.

obliteration To remove or make imperceptible by pressure. Often refers to the process of using fingers to put significant pressure over a pulse site so that the pulse can no longer be felt.

occult Hidden or difficult to observe.

oliguria Scant urinary output.

oncotic pressure gradient The pressure difference between the osmotic pressure of blood and that of tissue fluid or lymph. It is an important force in maintaining fluid balance between the vascular space and interstitium.

open bed Fanfolded top linens on a hospital bed for easy patient access.

oral hygiene Maintenance of tissues and structure of the mouth; includes brushing teeth, dental flossing, and cleaning of dentures.

orientation The awareness of one's physical environment with regard to time, place, and the identity of other persons; the ability to adapt to such an existing or new environment.

orthopneic A body position that enables a patient to breathe comfortably. Usually, the patient is sitting up and bent forward, with the arms supported on a table or chair arms.

orthostatic hypotension Abnormally low blood pressure occurring when an individual moves from a sitting or lying position to a standing position. Also called *postural hypotension.*

osmosis The movement of a pure solvent, such as water, through a semipermeable membrane from a solution that has a lower solute concentration to one that has a higher solute concentration.

osteoporosis A loss of calcium from the bone resulting in softening.

ostomate Person who has an ostomy.

ostomy Surgical procedure in which an opening is made into the abdominal wall to allow the passage of intestinal contents from the bowel (colostomy) or urine from the bladder (urostomy).

oxygen toxicity A condition of oxygen overdosage that can result in pathologic tissue changes, such as retinopathy of prematurity or bronchopulmonary dysplasia.

oxygenation The process of combining or treating with oxygen.

pain An unpleasant sensation caused by noxious stimulation of the sensory nerve endings.

palpation Method of physical examination whereby the fingers or hands of the examiner are applied to the client's body for the purpose of feeling body parts underlying the skin.

Papanicolaou test A simple smear method of examining stained exfoliative cells. It is used most commonly to detect cancers of the cervix, but it may be used for tissue specimens from an organ.

paracentesis A procedure in which fluid is withdrawn from a cavity of the body. It is most commonly performed to remove excessive accumulations of ascitic fluid from the abdomen.

paraplegia Paralysis of the legs below the level of injury to the spinal cord.

parasite An organism living in or on and obtaining nourishment from another organism.

parenteral Not in or through the digestive system.

parenteral therapy Fluids and medications introduced into the body other than through the gastrointestinal tract.

parenthood stage Stage of family life at the birth of a child.

partial bath A patient's incomplete bath; a nurse usually must bathe the back, legs, and feet.

passive euthanasia Deliberately bringing about the death of a person who has an incurable disease or condition by withholding treatment and allowing the person to die.

patent Open and unblocked, such as a patent airway or patent anus.

pathogen Any microorganism capable of producing disease.

patient teaching Teaching the patient from admission, throughout the hospital stay, and after discharge as needed. The nurse teaches self-care and independence as possible.

patient unit The space allotted to the patient in a health care facility; usually includes a bed, an overbed table, a bedside table, and possibly a chair or other furniture.

patient-controlled analgesia (PCA) Drug-delivery system that allows clients to self-administer analgesic medications when they want.

Patient's Bill of Rights A list of the patient's rights established by the American Hospital Association that protects the patient but is not a legally binding document.

patrilocal/patriarchal family Family in which a man has the main authority and power.

pediculosis Infested with sucking lice.

perception Person's mental image or concept of elements in each person's environment, including information gained through the senses.

percussion A technique in physical examination used to evaluate the size, borders, and consistency of some of the internal organs and to discover the presence and evaluate the amount of fluid in a cavity of the body.

perineal care Cleansing of the perineal region to remove normal secretions and prevent the growth of microorganisms.

perioperative blood salvage Collection of blood during surgery or up to 12 hours after surgery. This is accomplished by collecting the blood under sterile conditions using suction at the operative site or collecting blood from chest drains after surgery. This blood may be transfused directly after processing (washed) to the patient.

perioperative nursing Nursing care provided to surgery patients during the entire inpatient period from admission to discharge.

peristalsis The coordinated, rhythmic contraction of smooth muscle that forces food through the digestive tract.

peristomal Around a stoma.

phantom pain A phenomenon common after amputation of a limb in which sensation or discomfort is experienced in the missing limb. In some people, severe pain persists.

phlebitis Inflammation of a vein.

physical assessment Part of the health assessment representing a synthesis of the information obtained in a physical examination.

PIE A documentation format used for charting by exception. It is a problem-solving approach.

piggyback Added on to an established intravenous infusion.

planning (in five-step nursing process) The selection of appropriate nursing interventions to be taken to meet the patient's needs or resolve the problem.

plasma The liquid portion of blood.

pleural space The space between the layers of the pleura that contains pleural fluid.

pneumothorax The collapse of a lung due to pressure exerted from abnormal air or other gas into the pleural space.

poison Any substance that impairs health or destroys life when ingested, injected, inhaled, or absorbed by the body in relatively small amounts.

poisoning The physical condition produced by ingestion, injection, inhalation, or exposure to a poisonous substance.

polyuria Production and excretion of abnormally large amounts of urine. Also called *diuresis.*

portal of entry Route by which microorganisms enter the human body.

portal of exit When a microorganism finds an exit from the body, it can then enter another host and cause disease.

postanesthesia care unit (PACU) An area adjoining the operating room to which surgical patients are taken while still under anesthesia.

postmortem After death.

postural drainage Special positions into which a patient can be placed to induce drainage of fluid from the lungs.

posture The position of the body with respect to the surrounding space; determined and maintained by the coordination of various muscles that move the limbs.

practical/vocational nursing Person educated and trained in basic nursing techniques and direct patient care at an accredited school of practical/vocational nursing but not as in-depth and comprehensively as the professional nurse. The practical nurse practices under the supervision of a registered nurse, physician, or dentist and must pass a state board examination.

precipitate Particles separated from a solution.

pressure point A site that is extremely sensitive to pressure such as the areas of the body where a bone lies close to the surface of the skin.

pressure ulcer Skin that turns red and broken in patients who are immobile for a period of time.

primary care The first contact in a given episode of illness that leads to a decision regarding a course of action to resolve the health problem. Primary care usually is provided by a physician, but some primary care functions are also handled by nurses.

primary health care A basic level of health care that includes programs directed at the promotion of health, early diagnosis of disease or disability, and prevention of disease. Primary health care is provided in an ambulatory facility to limited numbers of people, often those living in a particular geographic area. It includes continuing health care, such as that provided by a family nurse practitioner.

primary intention Primary union of the edges of a wound, progressing to complete scar formation without granulation.

principle (1) A general truth or a settled rule of action; (2) a prime source or element from which anything proceeds; (3) a law on which others are founded or from which others are derived.

problem Question proposed for solution or consideration.

problem-oriented medical record (POMR) A method of recording data about the health status of a patient in a problem-solving system. Parts included are data base, problem list, initial plan, and progress notes.

process recording A system used for teaching nursing students to understand and analyze verbal and nonverbal interaction. The conversation between nurse and patient is written on special forms or in a special format. The student nurse is instructed to record observations, perceptions, thoughts, and feelings, as well as the words exchanged. The process recording is then studied by the nursing instructor to discover and to help the student nurse identify patterns of difficulty in communicating with the patient.

proctoscopy The examination of the rectum with an endoscope inserted through the anus.

productive cough A sudden expulsion of air from the lungs that effectively removes sputum from the respiratory tract and helps clear the airways.

prolapse Falling, sinking, or sliding of an organ from its normal position or location in the body, such as a prolapsed uterus.

proliferation The reproduction or multiplication of similar forms. The term is usually applied to increases of cells or cysts.

prone Being in the horizontal position when lying face downward.

prosthesis An artificial replacement for a missing part of the body, such as an artificial limb or total joint replacement.

protein Any of a large group of naturally occurring, complex, organic nitrogenous compounds.

proteinuria Albumin in the urine. Also called *albuminuria.*

proximodistal From the center of the body outward.

psychomotor learning The acquisition of ability to perform motor skills.

psychosexual theory Theory of development by Sigmund Freud that repressed sexual problems from childhood are the cause of problems later in life.

pulse The regular, recurrent expansion and contraction of an artery produced by the ejection of blood from the left ventricle of the heart as it contracts.

pulse deficit A condition that exists when the radial pulse is less than the apical pulse. The condition indicates a lack of peripheral perfusion for some of the heart contractions.

pulse pressure The difference between systolic and diastolic pressures.

purulent Containing or forming pus.

pyuria Pus in the urine.

quadriplegia Paralysis of the arms, legs, and trunk below the level of an associated injury of the spinal cord.

radiating pain Pain perceived at a source and extending to surrounding or nearby tissues.

radiography The production of shadow images on photographic emulsion through the action of ionizing radiation. The image is the result of the differential attenuation of the radiation in its passage through the object being radiographed.

radiopaque Not permitting the passage of x-rays or other radiant energy.

range of motion (ROM) The range of movement of a joint, from maximum extension to maximum flexion, as measured in degrees of a circle.

rapid eye movement (REM) Stage of sleep in which dreaming and rapid eye movements are prominent; important for mental restoration.

rebound effect Continuing heat therapy beyond the time needed that provides the opposite effect by constricting blood vessels, causing greater risk for burns.

reception Free nerve endings, constituting most of the pain receptors, that warn a person of harmful changes in the environment.

recording A written form of communication that permanently documents information relevant to the nursing care of the patient.

rectal tube A flexible tube inserted into the rectum to assist in the relief of flatus.

referred pain Pain felt at a site different from that of an injured or a diseased organ or part of the body.

registered nursing Health care profession in which a course of study has been completed at an accredited school of nursing and an examination administered by a state board of nursing has been passed.

renal calculi Calcium stones in the renal pelvis.

reservoir A nonhuman host that serves as a means of sustaining an infectious microorganism as a potential source of human infection.

residual urine Urine remaining in the bladder immediately after urinating.

respiration The exchange of oxygen and carbon dioxide between the atmosphere and body cells, including inspiration and expiration, diffusion of oxygen from the pulmonary alveoli to the blood, and diffusion of carbon dioxide from the blood to the alveoli.

respiratory arrest The cessation of breathing.

responsibility Carrying out duties associated with a particular role.

restraint Any of numerous devices used in aiding the immobilization of patients.

retention A resistance to movement or displacement; the inability to urinate or defecate.

retention enema A medicinal or nutrient enema specially formulated so that it will remain in the bowel without stimulating the nerve endings that would ordinarily result in evacuation.

reverse isolation Isolation procedures designed to protect a patient from infectious organisms that might be carried by the staff, other patients, or visitors or on droplets in the air or on equipment or materials.

Rh factor An antigenic substance present in the erythrocytes of 85% of the people. A person having the factor is Rh positive; a person lacking the factor is Rh negative.

rigor mortis The stiffening of muscles after death.

sanguineous Pertaining to blood or containing blood, such as full blooded.

secondary intention Wound closure in which the edges are separated, granulation tissue develops to fill the gap, and finally, epithelium grows in over the granulation, producing a larger scar than that resulting with primary intention.

self-actualization The fundamental tendency toward the maximal realization and fulfillment of one's human potential.

semi-Fowler's Placement of the patient in an inclined position, with the upper half of the body raised by elevating the head of the bed approximately 30 degrees.

sensitivity Susceptibility to a substance, such as a drug or an antigen.

separation anxiety Fear and apprehension caused by separation from familiar surroundings and significant persons.

sequential compression device (SCD) Special stockings that apply varying degrees of external compression to prevent deep vein thrombosis. The pressure on the vein walls causes the values to contract and increases blood flow.

serosanguineous Composed of serum and blood.

serous Pertaining to, resembling, or producing serum.

serum Any serous fluid that moistens the surface of serous membranes; also called *blood.*

shearing force An applied force or pressure exerted against the surface and layers of the skin as tissues slide in opposite but parallel planes.

sigmoidoscopy The inspection of the rectum and sigmoid colon by the aid of a sigmoidoscope.

Sims' A position in which the patient lies on the left side with the right knee and thigh drawn upward toward the chest. The chest and abdomen are allowed to fall forward. It is the position of choice for administering enemas or conducting rectal examinations.

single-parent family A family consisting of only the mother or father and one or more dependent children.

sitz bath A bath in which only the hips and buttocks are immersed in water or saline solution; the time allotted is usually 20 minutes.

skin graft A portion of skin implanted to cover areas where skin has been lost through burns or injury or by surgical removal of diseased tissue.

slander A false statement about another that harms the reputation.

sleep State marked by reduced consciousness, diminished activity of the skeletal muscles, and depressed metabolism.

sleep apnea A sleep disorder characterized by periods of an absence of attempts to breathe. The person is momentarily unable to move respiratory muscles or maintain airflow through the nose and mouth.

sleep deprivation Condition resulting from a decrease in the amount, quality, and consistency of sleep.

sleep terrors A condition occurring during stages 3 or 4 of nonrapid eye movement sleep that is characterized by repeated episodes of abrupt awakening, usually with a panicky scream, accompanied by intense anxiety, confusion, agitation, disorientation, unresponsiveness, marked motor movements, and total amnesia concerning the event.

sling A bandage or device used to support an injured part of the body.

small bowel x-ray series Examination in which the entire small bowel is visualized. Frequently ordered to diagnose tumors, obstruction, diverticulitis, and ulcerative colitis.

SOAPIE Acronym for subjective, objective, assessment, and planning (also implementation and evaluation), the four parts of the written account of a patient's health problem in a problem-oriented record.

somnambulism (1) A condition occurring during stages 3 or 4 of nonrapid eye movement sleep that is characterized by complex motor activity, usually culminating in leaving the bed and walking about, with no recall of the episode on awakening; (2) a hypnotic state in which the person has full possession of the senses but no recollection of the episode.

specific gravity The ratio of the density of a substance to the density of another substance accepted as a standard.

sphygmomanometer A device for measuring arterial blood pressure.

splinting The process of immobilizing, restraining, or supporting a body part.

spore A reproductive unit of some genera of fungi or protozoa. A spore is resistant to heat, drying, and chemicals.

sputum Material coughed up from the lungs and expectorated through the mouth. It contains mucus, cellular debris, or microorganisms, and it also may contain blood or pus.

standard A measure or guide that is recognized or acceptable, such as the nursing standards.

standards of practice A set of guidelines for providing quality care and a criteria for evaluating care. Such guidelines help assure patients that they are receiving high-quality care. The standards are important if a legal dispute arises over the quality of care provided to a patient.

staple A wound closure device made of stainless steel.

stasis A disorder in which the normal flow of a fluid through a vessel of the body is slowed or halted.

state board of nursing The state governing agency that has the power to enact laws regarding the practice of nursing; adopt rules and regulations concerning standards for nursing programs and curricula; license nurses; and suspend, deny, or revoke any persons who violate same.

step-parent family A blended family form whereby the family must try to adjust to having a different mother or father figure in the household.

sterilization Destruction of microorganisms using heat, water, chemicals, or gases.

stimulus Anything that excites or incites an organism or part to function, become active, or respond.

stoma An artificial opening of an internal organ on the surface of the body created surgically, such as for a colostomy, an ileostomy, or a tracheostomy.

stomatitis An inflammatory condition of the mouth.

subcutaneous Injection given into the connective tissue under the dermis. The subcutaneous tissue absorbs drugs more slowly than those injected into muscle. Injections are usually given at an angle of 45 degrees.

subcutaneous emphysema The presence of free air or gas in the subcutaneous tissues.

subjective data Information gathered from client statements; the client's feelings and perceptions. Not verifiable by another except by inference.

sublingual Beneath the tongue. Some medications are administered by this method.

sudden death Unexpected death.

sudden infant death syndrome (SIDS) The unexpected and sudden death of an apparently normal and healthy infant that occurs during sleep and with no physical or autopsic evidence of disease.

superego That part of the psyche functioning mostly in the unconscious that develops when the standards of the parents and of society are incorporated into the ego. The superego has two parts, the conscience and the ego ideal.

superficial pain Pain near the surface of the skin or another surface.

surface temperature Temperature of the skin.

surgical asepsis Protection against infection by destruction of all microorganisms and their spores or reproductive cells.

surgical bed The manner of making a bed in which the top bed linens are fanfolded to the bottom of the bed, the pillow is on top of the fanfold sheets, and a protective plastic sheet is on the bed at approximately the site of surgery.

susceptible host Sensitive to effects of an infectious disease; lacking immunity or resistance. When the body cannot fight off microorganisms.

suture Material used to close a wound; may be absorbable or nonabsorbable catgut, silk, wire, or synthetic material.

systolic pressure The blood pressure measured during the period of ventricular contraction (systole). In blood pressure readings, it is normally the higher of the two measurements.

tachycardia A rapid heartbeat, greater than 100 beats per minute.

tachypnea An abnormally rapid rate of breathing.

teaching Communication intended to produce learning by providing information, clarifying thinking, or demonstrating a skill.

tepid sponge bath The administration of lukewarm water to the skin for the purpose of reducing an elevated temperature.

testicular self-examination Procedure for detecting tumors or other abnormalities in the male testes.

theory An abstract statement formulated to predict, explain, or describe the relationships among concepts, constructs, or events. Theory is developed and tested by observation and research using factual data.

therapeutic nurse-patient relationship Patient-focused relationship between the nurse and the patient established to help the nurse give the patient the best possible nursing care. The four phases are preinteraction, orientation, working, and termination.

thoracentesis Surgical perforation of the chest wall and pleural space with a needle to aspirate fluid or obtain a specimen for diagnostic or therapeutic purposes.

threshold The point at which a stimulus is great enough to produce an effect; for example, a pain threshold is the point at which a person becomes aware of pain.

thrombophlebitis Inflammation of a vein accompanied by formation of a clot.

thrombus A blood clot in a vessel.

tidal volume The amount of air inhaled and exhaled during normal ventilation.

tolerance The ability to endure hardship, pain, or ordinarily injurious substances, such as drugs, without apparent physiologic or psychologic injury.

topical Pertaining to a drug or treatment applied topically.

tort Injurious act for which the injured party can bring civil action.

total parenteral nutrition (TPN) The administration of a nutritionally adequate hypertonic solution consisting of glucose, protein hydrolysates, minerals, and vitamins through an indwelling catheter into the superior vena cava. The high rate of blood flow results in a rapid dilution of the solution, and full nutritional requirements can be met indefinitely.

tracheostomy An artificial opening into the trachea. Most often a tube is inserted into the opening to maintain patency.

traction The process of putting a limb, bone, or group of muscles under tension by means of weights and pulleys to align or immobilize the part or to relieve pressure on it.

transcutaneous electrical nerve stimulation (TENS) A method of pain control by the application of electric impulses to nerve endings. It is performed through electrodes placed on the skin and attached to a stimulus by flexible wires.

transfer To relocate a patient from one location to another.

transfusion reaction A systematic response by the body to the administration of blood incompatible with that of the recipient.

transmission The transfer or conveyance of a thing or condition, such as a nerve impulse, infectious or genetic disease, or a hereditary trait, from one person or place to another.

Trendelenburg's Position in which the head is lower than the body and legs on an inclined plane.

T-tube A drain that may be inserted into the common bile duct during gallbladder surgery to remove bile until swelling of the duct subsides.

turgor Normal resiliency of the skin caused by the outward pressure of cells and interstitial fluid.

typing Determining a blood group, such as A, O, and ABO.

ultrasonography The process of imaging deep structures of the body by measuring and recording the reflection of pulsed or continuous high-frequency sound waves.

universal precautions CDC-recommended "universal blood and body fluid precautions." Precautions include preventing injury from needles and sharps, wearing protective devices during resuscitation, and avoiding patient and equipment contact if draining lesion exists in health care worker.

upper gastrointestinal series Pertaining to the

upper gastrointestinal tract from the esophagus to and including the duodenum. The term is commonly applied to radiographic or fluoroscopic diagnostic views after ingestion of a barium sulfate "milkshake."

ureterostomy Diversion of urine through a surgical opening in the abdomen.

urinal A plastic or metal receptacle for collecting urine.

urinalysis A physical, microscopic, or chemical examination of urine.

urinary incontinence Inability to control urination.

urinary tract infection (UTI) An infection of one or more structures in the urinary tract.

vaccine A suspension of attenuated or killed microorganisms administered intradermally, intramuscularly, orally, or subcutaneously to induce active immunity to an infectious disease.

validation The verification that data are free from misinterpretation, error, and bias.

value A personal belief about the worth of a given idea or behavior.

vaporizer A device that produces mist to increase humidity in the air.

vector (1) A quantity having direction and magnitude usually depicted by a straight arrow whose length represents magnitude and whose head represents direction; (2) a carrier, especially one that transmits disease; (3) a retrovirus that has been modified by alteration of its genetic component.

venipuncture Technique in which a vein is punctured transcutaneously by a sharp rigid stylet (such as a butterfly needle), a cannula (such as an angiocatheter), or a needle attached to a syringe.

veracity Truthfulness or honesty.

verbal communication The interchange of information using spoken or written words.

vial A container with a metal-enclosed rubber seal.

villi One of the many tiny projections barely visible to the naked eye clustered over the entire mucous surface of the small intestine.

visceral pain Abdominal pain caused by any abnormal condition of the viscera. It is characteristically severe, diffuse, and difficult to localize.

vital capacity A measurement of the amount of air that can be expelled at the normal rate of exhalation after a maximum inspiration, representing the greatest possible breathing capacity.

vital signs The measurements of pulse rate, respiration rate, and body temperature. Although not strictly a vital sign, blood pressure is also customarily included. May also be called *cardinal signs*.

vitamin An organic compound essential in small quantities for normal physiologic and metabolic functioning.

weight bearing Ability to apply full or partial weight on the lower extremities during ambulation.

wound Any physical injury involving a break in the skin, usually caused by an act or accident rather than by a disease.

Z-track injection A technique for injecting irritating preparations into muscle without tracking residual medication through sensitive tissues.

INDEX

B

N

P

Q

R